Case Studies Case studies encourage active learning and promote critical thinking skills in learners. Students can read about real-life scenarios, and then analyze the situation they are presented with. Case studies are available for completion online using the book's full suite of interactive resources.

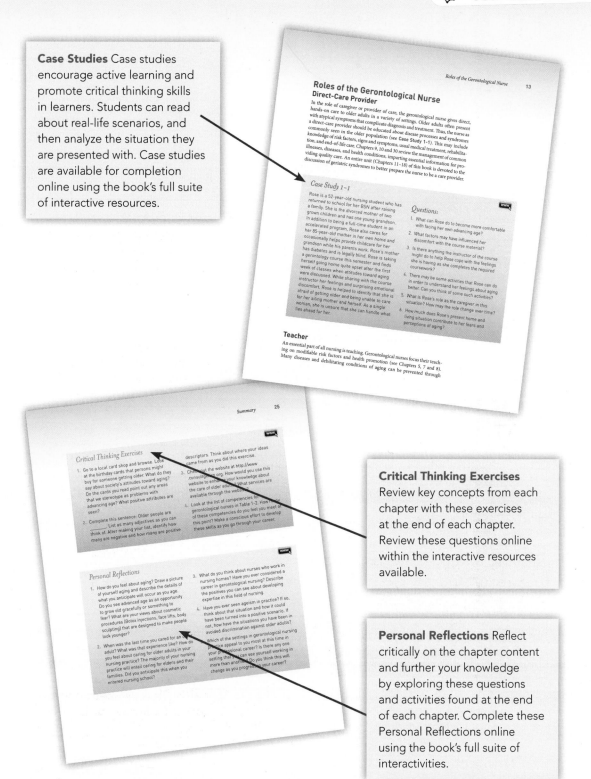

Roles of the Gerontological Nurse
Direct-Care Provider

In the role of caregiver or provider of care, the gerontological nurse gives direct, hands-on care to older adults in a variety of settings. Older adults often present with atypical symptoms that complicate diagnosis and treatment. Thus, the nurse as a direct-care provider should be educated about disease processes and syndromes commonly seen in the older population (see *Case Study 1-1*). This may include knowledge of risk factors, signs and symptoms, usual medical treatment, rehabilitation, and end-of-life care. Chapters 9, 10 and 30 review the management of common illnesses, diseases, and health conditions, imparting essential information for providing quality care. An entire unit (Chapters 11–18) of this book is devoted to the discussion of geriatric syndromes to better prepare the nurse to be a care provider.

Case Study 1–1

Rose is a 52-year-old nursing student who has returned to school for her BSN after raising a family. She is the divorced mother of two grown children and has one young grandson. In addition to being a full-time student in an accelerated program, Rose also cares for her 85-year-old mother in her own home and occasionally helps provide childcare for her grandson while his parents work. Rose's mother has diabetes and is legally blind. Rose is taking a gerontology course this semester and finds herself going home quite upset after the first week of classes when attitudes toward aging were discussed. While sharing with the course instructor her feelings and surprising emotional discomfort, Rose is helped to identify that she is afraid of getting older and being unable to care for her ailing mother and herself. As a single woman, she is unsure that she can handle what lies ahead for her.

Questions:

1. What can Rose do to become more comfortable with facing her own advancing age?
2. What factors may have influenced her discomfort with the course material?
3. Is there anything the instructor of the course might do to help Rose cope with the feelings she is having as she completes the required coursework?
4. There may be some activities that Rose can do in order to understand her feelings about aging better. Can you think of some such activities?
5. What is Rose's role as the caregiver in this situation? How may the role change over time?
6. How much does Rose's present home and living situation contribute to her fears and perceptions of aging?

Teacher

An essential part of all nursing is teaching. Gerontological nurses focus their teaching on modifiable risk factors and health promotion (see Chapters 5, 7 and 8). Many diseases and debilitating conditions of aging can be prevented through

Critical Thinking Exercises

1. Go to a local card shop and browse. Look at the birthday cards that persons might buy for someone getting older. What do they say about society's attitudes toward aging? Do the cards you read point out any areas that we stereotype as problems with advancing age? What positive attributes are seen?

2. Complete this sentence: Older people are think of. ... List as many adjectives as you can think of. After making your list, identify how many are negative and how many are positive

3. Check out the website at http://www .consultgerirn.org. How would you use this website to enhance your knowledge about the care of older adults? What services are available through the website

4. Look at the list of competencies for gerontological nurses in Table 1-2. How many of these competencies do you feel you meet at this point? Make a conscious effort to develop these skills as you go through your career.

descriptors. Think about where your ideas came from as you did this exercise.

Personal Reflections

1. How do you feel about aging? Draw a picture of yourself aging and describe the details of what you anticipate will occur as you age. Do you see advanced age as an opportunity to grow old gracefully or something to fear? What are your views about cosmetic procedures (Botox injections, face lifts, body sculpting) that are designed to make people look younger?

2. When was the last time you cared for an old adult? What was that experience like? How do you feel about caring for older adults in your nursing practice? The majority of your nursing practice will entail caring for elders and their families. Did you anticipate this when you entered nursing school?

3. What do you think about nurses who work in nursing homes? Have you ever considered a career in gerontological nursing? Describe the positives you can see about developing expertise in this field of nursing.

4. Have you ever seen ageism in practice? If so, think about that situation and how it could have been turned into a positive scenario. If not, how have the situations you have been in avoided discrimination against older adults?

Which of the settings in gerontological nursing practice appeal to you most at this time in your professional career? Is there any one setting that you can see yourself working in more than another? Do you think this will change as you progress in your career?

Critical Thinking Exercises Review key concepts from each chapter with these exercises at the end of each chapter. Review these questions online within the interactive resources available.

Personal Reflections Reflect critically on the chapter content and further your knowledge by exploring these questions and activities found at the end of each chapter. Complete these Personal Reflections online using the book's full suite of interactivities.

THIRD EDITION

Gerontological Nursing

COMPETENCIES FOR CARE

Edited by

Kristen L. Mauk, PhD, DNP, RN, CRRN, GCNS-BC, GNP-BC, FAAN
Professor of Nursing
Kreft Endowed Chair for the Advancement of Nursing Science
Valparaiso University
President
Senior Care Central, LLC
Valparaiso, Indiana

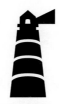

JONES & BARTLETT
LEARNING

World Headquarters
Jones & Bartlett Learning
5 Wall Street
Burlington, MA 01803
978-443-5000
info@jblearning.com
www.jblearning.com

Jones & Bartlett Learning books and products are available through most bookstores and online booksellers. To contact Jones & Bartlett Learning directly, call 800-832-0034, fax 978-443-8000, or visit our website, www.jblearning.com.

Substantial discounts on bulk quantities of Jones & Bartlett Learning publications are available to corporations, professional associations, and other qualified organizations. For details and specific discount information, contact the special sales department at Jones & Bartlett Learning via the above contact information or send an email to specialsales@jblearning.com.

Production Credits:
Executive Publisher: Kevin Sullivan
Acquisitions Editor: Amanda Harvey
Editorial Assistant: Sara Bempkins
Production Editor: Cindie Bryan
Senior Marketing Manager: Jennifer Stiles
VP, Manufacturing and Inventory Control: Therese Connell
Composition: diacriTech
Cover Design: Kristin E. Parker
Rights & Photo Research Assistant: Joseph Veiga
Cover Image: © George Doyle/Thinkstock
Printing and Binding: Courier Companies
Cover Printing: Courier Companies

To order this product, use ISBN: 1-978-1-2840-2719-8

Library of Congress Cataloging-in-Publication Data
Gerontological nursing : competencies for care / [edited by] Kristen L. Mauk. — 3rd ed.
       p. ; cm.
   Includes bibliographical references and index.
   ISBN 978-1-4496-9463-0 (pbk.) — ISBN 1-4496-9463-2 (pbk.)
   I. Mauk, Kristen L.
   [DNLM: 1. Geriatric Nursing—methods. 2. Aging—physiology. 3. Aging—psychology. WY 152]
   618.97'0231—dc23
                                                                    2012044937

6048

Printed in the United States of America
17 16 15 14   10 9 8 7 6 5 4

Gerontological
Nursing

COMPETENCIES FOR CARE

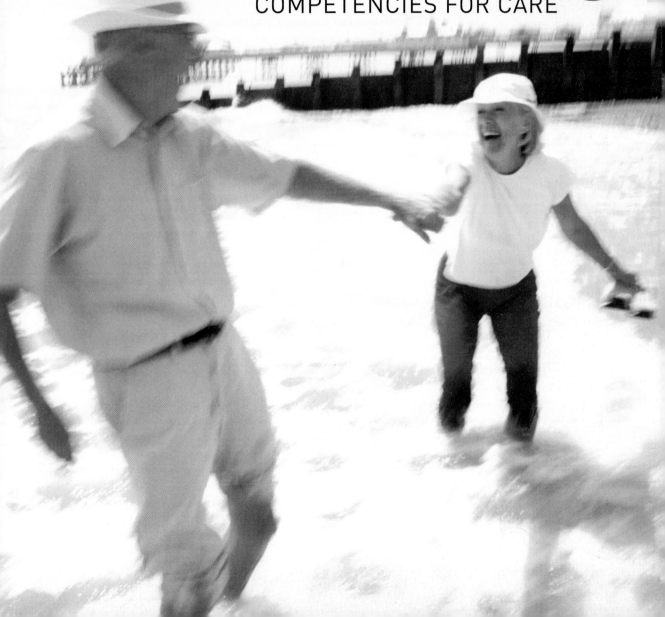

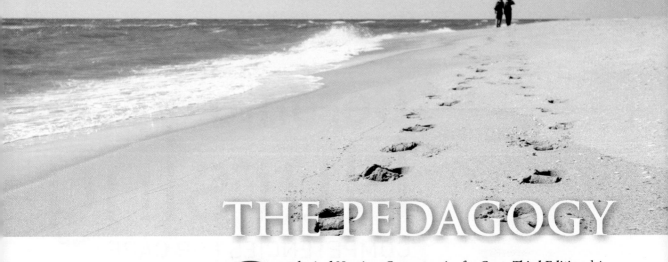

THE PEDAGOGY

Gerontological Nursing: Competencies for Care, Third Edition drives comprehension through various strategies that meet the learning needs of students, while also generating enthusiasm about the topic. This interactive approach addresses different learning styles, making this the ideal text to ensure mastery of key concepts. The pedagogical aids that appear in most chapters include the following:

Learning Objectives These objectives provide instructors and students with a snapshot of the key information they will encounter in each chapter. They serve as a checklist to help guide and focus study. Objectives can also be found within the text's online resources. Use the access code at the front of your book to view these additional resources.

Key Terms Found in a list at the beginning of each chapter, these terms will create an expanded vocabulary. The "www" icon directs students to the text's online resources to see these terms in an interactive glossary and use flashcards and word puzzles to nail the definitions. Use the access code at the front of your book to view these additional resources.

LEARNING OBJECTIVES

At the end of this chapter, the reader will be able to:

> Define important terms related to nursing and the aging process.
> Outline significant landmarks that have influenced the development of gerontological nursing as a specialty.
> Identify several subfields of gerontological nursing.
> Develop the beginnings of a personal philosophy of aging.
> Describe the unique roles of the gerontological nurse.
> Discuss the scope and standards of gerontological nursing practice.
> Examine core competencies in gerontological nursing.
> Compare the nine essentials of baccalaureate nursing education with the core competencies in gerontological nursing.
> Distinguish among the educational preparation, practice roles, and certification requirements of the various levels of gerontological nursing practice.

KEY TERMS

Ageism
Attitudes
Certification
Core competencies
Geriatrics
Gerontological nursing
Gerontological rehabilitation nursing
Gerontology
Gerocompetencies

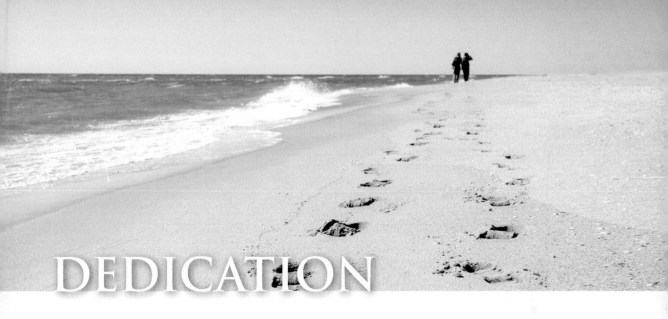

DEDICATION

For my husband, Jim, for being my friend and
partner in our many adventures.

And to all my wonderful children for their constant
encouragement, love, and support:

Rachel, Cowboy Jim, Kenny, Jennifer Ann, Big Daniel,
Elizabeth, Jordan, Vika, and Little Daniel.

You are the best family ever.

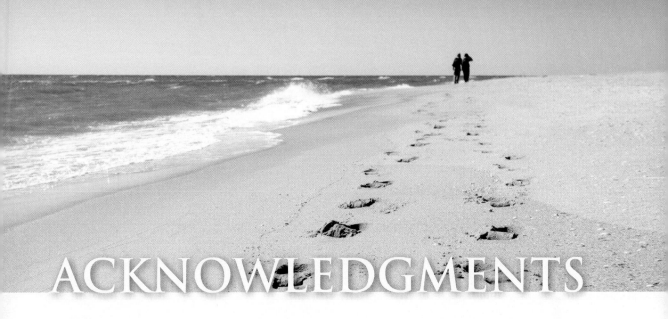

ACKNOWLEDGMENTS

Thanks to the parents and grandparents who have been a part of my life and the lives of my children:

Pat and Marvin Bell

Kenny and Norma Easton

Pete and Kay Gibson

Jim and Phyllis Hays

Larry and Gracie Mauk

Your legacies are a great gift to all the people in your lives, and you have each been influential in shaping mine.

I would also like to thank the excellent staff at Jones & Bartlett Learning for all their help, especially Sara Bempkins, Cindie Bryan, and Amanda Harvey.

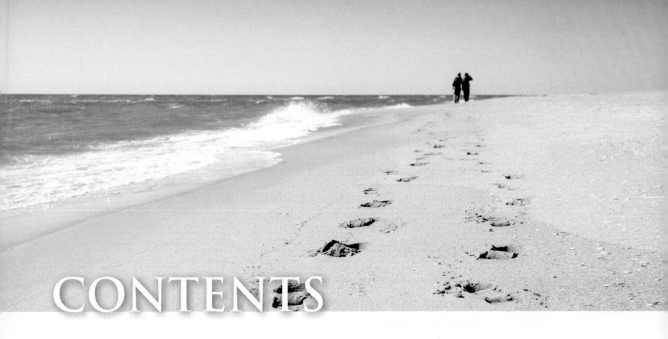

CONTENTS

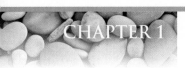

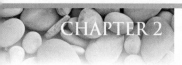

CHAPTER 2

The Aging Population   29

Cheryl A. Lehman

Andrea Wirt

(Competency 19)

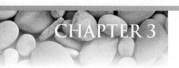

CHAPTER 3

Theories of Aging   63

Jean Lange

Sheila Grossman

(Competency 19)

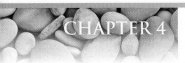
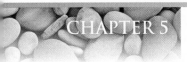

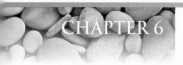

CHAPTER 6 Comprehensive Assessment of the Older Adult   149

Lorna Guse

(Competencies 3, 4, 6)

UNIT III Health Promotion, Risk Reduction, and Disease Prevention   185

(Competencies 3–5, 9, 17, 18)

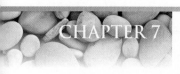

CHAPTER 7 Promoting Healthy Aging   187

David Haber

(Competencies 4, 5, 9, 17, 18)

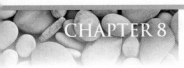

CHAPTER 8

Identifying and Preventing Common Risk Factors in the Elderly   223

Joan M. Nelson

(Competencies 3, 4, 9, 17)

UNIT IV   Illness and Disease Management   267
(Competencies 9, 15–18)

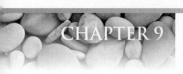

CHAPTER 9   **Management of Common Illnesses, Diseases, and Health Conditions   270**
Kristen L. Mauk

Patricia Hanson

Debra Hain

(Competencies 9, 5, 17, 18)

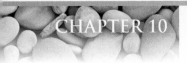

CHAPTER 10

Nursing Management of Dementia   377

Christine E. Schwartzkopf

Prudence Twigg

(Competencies 9, 15)

UNIT V   Management of Geriatric Syndromes   415

(Competencies 3, 7, 12, 17)

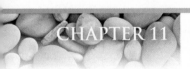

CHAPTER 11

Polypharmacy   417

Demetra Antimisiaris

Dennis J. Cheek

(Competencies 7, 17)

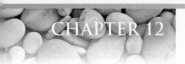
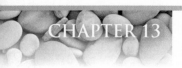

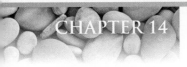
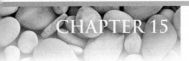
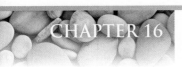

CHAPTER 17

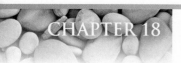

CHAPTER 18

CHAPTER 19

Dawna S. Fish

Marilyn Ter Maat

(Competencies 1, 11, 13)

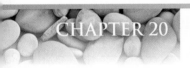

CHAPTER 20   **Ethical/Legal Principles and Issues**   **711**

Janice Edelstein

(Competencies 1, 11, 12)

UNIT VII   **Gerontological Care Issues**   **733**

(Competencies 3–6, 8–11, 13–16, 18)

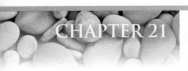

CHAPTER 21   **Culture and Spirituality**   **735**

MaryAnne Pietraniec Shannon

Linda J. Hassler

(Competencies 8, 10, 13, 18)

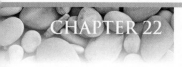

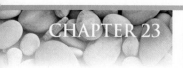

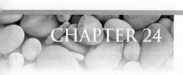

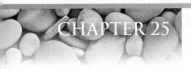

CHAPTER 25

Caring Across the Continuum 857

Carol Ann Amann

Raeann G. LeBlanc

(Competencies 4, 5, 8, 10, 14)

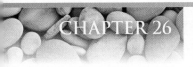

CHAPTER 26

End-of-Life Care 881

Patricia Warring

Luana S. Krieger-Blake

(Competencies 11, 16)

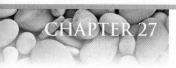

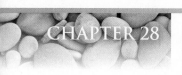

UNIT VIII   **eChapters**
Use the access code at the front of your book to view
these additional chapters online.

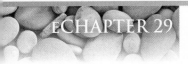

ECHAPTER 29   **Review of the Aging of Physiological Systems**
Janice Heineman

Jennifer Hamrick-King

Beth Scaglione Sewell

(Competencies 9, 19)

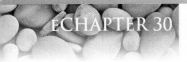

ECHAPTER 30   **Care of the Older Adult with Cancer**
Ashley Leak

Stephanie Lucas

(Competencies 9, 16)

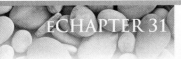

ECHAPTER 31   **Interdisciplinary Collaboration and Teams**
Deborah Dunn

Teresa L. Cervantez Thompson

(Competency 13)

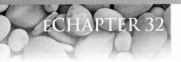

ECHAPTER 32   **Legal Aspects of Gerontological Nursing**
Mary Alice Kothe

(Competencies 1, 11, 13)

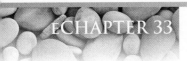

ECHAPTER 33   **Technology and Care of Older Adults**
Linda L. Pierce

Victoria Steiner

(Competencies 5, 18)

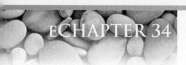
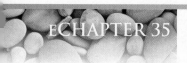
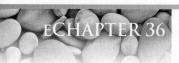

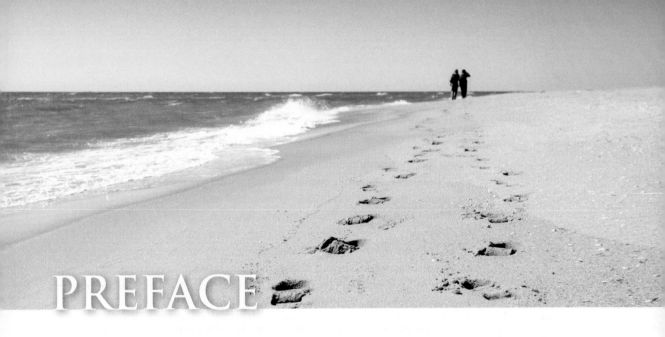

PREFACE

Although there are numerous excellent gerontological nursing texts on the market today, the approach to this book is unique in that the first and second editions were based on an essential document from the American Association of Colleges of Nursing and the John A. Hartford Foundation Institute for Geriatric Nursing (July 2000), entitled *Older Adults: Recommended Baccalaureate Competencies and Curricular Guidelines for Geriatric Nursing Care*. The new edition uses the updated document, *Recommended Baccalaureate Competencies and Curricular Guidelines for the Nursing Care of Older Adults* (September 2010), published by the same two organizations. This book is intended to be a basic baccalaureate-level gerontological nursing text, although much of the new edition is also appropriate for graduate level coursework, and it is structured to ensure that students will obtain the recommended competencies and knowledge necessary to provide excellent care to older adults. It can be used for a stand-alone course or in sections to be integrated throughout a nursing curriculum.

Using the recommended competencies as a guide, each chapter is written to assist students of gerontological nursing in acquiring the essential knowledge and skills to provide excellent care for older adults. Competencies as set forth in the AACN/Hartford Foundation document are listed at the beginning of each chapter to help direct students' learning.

This book has several outstanding features. First, the framework, as described, is unique. In addition, the text is an edited work with a diverse authorship of nearly 70 contributors and numerous reviewers who represent all areas of gerontological nursing, including management, education, quality assurance, clinical practice in a variety of settings, advanced practice roles, research, business, consulting, and academia. This third edition adds 40 new authors, with the vast majority of authors from the last edition continuing their work in the new edition. All chapters have been updated to include current resources and evidence-based clinical practice. Interdisciplinary collaboration of many chapters was accomplished by including nurse authors writing with colleagues whose backgrounds are in psychology, social work, pharmacy, speech therapy, gerontology, rehabilitation, biology, and sociology.

For this third edition, comments and recommendations of instructors who have used the text were carefully considered. In answer to requests, an entirely new unit was added on geriatric syndromes. There are 17 new chapters in the third edition, including chapters on polypharmacy, falls, delirium, depression and anxiety, incontinence, sleep disorders, dysphagia, pressure ulcers, culture and spirituality, elder abuse, pain management, care of the older adult with cancer, emergency care, caring across the continuum, current system models, and health policy. Healthy aging is a theme more heavily emphasized in the new edition. Many original photos and content portray older adults as actively aging.

The text has a user-friendly and comprehensive format. Several features were designed to appeal to students. The following pedagogical features are used:

> Learning objectives
> Key terms list (with terms highlighted in chapter)
> Tables that summarize key points
> Boxes to highlight interesting information and key practice points
> Web exploration and links
> Notable quotes of interest
> Pictures/diagrams/drawings
> Original photographs
> Research highlights with application to practice
> Evidence-based practice boxes and guidelines
> Critical thinking exercises
> Personal reflection exercises
> Case studies with questions
> Resource lists
> References (including websites)
> Recommended readings
> Glossary

Students will be delighted to have a glossary at the end of the text, as well as definitions of key terms within the chapters. The competencies recommended by the AACN/Hartford Foundation are threaded throughout the book. Students will also benefit from new online resources and educational materials available from the publisher.

Instructors will find the accompanying online instructor's manual to be a time-saving tool. It is designed to provide a complete curriculum for instructors and students, even for those who may lack a strong geriatric background. The instructor's manual suggests activities for learning and in-class exercises, and provides PowerPoint slides for lectures that coincide with student readings in the main text. A test bank is also provided. Most of the work for development of a gerontological nursing course or integration in portions into the curriculum has already been done for instructors.

This book is divided into sections that directly follow the AACN/Hartford Foundation Institute's Competencies *Recommended Baccalaureate Competencies and Curricular Guidelines for the Nursing Care of Older Adults* (September 2010, pp. 12–13). The 19 gerontological nursing competency statements shown here, with the corresponding Essential from the AACN Baccalaureate competencies, are those necessary to provide high-quality care to older adults and their families:

1. Incorporate professional attitudes, values, and expectations about physical and mental aging in the provision of patient-centered care for older adults and their families.
   Corresponding to Essential VIII

2. Assess barriers for older adults in receiving, understanding, and giving of information.
   Corresponding to Essentials IV & IX

3. Use valid and reliable assessment tools to guide nursing practice for older adults.
   Corresponding to Essential IX

4. Assess the living environment as it relates to functional, physical, cognitive, psychological, and social needs of older adults.
   Corresponding to Essential IX

5. Intervene to assist older adults and their support network to achieve personal goals, based on the analysis of the living environment and availability of community resources.
   Corresponding to Essential VII

6. Identify actual or potential mistreatment (physical, mental, or financial abuse; and/or self neglect) in older adults and refer appropriately.
   Corresponding to Essential V

7. Implement strategies and use online guidelines to prevent and/or identify and manage geriatric syndromes.
   Corresponding to Essentials IV & IX

8. Recognize and respect the variations of care, the increased complexity, and the increased use of healthcare resources inherent in caring for older adults.
   Corresponding to Essentials IV & IX

9. Recognize the complex interaction of acute and chronic comorbid physical and mental conditions and associated treatments common to older adults.
   Corresponding to Essential IX

10. Compare models of care that promote safe, quality physical and mental health care for older adults, such as PACE, NICHE, Guided Care, Culture Change, and Transitional Care Models.
    Corresponding to Essential II

11. Facilitate ethical, noncoercive decision making by older adults and/or families/caregivers for maintaining everyday living, receiving treatment, initiating advance directives, and implementing end-of-life care.
    Corresponding to Essential VIII

12. Promote adherence to the evidence-based practice of providing restraint-free care (both physical and chemical restraints).
    Corresponding to Essential II

13. Integrate leadership and communication techniques that foster discussion and reflection on the extent to which diversity (among nurses, nurse assistive personnel, therapists, physicians, and patients) has the potential to impact the care of older adults.
    Corresponding to Essential VI

14. Facilitate safe and effective transitions across levels of care, including acute, community-based, and long-term care (e.g., home, assisted living, hospice, nursing homes) for older adults and their families.
    Corresponding to Essentials IV & IX

15. Plan patient-centered care with consideration for mental and physical health and well-being of informal and formal caregivers of older adults.
    Corresponding to Essential IX

16. Advocate for timely and appropriate palliative and hospice care for older adults with physical and cognitive impairments.
    Corresponding to Essential IX

17. Implement and monitor strategies to prevent risk and promote quality and safety (e.g., falls, medication mismanagement, pressure ulcers) in the nursing care of older adults with physical and cognitive needs.
    Corresponding to Essentials II & IV

18. Utilize resources/programs to promote functional, physical, and mental wellness in older adults.
    Corresponding to Essential VII

19. Integrate relevant theories and concepts included in a liberal education into the delivery of patient-centered care for older adults.
    Corresponding to Essential I

By using this text and the instructor's manual as a curricular guide, instructors should be able to ensure that nursing students will meet the essential competencies that are recommended for excellent care of older adults.

REFERENCE

American Association of Colleges of Nursing and the John A. Hartford Institute for Geriatric Nursing (2010). Recommended baccalaureate competencies and curricula guidelines for nursing care of older adults, A supplement to the Essentials of baccalaureate education for professional nursing practice (pp. 12–13). Washington, DC: Author.

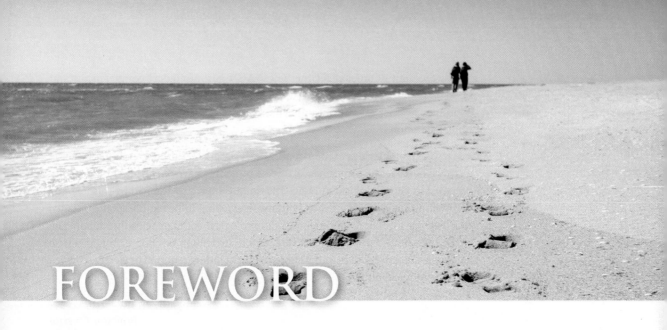

FOREWORD

The recently passed Patient Protection and Affordable Care Act has focused national attention on the importance of health in the well-being of all Americans. Nowhere is this more evident than for people 65 and over—the expanding aging population who now constitute the "core business" of our healthcare system: primary care, hospitals, home care, and nursing homes. With baby boomers having reached old age, and over one-half of older adults 75 years and older, the need for a health workforce capable of delivering quality care to older adults has never been more critical. As the largest group of healthcare providers, it is essential that nurses have the knowledge and skills commensurate to delivering competent care to older adults.

Baccalaureate nursing education has led nursing in assuring a nurse workforce prepared for care of older adults. Since 2000, with support from the John A. Hartford Foundation, the American Association of Colleges of Nursing (AACN) has taken major steps to assure the infusion of gerontological nursing into the curriculum of baccalaureate nursing programs. In 2008, AACN revised *The Essentials of Baccalaureate Education for Professional Nursing Practice* to include competencies in gerontological nursing. In collaboration with the Hartford Institute for Geriatric Nursing at New York University, AACN updated the document *Older Adults: Recommended Baccalaureate Competencies and Curricular Guidelines for Geriatric Nursing Care*. AACN and the Hartford Institute created a national initiative, the Geriatric Nursing Education Consortium (GNEC), to ensure that faculty were familiar with extensive online resources that provide a framework for baccalaureate nursing programs to structure curriculum to assure competencies in care of older adults in their graduates.

This much-expanded third edition of *Gerontological Nursing: Competencies for Care* reflects extensive and exemplary use of these resources. New chapters, such as those on management of geriatric syndromes, culture and spirituality, and caring across the continuum, reflect the new AACN gerontological competencies and build on GNEC resources. As was the case in the first and second editions, this text continues to offer faculty an authoritative resource to foster geriatric curricular implementation.

Despite major strides to prepare faculty in geriatrics, this text continues to serve a critical need because most baccalaureate programs have only a handful of faculty prepared in gerontological nursing. The unique approach adopted by this text can help gerontological nursing faculty transmit essential information to other faculty, thus helping to imbed and integrate gerontological competencies throughout the curriculum. It also provides the structure for curriculum development and course content for those schools seeking to create free-standing required or elective courses in gerontological nursing.

Mathy Mezey, EdD, RN, FAAN
Professor Emerita
Senior Research Scientist
Associate Director,
the Hartford Institute for Geriatric Nursing
College of Nursing
New York University

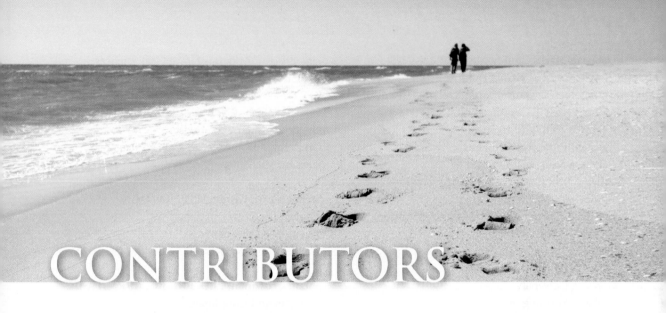

CONTRIBUTORS

Carol Ann Amann, BSN, MSN, RN-BC, CDP
Gannon University
Morosky College of Health Professions and
    Sciences
Erie, Pennsylvania

Demetra Antimisiaris, PharmD, CGP, FASCP
Associate Professor
University of Louisville Department of Family and
    Geriatric Medicine
Louisville, Kentucky

LaShonda Barnette, RNC
Case Manager, Gaston Memorial Hospital
Gastonia, North Carolina

Kathleen Blais, RN, MSN, EdD
Professor Emerita
Florida International University
College of Nursing and Health Sciences
Miami, Florida

Nora Bollinger, MSN, RN, CMSRN
Clinical Nurse Educator
Kennedy University Hospital
Cherry Hill, New Jersey

Lisa Byrd, PhD FNP-BC, GNP-BC
Gerontologist
Assistant Professor
University of Mississippi Medical Center
Jackson, Mississippi

Teresa Cervantez Thompson, PhD, RN, CRRN
Dean and Professor
College of Nursing and Health
Madonna University
Livonia, Michigan

Dennis J. Cheek, RN, PhD, FAHA
Abell-Hanger Professor
Texas Christian University
Harris College of Nursing and Health Sciences
Fort Worth, Texas

David Cheesebrow, RN, MAPA, MA, CEN, CCRN-A
Associate Professor
Bethel University
St. Paul, Minnesota

Audrey Cochran, MSN, GCNS-BC, CCCN
Care Planning and Education for the Elderly
Bakersfield, California

Deborah Marks Conley, MSN, APRN-CNS, GCNS-BC, FNGNA
Gerontological Clinical Nurse Specialist - AgeWISE and NICHE Coordinator
Nebraska Methodist Hospital
Assistant Professor of Nursing
Nebraska Methodist College
Omaha, Nebraska

Neva L. Crogan, PhD, GNP-BC, GCNS-BC, FNGNA, FAAN
Professor
School of Nursing
Gonzaga University
Spokane, Washington

Margaret Dean, RN, CS-BC, NP-C, MSN, FAANP
Assistant Professor of Nursing
Geriatric Nurse Practitioner
Associate Faculty School of Medicine
Texas Tech Health Sciences Center
Amarillo, Texas

B. Renee Dugger, DNP, RN, GCNS-BC
Associate Professor, Nursing
University of South Carolina Beaufort
Bluffton, South Carolina

Deborah Dunn, EdD, MSN, GNP-BC, ACNS-BC
Professor & Nurse Practitioner Program Director
College of Nursing and Health
Madonna University
Livonia, Michigan

Janice Edelstein, EdD, RN
Nebraska Methodist Health System
Omaha, Nebraska

Carol Enderlin, PhD, RN
Clinical Assistant Professor
College of Nursing

University of Arkansas for Medical Sciences
Little Rock, Arkansas

Dawna S. Fish, RN, BSN, COS-C
Quality Assurance Supervisor
Great Lakes Home Health and Hospice
Jackson, Michigan

Stephanie M. Grode, MSN, RN, OCN
Adjunct Faculty
Waynesburg University
Waynesburg, Pennsylvania

Sheila Grossman, PhD, FNP-BC, APRN, FAAN
Professor and Coordinator
Family Nurse Practitioner Program
School of Nursing
Fairfield University
Fairfield, Connecticut

Valerie Gruss, PhD, CNP-BC
Department of Biobehavioral Science
Institute for Health Care Innovation
UIC College of Nursing
Chicago, Illinois

Lorna Guse, PhD, RN
Associate Professor
Faculty of Nursing
University of Manitoba
Winnipeg, Manitoba, Canada

David Haber, PhD
NTT Assistant Professor of Gerontology
Western Oregon University
Monmouth, Oregon

Debra Hain, PhD, APRN, AGNP, BC
Assistant Professor/Lead AGNP Faculty
Florida Atlantic University
Christine E. Lynn College of Nursing
Boca Raton, Florida

Nurse Practitioner
Cleveland Clinic Florida
Department of Nephrology/Hypertension

Jennifer Hamrick-King, PhD
Graduate Center for Gerontology
College of Public Health
University of Kentucky
Lexington, Kentucky

Patricia Hanson, PhD, APRN, GNP
Professor
College of Nursing and Health
Madonna University
Livonia, Michigan

Melodee Harris, PhD, APN, GNP-BC
Associate Professor
Carr College of Nursing
Harding University
Searcy, Arizona

Barbara E. Harrison, PhD, FNP-BC, GNP-BC
Associate Professor
College of Health Sciences
University of Delaware
Newark, Delaware

Linda J. Hassler, RN, MS, GCNS-BC, FNGNA
Geriatric Program Manager
Cultural Ambassador Coordinator
Meridian Health Ann May Center for Nursing and
    Allied Health
Neptune, New Jersey
Adjunct Faculty, Georgian Court University
Lakewood, New Jersey

Janice M. Heineman, PhD
Senior Research Associate
Institute for the Future of Aging Services American
    Association of Homes and Services for the Aging
Washington, D.C.

Sandra J. Higelin, MSN, RN, CNS, CWCN, CLNC

Lisa Hutchison, PharmD, MPH, BCPS, FCCP
Associate Professor of Pharmacy Practice
University of Arkansas for Medical Sciences
Little Rock, Arkansas

Donald D. Kautz, RN, PhD, CRRN, CNE
Assistant Professor of Nursing
University of North Carolina at Greensboro
Greensboro, North Carolina

Annette Kelly, PhD, ARNP
Nursing Research Consultant
Adjunct Faculty
School of Nursing & Health Sciences
Florida Southern College
Lakeland, Florida

Mary Alice Kothe, MSN, RN, LNCC
Faculty
Western Governors University

Luana S. Krieger-Blake, MSW, LCSW
Social Worker
Pines Village Retirement Community
Valparaiso, Indiana

Cheryl Kruschke, EdD, MS, RN, CNE
Assistant Professor, Online Nursing
    Program
Loretto Heights School of Nursing
Regis University
Denver, Colorado

Jean W. Lange, PhD, RN, FAAN
Founding Dean and Professor
School of Nursing
Quinnipiac University
Hamden, Connecticut

Ashley Leak, PhD, RN-BC, OCN
Cancer Care Quality Training Post Doctoral
    Fellow
Gillings School of Global Public Health
Department of Health Policy and Management
Adjunct Assistant Professor, School of Nursing
The University of North Carolina at
    Chapel Hill
Chapel Hill, North Carolina

Raeann G. LeBlanc, DNP, ANP-BC, GNP-BC
Assistant Clinical Professor
School of Nursing
University of Massachusetts Amherst
Amherst, Massachusetts

**Cheryl A. Lehman, PhD, RN, CNS-BC, RN-BC,
    CRRN**
Clinical Associate Professor
The University of Texas Health Science Center, San
    Antonio
School of Nursing
Department of Health Restoration and Care Systems
    Management
San Antonio, Texas

Mary Beth Lochner, RN, DNP, FNP-C
Gerontologist – Owner and Chief Clinician
Journeys Health Clinic at the Voyager Resort
Tucson, Arizona
Adjunct Clinical Professor, College of Nursing
The University of Arizona

Patrick Luib, GNP-BC, RN
Manager
Geriatric Clinical Services
Visiting Nurse Service of New York

**Kristen L. Mauk, PhD, DNP, RN, CRRN,
    GCNS-BC, GNP-BC, FAAN**
Professor of Nursing
Kreft Endowed Chair

Valparaiso University
President
Senior Care Central, LLC
Valparaiso, Indiana

Kerry Mees, BA
Graduate Student, SLP
University of Kansas
Lawrence, Kansas

Michelle Moccia, MSN, ANP-BC, CCRN
Program Director, Senior ER
St. Mary Mercy Hospital
Livonia, Michigan

Joan Nelson, RN, MS, DNP
Associate Professor
University of Colorado Denver
College of Nursing
Denver, Colorado

Carole A. Pepa, PhD, RN
Professor of Nursing
Valparaiso University
Valparaiso, Indiana

**Linda L. Pierce, PhD, RN, CNS, CRRN, FAHA,
    FAAN**
Professor
College of Nursing
University of Toledo
Toledo, Ohio

Karen M. Rose, PhD, RN
Assistant Professor of Nursing
University of Virginia
Charlottesville, Virginia

**Susan Saboe Rose, PhD, PMHNP-BC, GCNS-BC,
    ARNP**
Legacy Medical Group
Portland, Oregon

Beth Scaglione Sewell, PhD
Associate Professor of Biology
Valparaiso University
Valparaiso, Indiana

Christine E. Schwartzkopf, MSN, RN, CRRN
Nursing Instructor
Dayton VAMC
Dayton, Ohio

MaryAnne Pietraniec Shannon, PhD, RN, GCNS-BC
Professor of Nursing
Sault College BScN Collaborative with Laurentian University
Sault Ste. Marie, Ontario, Canada

Jeanne St. Pierre, MN, RN, GCNS-BC
Gerontological Clinical Nurse Specialist
NICHE Program Coordinator
Fellow, Geriatric Nursing Leadership Academy
Salem Hospital
Salem, Oregon

Victoria Steiner, PhD
Associate Professor
College of Medicine
University of Toledo
Toledo, Ohio

Kathleen Stevens, PhD, RN, CRRN, NE-BC
Director of Nursing Education
Rehabilitation Institute of Chicago
Assistant Professor
Northwestern University, Feinberg School of Medicine
Chicago, Illinois

Deborah M. Strickland, MSN, RN
PhD Student, West Virginia University
Faculty
Penn State New Kensington Campus

Marilyn Ter Maat, MSN, CRRN-A, NEA, BC, FNGNA
Rehabilitation Nurse Consultant
Windcrest, Texas

Prudence Twigg, PhDc, RN, ANP-BC, GNP-BC
Visiting Lecturer
Department of Family Health
Indiana University School of Nursing at Indianapolis
Gerontological Nurse Practitioner
Advanced Healthcare Associates
Indianapolis, Indiana

Brenda Tyczkowski, RN, DNP
University of Wisconsin – Green Bay
Professional Program in Nursing
Assistant Professor
Academic Director – Health Information Management Technology (HIMT)

Kathleen Urban, MS, BSN, CRRN, CCM
Director, Rehabilitation Services
Nursing Administration, Nursing Safety Officer
Garden City Hospital
Garden City, Michigan

Karion Gray Waites, MSN, DNP, RN, FNP-BC, CRRN
Nurse Practitioner
Department of Physical Medicine and Rehabilitation
Department of Rehabilitation Nursing
University of Alabama at Birmingham Hospital
Birmingham, Alabama

Kristine Williams, RN, PhD, FNP-BC, FGSA, FAAN
Sally Mathis Hartwig Professor in Gerontological Nursing
Iowa City, Iowa

Patricia Warring, RN, MSN, ACHPN
Clinical Nurse Specialist
VNA of Porter County
Valparaiso, Indiana

Andrea Wirt, RN, MSN, GNP-C
Geriatric Nurse Practitioner
Department of Geriatrics

University of Texas Medical Branch
Galveston, Texas

Deanne Zwicker, DrNP, ANP/GNP- BC
Assistant Professor
George Mason University School of
    Nursing
Manassas, Virginia

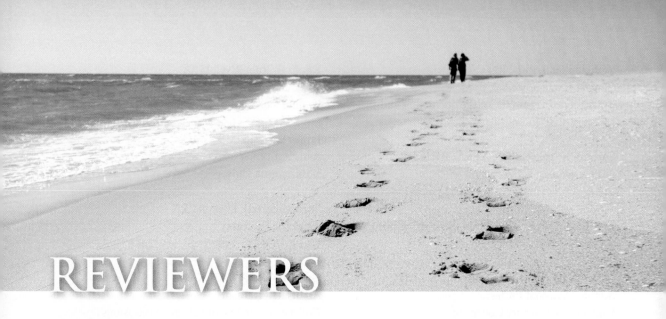

REVIEWERS

Helen Brantley, PhD
Associate Professor
South Carolina State University
Orangeburg, SC

Julie Britton RN-BC, MSN, GCNS, FGNLA
Genesis HealthCare

Glenda C. Broad, MSN, RN
Adjunct Instructor
Lancaster General College of Nursing and
    Health Sciences

**Kathryn M. Cacic, DNP, APNP, RN, ANP-BC,
    CCRN**
Nurse Practitioner
Clinical Research – University of Wisconsin

**Dia D. Campbell-Detrixhe, PhD, RN,
    FNGNA, CNE**
Assistant Professor of Nursing
Oklahoma City University, Kramer School of
    Nursing

Brenda Y. Cartwright, EdD, CRC, NCC, MHC
Professor and Program Director
University of Hawaii at Manoa

**Cassandra Sligh Conway, PhD,
    CRC, GCDF**
Chair/Associate Professor,
South Carolina State University
Orangeburg, SC

Charles W. Ewing, PhD, CLAS, CHES
University of North Texas, Department of
    Sociology/Gerontology

Kay Foland, PhD, RN, PMHNP-BC
Professor
South Dakota State University

Rita Gilpatrick, MSN, FNP-BC
Clinical Service Manger
Nurse Practitioner
Evercare/Optum Health

**Johannah Uriri Glover, PhD, MSN,
    MNSc, RN**
Arizona State University College of Nursing &
    Health Innovation
Clinical Associate Professor/Core Director
    of the ASU College of Nursing John
    Hartford Center for Nursing Excellence
    Integration Core

Kathleen Hall, PhD, RN
Clinical Instructor
University of Vermont College of Nursing and
    Health Sciences

Barbara A. Heise, PhD, APRN, BC, CNE
Brigham Young University
College of Nursing

Ann Kriebel-Gasparro, MSN, FNP-BC, GNP-BC,
    DrNP-c

Constance Lemley, MSN, RN, GCNS-BC
Adjunct Assistant Professor
Valparaiso University College of
    Nursing

Catherine T. Milne, MSN, APRN, ANP/ACNS-BC,
    CWOCN
Connecticut Clinical Nursing Associates, LLC
Bristol, Connecticut

Linda Miles, MSN, RN
Program Director for Center for Excellence in
    Gerontological Studies; Assistant Professor
Bryan College of Health Sciences

Linda Murphy, MSN, RN-BC, ONC
Associate Professor of Nursing
College of the Desert

Nancy Rowe, PhD, RN, CNS
Assistant Professor
Retired from Mount Carmel College of
    Nursing

Karen R. Rue, RNC, MBA
Gerontology Nurse, Certified
Hailind Consulting

James Siberski, MS, CMC
Assistant Professor
Misericordia University

Frances Sparti, DNP, APRN
Associate Professor
UALR DON

Gail Vitale, EdD, RN, CNS
Associate Professor
College of Nursing and Health Professions
Lewis University
One University Parkway
Romeoville, IL

Kimberly Walker-Daniels, RN, BSN, RN-BC,
    CMSRN, WCC

Marjorie G. Webb, DNP, RN, ACNP-BC
Associate Professor
Metropolitan State University

Teresa A. Wenner, MSN, RN-BC
Instructor of Nursing
DeSales University
Center Valley, Pennsylvania

Ellen Zisholtz
Director/Professor
South Carolina State University
Orangeburg, SC

Unit I
Foundations for Gerontological Nursing

(COMPETENCIES 1, 9, 19)

LEARNING OBJECTIVES

At the end of this chapter, the reader will be able to:

> Define important terms related to nursing and the aging process.
> Outline significant landmarks that have influenced the development of gerontological nursing as a specialty.
> Identify several subfields of gerontological nursing.
> Develop the beginnings of a personal philosophy of aging.
> Describe the unique roles of the gerontological nurse.
> Discuss the scope and standards of gerontological nursing practice.
> Examine core competencies in gerontological nursing.
> Compare the nine essentials of baccalaureate nursing education with the core competencies in gerontological nursing.
> Distinguish among the educational preparation, practice roles, and certification requirements of the various levels of gerontological nursing practice.

KEY TERMS

Ageism
Attitudes
Certification
Core competencies
Geriatrics

Gerontological nursing
Gerontological rehabilitation nursing
Gerontology
Gerocompetencies

Chapter 1

(Competencies 1, 19)

Introduction to Gerontological Nursing

Deborah Conley
Jeanne St. Pierre

The History of Gerontological Nursing

The history and development of gerontological nursing is rich in diversity and experiences, as is the population it serves. There has never been a more opportune time than now to be a gerontological nurse (see **Figure 1-1**)! No matter where nurses practice, they will at some time in their career care for older adults. Nurses must recognize gerontological nursing as a specialty and use the science within this specialty to guide their practice. The healthcare movement is constantly increasing life expectancy; therefore, nurses should expect to care for relatively larger numbers of older people over the next decades. With the increasing numbers of acute, chronic, and terminal health conditions experienced by older adults, nurses are in key positions to provide disease prevention and health promotion, promote positive aging, and assist this growing population in end-of-life decision making.

The National Gerontological Nursing Association (NGNA), the *American Journal of Nursing*, the American Nurses Association (ANA), Sigma Theta Tau International (STTI), and the John A. Hartford Foundation Institute for Geriatric Nursing at New York University contributed significantly to the development of the specialty of gerontological nursing. The specialty was formally recognized in the early 1960s when the ANA recommended a specialty group for geriatric nurses and the formation of a geriatric nursing division, and convened the first national nursing meeting on geriatric nursing practice. The growth of the specialty soared over the next three decades. In the early 1970s, the ANA *Standards for Geriatric Practice* and the *Journal of Gerontological Nursing* were first published (in 1970 and 1975, respectively). Following the enactment of federal programs such as Medicare and Medicaid, rapid growth in the healthcare

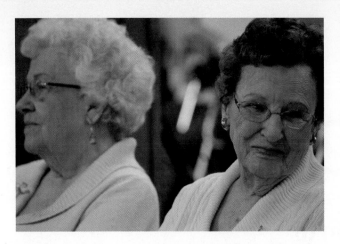

Figure 1-1 More nurses educated in gerontological nursing are needed to care for the growing number of older adults.

industry for elders occurred. In the 1970s, the Veterans Administration (VA) funded a number of Geriatric Research Education and Clinical Centers (GRECCs) at VA medical centers across the United States. Nurses were provided substantial educational opportunities to learn about the care of older veterans through the development of GRECCs. The Kellogg Foundation also funded numerous certificate nurse practitioner programs at colleges of nursing for nurses to become geriatric nurse practitioners. These were not master's in nursing-level programs, but they provided needed nurses who were educated in geriatrics to meet the growing needs of an aging population.

Terminology used to describe nurses caring for elders has included geriatric nurses, gerontic nurses, and gerontological nurses. These terms all have various meanings; however, gerontological nursing provides an all-encompassing view of the care of older adults. In 1976, the ANA Geriatric Nursing Division changed its name to the Gerontological Nursing Division and published the *Standards of Gerontological Nursing* (Ebersole & Touhy, 2006; Meiner, 2011).

The decade of the 1980s saw a substantial growth in gerontological nursing when the NGNA was established, along with the release of the revised ANA statement on the *Scope and Standards of Gerontological Nursing Practice*. Increased numbers of nurses began to obtain master's and doctoral preparation in gerontological nursing, and higher education established programs to prepare nurses as advanced practice nurses in the field (geriatric nurse practitioners and gerontological clinical nurse specialists). Thus, interest in theory to build nursing as a science grew and nurses were beginning to consider gerontological nursing research as an area of study **Box 1-1**. Implementation of five Robert Wood Johnson (RWJ) Foundation Teaching-Nursing Homes provided the opportunity for nursing faculty and nursing homes to collaborate to enhance care to institutionalized elders. An additional eight community-based RWJ grant-funded demonstration projects enabled older adults to remain in their homes and fostered cooperation between social services and healthcare agencies to partner in providing in-home care.

In the 1990s, the John A. Hartford Foundation Institute for Geriatric Nursing was established at the NYU Division of Nursing. It provided unprecedented momentum to improve nursing education and practice and increase nursing research in the care of older adults. In addition, it focused on geriatric public policy and consumer education. The Nurses Improving Care for Healthsystem Elders (NICHE) program gained a national reputation as the model of acute care for older adults.

BOX 1-1   Research Highlight

Aim: To demonstrate that implementation of cognitively stimulating activities is clinically feasible and has the potential to reduce delirium severity and duration and functional loss in postacute-care settings in participants who experience delirium superimposed on dementia.

Method/Sample: Participants were recruited and enrolled at the time of discharge from the hospital and admission to a postacute care/rehabilitation center. Written consent for participation was obtained from each participant's legally authorized representative. Sixteen participants met enrollment criteria and were randomly assigned to one of two conditions: cognitive stimulation (intervention; n = 11) or usual care (control; n = 5). On average, the age in both groups was 85 and the majority was female.

Intervention: The intervention group received routine care and rehabilitation therapies for their medical-surgical condition. They also received cognitive stimulation using simple recreational activities that was increasingly challenging and tailored to each person's interest and functional ability. The control group received routine care and rehabilitation therapies without the cognitive stimulation.

Measures: Daily blinded assessments of delirium, delirium severity, and functional status were measured for up to 30 days.

Findings: The ease of clinical feasibility of using the various tools and implementing interventions was demonstrated. All nursing facility staff reported they were satisfied with the implementation/interventions and would recommend it to other facilities. The control group had a statistically significant decrease in physical function and mental status over time as compared with the intervention group. Delirium, severity of delirium, and attention approached significance and improvement over time favored the intervention group. The control group had more days of delirium than the intervention group.

Application to practice: Nurses are in key positions to positively impact patient outcomes using nonpharmacological nursing interventions in this patient population. Assisting older adults to regain adequate function after hospitalization so they may return to their homes is enormous in terms of quality of life, caregiver burden, and costs.

Source: Kolanowski, A., Fick, D., Clare, L., Steis, M., Boustani, M., & Litaker, M. (2010). Pilot study of a nonpharmacological intervention for delirium superimposed on dementia. *Research in Gerontological Nursing, 20,* 1–7. doi:10.3928/19404921-20101001-98

The 21st century has provided a resurgence in interest in gerontological care. As the baby boomers, who began turning sixty-five years of age in 2011, continue to age, this cadre of individuals will not only expect but demand excellence in geriatric care.

In 2003, the collaborative efforts of the John A. Hartford Institute for Geriatric Nursing, the American Academy of Nursing, and the American Association of Colleges of Nursing (AACN) led to the development of the Hartford Geriatric Nursing Initiative (HGNI). This initiative substantially increased the number of gerontological nurse scientists and the development of evidence-based gerontological nursing practice. Today, there are multiple professional journals, books, websites, and organizations dedicated to the nursing care of older adults. One of the newest journals to emerge in 2008 was the *Journal of Gerontological Nursing Research*.

In 2008, the Honor Society of Nursing, Sigma Theta Tau International (STTI), recognized the ability of nurses to influence practice and patient outcomes in geriatric health care and developed the Geriatric Nursing Leadership Academy (GNLA). This 18-month mentored leadership experience for nurses is funded by the John A. Hartford Foundation and developed in partnership with the Hartford Foundation's Centers of Geriatric Nursing Excellence. GNLA is a premier opportunity for nurses dedicated to influencing policy and geriatric health outcomes. Fellows of the GNLA become active participants in the national network of gerontological nursing leaders. In 2011, this program received additional funding from Hill-Rom Inc. and the Northwest Health Foundation.

In 2009, the Geriatric Nursing Education Consortium (GNEC) was established by AACN and funded by the John A. Hartford Foundation to enhance gerontological nursing content in senior-level undergraduate nursing courses. To successfully incorporate content into the curriculum, faculty must be educated and have accessible evidence-based gerontological content, access to resources, and support from professional gerontological nursing colleagues.

A national Geropalliative Care nurse residency initiative in 2010 was spearheaded by Massachusetts General Hospital and funded in part by The Center to Champion Nursing in America, an initiative of the American Association of Retired Persons (AARP), the AARP Foundation, and the Robert Wood Johnson Foundation. Massachusetts General Hospital's Yvonne L. Munn Center for Nursing Research provided direction and oversight for the AgeWISE residency, which has been implemented in 13 acute care settings in the United States. More information about the AgeWISE residency may be found at http://championnursing.org/blog/nurse-residency-geropalliative-care.

The Advancing Care Excellence for Seniors (ACES) was established in 2010 and developed through a partnership between the National League for Nursing (NLN) and Community College of Philadelphia with funding from the John A. Hartford Foundation, Laerdal Medical, and the Independence Foundation. Implemented through the NLN, this nursing faculty development program has enhanced and empowered faculty to teach gerontological nursing content for undergraduate nursing students. ACES assist students to value the importance of individualized aging, complexity of care, and vulnerability during life transitions. Knowledge about care of older adults is framed around these ideas and guides selection of content in the nursing curriculum. More information on ACES can be found at http://www.nln.org/facultyprograms/facultyresources/aces/index.htm.

The development of gerontological nursing as a specialty is attributed to a host of nursing pioneers. The majority of these nurses were from the United States; however, two key trailblazers were from England. Florence Nightingale and Doreen Norton provided early insights into the "care of the aged." Nightingale was truly the first gerontological nurse, because she accepted the nurse superintendent position in an English institution comparable to our current nursing homes. She cared for wealthy women's maids and helpers in an institution called the Care of Sick Gentlewomen in Distressed Circumstances (Ebersole & Touhy, 2006). Doreen Norton summarized her thoughts on geriatric nursing in a 1956 speech at the annual conference of the Student Nurses Association in London. She later focused her career on care of the aged and wrote often about the unique and specific needs of elders and the nurses caring for them. She identified the advantages of including geriatric care in basic nursing education as: (1) learning patience, tolerance, understanding, and basic nursing skills; (2) witnessing the terminal stages of disease and the importance of skilled nursing care at that time; (3) preparing for the future, because no matter where one works in nursing, the aged will be a great part of the care; (4) recognizing the importance of appropriate rehabilitation, which calls upon all the skill that nurses possess; and (5) being aware of the need to undertake research in geriatric nursing (Norton, 1956).

Landmarks in the Development of Gerontological Nursing

Nurse scientists, educators, authors, and clinicians forged the way for the overall development of gerontological nursing as we know it today. The following is a summary of significant landmarks in the development of gerontological nursing as a specialty:

1902 *American Journal of Nursing* (*AJN*) publishes first geriatric article by an MD

1904 *AJN* publishes first geriatric article by an RN

1925 *AJN* considers geriatric nursing as a potential specialty
Anonymous column entitled "Care of the Aged" appears in *AJN*

1950 First geriatric nursing textbook, *Geriatric Nursing* (Newton), published
First master's thesis in geriatric nursing completed by Eleanor Pingrey
Geriatrics becomes a specialization in nursing

1952 First geriatric nursing study published in *Nursing Research*

1961 ANA recommends specialty group for geriatric nurses

1962 ANA holds first National Nursing Meeting on Geriatric Nursing Practice

1966 ANA forms a Geriatric Nursing Division
First Gerontological Clinical Nurse Specialist master's program begins at Duke University

1968 First RN (Gunter) presents at the International Congress of Gerontology

1970 ANA creates the *Standards of Practice for Geriatric Nursing*

1973 ANA offers the first generalist certification in gerontological nursing (74 nurses certified)

1975 First nursing journal for the care of older adults published: *Journal of Gerontological Nursing* by Slack, Inc.
First nursing conference held at the International Congress of Gerontology

1976 ANA Geriatric Nursing Division changes name to Gerontological Nursing Division
ANA publishes *Standards of Gerontological Nursing*

1977 Kellogg Foundation funds Geriatric Nurse Practitioner certificate education
First gerontological nursing track funded by the Division of Nursing at the University of Kansas

1979 First national conference on gerontological nursing sponsored by the *Journal of Gerontological Nursing*

1980 *AJN* publishes *Geriatric Nursing* journal
Education for Gerontic Nurses by Gunter and Estes suggests curricula for all levels of nursing education
ANA establishes Council of Long-Term Care Nurses

1980 First Robert Wood Johnson (RWJ) Foundation grants for health-impaired elders given (eight in the United States)

1981 First International Conference on Gerontological Nursing sponsored by the International Council of Nursing (Los Angeles, California)
ANA Division of Gerontological Nursing publishes *Statement on Scope of Practice*
John A. Hartford Foundation's Hospital Outcomes Program for the Elderly (HOPE) uses a Geriatric Resource Nurse (GRN) model developed at Yale University under the direction of Terry Fulmer

1982 Development of RWJ Foundation Teaching–Nursing Home Program (five programs in the United States)

1983 First endowed university chair in gerontological nursing (Florence Cellar Endowed Gerontological Nursing Chair) established at Case Western Reserve University

1984 National Gerontological Nursing Association (NGNA) established
ANA Division on Gerontological Nursing Practice becomes Council on Gerontological Nursing

1986 National Association for Directors of Nursing Administration in Long-Term Care established
ANA publishes *Survey of Gerontological Nurses in Clinical Practice*

1987 ANA revises *Standards and Scope of Gerontological Nursing Practice*

1988 First PhD program in gerontological nursing established (Case Western Reserve University)

1989 ANA certification established for Clinical Specialist in Gerontological Nursing

1990 ANA establishes Division of Long-Term Care within the Council of Gerontological Nursing

1992 Nurses Improving Care for Healthsystem Elders (NICHE) established at New York University (NYU) Division of Nursing, based on the HOPE programs

1996 John A. Hartford Foundation Institute for Geriatric Nursing established at NYU Division of Nursing; NICHE administered through the John A. Hartford Foundation Institute for Geriatric Nursing

1998 ANA certification available for geriatric advanced practice nurses as geriatric nurse practitioners or gerontological clinical nurse specialists

2000 American Academy of Nursing, the John A. Hartford Foundation, and the NYU Division of Nursing develop the Building Academic Geriatric Nursing Capacity (BAGNC) program

2002 American Nurses Foundation (ANF) and ANA fund the Nurse Competence in Aging (NCA) joint venture with the John A. Hartford Foundation Institute for Geriatric Nursing

2003 The John A. Hartford Foundation Institute for Geriatric Nursing, the American Academy of Nursing, and the American Association of Colleges of Nursing (AACN) combine efforts to develop the Hartford Geriatric Nursing Initiative (HGNI); John A. Hartford Foundation Institute for Geriatric Nursing at NYU awards Specialty Nursing Association Programs-in Geriatrics (SNAP-G) grants

2004 American Nurses Credentialing Center's first computerized generalist certification exam is for the gerontological nurse

2005 *Journal of Gerontological Nursing* celebrates 30 years

2007 NICHE program at John A. Hartford Foundation Institute for Geriatric Nursing at NYU receives additional funding from the Atlantic Philanthropies and U.S. Aging Program

2008 *Geriatric Nursing* journal celebrates 30 years

Journal of Gerontological Nursing Research emerges

2009 Geriatric Nursing Education Consortium (GNEC) faculty development initiative of AACN established: Sigma Theta Tau International (STTI) Geriatric Nursing Leadership Academy launches

2010 NLN's Advancing Care Excellence for Seniors (ACES), a nursing faculty development initiative, launches; AgeWISE Geropalliative Care Nurse Residency, a national initiative disseminated by Massachusetts General Hospital's Yvonne L. Munn Center for Nursing Research, is established

Attitudes Toward Aging and Older Adults

As a nursing student, you may have preconceived ideas about caring for older adults. Such ideas are influenced by your observations of family members, friends, neighbors, and the media, as well as your own experience with older adults. Perhaps you have a close relationship with your grandparents or you have noticed the aging of your own parents. For some of you, the aging process may have become noticeable when you look at yourself in the mirror. But for all of us, this universal phenomenon we call aging has some type of meaning, whether or not we have taken the time to consciously think about it.

The way you view aging and older adults is often a product of your environment and the experiences to which you have been exposed. Negative *attitudes* toward aging or older adults (*ageism*) often arise in the same way—from negative past experiences. Many of our attitudes and ideas about older adults may not be grounded in fact. Some of you may have already been exposed to ageism, which is often displayed in much the same way as sexism or racism—via attitudes and actions. This is one reason for studying the aging process—to examine the myths and realities, to separate fact from fiction, and to gain an appreciation for what older adults have to offer.

Population statistics show that the majority of your careers as nurses will include caring for older adults. As Mathy Mezey, director of the John A. Hartford Foundation Institute for Geriatric Nursing at NYU, stated, care of older adults is clearly the "core business" of our health care system (Mezey, 2010, p. xiii). Providing high-quality care to elders requires knowledge of the intricacies of the aging process as well as the unique syndromes and disease conditions that can accompany growing older.

As you read and study this text, you are encouraged to examine your own thoughts, values, feelings, and attitudes about growing older. Perhaps you already have a positive attitude toward caring for older adults—build on that value, and consider devoting your time and efforts to the practice of gerontological nursing. If, however, you are reading this chapter with the idea that gerontological nursing is a less-desirable field of nursing, or that working with older people would be an option of last resort, then you may need to reexamine these feelings. Equipped with the facts and positive experiences with older adults, you may change your mind.

Advocates for older adults, such as Nobel laureate Elie Wiesel, feel that older adults, as repositories of our collective memories, should be appreciated and respected. Because of the rapid growth in the numbers of older adults worldwide (see Chapters 2 and 19), gerontological nursing is the place to be! Caring for the largest number of older adults in history presents enormous opportunities. With the over-85 age group being the fastest growing portion of the population, the complexity of caring for so many people with multiple physical and psychosocial changes will present a challenge for even the most daring of nurses. New graduates of nursing programs must be competent in caring for older adults across multiple health settings (Institute of Medicine, 2008) (see Figure 1-1), and it is vital that nursing students understand how coordinating care during significant life transitions for older adults is fundamental to ensuring culturally competent, individualized, holistic care for the older adult and their caregivers (see **Figure 1-2**). However, this focus may not be sufficiently emphasized in today's nursing curricula, unless you are fortunate to be enrolled in a program that has a stand-alone gerontological nursing course. Will you be ready to care for this unique and challenging population?

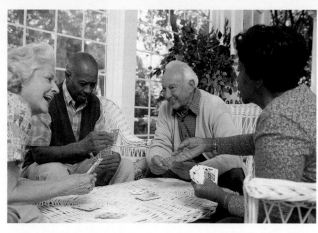

Figure 1-2 Assisted living facilities aid older people with activities of daily living.
Source: © Comstock Images/Alamy Images.

The purpose of this text is to provide the essential information needed by students of gerontological nursing to provide evidence-based care to older adults. In your study of this text, you will be presented with knowledge and insights from experienced professionals with expertise in various areas of gerontological nursing and geriatrics. Each chapter contains thought-provoking activities and questions for personal reflection. Case studies will help you to think about and apply the information. A glossary, divided by chapter, is included at the end of this text to help you master key terms, and plenty of tables and figures summarize key information. Websites are included as a means of expanding your knowledge. Use this text as a guidebook for your study. Use all the resources available, including your instructors, to immerse yourself in the study of gerontological nursing. By the end of this text, you will have learned about the essential competencies needed to provide quality evidence-based care to older adults and their families.

Definitions

Gerontology is the broad term used to define the study of aging and/or the aged. This includes the biopsychosocial aspects of aging. Under the umbrella of gerontology are several subfields, including geriatrics, social gerontology, geropsychology, geropharmacology, gerontological nursing, and gerontological rehabilitation nursing.

What is old and who defines old age? Interestingly, although "old" is often defined as over 65 years of age, this is an arbitrary number set by the Social Security Administration. Today, the older age group is often divided into the young old (ages 65–74), the middle old (ages 75–84), and the old old, very old, or frail elderly (ages 85 and up). However, these numbers merely provide a guideline and do not actually define the various strata of the aging population. Among individuals, vast differences exist between biological and chronological aging, and between the physical, emotional, and social aspects of aging. How and at what rate a person ages depends upon a host of factors that will be discussed throughout this book. The aging population as well as theories and concepts related to aging are discussed further in Chapters 2 and 3.

Geriatrics is often used as a generic term relating to older adults, but specifically refers to the medical care of the older adults. Geriatricians are physicians trained in geriatric medicine. For this reason, many nursing journals and texts have chosen to use the term gerontological nursing instead of geriatric nursing because gerontological denotes a holistic viewpoint, including both wellness and illness care of older adults.

Social gerontology is concerned mainly with the social aspects of aging versus the biological or psychological. "Social gerontologists not only draw on research from all the social sciences—sociology, psychology, economics, and political science—they also seek to understand how the biological processes of aging influence the social aspects of aging" (Quadagno, 2005, p. 4). Geropsychology is a branch of psychology concerned with helping older persons and their families maintain well-being, overcome problems, and achieve maximum potential during later life. Geropharmacology is the study of pharmacology as it relates to older adults. Financial gerontology is another emerging subfield that combines knowledge of financial planning and services with a special expertise in the needs of older adults. Cutler (2004) defines financial gerontology as "the intellectual intersection of two fields, gerontology and finance, each of which has practitioner and academic components" (p. 29).

Gerontological rehabilitation nursing combines expertise in gerontological nursing with rehabilitation concepts and practice. Nurses working in gerontological rehabilitation often care for older adults with chronic illnesses and long-term functional limitations such as stroke, head injury, multiple sclerosis, Parkinson's disease, spinal cord injury, arthritis, joint replacements, and amputations. The goal of gerontological rehabilitation nursing is to assist older adults to regain and maintain the highest level of function and independence possible while preventing complications and enhancing quality of life.

Gerontological nursing falls within the discipline of nursing and the scope of nursing practice. It involves nurses advocating for the health of older adults at all levels of prevention. The health status of older adults is diverse and complex. A key focus of health promotion and disease prevention in gerontological nursing is to minimize the loss of independence associated with functional decline and illness. Gerontological nurses work with healthy older adults in their communities, acutely ill elders requiring hospitalization and treatment, and chronically ill or disabled elders in long-term care facilities, skilled care, home care, and palliative and hospice care. The scope of practice for gerontological nursing includes all older adults from about 65 years of age until death. Gerontological nursing is guided by standards of practice that will be discussed later in this chapter.

Roles of the Gerontological Nurse
Direct-Care Provider

In the role of caregiver or provider of care, the gerontological nurse gives direct, hands-on care to older adults in a variety of settings. Older adults often present with atypical symptoms that complicate diagnosis and treatment. Thus, the nurse as a direct-care provider should be educated about disease processes and syndromes commonly seen in the older population (see **Case Study 1-1**). This may include knowledge of risk factors, signs and symptoms, usual medical treatment, rehabilitation, and end-of-life care. Chapters 9, 10 and 30 review the management of common illnesses, diseases, and health conditions, imparting essential information for providing quality care. An entire unit (Chapters 11–18) of this book is devoted to the discussion of geriatric syndromes to better prepare the nurse to be a care provider.

Case Study 1-1

Rose is a 52-year-old nursing student who has returned to school for her BSN after raising a family. She is the divorced mother of two grown children and has one young grandson. In addition to being a full-time student in an accelerated program, Rose also cares for her 85-year-old mother in her own home and occasionally helps provide childcare for her grandson while his parents work. Rose's mother has diabetes and is legally blind. Rose is taking a gerontology course this semester and finds herself going home quite upset after the first week of classes when attitudes toward aging were discussed. While sharing with the course instructor her feelings and surprising emotional discomfort, Rose is helped to identify that she is afraid of getting older and being unable to care for her ailing mother and herself. As a single woman, she is unsure that she can handle what lies ahead for her.

Questions:

1. What can Rose do to become more comfortable with facing her own advancing age?

2. What factors may have influenced her discomfort with the course material?

3. Is there anything the instructor of the course might do to help Rose cope with the feelings she is having as she completes the required coursework?

4. There may be some activities that Rose can do in order to understand her feelings about aging better. Can you think of some such activities?

5. What is Rose's role as the caregiver in this situation? How may the role change over time?

6. How much does Rose's present home and living situation contribute to her fears and perceptions of aging?

Teacher

An essential part of all nursing is teaching. Gerontological nurses focus their teaching on modifiable risk factors and health promotion (see Chapters 5, 7 and 8). Many diseases and debilitating conditions of aging can be prevented through lifestyle modifications in the areas of diet, smoking cessation, weight management, physical activity, and stress management, as well as routine healthcare screenings (see Chapter 7). Nurses have a responsibility to educate the older adult population about ways to decrease their risk of certain disorders such as heart disease, cancer, and stroke, the leading causes of death for this age group. Nurses may develop expertise in specialized areas and teach skills to other nurses in order to promote evidence-based care among older adults.

Leader

Gerontological nurses act as leaders during everyday practice as they balance the concerns of the patient, family, nursing, and the rest of the interprofessional team. All nurses must be skilled in leadership, time management, building relationships, communication, and managing change. Nurse leaders who are in management positions may supervise other nursing personnel including licensed practical nurses (LPNs), certified nursing assistants (CNAs), technicians, nursing students, and other unlicensed assistive personnel. The role of the gerontological nurse as manager and leader is further discussed in Chapter 19.

Advocate

As an advocate, the gerontological nurse acts on behalf of older adults to promote their best interests and strengthen their autonomy and decision making. Advocacy may take many forms, including active involvement at the political level or helping to explain medical or nursing procedures to family members on a unit level. Nurses may also advocate for patients through other activities such as helping family members choose the best nursing home for their loved one or supporting family members who are in a caregiving role. Whatever the situation, gerontological nurses must remember that being an advocate does not mean making decisions for older adults, but empowering them to remain independent and retain dignity, even in difficult situations.

Evidence-Based Clinician

The appropriate level of involvement for nurses at the baccalaureate level is implementation of evidence-based practice (EBP) principles. Gerontological nurses must remain abreast of current research literature, reading and translating into practice the results of reliable and valid studies. Using EBP, gerontological nurses can improve the quality of patient care in all settings. Although nurses with undergraduate degrees may be involved in research in some facilities, such as posing a clinical inquiry or assisting with data collection, their basic preparation is aimed primarily at using research in practice. All nurses should read professional journals specific to their specialty and continue their education by attending seminars and workshops, participating in professional organizations, pursuing additional formal education or degrees, and obtaining certification. By implementing evidence-based practice, gerontological nurses can improve the quality of patient care in all settings.

Expanded roles of the gerontological nurse may also include counselor, consultant, coordinator of services, administrator, collaborator, geriatric care manager, and others. Several of these roles are discussed in Chapters 19, 20, 31, and 32.

Certification

To provide competent, evidence-based care to older adults, nurses need to have gerontological nursing content in their basic undergraduate nursing curricula and are encouraged to become certified in gerontological nursing. Hospitalized older adults have multiple co-existing terminal and chronic health problems and a higher acuity level than their younger counterparts, requiring advanced nursing knowledge. Despite all the work that has been done to encourage gerontological nursing *certification*, less than 1% of nurses in the United States hold this designation. Adults age 65 and older utilize >48% of the nation's total healthcare resources and represent approximately 55% of all admissions to hospitals (Centers for Disease Control and Prevention [CDC], 2012). Patients and their families are knowledgeable about quality health care and patient safety and want the most expert clinicians at the bedside. Certification provides reassurance to patients and their families that the nurses caring for them are highly skilled and possess expert knowledge in providing excellence in gerontological nursing care (Hartford Institute for Geriatric Nursing, 2012).

Nurse certification is a formal process by which a certifying agency validates a nurse's knowledge, skills, and competencies through a computerized exam in a specialty area of practice. There are two levels of certification: generalist and advanced practice level **Table 1-1**. Each has different eligibility standards. The American Nurses Credentialing Center (ANCC) is the certifying body for both levels of gerontological nursing practice.

Generalist Certification

The generalist in gerontological nursing has completed a basic entry-level program in nursing, which can be a diploma in nursing, or an associate or bachelor of science degree in nursing. Before meeting additional eligibility requirements to become certified in gerontological nursing, the applicant must be a licensed registered nurse for at least 2 years. ANCC offers the generalist computerized exam in gerontological nursing at over 300 computer-based testing sites across the country. This exam was the first one to become computerized, increasing the convenience of sitting for gerontological nursing certification.

TABLE 1-1   Websites for Test Content Outlines
http://www.nursecredentialing.org/NurseSpecialties/Gerontological.aspx
http://www.nursecredentialing.org/NurseSpecialties/GerontologicalCNS.aspx
http://www.nursecredentialing.org/NurseSpecialties/GerontologicalNP.aspx

---

BOX 1-2   Web Exploration

Explore the following websites for further information on certification and gerontological associations of interest to nurses.

Educational Websites

American Nurses Association (ANA)
http://www.nursingworld.org

Hartford Geriatric Nursing Initiative, ConsultGeriRN.org
http://www.consultgeriRN.org

Associations

U.S. Administration on Aging
http://www.aoa.gov

American Geriatrics Society
http://www.americangeriatrics.org

American Nurses Credentialing Center (ANCC)
http://www.nursecredentialing.org

Gerontological Society of America
http://www.geron.org

Hospice and Palliative Nurses Association (HPNA)
http://www.hpna.org

John A. Hartford Foundation Institute for Geriatric Nursing
http://www.hartfordign.org

National Adult Day Services Association
http://www.nadsa.org

National Association of Professional Geriatric Care Managers
http://www.caremanager.org

National Council on the Aging
http://www.ncoa.org/

National Gerontological Nursing Association
http://www.ngna.org

National Institute on Aging
http://www.nia.nih.gov

Certification has been connected to decreased medical errors and increased job satisfaction. Piazza, Donahue, Dykes, Griffin, & Fitzpatrick (2006) noted that nurse managers have reported that certification validates a nurse's specialized knowledge and demonstrates clinical competence and credibility. Additionally, by meeting national standards, certification empowers nurses as professionals and aligns them with an organizational goal of promoting positive work experiences for nurses. Certification creates an intrinsic sense of professional pride and accomplishment and validates competence in a specialized area to colleagues, peers, and the public.

Certified gerontological nurses utilize principles of gerontological nursing and gerontological competencies as they implement the nursing process with patients. Gerontological certified nurses:

> Assess, manage, and deliver health care that meets the needs of older adults
> Evaluate the effectiveness of their care
> Identify the strengths and limitations of their patients
> Maximize patient independence
> Involve patients and family members (ANCC, 2012)

There are a number of compelling reasons for nurses to pursue gerontological nurse certification. Certified gerontological nurses:

> Experience a high degree of professional accomplishment and satisfaction
> Demonstrate a commitment to their profession
> Provide higher quality of care to older adults
> Act as resources for other nurses and interprofessional team members
> Demonstrate evidence-based gerontological nursing care
> Are recognized as national leaders in gerontological nursing care
> Create the potential for higher salaries and benefits
> Are actively recruited for employment as nursing faculty, in Magnet and Nurses Improving Care for Healthsystem Elders (NICHE) designated hospitals, in long-term care facilities, in acute rehab, and in community health agencies (ANCC, 2012; Hartford Institute for Geriatric Nursing, 2012)

See the ANCC website (http://www.nursecredentialing.org/certification.aspx# specialty) for eligibility requirements and information about gerontological nurse certification and recertification.

Advanced Practice Certification

The ANCC currently offers two separate advanced practice certification exams in gerontological nursing: the clinical specialist in gerontological nursing (GCNS-BC) and the gerontological nurse practitioner (GNP-BC). There are different eligibility requirements for each exam. The ANCC website http://www.nursecredentialing .org/certification.aspx#specialty has eligibility requirements and information on certification and recertification. Per the ANCC, current eligibility requirements for gerontological CNS certification include holding a current, active RN license in a state or territory of the United States or the professional, legally recognized equivalent in another country and holding a master's, postgraduate, or doctorate degree from a clinical nurse specialist in gerontology program accredited by the Commission on Collegiate Nursing Education (CCNE) or the National League for Nursing Accrediting Commission (NLNAC). A minimum of 500 faculty-supervised clinical hours in the Gerontological CNS role and specialty must be included in the educational program. This Gerontological CNS graduate program must include three separate courses in advanced physical/health assessment, advanced pharmacology, and advanced pathophysiology.

Eligibility requirements for gerontological NP certification are the same as for the CNS with the addition of graduate coursework in health promotion and disease prevention, and differential diagnosis and disease management.

The advanced gerontological specialty certification will be phased out by 2015 in favor of the Adult-Gerontology Clinical Nurse Specialist (expected launch 2014), Adult-Gerontology Acute Care Nurse Practitioner, and Adult-Gerontology Primary Care Nurse Practitioner (expected launch 2013). Only CNSs and NPs who are currently certified in gerontology will be able to maintain the current much-needed specialty certification, but the ANCC will no longer offer certification exams for the GNP and GCNS after the phase out.

Many states require advanced practice registered nurses (APRNs) to hold a separate license as an APRN. The advanced practice role encompasses education, consultation, research, case management, administration, and advocacy in the care of older adults. In addition, APRNs develop advanced knowledge of nursing theory, research, and clinical practice. The APRN is an expert in providing care for older adults, families, and groups in a variety of settings.

The GCNS focuses on three spheres of influence: patient/family care, developing nurses, and impacting organizations and systems. Gerontological clinical nurse specialists play important roles in acute care by developing and implementing gerontological nursing evidence-based practice. In addition, some roles involve a collaborative practice or consultative role with hospitals or long-term care facilities and interdisciplinary teams. In some states, GCNSs may obtain prescriptive authority and broaden their scope of practice. Gerontological CNSs have developed and managed clinics for common conditions in the older population such as incontinence, falls, wounds, or cognitive impairments. The ANCC describes the role of the gerontological CNS as follows:

> The Clinical Nurse Specialist in Gerontological Nursing (GCNS) is a registered nurse prepared in a graduate level gerontological clinical nurse specialist program to provide advanced care for older adults, their families, and significant others. The GCNS has an expert understanding of the dynamics, pathophysiology, and psychosocial aspects of aging. The GCNS uses advanced diagnostic and assessment skills and nursing interventions to manage and improve patient care. Using theory and research, the GCNS's practice considers all influences on a patient's health status and the related psychosocial and behavioral problems arising from the patient's altered physiological condition. The GCNS practices in diverse settings and is actively engaged in education (e.g., patient, staff, students, and colleagues), case management, expert clinical practice, consultation, research, and administration. (ANCC, 2008, p. 1)

The geriatric nurse practitioner (GNP) practices in acute or long-term care settings and in collaborative practice with physicians who maintain large geriatric practices. Geriatric nurse practitioners make regular visits to nursing homes where patients in their collaborative practice reside, and they also practice in rehabilitation facilities, working in outpatient clinics for rehabilitation patients after discharge or with specialty physicians, managing caseloads, and diagnosing and treating geriatric syndromes. The ANCC describes the role of the gerontological nurse practitioner as follows:

> The GNP is a registered nurse prepared in a graduate level geriatric nurse practitioner program to provide a full range of health care

services on the wellness-illness health care continuum at an advanced level to older adults. The GNP practice includes independent and inter-dependent decision making, and is directly accountable for clinical judgments. The graduate level preparation expands the GNP's role to include differential diagnosis and disease management, participation in and use of research, development and implementation of health policy, leadership, education, case management, and consultation. (ANCC, 2008, p. 1)

Scope and Standards of Practice

The scope of nursing practice is defined by state regulation, but is also influenced by the unique needs of the population being served. The needs of older adults are complex and multifaceted, and the focus of nursing care depends on the setting in which the nurse practices.

Gerontological nursing is practiced in accordance with standards developed by the profession of nursing. In 2010, the ANA Division of Gerontological Nursing Practice published the third edition of the *Scope and Standards of Gerontological Nursing Practice*, in collaboration with the National Gerontological Nursing Association, the National Association of Directors of Nursing Administrators in Long-Term Care, and the National Conference of Gerontological Nurse Practitioners. These standards are divided into clinical care and the role of the professional nurse, both at the generalist and advanced practice nurse level of practice. There are six standards, which include assessment, diagnosis, outcome identification, planning, implementation, and evaluation. The eight standards of professional gerontological nursing performance include quality of care, performance appraisals, education, collegiality, ethics, collaboration, research, resource utilization, and transitions of care. Students should note that these are the basic standards for professional nursing, but they are specifically developed for the care of older adults. Core competencies, discussed in the next section, provide specific guidelines for gerontological nursing care. A full description and copy of the scope and standards is available at http://www.ngna.org or http://www.nursesbooks.org/Main-Menu/Specialties/Gerontology/Gerontological-Nursing-Practice.aspx.

Core Competencies

Specific *core competencies* have been identified for gerontological nursing in addition to general professional nursing preparation. These competencies are influenced by the level at which the nurse will function and the role expectations of the nurse. Core competencies provide a foundation of added knowledge and skills necessary for the nurse to implement in daily practice. Common bodies of assumptions, knowledge, skills, and attitudes that are essential for excellent clinical nursing practice with older adults have been developed and provide the basic foundation for all levels of gerontological nursing practice.

The AACN and the John A. Hartford Foundation Institute for Geriatric Nursing at NYU College of Nursing assembled input from qualified gerontological nursing experts to publish *Recommended Baccalaureate Competencies and Curricular Guidelines for Geriatric Nursing Care* in 2008. These gerocompetency statements were updated in 2010 and are a supplement to *The Essentials of Baccalaureate Education for Professional Nursing Practice* (AACN, 2008). The gerocompetency statements provide the framework for this text. There are 19 gerocompetency statements, which are divided into the 9 *Essentials* identified in the AACN document, with associated rationale, suggestions for content, teaching strategies, resources, and glossary of terms (see **Table 1-2**). The purpose of this document specific to gerontological nursing was to use the AACN's *Essentials of Baccalaureate Education for Professional Nursing Practice* (2008) as a framework to help nurse educators integrate specific nursing content into their programs. These appear in **Table 1-3**. The *gerocompetencies* in Table 1-2 correlate with and were derived from the suggestions in the more general AACN document in Table 1-3. By using these published documents as guides, nursing faculty and others who educate in the area of gerontological nursing will be able to prepare students to be competent in providing gerontological best practices to older adults and their families. As students, we want you to understand the rationale for including gerocompetency content in your nursing education. It is essential for you to become competent in gerontological nursing concepts and principles as you move forward in your education and nursing practice, in order to be prepared for the tsunami of older adults you will be caring for (Stierle, et al., 2006).

TABLE 1-2   Gerontological Nursing Competency Statements
1.   Incorporate professional attitudes, values, and expectations about physical and mental aging in the provision of patient-centered care for older adults and their families. *Corresponding to Essential VIII*
2.   Assess barriers for older adults in receiving, understanding, and giving of information. *Corresponding to Essentials IV & IX*
3.   Use valid and reliable assessment tools to guide nursing practice for older adults. *Corresponding to Essentials IX*
4.   Assess the living environment as it relates to functional, physical, cognitive, psychological, and social needs of older adults. *Corresponding to Essential IX*
5.   Intervene to assist older adults and their support network to achieve personal goals, based on the analysis of the living environment and availability of community resources. *Corresponding to Essential VII*
6.   Identify actual or potential mistreatment (physical, mental, or financial abuse, and/or self-neglect) in older adults and refer appropriately. *Corresponding to Essential V*

7. Implement strategies and use online guidelines to prevent and/or identify and manage geriatric syndromes.
   Corresponding to Essentials IV & IX

8. Recognize and respect the variations of care, the increased complexity, and the increased use of healthcare resources inherent in caring for older adults.
   Corresponding to Essentials IV & IX

9. Recognize the complex interaction of acute and chronic comorbid physical and mental conditions and associated treatments common to older adults.
   Corresponding to Essential IX

10. Compare models of care that promote safe, quality physical and mental health care for older adults such as PACE, NICHE, Guided Care, Culture Change, and Transitional Care Models.
    Corresponding to Essential II

11. Facilitate ethical, noncoercive decision making by older adults and/or families/caregivers for maintaining everyday living, receiving treatment, initiating advance directives, and implementing end-of-life care.
    Corresponding to Essential VIII

12. Promote adherence to the evidence-based practice of providing restraint-free care (both physical and chemical restraints).
    Corresponding to Essential II

13. Integrate leadership and communication techniques that foster discussion and reflection on the extent to which diversity (among nurses, nurse assistive personnel, therapists, physicians, and patients) has the potential to impact the care of older adults.
    Corresponding to Essential VI

14. Facilitate safe and effective transitions across levels of care, including acute, community-based, and long-term care (e.g., home, assisted living, hospice, nursing homes) for older adults and their families.
    Corresponding to Essentials IV & IX

15. Plan patient-centered care with consideration for mental and physical health and well-being of informal and formal caregivers of older adults.
    Corresponding to Essential IX

16. Advocate for timely and appropriate palliative and hospice care for older adults with physical and cognitive impairments.
    Corresponding to Essentials IX

17. Implement and monitor strategies to prevent risk and promote quality and safety (e.g., falls, medication mismanagement, pressure ulcers) in the nursing care of older adults with physical and cognitive needs.
    Corresponding to Essentials II & IV

18. Utilize resources/programs to promote functional, physical, and mental wellness in older adults.
    Corresponding to Essential VII

19. Integrate relevant theories and concepts included in a liberal education into the delivery of patient-centered care for older adults.
    Corresponding to Essential I

Source: AACN/Hartford Foundation, 2010, p. 12–13. Retrieved from http://www.aacn.nche.edu/geriatric-nursing/AACN_Gerocompetencies.pdf

TABLE 1-3   The Nine Essentials of Baccalaureate Education for Professional Nursing Practice

Essential I: Liberal Education for Baccalaureate Generalist Nursing Practice

Essential II: Basic Organizational and Systems Leadership for Quality Care and Patient Safety

Essential III: Scholarship for Evidence-Based Practice

Essential IV: Information Management and Application of Patient Care Technology

Essential V: Healthcare Policy, Finance, and Regulatory Environments

Essential VI: Interprofessional Communication and Collaboration for Improving Patient Health Outcomes

Essential VII: Clinical Prevention and Population Health

Essential VIII: Professionalism and Professional Values

Essential IX: Baccalaureate Generalist Nursing Practice

Source: American Association of Colleges of Nursing [AACN]. (2008). The essentials of baccalaureate education for professional nursing practice. Washington, DC: Author.

Research in Gerontological Nursing

Nursing research can be defined as the "diligent, systematic inquiry or investigation to validate and refine existing knowledge and generate new knowledge" (Burns & Grove, 2011, p. 2). Research in gerontological nursing is robust as evidenced by the growth in recent years of gerontological nursing journals, books, and other medical and nursing publications. Many colleges and universities support research in gerontological nursing, particularly the nine academic centers that host Hartford Centers for Geriatric Nursing Excellence in Arizona, Arkansas, California, Iowa, Minnesota, Oregon, Pennsylvania, and Utah.

Using nursing research in practice is called evidence-based practice, defined as "the conscientious use of best research evidence in combination with a clinician's expertise, as well as patient preferences and values, to make decisions about the type of care that is provided" (Sackett, Straus, Richardson, Rosenberg, & Haynes, 2000, p. 1). Nursing practice based on the best available evidence ensures that optimal quality of care is provided by helping nurses to know what works and how evaluate outcomes.

Gerontological nursing research has made contributions to nursing science in many areas. Examples include delirium superimposed on dementia, medication issues at discharge for patients with heart failure, and older adult stereotypes among care providers (see **Boxes 1-4** and **1-5**).

BOX 1-3   Additional Resources

American Nurses Credentialing Center (ANCC)

P.O. Box 791333
Baltimore, MD 21279-1333
202-651-7000
800-284-2378

http://www.nursecredentialing.org

John A. Hartford Foundation

55 East 59th Street
16th Floor
New York, NY 10022-1178
212-832-7788

Email: mail@jhartfound.org
http://www.hartfordign.org

BOX 1-4   Research Highlight

Aim: To compare two categories of experiences—contact with older adults versus education about older adults—for their impact on ageist stereotypes.

Methods: Two hundred twenty-five caregivers assisting older adults at five residential care sites in Tasmania, Australia, most of whom were of European descent, participated in psychometric testing regarding prejudice and attitudes toward older adults.

Findings: Regular contact with older adults, especially if the contact underscores the older adult's dependency, may not reduce stereotypes; rather, it may even reinforce them. Higher levels of general education, as well as specific education about aging and older adults, seems to be associated with fewer stereotypes and more positive attitudes towards elders. This finding is also supported by other studies on ageism.

Application to practice: The researchers suggest that while contact with older adults may not improve ageist stereotypes, education shows promise as a starting point for developing more favorable care provider attitudes. In addition, the authors cite research in empathy education, which may also be an effective strategy for reducing prejudice.

Source: Reyna, C., Goodwin, E. J., & Ferrari, J. R. (2007). Older adult stereotypes among care providers in residential care facilities. *Journal of Gerontological Nursing, 33,* 50–55.

BOX 1-5   Research Highlight

Aim: To describe discharge medication reconciliation discrepancies in older adults with heart failure who were discharged to home from the hospital.

Methods: A secondary analysis of medical records collected during a randomized controlled trial testing transitional care interventions for older adults with heart failure.

Findings: Seventy-one percent of hospital discharges had at least one medication reconciliation problem, with an average of 1.3 per discharge. A majority of problems involved high-risk medications that have been shown to be associated with adverse drug events.

Application to practice: Nurses are usually involved in discharge teaching and can therefore make a positive impact by ensuring clear medication instructions that include the time the medication was last given, noting any changes to the patient's prior medication regimen, and clarifying vague terms, such as "take as directed."

Source: Foust J. B., Naylor, M. D., Bixby, M. B. & Ratcliffe, S. J. (2012). Medication problems occurring at hospital discharge among older adults with heart failure. *Research in Gerontological Nursing, 5*, 25–33.

Summary

Gerontological nursing is a specialty practice that focuses on the unique needs of older adults and their families. It builds on the theories and foundations of nursing practice with application of a growing body of literature generated by gerontological nursing scientists. It requires specialized knowledge in the art and science of nursing, coupled with gerontological nursing best practices, to manage the complex needs of this population. Caring for older adults is influenced by many factors, one of which is recognizing one's own attitude about aging. It is imperative, with the aging of today's population, that all nurses have basic gerontological nursing concepts and principles taught in their undergraduate program. With the growth of the older population, more nurses certified and specializing in gerontological nursing will be needed. Gerontological nurses practice in almost all settings and there are emerging subfields of this specialty that offer promise of future roles for nurses who care for older adults. Focusing on the individualization of the aging person, nurses should explore the multiple career options in this rewarding, exciting, creative, and uniquely innovative field of gerontological nursing.

Critical Thinking Exercises

1. Go to a local card shop and browse. Look at the birthday cards that persons might buy for someone getting older. What do they say about society's attitudes toward aging? Do the cards you read point out any areas that we stereotype as problems with advancing age? What positive attributes are seen?

2. Complete this sentence: Older people are _____. List as many adjectives as you can think of. After making your list, identify how many are negative and how many are positive

descriptors. Think about where your ideas came from as you did this exercise.

3. Check out the website at http://www .consultgerirn.org. How would you use this website to enhance your knowledge about the care of older adults? What services are available through the website?

4. Look at the list of competencies for gerontological nurses in Table 1-2. How many of these competencies do you feel you meet at this point? Make a conscious effort to develop these skills as you go through your career.

Personal Reflections

1. How do you feel about aging? Draw a picture of yourself aging and describe the details of what you anticipate will occur as you age. Do you see advanced age as an opportunity to grow old gracefully or something to fear? What are your views about cosmetic procedures (Botox injections, face lifts, body sculpting) that are designed to make people look younger?

2. When was the last time you cared for an older adult? What was that experience like? How do you feel about caring for older adults in your nursing practice? The majority of your nursing practice will entail caring for elders and their families. Did you anticipate this when you entered nursing school?

3. What do you think about nurses who work in nursing homes? Have you ever considered a career in gerontological nursing? Describe the positives you can see about developing expertise in this field of nursing.

4. Have you ever seen ageism in practice? If so, think about that situation and how it could have been turned into a positive scenario. If not, how have the situations you have been in avoided discrimination against older adults?

5. Which of the settings in gerontological nursing practice appeal to you most at this time in your professional career? Is there any one setting that you can see yourself working in more than another? Do you think this will change as you progress in your career?

References

American Association of Colleges of Nursing [AACN] (2008). *The essentials of baccalaureate education for professional nursing practice.* Washington, DC: Author.

American Association of Colleges of Nursing [AACN]. (2012). *GNEC.* Retrieved from http://www.aacn .nche.edu/geriatric-nursing/gnec

American Association of Colleges of Nursing [AACN] and the John A. Hartford Institute for Geriatric Nursing. (2010). Recommended baccalaureate competencies and curricula guidelines for nursing care of older adults, a supplement to the essentials of baccalaureate education for professional nursing practice. Washington, DC: Author.

American Nurses Association [ANA]. (2010). *Scope and standards of gerontological nursing practice.* Washington, DC: Author.

American Nurses Credentialing Center [ANCC]. (2008). *Clinical nurse specialist in gerontology.* Retrieved from http://www.nursecredentialing.org/Documents/Certification/Application/NursingSpecialty/ GerontologicalCNS.aspx

American Nurses Credentialing Center. (2012). Gerontological Nursing. Retrieved from http://www. nursecredentialing.org/NurseSpecialties/Gerontological.aspx

Burns, N. & Grove, S.K. (2011). Understanding nursing research: Building an evidence-based practice (4th ed.). St. Louis, MO: Elsevier Saunders.

Centers for Disease Control and Prevention [CDC]. (2012). Key aging statistics. Retrieved from http:// www.cdc.gov/nchs/nchs_for_you/older_americans.htm

Cutler, N. E. (2004). Aging and finance 1991 to 2004. *Journal of Financial Service Professionals, 58*(1), 29–32.

Ebersole, P., & Touhy, T. (2006). *Geriatric nursing: Growth of a specialty.* New York, NY: Springer.

Foust J. B., Naylor, M. D., Bixby, M. B. & Ratcliffe, S. J. (2012). Medication problems occurring at hospital discharge among older adults with heart failure. *Research in Gerontological Nursing, 5,* 25–33.

Hartford Institute for Geriatric Nursing. (2012). Retrieved from http://www.consultgerirn.org

Institute of Medicine. (2008). *Retooling for an aging America: Building the health care workforce.* Washington., DC: The National Academies Press.

Kolanowski, A., Fick, D., Clare, L., Steis, M., Boustani, M., & Litaker, M. (2010). Pilot study of a nonpharmacological intervention for delirium superimposed on dementia. *Research in Gerontological Nursing, 20,* 1–7. doi:10.3928/19404921-20101001-98

Meiner, S. (2011). *Gerontologic nursing* (3rd ed.). St. Louis, MO: Mosby.

Mezey, M. (2010). Foreword. In K. L. Mauk (Ed.) *Gerontological Nursing: Competencies for Care* (pp. xviii). Sudbury, MA: Jones and Bartlett Publishers, LLC.

National League of Nursing [NLN]. (2012). *Faculty resources.* Retrieved from http://www.nln.org/ facultyprograms/facultyresources/aces/index.htm

Norton, D. (1956, July 6). The place of geriatric nursing in training. *Nursing Times,* 264.

Piazza, I.M., Donahue, M., Dykes, P.C., Griffin, M. Q., & Fitzpatrick, J. J. (2006). Differences in perceptions of empowerment among nationally certified and non-certified nurses. *Journal of Nursing Administration, 36*(5), 277–283.

Quadagno, J. (2005). *Understanding the older client.* Boston, MA: McGraw-Hill.

Reyna, C., Goodwin, E. J., & Ferrari, J. R. (2007). Older adult stereotypes among care providers in residential care facilities. *Journal of Gerontological Nursing, 33,* 50–55.

Sackett, D. L., Straus, S. E., Richardson, W. S., Rosenberg, W., & Haynes, R. B. (2000). Evidence-based medicine: How to practice and teach EBM (2nd ed.). Edinburgh, UK: Churchill Livingstone.

Stierle, L. J., Mezey, M., Schumann, M. J., Esterson, J., Smolenski, M. C., Horsley, K. D., … Gould, E. (2006). Professional development. The Nurse Competence in Aging initiative: Encouraging expertise in the care of older adults. *American Journal of Nursing, 106*(9), 93–96.

For a full suite of assignments and additional learning activities, see the access code at the front of your book.

LEARNING OBJECTIVES

At the end of this chapter, the reader will be able to:

> Review statistics related to aging in the United States.
> Describe social and economic issues related to aging in the United States.
> Discuss aging across different cultures.
> Recognize differences between aging in the 21st century and aging in the past.
> Critically evaluate successful aging.

KEY TERMS www

Aging in place	Graying of America
Baby boomers	Native-born
Centenarian	Older adult
Chronic disease	Oldest old
Cohort	PACE
Demographic tidal wave	Pig in a python
Elderly	Seniors
Foreign-born	Silver tsunami

The Aging Population

Cheryl A. Lehman
Andrea Wirt

U.S. society, and indeed, U.S. families, will be greatly challenged by the *graying of America* over the next few decades. A steadily growing aging population has the potential to affect social policy, societal resources, businesses, and communities, not to mention healthcare systems.

The Numbers

More than one out of every eight Americans is age 65 or older. This older population numbered 40.4 million in 2010, an increase of 5.4 million or 15.3% since 2000. In this same decade, 2000–2010, the number of Americans ages 45–64—who will reach 65 over the next two decades—increased by 31%. The 65 or over population has increased from 35 million in 2000 to 40 million in 2010 (a 15% increase) and is projected to increase to 55 million in 2020 (a 36% increase for the decade). The population of the *oldest old* (85+ years) is projected to increase from 5.5 million in 2010 to 6.6 million in 2020 (a 19% increase for the decade) (Administration on Aging, 2011a). It is anticipated that by 2018, older adults will outnumber children under the age of 5 in the world for the first time in history (Kinsella & He, 2009).

Why the Increase in the Number of Older Adults?

The trend of increasing numbers of *older adults* in the United States can be attributed to two main causes: the increased life expectancy of our *seniors* and the fertility of the U.S. population at various points in time.

In 1935, when Social Security was enacted, the life expectancy for someone who was 65 years old was 12 additional years for males (or 77 years total) and 13 additional years for females (or 78 years total). This has risen to 17.9 and 20.3 additional years, respectively. By 2080, the additional life expectancy for a 65-year-old is expected to have increased to 20 years and 23 years, respectively (Centers for Disease Control and Prevention [CDC], 2009). There is less of a racial difference in life expectancy than in other parameters of aging. In 2006, life expectancy at birth was 5 years higher for Whites than for Blacks, but at age 65, Whites could expect to live for 1.5 years longer than Blacks. For those who live to age 85, the life expectancy for Black people is slightly higher than for Whites (Federal Interagency Forum, 2010).

Changes in life expectancy throughout the 20th century were mainly due to improved sanitation, advances in medical care, and the implementation of preventive health services (Merck Institute of Aging and Health [MIAH], CDC, & Gerontological Society of America, 2004). In the early 1900s, deaths were mostly due to infectious diseases and acute illnesses. The older population of today, however, must deal with challenges that would be unfamiliar to their own parents: dealing with *chronic disease* and affording healthcare services. The average 75-year-old now suffers from three chronic diseases and uses five prescription drugs (MIAH et al., 2004). Modern treatments for diseases that used to kill older adults, such as myocardial infarction and stroke, as well as the improved technical procedures for health services such as transplants and intensive care, have contributed to the increased longevity of the population. Healthcare costs, including medication costs, have thus become a primary issue for many seniors. The repercussions of rising healthcare costs have been felt within the state and federal governments, as they seek to help support their senior citizens' health. Nearly 95% of healthcare expenditures for older Americans are for chronic diseases (MIAH et al., 2004).

Fertility of the population also affects the number of older adults. The fertility rate in the United States has been steadily falling for the past 200 years. In 1800, the average woman had 7 children; by the end of World War II, this had decreased to 2.4 children. However, in the two decades after the war, the fertility rate increased to 3.5 children (Munnell, 2004). Of course, one could argue that some of these changes have less to do with fertility rate and more to do with the influence of other factors such as the acceptance and use of birth control as well as the changing values of different generations.

The growth of the older population slowed somewhat during the 1990s because of the relatively small number of babies born during the Great Depression of the 1930s. However, the older population will explode between 2010 and 2030, when the *baby boomer* generation reaches age 65. This extremely large segment of the U.S. population, who were born between 1946 and 1964, started turning 65 in 2011. This anticipated increase has been called both a *demographic tidal wave* (MIAH et al., 2004) and a *pig in a python* (meaning a bulge in population moving slowly through time) (Munnell, 2004).

Beginning in 2012, nearly 10,000 Americans will turn 65 every day (MIAH et al., 2004). By 2030, the older population will comprise 20% of the total population of the United States (which will comprise about 72 million people) (Federal Interagency Forum, 2010; MIAH et al., 2004). This group of older adults will be the "healthiest, longest lived, best educated, [and] most affluent in history" (Experience Corps, 2005). After 2030, the population of oldest old (those over 85 years) will grow the fastest. According to the Federal Interagency Forum (2010), the U.S. Census Bureau projects that the population of those 85 or older could grow from 5.7 million in 2008 to 19 million by 2050 (see **Figure 2-1**). Some research has raised new concerns about future increases in life expectancy in the United States as compared to other high-income countries. Poor lifestyle choices such as smoking and current obesity levels, especially for women age 50 and over, may negatively impact life expectancy of the current generation of older adults (National Research Council, 2011).

The Distribution of Seniors in the United States

The distribution of older Americans varies across the United States, due in part to patterns of migration after retirement. It is also caused by birth and death rates in the various states and regions. In 2010, one-half of persons age 65 or older lived in 11 states: California, Florida, New York, Illinois, Texas, Pennsylvania, Ohio, Michigan, North Carolina, Georgia and New Jersey. Persons aged 65+ constituted approximately 14% or more of the total population in 17 states in 2010: Florida (17.4%), West Virginia (16.1%), Maine (15.9%), Pennsylvania (15.5%), Iowa (14.9%), Montana (14.9%), Vermont (14.6%), Hawaii (14.5%), North Dakota (14.5%),

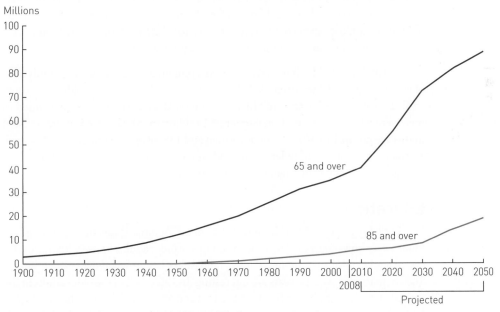

NOTE: Data for 2010–2050 are projections of the population.
Reference population: These data refer to the resident population.

Figure 2-1 Population age 65 and over and age 85 and over, selected years 1900–2008, and projected 2010–2050.

Source: Data from the U.S. Census Bureau. Decennial census. Population estimates and projection.

Rhode Island (14.4%), Arkansas (14.4%), Delaware (14.4%), South Dakota (14.3%), Connecticut (14.2%), Ohio (14.1%), Missouri (14.0%), and Oregon (14.0%). In 13 states, the 65+ population increased by 20% or more between 2000 and 2010: Alaska (50% increase), Nevada (47%), Idaho (32.5%), Arizona (32.1%), Colorado (31.8%), Georgia (31.4%), Utah (31.0%), South Carolina (30.4%), New Mexico (28.5%), North Carolina (27.7%), Delaware (26.9%), Texas (26.1%), and Washington (25.3%). Most persons aged 65+ lived in metropolitan areas in 2010 (78.9%). About 64% of older persons lived in the suburbs, 36% lived in central cities, and 20% lived in nonmetropolitan areas (Administration on Aging, 2011a).

The *elderly* are less likely to change residence than other age groups. From 2009 to 2010, only 5.8% of older persons moved, as opposed to 16.9% of the under-65 population. Most older movers (58.7%) stayed in the same county and 78.2% remained in the same state. Only 21.8% of the movers moved out of state or abroad (Administration on Aging, 2011a).

Issues of Gender

Women outnumber men in the United States, a trend that is expected to continue. In 2010, there were 23 million older women in the United States, compared to 17.5 million older men. This is a ratio of 132 women for every 100 men. The female to male sex ratio increases with age. For the age group 65–69, it is 112:100; for those 85+, it is 206:100 (with more than two females for every male). In 2009, a 65-year-old female could be expected to have an additional 20 years of life expectancy; for males, it was 17.3 years (Administration on Aging, 2011a).

In 2010, 72% of older men were married, compared to 42% of women. Only 37% of women ages 75–84 were married; this dropped to 15% in the 85 or older age group, while 55% of men 85 years and older were married. Four times as many women as men were widowed (8.7 million women; 2.1 million men). Divorce is more unusual in this age group. In 2010, 12% of older men and 13% of older women were divorced. A smaller proportion of older adults had never been married (Administration on Aging, 2010; Federal Interagency Forum, 2010).

Education

Level of education attained can affect the socioeconomic status of the older adult. **Figure 2-2** shows sources of income for groups of older adults. Those with more education tend to have more money, higher standards of living, and above-average health. The comparisons over the years are interesting. In 1965, 24% of the older adults in the United States had graduated from high school and 5% had at least a bachelor's degree. In 2010, however, 79.5% of older adults had graduated from high school, while 22.5% of older adults had at least a bachelor's degree. Differences also exist in education between ethnic groups. In 2010, 84.3% of older non-Hispanic Whites, 73.6% of older Asians, 64.8% of older Blacks, and 47% of older Hispanics had completed high school (Administration on Aging, 2010; Federal Interagency Forum, 2010).

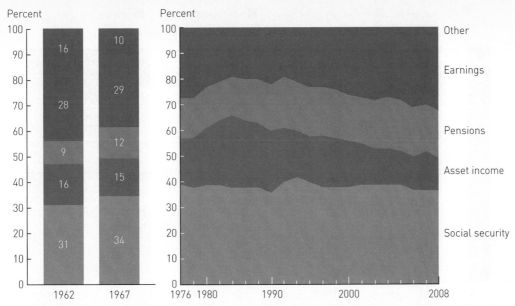

NOTE: A married couple is age 65 and over if the husband is age 65 and over or the husband is younger than age 55 and the wife is 65 and over. The definition of "other" includes, but is not limited to, public assistance, unemployment compensation, workers compensation, alimony, child support, and personal contributions.
Reference population: These data refer to the civilian noninstitutionalized resident population.

Figure 2-2 Sources for income for married couples and non-married people who are age 65 and over, percent distribution, selected years 1962–2008.

Source: Data from the U.S. Census Bureau, Current Population Survey, Annual Social and Economic Supplement, 1997–2009.

Living Arrangements

Living arrangements of older adults are linked to income, health status and the availability of caregivers. Older people who live alone are more likely than their married counterparts to live in poverty. Over one-half (55.1%) of noninstitutionalized older adults lived with their spouse in 2010. In that year, older men were more likely to be living with a spouse than were older women (69.9% compared to 41.3%; see **Figure 2-3** for statistics through 2008). Only 30.4% of women age 75 or older lived with a spouse, and older women were twice as likely as older men to be living alone (37.3% compared to 19.1%). The likelihood of living alone increases with age: among women age 75 or older, 47% lived alone in 2010.

A total of about 1.94 million older adults lived in households with a child present in the house in 2010. About 485,000 of these were grandparents over 65 years of age with the primary responsibility for their grandchildren who lived with them (Administration on Aging, 2010).

Although only a small percentage (4.1%) of older adults resided in nursing homes in 2009, the percentage increases with age. This ranges from 1.1% for persons

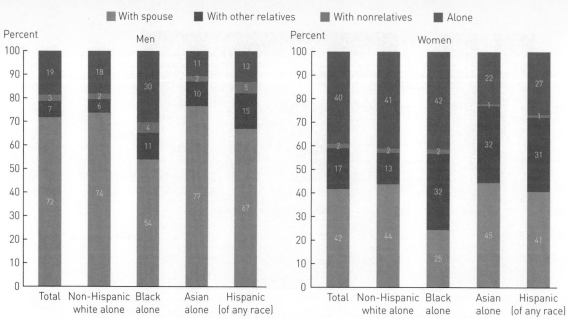

Figure 2-3 Living arrangements of the population age 65 and over, by sex and race and Hispanic origin, percent distribution, 2008.

Source: Data from the U.S. Census Bureau, Current Population Survey, Annual Social and Economic Supplement, 2008.

ages 65–74, to 3.5% for persons ages 75–84, and to 13.2% for persons ages 85+. Another 2.4% of older adults lived in "senior housing" in 2009, which often offers supportive services to residents (Administration on Aging, 2011a).

Living arrangements, like education, also vary by race and ethnicity. In 2008, older Asian women were more likely than older women of other races to live with relatives other than a spouse. Older non-Hispanic White and older Black females were more likely than others to live alone. Older Black men lived alone three times as much as older Asian men. Older Hispanic men were more likely than other races and ethnicities to live with relatives other than a spouse. The chance of living alone increases as age increases.

Older people who lived alone had higher poverty rates than those who lived with their spouse. In 2010, 16% of older persons who lived alone lived in poverty, but only 5% of older married men and women lived in poverty (Federal Interagency Forum, 2010).

Effects of Ethnicity

The growing aging population consists of a significantly increased proportion of minorities. Minority elders will make up 42% of the elderly population over the next 40 years (Vincent & Velkoff, 2010). The diversity as well as the vast increase in number of this group provides a distinct challenge to meeting healthcare needs. The losses (spouses, friends, independence, levels of function, status in society) often encountered in aging coupled with low socioeconomic status and lifetime racial discriminations put this group at increased risk for poor outcomes (Markides & Miranda, 1997). An understanding of cultural diversity and the unique challenges it poses is needed to address health issues and promote wellness.

The older population in the United States is growing more racially and ethnically diverse as it ages. In 2010, 80% of U.S. older adults were non-Hispanic Whites, 8.4% were Black, 3.4% Asian, and 6.9% Hispanic (see **Table 2-1**). By 2050, the composition of the older population will be 59.4% non-Hispanic White, 19.8% Hispanic, 11% Black, 8.6% Asian, and 1% American Indian and Native Alaskan (Administration on Aging, 2010; Federal Interagency Forum, 2010).

African Americans

The number of African American elders is projected to increase from 3.2 million in 2008 to over 9.9 million by 2050. In 2008, African Americans comprised 8.3% of the older population. By 2050, this is expected to increase to 11%. The poverty rate for older African Americans was 20% in 2008, compared to 9.7% for the total elderly population. Households containing families headed by African Americans age 65 years or older reported a median income of $35,025 in 2008, compared to $44,188 for all older households. The median personal income for African American men was $19,161, and $12,499 for African American women, compared to $25,503 for

TABLE 2-1 U.S. Population Age 65+ by Race and Hispanic Origin, 2010	Numbers	Percentage
Black Alone, Not Hispanic	3,374,381	8.4%
Native American Alone, Not Hispanic	179,819	0.4%
Native Hawaiian/Pacific Islander Alone, Not Hispanic	29,568	0.1%
Asian Alone, Not Hispanic	1,376,471	3.4%
Two or More Races, Not Hispanic	316,690	0.8%
Hispanic	2,781,624	6.9%
Total Minority Population Age 60 and Older	8,058,553	20.0%
White Alone, Not Hispanic	32,209,431	80.0%
U.S. Total 65 and over	40,267,984	100.0%

Source: Data from the U.S. Census Bureau, Administration on Aging.

all elderly men and $14,599 for all elderly women (Administration on Aging, 2010). There is also a great disparity in net worth between Black and White households headed by older Americans. In 2007, net worth among older Black households was estimated to be $46,000, compared to $280,000 among older White households (Federal Interagency Forum, 2010). The lack of economic resources and poor access to health care add to the increased incidence of disease with greater complications in this subgroup (see **Case Study 2-1**).

Higher rates of diabetes, hypertension, and chronic kidney disease are seen in African Americans (Ross, 2000). While 26.9% of older Americans aged 65 and over are estimated to have diabetes, there is a racial difference, with 10.2% of non-Hispanic Whites over age 20 and 18.7% of non-Hispanic Blacks over the age of 20 having diabetes (CDC, 2011). African American men have higher incidences of lung and prostate cancer as compared to Whites, and African Americans' overall risk to develop kidney disease is highest of the senior groups.

Among the most frequently occurring chronic conditions in the African American elderly in 2005–2007 were hypertension (84%), arthritis (53%), heart disease (27%), diabetes (29%), sinusitis (15%), and cancer (13%). This generally compares negatively to the following figures for all older persons in the United States: hypertension (71%), arthritis (49%), heart disease (31%), diabetes (18%), sinusitis (14%), and cancer (22%) (Administration on Aging, 2010).

African Americans often do not use routine preventive services at recommended rates and are less likely to have a regular provider of health care, opting instead for hospital outpatient departments, historically known for long waits and inconsistent providers (Markides & Miranda, 1997). The top five causes of death among African

---

Case Study 2-1

Mrs. Johnson is an 87-year-old African American female admitted to the hospital from her home. She is widowed and has no children. Her neighbors watch out for her, bringing her groceries and making sure that she's OK each day. Mrs. Johnson's neighbor, Mrs. Edwards, accompanies her to the hospital.

Mrs. Johnson is admitted for shortness of breath, attributed to nonadherence to her medication regimen for congestive heart failure. She is alert, oriented, and very pleasant.

Mrs. Edwards takes you aside and tells you that she is concerned about Mrs. Johnson's home situation.

Questions:

1. What might you suspect about Mrs. Johnson's financial situation?

2. What might you suspect about Mrs. Johnson's home situation?

3. How might these factors contribute to her hospital admission?

4. Based upon your suspicions, what questions might you ask Mrs. Johnson as you admit her to your unit?

Americans are heart disease, cancer, stroke, diabetes, and unintentional accidents (CDC, 2005). From these statistics, it is evident that preventive services have the potential to affect the longevity of this population.

Hispanics

The Hispanic population is now the largest ethnic minority in the United States (Porter, 2011). The over-65-year-old Hispanic population is the fastest growing segment of the total U.S. population; by 2019, the Hispanic population age 65 or older is projected to be the largest racial/ethnic minority in this age group (Administration on Aging, 2010). By 2050, Hispanic elderly will make up 19.8% of all U.S. elderly, adding up to 17 million Hispanics over the age of 65 (Administration on Aging, 2010). The Hispanic population in the United States consists of a diverse population from Mexico, Cuba, Puerto Rico, the Dominican Republic, and other countries of Central and South America. The poverty rate in 2008 for Hispanic elderly in the United States was nearly twice that of the total older population, 19.3% compared to 7.6% (Administration on Aging, 2010).

The chronic diseases of cardiovascular disease, diabetes, cancer, and cerebrovascular disease are seen in significant numbers in the Hispanic population. Centers for Disease Control and Prevention (2005) data show Hispanics are less likely to obtain preventive services such as flu and pneumonia vaccines and mammograms as compared to Whites. In 2008, 10.7% of Hispanics over 65 years old were diagnosed with diabetes, as compared to 6.9% of non-Hispanic Whites and 10.9% of African Americans (Administration on Aging, 2010). Hispanics also have higher rates of cervical, esophageal, gallbladder, and stomach cancer as compared to Whites. Poverty levels, only slightly lower than for African American elderly, and language barriers are often impediments to accessing healthcare coverage and healthcare services (Ross, 2000). The top five causes of death among Hispanics are heart disease, cancer, unintentional injuries, stroke, and diabetes (CDC, 2010).

In 2008, 70% of Hispanics age 65 or over lived in four states: California, Florida, New York, and Texas (Administration on Aging, 2010). Hispanics in general receive assistance in the home, versus long-term facilities, when functionally declining (Angel & Angel, 1997). Family members frequently act as their caregivers, and multigenerational families under one roof are common. On average, Hispanic families and households are larger than non-Hispanic families and households (Aranda & Miranda, 1997). Overall, the percentage of Hispanic elderly living alone is lower than that of the general population (Administration on Aging, 2010). Older Hispanics are more likely to be married and to rely on family over friends when compared to White elderly.

Asians and Pacific Islanders

This subgroup actually is composed of 40 different ethnic groups with various economic, educational, and health profiles (Ross, 2000). Some identified ethnicities include Chinese, Filipino, Japanese, Pacific Islander, and Hawaiian. National data, however, do not necessarily discern between ethnicities, which complicates identifying demographics and patterns for each culture. The Asian American and Pacific Islander population has been the fastest growing racial/ethnic group in the United States recently, having increased 141% between 1970 and 1980 and 99% between 1980 and 1990 (Elo, 1997). According to the U.S. Census Bureau, projections for the years 2010–2050 include population increases for Asian Americans and Pacific Islanders from 3.4% to 8.6% of the U.S. population (Administration on Aging, 2010).

Life expectancy data have historically shown an advantage for the Asian American and Pacific Islander population. Census data from 1995 showed life expectancy at birth of Asian Americans and Pacific Islanders to be 79.3 years for males and 84.9 years for females, as compared to 73.6 and 80.1 for White males and females, respectively. Elo (1997) questions inconsistencies in the data due to the heterogeneity of the group. The evaluation of mortality data did place Chinese, Japanese, and Filipinos well below White Americans. As a whole, cancer and heart disease contribute less to all-cause mortality in the Asian American and Pacific Islander population than in Whites. Cerebrovascular disease, however, is a more prominent cause of death for some subgroups of Asian Americans and Pacific Islanders (Elo, 1997). Discrepancies are seen in mortality causes depending on whether persons are native or foreign-born, pointing to the impact of acculturation in U.S. society. Overall, though, the top five causes of death among Asian Americans or Pacific Islanders are heart disease, cancer, stroke, unintentional injuries, and diabetes (CDC, 2010).

Kitano, Tazuko, and Kitano (1997) note the inconsistency of this minority group's use of community-based professional resources. Dependence on familial and informal ethnic resources is seen more often than use of traditional health resources. Length of the family's time in this country (recent arrival vs. present for a century) impacts comfort and ease of resource use. Healthcare providers will need to address not only the diversity within this minority group, but also the time or extent of acculturation and assimilation within each subgroup.

American Indians and Alaskan Natives

The category of American Indians and Alaskan Natives (AI/ANs) represents 500 nations, tribes, bands, and native villages in which 150 languages are used (Kramer, 1997). Overall, the 2005–2007 Current Population Survey found that the AI/AN population has larger families, less health insurance, and twice the level of poverty as the rest of the American population (Indian Health Service [IHS], 2012). The 2000 Census found that the AI/AN population is younger than all races of the United States, with a median age of 25 years, compared to the U.S. populations median of 35 years. This population is also living longer than in the past: In 1972–1974, the life expectancy at birth was 63.6 years; it is now 72.6 years, 5.2 years less than the general U.S population. Leading causes of death in this population are heart disease, cancer, unintentional injuries, diabetes, and cerebrovascular disease. "The American Indian and Native Alaskan older population (non-Hispanic and Hispanic) was 212,605 in 2007 and is projected to grow to almost 918,000 by 2050" (Administration on Aging, 2011b). See **Figure 2-4**.

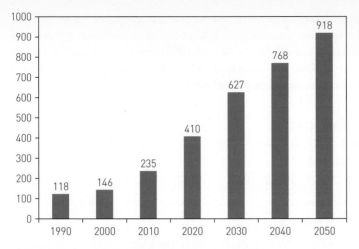

Figure 2-4 Past, present, and future: American Indian and Alaskan Native persons 65+, 1990–2050 (numbers in thousands).

Source: Data from the U.S. Census Bureau, Administration on Aging, Retrieved from: http://www.aoa.gov/AoARoot/Aging_Statistics/Minority_Aging/Facts-on-AINA-Elderly2008-plain_format.aspx

Historically, political developments forced the concentration of American Indians first onto reservations west of the Mississippi and then to more urban areas (Chapleski, 1997). Due to these relocation efforts, AI/ANs are not necessarily in close proximity to IHS facilities, and thus may have difficulty with accessing preventive care. In 2009, 50% of AI/AN elders lived in six states: California, Oklahoma, Arizona, New Mexico, Texas, and North Carolina (Administration on Aging, 2011b). Although many AI/ANs live in rural areas, many have moved to urban areas, where 57% of the population currently resides (IHS, 2012). Chronic disease prevalence in AI/AN increased significantly in the 20th century (see **Case Study 2-2**).

Case Study 2-2

Mr. Andrew Crow is a 67-year-old American Indian. He has been unemployed for the past 5 years. He lives on a reservation in Oklahoma with his wife and three teenage children. Mr. Crow came to the health clinic for a routine checkup. You note that he is overweight.

Questions:

1. How should you focus your physical assessment?

2. What chronic diseases might Mr. Crow be at high risk for?

3. What are the implications for his family?

4. Develop a plan of care for Mr. Crow and his family members.

Studies indicate that older AI/ANs have higher rates of hypertension, diabetes, back pain, and vision loss than the general U.S population. Nationally, more than one in five AI/AN elders has diabetes. Goins and Pilkerton (2010) found the following rates of disease in older American Indians compared to the general population (general population percentages in parenthesis):

> Diabetes 42% (16%)
> Hypertension 58% (47%)
> Vision loss 31% (14%)
> Back pain 37% (29%)

Goins and Pilkerton also found evidence that American Indians at age 55 were experiencing disease states such as cataracts more frequently found in the 70-year-old general population.

American Indians and Alaskan Natives have the highest rates of diabetes in the United States (IHS, 2012). Diabetes is seen very frequently in the younger age groups, with grave implications as the population ages. The AI/AN population also has higher rates of obesity, substance abuse, and mental health problems. According to the IHS, geographic isolation, economic factors, and suspicion toward traditional spiritual beliefs are some of the reasons why health among AI/ANs is poorer than other groups.

In the 2000 Census, AI/ANs reported the highest rates of functional limitation, particularly in the age 55–64-years group. Disability is one of the strongest predictors of the need for nursing home admission in the older adult. This trend is "becoming increasingly important because the number of AI/ANs aged 75 years or older who will need long-term care will double in the next 25 years" (Goins, Moss, Buchwald, & Guralnik, 2007, p. 690) and Congress has a history of providing poorer funding to the healthcare services for AI/ANs compared to other U.S populations.

Other Minorities

The Older Foreign-Born Population in the United States

The *foreign-born* are those people who are living in the United States who were not U.S. citizens at birth. The 2003 Annual Social and Economic Supplement to the Census found that 10.8% of the elderly population in the United States was foreign-born (He, Sengupta, Velkoff, & DeBarros, 2005). Thirty-five percent of these older adults were born in Europe, and 57.8% were born in Latin America or Asia. Nearly 70% of the older foreign-born population were naturalized citizens. The largest region of birth for this population (53%) was Latin America, while 28% were born in Asia, 12% in Europe, 4% in Africa, and 2% in North America. Of the Latin Americans, 55% were born in Mexico. Foreign-born persons comprised 12.4% of the over-65 population at the time of the 2010 Census. More than 28% of the population born in Europe was aged 65 and over (Grieco et al., 2010).

Nearly 66% of the older foreign-born in the United States have lived here for more than 30 years. The older foreign-born are twice as likely to be naturalized citizens as the foreign-born of all ages (see **Table 2-2**). Almost 50% of the older foreign-born have not completed high school (compared to 29% of *native-born* older Americans). Older foreign-born are more likely than native-born elders to live in multigenerational family households, and their poverty rate is also higher than for native-born U.S. citizens. They are also less likely to have health coverage (He, 2000). A language other than English is spoken in 12.6% of the homes of the foreign-born elderly. Less than one-half of the older adults who spoke another language at home spoke English very well (He et al., 2005).

U.S. Veterans

There are currently three *cohorts* of aging veterans: those who served in World War II, those who served in the Korean War, and those who served in Vietnam. Changes in the population of older Americans who are veterans of the armed services are expected to continue as the Vietnam-era cohort ages. In 2000, there were 9.8 million veterans age 65 or older in the United States—two of every three men 65 or older were veterans. More than 95% of these veterans were male. Between 1990 and 2000, the number of male veterans age 85 or older increased from 142,000 to 400,000 (**Figure 2-5**). There is a projected increase after 2010 as the Vietnam-era cohort ages. The number of veterans 85 or older is expected to increase steadily to a peak of 1.2 million in 2012 (Federal Interagency Forum, 2010). This increase in the number of veterans will challenge the U.S. Department of Veterans Affairs, which has traditionally supplied a major proportion of the health care that veterans receive.

> ### Notable Quotes
>
> "They are our storytellers—our elderly are meant to be those who share the secrets of wisdom and knowledge and life with our youth."
>
> —Cameron Diaz

TABLE 2-2   Population 65 and Over by Citizenship Status—March 2009

Age Group	Native Population	Foreign-Born	Naturalized Citizen	Not a Citizen
65 to 69 years	10,583	1,438	965	473
70 to 74 years	7,711	1,225	830	395
75 to 79 years	6,356	826	568	258
80 to 84 years	5,143	640	480	161
85 years and over	4,233	460	347	114

Source: Data from the U.S. Census Bureau.

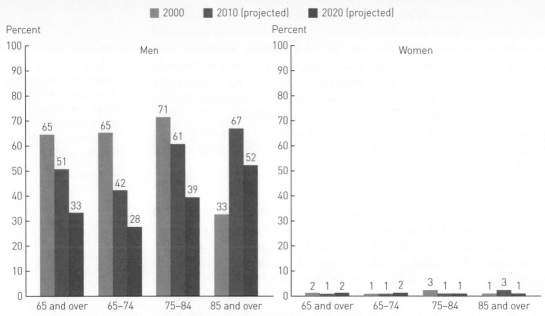

Reference population: These data refer to the resident population of the United States and Puerto Rico.

Figure 2-5 Percentage of population age 65 and over who are veterans, by sex and age group, United States and Puerto Rico, 2000 with projections for 2010 and 2020.

Source: Data from the U.S. Census Bureau, Decennial Census and Population Projections, Department of Veterans Affairs.

Changes in the healthcare systems of the military are currently being seen as a direct result of the Iraq and Afghanistan wars. It is unknown how the numbers of wounded military personnel from these wars will affect the U.S. Department of Veterans Affairs in the short or in the long term. It can be anticipated, however, that the number of veterans with significant physical and emotional disabilities will increase and that their needs for health care will also increase as this newest cohort ages. The greater incidence of those with polytraumatic injuries and multiple limb amputation who have survived the advanced weapons of war will pose an additional challenge to the healthcare system as they age. The impact on the healthcare system of the unusual deployment of older troops to Iraq and Afghanistan is also unknown.

The Aging Disabled Population

Advances in health care have increased the life span of persons with disabilities. These include those traumatically injured as well as those born with or who acquired a disability.

Traumatically injured persons are now more likely to receive expert emergency services at the time of their accident. Advances in intensive care services, surgical services, diagnostic services, and the knowledge and skills of healthcare workers have combined to prolong the lives of persons who used to die within days or months of their traumatic injuries. For the first time in history, persons with spinal cord injuries and brain injuries are living to become elderly. They are truly entering a time in their life that is unpredictable, because they are the first to reach these advanced ages. Unforeseen effects of aging in persons with spinal cord injury, for example, include shoulder injury (from repetitive movements related to wheelchair mobility) and increased risk of pressure ulcers.

Developmentally disabled individuals are another special aging group. Technological advances and improvements in health care are prolonging the lives of those with disabilities such as mental retardation. Twelve percent of persons with developmental disabilities are now 65 or older; this translates to between 200,000 and 500,000 people. There are great implications for the U.S. healthcare system as this population continues to age, grow, and outlive their parents. Unforeseen secondary health problems are beginning to be seen in this older population, including obesity, chronic skin problems, and early aging (Connolly, 1998).

Elderly Inmates

One oft-forgotten segment of the elderly population in the United States is the prisoners. As of 2010, there were 26,100 inmates over the age of 65 in federal and state prisons, a 63% increase from 2007 (Human Rights Watch, 2012). There are two older populations in our prisons: those serving long and/or life sentences who committed crimes when young and those who are older when the crime was committed. The length of incarceration is therefore different between these two groups, and the effects of incarceration on the aging process may be different as well. There is often little motivation and power to release aged and infirm prisoners before their sentence is completed, adding to the increasing numbers of elderly and disabled inmates in prisons in the United States (Human Rights Watch).

Not all elderly prisoners are violent offenders. California's three-strikes law has resulted in 4,431 nonviolent offenders in the system who will be serving sentences of 25 years to life; the average age of these prisoners is 36 years (Human Rights Watch, 2012). "Leandro Andrade is one. At 37 he was convicted of stealing $150 worth of videotapes from two different stores. These convictions counted as his 'third' strike and he received a sentence of two consecutive 25-years-to-life sentences. The earliest he can be released will be when he is 87 years old" (Human Rights Watch, p. 29).

Elderly even has a different connotation in the world of jail cells and prisons. Due to the stressors related to incarceration, as well as the increased likelihood of an unhealthy lifestyle preceding incarceration, prisoners aged 50–55 experience physical and mental changes normally associated with free-world citizens at least 10 years older. Substandard environment, nutrition, exercise, and medical care during incarceration likely helps to accelerate the aging process, as does the violence, anxiety, and stress associated with prison life (see **Case Study 2-3**).

A 50-year-old inmate may have a physiological age that is 10–15 years older than his or her biological age due to the use of illicit drugs, alcohol intake, and limited access to preventive care and health services. It can cost three times as much to

Case Study 2-3

Mr. Everett is a 62-year-old inmate in a state penitentiary, admitted to your unit for hypertension, heart failure, and chest pain. He is accompanied by a prison guard, who watches your every move. The guard has handcuffed Mr. Everett to the bed.

This is the first prisoner that you've ever cared for. You are surprised at how old Mr. Everett looks.

You complete your admission assessment and talk to him about the plans for his care.

Questions:

1. Why might this patient appear to be older than his stated age?

2. How could his social situation affect his plan of care, hospital stay, and recovery?

care for an older inmate as compared to a younger one. Inmates age 55 or older tend to have at least three chronic conditions, and up to 20% have a mental illness (Mitka, 2004). Aged inmates can require such complicated and costly procedures as dialysis three times weekly, special diets, and expensive medications. Adaptive equipment, such as walkers and wheelchairs, may also be needed for mobility. In 2003 in Texas, 1,159 inmates over the age of 65 required 24-hour skilled nursing care (McMahon, 2003).

Prisoners have been called the only population in the United States with a legal right to health care. Due to these legal rights and the expanding aging prison population, combined with tight federal and state budgets, it is no wonder that some think that the U.S. prison system is overdue for a healthcare crisis (Mitka, 2004). Some states, like Texas, have developed separate facilities for their geriatric prisoners. Others have integrated telemedicine into their facilities or developed chronic care clinics. Some, recognizing the likelihood of inmates not only aging in place in prison but also dying of chronic disease while in prison, have implemented hospice programs for their dying, elderly prisoners.

Health Disparities

Health disparities have been defined as "preventable differences in the burden of disease, injury, violence, or in opportunities to achieve optimal health experienced by socially disadvantaged racial, ethnic, and other population groups and communities" (CDC, 2012, p.1). Not all older adults in the United States have benefited from recent advances in health care because of factors such as age, gender, race, and economic circumstances.

Substantial disparities have been documented by the CDC (2012) in vaccine administration, colorectal cancer screening, coronary heart disease and stroke, preventable hospitalizations, hypertension, and hypertension control based on race, ethnicity, and gender. While funding (i.e. Medicare) expands healthcare access for the older adults, it does not address older adults who do not meet criteria for Medicare funding.

In one study, older women saw their physician as much as men did, but did not receive the flu vaccine and cholesterol screening as frequently as older males (Cameron, Song, Manheim, & Dunlop, 2010). Males in that study also tended to be admitted to the hospital more frequently. In other studies, when hospitalized, women tended to have shorter lengths of stay. While there may be social reasons for the healthcare discrepancies between genders, it is disturbing to think that older women as a group may not receive needed preventive services because of gender rather than lack of need.

Racial and ethnic disparities in health care have also been documented for the older adult population. The core of this issue is likely complex and multifaceted, with caregiver bias, poverty level, language, literacy, and other as-yet-unidentified factors playing a role.

Mortality and Morbidity

Causes of Death

The leading cause of death for older adults in 2006 was diseases of the heart, followed by malignant neoplasms, cerebrovascular diseases, chronic lower respiratory diseases, Alzheimer's disease, diabetes, and influenza and pneumonia (see **Table 2-3**). Death rates for diseases of the heart and cerebrovascular diseases decreased by 50% from 1981 to 2006, while age-adjusted death rates for diabetes mellitus increased by 29% and death rates for chronic lower respiratory diseases increased by 50% during the same time period. Diseases of the heart and malignant neoplasms are the top two causes of death for people age 65 or older in the United States, regardless of race, gender, or ethnic origin. Race and ethnicity do play a part in other causes of death, however. In 2001, diabetes mellitus was the fifth leading cause of death among Black men, the fourth among Hispanic men, and the sixth among White men and men of Asian or Pacific Islander origin. For women aged 65 or older, diabetes mellitus was the fourth leading cause of death for Hispanics and Blacks, and the seventh leading cause of death among Whites (Federal Interagency Forum, 2004).

Chronic Diseases

The prevalence of chronic diseases increases with age. Six of the seven leading causes of death among older Americans are chronic diseases such as heart disease, stroke, cancer, and diabetes. Older women report higher numbers of chronic diseases such as hypertension and arthritis, whereas men report more heart disease and cancer (see **Figure 2-6**). Ethnic and racial differences also exist in the prevalence of chronic diseases. Older Blacks report higher levels of hypertension and diabetes than non-Hispanic Whites, whereas Hispanics report higher levels of diabetes than

TABLE 2-3   Number and Share of Elderly Deaths Attributes to Leading Causes of Death, 1980 and 2004

Cause	1980		2004	
	Deaths	Percentage	Deaths	Percentage
Heart disease	595,406	44.4	533,302	30.4
Cancer	258,389	19.3	385,847	22.0
Stroke	146,417	10.9	130,538	7.4
Chronic lower respiratory disease	43,587	3.2	105,197	6.0
Alzheimer's disease	1,037	0.1	65,313	3.7
Diabetes	25,216	1.9	53,956	3.1
Influenza/pneumonia	45,512	3.4	52,760	3.0
Nephritis (renal conditions)	12,968	1.0	35,105	2.0
Accidents	24,844	1.8	35,020	2.0
Septicemia	6,843	0.5	25,644	1.5
Subtotal (top 10 causes of death)	*1,166,078[a]*	*86.9*	*1,422,682*	*81.0*
All causes	**1,341,848**	**100.0**	**1,755,669**	**100.0**

Source: CRS compilation from National Center for Health Statistics, Health, United States, 2006, available at http://www.cdc.gov/nchs/data/hus/hus06.pdf

non-Hispanic Whites. Both diabetes and hypertension are increasing among older Americans (Federal Interagency Forum, 2010).

Sensory impairments and oral health problems become more frequent with aging. Early detection can prevent or postpone the physical, social, and emotional effects that these changes have on a senior's life. In 2008, nearly 42% of older men and nearly 30% of older women reported difficulty with hearing. Those age 85 years or older reported more difficulty than those ages 65–74. Vision trouble affects about 18% of older adults. In 2008, 19% of women and 15% of men 65 or over reported trouble with vision. Common eye conditions resulting in vision loss include glaucoma, macular degeneration, and cataracts. Thirty-four percent of persons 85 years of age or older reported edentulism (lack of teeth). Poorer older adults were less likely to have teeth than those above the poverty threshold (42% compared to 23%) (Federal Interagency Forum, 2010). Glasses, hearing aids, and dentures can be difficult to obtain for financial reasons: They are expensive and they are not covered services under Medicare. Thus, many older adults may not possess these assistive devices, or may have out-of-date or ill-fitting devices, which can affect cognitive status (hearing aids and glasses), nutritional intake (dentures), and likelihood of falling (glasses).

Memory loss is not unusual in the older adult. Older men are more likely to experience moderate or severe memory impairment than older women. In 2002,

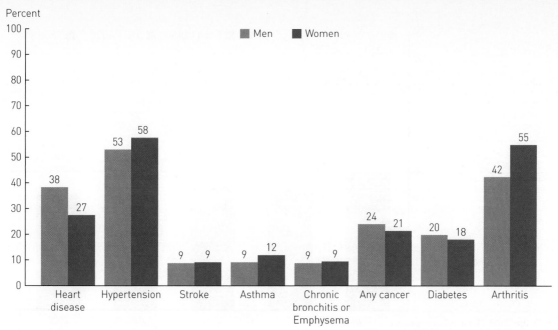

NOTE: Data are based on a 2-year average from 2007–2008. See Appendix B for the definintion of race and Hispanic origin in the National Health Interview Survey.
Reference population: These data refer to the civilian noninstitutionalized population.

Figure 2-6 Chronic health conditions among the population age 65 and over, by sex, 2007–2008.

Source: Data from the Centers for Disease Control and Prevention, National Center for Health Statistics, Nation Health Interview Survey.

15% of men age 65 or older and 11% of women of the same age experienced moderate to severe memory impairment. At age 85 or older, nearly 33% of both women and men suffered from this impairment. In 2002, the proportion of people age 85 or older with moderate or severe memory impairment was 32%, compared to 5% of people ages 65–69 (Federal Interagency Forum, 2004). As the elderly U.S. population grows, the number of individuals with dementia will also increase, making planning for the long-term care needs of those individuals increasingly important (Plessman et al., 2007)

Many people feel that older age is highly correlated with disability. The age-adjusted proportion of people in the United States age 65 or older with chronic disabilities actually declined from 1984 to 1999. Due to the population growth, however, the actual numbers of older persons with chronic disabilities increased from 6.2 million in 1984 to 6.8 million in 1999. Older women reported more difficulties in physical functioning than older men. In 2007, 32% of older women reported that they were unable to perform at least one of five activities, compared to 19% of men (see **Figure 2-7**). Those aged 85 years or older had more physical limitations

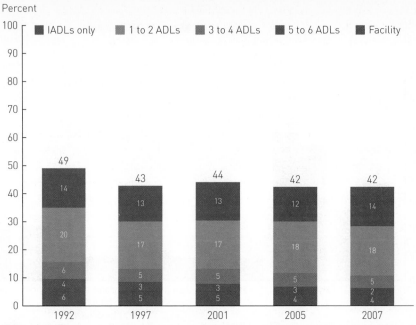

NOTE: A residence is considered a long-term care facility if it is certified by Medicare or Medicaid; has 3 or more beds and is licensed as a nursing home or other long-term care facility and provides at least one personal care service; or provides 24-hour, 7-day-a-week supervision by a caregiver. ADL limitations refer to difficulty performing (or inability to perform for a health reason) one or more of the following tasks: bathing, dressing, eating, getting in/our of chairs, walking, or using the toilet. IADL limitations refer to difficulty performing (or inability to perform for a health reason) one or more of the following tasks: using the telephone, light housework, heavy housework, meal preparation, shopping, or managing money. Rates are age adjusted using the 2000 standard population. Data for 1992, 2001, and 2007 do not sum to the totals because of rounding.
Reference population: These data refer to Medicare enrollees.

Figure 2-7 Percentage of Medicare enrollees age 65 and over who have limitations in activities of daily living (ADLs) or instrumental activities of daily living (IADLs), or who are in a facility, selected years 1992–2007.

Source: Centers for Medicare and Medicaid Services, Medicare Current Beneficiary Survey.

than those between 65 and 74 years. Physical functioning is also somewhat related to race and ethnicity. Nineteen percent of non-Hispanic White males were unable to perform at least one physical activity, compared to 26% of non-Hispanic Blacks. For women, no significant difference was noted among non-Hispanic Whites, non-Hispanic Blacks, and Hispanics in inability to perform at least one activity (Federal Interagency Forum, 2010).

Genetics and Genomics

Genomics is the identification of gene sequences in the DNA, while genetics is the study of heredity and the transmission of certain genes through generations. Both genomics and genetics play a role in health and longevity for older adults. Some studies in this field have to do with the origins of disease: Alzheimer's and asthma are two examples. Other studies are examining the aging process itself: Are there certain genes, or sequences of genes, that assure healthy aging? Yet others are examining the complex interactions between environment, genes, and aging.

One clinically relevant field of study concerns the enzyme systems that contribute to the metabolism of medications, the Cytochome P450 and related enzyme systems. It has been found that medications are metabolized by specific enzyme systems, and if the provider is aware of these systems, many drug interactions and adverse events could be prevented. This is especially important in the older adult population, which is much more likely to be prescribed multiple medications for multiple ailments. It is anticipated that during your own time as a nurse, this field will explode with knowledge that will directly affect your practice and your patients' health. Even now, genetic testing is becoming available, some of which is covered by insurance and Medicare, to ascertain the presence or absence of genetic variations that affect drug metabolism. One such test is for genetic variations affecting metabolism of warfarin (Coumadin).

Good Health in Aging?

Feeling depressed about aging and the aged? Although the statistics can sound grim, in actuality, aging is enjoyed by the vast majority of seniors. More than 72% of seniors report having good to excellent health (see **Figure 2-8** and **Table 2-4**). The number of seniors living in nursing homes declined from 5.2% in 1990 to 4.5% in 2000. Only 18.2% of those age 85 or older lived in nursing homes in 2000,

> ### Notable Quotes
>
> "We are not victims of aging, sickness, and death. These are part of scenery, not the seer, who is immune to any form of change. This seer is the spirit, the expression of eternal being."
>
> —Deepak Chopra

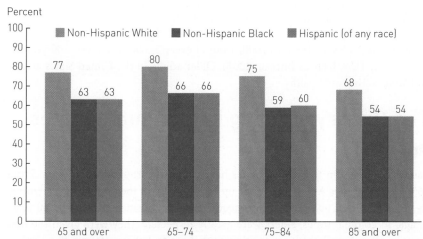

NOTE: Data are based on a 3-year average from 2006–2008. See Appendix B for the definition of race and Hispanic origin in the National Health Interview Survey.A
Reference population: These data refer to the civilian noninstitutionalized population.

Figure 2-8 Respondent-reported good to excellent health among the population 65 and older by age group, race, and Hispanic origin, 2006–2008.

Source: Data from the Centers for Disease Control and Prevention, National Center for Health Statistics, Nation Health Interview Survey.

TABLE 2-4   Percentage of Persons Age 65 or Older Who Reported Good to Excellent Health, by Age Group, Sex, and Race and Hispanic Origin, 2006 to 2008

Good to excellent health				
Both sexes				
65 and over	74.5	76.7	62.5	63.4
Men				
65 and over	74.8	76.4	65.2	64.8
65–74	77.6	79.6	67.5	67.2
75–84	72.5	74.1	61.6	62.1
85 and over	64.9	66.3	58.0	53.1
Women				
65 and over	74.4	76.9	60.7	62.5
65–74	77.7	80.5	64.8	65.6
75–84	72.5	75.3	56.9	58.7
85 and over	67.1	68.7	52.1	54.5

NOTE: Data are based on a 3-year average from 2006–2008. See Appendix B for the definition of race and Hispanic origin in the National Health Interview Survey.
Reference population: These data refer to the civilian noninstitutionalized population.

Source: Data from the Centers for Disease Control and Prevention, National Center for Health Statistics, Nation Health Interview Survey.

compared to 24.5% in 1990. In 2000, 1 out of every 5,578 people was 100 years of age or older (U.S. Census Bureau, 2001). Older adults in the United States are, by and large, active and healthy.

The History of Aging in the United States

Pre-1900

Patterns of aging in the United States have changed throughout the years. From 1650 to 1850, older Americans made up less than 2% of the population (Fleming, Evans, & Chutka, 2003). Old age in those times was considered to start at 60 years of age. In colonial times, elders were greatly respected: They were given the best seats in church and Puritans taught youth how to behave toward their elders (Egendorf, 2002). By 1870, older adults made up 3% of the U.S. population, and only 0.37% were over the age of 80. Some older adults lived with nuclear families and were treated with great respect. Among the upper classes, the older adults tended to control the family's land and wealth, thus maintaining authority over the family. Poor people in those times often did not live to old age—old age was a privilege of the rich. The elderly poor were seen as a burden on society, so if old age was attained by a poor person, it was accompanied by derision and scorn from other citizens (Fleming et al., 2003).

Youth came to be increasingly valued during the American Revolution, and older adults declined in status. Fashion favored a youthful look, and clothing flattered the younger frame. Claimed ages in the census drifted downward, because people did not want to acknowledge their actual age. Terms such as "old fogey," "codger," and "geezer" came into being. Retirement from public office became mandatory at age 60 or 70 in many states (Egendorf, 2002; Fleming et al., 2003).

By the end of the 19th century, age stratification was prevalent in American life. Activities like school attendance, marriage, and retirement became based on age. By the start of the 1900s there were increasing numbers of older adults. Cultural focus shifted to business, medicine, and scientific advances. Older adults were devalued (Fleming et al., 2003).

Throughout history, old age has often been associated with lack of income and dependency on others. Poverty was greater in the southern states, especially among widows and Blacks. Immigrants and Blacks were the least prepared for the lack of income after retirement. Here is a quote from a former slave:

> When my mother became old, she was sent to live in a lonely log-hut in the woods. Aged and worn out slaves, whether men or women, are commonly so treated. No care is taken of them, except, perhaps, that a little ground is cleared about the hut, on which the old slave, if able, may raise a little corn. As far as the owner is concerned, they live or die as it happens; it is just the same thing as turning out an old horse. (Fleming et al., 2003, p. 915)

Harriet Jacobs (1861) noted:

> Slaveholders have a method, peculiar to their institution, of getting rid of old slaves, whose lives have been worn out in their service. I knew an old woman, who for seventy years faithfully served her master. She had become almost helpless, from hard labor and disease. Her owners moved to Alabama, and the old black woman was left to be sold to any body who would give twenty dollars for her. (p. 27)

There were no national or state social supports for the poor in early America. Rather, the townships assisted the poor. In some communities, the rising taxes needed for relief of the poor led the communities to rid themselves of the poor by auctioning them off to farms for labor. Some communities even denied refuge to nonresidents, forcing the elderly to go from town to town in search of assistance. Citizens often divided the poor into two categories: the "worthy poor," who were unable to support themselves because of illness, disability, or old age, through no fault of their own, and the immoral, lazy, alcoholic poor. The elderly who had failed to save for their older years were also deemed by some to be unworthy of assistance by the community (Fleming et al., 2003; The Poorhouse Story, 2005). The poor were often sent to poorhouses, which were warehouses for the old, insane, widowed, unmarried mothers, criminals, and drunks. They were often filthy and unsafe. Physical abuse, lack of waste facilities, rats, and poor food made poorhouses dangerous places for the elderly, yet the poor elderly often ended up supported by the community and placed in the poorhouse.

The 1900s

Military pensions were initiated by the U.S. government in 1861. In 1904, President Theodore Roosevelt established old age as a disability. By 1910, 25% of the elderly U.S. population (Northern White soldiers and their widows) was receiving military pensions, which accounted for 43% of federal expenditures. This first pension system did not last—it dissolved after supporting the last Union veterans and their families (Fleming et al., 2003).

After the Civil War, elderly Blacks worked as sharecroppers or became dependent upon their extended families. Black, White, and Hispanic tenant farmers worked well into their old age, lacking the education and resources to do otherwise. Older Blacks migrated to the cities as the mechanical cotton picker forced them from their land. Those who did not migrate to the cities suffered ever-worsening poverty (Fleming et al., 2003).

By 1900, poorhouses had changed into old-age homes. The costs of old-age homes became a burden for many counties, so in these counties elders were transferred to state-funded mental institutions. Charitable homes came into being, run by religious organizations, benevolent societies, and ethnic organizations. For-profit homes also developed, serving the chronically ill or disabled. Standards and oversight on all of these facilities were minimal (Fleming et al., 2003).

By the 1920s, the elderly population in the United States was increasingly seen as obsolete. The workplace denigrated older workers, seeing them as less productive and with too few attributes for working in the factories. Older workers were more likely to be injured on the job, and unions pushed for older workers to leave to make room for younger workers. Firms began to introduce mandatory retirement. Persons over 45 years of age began to have trouble finding work. Older workers suddenly found themselves without work, health insurance, unemployment insurance, or retirement savings (Fleming et al., 2003).

The 1920s also brought the fall of the stock market and inflation, which led to the Great Depression of the 1930s. In 1920, 25% of older adults were impoverished. This increased to 30% before the Depression, to 50% in 1935, and to 66% by 1940 (Fleming et al., 2003). There was mass unemployment, and poor families could no longer afford to support their elders. Old people became dependent upon local and state governments for support.

Franklin Roosevelt signed the Social Security Act in 1935. This act provided income assistance for the elderly. Roosevelt's purpose was to enact a law that would give some measure of protection to the average U.S. citizen and his or her family against a poverty-ridden old age. However, medical costs began to rise, forcing the elderly to again rely on the government for assistance. Medicare and Medicaid were signed into law in 1965 by President Lyndon Johnson. These programs offered a form of health insurance to those who previously had been seen as uninsurable families (Fleming et al., 2003).

County "poor farms" continued to exist. The Social Security Act of 1935, however, denied funding to these facilities. Private care homes flourished in the 1940s, again with few standards or oversights. Social pressures begat the for-profit long-term care industry. In the 1950s, a federal relationship flourished with the providers. By 1960, however, there was still a shortage of 500,000 long-term care beds in the United States. By 1997, nearly 4% of the U.S. population was being cared for in nursing homes. Currently, about 55% of persons 85 or older are impaired and require long-term care (Carbonell, 2005).

In 1880, 75% of men 65 or older were employed, being too poor to retire. They only left work due to poor health or the inability to find work. With the emphasis on youth and the passage of the Social Security and Medicare/Medicaid bills, the number of older men who are employed has steadily dropped throughout the years. In 2003, less than 20% of men 65 or older worked full- or part-time (Carbonell, 2005).

Aging Today

Aging in place is defined as the ability to live in one's own home and community safely, independently, and comfortably, regardless of age, income, or ability level (CDC, 2011). Today, the majority of people would prefer to "age in place" because it promotes independence, autonomy, and connection to the social support of family and friends (Wiles et al., 2011). Remaining in one's homes and communities for as long as possible also avoids costly institutionalized care, an outcome favored by policymakers, health providers, and many older persons themselves (Wiles et al.) (see **Figure 2-9**). Challenges of aging in place include age-related changes (vision loss, hearing impairment, decreased strength, gait imbalance, mental process changes, and chronic diseases) impacting function and access to services. In order to meet these challenges, planning is crucial for the success of aging in place. Modifications to the home, utilization of assistive devices, and obtaining in-home services will be necessary with an increase in disability. Coordination of these needed adaptations can be overwhelming. Elderly individuals and their families will need to access assistance from social workers; geriatric care managers; and community, local, and federal government programs. The informal assistance from family, friends, and neighbors cannot be overlooked (National Institute on Aging [NIA], 2012).

Since the Older Americans Act (OAA) of 1965 was passed, the Administration on Aging (AOA) has provided elderly Americans services allowing them to age

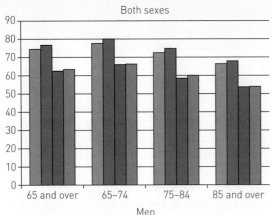

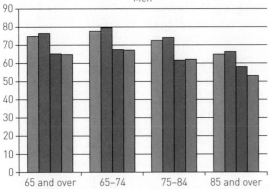

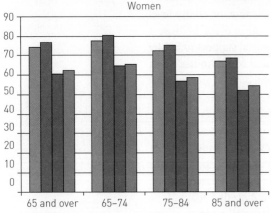

NOTE: Data are based on a 3-year average from 2006–2008. See Appendix B for the definition of race and Hispanic origin in the National Health Interview Survey.

Reference population: These data refer to the civilian non institutionalized population.

Figure 2-9 The majority of older adults are healthy, active, and continue to be engaged in society after retirement.

Source: Data from the Centers for Disease Control and Prevention, National Center for Health Statistics, Nation Health Interview Survey.

in their homes. Through the Aging Services Network, a range of community-based services such as home delivered and congregate meals, case management, transportation, and homemaker and caregiver support are funded, targeting the most vulnerable elderly (Barrett & Schimmel, 2010). One of the programs to provide comprehensive care for older adults trying to age in place is The Program of All-inclusive Care for the Elderly (*PACE*) model.

PACE was first developed in the 1970s and is a model focused on the concept that the well-being of seniors with chronic care needs and their families are best served in the community whenever possible. PACE serves individuals who are age 55 or older, certified by their state to need nursing home care, able to live safely in the community at the time of enrollment, and live in a PACE service area. Services include all medical and social supports, including: adult day care, medical evaluations, meals, prescription medications, therapies, in-home personal care and homemaking, respite care, and hospice. Eighty-two programs are now in place in 29 states (National PACE Association, 2002).

An inaugural survey conducted by National Council on Aging (NCOA) and United Healthcare examined seniors' outlook and preparedness for aging. The survey evaluated individual readiness for aging and perceptions of their community's ability to meet their needs as they aged. The survey sample had 40% of its respondents make low to moderate incomes ($30,000 or less per year). This group was most likely to have little confidence that they will be financially prepared for their long-term care; however, overall one-third of the survey respondents felt financially unprepared (NCOA, 2012). These data emphasize the need for those providers of care to the elderly to better educate elders on services available and that proactive measures must be taken in order to age in place successfully.

Centenarians

Centenarians make up the fastest-growing segment of our population in the United States, with the

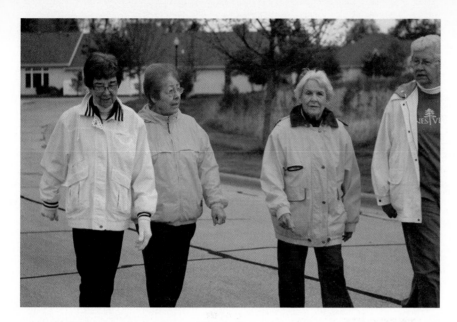

Figure 2-10 The majority of people are healthy, active, and continue to be engaged in society after retirement.

over-85-year-olds making up the second-fastest-growing segment (Figure 2-10). The U.S. Census Bureau (2011) estimates that there were 71,991 centenarians in the United States on December 1, 2010 and it is expected that there will be 601,000 centenarians in the U.S by 2050. The U.S. Census of 1990 found that four in five centenarians are women, and 78% of this age group are non-Hispanic White. African Americans make up the second largest group at 16%; this correlates with 76% and 12% of the total population, respectively. In the next 40 years, the number of centenarians may reach as many as 850,000, depending upon changes in life expectancy over these years. Hispanics and Asian Americans will share a greater percentage of this age group, with non-Hispanic Whites nearing 55%.

Centenarians were found to be a predominately lower educated, more impoverished, widowed, and more disabled population as compared to other elderly cohorts (U.S. Department of Health and Human Services, 1999). The lower education level of this cohort is not surprising considering the increase in levels of education noted over the span of the past century. The marital status of centenarians was overwhelmingly widowed, with 84% of 100-year-old women widowed as compared to 58% of men. Poverty status is more varied in this group and is dependent on race. Women generally were more likely to live in poverty in this age group. White centenarians were less likely than other races except Asian and Pacific Islanders to live in poverty. Disability, identified as having mobility and self-care limitations, was seen across all races. Not surprisingly, consistent with disability trends, all races of centenarians except American Indians and Alaskan Natives were noted to be not living alone. The increased likelihood of living in a nursing home at this age was noted in all race categories.

The New England Centenarian study was a population-based study conducted within the New England area. The researchers noted a surprising heterogeneity in this group, including a wide range of economic statuses, educational attainment, racial backgrounds, and origins of birth. Physical status varied widely as well. Fifteen percent of centenarians in this study were still living independently at home, while 50% lived in nursing homes and the remainder lived with family. Three-quarters of the study group suffered from some form of cognitive impairment. Health histories noted 95% of subjects enjoyed unimpaired health well into their ninth decade (Perls, Silver, & Lauerman, 1999). Most notable in this study is the observation that the older one gets, the healthier one has been. It is suspected the centenarians have not necessarily survived disease but have avoided chronic/acute diseases, successfully navigating through obstacles and the physical/psychosocial challenges of their lives (Griffith, 2004).

Summary

This chapter has reviewed some of the important facts and statistics about the aging population, a.k.a. the "*silver tsunami*." Aging in the United States will greatly impact society as the baby boomers enter the older age group. Health disparities already exist among minority elderly groups and are likely to continue (AHRQ, 2008). Other groups considered vulnerable older adults include U.S. veterans, those with disabilities, and prisoners. Finally, successful aging is thought to be possible with wise lifestyle choices and avoidance of risk factors. These are further discussed throughout this text.

Resource List

Aging Statistics

    Administration on Aging:

    http://www.aoa.gov/

    American Association of Retired Persons:

    http://www.aarp.org

    American Geriatrics Society:

    http://www.americangeriatrics.org

Centers for Disease Control and Prevention:

http://www.cdc.gov/aging/

Federal Interagency Forum on Aging-Related Statistics:

http://www.agingstats.gov

Gray Panthers:

http://www.graypanthers.org

Merck Manual of Health and Aging:

http://www.merck.com/pubs/mmanual_ha/sec1/ch03/ch03a.html

National Institute on Aging:

http://www.nia.nih.gov/

Online Journals

BMC Geriatrics:

http://www.biomedcentral.com/bmcgeriatr

Geriatrics:

http://www.geri.com/geriatrics/

Geriatrics and Aging:

http://www.geriatricsandaging.com

Longevity

Estimate your longevity potential by accessing the Life Expectancy Calculator at:

http://www.livingto100.com

CDC/National Center for Health Statistics:

http://www.cdc.gov/nchs/fastats/lifexpec.htm

Critical Thinking Exercises

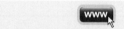

1. **You will be one of the nurses caring for the baby boomers as they age**. How will the prevalence of aged patients affect your nursing practice? What are the implications for your ongoing nursing education?

2. **Healthful living becomes ever more important to prevent the chronic diseases** of the aged. Fewer chronic diseases in the aged could mean that more healthcare services are available for those without chronic diseases. What is healthful living? What will your role be in promoting healthful living to your patients? Should nurses be responsible for promoting healthful living when they could be caring for sick patients?

3. **The health care of the baby boomers will likely be affected by changes in Social Security, Medicare, and Medicaid.** What implications does this have for your nursing practice? How might you address this issue as a nurse? How might you address this issue as a citizen?

4. **The population of the United States is becoming ever more ethnically and culturally diverse.** What healthcare issues can you foresee as this ethnically diverse population ages?

5. **Think about older celebrities in the United States and abroad,** and compare your thoughts about them to your thoughts about older people in general. Do you have different thoughts and feelings about Bill Clinton and George W. Bush (former presidents, both age 65 in 2012) than you do about a nursing home patient? How about those celebrities who are growing older—Cher (singer, age 65), Barbra Streisand (singer, age 70), Colin Powell (general, age 75), Dan Rather (newsman, age 80), Cloris Leachman (actress, age 85)? Compare and contrast a well-known senior celebrity with an aged patient you have recently met.

Personal Reflection   www.

The aging of America will affect you both personally and professionally. Government resources will become more and more strained as the baby boomers become elders and begin to use these resources. Medicare, Medicaid, and Social Security may not continue to exist as we know them. There will be fewer beds available in both acute and chronic care facilities to care for the growing aged population. There may not be enough geriatric specialty physicians and nurses to care for the vast numbers of older adults. How could these circumstances affect you and your family? What are your personal plans for your own aging? Have you started to save money for retirement? Are you living a healthy lifestyle, eating "right," and exercising? Are you or your children overweight? Do you smoke or drink alcohol excessively? Are you ready to become involved in the political process so that your opinion is heard?

References

Administration on Aging, Department of Health and Human Services. (2010). *A profile of older Americans: 2010.* Retrieved from http://www.aoa.gov/AoAroot/Aging_Statistics/Profile/2010/index.aspx

Administration on Aging, Department of Health and Human Services. (2011a). *A profile of older Americans: 2011.* Retrieved from http://www.aoa.gov/AoARoot/Aging_Statistics/Profile/2011/docs/2011profile.pdf

Administration on Aging, Department of Health and Human Services. (2011b). *A statistical profile of American Indian and Native Alaskan elderly.* Retrieved from http://www.aoa.gov/AoARoot/Aging_Statistics/Minority_Aging/Facts-on-AINA-Elderly2008-plain_format.aspx

AHRQ. (2008). National Healthcare Disparities report, 2008. Retrieved from http://www.ahrq.gov/qual/nhdr08/Chap4c.htm

Angel, R. J., & Angel, J. L. (1997). Health service use and long-term care among Hispanics. In K. S. Markides & M. R. Miranda (Eds.), *Minorities, aging and health* (pp. 343–366). Thousand Oaks, CA: Sage.

Aranda, M. P., & Miranda, R. M. (1997). Hispanic aging, social support, and mental health: Does acculturation make a difference? In K. S. Markides & M. R. Miranda (Eds.), *Minorities, aging, and health* (pp. 271–294). Thousand Oaks, CA: Sage.

Barrett, A. & Schimmel, J. (2010). Multiple Service Use Among OAA Title III Program Participants. Washington, DC: Mathematica Policy Research.

Cameron, K.A., Song, J., Manheim, L.M. & Dunlop, D.D. (2010). *Gender disparities in health and healthcare among older adults.* Retrieved from http: //www.ncbi.nlm.nih.gov/pmc/articles/PMC2965695/

Carbonell, J. (May 17, 2005). Testimony before the Subcommittee on Retirement Security and Aging, Committee on Health, Education, Labor and Pensions, United States Senate. Retrieved from http://www.aoa.gov/press/speeches/2005/05_May/HHS%20Statement%20May%2017.pdf

Centers for Disease Control and Prevention [CDC]. (2005). Health disparities experienced by Black or African Americans—United States. *Morbidity and Mortality Weekly Report, 54*(1), 1–3.

Centers for Disease Control and Prevention [CDC]. (2009). *Fast stats: Life expectancy.* Retrieved from http://www.cdc.gov/nchs/fastats/older_americans.htm

Centers for Disease Control and Prevention [CDC]. (2010). *Office of Minority Health and Health Disparities.* Retrieved from http://www.cdc.gov/omhd/Populations/HL/HL.htm#Ten

Centers for Disease Control and Prevention [CDC]. (2011). *Fact sheet: CDC health disparities and inequalities report.* Retrieved from http://www.cdc.gov/minorityhealth/reports/CHDIR11/FactSheet.pdf

Chapleski, E. E. (1997). Long term care among American Indians: A broad lens perspective on service preference and use. In K. S. Markides & M. R. Miranda (Eds.), *Minorities, aging, and health* (pp. 367–394). Thousand Oaks, CA: Sage.

Connolly, B. H. (1998). General effects of aging on persons with developmental disabilities. *Topics in Geriatric Rehabilitation, 13*(3), 1–18.

Egendorf, L. (Ed.). (2002). *An aging population.* San Diego, CA: Greenhaven Press. Retrieved from http://www.enotes.com/aging-population-article

Elo, I. (1997). Adult mortality among Asian Americans and Pacific Islanders: A review of the evidence. In K. S. Markides & M. R. Miranda (Eds.), *Minorities, aging, and health* (pp. 41–78). Thousand Oaks, CA: Sage.

Experience Corps. (2005). *Fact sheet on aging in America.* Retrieved from http://www.experiencecorps.org/research/factsheet.html

Federal Interagency Forum on Aging-Related Statistics. (November 2004). *Older Americans 2004: Key indicators of well-being.* Washington, DC: U.S. Government Printing Office. Retrieved from http://www.agingstats.gov/Agingstatsdotnet/Main_Site/Data/Data_2004.aspx

Federal Interagency Forum on Aging-Related Statistics. (November 2010). *Older Americans 2010: Key indicators of well-being.* Washington, DC: U.S. Government Printing Office. Retrieved from http://www.agingstats.gov/agingstatsdotnet/Main_Site/Data/2010_Documents/Docs/OA_2010.pdf

Fleming, K., Evans, J. M., & Chutka, D. S. (2003). A cultural and economic history of old age in America. *Mayo Clinic Proceedings, 78*(7), 914–921.

Goins, R. T., Moss, M., Buchwald, D., & Guralnik, J. M. (2007). Disability among older American Indians and Alaska Natives: An analysis of the 2000 Census public use microdata sample. *Gerontologist, 47*(5), 690–696.

Goins, R. T. & Pilkerton, C. S. (2010). Comorbidity among older American Indians: The Native Elder Care Study. *Journal of Cross-Cultural Gerontology, 25*(4), 343–354.

Grieco, M., Acosta, Y. D., de la Cruz, G. P., Gambino, C., Gryn, T., Larsen, L. J., … Walters, N. P. The foreign-born population in the United States; 2010: *American Community Survey Reports.* Retrieved from http://www.census.gov/prod/2012pubs/acs-19.pdf

Griffith, R. W. (2004). The centenarian study. Retrieved from http://www.healthandage.com

He, W. (2000). *The older foreign-born population of the United States: 2000.* Washington, DC: U.S. Census Bureau, U.S. Department of Health and Human Services, U.S. Department of Commerce.

He, W., Sengupta, M., Velkoff, V., & DeBarros, K.A. (2005). *65+ in the United States.* Retrieved from http://www.census.gov/prod/2006pubs/p23-209.pdf

Human Rights Watch. (2012). Old behind bars: The aging prison population in the United States. Retrieved from http://www.hrw.org/sites/default/files/reports/usprisons0112webwcover_0.pdf

Indian Health Service [IHS]. (2012). *Fact sheets.* Retrieved from http://www.ihs.gov/PublicAffairs/IHSBrochure/

Jacobs, H. (1861). Incidents in the life of a slave girl: Written by herself. Child, M. L. (Ed.). Boston, MA: Published for the author. Retrieved from http://docsouth.unc.edu/fpn/jacobs/jacobs.html

Kinsella, G, & He, W. (2009). *An aging world, 2008.* U.S. Census Bureau, International Population Reports, P95/09-1. Washington, DC: U.S. Government Printing Office.

Kitano, H. H., Tazuko, S., & Kitano, K. J. (1997). Asian American elderly mental health. In K. S. Markides & M. R. Miranda (Eds.), *Minorities, aging, and health* (pp. 295–315). Thousand Oaks, CA: Sage.

Kramer, B. J. (1997). Chronic diseases in American Indian populations. In K. S. Markides & M. R. Miranda (Eds.), *Minorities, aging, and health.* (pp. 181–202). Thousand Oaks, CA: Sage.

Markides, K. S. & Miranda, M. R. (Eds.). (1997). *Minorities, aging, and health.* Thousand Oaks, CA: Sage.

McMahon, P. (2003). Aging inmates present prison crisis. *USA Today.* Retrieved from http://www.usatoday.com/news/nation/2003-08-10-prison-inside-usat_x.htm

Merck Institute of Aging and Health (MIAH), Centers for Disease Control and Prevention, & Gerontological Society of America. (2004). *The state of aging and health in America 2004.* Retrieved from http://www.cdc.gov/aging/pdf/State_of_Aging_and_Health_in_America_2004.pdf

Mitka, M. (2004). Aging prisoners stressing the health care system. *Journal of the American Medical Association, 292*(4), 423–424.

Munnell, A. H. (2004). Population aging: It's not just the baby boom. *An Issue in Brief: Center for Retirement Research at Boston College, 16*, 1–7.

National Institute on Aging. (2012). Health and aging. Retrieved from http://www.nia.nih.gov/health/featured/healthy-aging-longevity

National Research Council. (2011). *Past smoking rates are a major reason for shorter lifespans in U.S. compared to other high-income countries; Obesity also appears to be significant factor*. Retrieved from http://www8.nationalacademies.org/onpinews/newsitem.aspx?RecordID=13089

National Council on Aging. (2012). Inaugural United States of Aging Survey Finds Most Older Adults Upbeat about Aging, But Some Are Uncertain about Long-Term Outlook for their Health and Finances. Retrieved from http://www.ncoa.org/press-room/press-release/inaugural-united-states-of.html

National PACE Association. (2002). Retrieved from www.npaonline.org

Perls, T., Silver, M., & Lauerman, J. (1999). *Living to 100: Lessons in living to your maximum*. New York, NY: Basic Books.

The Poorhouse Story. (2005). Retrieved from http://www.poorhousestory.com/index.htm

Plessman, B. L., Langa, K. M., Fisher, G. G., Heeringa, S. G., Weir, D. R. Ofstedal, M. B., … Wallace, R. B. (2007). Prevalence of dementia in the United States: The Aging, Demographics, and Memory Study. *Neuroepidemiology, 29*, 125–137.

Porter, C. (2011). *Hispanics are largest minority group in United States*. Embassy of the United States, Brussels, Belgium. Retrieved from: http://www.uspolicy.be/headline/hispanics-are-largest-minority-group-united-states

Ross, H. (2000). *Growing older: Health issues for minorities: Closing the gap. Newsletter of the Office of Minority Health*. Washington, DC: U.S. Department of Health and Human Services.

U.S. Census Bureau. (2001). T*he 65 years and over population: 2000. Census 2000 Brief*. Washington, DC: U.S. Department of Commerce, Economics and Statistics Administration.

U.S. Census Bureau. (2011). *Older Americans Month: May, 2011*. Retrieved from http://www.census.gov/newsroom/releases/archives/facts_for_features_special_editions/cb11-ff08.html

U.S. Department of Health and Human Services. (1999). *Centenarians in the United States*. Available at http://www.census.gov/prod/99pubs/p23-199.pdf

Vincent, G.K. & Velkoff, V. A. (2010). *The next four decades: The older population in the United States: 2010–2050*. Retrieved from http://www.census.gov/prod/2010pubs/p25-1138.pdf

Wiles, J. L., Leibing, A., Guberman, N., Reeve, J., & Allen, R. E. S. (2011). The Meaning of "Ageing in Place" to Older People. The Gerontologist. Retrieved from http://gerontologist.oxfordjournals.org/content/early/2011/10/07/geront.gnr098.full.pdf+html. doi:10.1093/geront/gnr098

For a full suite of assignments and additional learning activities, see the access code at the front of your book.

At the end of this chapter, the reader will be able to:

> Identify the major theories of aging.
> Compare the similarities and differences between biological and psychosocial theories.
> Describe the process of aging using a biological and a psychosocial perspective.
> Analyze the rationale for using multiple theories of aging to describe the complex phenomenon of aging.
> Describe a general theoretical framework, taken from all of the aging theories, that will assist nurses in making clinical decisions in gerontology.

KEY TERMS

Apoptosis	Nonstochastic theories of aging
Free radicals	Reactive oxygen species (ROS)
Immunomodulation	Senescence
Lipofuscin	Stochastic theories of aging
Melatonin	Telomerase
Mitochondria	Telomere

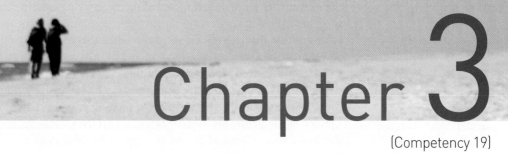

Chapter 3

Theories of Aging

Jean Lange
Sheila Grossman

From the beginning of time, the elusive phenomenon of preserving youth has been a topic of discussion in science, health care, technology, and everyday life. Is there anyone who would not be interested in knowing how the human organism ages? Doesn't everyone want to live a long and healthy life? There are few who would not want to see what the future holds for our bodies and minds; even more curiosity surrounds what advances have been made or will possibly be made to alter and slow the aging process. Understanding what knowledge theories of aging have generated and reviewing the validity of these findings and how they impact evolution and scientific advances is a first step toward understanding the mystery of aging. Troen (2003) suggested, "The beneficial paradox may be that the maximum lifespan potential of humans may have been achieved, in part, due to our ability to grow old" (p. 5).

Complex physiological, social, economic, and psychological challenges present themselves as we age. Older adults may face declines in health and physical functioning that may necessitate moving to supportive care environments that drain financial resources. The death of friends or loved ones, grappling with questions about the meaning of life, maintaining a satisfactory quality of life in the face of increasing disability, adapting to retirement, and contemplating death are just a few of the psychological challenges that aging adults may face. Theories that can effectively guide nursing practice with older adults must be comprehensive yet consider individual differences. Cultural, spiritual, regional, socioeconomic, educational, and environmental factors as well as health status impact older adults' perceptions and choices about their healthcare needs. According to Haight and colleagues, "a good gerontological theory integrates knowledge, tells how and why phenomena are related, leads to prediction, and provides process and understanding. In addition, a good theory must be holistic and take into account all that impacts on a person throughout a lifetime of aging" (Haight, Barba, Tesh, & Courts, 2002, p. 14).

Since the early 1950s, sociologists, psychologists, and biologists have proposed varied theories about the aging process. Although there is increased emphasis in the nursing literature on issues regarding the growing elderly population, limited work has been done to develop nursing-specific aging theories. Increasingly, there is recognition that aging is a distinct discipline that requires aging theories having an interdisciplinary perspective. A model by Alkema and Alley (2006) attempts to address this need. The purpose of this chapter is to review the chronological development of biopsychosocial aging theories, the evidence supporting or refuting these theories, and their application to nursing practice. CINAHL, the National Library of Medicine, the Web of Science, PsycINFO, and Sociological Abstracts databases were reviewed to assess support for and clinical application of the theories of aging.

TABLE 3-1 Psychosocial Theories of Aging	
Theory	**Description**
Sociological Theories	Changing roles, relationships, status, and generational cohort impact the older adult's ability to adapt.
Activity	Remaining occupied and involved is necessary to a satisfying late life.
Disengagement	Gradual withdrawal from society and relationships serves to maintain social equilibrium and promote internal reflection.
Subculture	The elderly prefer to segregate from society in an aging subculture sharing loss of status and societal negativity regarding the aged. Health and mobility are key determinants of social status.
Continuity	Personality influences roles and life satisfaction and remains consistent throughout life. Past coping patterns recur as older adults adjust to physical, financial, and social decline and contemplate death. Identifying with one's age group, finding a residence compatible with one's limitations, and learning new roles postretirement are major tasks.
Age stratification	Society is stratified by age groups that are the basis for acquiring resources, roles, status, and deference from others. Age cohorts are influenced by their historical context and share similar experiences, beliefs, attitudes, and expectations of life course transitions.
Person-Environment-Fit	Function is affected by ego strength, mobility, health, cognition, sensory perception, and the environment. Competency changes one's ability to adapt to environmental demands.
Gerotranscendence	The elderly transform from a materialistic/rational perspective toward oneness with the universe. Successful transformation includes an outward focus, accepting impending death, substantive relationships, intergenerational connectedness, and unity with the universe.

Psychosocial Theories of Aging

The earliest theories on aging came from the psychosocial disciplines (see **Table 3-1**). Psychosocial theories attempt to explain aging in terms of behavior, personality, and attitude change. Development is viewed as a lifelong process characterized by transitions. Psychological theories are concerned with personality or ego development and the accompanying challenges associated with various life stages. How mental processes, emotions, attitudes, motivation, and personality influence adaptation to physical and social demands are central issues.

Sociological theorists consider how changing roles, relationships, and status within a culture or society impact the older adult's ability to adapt. Societal norms can affect how individuals envision their role and function within that society, and

Theory	Description
Psychological Theories	Explain aging in terms of mental processes, emotions, attitudes, motivation, and personality development that is characterized by life stage transitions.
Human needs	Five basic needs motivate human behavior in a lifelong process toward need fulfillment.
Individualism	Personality consists of an ego and personal and collective unconsciousness that views life from a personal or external perspective. Older adults search for life meaning and adapt to functional and social losses.
Stages of personality	Personality develops in eight sequential stages with corresponding life development tasks. The eighth phase, integrity versus despair, is characterized by evaluating life accomplishments; struggles include letting go, accepting care, detachment, and physical and mental decline.
Life-course/life span	Life stages are predictable and structured by roles, relationships, values, development and goals. Persons adapt to changing roles and relationships. Age-group norms and characteristics are an important part of the life course.
Selective optimization	Individuals cope with aging losses through activity/role selection, optimization, and compensation. Critical life points are morbidity, mortality, and quality of life. Selective optimization with compensation facilitates successful aging.

thus impact role choices as well as how roles are enacted. The role of women in the United States has been redefined greatly since the 1960s. Such cohort or generational variables are a key component of sociological theories of aging.

Sociological Theories of Aging

Activity Theory

Sociological theorists have attempted to explain older adult behavior in relationship to society with such concepts as disengagement, activity, and continuity. One of the earliest theories addressing the aging process was begun by Havighurst and Albrecht in 1953 when they discussed the concept of activity engagement and positive adaptation to aging. From studying a sample of adults, they concluded that society expects retired older adults to remain active contributors. Activity theory was conceived as an actual theory in 1963 and purports that remaining occupied and involved is a necessary ingredient to a satisfying late-life (Havighurst, Neugarten, & Tobin, 1963) (see **Figure 3-1**). The authors do not qualify the activity characteristics that are most directly linked to life satisfaction. Havighurst and Albrecht associate activity with psychosocial health and suggest activity as a means to prolong middle age and delay the negative effects of old age. An assumption of this theory is that inactivity negatively impacts one's self-concept and perceived quality of life and hastens aging.

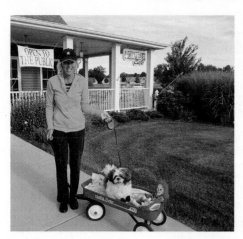

Figure 3-1 Activity theory suggests that remaining involved and engaged is a needed ingredient to a satisfying late life.

Arguments against this point of view are that it fails to consider that activity choices are often constrained by physical, economic, and social resources. Furthermore, roles assumed by older adults are highly influenced by societal expectations (Birren & Schroots, 2001). Maddox (1963) suggested, however, that leisure time presents new opportunities for activities and roles, such as community service, that may be more consistent with these limitations. A second criticism of activity theory is the unproven assertion that continued activity delays onset of the negative effects of aging.

Despite these criticisms, the central theme of activity theory—that remaining active in old age is desirable—is supported by most research. Lemon and colleagues found a direct relationship between role and activity engagement and life satisfaction among older adults (Lemon, Bengston, & Peterson, 1972). The authors also observed that the quality of activities, as perceived by older adults, is more important than the quantity. Other investigators added that informal activities such as meeting friends for lunch or pursuing hobbies through group activities are more likely to improve life satisfaction than formal or solitary activities (Longino & Kart, 1982). In a study of older Americans, participation in shared tasks was an important predictor of life satisfaction, particularly among retirees (Harlow & Cantor, 1996). According to Schroots (1996), successful aging means being capable of doing activities that are important to the older adult despite limitations. One study, however, found that in a convenience sample of 386 older women, engaging in the social activity of shopping was not predictive of life satisfaction (Hyun-Mee & Miller, 2007). This suggests that the type of activity may be an important consideration rather than merely the frequency of engagement.

Disengagement Theory

In stark contrast to activity theorists, sociologists Cumming and Henry (1961) assert that aging is characterized by gradual disengagement from society and relationships. The authors contend that this separation is desired by society and older adults, and that it serves to maintain social equilibrium. Persons are freed from social responsibilities and gain time for internal reflection, while the transition of responsibility from old to young promotes societal functioning without interruption from lost members. Diminishing social contacts leads to further disengagement in a cyclical process that is systematic and inevitable. The outcome of disengagement, authors propose, is a new equilibrium that is ideally satisfying to both the individual and society. In support of this theory, an instrument measuring change in activity among older adults supports a tendency for less social contact among those over age 75 (Adams, 2004). The author reports, "In almost all instances, the group 75 years old and older reported a higher proportion of disengaged responses; they were particularly less invested than their younger counterparts in keeping up with hobbies, making plans for the future, making and creating things, and taking care of others" (p. 102).

The emphasis this theory places on social withdrawal has been challenged by other theorists who argue that a key element of life satisfaction among older adults appears to be engagement in meaningful relationships and activities (Baltes, 1987; Lemon et al., 1972; Neumann, 2000; Schroots, 1996). Others contend that the decision to withdraw varies across individuals and that disengagement theory fails to account for differences in sociocultural settings and environmental opportunities (Achenbaum & Bengtson, 1994; Marshall, 1996). Rapkin and Fischer (1992) found that demographic disadvantages and age-related transitions were related to a greater desire for disengagement, support, and stability. Elders who were married and healthy were more likely to report a desire for an energetic lifestyle. Cumming and Henry's notion of a necessary fit between society's needs and older adult activity is supported, however (Back, 1980; Birren & Schroots, 2001; Riley, Johnson, & Foner, 1972). Until recently, Social Security laws placed economic barriers against retirement before the mid-60s, but as years of healthy life expectancy increase, society is reframing its notions about the capability of older adults to make valuable contributions (Uhlenberg, 1992). Many adults are working past retirement age or begin part-time work in a new field. Others are actively engaged in a variety of volunteer projects that may substantially benefit their communities. The many examples of what is now termed "successful aging" are challenging the common association of aging with disease.

Subculture Theory

Unlike activity theorists, Rose (1965) viewed older adults as a unique subculture within society formed as a defensive response to society's negative attitudes and the loss of status that accompanies aging. As in disengagement theory, Rose proposed that although this subculture segregates the elderly from the rest of society, older adults prefer to interact among themselves. Rose contended that in the United States, one's degree of health and mobility is more critical in defining social status than occupation, education, or income. Older adults have a social disadvantage regarding status and associated respect because of the functional decline that accompanies aging.

Rose's theory argues for social reform. Growing numbers of older adults make it necessary to pay more attention to the needs of this age group and are challenging the prevailing view of aging as negative, undesirable, burdensome, and lacking status. Questions are beginning to be asked about whether society should be more supportive of older adults in terms of their environment, health care, work opportunities, and social resources. The emphasis on whether societal or older adults' needs take precedence is beginning to shift in favor of older adults. McMullin (2000) argued that sociological theories need to more clearly address the diversity among older adults as well as the disparity from other age groups. Research that supports or refutes Rose's theory is needed.

Continuity Theory

In the late 1960s, Havighurst and colleagues recognized that neither activity nor disengagement theories fully explain successful aging from a sociological point of view (Havighurst, Neugarten, & Tobin, 1968). Borrowing from psychology, they hypothesized that personality influences the roles one assumes, how roles are enacted, and one's satisfaction with living. They explained their new perspective in the continuity theory, also known as development theory. Continuity theory suggests that personality is well developed by the time one reaches old age and tends to remain consistent across the life span. Coping and personality patterns provide clues as to how an aging individual will adjust to changes in health, environment, or socioeconomic conditions, and what activities he or she will choose to engage in; thus, continuity theory acknowledges that individual differences produce varied responses to aging.

Havighurst and associates (1963) identified four personality types from their observations of older adults: integrated, armored-defended, passive-dependent, and unintegrated. Integrated personality types have adjusted well to aging, as evidenced by activity engagement that may be broad (reorganizers), more selective (focused), or disengaged. Armored-defended individuals tend to continue the activities and roles held during middle age, whereas passive-dependent persons are either highly dependent or exhibit disinterest in the external world. Least well-adjusted are unintegrated personality types who fail to cope with aging successfully. Havighurst (1972) later defined adjusting to physical, financial, and social decline; contemplating death; and developing a personal and meaningful perspective on the end of life as the tasks of older adulthood (**Box 3-1**). Successful accomplishment of these tasks is evidenced by identifying with one's age group, finding a living environment that is compatible with physical functioning, and learning new societal roles postretirement.

Research suggests that self-perception of personality remains stable over time, and attitude and degree of adaptation to old age are related to life satisfaction. When older adults were asked how they thought they had changed over the years, almost all respondents thought they were still essentially the same person. Degree of continuity was related to a more positive affect in these subjects (Troll & Skaff, 1997). In another study, Efklides and colleagues investigated effects of demographics, health status, attitude, and adaptation to old age on quality of life perceptions among older adults. The authors reported that positive attitude and adaptation to old age were associated with better perceptions about quality of life in this Greek sample (Efklides, Kalaitzidou, & Chankin, 2003). Agahi, Ahacic, and Parker (2006)

BOX 3-1   Research Highlight

Aim: This study investigated the relationship between social support and psychological distress in older adults over an 8-year period.

Methods: Canadian National Population Health Survey telephone survey data from 1998 and 2007 regarding residents' health, sociodemographic status, health services utilization, predictors of health, chronic conditions, and activity restrictions were analyzed. Respondants included 2,564 adults aged 55 to 89 years (mean age 64 yeras). Bivariate autoregressive cross-lagged models were used to analyze the data. Four dimensions of social support (emotional/informational support, tangible support, positive social interactions, and affectionate support) were examined in relationship to psychological distress, defined as a nonspecific negative psychological state that includes feelings of depression and anxiety. Structural equation modeling was used to analyze relationships among the variables.

Findings: Emotional/informational support, positive social interactions, and affectionate support were directly related to psychological distress. Higher psychological distress was related to subsequently higher levels of positive social interaction and emotional/informational support. Prior affectionate support predicted later support, and prior psychological distress predicted later levels of distress.

Application to practice: Psychological distress among older adults may predict subsequent levels of social support. Implications for these findings include the need for a greater awareness of the bidirectional nature of the relationship between social support and psychological distress among those who develop programs targeting older adults.

Source: Robitaille, A., Orpana, H., & McIntosh, C. N. (2012). Reciprocal relationship between social support and psychological distress among a national sample of older adults: An autoregressive cross-lagged model. *Canadian Journal on Aging—La Revue Canadienne Du Vieillissement, 31*(1), 13.

used continuity theory to examine patterns of change in older adults' participation in leisure activities over time. Consistent with continuity as well as activity and disengagement theories, the authors found that active participation tends to decline over time, and lifelong participation patterns predict involvement later in life. Critics of continuity theory, however, caution that the social context within which one ages may be more important than personality in determining what and how roles are played (Birren & Schroots, 2001).

Age Stratification Theory

In the 1970s, sociologists began to examine the interdependence between older adults and society, recognizing that aging and society are interrelated and cause reciprocal changes to individuals, age group cohorts, and society (Riley et al., 1972). Riley and colleagues observed that society is stratified into different age categories that are the basis for acquiring resources, roles, status, and deference from others in society. In addition, age cohorts are influenced by the historical context in which they live; thus, age cohorts and corresponding roles vary across generations. People born in the same cohort have similar experiences with shared meanings, ideologies, orientations, attitudes, and values as well as expectations regarding the timing of life course transitions. Individuals in different generations have different experiences that may cause them to age in different ways (Riley, 1994).

Age stratification transitioned aging theory from a focus on the individual to a broader context that alerted gerontologists to the influence of cohort groups and the socioeconomic and political impact on how individuals age (Marshall, 1996). Uhlenburg (1996) borrowed from age stratification theory in developing a framework for understanding what social changes are needed to reduce the burden that aging cohorts place on society in terms of their care needs at different stages of later life.

Newsom and Schulz (1996) demonstrated that physical impairment is associated with fewer social contacts, less social support, depression, and lower life satisfaction. This finding suggests that social networks are an important element in how individuals age. Yin and Lai (1983) used age stratification theory to explain the changing status of older adults due to differences among cohort groups. Investigators studying age segregation versus integration in residential settings learned that outcomes were less favorable among settings with single cohort groups (Hagestad & Dannefer, 2002; Uhlenberg, 2000).

Person-Environment-Fit Theory

In addition to the broadened view of aging that emerged in the 1970s, another shift in aging theory in the early 1980s blended existing theories from different disciplines. Lawton's (1982) person-environment-fit theory introduced functional competence in relationship to the environment as a central theme. Functional competence is affected by multiple intrapersonal conditions such as ego strength, motor skills, biologic health, cognitive capacity, and sensori-perceptual capacity, as well as external conditions posed by the environment. The degree of competency may change as one ages, affecting functional ability in relationship to environmental demands. A person's ability to meet these demands is affected by his or her level of functioning and influences the ability to adapt to the environment. Those functioning at lower levels can tolerate fewer environmental demands.

Lawton's (1982) theory is useful for exploring optimal environments for older adults with functional limitations and identifying needed modifications in older adult residential settings. Building on Lawton's work, Wahl (2001) developed six models to explain relationships between aging and the environment, home, institution, and relocation decision making. O'Connor and Vallerand (1994) used Lawton's theory to examine the relationship between long-term care residents' adjustment and their motivational style and environment. Older adults with self-determined motivational styles were better adjusted when they lived in homes that provided opportunities for freedom and choice, whereas residents with less self-determined motivational styles were better adjusted when they lived in high-constraint environments. The authors concluded that their findings supported the person-environment-fit theory of adjustment in old age.

In a more recent study, Iwarsson's (2005) findings partially supported a relationship between environmental fit and functioning. Dependence with activities of daily living (ADLs) was significantly related to activities of daily living among only the frailest older adults in his longitudinal study.

Gerotranscendence Theory

One of the newest aging theories is Tornstam's (1994) theory of gerotranscendence. This theory proposes that aging individuals undergo a cognitive transformation from a materialistic, rational perspective toward oneness with the universe. Characteristics of successful transformation include a more outward or external focus, accepting impending death without fear, an emphasis on substantive relationships, a sense of connectedness with preceding and future generations, and spiritual unity with the universe. Gerotranscendence borrows from disengagement theory but does not accept the idea that social disengagement is a necessary and natural development. Tornstam asserted that activity and participation must be the result of one's own choices, which differ from one person to another. Control over one's life in all situations is essential for the person's adaptation to aging as a whole.

Gerotranscendence has been tested in several studies. In an ongoing longitudinal study based on the principles of gerodynamics, Schroots (2003) is investigating how people manage their lives, cope with transformations, and react to affective-positive and negative life events. In nursing, Wadensten (2002) used the theory of gerotranscendence to develop guidelines for care of older adults in a nursing home. The results indicate that these guidelines may be useful for facilitating the process of gerotranscendence in nursing home residents.

Psychological Theories of Aging

Human Needs Theory

At the same time that activity theory was being developed, Maslow (1954), a psychologist, published the human needs theory. In this theory, Maslow surmised that a hierarchy of five needs motivates human behavior: physiologic, safety and security, love and belonging, self-esteem, and self-actualization. These needs are prioritized such that more basic needs like physiological functioning or safety take precedence over personal growth needs (love and belonging, self-esteem, and self-actualization). Movement is multidirectional and dynamic in a lifelong process toward need fulfillment. Self-actualization requires the freedom to express and pursue personal goals and be creative in an environment that is stimulating and challenging.

Although Maslow does not specifically address old age, it is clear that physical, economic, social, and environmental constraints can impede need fulfillment of older adults. Maslow asserted that failure to grow leads to feelings of failure, depression, and the perception that life is meaningless. Since inception, Maslow's theory has been applied to varied age groups in many disciplines. Ebersole, Hess, and Luggen (2004) linked the tasks of aging described by several theorists (Butler & Lewis, 1982; Havighurst, 1972; Peck, 1968) to the basic needs in Maslow's model. Jones and Miesen (1992) used Maslow's hierarchy to present a nursing care model for working with aged persons with specific needs in an attempt to relate all patient needs to universal, rather than exceptional, needs. The model is designed to be used by caregivers in residential settings.

Theory of Individualism

Like Maslow's theory, Jung's theory of individualism is not specific to aging. Jung (1960) proposed a lifespan view of personality development rather than attainment of basic needs. Jung defined personality as being composed of an ego or self-identity with a personal and collective unconsciousness. Personal unconsciousness is the private feelings and perceptions surrounding significant persons or life events. The collective unconscious is shared by all persons and contains latent memories of human origin. The collective unconscious is the foundation of personality on which the personal unconsciousness and ego are built. Individual personalities tend to view life primarily either through the self or through others; thus, extroverts are more concerned with the world around them, whereas introverts interpret experiences from the personal perspective. As individuals age, Jung proposed that elders engage in an "inner search" to critique their beliefs and accomplishments. According to Jung, successful aging means acceptance of the past and an ability to cope with functional decline and loss of significant others. Neugarten (1968) supported Jung's association of aging and introspection and asserts that "interiority" promotes positive inner growth. Subsequent theorists also describe introspection as a part of healthy aging (Erikson, 1963; Havighurst et al., 1968).

Stages of Personality Development Theory

Similar to other psychologists' theories at the time, Erikson's theory focuses on individual development. According to Erikson (1963), personality develops in eight sequential stages that have a corresponding life task that one may succeed at or fail to accomplish. Progression to a subsequent life stage requires that tasks at prior stages be completed successfully. Older adults experience the developmental stage known as "ego integrity versus despair." Erikson proposed that this final phase of development is characterized by evaluating one's life and accomplishments for meaning. In later years, Erikson and colleagues expanded upon his original description of integrity versus despair, noting that older adults struggle with letting go, accepting the care of others, detaching from life, and physical and mental decline (Erikson, Erikson, & Kivnick, 1986).

Several authors have expanded upon Erikson's work. Peck (1968) refined the task within Erikson's stage of ego integrity versus despair into three challenges: ego differentiation versus work role reoccupation, body transcendence versus body preoccupation, and ego transcendence versus ego preoccupation. Major issues such as meaningful life after retirement, the empty nest syndrome, dealing with the functional decline of aging, and contemplating one's mortality are consistent with Peck's conceptualization. Butler and Lewis (1982) later defined the challenges of late life as adjusting to infirmity, developing satisfaction with one's lived life, and preparing for death, mirroring those tasks described earlier by Peck.

Erikson's theory is widely employed in the behavioral sciences. In nursing, Erikson's model is often used as a framework for examining the challenges faced by different age groups. In a study of frail elderly men and women, Neumann (2000) used Erikson's theoretical framework when asking participants to discuss their perceptions about the meaning of their lives. She found that older adults who expressed higher levels of meaning and energy described a sense of connectedness, self-worth, love, and respect that was absent among participants who felt unfulfilled. This finding is consistent with the potential for positive or negative outcomes described by Erikson and colleagues (1986) in his stage of "integrity versus despair." In a qualitative study with six participants, five of whom were women, Holm and colleagues examined the value of storytelling among dementia patients. The investigators told stories linked to Erikson's developmental stages to stimulate sharing among the participants. The authors report that these stages were clearly evident among the experiences related by the participants (Holm, Lepp, & Ringsberg, 2005).

Life-Course (Life Span Development) Paradigm

In the late 1970s, the predominant theme of behavioral psychology moved toward the concept of "life course," in which life, although unique to each individual, is divided into stages with predictable patterns (Back, 1980). The significance of this shift was the inclusion of late as well as early life. Most theorists up to this point had focused primarily on childhood in their research. The substance of the life-course paradigm drew from the work of a European psychologist in the 1930s (Bühler, 1933). This new emphasis on adulthood occurred because of a demographic shift toward increasing numbers of older adults, the emergence of gerontology as a specialty, and the availability of subjects from longitudinal studies of childhood begun during the 1920s and 1930s (Baltes, 1987).

The central concepts of the life-course perspective blend key elements in psychological theories such as life stages, tasks, and personality development with sociological concepts such as role behavior and the interrelationship between individuals and society. The central tenet of life-course is that life occurs in stages that are structured according to one's roles, relationships, internal values, and goals. Individuals may choose their goals but are limited by external constraints. Goal achievement is associated with life satisfaction (Bühler, 1933). Individuals must adapt to changed roles and relationships that occur throughout life, such as getting married, finishing school, completing military service, getting a job, and retiring (Cunningham & Brookbank, 1988). Successful adaptation to life change may necessitate revising beliefs in order to be consistent with societal expectations. The life-course paradigm is concerned with understanding age group norms and their characteristics. Since the 1970s, the work of many behavioral psychologists such as Elder, Hareven, and Jackson has emerged from the life-course perspective, which remains a dominant theme in the psychology literature today. Selective optimization with compensation, discussed in the following section, is one example of a theory that emerged from the life-course perspective.

Selective Optimization with Compensation Theory

Baltes's (1987) theory of successful aging emerged from his study of psychological processes across the lifespan and, like earlier theories, focuses on the individual. He asserts that individuals learn to cope with the functional losses of aging through processes of selection, optimization, and compensation. Aging individuals become more selective in activities and roles as limitations present themselves; at the same time, they choose those activities and roles that are most satisfying (optimization). Finally, individuals adapt by seeking alternatives when functional limits prohibit sustaining former roles or activities. As people age, they pass through critical life points related to morbidity, mortality, and quality of life. The outcome of these critical junctures may result in lower- or higher-order functioning that is associated with higher or lower risk, respectively, for mortality. Selective optimization with compensation is a positive coping process that facilitates successful aging (Baltes & Baltes, 1990).

Much of the research testing psychosocial theories centers on life-course concepts (Baltes, 1987; Caspi, 1987; Caspi & Elder, 1986; Quick & Moen, 1998; Schroots, 2003). In an ongoing longitudinal study called "Life-Course Dynamics," Shroots examines the self-organization of behavior over the course of life. He has found that life structure tends to be consistent over time and is influenced by life events and experiences. The relationship of life events to structure does change, however, as we age. In an effort to outline the temporal and situational parameters of social life,

Caspi (1987) developed a model for personality analysis using life-course concepts such as interactions among personality, age-based roles, and social transitions in a historical context. Life-course principles have also been used to examine gender differences in retirement satisfaction. Quick and Moen (1988) report that retirement quality for women is associated with good health, a continuous career, earlier retirement, and a good postretirement income.

For men, good health, an enjoyable career, low work-role prominence, preretirement planning, and retiring voluntarily impacted satisfaction. The authors concluded that a gender-sensitive life-course approach to life transitions is essential.

Caspi and Elder (1986) criticized the life-course perspective of aging because it assumes that adaptation is governed by factors beyond the immediate situation. In a small sample of women, the authors examined how social and psychological factors experienced by women in the 1930s relate to life satisfaction in their older age. They reported relationships among intellect, social activity, and life satisfaction in older, working-class women, but emotional health was a better predictor of life satisfaction among older women from higher class origins. Differences in how the Depression impacted adaptation to old age among women from distinct social classes were described. The authors concluded that the influence of social change on life course is intertwined with individual factors.

Biological Theories of Aging

The biological theories explain the physiologic processes that change with aging. In other words, how is aging manifested on the molecular level in the cells, tissues, and body systems; how does the body–mind interaction affect aging; what biochemical processes impact aging; and how do one's chromosomes impact the overall aging process? Does each system age at the same rate? Does each cell in a system age at the same rate? How does chronological age influence an individual who is experiencing a pathophysiological disease process—how does the actual disease, as well as the treatment, which might include drugs, *immunomodulation*, surgery, or radiation, influence the organism? Several theories purport to explain aging at the molecular, cellular, organ, and system levels; however, no one predominant theory has evolved. Both genetics and environment influence the multifaceted phenomenon of aging.

Some aging theorists divide the biological theories into two categories:

1. A stochastic or statistical perspective, which identifies episodic events that happen throughout one's life that cause random cell damage and accumulate over time, thus causing aging.
2. The nonstochastic theories, which view aging as a series of predetermined events happening to all organisms in a timed framework.

Others believe aging is more likely the result of both programmed and stochastic concepts as well as allostasis, which is the process of achieving homeostasis via both behavioral and physiological change (Carlson & Chamberlain, 2005; Miquel, 1998). For example, there are specific programmed events in the life of a cell, but cells also accumulate genetic damage to the *mitochondria* due to free radicals and the loss of self-replication as they age. The following discussion presents descriptions of the different theories in the stochastic and nonstochastic theory categories, and also provides studies that support the various theoretical explanations.

Stochastic Theories

Studies of animals reflect that the effects of aging are primarily due to genetic defects, development, environment, and the inborn aging process (Harman, 2006; Goldsmith, 2011). There is no set of statistics to validate that these same findings are true with human organisms. The following *stochastic theories of aging* are discussed in this section: free radical theory, Orgel/error theory, wear and tear theory, and connective tissue theory.

Free Radical Theory

Oxidative free radical theory postulates that aging is due to oxidative metabolism and the effects of *free radicals*, which are the end products of oxidative metabolism. Free radicals are produced when the body uses oxygen, such as with exercise. This theory emphasizes the significance of how cells use oxygen (Hayflick, 1985). Also known as superoxides, free radicals are thought to react with proteins, lipids, deoxyribonucleic acid (DNA), and ribonucleic acid (RNA), causing cellular damage. This damage accumulates over time and is thought to accelerate aging.

Free radicals are chemical species that arise from atoms as single, unpaired electrons. Because a free radical molecule is unpaired, it is able to enter reactions with other molecules, especially along membranes and with nucleic acids. Free radicals cause:

> Extensive cellular damage to DNA, which can cause malignancy and accelerated aging due to oxidative modification of proteins that impact cell metabolism
> Lipid oxidation that damages phospholipids in cell membranes, thus affecting membrane permeability
> DNA strand breaks and base modifications that cause gene modulation

This cellular membrane damage causes other chemicals to be blocked from their regularly friendly receptor sites, thus mitigating other processes that may be crucial to cell metabolism. Mitochondrial deterioration due to oxidants causes a significant loss of cell energy and greatly decreases metabolism. Ames (2004) and Harman (1994) suggested some strategies to assist in delaying the mitochondrial decay, such as:

> Decrease calories in order to lower weight.
> Maintain a diet high in nutrients, including antioxidants.

> Avoid inflammation.
> Minimize accumulation of metals in the body that can trigger free radical reactions.

Additionally, studies are in process that demonstrate that mitochondrially targeted antioxidant treatments may decrease the adverse effects of Alzheimer's disease (Reddy, 2006).

Dufour and Larsson (2004) cite evidence of mitochondrial DNA damage accumulation and the aging process in mice. With the destruction of membrane integrity comes fluid and electrolyte loss or excess, depending on how the membrane was affected. Little by little there is more tissue deterioration. The older adult is more vulnerable to free radical damage because free radicals are attracted to cells that have transient or interrupted perfusion. Many older adults have decreased circulation because they have peripheral vascular, as well as coronary artery, disease. These diseases tend to cause heart failure that can be potentially worsened with fluid overload and electrolyte imbalance.

The majority of the evidence to support this theory is correlative in that oxidative damage increases with age. It is thought that people who limit calories, fat, and specific proteins in their diet may decrease the formation of free radicals. Roles of *reactive oxygen species (ROS)* are being researched in a variety of diseases such as atherosclerosis, vasospasms, cancers, trauma, stroke, asthma, arthritis, heart attack, dermatitis, retinal damage, hepatitis, and periodontitis (Lakatta, 2000; Gans, Putney, Bengtson, & Silverstein, 2009). Lee, Koo, and Min (2004) reported that antioxidant nutraceuticals are assisting in managing and, in some cases, delaying some of the manifestations of these diseases. Poon and colleagues described how two antioxidant systems (glutathione and heat shock proteins) are decreased in age-related degenerative neurological disorders (Poon, Calabrese, Scapagnini, & Butterfield, 2004). They also cited that free radical-mediated lipid peroxidation and protein oxidation affect central nervous system function. And now, for the first time, there is the possibility of investigating genetically altered animals to determine the impact of oxidative damage in aging (Bokov, Chaudhuri, & Richardson, 2004).

Examples of some sources of free radicals are listed in **Box 3-2**. In some instances, free radicals reacting with other molecules can form more free radicals, mutations, and malignancies. The free radical theory supports that as one lives, an accumulation of damage has been done to cells and, therefore, the organism ages. Grune and Davies (2001) go so far as to describe the free radical theory of aging as "the only aging theory to have stood the test of time" (p. 41). They further described how free radicals can generate cellular debris rich in lipids and proteins called lipofuscin, which older adults have more of when compared to younger adults. It is thought that *lipofuscin*, or age pigment, is a nondegradable material that decreases lysosomal function, which in turn impacts already disabled mitochondria (Brunk & Terman, 2002). Additionally, lipofuscin is considered a threat to multiple cellular systems including the ubiquitin/proteasome pathway, which leads to cellular death (Gray & Woulfe, 2005).

BOX 3-2   Exogenous Sources of Free Radicals

Tobacco smoke	Organic solvents	Ozone
Pesticides	Radiation	Selected medications

Orgel/Error Theory

This theory suggests that, over time, cells accumulate errors in their DNA and RNA protein synthesis that cause the cells to die (Orgel, 1970). Environmental agents and randomly induced events can cause error, with ultimate cellular changes. It is well known that large amounts of X-ray radiation cause chromosomal abnormalities. Thus, this theory proposes that aging would not occur if destructive factors such as radiation did not exist and cause "errors" such as mutations and regulatory disorders.

Hayflick (1996) did not support this theory, and explained that all aged cells do not have errant proteins, nor are all cells found with errant proteins old.

Wear and Tear Theory

Over time, cumulative changes occurring in cells age and damage cellular metabolism. An example is the cell's inability to repair damaged DNA, as in the aging cell. It is known that cells in heart muscle, neurons, striated muscle, and the brain cannot replace themselves after they are destroyed by wear and tear. Researchers cite gender-specific effects of aging on adrenocorticotropic activity that are consistent with the wear and tear hypothesis of the ramifications of lifelong exposure to stress (Van Cauter, Leproult, & Kupfer, 1996). There is some speculation that excessive wear and tear caused by exercising may accelerate aging by increasing free radical production, which supports the idea that no one theory of aging incorporates all the causes of aging, but rather that a combination of factors is responsible.

Studies of people with osteoarthritis suggest that cartilage cells age over time, and this degeneration is not due solely to strenuous exercise but also to general wear and tear. The studies point out that aged cells have lost the ability to counteract mechanical, inflammatory, and other injuries due to their *senescence* (Aigner, Rose, Martin, & Buckwalter, 2004).

Connective Tissue Theory

This theory is also referred to as cross-link theory, and it proposes that, over time, biochemical processes create connections between structures not normally connected. Several cross-linkages occur rapidly between 30 and 50 years of age. However, no research has identified anything that could stop these cross-links from occurring. Elastin dries up and cracks with age; hence, skin with less elastin (as with the older adult) tends to be drier and wrinkled. Over time, because of decreased extracellular fluid, numerous deposits of sodium, chloride, and calcium build up in the cardiovascular system. No clinical application studies were found to support this theory.

Nonstochastic Theories

The *nonstochastic theories of aging* are founded on a programmed perspective that is related to genetics or one's biological clock. Goldsmith (2004) suggests that aging is more likely to be an evolved beneficial characteristic and results from a complex structured process and not a series of random events. The following nonstochastic theories are discussed in this section: programmed theory, gene/biological clock theory, neuroendocrine theory, and immunologic/autoimmune theory.

Programmed Theory

As people age, more of their cells start to decide to commit suicide or stop dividing. The Hayflick phenomenon, or human fibroblast replicative senescence model, suggests that cells divide until they can no longer divide, whereupon the cell's infrastructure recognizes this inability to further divide and triggers the *apoptosis* sequence or death of the cell (Gonidakis & Longo, 2009; Sozou & Kirkwood, 2001). Therefore, it is thought that cells have a finite doubling potential and become unable to replicate after they have done so a number of times. Human cells age each time they replicate because of the shortening of the telomere. *Telomeres* are the most distal appendages of the chromosome arms. This theory of programmed cell death is often alluded to when the aging process is discussed. The enzyme *telomerase*, also called a "cellular fountain of youth," allows human cells grown in the laboratory to continue to replicate long past the time they normally stop dividing. Normal human cells do not have telomerase.

It is hypothesized that some cancer, reproductive, and virus cells are not restricted, having a seemingly infinite doubling potential, and are thus immortal cell lines. This is because they have telomerase, which adds back DNA to the ends of the chromosomes. One reason for the Hayflick phenomenon may be that chromosome telomeres become reduced in length with every cell division and eventually become too short to allow further division. When telomeres are too short, the gene notes this and causes the cell to die or apoptosize. Shay and Wright (2001) suggest that telomerase-induced manipulations of telomere length are important to study to define the underlying genetic diseases and those genetic pathways that lead to cancer.

Although it is unknown what initial event triggers apoptosis, it is generally acknowledged that apoptosis is the mechanism of cell death (Thompson, 1995). Henderson (2006) reviewed how fibroblast senescence is connected to wound healing and discussed the implications of this theory for chronic wound healing. Increased cell apoptosis rates do cause organ dysfunction, and this is hypothesized to be the underlying basis of the pathophysiology of multiple organ dysfunction syndrome (MODS) (Papathanassoglou, Moynihan, & Ackerman, 2000).

Gene/Biological Clock Theory

This theory explains that each cell, or perhaps the entire organism, has a genetically programmed aging code that is stored in the organism's DNA. Slagboom and associates describe this theory as comprising genetic influences that predict physical condition, occurrence of disease, cause and age of death, and other factors that contribute to longevity (Slagboom, Bastian, Beekman, Wendendorf, & Meulenbelt, 2000).

A significant amount of research has been done on circadian rhythms and their influence on sleep, melatonin, and aging (Ahrendt, 2000; Moore, 1997; Richardson & Tate, 2000). These rhythms are defined as patterns of wakefulness and sleep that are integrated into the 24-hour solar day (Porth, 2009). The everyday rhythm of this cycle of sleep–wake intervals is part of a time-keeping framework created by an internal clock. Research has demonstrated that people who do not have exposure to time cues such as sunlight and clocks will automatically have sleep and wake cycles that include approximately 23.5 to 26.5 hours (Moore, Czeisler, & Richardson, 1983). This clock seems to be controlled by an area in the hypothalamus called the suprachiasmatic nucleus (SCN), which is located near the third ventricle and the optic chiasm. The SCN, given its anatomic location, does receive light and dark input from the retina, and demonstrates high neuronal firing during the day and low firing at night. The SCN is connected to the pituitary gland, explaining the diurnal regulation of growth hormone and cortisol. Also because of the linkage with the hypothalamus, autonomic nervous system, and brain stem reticular formation, diurnal changes in metabolism, body temperature, and heart rate and blood pressure are explained (Porth, 2009). It is thought that biological rhythms lose some rhythmicity with aging.

Melatonin is secreted by the pineal gland and is considered to be the hormone linked to sleep and wake cycles because there are large numbers of melatonin receptors in the SCN. Researchers have studied the administration of melatonin to humans and found a shift in humans' circadian rhythm similar to that caused by light (Ahrendt, 2000). The sleep–wake cycle changes with aging, producing more fragmented sleep, which is thought to be due to decreased levels of melatonin.

This theory indicates that there may be genes that trigger youth and general well-being as well as other genes that accelerate cell deterioration. Why do some people have gray hair in their late 20s and others live to be 60 or beyond before graying occurs? It is known that melanin is damaged with ultraviolet light and is the ingredient that keeps human skin resilient and unwrinkled. People who have extensive sun exposure have wrinkles earlier in life due to damage to collagen and elastin. But why, if we know that people have a programmed gene or genes that trigger aging, wouldn't we prevent the gene(s) from causing the problems they are intending to promote?

For example, hypertension, arthritis, hearing loss, and heart disease are among the most common chronic illnesses in older adults (Cobbs, Duthie, & Murphy, 1999).

Each of these diseases has a genetic component to it. So if the healthcare profession can screen people when they are younger before they develop symptoms of target organ disease due to hypertension, loss of cartilage and hearing, and aspects of systolic and diastolic dysfunction, it is possible for people to live longer without experiencing the problems connected to these chronic illnesses.

The knowledge being acquired from the genome theory is greatly impacting the possibility of being able to ward off aging and disease. Studies of tumor suppressor gene replacement, prevention of angiogenesis with tumor growth, and regulation of programmed cell death are in process (Daniel & Smythe, 2003). Parr (1997) and Haq (2003) cited that caloric restriction extends mammalian life. By restricting calories there is a decreased need for insulin exposure, which consequently decreases growth factor exposure. Both insulin and growth factor are related to mammals' genetically determined clock, controlling their life span, so there is more evidence supportive of aging being influenced by key pathways such as the insulin-like growth factor path (Haq, 2003). More and more genetic findings are being related to aging and disease, such as the significance of the apolipoprotein E gene and correlations of more or less inflammation and DNA repair to aging (Stessman et al., 2005; Christenson, Johnson, & Vaupel, 2006).

Neuroendocrine Theory

This theory describes a change in hormone secretion, such as with the releasing hormones of the hypothalamus and the stimulating hormones of the pituitary gland, which manage the thyroid, parathyroid, and adrenal glands, and how it influences the aging process. The following major hormones are involved with aging:

> Estrogen decreases the thinning of bones, and when women age, less estrogen is produced by the ovaries. As women grow older and experience menopause, adipose tissue becomes the major source of estrogen.
> Growth hormone is part of the process that increases bone and muscle strength. Growth hormone stimulates the release of insulin-like growth factor produced by the liver.
> Melatonin is produced by the pineal gland and is thought to be responsible for coordinating seasonal adaptations in the body.

There is a higher chance of excess or loss of glucocorticoids, aldosterone, androgens, triiodothyronine, thyroxine, and parathyroid hormone when the hypothalamus-pituitary-endocrine gland feedback system is altered. When the stimulating and releasing hormones of the pituitary and the hypothalamus are out of synch with the endocrine glands, an increase in disease is expected in multiple organs and systems. Of significance are the findings of Rodenbeck and Hajak (2001), who cited that, with physiological aging and also with certain psychiatric disorders, there is increased activation of the hypothalamus-pituitary-adrenal axis, which causes increased plasma cortisol levels. The increased cortisol levels can be linked with several diseases.

Holzenberger, Kappeler, and De Magalhaes Filho (2004) stated that by inactivating insulin receptors in the adipose tissue of mice, the life span of the mice increases because less insulin exposure occurs. This further supports the idea that the neuroendocrine system is connected to life span regulation. Thyagarajan and Felten (2002) suggest that as one ages, there is a loss of neuroendocrine transmitter function that is related to the cessation of reproductive cycles as well as the development of mammary and pituitary tumors.

Immunologic/Autoimmune Theory

This theory was proposed 40 years ago and describes the normal aging process of humans and animals as being related to faulty immunological function (Effros, 2004). There is a decreased immune function in the elderly. The thymus gland shrinks in size and ability to function; thymus hormone levels are decreased at the age of 30 and are undetectable by the age of 60 (Williams, 1995). Involution of the thymus gland generally occurs at about 50 years. The elderly are more susceptible to infections as well as cancers. There is a loss of T-cell differentiation, so the body incorrectly perceives old, irregular cells as foreign bodies and attacks them.

There is also an increase in certain autoantibodies such as rheumatoid factor and a loss of interleukins. Some think that this change increases the chance of the older adult developing an autoimmune disease such as rheumatoid arthritis. Concurrently, resistance to tumor cells declines as one ages (Williams, 1995). Older adults are more prone to infection such as wound and respiratory infections, as well as to nosocomial infections if they are hospitalized.

Venjatraman and Fernandes (1997) cite that active and healthy older adults who participated in endurance exercises had a significantly increased natural killer cell function that, in turn, caused increased cytokine production and enhanced T-cell function, which improves general well-being. In contrast, those not exercising see a loss of immunological function as they age. The idea that increased exercise causes new growth of muscle fibers is not new, but that it also causes an increased immunological function, sense of well-being, and level of general health is significant. It is supportive of the fact that there is a combination of factors that influence the prevention or, in some cases, the promotion of aging. Also important to note is that there should be a balance of exercising and resting because overdoing exercise can lead to injuries, and this would support the wear and tear theory of aging.

Table 3-2 summarizes the major theories of aging originating from a biological perspective. It seems that no one theory fully describes the etiology of aging. Kirkwood (2000) cited the impact that single gene mutations and various environmental interventions such as diet and stress have on aging. Of all the theories discussed in this section, it appears that the gene theory and free radical theory seem to have the most support.

TABLE 3-2	Biological Theories of Aging
Theory	**Description**
Stochastic Theories	Based on random events that cause cellular damage that accumulates as the organism ages.
Free radical theory	Membranes, nucleic acids, and proteins are damaged by free radicals, which causes cellular injury and aging.
Orgel/error theory	Errors in DNA and RNA synthesis occur with aging.
Wear and tear theory	Cells wear out and cannot function with aging.
Connective tissue/ cross-link theory	With aging, proteins impede metabolic processes and cause trouble with getting nutrients to cells and removing cellular waste products.
Nonstochastic Theories	Based on genetically programmed events that cause cellular damage that accelerates aging of the organism.
Programmed theory	Cells divide until they are no longer able to, and this triggers apoptosis or cell death.
Gene/biological clock theory	Cells have a genetically programmed aging code.
Neuroendocrine theory	Problems with the hypothalamus-pituitary-endocrine gland feedback system cause disease; increased insulin growth factor accelerates aging.
Immunological theory	Aging is due to faulty immunological function, which is linked to general well-being.

Implications for Nursing

For many years, nursing has incorporated psychosocial theories such as Erikson's personality development theory into its practice (Erikson, 1963). Psychological theories enlighten us about the developmental tasks and challenges faced by older adults and the importance of finding and accepting meaning in one's life. From sociologists, nursing has learned how support systems, functionality, activity and role engagement, cohorts, and societal expectations can influence adjustment to aging and life satisfaction. These broadly generalized theories, however, lack the specificity and holistic perspective needed to guide nursing care of older adults who have varied needs and come from different settings and sociocultural backgrounds (see **Case Study 3-1**).

Case Study 3-1

Mr. Ronald Dea, 64 years old, had been planning for many years to retire from his position as an accountant at a software company at his 65th birthday. Then his wife of 40 years died of lymphoma last year. He now finds that he only gets out of his house to work. He has let his racquetball membership, swimming club, and night out with his neighborhood friends slide. He finds he does not go out socially at all anymore except for visiting his two children and their families, who live out of town, when invited. He is no longer active in the Lions Club nor does he regularly attend his church where he and his wife used to be very involved.

Now he is deliberating whether to retire or not because he is aware that his work has become the only thing in his life. He is finding he does not have the energy he used to and that he is not excited about the weekend time he used to enjoy so much. He also has found he does not enjoy food shopping, so Mr. Dea generally buys his main meal at work and then snacks on crackers and cheese at night. He generally eats a donut or a bagel for breakfast. On the weekends, Mr. Dea stays in bed until noon and does not eat anything until night when he goes to the nearby fast food drive-in window to pick up fried chicken or has a pizza delivered.

He has not changed anything in his bedroom since his wife died nor removed any of his wife's belongings from the home. Mr. Dea has been delaying his regularly scheduled visits to his hematologist for management of his hemochromatosis. He has been gaining weight, approximately 14 pounds, since his wife was first diagnosed with cancer about 2.5 years ago. He has also started smoking a cigar just about every evening. It was after his nightly smoke, when he was walking up the hill in his backyard one evening, that he fell and fractured his hip.

Mr. Dea has just been discharged home from the rehabilitation center, and you are the visiting nurse assigned to him. He has planned judiciously for his retirement but has been afraid to prepare the paperwork. Mr. Dea confides in you that he wants to remain independent as long as possible. He shares his concerns with you and inquires what your opinion is of how he should proceed. One of his daughters is at his home for the next 2 weeks to assist him and is pushing him to retire and move in with her and her family.

Drawing from aging theory, what are some of the challenges you believe Mr. Dea is dealing with? What would you, given the knowledge you have learned regarding aging theories, recommend to Mr. Dea regarding retirement? Would you recommend he sell his house and move out of the town he has lived in for so many years? What other living arrangements might be conducive for Mr. Dea? Who would you suggest he and his daughter talk with regarding his everyday needs if he chooses to stay in his house during his convalescence? What are his priority needs for promoting his health? How would these be best managed? Use aging theory to support your responses.

In a quest for a theoretical framework to guide caregiving in nursing homes, Wadensten (2002) and Wadensten and Carlsson (2003) studied 17 nursing theories that were generated from the 1960s to the 1990s and found that none of the theorists discussed what aging is, nor did the theorists offer advice on how to apply their theory to caring for the older adult. Wadensten wrote that existing "nursing theories do not provide guidance on how to care for older people or on how to support them in the developmental process of aging. There is a need to develop a nursing care model that, more than contemporary theories, takes human aging into consideration" (p. 119). Others concur that nursing needs to develop more situation-specific theories of aging to guide practice (Bergland & Kirkevold, 2001; Haight et al., 2002; Miller, 1990; Putnam, 2002). Two new theories, the functional consequences theory (Miller) and the theory of thriving (Haight et al.), are nurse-authored and attempt to address this need.

Nursing Theories of Aging

Functional Consequences Theory

Functional consequences theory (see **Table 3-3**) was developed to provide a guiding framework that would address older adults with physical impairment and disability (Miller, 1990). Miller's theory borrows from several nursing and nonnursing theories including functional health patterns; systems theory; King's (1981) conceptualization of person, health, environment, and the nurse–client transaction; Lawton's (1982) person-environment fit; and Rose and Killien's (1983) conceptual work defining risk and vulnerability. Miller asserts that aging adults experience environmental and biopsychosocial consequences that impact their functioning. The nurse's role is to assess for age-related changes and accompanying risk factors, and to design interventions directed toward risk reduction and minimizing age-associated disability. Nursing's goal is to maximize functioning and minimize dependency to improve the safety and quality of living (Miller, 1990).

Functional consequences theory assumes that quality of life is integrated with functional capacity and dependency needs, and that positive consequences are possible despite age-related limitations. In addition to those experiencing negative functional consequences, Miller (1990) applied her theory to highly functioning older adults as well as to adult caregivers. She distinguished the focus and goal of nursing interventions in varied settings (inpatient, outpatient, acute, or long-term care); thus, her theory can be used in many settings. Interventions are broadly interpreted as those of nurses, other healthcare providers, older adults, or

TABLE 3-3 Nursing Theories of Aging	
Theory	**Description**
Functional consequences theory	Environmental and biopsychosocial consequences impact functioning. Nursing's role is risk reduction to minimize age-associated disability in order to enhance safety and quality of living.
Theory of thriving	Failure to thrive results from a discord between the individual and his or her environment or relationships. Nurses identify and modify factors that contribute to disharmony among these elements.

BOX 3-3   Web Exploration

End-of-Life Nursing Education Consortium
(http://www.aacn.nche.edu/elnec)

The core curriculum in end-of-life consists of nine content modules with a syllabus, objectives, student note-taking outlines, detailed faculty content outlines, slide copies, reference lists, and supplemental teaching materials available in hard copy and CD-ROM.

The Geriatric Nursing Education Project
(www.aacn.nche.edu/Education/Hartford)

Offers faculty development institutes, online interactive case studies, a guide for integrating gerontology into nursing curricula, and a complimentary catalog of geriatric nursing photos that may be used free of charge for print or Web-based media by schools of nursing.

Consult GeriRN
(http://consultgerirn.org/)

An evidence-based online resource for nurses in clinical and educational settings. Includes many resources on a wide variety of topics related to aging including evidence-based geriatric protocols, hospital competencies for older adults, continuing education contact hours, the "Try This" series of assessment tools, information related to common geriatric problems, and links to additional age-related agencies and references.

The John A. Hartford Foundation Institute for Geriatric Nursing
(www.hartfordign.org)

A wealth of resources including core curriculum content for educators in academic and practice settings, consisting of detailed content outlines, case studies, activities, resources, PowerPoint slides, an online gerontological nursing certification review course, research support programs, best practice guidelines, consultation services, and geriatric nursing awards.

Mather LifeWays Institute on Aging
(http://www.matherlifeways.com/re_researchandeducation.asp)

Offers programs for faculty development (Web-based), long-term care staff, and family caregivers.

National Institute on Aging
(http://newcart.niapublications.org)

Free publications about older adults for health professionals and patients.

Toolkit for Nurturing Excellence at End-of-Life Transition
(www.tneel.uic.edu/tneel.asp)

A package for palliative care education on CD-ROM that includes audio, video, graphics, PowerPoint slides, photographs, and animations of individuals and families experiencing end-of-life transitions. An evidence-based self-study course on palliative care will soon be available for the national and international nursing community.

significant others, so this theory may be useful in other healthcare disciplines. This theory was used to create an assessment tool for the early detection of hospitalized elderly patients experiencing acute confusion and to prevent further complications (Kozak-Campbell & Hughes, 1996). Additional testing is needed to determine the utility of the functional consequences theory in other settings.

Theory of Thriving

The theory of thriving (Haight et al., 2002) is based on the concept of failure to thrive and Bergland and Kirkevold's (2001) application of thriving to the experience of well-being among frail elders living in nursing homes. They discuss the concept in three contexts: an outcome of growth and development, a psychological state, and an expression of physical health state. Failure to thrive first appeared in the aging literature as a diagnosis for older adults with vague symptoms such as fatigue, cachexia, and generalized weakness (Campia, Berkman, & Fulmer, 1986). Other disciplines later defined undernutrition, physical and cognitive dysfunction, and depression as its major attributes (Braun, Wykle, & Cowling, 1988). In their concept analysis of failure to thrive, Newbern and Krowchuk (1994) identified attributes under two categories: problems in social relatedness (disconnectedness and inability to find meaning in life, give of oneself, or attach to others) and physical/cognitive dysfunction (consistent unplanned weight loss, signs of depression, and cognitive decline).

Haight and colleagues (2002) view thriving in a holistic, life-span perspective that considers the impact of environment as people age. They assert that thriving is achieved when there is harmony among a person and his or her physical environment and personal relationships. Failure to thrive is because of discord among these three elements. Nurses caring for patients can use this theory to identify factors that may impede thriving and plan interventions to address these concerns.

Theory of Successful Aging

Twenty-first century literature has focused on what it means to age well. Flood (2006) proposed that aging well is defined by the extent to which older adults adapt to the cumulative physical and functional changes they experience. Moreover, the individual's perception about how well they have aged is fundamentally connected to believing that one's life has meaning and purpose. Thus, spirituality is a central ingredient of Flood's theory. A prerequisite to applying this theory is the capacity for reflection and responsiveness to changes internally and in the environment. Flood proposed the following assumptions:

1. Aging is a progressive process of simple to increasingly complex adaptation.
2. Aging may be successful or unsuccessful, depending upon where a person is along the continuum of progression from simple to more complex and their extensive use of coping processes.
3. Successful aging is influenced by the aging person's choices.
4. Aging people experience changes, which uniquely characterize their beliefs and perspectives as different from those younger adults (Flood, 2006).

Outcomes of aging successfully, according to this theory, include remaining physically, psychologically, and socially engaged in meaningful ways that are individually defined. Achieving a comfortable acceptance of the finality of life is also considered a hallmark of successful aging. The inclusion of more interdisciplinary exercises with

Notable Quotes

Some people, older people especially, tend to draw into themselves...they grow isolated. That's a big mistake! You never know when you might need other people, but you need to earn their help. You have to contribute to your community."

—Bessie Delany in *Having Our Say: The Delany Sisters' First 100 Years*, 1994, p. 89.

Notable Quotes

I'd say one of the most important qualities to have is the ability to create jobs in you life...we all have to do it for ourselves.

—Bessie Delany in *Having Our Say: The Delany Sisters' First 100 Years*, 1994, pp. 32–33.

nursing, medical, and other healthcare students, such as "Healthy Aging Rounds" (Mohler, D'Huyvetter, Tomasa, O'Neill, & Fain, 2010), has demonstrated that education can improve healthcare providers' attitudes and understanding of healthy aging.

Summary

Nursing theories of thriving and functionality contribute to our understanding of aging; however, neither encompasses all of the holistic elements (cultural, spiritual, geographic, psychosocioeconomic, educational, environmental, and physical) of concern to nursing. Flood's theory of successful aging provides a more comprehensive theoretical framework to guide nursing practice, but it has yet to be tested in practice. Given the diversity of older adults living in independent, assisted, and residential care settings there remains much that can be useful from the theories of other disciplines. From the stochastic and programmed biological theories of aging, nurses can better manage nutrition, incontinence, sleep rhythms, immunological response, catecholamine surges, hormonal and electrolyte balance, and drug efficacy for older adults with chronic illnesses. Using psychosocial aging theories, nurses can assist both the older adult and his or her family in recognizing that the life they have lived has been one of integrity and meaning and facilitate peaceful death with dignity. Ego integrity contributes to older adults' well-being and reduces the negative psychological consequences that are often linked to chronic illness and older age. Finally, being cognizant of older adults' socioeconomic resources will assist the nurse and older adult in planning cost-effective best practices to improve symptom management and treatment outcomes.

Using knowledge gained from aging theories, nurses can:

> Help people to use their genetic makeup to prevent comorbidities
> Facilitate best practices for managing chronic illnesses
> Maximize individuals' strengths relative to maintaining independence
> Facilitate creative ways to overcome individuals' challenges
> Assist in cultivating and maintaining older adults' cognitive status and mental health

In conclusion, aging continues to be explained from multiple theoretical perspectives. Collectively, these theories reveal that aging is a complex phenomenon still much in need of research. How one ages is a result of biopsychosocial factors. Nurses can use this knowledge as they plan and implement ways to promote health care to all age groups. As in other disciplines, the state of the science on aging is rapidly improving within the nursing profession. Nursing is developing a rich body of knowledge regarding the care of older adults. Programs and materials developed by the Hartford Institute for Geriatric Nursing, the End of Life Nursing Education Consortium, the American Association of Colleges of Nursing, and the Mather Institute provide a strong foundation for developing and disseminating our current knowledge. Nursing research must continue to span all facets of gerontology so that new information will be generated for improved patient outcomes.

BOX 3-4 Recommended Reading

Azinet. (2003). Resources on aging information: How do we age?. Retrieved from http://www.azinet.com/aging/

Bragg, E. J., Warshaw, G. A., van der Willik, O., Meganathan, K., Weber, D. Cornwall, D. & Leonard, A. C. (2011). Paul B. Beeson career development awards in aging research and United States medical schools aging and geriatric medical programs. *Journal of American Geriatric Society, 59*(9), 1730–1738.

Critical Thinking Exercises

1. **Mrs. Smith, 72 years old and recently diagnosed with a myocardial infarction**, asks why she should take a cholesterol-lowering drug for her hyperlipidemia at her age. Why should she engage in the lifestyle changes her nurse is recommending?

2. **Your 82-year-old patient, Rodney Whitishing, has been healthy most of his life** and now is experiencing, for the second winter in a row, an extremely severe case of influenza. He has never received a flu shot as a preventive measure because he felt he was very strong and healthy. Explain how you would describe the older adult's immune system and why older adults seem to be more vulnerable to influenza.

3. **John, an 85-year-old man with emphysema**, is brought to your clinic by his family because of increasing complaints about shortness of breath. John uses oxygen at home, but states that he is afraid to walk more than a few steps or show any emotion because he will become unable to get enough air. John tells you that he feels his life is not worth living. Using the theories of aging, how might you respond to this situation?

Personal Reflections

1. Develop a philosophy of how theories of aging can support or refute the idea of categorizing people in the young-old, middle-old, and old-old classifications according to chronological age. What other characteristics could be used to categorize people as they age? Give an example of how you would perceive a relative or friend of yours who is in the sixth or seventh decade of life.

2. Comparable to infant–child development stages, generate five or six stages of development for older adults to accomplish as they complete their work stage and begin their retirement era.

3. Using theories of aging with biological, psychological, and sociological perspectives, hypothesize how these frameworks influence the older adult's development.

References

Achenbaum, W. A., & Bengtson, B. L. (1994). Re-engaging the disengagement theory of aging: On the history and assessment of theory development in gerontology. *Gerontologist, 34*, 756–763.

Adams, K. B. (2004). Changing investment in activities and interests in elders' lives: Theory and measurement. *International Journal of Aging & Human Development, 58*(2), 87–108.

Agahi, N., Ahacic, K., & Parker, M. G. (2006). Continuity of leisure participation from middle age to old age. *The Journals of Gerontology, 61B*(6), S340–S346.

Ahrendt, J. (2000). Melatonin, circadian rhythms, and sleep. *New England Journal of Medicine, 343*, 1114–1115.

Aigner, T., Rose, J., Martin, J., & Buckwalter, J. (2004). Aging theories of primary osteoarthritis: From epidemiology to molecular biology. *Rejuvenation Research, 7*(2), 134–145.

Alkema, G. E., & Alley, D. E. (2006). Gerontology's future: An integrative model for disciplinary advancement. *The Gerontologist, 46*, 574–582.

Ames, B. (2004). Mitochondrial decay, a major cause of aging, can be delayed. *Journal of Alzheimer's Disease, 6*(2), 117–121.

Back, K. (1980). *Life course: Integrated theories and exemplary populations.* Boulder, CO: Westview Press.

Baltes, P. B. (1987). Theoretical propositions of life-span developmental psychology: On the dynamics between growth and decline. *Developmental Psychology, 23*, 611–626.

Baltes, P. B., & Baltes, M. M. (1990). Psychological perspectives on successful aging: The model of selective optimization with compensation. In P. B. Baltes & M. M. Baltes (Eds.), *Successful aging: Perspectives from the behavioral sciences* (pp. 1–34). New York, NY: Cambridge University Press.

Bergland, A., & Kirkevold, M. (2001). Thriving: A useful theoretical perspective to capture the experience of well-being among frail elderly in nursing homes? *Journal of Advanced Nursing, 36*, 426.

Birren, J. E., & Schroots, J. J. F. (2001). History of gero-psychology. In J. E. Birren (Ed.), *Handbook of the psychology of aging* (5th ed., pp. 3–28). San Diego, CA: Academic Press.

Bokov, A., Chaudhuri, A., & Richardson, A. (2004). The role of oxidative damage and stress in aging. *Mechanisms of Ageing Development, 125*(10–11), 811–826.

Braun, J. V., Wykle, M. N., & Cowling, W. R. (1988). Failure to thrive in older persons: A concept derived. *Gerontologist, 28*, 809–812.

Brunk, U., & Terman, A. (2002). The mitochondrial-lysosomal axis theory of aging—Accumulation of damaged mitochondria as a result of imperfect autophagocytosis. *European Journal of Biochemistry, 269*(8), 1996–2002.

Bühler, C. (1933). *Der menschliche Lebenslauf als psychologisches Problem [Human life as a psychological problem].* Oxford, England: Hirzel.

Butler, R. N., & Lewis, M. I. (1982). *Aging & mental health* (3rd ed.). St. Louis, MO: Mosby.

Campia, E., Berkman, B., & Fulmer, T. (1986). Failure to thrive for older adults. *Gerontologist, 26*(2), 192–197.

Carlson, E., & Chamberlain, R. (2005). Allostatic load and health disparities: A theoretical orientation. *Research in Nursing & Health, 28*(4), 306–315.

Caspi, A. (1987). Personality in the life course. *Journal of Personality and Social Psychology, 53*, 1203–1213.

Caspi, A., & Elder, G. H. (1986). Life satisfaction in old age: Linking social psychology and history. *Psychology and Aging, 1*, 18–26.

Christensen, K., Johnson, R. E. & Vaupel, J.W. (2006). The quest for genetic determinants of human longevity: Challenges and insights. *National Review of Genetics. 7*, 436–448.

Cobbs, E., Duthie, E., & Murphy, J. (Eds.). (1999). *Geriatric review syllabus: A core curriculum in geriatric medicine* (4th ed.). Dubuque, IA: Kendall/Hunt for the American Geriatric Society.

Cumming, E., & Henry, W. (1961). *Growing old.* New York, NY: Basic Books.

Cunningham, W., & Brookbank, J. (1988). *Gerontology: The physiology, biology and sociology of aging.* New York, NY: Harper & Row.

Daniel, J., & Smythe, W. (2003). Gene therapy of cancer. *Seminars of Surgical Oncology, 21*(3), 196–204.

Dufour, E., & Larsson, N. (2004). Understanding aging: Revealing order out of chaos. *Biochimica et Biophysica Acta-Bioenergetics, 1658*(1–2), 122–132.

Ebersole, P., Hess, P., & Luggen, A. S. (2004). *Toward healthy aging: Human needs and nursing response* (3rd ed.). St. Louis, MO: Mosby.

Effros, R. (2004). From Hayflick to Walford: The role of T cell replicative senescence in human aging. *Experimental Gerontology, 39*(6), 885–890.

Efklides, A., Kalaitzidou, M., & Chankin, G. (2003). Subjective quality of life in old age in Greece: The effect of demographic factors, emotional state, and adaptation to aging. *European Psychologist, 8,* 178–191.

Erikson, E. (1963). *Childhood and society.* New York, NY: W. W. Norton.

Erikson, E. H., Erikson, J. M., & Kivnick, H. Q. (1986). *Vital involvement in old age: The experience of old age in our time.* New York, NY: W. W. Norton.

Flood, M. (2006). A mid-range theory of successful aging. *Journal of Theory Construction and Testing, 9*(2), 35–39.

Gans, D., Putney, N. M., Bengtson, V.L., & Silverstein, M. (2009). The future of theories of aging. In V. Bengtson, M. Silverstein, N. Putney, & D. Gans (Eds.), *Handbook of theories of aging.* (pp. 723–738). New York, NY: Springer,

Goldsmith, T. (2004). Aging as an evolved characteristic—Weismann's theory reconsidered. *Medical Hypotheses, 62*(2), 304–308.

Goldsmith, T. C. (2011). *Theories of aging and implications for public health.* Crownsville, MD: Azinet.

Gonidakis, S., & Longo, V. D. (2009). Programmed longevity and programmed aging theories. In V. Bengtson, M. Silverstein, N. Putney, & D. Gans (Eds.), *Handbook of theories of aging.* (pp. 215–228). New York, NY: Springer.

Gray, D., & Woulfe, J. (2005). Lipofuscin and aging: A matter of toxic waste. *Science of Aging Knowledge Environment, 5,* 1.

Grune, T., & Davies, K. (2001). Oxidative processes in aging. In E. Masoro & S. Austad (Eds.), *Handbook of the biology of aging* (5th ed., pp. 25–58). San Diego, CA: Academic Press.

Hagestad, G. O., & Dannefer, D. (2002). Concepts and theories of aging: Beyond microfication in social sciences approaches. In R. H. Binstock & L. K. George (Eds.), *Handbook of aging and the social sciences* (5th ed., pp. 3–21). San Diego: Academic Press.

Haight, B. K., Barba, B. E., Tesh, A. S., & Courts, N. F. (2002). Thriving: A life span theory. *Journal of Gerontological Nursing, 28*(3), 14–22.

Haq, R. (2003). Age-old theories die hard. *Clinical Investigative Medicine, 26*(3), 116–120.

Harlow, R. E., & Cantor, N. (1996). Still participating after all these years: A study of life task participation in later life. *Journal of Personality and Social Psychology, 71,* 1235–1249.

Harman, D. (1994). Aging: Prospects for further increases in the functional life-span. *Age, 17*(4), 119–146.

Harman, D. (2006). Understanding and modulating aging: An update. *Annals of the New York Academy of Sciences, 1067,* 10–21.

Havighurst, R. (1972). *Developmental tasks and education.* New York, NY: David McKay.

Havighurst, R. J., & Albrecht, R. (1953). *Older people.* Oxford, England: Longmans, Green.

Havighurst, R. J., Neugarten, B. L., & Tobin, S. S. (1963). Disengagement, personality and life satisfaction in the later years. In P. Hansen (Ed.), *Age with a future* (pp. 419–425). Copenhagen, Denmark: Munksgoasrd.

Havighurst, R. J., Neugarten, B. L., & Tobin, S. S. (1968). Disengagement and patterns of aging. In B. L. Neugarten (Ed.), *Middle age and aging* (pp. 67–71). Chicago, IL: University of Chicago Press.

Hayflick, L. (1985). Theories of biologic aging. *Experimental Gerontology, 10,* 145–159.

Hayflick, L. (1996). *How and why we age.* New York, NY: Ballantine Books.

Henderson, E. (2006). The potential effect of fibroblast senescence on wound healing and the chronic wound environment. *Journal of Wound Care, 15*(7), 315–318.

Holm, A. K., Lepp, M., & Ringsberg, K. C. (2005). Dementia: Involving patients in storytelling—a caring intervention. A pilot study. *Journal of Clinical Nursing, 14*(2), 256–263.

Holzenberger, M., Kappeler, L., & De Magalhaes Filho, C. (2004). IGF-1 signaling and aging. *Experimental Gerontology, 39*(11–12), 1761–1764.

Hyun-Mee, J., & Miller, N. J. (2007). Examining the effects of fashion activities on life satisfaction of older females: Activity theory revisited. *Family & Consumer Sciences Research Journal, 35*(4), 338–356.

Iwarsson, S. (2005). A long-term perspective on person-environment fit and ADL dependence among older Swedish adults. *Gerontologist, 45*(3), 327–336.

Jones, G. M., & Miesen, B. L. (Eds.). (1992). *Care-giving in dementia: Research and applications.* New York, NY: Tavistock/Routledge.

Jung, C. G. (1960). The *structure and dynamics of the psyche. Collected works (Vol. VIII).* Oxford, England: Pantheon.

King, I. M. (1981). *A theory for nursing.* New York, NY: John Wiley & Sons.

Kirkwood, T. (2000). Molecular gerontology: Bridging the simple and complex. *Annals of the New York Academy of Sciences, 908,* 14–20.

Kozak-Campbell, C., & Hughes, A. M. (1996). The use of functional consequences theory in acutely confused hospitalized elderly. *Journal of Gerontological Nursing, 22*(1), 27–36.

Lakatta, E. (2000). Cardiovascular aging in health. *Clinical Geriatric Medicine, 16,* 419–444.

Lawton, M. P. (1982). Competence, environmental press, and the adaptation of older people. In M. P. Lawton, P. G. Windley, & T. O. Byerts (Eds.), *Aging and the environment: Theoretical approaches* (pp. 33–59). New York, NY: Springer.

Lee, J., Koo, N., & Min, D. (2004). Reactive oxygen species, aging, and antioxidative nutraceuticals. *Comprehensive Reviews in Food Science and Food Safety, 3*(1), 21–33.

Lemon, B. W., Bengston, V. L., & Peterson, J. A. (1972). An exploration of the activity theory of aging: Activity types and life satisfaction among in-movers to a retirement community. *Journal of Gerontology, 27,* 511–523.

Longino, C. F., & Kart, C. S. (1982). Explicating activity theory: A formal replication. *Journal of Gerontology, 35,* 713–722.

Maddox, G. L. (1963). Activity and morale: A longitudinal study of selected elderly subjects. *Social Forces, 42,* 195–204.

Marshall, V. W. (1996). The stage of theory in aging and the social sciences. In R. H. Binstock & L. K. George (Eds.), *Handbook of aging and the social sciences* (4th ed., pp. 12–26). San Diego, CA: Academic Press.

Maslow, A. H. (1954). *Motivation and personality.* New York, NY: Harper & Row.

McMullin, J. A. (2000). Diversity and the state of sociological aging theory. *Gerontologist, 40,* 517–530.

Miller, C. A. (1990). *Nursing care of older adults: Theory and practice.* Glenview, IL: Scott, Foresman/Little, Brown Higher Education.

Miquel, J. (1998). An update on the oxygen stress-mitochondrial mutation theory of aging: Genetic and evolutionary implications. *Experimental Gerontology, 33*(1–2), 113–126.

Mohler, M. J., D'Huyvetter, K., Tomasa, L., O'Neil, L., & Fain, M. (2010). Healthy aging rounds: Using healthy-aging mentors to teach medical students about physical activity and social support assessment, interviewing, and prescription. *Journal of American Geriatric Society, 58,* 2407–2411.

Moore, M., Czeisler, C., & Richardson, G. (1983). Circadian time-keeping in health and disease. *New England Journal of Medicine, 309,* 469–473.

Moore, R. (1997). Circadian rhythms: Basic neurobiology and clinical application. *Annual Review of Medicine, 48,* 253–266.

Neugarten, B. L. (1968). Adult personality: Toward a psychology of the life cycle. In B. L. Neugarten (Ed.), *Middle age and aging: A reader in social psychology* (pp. 137–147). Chicago, IL: University of Chicago Press.

Neumann, C. V. (2000). *Sources of meaning and energy in the chronically ill frail elder.* Unpublished paper prepared for the Ronald E. Mcnair Research Program, University of Wisconsin-Milwaukee.

Newbern, V. B., & Krowchuk, H. V. (1994). Failure to thrive in elderly people: A conceptual analysis. *Journal of Advanced Nursing, 19,* 840–849.

Newsom, J. T., & Schulz, R. (1996). Social support as a mediator in the relation between functional status and quality of life in older adults. *Psychology, 3*, 34–44.

O'Connor, B. P., & Vallerand, R. J. (1994). Motivation, self-determination, and person-environment fit as predictors of psychological adjustment among nursing home residents. *Psychology and Aging, 9*(2), 189–194.

Orgel, L. (1970). The maintenance of the accuracy of protein synthesis and its relevance to aging: A correction. *Proceedings of the National Academy of Sciences, 67*, 1476.

Papathanassoglou, E., Moynihan, J., & Ackerman, M. (2000). Does programmed cell death (apoptosis) play a role in the development of multiple organ dysfunction in critically ill patients? A review and a theoretical framework. *Critical Care Medicine, 28*(2), 537–549.

Parr, T. (1997). Insulin exposure and aging theory. *Gerontology, 43*(3), 182–200.

Peck, R. C. (1968). Psychological development in the second half of life. In B. L. Neugarten (Ed.), *Middle age and aging: A reader in social psychology* (pp. 88–92). Chicago, IL: University of Chicago Press.

Poon, H., Calabrese, V., Scapagnini, G., & Butterfield, D. (2004). Free radicals in brain aging. *Clinics in Geriatric Medicine, 20*(2), 329–359.

Porth, C. (2009). Pathophysiology: *Concepts of altered health states* (8th ed.). Philadelphia, PA: Lippincott Williams & Wilkins.

Putnam, M. (2002). Linking aging theory and disability models: Increasing the potential to explore aging with physical impairment. *Gerontologist, 42*, 799–806.

Quick, H. E., & Moen, P. (1998). Gender, employment, and retirement quality: A life course approach to the differential experiences of men and women. *Journal of Occupational Health Psychology, 3*, 44–64.

Rapkin, B. D., & Fischer, K. (1992). Personal goals of older adults: Issues in assessment and prediction. *Psychology and Aging, 7*, 127–137.

Reddy, P. H. (2006). Mitochondrial oxidative damage in aging and Alzheimer's disease: Implications for mitochondrially targeted antioxidant therapeutics. *Journal of Biomedicine and Biotechnology. 2006*, 1–13. doi: 10.1155/JBB/2006/31372.

Richardson, G., & Tate, B. (2000). Hormonal and pharmacological manipulation of the circadian clock: Recent developments and future strategies. *Sleep, 23*(Suppl. 3), S77–S88.

Riley, M. W. (1994). Age integration and the lives of older people. *Gerontologist, 34*, 110–115.

Riley, M. W., Johnson, M., & Foner, A. (1972). *Aging and society: A sociology of age stratification (Vol. 3)*. New York, NY: Russell Sage Foundation.

Robitaille, A., Orpana, H., & McIntosh, C. N. (2012). Reciprocal relationship between social support and psychological distress among a national sample of older adults: An autoregressive cross-lagged model. *Canadian Journal on Aging—La Revue Canadienne Du Vieillissement, 31*(1), 13.

Rodenbeck, A., & Hajak, G. (2001). Neuroendocrine dysregulation in primary insomnia. *Reviews of Neurology, 157*(11 Pt 2), S57–S61.

Rose, A. M. (1965). The subculture of the aging: A framework for research in social gerontology. In A. M. Rose & W. Peterson (Eds.), *Older people and their social worlds* (pp. 3–16). Philadelphia, PA: F. A. Davis.

Rose, M. H., & Killien, M. (1983). Risk and vulnerability: A case for differentiation. *Advances in Nursing Science, 5*, 60–73.

Schroots, J. J. F. (1996). Theoretical developments in the psychology of aging. *Gerontologist, 36*, 742–748.

Schroots, J. J. F. (2003). Life-course dynamics: A research program in progress from the Netherlands. *European Psychologist, 8*, 192–199.

Shay, J., & Wright, W. (2001). Telomeres and telomerase: Implications for cancer and aging. *Radiation Research, 155*(1), 188–193.

Slagboom, P., Bastian, T., Beekman, M., Wendendorf, R., & Meulenbelt, I. (2000). Genetics of human aging. *Annals of the New York Academy of Science, 908*, 50–61.

Sozou, P., & Kirkwood, T. (2001). A stochastic model of cell replicative senescence based on telomere shortening, oxidative stress, and somatic mutations in nuclear and mitochondrial DNA. *Journal of Theoretical Biology, 213*(4), 573–586.

Stessman, J., Maaravi, Y., Hammerman-Rozenberg, R., Cohen, A., Nemanov, L., Gritsenko, I., … Ebstein, R. P. (2005). Candidate genes associated with ageing and life expectancy in the Jerusalem longitudinal study. *Mechanisms of Ageing Development. 126*, 333–339.

Thompson, C. (1995). Apoptosis in the pathogenesis and treatment of disease. *Science, 267*, 1456–1462.

Thyagarajan, S., & Felten, D. (2002). Modulation of neuroendocrine-immune signaling by L-deprenyl and L-desmethyldeprenyl in aging and mammary cancer. *Mechanisms of Ageing Development, 123*(8), 1065–1079.

Tornstam, L. (1994). Gerotranscendence: A theoretical and empirical exploration. In L. E. Thomas & S. A. Eisenhandler (Eds.), *Aging and the religious dimension* (pp. 203–226). Westport, CT: Greenwood.

Troen, B. (2003). The biology of aging. *Mount Sinai Journal of Medicine, 70*(1), 3–22.

Troll, L. E., & Skaff, M. M. (1997). Perceived continuity of self in very old age. *Psychology and Aging, 12*, 162–169.

Uhlenberg, P. (1992). Population aging and social policy. *Annual Review of Sociology, 18*, 449–474.

Uhlenberg, P. (1996). The burden of aging: A theoretical framework for understanding the shifting balance of care giving and care receiving as cohorts age. *Gerontologist, 36*, 761–767.

Uhlenberg, P. (2000). Why study age integration? *Gerontologist, 40*, 261–266.

Van Cauter, E., Leproult, R., & Kupfer, D. (1996). Effects of gender and age on the levels and circadian rhythmicity of plasma cortisol. *Journal of Clinical Endocrinology Metabolism, 81*(7), 2468–2473.

Venjatraman, F., & Fernandes, G. (1997). Exercise, immunity and aging. *Aging, 9*(1–2), 42–56.

Wadensten, B. (2002). *Gerotranscendence from a nursing perspective: From theory to implementation.* Uppsala University. Retrieved from http://www.samfak.uu.se/Disputationer/Wadensten.htm

Wadensten, B., & Carlsson, M. (2003). Nursing theory views on how to support the process of ageing. *Journal of Advanced Nursing, 42*(2), 118–124.

Wahl, H. W. (2001). Environmental influences on aging and behavior. In J. E. Birren & K. W. Schaie (Eds.), *Handbook of the psychology of aging* (5th ed., pp. 215–237). San Diego, CA: Academic Press.

Williams, M. (1995). *The American Geriatric Society's complete guide to aging and health.* New York, NY: Harmony Books.

Yin, P., & Lai, K. H. (1983). A reconceptualization of age stratification in China. *Journal of Gerontology, 38*, 608–613.

For a full suite of assignments and additional learning activities, see the access code at the front of your book.

Unit II
Communication and Assessment

(COMPETENCIES 2–6, 13, 15)

LEARNING OBJECTIVES

At the end of this chapter, the reader will be able to:

> State the importance of communication with older adults.
> Identify effective and ineffective communication strategies.
> Understand how normal and pathological changes of aging effect communication.
> Describe communication strategies for older adults with common normal and pathological changes of aging.
> Describe person-centered communication.

KEY TERMS

Active memory
Alzheimer's disease
Anomia
Aphasia
Apraxia
Background noise
Broca's aphasia
Cataract
Chronic obstructive pulmonary disorder (COPD)
Cognition
Communication Enhancement Model
Communication in end-of-life care
Communication Predicament of Aging Model
Compensatory strategies
Conductive hearing loss
Declarative memory
Dementia

Depression
Diabetic retinopathy
Dry eyes
Dual sensory impairment
Dysarthria
Elderspeak
Environmental factors
Episodic memory
Frequency
Glaucoma
Global aphasia
Hearing Aid
Isolation
Lack of opportunities
Language
Lexical memory
Long-term memory
Macular degeneration
Mixed hearing loss
Nondeclarative memory
Nonverbal communication

Parkinson's disease
Patient-centered communication
Person-first language
Personal amplification device
Presbycusis
Presbyopia
Restorative strategies
Semantic memory
Sensorineural hearing loss
Short-term memory
Situational factors
Social networks
Speech
Successful aging
Task talk
Teach-back method
Tinnitus
Verbal communication
Wernicke's aphasia
Working memory

Chapter 4

(Competencies 2, 5, 15)

Therapeutic Communication with Older Adults, Families and Caregivers

Kristine Williams
Kerry Mees

Communication Basics

Communication links human beings to others and the environment, and it is an important part of life for people of all ages, including older adults. The ability to relate to others is a unique human characteristic with importance that continues into old age. Humans use communication to provide and receive information from others. Successful communication involves conveying a message between a sender and a receiver. Effective communication is a dynamic process that includes ongoing exchange of information with feedback between the sender and receiver. Communication relies heavily upon intact senses, such as hearing and vision, and physical and cognitive processes, all of which are required to send and receive messages. In addition, the environment must be conducive to permitting message transmission between the sender and receiver. Communication is complex, encompassing both verbal and nonverbal aspects and is a learned skill that relies on physical and cognitive abilities and multiple senses. *Verbal communication* relies on knowledge of a common language as well as the ability to produce words, while *nonverbal communication* includes tone of voice and physical behaviors such as body language and eye contact. Communication failures occur when barriers to communication exist in any component of this interactive system.

Communication is an integral part of quality health care, as identified in the 2001 Institute of Medicine report *Crossing the Quality Chasm*, which identified patient-centeredness and *patient-centered communication* as key characteristics of quality health care. Dimensions of patient centeredness include respect for patient values, preferences, and expressed needs, along with a focus on information, communication, and education of patients in clear terms. Consistent and effective communication between patient and clinician has been associated with improved patient satisfaction and safety, better health outcomes, and lower healthcare costs. In contrast, communication break-down has been implicated in healthcare disparities and medical errors. Professional standards include respectful and effective communication as key factors in informed consent and a trusting relationship (Paget et al., 2011).

Communication is essential for the giving and receiving of information and the exchange of ideas, thoughts, and feelings. We communicate to exchange information and to meet our physical, social, and emotional needs, as well as to meet the needs of others. The Joint Commission on American Hospitals has recognized and mandated attention to effective communication in healthcare settings to prevent errors and safety issues (The Joint Commission, 2010). Social interaction has been found to have protective health effects (Kiely, Simon, Jones, & Morris, 2000), can save time and be therapeutic for patients, and can encourage self-care and autonomy. Research indicates that older adults cite their ability to relate to nurses as a primary predictor of satisfaction with care and nurses who establish close nurse–patient relationships report higher levels of job satisfaction (Grau, Chandler, & Saunders, 1995; Parsons, Simmons, Penn, & Furlough, 2002).

Communication and Older Adults

Successful aging is a concept to which both young and old aspire. Successful aging includes not only maintaining physical, cognitive, and functional abilities, but also maintaining engagement with others, through communication (Rowe & Kahn, 1997). Thus, assisting older adults to maintain their connection to others through communication is an important focus for nursing, in addition to the fact that communication is a critical part of the nursing process (Benner, 2004).

A number of physical and psychological changes occur with aging that influence both communication abilities and opportunities. In this chapter, effective communication and common normal and pathological changes of aging that challenge communication for older adults will be discussed. Environmental influences on communication for older adults and strategies to improve nursing communication with older adults, their families, and caregivers will be explored.

Effective communication depends on a number of factors, including a shared language and frame of reference, a conductive environment, mental abilities (perception, attention, intellectual understanding, and memory), respect and trust, and expectation of a response. Verbal strategies that support communication include addressing the older adult by name, listening and responding on topic, reflecting on feelings, and validating and asking for more information. Nonverbal communication can provide a stronger message than actual spoken words, so attention should be given to one's posture, eye contact, and tone of voice.

Environmental and situational factors influence nursing communication with older adults. These include the institutional context of communication, the focus on care tasks, lessened opportunities for communication, and intergenerational communication issues. Additional situations that affect communication include the normal and pathological conditions of aging.

Healthcare settings were historically institutions where patients received health care under the control of healthcare providers. Accordingly, staff in care facilities may control communication and focus on care tasks instead of to using a person-centered approach to care.

Task talk also predominates in nurse–patient conversations in healthcare settings where heavy workloads and staffing shortages contribute to the communication with patients being almost exclusively about care tasks. Communicating and involving older adults in their nursing care is beneficial. However, older adults also value talk on an interpersonal level; this person-centered communication is described in more detail below. Person-centered talk acknowledges the older adult as a unique person and indicates a willingness to interact with that individual.

Person-Centered Communication

Person-centered communication is an integral part of person-centered care and reflects a focus on the patient and their unique perceptions and experiences with health and illness. Nursing interventions include providing information to promote health and healing and to engage patients in self-care. Thus, person-centered care confirms the uniqueness of the patient and allows the patient to participate in his or her own care.

Communication Obstacles Faced by Older Adults

Lack of Opportunities

Older adults experience an increased *lack of opportunities* for communication. As age advances, *social networks* decline as children leave home and spouses and significant others die. Many older adults live alone and may be isolated, leading to fewer opportunities to communicate with peers and loved ones. For older adults who are hospitalized or who live in supportive care settings such as nursing homes, opportunities to talk with significant others decline further and most opportunities to communicate rely on nursing staff as communication partners. Many of the healthcare workers who provide direct care to older adults are paraprofessionals who may have limited training in communication skills and lack specialized skills for communication with older adults who suffer from aphasia or the communication challenges that accompany dementia (see **Table 4-1**).

Direct care staff frequently work in teams, another factor with potential implications for communication with older adults. Staff members working in teams tend to talk to other staff, frequently leaving the patient out of the conversation. This type of ignoring talk also occurs during office visits and clinic appointments. For example, it is common for a son or daughter to take their parent to a healthcare appointment.

TABLE 4-1   Strategies for Communication with Persons with Dementia that Support Personhood

Strategy	Definition	Example
Recognition	Acknowledge the person, know their name, affirm uniqueness.	"Come along Mrs. Jones, your dinner is being served."
Negotiation	Consult the person about preferences, desires, needs.	"That was a nice bit of fresh air. I'm ready for my dinner now; would you like to join me?"
Validation	Acknowledge the person's emotions/feelings and respond.	"Mrs. Johnson, it sounds like you would like to wait for your bath."
Facilitation/ Collaboration	Work together, involve the person. Enable the person to do what otherwise he/ she wouldn't be able to do by providing the missing parts of the action.	"What is it you are looking for Mrs. Smith? Can I help? Tell me what it is and we can look for it together."

Source: Adapted from Ryan, E.B., Byrne, K., Spykerman, H., & Orange, J.B. Evidencing Kitwood's Personhood Strategies: Conversation as Care in Dementia (2005) in *Alzheimer's Test, Talk, and Context: Enhancing Communication.* Edited by Boyd Davis, Palgrave, McMillan, New York.

Typically, the younger adult and the healthcare provider will talk above or around the older adult, often excluding them from the conversation about their health and treatment plan.

Intergenerational Communication

Nurses are typically younger than older adult patients, creating an intergenerational relationship when it comes to communication. Society has adopted negative stereotypes of aging with beliefs that older adults are less competent at communication as well as in other functional areas. Because of this, younger persons often modify their speech when they talk to older adults. Modifications include simplification—measurable reductions in complexity of grammar and vocabulary—and clarification strategies, which include adding repetitions and stressing and altering the pitch of one's speech, resulting in speech that is overly caring and controlling and less respectful than normal adult-to-adult speech. This type of speech has been called *elderspeak* and is widespread in community and elder-care settings. Elderspeak is similar to babytalk—in fact, the early social scientists who described elderspeak played audio recordings from a children's day care center and from a nursing home, and research study volunteers were unable to tell these apart (Caporael, 1981). Common features of elderspeak include terms of endearment (such as "honey," "dearie," and "sweetie") and tag questions that prompt the older adult to respond as the younger person wishes (for example, "You're ready for lunch now, aren't you?") (see **Figure 4-1**).

The *Communication Predicament of Aging Model* describes how these speech modifications occur and lead to negative outcomes for older adults (Ryan, Hummert, & Boich, 1995). Aging individuals who receive elderspeak messages may recognize they are being talked down to and respond by withdrawing from engagement in patronizing conversations, or they may suffer increased depression or decreased self-esteem. Older adults may also respond by enacting behaviors consistent with their own negative stereotypes of a frail elder and may avoid self-care activities.

The *Communication Enhancement Model* (Ryan, Meredith, Maclean, & Orange, 1995) provides direction for effective healthcare-provider communication. This model directs that the younger adult healthcare provider make an individualized assessment of the communication abilities of each older adult and only modify speech as needed to support effective communication with that individual. For example, many younger adults assume that all older adults have hearing loss and speak loudly and slowly to all elders. For older adults with intact hearing, excessively loud and high-pitched speech can be distorted, making it harder for them to understand.

Diminutives (inappropriately intimate terms of endearment; imply parent–child relationship)

Example	**Alternative Strategy**
Referring to residents as honey, sweetie, dearie, or grandma	Refer to residents by their full name (i.e., Mrs. Robinson) or by their preferred name

Inappropriate Plural Pronouns (substituting a collective or "we" pronoun when referring to an independent older adult)

Example	**Alternative Strategy**
Are *we* ready for *our* medicine?	Are *you* ready for *your* medicine?
Let's take *our* bath now.	*Let me* help *you* take *your* bath now.

Tag Questions (prompts the answer to the question and implies the older adult can't act alone)

Example	**Alternative Strategy**
You would rather wear the blue socks, *wouldn't you?*	Would you like to wear the blue socks?

Figure 4-1 Examples of elderspeak communication with alternative strategies.

Cultural Competence and Health Literacy

Older adults may have limited education and different cultural backgrounds from nurses, and these factors can be barriers to effective communication. The Joint Commission (2010) has issued standards related to these factors, including requiring use of professional interpreters. Nurses must be aware of medical jargon and avoid its use in communication with older adults. A good practice is the ***teach-back method*** (NC Health Literacy Program, nd.). After providing health information, nurses should have patients repeat back to them what information they have received. This is an easy and effective method to assess comprehension of health teaching.

Communication in end-of-life care is of critical importance and may be complicated by emotional distress and prior relationships with family and significant others. Providing information may be especially difficult for healthcare workers when the news is bad or when listening skills of patients and families are poor. Chapter 26 provides a thorough discussion of end-of-life care.

Changes Throughout the Typical Aging Process

There are numerous age-related factors that affect communication in normal-aging adults. Vision, hearing, and cognitive processing gradually decline as the aging process occurs. In addition, speech and language skills, social networks, and environmental factors often change, which can promote or inhibit communication. Psychological elements such as depression, which has a negative impact on memory, also play a role in one's ability to effectively communicate.

Vision

Normal-Aging Changes in Vision

As people age, functioning of anatomical structures decreases, which is true in respect to vision. Age-related changes can start occurring in one's 30s. Over time, the cornea become less sensitive and the pupils decrease to about one-third of their size during young adulthood (Dugdale, 2011). It also takes longer for one's eyes to adjust from light to dark environments, such as walking out of a movie theater on a sunny day. The lenses become less flexible and slightly yellowed and cloudy (Dugdale). Visual acuity also decreases as age increases. In the normal aging process, *presbyopia* ("aging-eye") occurs (National Eye Health Education Program [NEHEP], 2006). Presbyopia is the decreased ability of the eye lens to focus on nearby objects due to normal aging. Typically, people become aware of this loss of visual focus around the age of 45 years. Although the age that presbyopia becomes apparent may vary from person to person, it will affect everyone at some point in their lives (NEHEP). This type of vision impairment may be corrected by wearing glasses or contact lenses. However, presbyopia increases as age increases, so glasses and lenses should be adjusted regularly.

In addition, it is common for older adults to experience an increase in sensitivity to light and glare (Ayalon, Feliciano, & Arean, 2006). Too little or too much light may hinder vision. This will vary from person to person, but typically older individuals require more light to be able to see adequately. On the other hand, bright lights, such as headlights, may temporarily blind a person and impair his/her ability to drive at night (Ayalon et al., 2006). Reading material with a glossy cover, such as magazines or laminated paper, may reflect light and make it more difficult to read. Changes also occur in the cones of the eyes, which affects how a person sees colors. For older adults, it is more difficult to differentiate between greens and blue than between reds and yellows. Contrasting warm and cool colors should be used when creating visuals such as calendars, instructions, and signs. Overall eye movement and peripheral vision is reduced as well, which causes the visual field to become smaller.

Pathological Changes That Affect Vision

Visual impairments in the aging population may be related to pathological issues such as age-related *macular degeneration, cataracts, glaucoma, diabetic retinopathy,* and *dry eyes*. Macular degeneration is a progressive degeneration of eye tissue and the effects are irreversible. Cataracts, or opaqueness of the lens, is the most common age-related eye disease and is reversed through surgical treatment. Glaucoma is the slow and progressive deterioration of optic nerve fibers; peripheral vision is impaired first, followed by central vision. Early detection can reduce the progression of the disease, as glaucoma is the number one disease that causes blindness. Diabetic retinopathy, or changes in the eye as a result of diabetes, can also cause blindness. Early detection and treatment help to prevent blindness (NEHEP, 2006).

Vision and Communication

Although vision is not the first thing we typically think of when discussing communication, impaired vision can lead to communication complications. Adequate vision supports interaction with the physical environment as well as participation in activities such as reading books, watching films, and socializing. Depending on the severity of the vision impairment, some people are able to compensate and continue daily activities without additional challenges. However, for most people, reading becomes more difficult. The person may hold the text further away in order for it to be clearer, ask someone else to read it aloud to him/her, or may simply refuse to read it. Vision issues affect the ability to read for enjoyment as well as for necessary activities such as reading and paying a bill, being able to see what to order off a menu, reading a calendar of appointments, or finding a phone number in the phonebook. Individuals with visual impairments may have not hearing, comprehension, or speech issues, but they miss out on one important aspect of communication: nonverbal communication. Nonverbal communication is often the way we communicate our emotional state (e.g., a smile when happy, a glare when angry). However, aspects of our emotions can also be communicated through our pitch, loudness, vocal quality, and intonation. These vocal changes can help those with visual impairments understand the other person. For example, when upset or stressed, often a person's voice increases in pitch, loudness, and may be more strained. In addition, the person may talk in short, quick phrases and overemphasize words to get the point across.

These vocal cues would help a person with visual impairments to understand the emotions of the other person without being able to see their facial expressions or actions. But let's say you point to an object across the room and begin to talk about it. Does the person have any clue as to what you are talking about? Did you say what it was? Did you describe it? Unfortunately, gestures rely on adequate vision, though touch could be used to help the person understand the gesture. Overall, the communication partner needs to provide clear speech to help compensate for the inability to see nonverbal communication.

Depression and *isolation* are common for individuals with vision impairments. These individuals may require more support and encouragement to attend social gatherings. Even if they have no hearing loss, cognitive decline, or speech and language impairments, individuals may avoid interacting with the "seeing" world. It is a great adjustment to transition from being able to see to no longer being able to rely on one's vision. The person may be more reliant on others to assist him/her in social engagements as well as daily activities. However, some people may feel embarrassed about having to rely on others, which could lead to them trying to avoid these certain situations and activities all together.

Hearing

There are three types of hearing loss: conductive, sensorineural, and mixed. *Conductive hearing loss* occurs when the cause of hearing loss is located in the outer and/or middle ear. The sound wave cannot effectively reach the inner ear, where the sound signal is sent to the brain (Norrix & Harris, 2008). Ear infections, punctured tympanic membrane (eardrum), otitis media (ear infections), broken bones in the ear (malleus, incus, stapes), scarred eardrum, fluid in the middle ear, earwax buildup, birth defects, and genetic conditions can all cause a conductive hearing loss (Vorvick & Schwarz, 2011). *Sensorineural hearing loss* (see **Box 4-1**) is damage that occurs in the inner ear and/or auditory nerve fiber. This type of hearing loss is the most common in older adults. Causes include short- or long-term exposure to loud noises, otoxicity, Meniere's disease, and tumors. When both conductive and sensorneural hear loss are present, it is called a *mixed hearing loss* (Norrix & Harris, 2008).

Normal-Aging Changes in Hearing

Like vision, hearing declines as people age. One in three adults aged 60 years and older and one in two adults over the age of 85 are reported to have some level of hearing loss. *Presbycusis* is a gradual hearing loss in both ears that typically begins in one's 50s (Lin, 2012). There are several possible factors that may contribute to presbycusis, including noise exposure over the course of a lifetime, illness and progression of diseases, ototoxins (exposure to certain medications), genetic predisposition, and natural deterioration of the inner ear (Norrix & Harris, 2008).

Normal hearing loss in older adults begins with the inability to hear higher frequencies. Microscopic hair cells within the cochlea (in the inner ear) detect frequencies from sound waves and then send signals to the brain. The hair cells that detect high *frequency* sounds are the most vulnerable to damage. Once the hair cells

BOX 4-1   Research Highlight

Aim: The researcher wished to examine the range of variability for vowel intelligibility among talkers during clear versus conversational speech for older adults with hearing loss.

Purpose: To establish the range of talker variability for vowel intelligibility in clear versus conversational speech for older adults with hearing loss and to determine whether talkers who produced a clear speech benefit for young listeners with normal hearing also did so for older adults with hearing loss.

Method: Clear and conversational vowels produced by 41 talkers were presented for identification by 40 older (ages 65–87 years) adults with sensorineural hearing loss. The researcher looked at the variables of age, gender, speaking style, and experience among talkers and their benefit on hearing among hearing-impaired older adults.

Results: "Vowel intelligibility within each speaking style and the size of the clear speech benefit varied widely among talkers. The clear speech benefit was equivalent to that enjoyed by young listeners with normal hearing in an earlier study. Most talkers who had produced a clear speech benefit for young listeners with normal hearing also did so for the older listeners with hearing loss in the present study. However, effects of talker gender differed between listeners with normal hearing and listeners with hearing loss" (Ferguson, 2012, p. 779). While the results varied somewhat, it was found that talkers who benefited normal hearing younger persons also showed benefit for older persons with hearing loss.

Application to practice: These results would suggest that talkers who produce clear speech to younger adults with normal hearing will also produce similar results with hearing-impaired older adults, at least with regard to vowel pronunciation. Reading and speaking clearly with normal articulation of vowels can benefit hearing impaired elders.

Source: Ferguson, S. H. (2012). Talker differences in clear and conversational speech: Vowel intelligibility for older adults with hearing loss. *Journal of Speech, Language, and Hearing Research, 55*, 779–790.

are damaged, they do not repair themselves nor do new hair cells grow, so hearing loss is permanent. The most common complaint from someone with presbycusis is that the person can hear what was said, but does not understand what was said (Norrix & Harris, 2008). This occurs because speech sounds are produced at different frequencies; since hair cells have been damaged, the high frequency sounds are not heard. Several consonants (p, t, k, f, s, th, sh, ch) that produced high-frequency and low-intensity sounds are not heard, which greatly impacts the meanings of words. When all the frequencies of a word are not present, the word does not sound like a true word or it sounds unclear. People with high-frequency hearing loss often claim that the speaker is mumbling. As presbycusis advances, hearing loss in the lower frequencies will occur (Norrix & Harris, 2008). At this point, the ability to understand speech, listen to music, and hear environmental noises is impaired.

Tinnitus is also fairly common in older individuals. This is a continual, abnormal sound in one or both ears. It is similar to the internal noise one hears after being exposed to loud noise, such as at a concert. Tinnitus is generally caused by some mild hearing loss and can be extremely annoying to the person. For some individuals, the symptoms are temporary, but others may experience this long-term (Vorvick & Schwarz, 2011). This interferes with being able to adequately hear speech.

Hearing and Communication

Hearing loss has a great impact on individuals' daily activities, relationships, cognition, psychological health, and quality of life. Work environments often rely on communication between people. Whether it is the employer and employees, therapist/doctor and patients, teacher and students, or clerk and customers, good communication is fundamental to work relationships as well as the organization, company, or group as a whole. Some individuals who have difficulty hearing leave jobs because they feel they can no longer do their job or because they become frustrated with the situation. People may feel embarrassed about having a hearing loss and do not want to address it with coworkers, family, or friends. Hearing loss can also put a strain on martial and familial relationships. If a spouse or family member continually repeats him/herself, frustration and increased stressed are likely to occur. If hearing loss is severe, warnings, alarms, and environmental noises important for safety are not heard—for example, a tornado siren warning people to take cover may sound like a soft noise in the background or may not be heard at all. Another example involves pedestrian safety: The sound of car approaching may not heard when an individual is crossing the street. These sounds provide important information about the surrounding environment and influences the choices people make. In addition, the person with hearing loss may no longer participate in the activities that he/she once did. If the person enjoyed going to movies or talking friends on the phone, hearing difficulties may hinder him/her from participating. Being able to understand conversation over the phone is one of the most difficult situations for individuals with hearing loss.

When communicating over the phone, there are no visual cues to help the person fill in what he/she cannot hear as one could if the conversation took place face-to-face. Social situations may also be avoided. Restaurants, parties, meetings, and family celebrations are just a few social situations in which there are lots of competing sounds. If there is music or television on in the background, multiple people talking, dim lighting, and dishes clanging, it makes it more difficult for the person to hear and understand conversation. This may lead to feelings of isolation even though there are people all around. Feeling isolated can lead to the avoidance of social situations, which perpetuates the isolation. People with hearing loss also may experience depression, loneliness, and decreased quality of life (Ayalon et al., 2006). In addition, hearing loss has shown to have a negative impact on cognitive functioning and it increases the risk of dementia (Oyler, n.d.). Not being able to hear adequately can lead to social isolation, a reduction of verbal communication, and an increase of cognitive load while listening.

Although hearing declines as part of the aging process, the majority of individuals do not seek options to compensate for hearing loss. In 2012, 26.7 million U.S. adults

Notable Quotes

"Hearing impairment of any type and degree is a barrier to incidental learning."

—Carol Flexer, PhD, audiologist, author, and distinguished professor

aged 50 years or older were reported to have significant hearing loss, but less than 15% used hearing aids (Lin, 2012). When evaluated by an audiologist, *hearing aids* amplify the frequencies in which hearing loss in present. They do not amplify all frequencies unless that person displays hearing loss across all frequencies. If hearing aids are not a viable option due to financial constraints or noncompliance from the client, there are *personal amplification devices* that can aid in hearing and are less expensive. These not only amplify the speaker's message, but also reduce *background noise.*

Dual Sensory Impairment

Dual sensory impairment is when one experiences a loss in both vision and hearing. Research indicates that 21% of individuals over the age of 70 experience dual sensory impairment (Lighthouse International, 2001). As age increases, the prevalence increases. This has a significant effect on functioning and overall quality of life: One system is unable to compensate for the impaired system, since both are impaired. For example, if only a hearing loss is present, then information can be given in written form to help compensate for the hearing loss, or if vision is impaired, then the individual relies on auditory input for communication. When both hearing and vision are impaired, it is more difficult for the message to be received. It has been predicted, but not tested, that this dual impact has a greater effect on quality of life and function compared to a single impairment (Saunders & Echt, 2011).

Cognition

As people age, there is a gradual decrease in brain mass and neuronal function that results in cognitive changes. Long-term and short-term memory declines as people age. *Short-term memory* is limited in capacity and information remains for only a few seconds. Older adults can hold approximately 5–9 pieces of information in short-term memory, such as a phone number. Some information in the short-term memory is then encoded to be stored in *long-term memory.* Long-term memory is much more expansive than short-term memory and there is no limit as to how long information can be stored here. There are two subgroups of long-term memory: declarative and nondeclarative. *Declarative memory* is factual information that can be declared and is divided into three types: *episodic* (events), *semantic* (concepts), and *lexical* (word) *memory* (Bayles & Tomoeda, 2007). For example, think of the word "park." If you picture a park and perhaps think of swing sets, flowers, grass, or a sunny day, all of which requires semantic memory. If you thought of a specific time that you went to a park, then you used episodic memory. Lexical memory is the memory of words including meanings, spellings, and pronunciations (Bayles & Tomoeda, 2007). If you decided to write about going to the park or tell a friend what you did, then you would be using lexical memory to select and say/write those words. *Nondeclarative memory* includes motor skills, cognitive skills, reflex responses, priming, and condition responses (Bayles & Tomoeda, 2007). Repetition typically strengthens nondeclarative memory. *Working memory* includes executive functions such as planning, attention, inhibition, encoding, and monitoring, while *active memory* is what you are thinking at any given moment (Bayles & Tomoeda, 2007).

Normal-Aging Changes in Cognition

As people age, certain types of memory are more vulnerable to declination than others. Episodic memory and working memory are the most affected in the aging processes, while semantic, lexical, and nondeclarative memory are preserved more (Bayles & Tomoeda, 2007). It may be difficult for the person to recall what he/she did the day before or what he/she ate for breakfast (episodic memory), and there may be difficulty with multitasking (e.g., talking and writing a check) because of declines in working memory (attending to information, encoding, etc.). More recent memories are especially difficult to recall. It is much easier for an older adult to recall a story that happened decades ago than perhaps something that happened earlier that day. Writing appointments in calendars and journaling about daily events are just a couple of ways to help aid a person with typical memory decline. In addition to the changes in episodic and working memory, there is a gradual decline in being able to recall names and faces. Repeating new names or developing an association with the name and person can help people remember more accurately. An association is connecting the person's name with something already established in one's mind. For example, you meet a new student in class, Lauren, and your favorite cousin's name is also Lauren. When you see your new classmate, a picture of your cousin's face pops into your head and then you remember your classmate's name is Lauren. Nondeclarative memory may be slower, yet still accurate (Bayles & Tomoeda, 2007). For example, an older individual who has played golf for many years can still play at the same level as he/she did at a younger age, but may it may take more time to complete one round.

With normal aging, cognitive processing slows and abstract reasoning becomes more difficult. Also, new information becomes harder to remember (Lubinski, 2010). Attending to daily tasks may be mildly impaired, especially when there are distracting factors such as the phone ringing or television noise (Schreck, 2010). On a day-to-day basis, older individuals may show that they have challenges with following conversations, managing money, driving, safety, and complex tasks (Schreck, 2010). Because of brain changes, individuals over 65 "are slower in perceiving, processing, and reacting especially when the situation requires rapid processing of complex information" (Bayles & Tomoda, 2007, p. 49). The overall knowledge a person has does not diminish; however, the time that is takes to process and retrieve that information does increase. This can appear to family members and care providers that knowledge is impaired, so it is important to provide adequate time for older individuals to process and respond.

Pathological Changes that Affect Cognition, Speech, and/or Language

Dementia is defined as memory loss accompanied by speech and language impairments and/or decline in executive functioning (Bayles & Tomoeda, 2007). Because changes in memory occur with normal aging, the symptoms have to be significant enough to interfere with social, occupational, or daily activities. Types of dementia include Alzheimer's disease, vascular dementia, dementia with Lewy bodies, mixed dementia, and frontotemporal dementia. Dementia can be present in numerous other conditions such as Parkinson's disease, Huntington's disease, Creutzfeldt–Jakob disease, Wernicke–Korsakoff syndrome, and normal pressure hydrocephalus (Alzheimer's Association, n.d.). *Alzheimer's disease* is the most common form of dementia and accounts for 60–80% of dementia cases (Alzheimer's Association, n.d.). Alzheimer's disease is a progressive degenerative brain disease that first affects memory (Bayles & Tomoeda, 2007). As it progresses, physical movement, communication, *cognition*, personality, and emotional/mental health are affected. In the United States, 1 out of 8 people over the age of 65 have Alzheimer's disease (Alzheimer's Association, 2012). Individuals 85 and over are at greater risk of having the disease; current research says and 1 out of 2 people over the age of 85 have Alzheimer's disease (Alzheimer's Association, 2012).

The Effect of Cognitive Issues on Communication.

Effective communication heavily relies on an intact memory. When we are listening, we first have to attune to the speaker and then use our memory to recall what the person said in order to make an appropriate response. When speaking, we use our memory to recall stories and information as well as to select the right words to convey what we mean. As with the aging process, episodic memory is the first to be affected in individuals with Alzheimer's disease (Bayles & Tomoeda, 2007). The difference between age-related changes and Alzheimer's disease-related change in episodic memory is the rapidness with which one forgets the information. Individuals with Alzheimer's disease as well as individuals with Parkinson's disease with dementia quickly forget, within seconds. In addition to short-term memory issues, they also experience long-term memory problems. Because of short-term memory impairments, people with dementia will repeat the same stories and/or ask the same questions. If a person with a memory impairment is asked what he/she did yesterday, common responses include "I don't remember," "I don't know," or say something vague such as "Oh, you know, the usual." Long-term memories from distant times, such as events that happened in childhood through young adulthood, are easier to recall and talk about than events that recently occurred. Reminiscent activities use pictures and objects from earlier in the individual's lifetime to facilitate conversation. This activity allows for individuals to practice communicating without having to rely on memory that is impaired. The aim is to reduce individuals' frustration when communicating by minimizing the demands on memory and to provide enjoyable communicative opportunities.

Eventually, speech and language are affected by the progressive nature of dementia. Difficulty in naming objects, recalling words, and recalling people's names are first impaired because these are memory-dependent skills (Bayles & Tomoeda, 2007). Often, individuals with dementia will use vague terms such as *thing*, *there*, *that*, or *them* instead using a specific word for a person or an object (Bayles & Tomoeda, 2007). Confrontation naming (e.g., pointing to a picture of an apple and asking "What is this?") is the most difficult task to fulfill because it demands adequate memory and language skills. Besides the picture of the object, there are no additional cues to help the person retrieve the information. Questions that incorporate confrontation naming should be avoided with those who have memory issues. For example, when looking at family pictures in a patient's room, refrain from asking, "Who is this?" or "What's her name?" Earlier on in the disease progression, individuals are typically aware that they should know the information, but simply cannot remember. This can lead to frustration, anger, guilt, and sadness. Instead, make a comment about that picture or ask multiple choice or yes/no questions—for example, "This is a beautiful picture. Is this your daughter?"

In the early stages, sentences are typically grammatically correct, but fragmented and repetitious (Bayles & Tomoeda, 2007). At this point, there are signs of declining vocabulary and words may be substituted with similar words (e.g., "look" for "took"). In addition, the person may perseverate on an idea or a topic (Bayles & Tomoeda, 2007). In the middle stages, attention, memory, speech, and language skills continue to decline. Speech becomes slower and more repetitive and the content becomes less cohesive. At this point, comprehension of written and spoken language is typically impaired. In the early states of cognitive decline, reading comprehension skills are often still intact, though this is influenced by several factors such as reading skills prior to the onset of dementia, education level, and current amount of opportunities to read. In the later stages, expressive and receptive communication is greatly affected. Reading of single words aloud is sometimes still a skill, but comprehension is severely impaired. Meaningful spoken sentences and phrases diminish as well as writing skills (Bayles & Tomoeda, 2007). It becomes very difficult for the person to communicate what he/she wants or needs. Nonverbal communication (facial expressions, behaviors, eye contact) may be the primary way for the patient to communicate his/her desires.

To effectively communicate with patients who have speech, language, and/or cognitive impairments, it is imperative to use a multitude of modalities to aid in communication. Although oral communication is what we generally think of most often when we think of communication, written information, pictures, drawings, concrete symbols (such as letters and numbers), gestures, and facial expressions all aid in effectively communicating a message. Some approaches will help patients communicate better than others. It is important to collaborate with the patient, family members, caregivers, and speech-language pathologists to determine approaches that work best for that specific person.

Speech and Language

Speech is the production of sounds used for communicate and *language* (spoken, written, or signed) is the symbol system used by a shared group of people for communication (Plante & Beeson, 2008). Both influence the ability to effectively communicate; however, speech does not have an impact on comprehension of verbal and nonverbal language, writing, and reading since it refers to speaking only. Language abilities influence receptive communication (e.g., auditory comprehension, reading comprehension) as well as expressive communication (e.g., speaking, writing).

Normal-Aging Changes in Speech and Language.

One area of language that has shown to improve with age is vocabulary. The longer one lives, the more that person is exposed to a variety of words and meanings, thus their vocabulary continues expand. When verbal knowledge was compared between 20 year olds and 80 year olds, the 80-year-old group had better scores than the 20-year-old group (Park et al., 2002). Syntax (the structure of sentences) remains intact throughout the process as well. Pragmatics (how we use language to interact) also remains relatively strong, but people tend to be more verbose and/or drift off topic in older adulthood. The rate of speech slows and articulation (pronunciation of sounds) becomes less clear because of the slowing rate of cognitive processing as well as declining strength and range of movement of the mouth, tongue, and jaw. Poor detention (loss of teeth) or dentures that do not fit properly are also factors that influence articulation.

Complex and lengthy verbal and written information may be more difficult to understand (Lubinski, 2010). Comprehension during conversation may be more challenging because of hearing, vision or sensory loss, cognitive changes, and emotional factors. As compared to younger adults, a study by Haro and Isaki (2009) found that older adults had more cohesive and organized speech and used less fillers (e.g., like, um, uh). Older individuals continue to display abilities to learn and retain world knowledge as well (Haro & Isaki, 2009). Appropriate content of sentences, vocabulary, and grammar remain strengths for normal-aging older adults; however, the length and complexity of sentences is reduced (Schreck, 2010). Nonspecific language (she, they, thing) becomes more prevalent without information as to who or what the speaker is referring to—for example, there person might say, "She's coming later," but does not say who *she* is. Although there are changes in being able to recall names of people, places, and objects and sentence complexity decreases, the ability to functionally communicate remains intact.

Aphasia is an acquired (not present at birth) language impairment and occurs when there is damage to language center in the brain. Although most people's language center is located in the left hemisphere of the brain, some individuals' language centers are located in the right hemisphere (Bayles & Tomoeda, 2007). Aphasia is most often a result of a stroke, but can result from trauma and illness as well (Bayles & Tomoeda, 2007). Although other conditions and diseases can cause language impairments, the term aphasia is used if it is primarily a language deficit. If cognition, personality, or speech is impaired, then it does not fit the diagnosis of aphasia. There are several types of aphasia that are categorized by fluency, comprehension, and repetition abilities. All types of aphasia share one common feature: *anomia*, which is a naming impairment (Bayles & Tomoeda, 2007).

When damage occurs to Broca's area of the brain, it is called *Broca's aphasia*. With this type of aphasia, comprehension remains intact, but spoken communication is nonfluent. Speech is slow, effortful, and choppy and often lacks proper grammatical markers, such as "-ed" at the end of a verb to indicate past tense. Individuals have difficulty initiating speech, but they provide good content. Repetition is moderately to severely impaired. Most people with Broca's aphasia are aware of their impairments and try to self-correct (Bayles & Tomoeda, 2007). Another nonfluent type of aphasia is *global aphasia*. With this type, the damage to the left hemisphere is greater than with Broca's, so the effects on communication are more devastating. A person with global aphasia has very limited spoken language and may only use single words, which can sound like nonsense words. Unlike Broca's aphasia, comprehension of written and spoken information is significantly impaired. In addition, written expression is as equally impaired as the spoken form. A common fluent type of aphasia is *Wernicke's* (pronounced Ver-nick-e) *aphasia*, which is caused by damage to Wernicke's area of the brain. People with this aphasia have fluent speech with low content. Individuals will say real or nonsense words, but the string of words has no clear meaning. Comprehension of spoken and written information is impaired, as is repetition. Unlike Broca's aphasia, those with Wernicke's are generally unaware of their communication deficits (Bayles & Tomoeda, 2007).

Dysarthria and *apraxia* are motor speech impairments caused by neurological changes in the body. Apraxia is an impairment with motor planning, while dysarthria refers to difficulties with executing speech movements (Yorkston, Beukelman, Strand, & Hakel, 2010). Some adults who have had a stroke will have aphasia (a language impairment) and dysarthria or apraxia (a speech impairment). In addition, individuals with Parkinson's disease often experience dysarthria. *Parkinson's disease* is a progressive degenerative condition that includes symptoms such as tremors (at rest), slow movements, rigidity of limbs or trunk, and an unstable balance (National Parkinson's Foundation, 2012a). Research estimates that in the United States, 50,000 to 60,000 people are diagnosed with Parkinson's disease each year (National Parkinson's Foundation, 2012b.) and there is a higher prevalence in individuals over the age of 60 (American Parkinson Disease Association, n.d.). Approximately 15% of individuals with Parkinson's disease develop dementia as the condition progresses (Yorkston et al., 2010). Slow movements and rigidity have a negative impact when producing speech. Because of rigidity of the trunk, people with Parkinson's have a reduction of air pressure needed to adequately support speech. Reduced vocal volume or a weak voice is common in the early stages. Other common problems include hoarse voice, monotonous voice, difficulty initiating speech, and reduced precision of articulation (Yorkston et al., 2010). When reduction in the precision of articulation occurs, the person is more difficult to understand when he or she is speaking to unfamiliar listeners. Rigidity also prevents a full range of motion of the articulators (jaw, tongue, etc.) and may contributing to reduced intonation and monoloudness (Yorkston et al., 2010). In addition, individuals often appear with a flat affect (no facial expression), which impacts aspects of nonverbal communication. When cognition is impaired in addition to speech issues, language issues are typically also impaired.

Symptoms of ***chronic obstructive pulmonary disorder*** (COPD) include shortness of breath, fatigue, chronic cough, and limited physical activity (Alexander, 2009). Speech is more difficult to maintain due to many of these symptoms. Individuals with COPD tend to have hoarse voices and speak at reduced volume because of continual shortness of breath. To prevent fatigue, other forms of communication such as writing, gestures, sign language, and speech-generating devices (e.g., iPad) can be used to supplement oral speech.

Social Networks

As mentioned previously, individuals with hearing and/or vision impairments often become isolated from social engagements. A hearing loss makes it difficult for the person to feel like part of the conversation or activity at hand. Individuals may feel embarrassed about the hearing loss and not ask for the message to be repeated, but instead pull away from situations in which he/she will not be able to hear. Lin (2012) wrote, "social engagement in older adults is the key determinant of overall morbidity and mortality in later life" (p. 1148). Many changes occur as people age. Although one's ability to communicate maybe intact, there may be few opportunities to communicate with others. One change in the social network as we age is retirement. People go from interacting with colleagues, clients, friends, and/or students 5 days a week to not necessarily interacting with anyone in a given day. The work environment is set up so that communication, whether it is through talking, emailing, or listening to presentations, occurs constantly throughout the day. Postretirement, individuals may have fewer day-to-day opportunities for interacting with others. In addition, as people continue to age, living situations have to be adapted. For some people, this means moving to a smaller home, perhaps in a less familiar neighborhood or a different city in order to be closer to family. It may mean moving into a retirement community, assisted living facility, or long-term care facility. This may cause the individual to be removed from his/her established social network. Many older adults are homebound or unable to drive or walk to places; this requires communication partners to come to him/her. Homebound adults have few opportunities to interact with people, which has a negative impact on quality of life and depression. Living facilities often provide programs and social events for residents to participate in; however, usually only a portion of the residents elect to participate. Hearing, vision, cognitive, and emotional issues all play a factor in one's desire and ability to socially engage.

Strategies to Aid Communication with Individuals with Communication Impairments

There are two types of strategies to help with communication issues: compensatory and restorative. ***Compensatory strategies*** focus on providing mechanisms to assist the person with the physical or neurological impairment. There are several types of compensatory strategies used with older adults such as adapting the environment; using alternative augmentative communication (AAC), technological devices, or memory aids; and having communication partners alter how they communicate with the person. *Restorative strategies* address rebuilding skills that are impaired. For example, a man with nonfluent aphasia might focus on saying common single-words to help communicate his wants and needs. As his ability to say these words increases, more words are taught. A person needs to be assessed by a speech-language pathologist to determine appropriate evidence-based strategies to implement. Below are some strategies for nurses as well as other professionals, caregivers, and family members to use to help facilitate effective communication with older adults (see **Table 4-2**).

Use person-first language. When referring to the patient, whether or not the patient is present, use *person-first language*. This stresses the person as an individual who has some condition or disease instead the condition or disease as a defining factor of the individual. For example, say or write *person*

TABLE 4-2 Strategies for Effective Communication with Persons with Vision, Hearing, Cognitive, and/or Speech/Language Impairments

Impairment Type	Communication Strategies
Vision	• Person-first language • Include the patient • Provide written information in large, easy to read print • Position yourself in the person's direct line of vision • Make sure glasses are or contacts are worn
Hearing	• Person-first language • Slower speaking rate and pause between phrases • Include the patient • Provide additional time for the person to respond • Summarize • Speak into the ear with less hearing loss • Write out information • Eliminate or minimize background noise • Limit the number of speakers • Position yourself in the person's direct line of vision • Make sure the hearing aid(s) or assistive listening device is on and working • Say names • Use touch to gain attention
Cognition	• Person-first language • Slower speaking rate and pause between phrases • Include the patient • Provide additional time for the person to respond • Simplify vocabulary and avoid jargon

with dementia instead of dementia or demented patient and a *person with a hearing loss,* not a hearing-impaired person. This communicates respect for the individual.

Include the patient. In some situations, family members and caregivers speak as if the person being talked about is not in the room. Be sure to include the individual in the conversation. If conversations that are taking place with the patient in the room, speak as though the person can understand you. Do not have conversations about the person in front of him/her and not include him/her, especially if you say something that might be hurtful or embarrassing to the person (e.g., *She doesn't remember anything anymore*).

Speak slower and pause between phrases. Slowing down the rate at which you speak allows you to speak clearer and provides distinct separation of words for better comprehension. Pause time between sentences allows for older adults whose retrieval and processing has decreased in speed to process and respond. This also helps individuals with hearing loss as well.

Impairment Type	Communication Strategies
Cognition	• Summarize • Write out information • Eliminate or minimize background noise • Limit the number of speakers • Say names • Encourage use of clues for word-finding difficulty • Use touch to communicate to gain attention • Request clarification
Speech and Language	• Person-first language • Slower speaking rate and pause between phrases • Include the patient • Provide additional time for the person to respond • Simplify vocabulary and avoid jargon • Summarize • Write out information • Eliminate or minimize background noise • Limit the number of speakers • Position yourself in the person's direct line of vision • Make sure the AAC device is on and working • Say names • Encourage use of clues for word-finding difficulty • Request clarification

Provide additional time for the person to respond. After asking a question or making a comment that you expect a response from, wait 5–10 seconds for a response. Since processing time slows in adults with and without pathological conditions, providing additional time allows for the person to process what was said, plan what to say, and then provide an oral or written response.

Simplify vocabulary and avoid jargon. Try to use language that is easy to understand; refrain from using slang and medical jargon, especially. Watch to see if the person understands what you are saying. If you think he/she did not understand or he/she says that do not understand, rephrase your sentence.

Summarize. If the person forgets the topic being discussed, summarize what has been said to help guide the person back into the conversation.

Use short, direct, clear phrases. Comprehension of complex sentences becomes more difficult as people age. Use short phrases, but remember to still use respectful language. Limit instructions to one or two steps at a time. Using short, clear phrases may help reduce the number of times you repeat the information.

Use touch to communicate. Some individuals have difficulty with attention and alertness due to cognitive issues, medication side effects, and/or medical health problems. Gently touch the person on the hand, shoulder, arm, or leg to help gain his/her attention. If you start speaking when the person is not attending, then you'll likely have to repeat your message.

Speak in the direction of the person. Make sure you are in the same room and are looking at the individual. This will help the person to prepare to listen. Being in the same room eliminates an environmental barrier, as talking to a person in another room or across the room leads to a reduced speech signal to the listener.

Speak into the ear with less or no hearing loss. For those who have hearing impairments, be sure look in their charts for information about their hearing. If one ear has better hearing, position yourself so that you are speaking in the direction of that ear.

Write out information. If the person does not understand you, write down key words, phrases, or sentences so the person can read the information. This will help ensure that the message is clearly communicated.

Provide written information in large, easy-to-read print. For individuals who have difficulty seeing written text, make sure that text is in an easy-to-read, large font. Stick to high-contrasting colors (e.g., black ink on white paper) and avoid using blue and green ink.

Request clarification. If you did not understand the intent of the person's message, ask questions that help he/she to clarify. Another option is to say what you think was said and ask the person if you understood correctly.

Encourage use of clues. There are times when we all struggle with finding the word we want to say. Since this typically occurs more often in older adults, encourage them to provide clues so that you can then guess the word. For example, you should suggest for them to describe appearance, function, and/ or location.

Eliminate or minimize background noise. Additional sounds compete with the speech sounds, making it more difficult to determine what was said. Music, television, and other conversations all makes it more difficult to attend to the conversation at hand.

Limit the number of speakers. Typically, group settings and social events have numerous people speaking at the same time or rapidly taking turns. This requires quick processing to be able to understand and keep up with the conversation. Because older adults are slower to process and respond to the information, it is best to limit the number of people speaking. This is less cognitively demanding for the individual.

Position yourself in the person's direct line of vision. This will let the person know that you are engaging in communication with him/her. Also, it provides visual information about what is being said. The person will be able to look at your lips and perhaps fill in what he/she does not understand simply by hearing. If understanding of nonverbal communication is still intact, positioning yourself in front of the person will allow for him/her to tune into the nonverbal communication (posture, facial expressions, gestures). Another element to keep in the mind is lighting: Be sure that there is adequate lighting so the person can see you. Individuals with vision impairments often require more lighting than those without vision issues.

Use gestures to aid in communication. Gestures help clarify the message when perhaps not all of it was understood. Pointing and demonstrating actions may help to aid understanding.

Say names. Say the person's name before providing instructions to get his/her attention. If memory is an issue, state your name as you enter the room so that the person does not have to guess who you are. When possible, use proper names instead of pronouns.

Make sure any assistive devices are on and working. This includes hearing aids (see **Figure 4-2**), assistive listening devices, and electronic AAC devices. If the person needs glasses to see, make sure he/she has easy access to them. If the person has difficulty hearing, ask the person to wear their hearing aids or properly place hearing aids before speaking (see **Figure 4-3**).

Communicating with Families and Significant Others

Nurses can support family members caring for older adults by assisting them to overcome communication barriers that occur as a normal part of aging and with pathological conditions such as terminal illness, stroke, and dementia. Healthcare providers must be aware of the need to include the older adult in communication regarding health matters as much as possible. This includes avoiding excluding the older adult patient from communication about their health care. Permission to communicate about the health condition with family and significant others is a key privacy issue that may be complicated if older adults become infirm or unable to communicate.

Notable Quotes

"Tell me and I'll forget. Show me and I'll remember. Involve me and I'll understand."

—Confucius

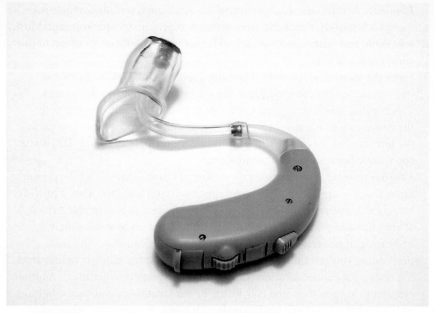

Figure 4-2 An example of a hearing aid.

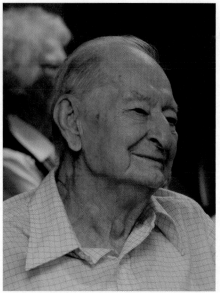

Figure 4-3 When teaching older adults, be sure to consider and address communication barriers.

Nurses can also help significant others to understand their role in care giving as well as their need to recognize stress they may encounter and resources to aid them in providing care. Nurses frequently counsel family caregivers, make referrals for resources such as respite care, and serve as role models for caregiver communication practices.

Communicating with the Professional and Nonprofessional Caregivers

In many settings, the nurse provides communication to the physician or other healthcare provider about the status of older adult patients. Nurses rely on effective communication and patient advocacy to describe a patient's condition that may require a change in the treatment plan. Nursing communication is also important to inform additional healthcare professionals such as speech-language pathologists and physical and occupational therapists, who may be needed to provide suggestions to improve patient well-being. Nurses may also communicate about patient care with paraprofessional providers, such as home health aides and certified nursing assistants, who provide the majority of direct care in assisted living and nursing home settings. In these situations, the nurse is the expert source of information and care should be taken to communicate clearly and with respect for other providers; nurses must be aware of their role as role models for paraprofessional providers.

Summary

The content in this chapter has focused on the importance of communication. Although many older adults may have significant sensory or cognitive impairments that affect their ability to communicate, nurses can use the techniques discussed in this chapter to facilitate appropriate communication. Health literacy should also be taken into account when planning teaching or educational materials. By choosing the most applicable strategies for information exchange, nurses can positively influence the communication process with older adults.

Case Study 4–1: Improving Communication

Mrs. W., a new resident in the nursing home, is walking toward another resident's room and is about to enter. Her caregiver observes her from the nursing station.

Please select example A or B below and change the words to improve the nurse's communication to show respect for the older adult.

A. Overly Nurturing Talk (highly caring, not controlling, inappropriately intimate)

Caregiver: "Where do you think you're going? That's not your room you silly girl."

Mrs. W. continues to enter the room.

Caregiver: "Well goodness, honey, you really are lost, aren't you? We can't have that now can we? Give me your hand and we'll find your room. Come on sweetie."

B. Directive Talk (high degree of control, little recognition of autonomy of the listener, little caring)

Caregiver: "That's not your room. You have no business being there. Residents can't go in the rooms of other residents."

Mrs. W. looks worried and pauses.

Caregiver: "Move along now and find your own room."

Critical Thinking Exercises

1. **Learn more about the Joint Commission standards related to communication** and safety in this 7-minute webcast. Consider how you can implement these standards in practice. http://www.jointcommission.org/multimedia/improving-patient-provider-communication---part-1-of-4/

2. **Watch a video presentation of the teach-back method** and see how to incorporate this technique into your practice. http://www.nchealthliteracy.org/teachingaids.html

Personal Reflections

1. Have you ever experienced hearing loss? Have you ever cared for someone who has hearing problems? Take the unfair hearing test and experience hearing deficits: http://www.youtube.com/watch?v=xzUwgJCZ1Gc

2. How would you feel not to be able to hear clearly? What would the world be like without complete hearing or sight? How would your communication on a daily basis change?

References

Alexander, J. E. (2009). Assessment and treatment approaches for the patient with COPD. *Perspectives on Gerontology*, *14*(2), 33–36.

Alzheimer's Association. (n.d.). *Key types of dementia*. Retrieved from http://www.alz.org/alzheimers_disease_related_diseases.asp

Alzheimer's Association. (2012). 2012 Alzheimer's disease facts and figures. *Alzheimer's and Dementia: The Journal of the Alzheimer's Association*, *8*, 131–168.

American Parkinson's Disease Association. (n.d.). *Basic info about PD*. Retrieved from http://www.apdaparkinson.org/publications-information/basic-info-about-pd/

Ayalon, L., Feliciano, L., & Arean, P. A. (2006). Aging changes that affect communication. In K. L. Mauk (Ed.), *Gerontological Nursing: Competencies for Care* (pp. 76–105). Sudbury, MA: Jones and Bartlett.

Bayles, K. A., & Tomoeda, C. K. (2007). *Cognitive-communication disorders of dementia*. San Diego, CA: Plural.

Benner, P. (2004). Relational ethics of comfort, touch, and solace — Endangered arts? *American Journal of Critical Care*, *13*(4), 346–349.

Caporael, L. (1981). The paralanguage of caregiving: Baby talk to the institutionalized aged. *Journal of Personality and Social Psychology*, *40*(5), 876–884.

Dugdale III, D. C. (2011). Aging changes in the senses. *Medline Plus, National Library of Medicine, National Institutes of Health*. Retrieved from http://www.nlm.nih.gov/medlineplus/ency/article/004013.htm

Ferguson, S. H. (2012). Talker differences in clear and conversational speech: Vowel intelligibility for older adults with hearing loss. *Journal of Speech, Language, and Hearing Research, 55*, 779–790.

Grau, L., Chandler, B., & Saunders, C. (1995). Nursing home residents' perceptions of the quality of their care. *Journal of Psychosocial Nursing, 33*(5), 34–41.

Haro, S., & Isaki, E. (2009). Age effects on language: Differences between young and normal aging adults. Retrieved from http://www.asha.org/Events/convention/handouts/2009/2386_Isaki_Emi/

Kiely, D. K., Simon, M. A., Jones, R. N., & Morris, J. N. (2000). The protective effect of social engagement on mortality in long-term care. *Journal of the American Geriatrics Society, 48*(12), 1367–1372.

Lighthouse International. (2001). Dual sensory impairment among the elderly. Retrieved from http://www.lighthouse.org/research/archived-studies/dual/

Lin, F. R. (2012). Hearing loss in older adults: Who's listening? *The Journal of the American Medical Association, 307*(11), 1147–1148.

Lubinski, R. (2010). Communicating effectively with elders and their families. *The ASHA Leader*. Retrieved from http://www.asha.org/Publications/leader/2010/100316/CommunicatingEffectivelyWithElders.htm

National Eye Health Education Program [NEHEP]. (2006). Eye health needs of older adults literature review. In: *NEHEP 5-year agenda* (pp. 32–50). Retrieved from http://www.nei.nih.gov/nehep/research/The_Eye_Health_needs_of_Older_Adult_Literature_Review.pdf

National Parkinson's Foundation. (2012a). What are the symptoms of Parkinson's disease? Retrieved from http://www.parkinson.org/Parkinson-s-Disease/PD-101/How-do-you-know-if-you-have-PD-.aspx

National Parkinson's Foundation. (2012b). What is Parkinson's disease? Retrieved from http://www.parkinson.org/Parkinson-s-Disease/PD-101/What-is-Parkinson-s-disease

NC Health Literacy Program. (n.d). Teach-back method Tool 5. Retrieved from http://www.nchealth-literacy.org/toolkit/tool5.pdf.

Norrix, L., & Harris, F. P. (2008). Disorders of hearing in adults. In E. Plante & P.M. Beeson, *Communication and Communication Disorders: A Clinical Introduction* (3rd ed.). Boston, MA: Pearson Education.

Oyler, A. L. (n.d.). Untreated hearing loss in adults – A growing national epidemic. Retrieved from http://www.asha.org/Aud/Articles/Untreated-Hearing-Loss-in-Adults/

Paget, L., Han, P., Nedza, S., Kurtz, P., Racine, E., Russell, S., … Von Kohorn, I. (2011). Patient-clinician communication: Basic principles and expectations. Washington D.C.: Institute of Medicine. Retrieved from http://www.iom.edu/pcc

Park, D. C., Lautenschlager, G., Hedden, T., Davidson, N. S., Smith, A. D., & Smith, P. K. (2002). Models of visuospatial and verbal memory across the adult life span. *Psychology and Aging, 17*(2), 299–320.

Parsons, S. K., Simmons, W. P., Penn, K., & Furlough, M. (2002). Determinants of satisfaction and turnover among nursing assistants. *Journal of Gerontological Nursing, 29*(3), 51–58.

Plante, E. & Beeson, P.M. (2008). *Communication and communication disorders: A clinical introduction, Third Edition*. Needham Heights, MA: Allyn & Bacon.

Rowe, J. W., & Kahn, R. L. (1997). Successful aging. *The Gerontologist, 37*, 433–440.

Ryan, E. B., Hummert, M. L., & Boich, L. H. (1995). Communication predicaments of aging; Patronizing behavior toward older adults. *Journal of Language and Social Psychology, 14*(1-2), 144–166.

Ryan, E. B., Meredith, S. D., Maclean, M. J., & Orange, J. B. (1995). Changing the way we talk with elders: Promoting health using the communication enhancement model. *International Journal of Aging and Human Development, 41*(2), 89–107.

Saunders, G. H., & Echt, K. (2011). Dual sensory impairment in an aging population. *The ASHA Leader*. Retrieved from http://www.asha.org/Publications/leader/2011/110315/Dual-Sensory-Impairment-in-an-Aging-Population.htm

Schreck, J. (November 2010). *The impact of "normal" aging on cognitive-communication skills*. Paper presented at the ASHA Annual Convention, Philadelphia, PA.

The Joint Commission. (2010). *Advancing effective communication, cultural competence, and patient-and-family-centered care: A roadmap for hospitals*. Oakbrook, Terrace, IL: Author.

Vorvick, L. J., & Schwartz, S. (updated 5/2011). Hearing loss. *Medline Plus, National Library of Medicine, National Institutes of Health*. Retrieved from http://www.nlm.nih.gov/medlineplus/ency/article/003044.htm

Yorkston, K. M., Beukelman, D. R., Strand, E. A, & Hakel, M. (2010). *Management of motor speech disorders in children and adults* (3rd ed.). Austin, TX: Pro-ed.

For a full suite of assignments and additional learning activities, see the access code at the front of your book.

LEARNING OBJECTIVES

WWW

On completion of this chapter, the reader will be able to:

> Apply key principles of adult learning to teaching older adults.
> Discuss how changing demographics of the United States influences various aspects of the teaching–learning process.
> Describe settings where health education for older adults can take place.
> Describe the influence of cultural diversity on learning styles of older adults.
> Discuss how health literacy influences teaching strategies used when educating older adults.
> Compare the effect of normal physiologic changes and chronic illness on the learning process.
> Apply strategies for enhancing teaching and learning of older adults.

KEY TERMS

WWW

Adult learning
Andragogy
Baby boomers
Cultural diversity
Gerogogy
Health disparity

Health literacy
Lifelong learning
Literacy
Social cognitive theory
Theory of adult learning
Theory of self-efficacy

Chapter 5

Teaching Older Adults and Their Families

Kathleen Blais
Nora Bollinger

The population of the United States is living longer as a result of advances in health care, willness/injury prevention programs, early identification and management of chronic illnesses, advanced technology in disease management, and improved treatments and healthcare delivery methods. To help these older Americans manage their health and well-being, nurses will need to teach an assortment of skills and knowledge to their clients. A wide variety of factors influence the strategies needed for effective teaching with these older adults. Similarly, a combination of factors influence the ability of older adult learners.

Changing Demographics

Individuals reaching age 65 have an average life expectancy of another 18.4 years (19.8 for females, 16.8 for males). By 2035, 77.5 million people (19.9% of the U.S. population) will be 65 years of age or older (U.S. Census Bureau, 2008b). The 85 and older population is projected to increase to 6.3 million by 2015, and 105,000 U.S. residents will be 100 years of age or older (U.S. Census Bureau, 2008b). The older population will require more educational opportunities to prepare them for retirement and life after retirement, including strategies for increasing personal responsibility for health and wellness, for improving or maintaining good health, and for managing declining health and limitations in function.

Gender differences will also affect the needs of the aging population. In 2010, older women outnumbered older men (130:100), and the female/male ratio increases with age. The diversity of the United States is also changing, and is expected to continue to change with the White non-Hispanic percentage of the population decreasing, and the percentage of Hispanic, Black, Asian, and American Indian/Alaskan Native population groups increasing. According to the U.S. Census Bureau (2008a), minorities will become the majority in 2042. Nurse educators will need to develop educational programs that address health disparities among minorities to improve the overall health of these groups.

Health Promotion and Illness/Injury Prevention

Healthy People 2020

The Federal Government recognized the need for renewed focus on the healthcare needs of the elderly by adding a specific topic area of Older Adults to Healthy People 2020 that identifies health objectives relevant to this population. Some of the objectives have implications for the education of older adults and their families, while other objectives are specifically geared toward health education and reaching educational objectives. **Table 5-1** lists Healthy People topic areas and objectives that can be used in health education programs appropriate for older adults. In addition to health-related educational topics, older adults often want information about second

TABLE 5-1	Healthy People 2020 Topics and Objectives That Have Implications for Older Adults
Topic	**Objectives**
Older Adults (OA)	• Increase the proportion of older adults who use the Welcome to Medicare benefit. • Increase the proportion of older adults with one or more chronic health conditions who report confidence in managing their conditions. • Increase the proportion of older adults who receive Diabetes Self-Management Benefits. • Reduce the proportion of older adults who have moderate to severe functional limitations. • Increase the proportion of older adults with reduced physical or cognitive function who engage in light, moderate, or vigorous leisure-time physical activities.
Arthritis, Osteoporosis, and Chronic Back Conditions (AOCBC)	• Reduce the proportion of adults with doctor-diagnosed arthritis who experience a limitation in activity due to arthritis or joint symptoms. • Reduce the proportion of adults with doctor-diagnosed arthritis who have difficulty in performing two or more personal care activities, thereby preserving independence. • Increase the proportion of adults with doctor-diagnosed arthritis who receive healthcare provider counseling. • Increase the proportion of adults with doctor-diagnosed arthritis who have had effective, evidence-based arthritis education as an integral part of the management of their condition. • Reduce hip fractures among older adults.
Cancer (C)	• Increase the proportion of adults who were counseled about cancer screening consistent with current guidelines.

career choices, exercise, hobbies, retirement, employment issues, volunteerism, financial management, legal concerns, and quality-of-life.

The Patient Protection and Affordable Care Act of 2010

The Patient Protection and Affordable Care Act of 2010 provides specific benefits to Medicare recipients, including educational interventions such as tobacco use cessation counseling and medical nutrition therapy to help people with diabetes or kidney disease manage their diet and care (U.S. Department of Health and Human Services [U.S. DHHS], 2012d). Older adults will need to be made aware of health promotion and medical screening options that are available to them under changing healthcare legislation. Programs should be developed to teach older adults basic computer skills so that they can access information on the Internet that will enhance their health.

Topic	Objectives
Diabetes (D)	• Increase the proportion of persons with diagnosed diabetes who receive formal diabetes education. • Increase prevention behaviors in persons at high risk for diabetes with prediabetes.
Disability and Health (DH)	• Reduce the proportion of older adults with disabilities who use inappropriate medications.
Educational and Community-Based Programs (ECBP-1)	• Increase the number of community-based organizations providing population-based primary prevention services.
Food Safety (FS)	• Increase the proportion of consumers who follow key food safety practices.
Heart Disease and Stroke (HDS)	• Increase the proportion of adults with elevated LDL cholesterol who have been advised by a healthcare provider regarding cholesterol-lowering management, including lifestyle changes and, if indicated, medication. • Increase the proportion of adults aged 20 years and older who are aware of, and respond to, early warning symptoms and signs of a heart attack. • Increase the proportion of adults aged 20 years and older who are aware of and respond to early warning symptoms and signs of a stroke.
Nutrition and Weight Status (NWS)	• Increase the proportion of physician office visits that include counseling or education related to physical activity.
Respiratory Diseases (RD)	• Increase the proportion of persons with current asthma who receive formal patient education.
Tobacco Use (TU)	• Increase tobacco cessation counseling in healthcare settings.

Educating tomorrow's older adults presents significant challenges to healthcare providers. When one considers that the span of years of older adulthood generally starts at age 65 and can continue to 100+ years of age, many factors can affect the ability of individual older adults to learn. Differences in age cohorts' educational levels, gender roles, work experiences, cultural and spiritual values and beliefs, and physical health can influence both motivation and ability to learn.

Gerontological Nursing: Scope and Standards

Nurses in all settings are expected to educate patients and their families. The American Nurses Association in collaboration with the National Gerontological Nursing Association developed the document *Gerontological Nursing: Scope and Standards of Practice* (2010), which identifies two standards that require nurses working with older adults to include health education of patients/clients, their families, consumers, and other health professionals in their practice. Standards of Practice standard 5B addresses health teaching and health promotion for patients, their families, and the community, and Standards of Professional Performance standard 9 addresses the nurse's responsibility for continuing her/his own knowledge development in the specialty and the knowledge of other healthcare providers.

The demographic factors discussed below influence how healthcare providers should structure education for older adults. Nurses must refocus on issues of education in gerontology and the effect of educational interventions on healthcare outcomes. Healthcare educators in industry, the community, rural and urban settings, colleges and universities, adult daycare centers, senior centers, hospices, continuing care retirement centers, and assisted living centers are expected to provide information on topics of interest not only to older adults, but also to adults who are anticipating and planning for their retirement years. Educational topics may include health promotion and illness/injury prevention, management of chronic disease, nutrition, exercise, retirement, employment issues, intergenerational issues, second career choices, financial management, legal concerns, and quality-of-life issues.

Principles of Adult Learning

Historically, formal education and learning were considered of little value for anyone over 50 years old. With few people living many years beyond the retirement age of 65, formal education was not considered necessary or beneficial. Learning in past decades may have been considered a selfish, self-centered desire. Working past 65 years of age was unwarranted unless financial strains dictated it. Social attitudes about learning after a certain age were gauged by how much time was left to live after retirement (Crawford, 2005).

Changes in thinking about *adult learning* began in the post-World War II era when the GI Bill of Rights resulted in millions of veterans being given the opportunity to attend college, promoting the idea that college degrees were not only for the wealthy, but also for the common person (Sheppard, 2002; U.S. Department of Veterans Affairs, 2012). This generation began to change people's way of thinking about adult learning and introduced the concept of *lifelong learning*, which resulted in an educational culture shift. The increased number of educated adults fostered economic productivity as well as improved the quality of life of adults (Crawford, 2005).

Beyond Age 65

With increasing life expectancy for both men and women, retirement at age 65 seems to be early for many older adults, given that people live 20 to 30 years beyond the usual retirement age. Adding to the generation of older adults who were born between 1920 and 1945 (considered the "silent generation" or "veteran generation") are the *baby boomers*, those born between 1946 and 1964, who currently account for millions of Americans in the workforce. It is predicted that as baby boomers retire there will be a labor shortage, with many choosing to return to the workforce either full- or part-time in the same career or in a second career after "retirement." These events may increase the need for new formal and informal educational opportunities for older adults (see **Figure 5-1**). Education for older adults will also be encouraged by the increasing availability of educational offerings, more grants and scholarships, and the change in societal norms where lifelong learning is socially acceptable and used for a variety of reasons including socialization, self-enrichment, and training for new skills.

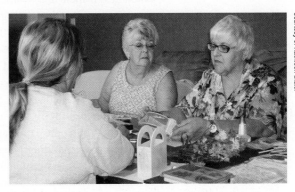

Courtesy of Kathleen Blais.

Figure 5-1 Older ladies meeting to learn a new craft and socialize.

Educational needs of older adults can be met in formal and informal settings including secondary schools, vocational/technical education programs, colleges and universities; university campus-based senior living and learning communities; in community settings such as homes, healthcare facilities, civic organizations, senior centers, support and social groups, and long-term care facilities; elder travel groups; and on the Internet. Because lifelong learning and education have been correlated with a delay in cognitive impairment with aging, their importance is relevant not only for the reasons cited earlier, but also for improved health and cognition (Diamond, 2001).

Theory of Adult Learning

Malcolm Knowles's *theory of adult learning* (1988), which is often used in the development, planning and implementation of adult educational programs, identifies motivation and relevance as key concepts in adults' learning. The term *androgogy* was coined to describe the unique characteristics of teaching and learning of adults. Adults expect respect for their abilities and experience; are autonomous, self-directed, independent learners; are goal oriented; and need to know that what they are learning is relevant and practical to their daily lives. They expect to actively participate in learning and build on previous life experiences. Adults derive much of their self-identity from past experiences, and nurses should use this knowledge when planning and implementing educational programs.

Theory of Self Efficacy

Another theory that may be useful in planning educational programs for older adults is the *theory of self-efficacy*. Bandura (1994) defines self-efficacy as "people's beliefs about their capabilities to produce designated levels of performance that exercise influence over events that affect their lives" (p. 71). Self-efficacy theory suggests that persons' self-efficacy is related to their belief that their actions influence outcomes in their life. Resnick (2002) elaborated on the self-efficacy theory from a nursing perspective stating that "self-efficacy and outcome expectations affect behavior, motivational level, thought patterns, and emotional reactions in response to any situation" (p. 1). The concept of self-efficacy includes behavior, cognitive factors, the environment, and the outcomes desired. Older adults can learn to compensate for declines in physical health by maximizing their intellectual capabilities of increased knowledge, skill, and experience. Self-efficacy theory is based on *social cognitive theory* (SCT), also called social learning theory. Social cognitive theory teaches that outcome expectations are the beliefs that certain outcomes will result if certain corresponding behaviors are performed (Billek-Sawhney & Reicherter, 2004). For example, in using SCT in the education of an older adult with a hip fracture, therapists found that a woman attending and participating in physical therapy (the behavior) saw improvement in her physical status that produced a positive belief (cognitive factor) that she could be successful. She continued an exercise class after discharge that was focused toward seniors (the environment), and this further strengthened her belief that her actions made a difference in her health outcomes as she participated and saw positive results in her physical strength and flexibility (Billek-Sawhney & Reicherter, 2004).

Older adults may need extra encouragement to engage in learning activities. *Gerogogy* is defined by Martha Tyler John (1988) as "the process involved in stimulating and helping older persons to learn" (p. 12). It is further described as the art and science of teaching older adults, involving teaching strategies that lead them to higher levels of empowerment and emancipation (Formosa, 2001; Thomas, 2007). Older adults can benefit from adjustments to teaching methods that consider impairments in the sensory, psychomotor, cognitive, and affective learning domains (Reynolds, 2005).

In addition, preferences for instructional methods relate to how individuals feel they learn best. For example, an older adult who is a visual learner may prefer to view posters or bulletin boards with educational information so that they may learn at their own pace (Thomas, 2007). Self-monitoring has been shown to improve the effectiveness of learning, and it reinforces the principle that adults are independent learners (Dunlosky et al., 2007). Conversely, an older adult who learns best through auditory means may prefer listening to a lecture or audiotapes. Someone who relates to learning using a more hands-on approach may retain knowledge best when there are experiential activities that require demonstration and return demonstration. For older adults with sensory impairments in vision or hearing or other physical limitations that affect learning, using multiple approaches can help compensate for limitations. For example, an older woman who describes herself as a visual learner but has visual limitations may benefit from a combination of visual materials created specifically for the visually impaired and listening to an audiotape that aligns with the visual presentation. Any and all of these means for educating older adults should be considered, keeping in mind that all learners may have unique preferences and learning styles.

Older Adults and Lifelong Learning

As the number of older adults increases and many are more visibly engaged in the daily recreational, cultural, and civic activities of the community, attitudes about aging have changed. Older adults are increasingly participating in retirement planning workshops to prepare for the next stage of life. Although older adults still expect the traditional retirement, 70% plan to work post-retirement in positions related to teaching, office support, crafts, retail sales, or health care (American Association for Retired Persons [AARP], 2008). Reasons cited by those planning to work into retirement are financial, enjoyment derived from working, and having something interesting to do. Many businesses provide training, retraining, cross-training, mentoring, shadowing, and career counseling for retirees who want to continue in the workplace. Despite the trends that support post-retirement employment, 60% of older adults have concerns that age discrimination will be a major barrier in the workplace. The Age Discrimination in Employment Act of 1967 was passed to protect workers older than 40 from discrimination in the workplace, including discrimination in hiring, promotion, and early retirement based on age (U.S. Equal Employment Opportunity Commission, 2012).

Learning in Late Life

Older adults have very specific ideas concerning how and what they want to learn (see **Boxes 5-1** and **5-2**).

For older adults who desire more formal education, many colleges or universities offer discounted or tuition-free courses. These courses may be in the traditional schedule format or on a less traditional schedule; they may be onsite or online. Other educational programs are often offered at no charge through alumni organizations, healthcare facilities, local school districts, labor organizations, banks/investment organizations, and specific industries. Industries offer workforce-related education and training. In addition, a variety of educational programs are offered for the older adult through national organizations (see **Table 5-2**)

BOX 5-1 Learning Preferences of Older Adults

Older adults prefer:

- Methods that are easy to access, require small investments of time and money to get started, and allow learning to begin immediately.

- Methods that are direct, hands-on experiences—putting hands on something, playing with it, listening to it, watching it, and thinking about it.

- Newspapers, magazines, books, and journals are the most frequently used tools for gathering information.

- Methods that enable them to keep up with what's going on in the world, for their own spiritual or personal growth, and/or for the simple joy of learning something new.

- Subjects that will improve the quality of their lives, build upon a current skill, or enable them to take better care of their health.

- Ability to use what they have learned right away or in the near future.

Source: Adapted from AARP Survey on Lifelong Learning. (2000). Retrieved from assets.aarp.org/rgcenter/general/lifelong.pdf

BOX 5-2 Learning Interests of Older Adults

- Retirement planning

- Financial planning

- Diet, nutrition, cooking

- Exercise, sport

- Weight control

- Stress management and relaxation activities

- Health and medicine

- Complementary and alternative therapies

- Creative activities, e.g., woodworking, sculpture, painting, craft

- Spirituality, re-creation, and personal growth

- Recreation

- Life skills, e.g., reading, writing

- Computer and other technology skills

- Art and cultural activities

- Travel for pleasure and learning

- Volunteering and community involvement

- Political activity

TABLE 5-2 Educational Programs and Internet Sites for Older Adults

Program	Web Address	Description
Elderhostel	http://www.roadscholar.org	A nonprofit organization dedicated to providing learning adventures for individuals 65 and older. Programs are available locally, nationally and internationally.
Administration on Aging (AoA)	http://www.aoa.gov	Provides a comprehensive overview of a wide variety of topics, programs, and services related to aging.
USA.gov for seniors	http://www.usa.gov/topics/seniors.shtml	Official U.S. gateway to all government information specific to the older adult
OASIS	http://www.oasisnet.org	A national nonprofit educational organization designed to enhance the quality of life for mature adults; offers challenging programs in the arts, humanities, wellness, technology, and volunteer service. Creates opportunities for older adults to continue their personal growth and provide meaningful service to the community.
Seniornet	http://www.seniornet.org	A nonprofit organization whose mission is "to provide older adults education for and access to computer technologies."
Shepherd's Centers	http://www.shepherdcenters.org	A network of interfaith community volunteer organizations that serves the needs of older adults in four areas: life maintenance, life enrichment, life reorganization, and life celebration.
AARP	http://www.aarp.org	The American Association of Retired Persons shares information to adults 55 and older on retirement, government programs, and educational opportunities. To benefit from sponsored programs, one must have a membership.

Barriers to Older Adults' Learning

Older adults may experience some unique barriers to learning. These include chronic illness, normal physiologic changes that occur with aging, *health disparities*, and other factors related to *cultural diversity*.

Chronic Illness

Chronic illnesses increase with advanced age and can present barriers to learning among older adults. Some type of disability (i.e., difficulty in hearing, vision, cognition, ambulation, self-care, or independent living) was reported by 37% of older persons in 2010. Some of these disabilities may be relatively minor, but others cause people to require assistance to meet important personal needs (Administration on Aging, 2011). In 2005, about 34 million persons reported being limited in their daily activities due to one or more chronic health problems. The National Health Interview Survey of 2005 reported that 44% of adults age 75 years or older felt they had limitations in their usual activities, and nearly one-third of adults over age 75 rated their health as fair or poor (Adams, Dey, & Vickerie, 2007). Heart attack and stroke are two of the chronic problems resulting in early retirement among Americans (National Institute on Aging/National Institutes of Health [NIA/NIH], 2007). Almost three-fourths (73.6%) of those age 80 and older report at least one disability. Healthcare providers must be aware of the challenges that chronic health conditions may place on a person's motivation and ability to learn. Strategies to facilitate learning and overcome the obstacles that chronic illness may cause must be considered; these may include having large print handouts for older adults with visual impairment or providing frequent breaks for older adults with arthritis, respiratory disease, or urinary frequency.

Specific barriers to education may include cognitive, affective, sensory, and psychomotor barriers. Older adults may have unique physical or cognitive limitations that affect learning ability. Physical and psychological changes that can affect learning are listed in **Box 5-3**. Cognitive barriers may include illnesses like Alzheimer's disease, dementia, or memory loss after a stroke. Ten percent of persons over age 70 have moderate or severe cognitive decline (NIA/NIH, 2007). Affective disorders may include depression and mood disorders. Sensory barriers can include hearing loss (presbycusis), visual changes (presbyopia), glaucoma, and cataracts. Psychomotor barriers may include decreased mobility related to chronic illnesses such as arthritis, or problems such as Parkinson's disease, stroke, and pulmonary diseases that affect the use of teaching tools or computers. Strategies for working with persons with memory problems such as those that occur with dementia are discussed in Chapters 4 and 10.

BOX 5-3   Physical and Psychological Changes in the Older Adult That Can Affect Learning

- Impaired vision
- Impaired hearing
- Decreased sense of taste and smell
- Limited mobility or range of motion
- Decreased reflexes
- Chronic illness

- Chronic pain
- Fatigue
- Stress
- Dementia
- Depression

Multidimensional motor sequence learning may be impaired in older adults. Boyd, Vidoni, and Siengsukon (2008) examined task sequencing that involved repeated tests of motor, spatial, and temporal dimensions and retention and found that the motor element was the most important for motor learning. Their results suggested "an age-related impairment in motor learning" (p. 351) that was found among healthy elderly in the study. Older adults did not seem to benefit from practicing a repeated sequence to improve motor performance.

Literacy

The literacy levels of older adults may be an additional barrier to learning. The National Literacy Act of 1991 defines *literacy* as "an individual's ability to read, write, and speak in English, and compute and solve problems at levels of proficiency necessary to function on the job and in society, to achieve one's goals, and develop one's knowledge and potential" (The Talking Page Literacy Organization, n.d., p. 2).

In a 1996 study of literacy in older adults (National Center for Educational Statistics [NCES], 1997), 71% of adults age 60 or over had limited reading skills, 68% had difficulty in quantitative skills, and 80% had difficulty in filling out forms. Younger Americans had better literacy skills than older Americans, and native English speakers had better literacy skills than non-native English speakers. Older adults in the study were more likely to have visual impairments that affected their ability to read and process printed information. In 2004 it was estimated that about 90 million people (or 74% of older American adults) had some problem accessing, reading, interpreting, or using healthcare information (Billek-Sawhney & Reicherter, 2005; Hixon, 2004).

However, given that literacy levels increase as the level of education increases, this dynamic is changing. According to the U.S. Census Bureau (2012), it is now estimated that the percentage of older persons who completed high school increased from 28% to 79.5%, and 22.5% of older adults had a bachelor's degree or higher. The percentage who had completed high school varied considerably by race and ethnic origin in 2010: 84.3% of Whites, 73.6% of Asians, 64.8% of Blacks, and 47.0% of Hispanics had at least a high-school diploma. The increase in educational levels is also evident within these groups; in 1970, for example, only 30% of older Whites and 9% of older Blacks were high school graduates (U.S. Census Bureau, 2012).

Health Literacy

The U.S. Department of Health and Human Services (2012a) defines *health literacy* as, "The degree to which individuals have the capacity to obtain, process, and understand basic health information and services needed to make appropriate health decisions" (p. 1). Older adults have a higher incidence of low health literacy, especially those of minority populations, low socioeconomic status, or who are medically underserved. People who have low health literacy may have greater difficulty in "locating providers and services, filling out complex health forms, sharing their medical history with providers, seeking preventive health care, knowing the connection between risky behaviors and health, managing chronic health conditions, and understanding directions on medicine" (U.S. DHHS, 2012c, p. 1). Healthy People 2020 identified a topic area of Health Communication and Health Information Technology, which includes the objective "to increase the health literacy of the population" (U.S. DHHS, 2012b, p.1). Given the extensive list of topics and objectives in Healthy People 2020 related to the health education needs of older adults, the ability of the individual to understand instructions on over-the-counter and prescription drug bottles; appointment slips; health education brochures; written and verbal instructions on medications, diet, and illness management; consent forms; and advance directives, along with the ability to negotiate complex healthcare systems, becomes necessary if one is to take advantage of educational opportunities in one's older years. The skills needed for health literacy are similar to the skills for general literacy, but with specific knowledge and skill sets specific to health care. Patients are often asked to analyze information, calculate medication doses, interpret information given by healthcare providers, and make life and death decisions with terminology that sounds like a foreign language. To accomplish these tasks, the individual must be able to read, complete simple math calculations, ask appropriate questions of the healthcare provider, and evaluate their own care needs.

Low literacy is correlated with poorer health status (per self-report) and increased knowledge deficit about health status. Acknowledging low literacy skills can be

---

BOX 5-4   Research Highlight

Purpose: The purpose of this study was to determine if an association existed among health literacy, memory performance, and performance-based functional ability in community-residing older adults.

Methods: The sample consisted of 45 adults whose mean age was 77.11 years and average number of years of education was 15.33. The Rivermead Behavioral Memory Test (RBMT), which classifies individuals into four categories of memory (normal, poor, mildly impaired, severely impaired), was used to recruit participants in two categories: normal (n=31) or impaired (n=14). Health literacy scores were measured using the Rapid Estimate of Adult Literacy in Medicine.

Findings: Health literacy scores were high (M=65.09, SD=2.80) with 34 (76%) of the

participants scoring 66 out of a possible 80. Pearson correlations demonstrated a significant relationship with health literacy scores and education and cognition, memory performance, and performance-based instrumental activities.

Application to practice: Nurses must be aware of both literacy and health literacy levels in their patient population and ensure that effective means of patient education are developed that consider the individual client's potential for understanding health information.

Source: McDougall, G. J. Jr., Mackert, M., and Becker, H. (2012). Memory performance, health literacy, and instrumental activities of daily living of community residing older adults. *Nursing Research, 61*(1), 70–75.

embarrassing to patients; therefore, educators must determine the scope of the problem in their own communities and patient populations and develop culturally sensitive strategies to assist in improving knowledge and enhancing health outcomes. Older adults may be literate in their work environment, but when confronted with "health" issues, have low literacy. For these reasons, it is recommended that nurses currently working with older adults use educational materials that are geared toward the fifth-grade level or lower. Strategies to improve readability of materials for older adults include:

> Keep the format and content simple, teaching one topic at a time.
> Use shorter words and sentences (try to substitute one- to two-syllable words for multisyllabic words where possible). Test paragraph literacy using the SMOG test.
> Use lay language for complex medical terms and ensure that translation is accurate.
> Increase the use of illustrations, pictures, and diagrams.
> Use larger font size (14 or greater) and plain type (e.g., Times New Roman, Arial, Calibri).
> Select contrasting colors for text and background—darker colors for text and lighter colors for background. Dark blue on pale yellow is preferable to black on white.
> Use the active voice in brochures or pamphlets

However, in addition to these general guidelines, nurses need to assess the learning needs of the particular individual or group with whom they are working in order to adapt teaching appropriately.

Technology for Older Adults' Lifelong Learning

According to a 2008 Pew Internet Survey on older adults and use of the Internet, 70% of those age 50–64 and 38% of adults 65 or older reported using the Internet. The fastest growing group of people learning to use the Internet is those 55 and older. Madden (2010) found that social networking use among Internet users 50 years of age and older nearly doubled between 2009 and 2010, so that now one-half of Internet users between the ages 50 and 64 and 26% of users age 65 and older used social networking sites. Older adults are more likely to use email than social networking, with 89% of adults 65 and over who use the Internet sending or receiving an email on a typical day. Additionally, "among Internet users ages 65 and older, 62% look for news online" (Madden, p. 4), with 34% doing so on a typical day. Older adults who were living with chronic disease used the Internet for blogging and participating in online health discussions. The process of aging may present challenges to older adults who wish to use computers to enhance learning, but it is clear that many older adults are embracing the use of computers and the Internet in some aspect of their lives. Barriers to the use of computers and the Internet for older adults include the cost of computers and

Case Study 5-1

Marjorie Hanes is 70 years old. She always wanted to learn how to speak Spanish and enrolled in the local college, despite having a hearing impairment. She was enjoying her classes as she continued her responsibilities in her home, including caring for her husband who had hypertension. Unfortunately, her husband suffered a stroke and Ms. Hanes had to assume the responsibility of primary caregiver for him, resulting in her withdrawing from college. She purchased some audiovisuals to help her practice her Spanish. When her husband recovered from his stroke, Ms. Hanes was able to reenroll at the college; however, her hearing loss had become worse over time, which made it difficult to continue learning a language in class. Ms. Hanes decided to continue using books and audiotapes to learn Spanish but she also had a new interest in plants and used educational programs on television to learn more about horticulture and working in her garden.

These activities provided Ms. Hanes with educational activities in the home while she continued to care for her husband, who died 3 years later. After her husband's death, Ms. Hanes was feeling isolated and decided to go back to the college and continue her learning. She found a cohort of older adults who were also interested in continuing their education in a variety of ways. At this time, Ms. Hanes was enjoying art and took a class in art history—something she had always wanted to learn more about. Taking this class was not hindered by her hearing loss. She visited art galleries and was involved in group discussions that were led by the class participants under supervision of the instructor. As an older adult, Ms. Hanes was engaged in a variety of learning experiences that changed over time because of circumstances in her life.

Questions:

1. How has Ms. Hanes incorporated lifelong learning into her older years?

2. How has Ms. Hanes adapted to the challenges she has faced to overcome barriers and continue her lifelong learning?

3. How might technology have been used to help Ms. Hanes continue her learning when her husband became ill?

4. In your role as a nurse educator, what would you recommend to Ms. Hanes to enhance her education or to meet her lifelong learning needs?

access to the Internet, concerns about being able to learn how to use a computer, and fears about privacy and security of computers and the Internet. Some of the challenges associated with the use of computer technology can be overcome (see **Table 5-3**).

As the baby boomers enter the 65-and-older age group, these statistics will change because of this generation's comfort with technology. Prior and continued experience in the use of computers and other modern technology affects attitudes and improves outcomes of subsequent training, so the learning needs of the computer literate will change over time. New challenges in technology use for older adults include use of cell phones, smart phones, and tablets as they integrate these devices into improved health care (see **Figure 5-2**). Seniors can often learn how to use computer technology at public libraries, learning centers, and commercial businesses that sell electronic

TABLE 5-3   Aging Alterations That Can Be Overcome By Using Computer Technology

Alteration	Effect On Computer Use	Possible Solutions
Decreased hearing	Sound from computer may not be heard	Use of external speakers and headphones to enhance sound
Decreased visual acuity	Need for bifocals, viewing monitor size may be too small, alteration in light/color distinction due to glaucoma &/or cataracts	Adjust monitor tilt to decrease glare Get larger monitor Change size of font to 14–16 Adjust contrast to assure clarity Adjust screen resolution to promote color contrast
Motor control or tremors Arthritis	May affect use of keyboard or control of mouse	Use "larger" mouse Use control arrows to move through text Purchase "touch screen" or voice-activated computer
Attention span	Inability to focus for extended periods of time and to comprehend new informational subjects	Programs contain small modules of information Repetition of last concept in each new module Utilization of multimedia presentations (PowerPoint, streaming video, summary sheets)

devices. Telemedicine services, which utilize technology to connect clients with healthcare providers, are another promising option to increase access to healthcare services for older adults, especially those living in rural areas or those who have limited mobility. These are discussed in detail in Chapter 33.

Technologic Aids to Learning

Many healthcare agencies have developed their own Web pages and health portals to adapt education for older adult viewers (**Box 5-5**). Web pages can be developed in different languages to provide health information to people whose primary language is not English. Web page usability issues related to the older adult include design, font size, colors, and clear instructions (Table 5-3; see Chapter 33 for further information). Navigation tasks and the format of the Web page may challenge cognitively impaired persons. The organization of the Web page should be consistent, with small segments and simple language. Instructions to website developers for the

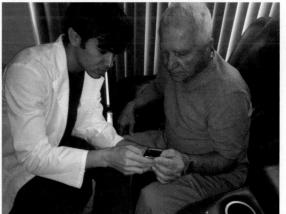

Courtesy of Sergio Medina.

Figure 5-2 Nurse teaching older patient to program his smart phone with a medication reminder.

development of multimedia for health education purposes should be clearly stated, and plain text should be available as an option. Tips for designing a Web page for older adults are listed in Chapter 33. Application of these principles can be seen at http://nihseniorhealth.gov.

BOX 5-5   Recommended Internet Resources for Teaching Older Adults

Administration on Aging (AoA):

http://www.AoA.gov

American Association for Retired Persons (AARP):

http://www.aarp.org

American Society on Aging (ASA):

http://www.asaging.org

Association for Continuing Higher Education:

http://www.acheinc.org

Association for Gerontology in Higher Education (AGHE):

http://www.aghe.org

Gerontological Society of America (GSA):

http://www.geron.org

The John A. Hartford Foundation Institute for Geriatric Nursing:

http://www.hartfordign.org

National Council on Aging (NCOA):

http://www.ncoa.org

National Gerontological Nurses Association (NGNA):

http://www.ngna.org

National Institute on Aging (NIA):

http://www.nia.nih.gov

Osher Lifelong Learning Institute:

http://www.olli.gmu.edu

Additional web resources for health education are available for specific disease processes from focused organizations including the American Heart Association, American Diabetes Association, Alzheimer's Association, etc.

Cultural Diversity and Health Disparities Among Older Adults

The issues of cultural diversity and health disparities cannot be ignored when considering educational issues for older adults. Diversity in terms of age, race, ethnicity, gender, sexual orientation, and socioeconomic status is an important factor to consider. By 2050, more than one-third of Blacks (12%), Hispanics (20%), and Asians (9%) combined will be 65 years of age or older and will need health education consistent with their cultural values and beliefs (Federal Interagency Forum on Aging-Related Statistics, 2010). Of particular significance is that the proportion of Hispanic individuals age 65 and older is expected to triple in the next decades. Older White Americans are twice as likely to report very good or excellent health as elderly Hispanics or Blacks (NIA/NIH, 2007). According to U.S. DHHS (2010), racial and ethnic minorities have higher rates of obesity, cancer, diabetes, and AIDS than their White counterparts. Forty-eight percent of Black adults have a chronic illness compared to 39% of the general population. Hispanic and Vietnamese women have twice the rate of White women for rates of cervical cancer. For groups where English is a second language, public health information is limited, and there are few bilingual healthcare providers. Strategies found to be effective for educating Hispanic adults with diabetes have included educational sessions, written materials in both English and Spanish (especially fact sheets), including family in teaching sessions, and using culturally appropriate interventions (Whittemore, 2007). These same strategies may be useful for older persons of other racial/ethnic groups. As the diversity of America increases, nurses must become better educated in the cultural norms and health needs of persons from various ethnic groups. A discussion of diversity and health disparities among the major ethnic groups appears in Chapter 2.

The disparities in disease incidence of racially diverse older populations suggest that there may be additional social and economic disadvantages related to minority groups that deserve special attention. There are greater disparities in healthcare access and delivery in later life among diverse groups. Culture and race influence how and what older adults from minority groups will want to learn. Of great concern is that many minority elderly do not use English as a first language. With this in mind, many print materials and Internet educational pages now are provided in a variety of languages. Nurses should learn about the literacy and education levels of all elders in the community where they serve (see **Figure 5-3**).

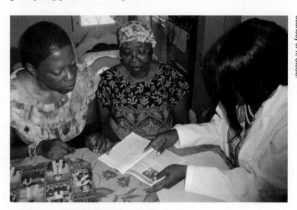

Courtesy of K. Steele.

Figure 5-3 Nurse teaching older patient and her daughter about her chronic illness.

Implications for Gerontological Educators

Education must meet the needs of the older adult, and these needs change depending on many factors including diversity, development of additional chronic diseases and the resulting limited functional abilities as one ages, availability of social support systems including family, and financial resources. The older adult cohort is not a homogeneous group, but is composed of persons of different cultures, races, educational levels, and socioeconomic statuses, all of which are factors that can influence learning. A rapidly growing pool of college-educated adults is reaching their retirement years. This is an exciting period for lifelong learning, which is now viewed as helping older adults improve their quality of life and adding meaning and creativity to their retirement years (Timmermann, 2005). As people live longer with chronic illness, there is a need to learn new life skills related to illness/injury prevention, health promotion, disease management, managing finances, and improving or maintaining quality of life. Educators must be able to evaluate individual and group educational requirements and develop programs that make appropriate use of technology.

Strategies for Teaching Older Adults and Their Caregivers

Education of older adults must be flexible. Nurses may teach at the bedside in acute care, in the home with individual patients and their families, or in group classes provided by healthcare organizations.

Strategies for Teaching Older Adults Individually

Older adults need to have a motivation to learn, so be certain to explain the purpose of the educational session at the beginning. In order to make the purpose of the education obvious, the objectives for any presentation must be clear and the content appropriate to the needs of the learner. Scheduling teaching time in advance with clear explanations of what will be taught will allow the learner time to mentally prepare for the session. It is best to let the learner(s) know when the teaching will take place; this allows the learner and family members to write down questions they may have in advance so they don't leave the session with their questions unanswered.

To assure success in any educational encounter with older adults, it is important to be respectful and helpful: respectful of what they have experienced and already know, and helpful in providing for what they do not know. Establishing a rapport with the learner and his/her family can be done by discussing what they expect from the session, what they already know about the topic, and how they prefer to learn. It is always necessary to evaluate the learner's readiness to learn by determining if there is any immediate stress or anxiety present, as these can interfere with the ability to take in and remember new information. If the learner is experiencing chronic pain, ensure that he/she has received medication prior to the learning session. Assure that the environment is free from distractions, is private and comfortable, and as conducive to learning as possible.

During the learning session, sit facing the older adult (and family members) and make sure that any personal adaptive equipment (hearing aids, glasses) is in place prior to starting the session. Allow sufficient time for questions. Have the learners repeat back to you what they have learned to ensure accurate understanding of the material. Have written materials available that are appropriate to the topic, learning style, and have been literacy tested. After presenting the information and allowing time for discussion, use the "teach-back technique" to evaluate understanding—this process allows the teacher to confirm that he/she has given clear instruction and re-teach material that is not understood. Provide written materials that the learner may take with them to reinforce the instruction. When the session is completed, document the teaching that has been done in the appropriate patient document and include copies of all handouts provided.

Strategies for Teaching Older Adults in Groups

Presentations to older adults and their families can take place in a variety of locations that include, but are not limited to, senior centers, independent living, assisted living, places of religious worship, hospital conference rooms, long-term care facilities, and libraries. Nurse educators should prepare for the sessions so that learners get the most from the presentation. **Box 5-6** highlights some ways to assure success in such a presentation. Some facilities have already gathered information from the participants on the topics of choice. It is always good to know the average age of the learners, any specific health concerns of the group, expected attendance, and any special needs of the participants. If possible, try to observe the participants at the facility where you will be teaching. Make sure the setting of the presentation is conducive to learning. If the attendees are known to have chronic illness such as chronic obstructive pulmonary disease (COPD), arthritis, or cardiac disease, make sure that the location can support comfortable seating and, if needed, allows oxygen in the room. Visit the location/facility ahead of time whenever possible to assess the learning environment. Talk to the facility director/group leader/learners to identify exactly what topic they expect you to present. Make sure that the date is publicized so the greatest number of learners can be present. Use brochures, community newsletters, newspaper bulletin boards, signs, and posters to advertise the program within the facility and, if permitted, in the community. Make sure that the time is convenient and does not interfere with other planned activities (e.g., games, crafts, exercise groups, meals). When considering the topic and needs of the learners, check that the time of the presentation is not too long. If there is a great deal of information to present, consider breaking the presentation into two or three sessions of 30 minutes to an hour; each session can briefly review prior learning and add new content.

BOX 5-6   Web Exploration

Visit http://nihseniorhealth.gov and evaluate its friendliness to an older adult user. Consider the font size, readability, and literacy level of the health education materials. Note the various teaching modalities for older adults.

Arrive early to greet attendees as they enter. Older adults feel more at ease if they get to meet the presenter and are more likely to ask questions if they see the speaker as approachable. Make sure everyone is settled and comfortable before starting. The atmosphere should be conducive to the older adult, including maintaining a comfortable temperature, lack of external noise and distractions, accessible bathroom facilities, and frequent breaks built into the time frame. If necessary, use a microphone so all participants can hear.

Assure enough time for questions. It is a good idea to provide paper and pencils so questions can be written down. Don't wait until the end for opening up to questions—answering questions during the presentation can not only be a gauge for measuring understanding of the material, but can also lead the speaker to reframe the content to meet the immediate needs of the group.

Confirm that your teaching materials are elder-friendly. Use multimedia teaching aides and, whenever possible, plan takeaway items that enhance the topic presented—for example, if talking about medication safety, give medication organizers. Handouts should be reviewed to make sure they are at the proper literacy level (as discussed earlier in this chapter). It is also a good idea to give sources for the material presented. If talking about heart health, for example, give the most current American Heart Association information handouts.

If planning group activities, keep them short and appropriate to the topic. If a game is appropriate (bingo, Jeopardy-like questions), assure all participants have the chance to "play." It is a good idea to make sure everyone leaves with something, whether it is a handout on the topic or a small item such as a pill organizer or some other useful item.

BOX 5-7   Preparing a Short Educational Program for Older Adults and Families

1. Assure that the goal of the presentation is to provide information that the group is interested in. Work with the facility to be certain that the date and time of the presentation does not interfere with other regularly planned activities.

2. If the program being presented is for a regularly scheduled support group for elders with chronic disease and their families, make sure that the information is specific to the needs of the group. For example, if the session is about coping with COPD, assure that the content is specific to the needs of the elder (medications, activity, oxygen use) as well as the family in assisting them to cope with the challenges that the disease presents.

3. The information presented should be relevant to the group both in content and format. Ask older adults who may attend what topics they are interested in and want to know more about.

4. The more current research done on the subject, the more comfortable the presenter will be. If a health-related topic, assure application of the principles of health literacy.

5. For the program itself, employ strategies appropriate to teaching older adults (Box 5-8).

6. Plan at least one interactive activity to increase group participation; this can aid in overall understanding of the presented material.

7. Intersperse questions throughout the class to:

    a. Evaluate understanding by learners and allow changes in presentation.

    b. Allow learners to feel connected to the presentation by answering questions and making them feel that each question is important and will add to the material already presented.

    c. Encourage participants to share their personal stories, as this will make the presentation more realistic to those participants.

8. Be flexible. Allow extra break time if needed and plan to stay after the program to answer individual questions as necessary.

BOX 5-8 Strategies for Teaching Older Adults

Use the principles of adult learning theory.

- Assess readiness to learn
- Involve the audience in the presentation
- Draw the learners into the discussion
- Provide reasons for them to learn by pointing out the significance of the topic

Use multiple teaching modalities to keep the material interesting and maintain attention.

- PowerPoint slides
- DVDs
- Handouts, brochures, or pamphlets
- Posters
- Demonstration/samples
- Quizzes/games
- Social media, e.g., YouTube
- Internet websites

Remember to accommodate any unusual physical needs.

- Avoid glare; control environmental temperature and noise level
- Use a microphone and speak slowly
- Face the audience as many elders lip read to fill in what they cannot hear

- Limit content to 30–40 minutes so questions can be answered
- Handouts should be in large font
- Make sure the room is large enough for the number of learners and their adaptive equipment
- If possible, have a helper to assist learners who need to leave for any reason or who come late

Make presentations elder-friendly

- Choose content that elders are interested in, such as advance directives, nutrition, heart health, medication safety, etc.
- Create a catchy title that will pique interest
- Use the principles of literacy and avoid "jargon" that may confuse the learner, but don't talk down to them. If you ask a few questions you should be able to judge the literacy level and speak at that level.
- Invite special speakers who are well known in the area to promote attendance.
- Provide a take-home item for all participants (e.g., handouts, pill organizers, etc.)

Summary

Nurses need to be prepared to meet the unique educational needs of the growing population of older adults who increasingly reflect a diversity of ethnicity, race, religion, gender, sexual orientation, and socioeconomic status. In addition to these factors, the older adult population also represents a wide diversity in age, ranging from 65 to 100+ years of age. The increased longevity and diversity indicates that there will be greater needs for health teaching related to health promotion; illness/injury prevention and chronic disease management for older adults, especially those over age 85; and minority groups. Older adults need to have a reason to engage in learning activities that is relevant to their lives and situation. Older adults are becoming more comfortable with technology and are accessing health information from the Internet. Nurses will need to be flexible and adaptable to meet the needs of the older adult group and use a variety of teaching modalities to make learning appealing and interesting. Nurses will need to provide accurate and reliable website resources for older patients and their families. Advance preparation including familiarization with the instructional setting and the expected learners is an important strategy in preparing educational programs for older adults. Nurses should also consider the physical, cognitive, and sensory changes that occur with normal aging, as well as chronic disease states, and adapt educational programs and materials to the unique needs of older adults.

Critical Thinking Exercises

`WWW`

1. **You have been approached by the Chief Nursing Officer at a long-term care facility to present an educational program on a "topic of interest"** to an expected group of 10 older adults in the assisted living unit. How would you determine an appropriate topic? How would you prepare for this presentation? What teaching modalities would you use? How would you adapt the environment to enhance learning for this group? How would you advertise the program? What Internet resources might you recommend to reinforce your instruction?

2. **On the medical-surgical floor of the hospital where you work as a graduate nurse,** the charge nurse asks you to do some one-on-one teaching with a 78-year-old widower who must learn to give himself insulin injections for newly diagnosed diabetes. How long do you think it will take for this patient to learn such a skill? What factors would you need to assess prior to beginning your instruction? What strategies will you use to prepare for this teaching session? What tools or teaching aids would be appropriate? What Internet resources might you recommend to reinforce your instruction?

3. **As a home health nurse, you are assigned to visit a diabetic patient** who was recently discharged following treatment for peripheral vascular disease and decubitus ulcers on the ankles. The patient lives with her adult daughter and her family. What educational interventions will you plan for this patient? Who will you include in the instruction? What will you need to assess prior to beginning your instruction? What strategies will you use to prepare for this teaching session? What tools or teaching aids would be appropriate? What Internet resources might you recommend to reinforce your instruction?

Personal Reflections

1. How do you employ teaching of older adults in your daily nursing care? How important is the role of teacher among the nurse's many roles? Have you ever considered a career in health education, and specifically in health education for older adults and their families? If so, how do you visualize yourself 5 or 10 years from now in such a position? What type of setting would you most like to work in if your primary job was related to health education of older adults?

2. Have you ever provided care for an older adult who did not speak English or for whom English was a second language? How did you feel when you tried to explain something to him/her? How do you think the client felt when he/she had difficulty understanding? What was the overall health status of this client? How did he/she cope with illness? What strategies would you employ to overcome the language barrier?

References

Adams, P. F., Dey, A. N., & Vickerie, J. L. (2007). Summary health statistics for the U.S. population: National Health Interview Survey. National Center for Health Statistics. *Vital Health Statistics Series 10, 233*, 1–104.

Administration on Aging. (2011). *A profile of older Americans: 2011*. Retrieved from http://www.aoa .gov/aoaroot/aging_statistics/Profile/2011/docs/2011profile.pdf

American Association of Retired Persons [AARP]. (2000). *AARP survey on lifelong learning*. Retrieved from assets.aarp.org/rgcenter/general/lifelong.pdf

American Association for Retired Persons [AARP]. (2008). *Staying ahead of the curve 2007: The AARP work and career study*. Retrieved from http://www.aarp.org/work/work-life/info-10-2008/2007_ Staying_Ahead_of_the_Curve.html

American Nurses Association. (2010). *Gerontological nursing: Scope and standards of practice*. Washington, DC: Author.

Bandura, A. (1994). Self-efficacy. In V. S. Ramachaudran (Ed.), *Encyclopedia of human behavior* (Vol. 4, pp. 71–81). New York, NY: Academic Press. Retrieved from http://www.des.emory.edu/mfp/BanEncy. html

Billek-Sawhney, B., & Reicherter., E.A. (2004). Social cognitive theory: Use by physical therapists in the education of the older adult client. *Topics in Geriatric Rehabilitation, 20*(4), 319–323.

Boyd, L. A., Vidoni, E. D., & Siengsukon, C. F. (2008). Multidimensional motor sequence learning is impaired in older but not younger or middle-aged adults. *Physical Therapy, 88*(3), 351–362.

Crawford, D. L. (2005). *The role of aging in adult learning: Implications for instructors in higher education*. Retrieved from http://education.jhu.edu/newhorizons/lifelonglearning/higher-education/ implications/index.html

Diamond, M. C. (2001, March 10). *Successful aging of the healthy brain*. Paper presented at the Conference of the American Society on Aging and the National Council on the Aging. New Orleans, LA. Retrieved from http://education.jhu.edu/newhorizons/Neurosciences/articles/Successful%20Aging/ index.html

Dunlosky, J., Cavallini, E., Roth, H., McGuire, C. L., Vecchi, T., & Hertzog, C. (2007). Do self- monitoring interventions improve older adult learning? *Journals of Gerontology, Series B: Psychological Sciences & Social Sciences, 62B*(special issue 1), 70–76.

Federal Interagency Forum on Aging-Related Statistics. (2010). *Older Americans 2010: Key Indicators of Well-Being*. Federal Interagency Forum on Aging-Related Statistics, Washington, DC: U.S. Government Printing Office Retrieved from http://agingstats.gov/agingstatsdotnet/Main_Site/Data/2010_ Documents/docs/OA_2010.pdf

Formosa, M. (2002). Critical gerogogy: Developing practical possibilities for critical educational gerontology. *Education and Ageing, 17*(1), 73–85.

Hixon, A. (2004). Functional health literacy: Improving health outcomes. *American Family Physician, 69*(9), 2077–2078.

John, M. T. (1988). *Geragogy: A theory for teaching the elderly*. Binghamton, NY: Haworth Press.

Knowles, M. (1988). *The adult learner: A neglected species* (3rd ed.). Houston, TX: Gulf.

Madden, M. (2010). *Older adults and social media*. Washington, DC: Pew Research Center. Retrieved from http://pewinternet.org/~/media//Files/Reports/2010/Pew%20Internet%20-%20Older%20Adults%20and%20Social%20Media.pdf

McDougall, G. J. Jr., Mackert, M., and Becker, H. (2012). Memory performance, health literacy, and instrumental activities of daily living of community residing older adults. *Nursing Research, 61*(1), 70–75.

National Center for Educational Statistics [NCES]. (1997). *Literacy of older adults in America*. Washington, DC: U.S. Department of Education, Office of Educational Research and Improvement.

National Institute on Aging/National Institutes of Health [NIA/NIH]. (2007). *Growing old in American: The health and retirement study*. Retrieved from http://www.nia.nih.gov/health/publication/growing-older-america-health-and-retirement-study/chapter-1-health

National Institutes of Health. (2011). *NIHSeinorHealth*. Retrieved from http://nihseniorhealth.gov

Resnick, B. (2002). The impact of self-efficacy and outcome expectations on functional status in older adults. *Topics in Geriatric Rehabilitation, 17*(4), 1–10.

Reynolds, S. (2005). Teaching the older adult. *Journal of the American Geriatric Society, 53*(3), 554–555.

Sheppard, T. (2002). The learning journey. *Navy Supply Corps Newsletter*. Retrieved from http://findarticles.com/p/articles/mi_m0NQS/is_3_65/ai_90624361/?tag=content;col1

The Talking Page Literacy Organization. (n.d.). National Illiteracy Action Project 2007–2012. Retrieved from http://www.talkingpage.org/NIAP2007.pdf

Thomas, C. M. (2007). Bulletin boards: A teaching strategy for older audiences. *Journal of Gerontological Nursing, 33*(3), 45–52.

Timmermann, S. (2003). Older adult learning: Shifting priorities in the 21st century. *Aging Today, 24*(4), p. 1.

U.S. Census Bureau. (2008a). *Projections of the population by selected age groups and sex for the United States: 2010 to 2050*. Retrieved from www.census.gov/population/www/projections/summary tables.html

U.S. Census Bureau. (2008b). *An older and more diverse nation by midcentury*. Retrieved from www.census.gov/newsroom/releases/archives/population/cb08-123.html

U.S. Census Bureau. (2012). *American factfinder*. Retrieved from http://factfinder2.census.gov/faces/tableservices/jsf/pages/productview.xhtml?pid=ACS_10_1YR_B15001&prodType=table

U.S. Department of Health and Human Services [U.S. DHHS]. (2010). *Health disparities: A case for closing the gap*. Retrieved from http://www.healthreform.gov/reports/healthdisparities/disparities_final.pdf

U.S. Department of Health and Human Services [U.S. DHHS]. (2012a). *About health literacy*. Retrieved from http://hrsa.gov/publichealth/healthliteracy/healthlitabout.html

U.S. Department of Health and Human Services [U.S. DHHS]. (2012b). *Healthy People 2020*. Retrieved from http://www.healthypeople.gov

U.S. Department of Health and Human Services [U.S. DHHS]. (2012c). *Healthy People 2020: Health communication and health information technology*. Retrieved from http://healthypeople.gov/2020/topicsobjectives2020/overview.aspx?topicid=18

U.S. Department of Health and Human Services [U. S. DHHS]. (2012d). *The health care law and you; Key features of the law: 65 and over*. Retrieved from http://www.healthcare.gov/law/features/65-older/index.html

U.S. Department of Veterans Affairs. (2012). *The GI Bill's history: Born of controversy: The GI Bill of Rights*. Retrieved from http://www.gibill.va.gov/benefits/history_timeline/index.html

U.S. Equal Employment Opportunity Commission. (2012). *The Age Discrimination in Employment Act of 1967*. Retrieved from http://www.eeoc.gov/laws/statutes/adea.cfm

Whittemore, R. (2007). Culturally competent interventions for Hispanic adults with type 2 diabetes: A systemic review. *Journal of Transcultural Nursing, 18*, 157–166.

For a full suite of assignments and additional learning activities, see the access code at the front of your book.

LEARNING OBJECTIVES

At the end of this chapter, the reader will be able to:

> Identify the major components of comprehensive assessment of older adults, including functional, physical, cognitive, psychological, social, and spiritual assessments.
> Name tools that are frequently used in the assessment of older adults.
> Recognize the challenges of conducting comprehensive assessments of older adults.
> Value the role of other health professionals in the assessment of older adults.
> Describe some of the issues in relation to comprehensive assessment of older adults.

KEY TERMS

Agnosia

Aphasia

Apraxia

Cataracts

Cerumen

Dysphagia

Excess disability

Functional incontinence

Glaucoma

Health literacy

Ketones

Longevity

Macular degeneration

Osteoarthritis

Osteoporosis

Otosclerosis

Overflow incontinence

Personhood

Polydipsia

Polyphagia

Polyuria

Presbycusis

Presbyopia

Stress incontinence

Urge incontinence

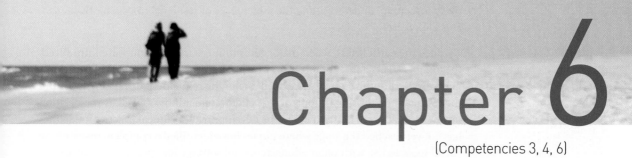

Chapter 6

(Competencies 3, 4, 6)

Comprehensive Assessment of the Older Adult

Lorna Guse

The basis of an individualized plan of care for an older adult is a comprehensive assessment. Enhanced skills in comprehensive geriatric assessment can improve health outcomes, increase nursing assessment confidence, and provide a role model for health-care teams (Stolee et al., 2003). Assessment has been described as the cornerstone of gerontological nursing, and the goal is to conduct a systematic and integrated assessment (Olenek, Skowronski, & Schmaltz, 2003). The health and healthcare needs of older adults are complex, deriving from a combination of age-related changes, age-associated and other diseases, heredity, and lifestyle. Assessment requires knowledge and an understanding of these complex factors, and a comprehensive baseline assessment is necessary in order to recognize changes that occur in relation to these complex factors. In assessing and providing care to older adults, nurses are members of a healthcare team that includes physicians, therapists, social workers, spiritual care workers, pharmacists, nutritionists, and others. Each member of the team has a contribution to make, and nurses should draw upon the knowledge of other team members to enhance the assessment process.

Comprehensive assessments can be lengthy, and this presents a challenge to nurses because depending on health status and energy level, the older adult may not be well or strong enough for an extensive physical or verbal-based assessment. If the older adult is experiencing memory problems, the reliability of question-based assessment may be suspect. The role of the family and particularly family caregivers (often spouses and adult children) adds another dimension. The literature suggests that when family members act as proxies for health information, there can be underestimates and overestimates of functional ability, cognition, and social functioning (Ostbye, Tyas, McDowell, & Koval, 1997). Assessment tools do not always identify the source of information, and even experienced nurses sometimes rely too much on secondary sources such as family members and caregivers rather than focusing on the older adult as the primary source of information (Luborsky, 1997). This is important to note, as a study compared preferences of nursing home residents with dementia with those as reported by their family members and nursing staff; the authors found that family and staff were relatively inaccurate in determining the preferences of residents (Mesman, Buchanan, Husfeldt, & Berg, 2011).

Since the early 1960s, when major tools to measure function were introduced, the number of assessment tools from which nurses can choose has increased exponentially. Part of this increase has been due to the refinement of existing tools and the testing and tailoring of tools across client populations, as well as the creation of new tools. The current growth in the development of clinical practice guidelines has not yet reached the stage where nurses have identified a complete roster of the "best" tools to use with older adults across all settings for specific areas of assessment (see http://www.consultgerirn.org for examples). However, certain tools are used by nurses because they have been used traditionally to provide a foundation for decision making and intervention strategies. In this chapter, we will identify these common tools and provide guidelines for assessment. In addition, several of the chapters in this text give examples of assessment tools related to specific content.

A cautionary note is needed. Comprehensive assessment is not a neutral process; the sources of information and tools used as well as the nurse's skill level have consequences for the older adult's individualized plan of care. The physical and social environment can support or suppress an older adult's abilities. Comprehensive assessment consists of objective and subjective elements, and how the assessment data are interpreted is of major importance. As Kane (1993) has suggested, interpretation is an art, and it is an art that nurses must aspire to master both as students and as practitioners.

Functional Assessment

Nurses typically conduct a functional assessment in order to identify an older adult's ability to perform self-care, self-maintenance, and physical activities, then plan appropriate nursing interventions based on the results. There are two approaches: One approach is to ask questions about ability, and the other approach is to observe ability through evaluating task completion. However, although we tend to speak of "ability," our verbal and observational tools tend to screen for "disability." Disability refers to the impact that health problems have on an individual's ability to perform tasks, roles, and activities, and it is often measured by asking questions about the performance of activities of daily living (such as eating and dressing) and instrumental activities of daily living (such as meal preparation and hobbies) (Verbrugge & Jette, 1994). The basis of our understanding of ability, disability, physical function, activities of daily living, and any contextual factors comes from work initiated by the World Health Organization (WHO) almost 30 years ago.

The International Classification of Impairment, Disability and Handicap (ICIDH) was first published by the WHO in 1980. It suggested relationships among impairment, disability, and handicap. In attempting to move away from a disease perspective and toward a health perspective, the WHO discontinued using the term handicap and made definitional changes, creating a new International Classification of Functioning, Disability, and Health (ICIDH-2) in 2001. The ICIDH-2 uses the term *disability* to reflect limitations in activities based on an interaction between the individual's health (including impairment, or problems in body function or structure) and the physical, social, and attitudinal environment. This broader perspective on health, activity, and environment is illustrated in the WHO definitions provided in **Box 6-1**. Kearney and Pryor (2004) have suggested that nursing has not yet integrated the ICIDH-2 framework into research, practice, and education; specifically, they suggest that the ICIDH-2 framework provides nurses with a broad structure "to address more fully, activity limitations and participation restrictions associated with impairment" (2004, p. 166). Moreover, they argue that in nursing education, students should be encouraged to develop "a healthcare plan that outlines strategies to promote maximum health, function, well-being, independence and participation in life for the individual" (2004, p. 167). Kearney and Pryor are, in fact, promoting an "ability" perspective rather than emphasizing deficits.

Taking an ability perspective on comprehensive assessment of older adults builds upon the ICIDH-2 framework and is informed by the work of Kearney and Pryor (2004) and others. Functional assessment should first emphasize an older adult's ability and the appropriate nursing interventions to support, maintain, and maximize ability; second, it should focus on an older adult's disability and the appropriate nursing interventions to compensate for and prevent further disability. Nursing interventions that create excess disability are not appropriate. *Excess disability* is defined as "functional disability greater than that warranted by actual physical and physiological impairment of the individual" (Kahn, 1964, p. 112). For example, assisting an older adult in a nursing home to get dressed in the morning when that individual is mentally and physically able to do this task creates excess disability, curbs independence, and discourages optimal wellness.

BOX 6-1   World Health Organization (2001) ICIDH-2 Definitions

In the context of health:

Body functions are the physiological functions of body systems (including psychological functions).

Body structures are anatomical parts of the body such as organs, limbs, and their components.

Impairments are problems in body function or structure such as significant deviation or loss.

Activity is the execution of a task or action by an individual.

Participation is involvement in a life situation.

Activity limitations are difficulties an individual may have in executing activities.

Participation restrictions are problems an individual may experience in involvement in life situations.

Environmental factors make up the physical, social, and attitudinal environment in which people live and conduct their lives.

Tools to assess functional ability tend to address self-care (basic activities of daily living, or ADLs), higher-level activities necessary to live independently in the community (instrumental activities of daily living, or IADLs), or highest-level activities (advanced activities of daily living, or AADLs) (Adnan, Chang, Arseven, & Emanuel, 2005). Advanced activities of daily living include societal, family, and community roles, as well as participation in occupational and recreational activities.

In selecting or using tools to measure functional ability, the nurse must be clear on two questions. First, is performance or capacity being assessed? Some tools ask, "Do you dress without help?" (performance) whereas others ask, "Can you dress without help?" (capacity). Asking about capacity places the emphasis on ability. The second question is, "Who is the source of information on functional ability?" Is information gained verbally from the family or from the older adult? Does the nurse assess functional ability by direct observation or by relying on the observations of others?

In 1987, the Omnibus Budget Reconciliation Act (OBRA) mandated the use of the Minimum Data Set (MDS) in all Medicaid- and Medicare-funded nursing homes. This assessment tool attempted to identify a resident's strengths, preferences, and functional abilities in a systematic way in order to better address his or her needs. The MDS was revised in 1995 and a home-based version was also later developed. In this chapter, we will not be looking at this particular assessment tool. Instead, examples of tools to assess functional ability will be presented in relation to ADL, IADL, and AADL. In addition, the use of physical performance measures will be discussed in relation to functional assessment.

Activities of Daily Living

The original ADL tool was developed by Katz and his colleagues during an 8-year period at the Benjamin Rose Hospital, a geriatric hospital in Cleveland, Ohio, using observations of patients with hip fractures and their performance of activities during recovery (Katz, Ford, Moskowitz, Jackson, & Jaffee, 1963). The Katz Index of ADL (Katz, Down, Cash, & Grotz, 1970) distinguished between independence and dependence in activities and created an ordered relationship among ADLs. It addressed the need for assistance in bathing, eating, dressing, transfer, toileting, and continence.

Other similar tools followed the Katz Index of ADL and are still being developed and refined. These tools can be divided into those that are generic and those that are disease- or illness-specific. Some tools are designed to provide a more sensitive assessment of ability for older adults with cognitive limitations. Such tools attempt to separate disability stemming from cognitive limitations from those caused by physical limitations. Generally speaking, since the early work of Katz and his colleagues, there has been an emphasis on more detailed assessments of ADL. Unfortunately, the development of different tools with different foci (for example, performance versus capacity) has tended to create confusion because these differences can lead to varying outcomes (Parker & Thorslund, 2007).

One widely used ADL tool is the Barthel Index (Mahoney & Barthel, 1965). This index was designed to measure functional levels of self-care and mobility, and it rates the ability to feed and groom oneself, bathe, go to the toilet, walk (or propel a wheelchair), climb stairs, and control bowel and bladder. Tasks typically assessed with ADL tools are listed in **Box 6-2**. In using the Barthel Index or any ADL assessment tool, it is critical that the assessment be detailed and individualized. For example, the Barthel item for "personal toilet" includes several tasks (wash face, comb hair, shave, clean teeth), and the older adult may be independent in some but not all of them and may require an assistive device for some but not all of them. A detailed assessment will provide information for appropriate nursing interventions—that is, those designed to promote ability and compensate for and prevent further disability for that individual.

Some older adults, specifically those with cognitive limitations but with good physical abilities, can manage their ADLs with direction and support (cueing and supervising). As pointed out by Tappen (1994), most ADL assessment tools were developed for physically impaired individuals and "are not sensitive to the functional difficulties experienced by the persons with Alzheimer's disease and related dementia" (1994, p. 38). The Refined ADL Assessment Scale is composed of 14 separate tasks within 5 selected ADL areas (toileting, washing, grooming, dressing, and eating) (Tappen, 1994). This scale represents an approach to ADL assessment known as "task segmentation," which means breaking down the ADL activity into smaller steps (Morris & Morris, 1997). For example, the steps of washing one's hands or getting dressed in the morning are fairly complex for someone with cognitive limitations. However, by cueing as needed, the nurse can assess which of the steps are challenging and which are not. In getting dressed in the morning, some older adults with cognitive limitations will require help in selecting clothing, but once these clothing pieces are selected and laid out, the older adult may require limited cueing to progress through the complex task of dressing. Beck (1988) has developed a dressing assessment tool for persons with

BOX 6-2 Tasks Typically Assessed with ADL Assessment Tools	
Eating	Ascending/descending stairs
Dressing	Communication
Bathing/washing	Transferring (e.g., from bed to chair)
Grooming	Toileting (bowel and bladder)
Walking/ambulation	

cognitive limitations that is particularly detailed. Another consideration for assessment is the use of assistive devices to support older adults and their activities of daily living. The development and use of assistive devices has increased among all segments of the older adult population, from those in nursing homes to those living in the community. It is important to ask about such devices and how they are used to perform activities of daily living. More detailed content on the use of assistive technology is presented in Chapter 14.

The most common ADL scale used in rehabilitation of older adults is the Uniform Data System for Medical Rehabilitation (UDSMR) Functional Independence Measure (FIM). The FIM instrument scores a person from 1 (needing total assistance or not testable) to 7 (complete independence) and is considered a reliable and valid tool. Categories measured include self-care, bowel and bladder, transfer, locomotion, communication, and social cognition (UDSMR, 1996). This measure is done at admission, discharge, and several times in between to assess progress in rehabilitation.

Instrumental Activities of Daily Living

Instrumental activities of daily living include a range of activities that are considered to be more complex compared with ADLs and address the older adult's ability to interact with his or her environment and community. It is readily apparent that items in IADL assessment tools are geared more for older adults living in the community; for example, items often ask about doing the laundry or shopping for groceries. It has also been suggested that IADL tools emphasize tasks traditionally associated with women's work in the home (Lawton, 1972). IADLs include the ability to use the telephone, cook, shop, do laundry and housekeeping, manage finances, take medications, and prepare meals. Missing from most IADL tools are activities that may be more associated with men, such as fixing things around the house or lawn care. One of the earliest IADL measures was developed by Lawton and Brody (1969). Tasks typically assessed with IADL tools are listed in **Box 6-3.**

BOX 6-3   Tasks Typically Assessed with IADL Assessment Tools

Using the telephone	Light or heavy housekeeping
Taking medications	Light or heavy yard work
Shopping	Home maintenance
Handling finances	Using transportation
Preparing meals	Leisure/recreation
Laundry	

Advanced Activities of Daily Living

Advanced activities of daily living include societal, family, and community roles, as well as participation in occupational and recreational activities. AADL assessment tools tend to be used less often by nurses and more often by occupational therapists and recreation workers to address specific areas of social tasks. One tool that seems to combine elements of ADLs, IADLs, and AADLs is the Canadian Occupational Performance Measure (COPM) (Chan & Lee, 1997). Developed by Law and colleagues (1994), this tool is designed to detect changes in self-perception of occupational performance over time.

The COPM asks older adults to identify daily activities that are difficult for them to do but, at the same time, are self-perceived as being important to do. The tool asks about self-care activities (personal care, functional mobility, and community management), productivity (paid/unpaid work, household management, and play/school), and leisure (quiet recreation, active recreation, and socialization). Consequently, interventions to enhance and support ability are planned to address those activities of importance to the older adult. The strength of the COPM is that it focuses on the older adult's functional priorities by asking about importance so that interventions can be tailored to enhance those priority activities and increase satisfaction.

Physical Performance Measures

One of the criticisms directed toward ADL and IADL assessment tools is that they are highly subjective, relying on the perspectives of older adults (and sometimes their family members) or on healthcare professionals who may tend to be more conservative in estimating ability (Guralnik, Branch, Cummings, & Curb, 1989). In contrast, physical performance measures involve direct observation of activities, such as observing the older adult prepare and eat a meal, but also include tasks related to balance, gait, and the ability to reach and bend. The Physical Performance Test (PPT) is one example of a physical performance assessment tool (Reuben & Sui, 1990). The seven-item version asks the individual to write a sentence, transfer five kidney beans from an emesis basin to a can (one at a time), put on and remove a jacket, pick up a penny from the floor, turn 360 degrees, and walk 50 feet (Reuben, Valle, Hays, & Sui, 1995).

The benefit of using physical performance measures is related to a potential relationship between physical ability and functional ability. The question is, does assessment of physical performance relate meaningfully to the ADL and IADL abilities of older adults? Does difficulty with walking and climbing stairs, for example, go hand-in-hand with ADL and IADL abilities such as toileting or grocery shopping? Findings have been inconsistent due at least in part to the several ways of measuring physical performance and functional ability. Some studies have suggested that physical performance measures provide good information to identify older adults who may be at risk for losing functional ability in ADL and becoming prone to falls (Gill, Williams, & Tinetti, 1995; Tinetti, Speechley, & Ginter, 1988).

Physical Assessment

Conducting a physical assessment of an older adult is based on technical competence in physical assessment, knowledge of the normal changes (Chapter 5) and diseases associated with aging, and good communication skills (Chapter 4). In this chapter, a basis in technical competence is taken for granted and the emphasis is on presenting physical assessment information that is particularly relevant to the older adult (see **Case Study 6-1**). Physical assessment with a "systems" approach reviews each body

Case Study 6-1

You are visiting an older couple in the community in order to assess the couple's functional ability and the potential for their needing assistance with ADLs or IADLs. Mr. and Mrs. Boyd are 72 and 67 years old, respectively, and have been married for 45 years. They have lived in the same neighborhood since Mr. Boyd retired from his bank manager job 12 years ago. Mrs. Boyd has been a housewife since her marriage. Mr. and Mrs. Boyd have one child, a son who lives in another city about 500 miles away. There are no other family members in their community.

As you sit with both of them at the kitchen table, Mrs. Boyd tells you to direct all your questions to her because Mr. Boyd has trouble understanding questions. She goes on to explain that Mr. Boyd used to garden and maintain the yard but no longer seems interested in doing anything. He sleeps a great deal, seems to be eating less, and is often uncommunicative when she speaks to him. She says that her husband is getting quite forgetful and that this worries her because he was always socially engaging and a man who could speak on several subjects.

Mrs. Boyd tells you that she makes all the decisions and spends most of her time planning meals, doing housework, and attending her ladies' church group. She says that she could really use some help with outdoor tasks because these tasks had been handled by Mr. Boyd until just recently. When you ask what she means by

"recently," Mrs. Boyd replies that a change seems to have occurred within the last 6 months.

You thank Mrs. Boyd for sharing this information with you, and you indicate that most of the questions can be directed to her but that you will be asking Mr. Boyd some questions as part of the assessment. Mrs. Boyd seems concerned by this but agrees to give you an opportunity to try and ask some questions of Mr. Boyd. You begin your assessment by asking Mrs. Boyd about her functional abilities, including ADLs and IADLs, indicating that you will be asking the same questions of Mr. Boyd.

Questions:

1. Drawing from the 10 principles of comprehensive assessment and your knowledge of functional, physical, cognitive, psychological, social, and spiritual assessment of older adults, what are the areas of assessment that you think should be explored first with Mr. and Mrs. Boyd?

2. Will you be relying on self-report, proxy report, performance measures, or all of these for the assessment?

3. Mrs. Boyd seems to want to dominate the interview. How will this affect the assessment process?

4. Which other health professionals do you think should be involved directly or in consultation in relation to your assessment?

system by first taking a history and then conducting a physical examination. It is important to ask questions that produce an accurate description of the older adult's physical health status, and furthermore, explore the meaning and implications of physical health status on an individual basis. The same changes in visual acuity for two older adults may have quite different meanings and implications—for one older adult, the changes may not affect their everyday activities whereas for the other, they may mean the loss of a driver's license and accompanying distress and hardship in relation to unmet transportation needs and decreased social contact.

Physical assessment by body systems usually involves a healthcare team approach. Physicians, including specialists such as a cardiologist, and nurses are key members of the team. Nurses often do an initial assessment or act as case finders in the community and in clinics. Other members of the healthcare team include a nutritionist, respiratory therapist, social worker, kinesiologist, physical therapist, and psychologist.

Circulatory Function

Several factors play a role in older adults and their circulatory status. Age-related changes in the heart muscle and blood vessels result in overall decreased cardiac function. These changes plus lifestyle, including limited exercise and physical activity, increase the likelihood that older adults will experience diminished circulatory function. Other lifestyle factors that have an impact on circulatory function are smoking behaviors and the consumption of alcohol. When the current cohort of older adults was young, the benefits of exercise and physical activity and the detrimental effects of smoking were not common knowledge. The social context was different compared with our current one.

The cumulative effects of age-related changes, heredity, and lifestyle mean that there can be great variation among older adults in relation to their circulatory function. In addition, through the use of medications and assistive devices, diminished circulatory function may have a greater or lesser impact on their day-to-day life. Although diseases of the circulatory system can occur at all ages, these diseases are associated with people in their older years, and comprehensive assessment will include taking a cardiac history and performing a physical examination.

The circulatory health assessment should address family history; current problems with chest pain or discomfort, especially if associated with exertion; current diagnoses and associated medications as well as over-the-counter and herbal medicines; sources of stress; and adherence to current medical regimens. The assessment should also include a physical examination, assessing blood pressure, listening to chest sounds, and taking a pulse rate. Other assessment protocols may include an exercise stress test, blood and serum tests, electrocardiograms, and other tests for imaging and assessing the condition of the heart and blood vessels. These advanced laboratory assessment protocols are usually ordered by physicians and the results are shared by the healthcare team as detailed assessment information.

Respiratory Function

Age-related changes to bones, muscles, lung tissue, and respiratory fluids all contribute to the respiratory difficulties experienced by some older adults. Older adults are particularly susceptible to respiratory diseases, and the signs of infection may not be as obvious as they are in younger adults; therefore, assessment of respiratory function should occur more often, particularly with older adults who may have compromised respiratory function because of disease, injury, or previous exposure to occupational or environmental pollutants. Older adults who have restricted mobility and are on extended bed rest are especially at risk for respiratory infections and serious sequential complications.

The respiratory assessment should ask about current medications (including prescribed, over-the-counter, and herbal) and take a history of smoking behavior and exposure to environmental pollutants during the life span. Other areas for assessment include current difficulties and anxieties associated with breathing, decreased energy to complete everyday tasks, frequent coughing, and production of excessive sputum. Physical examination includes observation of posture and breathlessness, and listening to chest sounds. Other assessment protocols include blood and pulmonary function tests, chest X-rays, and sputum analysis. Information from these tests assists the nurse in a total assessment of respiratory function.

Gastrointestinal Function

Age-related changes in the gastrointestinal system are not dramatic and therefore may not be noticed by most older adults. Smooth muscle changes mean decreased peristaltic action and reduced gastric acid secretion, which may affect gastric comfort and appetite. A concern of many older adults is constipation, which is usually defined as the lack of a bowel movement for 3 or more days. A lack of dietary fiber, low levels of physical activity, and lack of fluid are associated with constipation among healthy older adults (Annells & Koch, 2003). Constipation is also associated with Parkinson's disease and irritable bowel syndrome or as a side effect of medications, so it should always be investigated (Woodward, 2012). Although the problem of constipation does not always receive serious attention, a review reported that chronic constipation was associated with serious consequences including fecal impaction, incontinence, and delirium, leading to severe curtailment in ADLs and, in some cases, necessitating hospitalization (Tariq, 2007).

Assessment of gastrointestinal function begins with asking about the older adult's usual diet; appetite and changes in appetite; occurrence of nausea, vomiting, indigestion, or other stomach discomforts; and problems with bowel function, including constipation and diarrhea. In relation to constipation, the nurse should ask about exercise, diet, and fluid intake, and whether the older adult is using prescribed, over-the-counter, or herbal remedies to deal with constipation. A 3- to 7-day meal diary can illustrate eating habits that might have an impact on constipation. Older adults with limited incomes may be less likely to purchase fresh fruit and vegetables because of cost; this can lower the ingestion of fresh fruits and vegetables and fluids, which contributes to constipation, as does limited exercise and mobility. Older adults have a diminished sense of thirst, and fluid intake may be inadequate to maintain normal bowel function. Diagnostic testing can include barium enemas and X-rays, stool analysis, and examination of the colon. Older adults residing in nursing homes are especially at risk for dehydration and associated consequences for bowel function (Mentes & Wang, 2011).

Special attention should be directed to changes in appetite and specifically to loss of appetite. Poor appetite with related declines in body weight and energy is often seen as a warning sign that signals future health problems (Morley, 2003). Decreased body weight is associated with negative changes to the skin, making it prone to injury, and reduced caloric intake affects energy levels needed for mobility and other activities of daily living. Poor appetite is not solely embedded in gastrointestinal function and instead includes aspects of social and psychological function. Mealtime is also a social experience and often involves interaction with others. One study of community-dwelling older adults reported that impaired appetite was associated with depression, poor self-rated health, smoking, chewing problems, visual impairment, and weight loss (Lee et al., 2006).

Oral health assessment is an area often overlooked with older adults, and nurses should routinely ask about oral health practices including brushing, flossing, and regular contact with a dentist. Poor oral care leads to dental caries, dry mouth, and mouth infections as well as systematic infections that can affect cardiac and respiratory function. Examination of the mouth should include observing the condition of the tongue, teeth, and gums for dehydration, infection, and poor oral hygiene. Check dentures to be sure they are well-fitting, particularly if a weight change has occurred. Especially at risk for oral health problems are older adults with limited incomes who cannot manage regular contact with a dentist and older adults in long-term care facilities who lack the physical or cognitive ability to maintain self-care in oral health (Bawden, 2006).

Genitourinary Function

Age-related changes in the genitourinary system along with age-related diseases such as diabetes and hypertension can have a major impact on everyday life. Bladder muscles weaken and bladder capacity is lessened. Difficulties in sensing that the bladder has not emptied may mean that residual urine stays within the bladder, creating a medium for potential infection. Older women are more likely to experience incontinence, which is often related to a history of childbirth or gynecologic surgeries. Gynecologic assessment of older women is an area of assessment that is sometimes neglected. Older women and their caregivers may mistakenly believe that because the childbearing years have passed or because of sexual inactivity, a gynecologic exam is no longer needed (Richman & Drickamer, 2007). The nurse should be asking questions about abnormal bleeding, vaginal discharge, and any urinary symptoms. Pelvic examinations and Pap smears are usually carried out by physicians, but nurses have an important role in identifying the need for this further assessment.

Older men may develop problems with an enlarged prostate that impedes the flow of urine through the urethra. Incontinence is not a normal part of aging; when incidents of incontinence occur regularly, this can lead to embarrassment, restricted social activity, and skin problems. Urinary incontinence can be managed and improved by nursing interventions that involve behavioral treatment options (McGuire, 2006). More detailed content on urinary incontinence, assessment, and nursing interventions are presented in Chapter 12. Unmanaged incontinence can have significant consequences to daily life, and unmanaged incontinence in the home environment is a major factor in the decision for nursing home placement.

A serious medical problem, chronic renal failure can arise as a complication of age-related diseases such as diabetes and hypertension. This is a potentially life-threatening illness that requires specialized care and may ultimately mean support through kidney dialysis.

Health history questions should attend to any previous or current difficulties related to the frequency and voluntary flow of urine during either the day or night. If incontinence is a problem, then questions should focus on the type of incontinence: *stress*, *urge*, *functional*, or *overflow* (see Chapter 12). Older adults who have problems with continence may restrict their fluid intake, which will have implications for other body systems, including skin condition and the gastrointestinal system. The nurse should ask about fluid intake, especially caffeine and alcohol (because these substances affect bladder tone) and observe the skin for dehydration. The nurse also should ask about medication use (prescribed, over-the-counter, and herbal remedies). Diagnostic tests include urine analysis tests for blood, bacteria, and other components such as *ketones*. Other diagnostic tests may be ordered by the physician to assess bladder muscle tone and function and prostate size and potential obstructions.

Sexual Function

Two of the prevailing myths in our society are that older adults are neither sexually active nor interested in sexual relationships. This is not the case; however, several factors associated with aging do have an impact on sexual activity, including lack of partner (often through widowhood), chronic illnesses, and medication use that may negatively affect performance and sexual satisfaction. In conducting a comprehensive assessment with an older adult, asking about sexual function is appropriate. However, it is important to be knowledgeable about age-related and disease-associated changes in relation to sexual function and to be sensitive and respectful of privacy because this is clearly a very personal area of human function.

Age-related changes for men include a decrease in the speed and duration of erection; in women there is a decrease in vaginal lubrication. Health and social factors may have a great impact on sexual activity among older adults; chronic illness such as osteoarthritis and diminished positive self-image because of a societal emphasis on youthful beauty are two such factors. Lack of privacy inhibits the expression of sexuality; this in particular can be a deterrent in residential long-term care facilities (Richman & Drickamer, 2007).

Assessment questions should focus on sexual function and whether there have been any changes or concerns. Do not assume that older adults are sexually inactive. Instead, ask about sexual activity and whether there have been changes or concerns in relation to sexuality and sexual activity. Asking these questions can open the door to further dialogue. In the past few years, there has been a great deal of advertising by pharmaceutical companies for erectile dysfunction drugs. The advertising is aimed at middle-aged and older adults, and there may be some natural curiosity about these new drugs. An older adult's questions about enhancement medications might be best answered in consultation with a pharmacist because of potential side effects and interactions with other medications.

Neurological Function

The neurological system affects all other body systems. Age-related changes involve declines in reaction time, kinetic and body balance problems, and sleep disturbances. Age-related diseases such as Alzheimer's disease and Parkinson's disease and other health problems such as stroke can lead to cognitive changes including memory loss, lack of spatial orientation, *agnosia*, *apraxia*, *dysphagia*, *aphasia*, and delirium. Dementia is a collection of diseases where the changes in brain cells and activity lead to progressive loss of mental capacity. Alzheimer's disease is the most common disease of dementia. Cognitive assessment for dementia will be discussed in a later section of this chapter.

Neurological assessment of older adults includes several components. The nurse should ask about medications (prescribed, over-the-counter, and herbal remedies) and any medical diagnosis related to the neurological system, such as history or family history of stroke. The nurse should observe and ask about previous and current impairments in speech, expression, swallowing, memory, orientation, energy level, balance, sensation, and motor function. Other areas of assessment relate to the occurrence of sleep disturbance, tremors, and seizures.

Musculoskeletal Function

Several age-related changes occur in the musculoskeletal system and lead to decreased muscle tone, strength, and endurance. The stiffening of connective tissue (ligaments and tendons) and erosion of articular surfaces of joints create restrictions in joint mobility. Declines in hormone production contribute to bone loss, and the ability to heal is reduced. Common musculoskeletal health problems include *osteoarthritis* and *osteoporosis*. Of particular concern are the risk of falls and the potential for fractures with their associated morbidity and mortality. One commonly used assessment tool for the risk of falls is the Morse Fall Scale; a description of this scale is provided in Chapter 12. In assessing older adults who have a history of falls, the use of fall diaries is recommended, along with training to complete the diaries (Perry et al., 2012).

The most commonly reported illness among older adults is osteoarthritis, and it is more likely to occur in the weight-bearing joints, especially the hips and knees. Because sore and stiff joints are universally associated with aging, older adults and healthcare professionals often take an accepting attitude about these complaints. The nurse should be asking about the history of sore joints: Which joints are affected? How long has there been pain? What kind of pain is it? Does it interfere with everyday activities? Is the pain managed? If so, how is it managed? Is there a history of bone and muscle injuries? Has there been surgery? Have alternative and complementary therapies such as acupuncture or herbal remedies been explored? What are the pertinent lifestyle factors for this older adult, including participating in exercise and physical activity?

Observation of posture, stance, and walking can assist in asking the appropriate questions: Does the older adult favor one side of the body while walking? Are assistive devices such as canes and walkers being used? Canes and walkers should be at the appropriate height in relation to body height. Ask whether an assessment was done by a therapist in selecting the height, weight, and type of cane or walker. In observing walking and rising from a chair, attend to body language and facial expressions that indicate discomfort. Observe and examine the kind of footwear being worn. Does the footwear offer adequate support while promoting good circulation?

The Up and Go Test provides a quick assessment of an older person's mobility and overall function. The nurse should measure a distance of 10 feet from the person's chair and ask the client to rise, walk to the line, turn, walk back, and sit down. An average time to do this is 10 seconds; greater than 10 seconds may indicate functional problems with ambulation (Reuben et al., 2008).

Osteoporosis is a major health problem and has an increasingly large impact on disability and the need for supportive and rehabilitative health services (Stone & Lyles, 2006). Osteoporosis causes a gradual loss of bone mass, and bones become porous and vulnerable to fracture. It is associated with aging, heredity, poor calcium intake, hormonal changes, and a sedentary lifestyle. Older adults with osteoporosis experience symptoms of chronic back pain, muscle weakness, joint pain, loss of height, and decrease in mobility. Bone density tests can compare bone mass with individuals of comparable or younger ages as a marker. If needed, calcium intake can be increased through diet or supplements. The nurse should ask about symptoms and whether a bone density test has been carried out; if so, what were the subsequent recommendations? Often the plan of care for osteoporosis is pain control and treatment, so it is important to assess current pain management strategies.

Sensory Function

Age-related and disease-related changes in sensory function can have profound effects on older adults and their day-to-day functioning. Of the five senses—hearing, vision, smell, taste, and touch—it is the occurrence of diminished vision and hearing that seems to have the greatest impact on older adults. Problems with vision or hearing can have negative effects on social interaction and hence on social and psychological health. A study sited in complex continuing care facilities demonstrated that hearing impairment and mood were associated, and that improved hearing was directly related to improved mood and quality of life (Brink & Stones, 2007).

Presbyopia refers to an age-related change in vision. The lens of the eye becomes less elastic and this creates less efficient accommodation of near and distant vision. *Presbycusis* refers to age-related progressive hearing loss. Decrements in vision and hearing can affect communication ability, with potential consequences to older adults' health, safety, everyday activities, socialization, and quality of life. Screening tools for vision and hearing are of two types: self-report and performance-based.

Specifically for vision, difficulty in reading has implications for *health literacy* and safety in relation to reading instructions on prescription bottles and following other written directions for health care. Age-related *macular degeneration*, the deterioration of central vision, is the leading cause of severe vision loss in older adults in the United States. Older adults should undergo regular eye examinations for changes in vision (including the formation of *cataracts*) and screening for ocular pressure (for *glaucoma*). The American Academy of Ophthalmology recommends periodic eye examinations at 1- to 2-year intervals for older adults who do not experience symptoms or high risk factors (Jung, Coleman, & Weintraub, 2007). These performance-based tests are conducted by other health professionals—optometrists and ophthalmologists—but nurses are often in a key position to screen for vision problems and to encourage older adults to initiate and maintain regular visits with other health professionals to assess vision changes.

The following two screening procedures are simple tests for functional vision:

1. Ask the older adult to read a newspaper headline and story and observe for difficulty and accuracy.
2. Ask the older adult to read the prescription bottle and, again, observe for difficulty and accuracy.

It is important to follow up with specific questions that explore the vision problem from the perspective of the individual: Is vision a problem? Does it interfere with everyday activities or with hobbies and social life? Are magnification aids or enlarged printed material useful strategies? Is home lighting contributing to the problem? Is it more difficult to see in the evening compared with other times of the day?

Hearing loss is a major concern for many older adults. Furthermore, the perceived stigma of hearing loss and attendant shame may lead some older adults to deny this loss and reject hearing assessment and the use of hearing aids (Wallhagen, 2009). According to the U.S. Census Bureau (Bureau of the Census, 1997), about 30% of older adults between 65 and 74 years of age and 50% of those between 75 and 79 years of age experience some hearing loss. Most hearing loss in older adults is both symmetric and bilateral, and hearing problems are exacerbated in a noisy environment. Non-aging-related hearing loss can be attributed to *cerumen* impaction, infection, occurrence of a foreign body, or *otosclerosis*. Assessment questions should ask about any hearing problems and how these problems affect the older adult's everyday life. The following question is useful in assessing ear and hearing problems: Are you experiencing a hearing problem or any ear pain, ringing in the ears, or ear discharge? One study reported that asking, "Do you have a hearing problem now?" was effective in screening for hearing loss among older adults (Gates, Murphy, Rees, & Fraher, 2003). An initial assessment question might be, "When is your hearing loss the biggest problem for you?" The nurse who assesses hearing function is in a good position to recommend further diagnostic testing with an audiologist.

For older adults who wear hearing aids, the condition and working order of these aids is often overestimated and should be regularly assessed and monitored. One study conducted in a retirement community reported that for most of those wearing hearing aids, a visual check indicated problems with either broken or missing components, inappropriate volume setting, or weak or dead batteries, and this was especially true for those older adults who were relatively dependent on nursing care (Culbertson, Griggs, & Hudson, 2004).

The other senses are taste, smell, and touch. Taste and smell are interrelated; the sense of smell influences the sense of taste for food as well as appetite. Although there are some age-related changes (for example, fewer taste receptors), older adults who are experiencing a noticeable loss of taste and smell generally have other medical conditions (Ferrini & Ferrini, 2012). Medical conditions, especially those affecting the nose; medication side effects; nutritional deficiencies; poor oral hygiene; alcohol use; and smoking can all detrimentally affect the senses of smell and taste. Assessments should ask generally about satisfaction with taste and smell, the duration and extent of the problem, and the impact of the problem on everyday life.

Integumentary Function

Age-related changes to the skin include loss of elasticity, slower regeneration of cells, diminished gland secretion, reduced blood supply, and structural changes, including loss of fat. This means that the skin of older adults is more susceptible to injury and infection and less resilient in terms of repair. Older adults with decreased mobility and extended bed rest are at high risk for skin damage and breakdown. For many older adults, skin dryness and itching are two common complaints. Emollients and powders can bring relief for most minor skin conditions.

Asking questions about skin problems and concerns and inspecting the skin are basic elements of assessment and should be done on a regular basis. If skin injury has already occurred, close monitoring and treatment are essential. The nurse should ask about rashes, itching, dryness, frequent bruising, and any open sores. Skin conditions can be linked with nutritional status and body weight, and the nurse can work with a nutritionist to promote a healthy diet and appropriate weight. Any loss of sensation, particularly in extremities, is a cause of concern. Impeded circulation with lack of sensation can lead to untreated skin breakdown, and prevention is preferable to the more serious consequences of infection and disability. In the event of wounds, there are assessment tools to gauge the extent and level, such as the Braden Wound Index, which is described in more detail in Chapter 12. Nurses with expertise in wound care, a specialized area of nursing practice, are usually available in acute and long-term care for consultation and advice.

The older adult's skin should be observed for color, hydration, circulation, and intactness. Fluid intake may be less than optimal and result in severe dryness. The nurse should be asking questions about skin changes, signs and symptoms of infection, usual skin care, and problems with healing. The nurse should also observe the fingernails and toenails for splitting and tears.

Endocrine and Metabolic Function

Age-related changes in endocrine function include decreased hormone secretion and breakdown of metabolites. Of special concern for older adults is the onset of diabetes mellitus or thyroid disease because these diseases can be insidious and silent: Much damage to the body can occur even before these conditions are diagnosed. Diabetes mellitus becomes more prevalent with age, but the symptoms of *polydipsia*, *polyphagia*, and *polyuria* may go unnoticed for several years. Because the thirst sensation diminishes with age, older adults may not be aware of their polydipsia. By the time the disease is diagnosed, more serious complications such as impaired circulation, foot ulcers, and vision disturbances may have ensued.

The more common form of diabetes mellitus among older adults is type 2 or non-insulin-dependent diabetes mellitus. With age, there is an increased resistance to the action of insulin within the body, and this change, in combination with lifestyle choices, places some older adults at inordinate risk for developing this disease. Age-related changes, heredity, obesity, poor nutrition, inadequate physical activity, and other illnesses increase the likelihood of type 2 diabetes among older adults. Given that the disease may be silent for many years, it is critical that nurses be attuned to assessing for the risk for developing diabetes among older adults and monitor changes and symptoms at every opportunity. As part of the health history, the following areas should be addressed:

> Family history of diabetes
> Changes in weight and appetite
> Fatigue

> Increased thirst and fluid intake
> Vision problems
> Slow wound healing
> Headache
> Gastrointestinal problems

More specific symptoms should be further assessed, including occurrence of polyphagia, polydipsia, and polyuria. Diagnostic tests such as fasting blood sugar can provide a definitive diagnosis. The oral glucose tolerance test is of little value by itself because the older adult may have impaired glucose tolerance but not diabetes (Armetta & Molony, 1999).

In terms of thyroid disease, the formation of nodules that interfere with normal thyroid functioning becomes more common with age. Unfortunately, hypothyroidism and associated symptoms of fatigue, forgetfulness, and cold sensitivity may be seen as normal "slowing down" with age and go undetected. Hyperthyroidism is much more likely in the older years, but among older adults, the typical symptoms of restlessness and hyperactivity may be lacking.

For older adults, hyperthyroidism, or an overproduction of thyroid hormone, does not usually mean major changes to everyday life. Nursing observation and assessment questions should address the occurrence of nervousness, heat intolerance, weight loss, tremor, and palpitations. Hypothyroidism, or below normal levels of thyroid hormone, causes several changes that can be uncomfortable and distressing. In the health history, the nurse should be assessing for skin changes (dry, flaky), fluid retention (edema and weight gain), fatigue, forgetfulness, constipation, and unusual sensitivity to the cold. Diagnostic tests (TSH test, TRH test, and radioimmunoassay) provide definitive diagnosis.

Hematologic and Immune Function

Several factors affect older adults' hematologic and immune systems. In relation to hematologic function, anemia is a common disorder among older adults, especially among those in nursing homes: About 40% of adults age 60 or older have iron-deficiency anemia. Although a slight decrease in hemoglobin occurs with aging, more often the anemia is attributable to an iron deficiency or another illness. Assessment should focus on observation of the color and quality of the skin and nail beds, and address food choices and food habits. Of a more serious nature, iron deficiency can occur because of blood loss, and the nurse should ask questions about occurrence of blood in stools. Diagnostic tests include hemoglobin, hematocrit, complete blood count (CBC), and red blood cell (RBC) count.

The immune system functions to protect the body from bacteria, viruses, and other microorganisms. Age-related changes to the immune system include diminished lymphocyte function and antibody immune responses. These changes put older adults at risk for infections. Vaccines for influenza and pneumonia are given in the fall and are available in physicians' offices, public health agencies, and other sites. As part of the assessment, the nurse should ask about recent and current infections and access to and use of vaccines to prevent infections. In terms of the symptoms of infection, it is important to remember that when evaluating vital signs, older adults tend to have a diminished febrile response to infection.

Some nurses are uncomfortable talking with older adults about sexual activity, prophylaxis, and sexually transmitted diseases (STDs), but these questions are an essential part of the health assessment process. Sexually active older adults, particularly those with more than one partner, are at risk for STDs. Of particular concern is the lack of STD education ("safe sex") programs focused on older adults, specifically HIV education. Human immunodeficiency virus (HIV) is a human retrovirus that causes acquired immune deficiency syndrome (AIDS). The disease is spread through parenteral and body fluids. It can be sexually transmitted through anal, oral, and vaginal intercourse.

AIDS is an epidemic in the United States, and the Centers for Disease Control and Prevention (CDC) reports that 11% of those infected are 50 years of age or older. Older adults may not be tested for HIV because they do not believe that they are at high risk or they may be unwilling to discuss their risky sexual behaviors. In terms of assessment, it is important to address the topic of sexual activity and ask the same questions that would be asked of a younger person. Open-ended questions are preferable, and it will be more productive to say, "Tell me about your sex life" rather than simply asking, "Do you have sex?" (Anderson, 2003). Depending on the status of sexual activity, other questions related to sexual preference and number of partners should be pursued. Signs and symptoms associated with HIV, such as weight loss, dehydration, ataxic gait, or fatigue, may go unnoticed or be attributed to age-related changes. However, once risk factors are identified, diagnostic testing will confirm a diagnosis.

Cognitive Assessment

Changes in cognitive function with age vary among older adults and are difficult to separate from other comorbidities (physical and psychological conditions), other age-related changes (for example, hearing) (see **Box 6-4**), the side effects of medications, and changes in intellectual activity. Generally speaking, older adults manifest a gradual and modest decline in short-term memory and experience a reduction in the speed with which new information is processed.

Cognitive function is usually understood in relation to the qualities of attention, memory, language, visuospatial skills, and executive capacity. The most extensively used cognitive assessment tool is the Mini Mental State Examination (MMSE) (Folstein, Folstein, & McHugh, 1975). The MMSE was originally developed to differentiate organic from functional disorders and to measure change in cognitive impairment, but it was not intended to be used as a diagnostic tool. It measures orientation, registration, attention and calculation, short-term recall, language, and

BOX 6-4   Research Highlight

Aim: To explore health literacy issues using the healthcare experiences of women with permanent visual impairments, including macular degeneration and other forms of retinopathy.

Methods: A sample of 15 community-dwelling women (aged 44–70 years) were interviewed and asked about how they had taken care of themselves since the onset of their visual problems. The qualitative content analysis was guided by the definition of health literacy from the Institute of Medicine (2004) as the ability to "obtain, process, and understand basic health-related information and services needed to make appropriate health decisions."

Findings: The women reported that healthcare workers made the following assumptions: that they could not provide their own self-care, that they were being cared for by personal caregivers, and they were dependent on government assistance. In addition, women reported that healthcare workers focused on their disability and not on them as persons.

Application to practice: In assessing the health literacy of older adults with visual impairment, nurses should ensure that the assessment is based on identifying ability, respecting personhood, and not making assumptions related to independence and pathology.

Source: Harrison, T. C., Mackert, M., & Watkins, C. (2010). Health literacy issues among women with visual impairments. *Research in Gerontological Nursing, 3*(1), 49–60.

BOX 6-5   Sample Items from the MMSE

Orientation to Time:

"What day is it?"

Registration:

"Listen carefully. I am going to say three words. You say them back after I stop.

"Ready? Here they are ...

"APPLE (pause), PENNY (pause), TABLE (pause). Now repeat those words back to me."

[Repeat up to five times, but score only the first trial.]

Naming:

"What is this?" [Point to a pencil or pen.]

Reading:

"Please read this and do as it says." [Show examinee the words on the stimulus form.]

CLOSE YOUR EYES

visuospatial function. It does not measure executive function, and the results of the MMSE can vary by age and education, with older individuals and those with fewer years of formal education having lower scores (Crum, Anthony, Bassett, & Folstein, 1993). In addition, some of the MMSE items may be less relevant for older adults who are hospital inpatients or who are living in long-term care facilities (Stewart, O'Riley, Edelstein, & Gould, 2012). For example, orientation-based questions regarding dates and day or time may be less relevant for long-term care residents compared with questions that ask about location of their room in the facility. A sample of items from the MMSE is given in **Box 6-5.** The entire MMSE is purchased by agencies and facilities as part of the assessment process. It is also available in the document

"Screening for Delirium, Dementia and Depression in Older Adults" (Registered Nurses' Association of Ontario, 2003) at: http://www.rnao.org

The Mini-Cog is another screening tool that can be administered in 5 minutes or less and requires minimal training (Doerflinger, 2007). The screening consists of a three-item recall and a clock-drawing test. This reliable tool can assist nurses with early detection of cognitive problems. A full-text article about the Mini-Cog can be accessed through http://www.consultgerirn.org

Dementia is a permanent progressive decline in cognitive function, and Alzheimer's disease is the most common form of dementia. The Diagnostic and Statistical Manual of Mental Disorders, 4th edition (DSM-IV), used by both the psychiatric and psychological communities, states that dementia of the Alzheimer's type typically is manifested by both impaired memory (long- or short-term) and inability to learn or recall new information, and is distinguished by one (or more) of the following cognitive disturbances: aphasia, apraxia, agnosia, or disturbance in executive functioning (i.e., planning, organizing, sequencing, abstracting). These cognitive limitations have broad and major implications for occupational and social interaction, as well as safety. The declines associated with Alzheimer's disease are progressive and irreversible. Definitive diagnosis is possible only on autopsy, but diagnosis is made in the absence of alternatives (for example, brain tumor and other neurological conditions or diseases). Several tools are available to assess cognitive function, and the common element of most is the assessment of memory function (see **Box 6-6**).

For nurses, assessing cognitive function is a challenging task because of the combination of factors that may be interacting: physical and psychological comorbidities, age-related changes, the side effects of medications, and changes in environment, as some examples. Added to this is the concern that for older adults and their families, even the suspicion of Alzheimer's disease can be a frightening and discouraging experience. The behaviors associated with dementia are stigmatizing and concerns arise related not only to the loss of memory, but even more so to the potential loss of the "person" as the disease progresses (Dupuis, Wiersma, & Loiselle, 2012). An influential individual in our understanding of the course and nature of cognitive

Notable Quotes

"Healthcare providers' lack of awareness of current geriatrics practice and persistence in holding the outdated belief that confusion is a normal part of aging contribute to significant underrecognition of dementia in all settings. Early recognition and diagnosis are critical to carrying out best practices in the care of older patients."

—Deirdre Mary Carolan Doerflinger, PhD, CRNP (2007), in *American Journal of Nursing*, p. 62.

BOX 6-6   Recommended Readings

American Geriatrics Society, AGS Panel. (Updated annually). Geriatrics at your fingertips. New York, NY: Blackwell.

Baldwin, S., & Capstick, A. (2007). *Tom Kitwood on dementia: A reader and critical commentary*. Buckingham, UK: McGraw-Hill Open University Press.

Kane, R. L., Ouslander, J. G., Abrass, I. B., & Resnick, B. (2008). *Essentials of clinical geriatrics* (6th ed.). New York, NY: McGraw-Hill.

Mast, B. T. (2011).*Whole person dementia assessment*. Baltimore, MD: Health Professionals Press.

decline in dementia was Tom Kitwood, who defined *personhood* and pioneered the theory and practice of "person-centered care." Personhood is "a standing or status that is bestowed upon one human being by others, in the context of relationship and social being…it implies recognition, respect and trust" (Kitwood, 1997). Kitwood and Bredin (1992) argued that older persons with dementia should be recognized for their uniqueness, their experiential being, and their relatedness with others. Taking this perspective, nursing assessment emphasizes individualization, asking about and taking into account previous preferences for care directly expressed by the older adult with dementia or from family members as proxies, when necessary.

Another area of assessment of older adults with dementia is that of "social ability." Social abilities include giving and receiving attention, participating in conversation, recognizing social stimuli, appreciating humor, and being helpful to others (Baum, Edwards, & Morrow-Howell, 1993; Dawson, Wells, & Kline, 1993; Sabat & Collins, 1999). Dawson and her colleagues have developed and validated a social abilities assessment subscale that can be used as a basis for supporting and maintaining ability in social life as much as possible. The entire tool (Abilities Assessment for the Nursing Care of Persons with Alzheimer's Disease and Related Disorders) is available in the document "Caregiving Strategies for Older Adults with Delirium, Dementia and Depression" (Registered Nurses' Association of Ontario, 2004) at http://www.rnao.org.

Psychological Assessment

Psychological assessment of older adults presents a wide continuum from positive mental health to mental health problems, and the tendency seems to be weighted toward assessment of mental health disorders. In this chapter we will be looking at two areas of psychological assessment: quality of life, which may include several positive mental health constructs, and depression, a common mental health problem.

Quality of Life

Quality of life and successful aging are two central concepts in assessment and care of older adults. Broadly speaking, quality of life encompasses all areas of everyday life: environmental and material components as well as physical, mental, and social well-being (Fletcher, Dickinson, & Philp, 1992). Quality of life among older adults is highly individualistic, subjective, and multidimensional in scope. With respect to what constitutes quality of life, what is important to one person may be quite unimportant to another. Related to quality of life is the concept of successful aging. Long associated with community living, successful aging has traditionally been linked with physical health, independence, functional ability, and *longevity*. However, other elements such as engagement in social life, self-mastery, optimism, personal meaning in life, and attainment of goals have been suggested as vital to the idea of successful aging (Reker, Peacock, & Wong, 1987; Rowe & Kahn, 1997). Elements of successful aging can include self-acceptance, positive relationships with others, and personal growth. A broad conceptualization of successful aging means broad applicability to older adults with varying abilities and disabilities. If we can go beyond the idea of physical health as the primary criterion for successful aging, then we can remove the labeling of frail older adults as being "unsuccessful" in their aging (Guse & Masesar, 1999).

Assessment of quality of life and successful aging can assist in better understanding the psychological health of older adults. Simply put, the following assessment questions will open dialogue on attitude, beliefs, and feelings about aging and mental health (see **Figure 6-1**). For example, the nurse can ask, "How would you describe your quality of life?" and "What would add to your quality of life?" Questions on successful aging are also informative. For example, "Would you describe yourself as someone who is aging successfully?" and "What would help you to age successfully?"

Depression

Clinical depression is the most common mental health problem among older adults, and it often goes undetected because clinicians attribute depressive symptoms to age-associated changes, chronic physical illness, medication side effects, or pain. The consequences of clinical depression can be serious and include suicidal ideation and suicide attempts. The prevalence of clinical depression in older Americans is estimated to be 14–20% among community-dwelling individuals, 30–40% among recently hospitalized individuals, and 15–30% among older persons residing in long-term care facilities (Anstey, von Sanden, & Sargent-Cox, 2007; Lebowitz et al.,

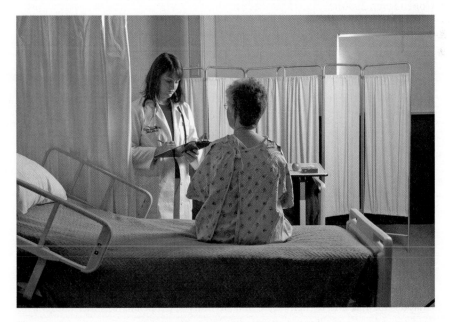

Figure 6-1 Quality care begins with comprehensive assessment.
Source: Photo courtesy of Don Battershall (Hartford Foundation)

1997; Wilson, Mottram, & Sexsmith, 2007). Minor depression can precede clinical or major depression and can be a response to stressors such as widowhood, loss of independence, or other losses. Older Americans may experience minor depression on a chronic basis but not meet the established criteria for clinical or major depression as outlined in the DSM-IV. To meet the DSM-IV criteria, an older adult must experience five or more of the following symptoms during a 2-week period (American Psychiatric Association, 2000):

> Sadness
> Lack of enjoyment of previously enjoyed activities
> Significant weight loss
> Sleep disturbance
> Restlessness
> Fatigue
> Feelings of worthlessness
> Impaired ability to think clearly or concentrate
> Suicide ideation or attempt

Depressed older adults may experience difficulty with sleeping, loss of appetite, physical discomfort, anxiety, hopelessness, bouts of crying, and thoughts of suicide. They may feel uncomfortable in social situations and curtail their usual social contacts and events, creating a downward spiral of depression and isolation. A study conducted among rural older adults in public housing facilities reported an association among symptoms of depression, poverty, and social isolation (Fisher & Copenhaver, 2006).

Depression is associated with cognitive limitations, and depressed older adults can experience disorientation, shortened attention span, emotional outbursts, and difficulty in intellectual functioning. Differentiating between dementia and depression when several of the same symptoms are present is a challenge for nurses. An excellent source is the document "Screening for Delirium, Dementia and Depression in Older Adults" (Registered Nurses' Association of Ontario, 2003), found at the website http://www.rnao.org, and Chapter 11 provides more information on the relationship among dementia, depression, and delirium.

The Geriatric Depression Scale (GDS) is widely used by nurses to assess symptoms of depression. The interviewer asks the older person a set of 30 questions with possible answers of yes or no. A "negative" response, which depending on the question may be a yes or no answer, is scored as one point; a higher score indicates more symptoms of depression. A score of 0–30 is possible, with 0–9 being normal, 10–19 indicating mild depression, and 20–30 indicating severe depressive symptoms. The 30-item GDS is provided in **Box 6-7**, and the capitalized responses are to be used in the scoring of responses. A shortened version of the GDS is presented in Chapter 30, and this 15-item scale may be more appropriate for older adults who are fatigued or have a limited attention span.

BOX 6-7   Geriatric Depression Scale (1983)

1. Are you basically satisfied with your life? Yes/NO

2. Have you dropped many of your activities or interests? YES/No

3. Do you feel that your life is empty? YES/No

4. Do you often get bored? YES/No

5. Are you hopeful about the future? Yes/NO

6. Are you bothered by thoughts you can't get out of your head? YES/No

7. Are you in good spirits most of the time? Yes/NO

8. Are you afraid that something bad is going to happen to you? YES/No

9. Do you feel happy most of the time? Yes/NO

10. Do you often feel helpless? YES/No

11. Do you often get restless and fidgety? YES/No

12. Do you prefer to stay at home, rather than going out and doing new things? YES/No

13. Do you frequently worry about the future? YES/No

14. Do you feel that you have more problems with memory than most? YES/No

15. Do you think that it is wonderful to be alive now? Yes/NO

16. Do you often feel downhearted and blue? YES/No

17. Do you feel pretty worthless the way you are now? YES/No

18. Do you worry a lot about the past? YES/No

19. Do you find life very exciting? Yes/NO

20. Is it hard to you to get started on new projects? YES/No

21. Do you feel full of energy? Yes/NO

22. Do you feel that your situation is hopeless? YES/No

23. Do you think that most people are better off than you are? YES/No

24. Do you frequently get upset over little things? YES/No

25. Do you frequently feel like crying? YES/No

26. Do you have trouble concentrating? YES/No

27. Do you enjoy getting up in the morning? Yes/NO

28. Do you prefer to avoid social gatherings? YES/No

29. Is it easy for you to make decisions? Yes/NO

30. Is your mind as clear as it used to be? Yes/NO

Source: Yesavage, J. A., Brink, T. L., Rose, T. L. Lum, O., Huang, V., Adey., M. M., & Leirer, V. O. (1983). Development and validation of a geriatric depression scale: A preliminary report. *Journal of Psychiatric Research, 17,* 37–49. (Reprinted with permission.)

Clinical depression may be chronic or have a shorter duration, and it is not the same as experiencing temporary feelings of unhappiness, confused thinking, and somatic complaints. Nurses are in a good position, whether it be in community, acute care, or long-term care practice, to screen for potential depression (Bruno & Ahrens, 2003). One study found that questions asking about functional ability decline, visual impairment, memory impairment, and using three or more medications provided a reasonably good screen for depressive symptoms and consequential health service utilization (Dendukuri, McCusker, & Belzile, 2004). Even asking the question, "Do you often feel sad or depressed?" is likely to open discussion and lead to further assessment of feelings of depression (Mahoney et al., 1994). Treatment of depression requires the input and knowledge base of several disciplines (Wang, 2011).

Social Assessment

Social functioning affects health and disease outcomes, and health status affects the ability to socialize and interact with others (Tomaka, Thompson, & Palacios, 2006). As people age, they may find that their social networks become smaller, and this may place them at risk in several ways. Decades of research have told us that individuals with low quantity and quality of social relationships have a higher morbidity and mortality risk compared with those who have a good quantity and quality of social contacts. A supportive social network and in particular the presence of a spouse can act to maintain an older adult in the community; the lack of a partner is a predictor of nursing home placement.

Social assessment of older adults includes collecting information on the presence of a social network and on the interaction between the older adult and family, friends, neighbors, and community. Kane, Ouslander, and Abrass (1989) developed a broad-based social assessment that includes asking questions about recent life events (such as death of a spouse), living arrangements, everyday activities requiring help (and who usually provides help), potential isolation (frequency of leaving the house and having visitors), adequacy of income, and sources of healthcare coverage (see **Box 6-8** for additional resources). Posed by the nurse, these general questions can identify areas of limitation in social contact and social support.

Having a social network of friends and family does not necessarily mean that there are social supports. However, the Lubben Social Network Scale contains 10 items, 3 of which have been found to differentiate those who are isolated from those who are not (Kane, 1995). These questions are:

> Is there any one special person you could call or contact if you needed help?
> In general, other than your children, how many relatives do you feel close to and have contact with at least once a month?
> In general, how many friends do you feel close to and have contact with at least once a month?

The more important aspects of social support may be the number of supportive persons and the various types of support (emotional, instrumental, and informational) that are available. Seeman and Berkman (1988) have identified four questions that assess the adequacy of social support. These questions are:

> When you need help, can you count on anyone for house cleaning, groceries, or a ride?
> Could you use more help with daily tasks?

BOX 6-8   Resource List

Hospital Elder Life Program (http://www. hospitalelderlifeprogram.org): The Hospital Elder Life Program (HELP) is a patient-care program, developed by doctors and nurses at the Yale School of Medicine, that is designed to prevent delirium among hospitalized older patients.

The John A. Hartford Foundation Institute for Geriatric Nursing (http://www.hartfordign.org and http://www.consultgerirn.org): These websites offer links to several assessment tools, including SPICES (an overall assessment tool), Fall Risk Assessment, and the Geriatric Depression Scale.

National Institute for Health and Clinical Excellence (NICE) (http://www.nice.org.uk): This agency is an excellence-in-practice organization

responsible for providing national guidance on the promotion of good health and the prevention and treatment of ill health in the United Kingdom. The website offers assessment and prevention tools in relation to falls and older adults.

Registered Nurses' Association of Ontario (http://www.rnao.org/bestpractices): This is the professional association of registered nurses in Ontario, Canada. It provides several best practices including assessment guidelines, for example, in the areas of pain; stage I to IV pressure ulcers; foot ulcers for people with diabetes; and screening for delirium, dementia, and depression in older adults.

> Can you count on anyone for emotional support (talking over problems or helping you make a decision)?
> Could you use more emotional help (receiving sufficient support)?

Asking these kinds of questions will help assess the adequacy and range of support available to an older adult. Nurses should be asking questions about social support and social function as part of the comprehensive assessment. The questions developed by Lubben can be used with older adults generally across settings (community and acute and long-term care settings), whereas some of the questions posed by Seeman and Berk clearly relate to older adults living in the community.

Spiritual Assessment

Spiritual assessment is an integral part of comprehensive assessment and provides a basis for an individualized plan of care (Forbes, 1994). Although there is a link between religiosity and spirituality, the two concepts are not synonymous. Religiosity refers to believing in God, organized rituals, and specific dogma; spirituality refers more broadly to ideas of belief that encompass personal philosophy and an understanding of meaning and purpose in life. Having religious beliefs may foster spirituality, but those without formal religious beliefs still can experience spirituality. Most health service intake forms have a place for collecting information on formal religious affiliation, but this does not necessary mean that the older adult is practicing his or her faith, or is active in a place of worship.

One of the earliest guidelines for spiritual assessment was developed by Stoll (1979), and it contains questions that address both religiosity and spirituality. The guidelines are divided into four areas:

1. The concept of God or deity (for example, "Is religion or God significant to you?")
2. Personal source of strength and hope (for example, "What is your source of strength and hope?")
3. Significance of religious practices and rituals (for example, "Are there any religious practices that are important to you?")
4. Perceived relationship between spiritual belief and health (for example, "Has being sick made any difference in your feelings about God or the practice of your faith?")

Nurses may not be comfortable conducting a spiritual assessment because it may seem inappropriately invasive or because it is an area that some nurses do not feel adequately prepared to address as an unmet need. If the intake record indicates a formal religious affiliation, then it is fairly straightforward to ask, "Do you have any religious needs?" or "Would you like to speak with a pastoral care worker?" Questions that address spirituality can begin by asking, "Are you having a spiritual need? Is there some way that I might help with your spiritual needs?" Another spiritual assessment question asks, "Have your health problems affected your feelings of meaning or purpose?" Spiritual assessment is an area that would benefit greatly from more research.

Other Assessment: Obesity

Obesity has become a major health problem among Americans, including older Americans, and it is associated with chronic disease and disability (Jensen, 2005). Given the obesity prevalence in middle-aged adults, the proportions and numbers of obese older adults are expected to increase substantially over the next decade (Arterburn, Crane, & Sullivan, 2004). Providing care to obese persons places caregivers, both family and staff members, at risk for injury. In 1998, the National Institutes of Health released the first federal overweight and obesity guidelines, which are based on the body mass index (BMI), a ratio of weight (in pounds) to height (in inches squared), as an assessment tool. The BMI is a number usually between 16 and 40; a BMI between 25 and 29 is considered "overweight" and more than 30 is considered "obese." For instructions on how to calculate a BMI, go to the Centers for Disease Control and Prevention (CDC) website: www.cdc.gov/nccdphp/dnpa/healthyweight/assessing/bmi.

The adverse effects of obesity in relation to cardiovascular disease, diabetes, osteoarthritis, and gallbladder disease are well documented (Fields & Strano 2005). Obese older adults are likely to experience balance and mobility problems that place them at risk for falls. One study reported obesity as being a risk factor for decline in functional ability (as assessed by needing assistance with ADLs and IADLs) (Jensen & Friedmann, 2002). Unfortunately, there has been little research conducted on obese older adults, and this remains an area for further research and tool refinement. It is not clear whether the markers for overweight and obesity are relevant to older adults who may experience illness-related weight gain or loss. It has been suggested that for many older adults, an emphasis on weight maintenance might be the best approach until more evidence is accumulated through research (Jensen & Friedmann, 2002).

Nurses can assess for overweight and obesity using the BMI and by asking about a history of weight change. If food intake is a concern, a common approach is to begin with a 3- to 7-day meal diary. This information can assist in determining a person's food habits. This is an area of assessment where nurses could benefit from working with the nutritionist and the dietician, who have a specialized knowledge base.

Developing an Individualized Plan of Care

At the beginning of this chapter, we indicated that the basis of an individualized plan of care for an older adult is a comprehensive assessment, and we have reviewed functional, physical, cognitive, psychological, social, and spiritual assessment. **Box 6-9** provides 10 guidelines for comprehensive assessment that form a basis with which to develop an individualized plan of care. Additionally, **Box 6-10** provides a

---

BOX 6-9   Ten Principles of Comprehensive Assessment

1. The cornerstone of an individualized plan of care for an older adult is a comprehensive assessment.

2. Comprehensive assessment takes into account age-related changes, age-associated and other diseases, heredity, and lifestyle.

3. Nurses are members of the healthcare team, contributing to and drawing from the team to enhance the assessment process.

4. Comprehensive assessment is not a neutral process.

5. Ideally, the older adult is the best source of information to assess his or her health. When this is not possible, family members or caregivers are acceptable as secondary sources of information. When the older adult cannot self-report, physical performance measures may provide additional information.

6. Comprehensive assessment should first emphasize ability and then address disability. Appropriate interventions to maintain and enhance ability and to improve or compensate for disability should follow from a comprehensive assessment.

7. Task performance and task capacity are two difference perspectives. Some assessment tools ask, "Do you dress without help?" (performance) whereas others ask, "Can you dress without help?" (capacity). Asking about capacity will result in answers that emphasize ability.

8. Assessment of older adults who have cognitive limitations may require task segmentation, or the breaking down of tasks into smaller steps.

9. Some assessment tools or parts of assessment tools may be more or less applicable depending on the setting, that is, community, acute care, or long-term care settings.

10. In comprehensive assessment, it is important to explore the meaning and implications of health status from the older adult's perspective. For example, the same changes in visual acuity for two older adults may have quite different meanings and implications for everyday life.

BOX 6-10   Assessment Tools Available Through The Try This Series

The following are available via http://consultgerirn.org/resources:

- SPICES: An Overall Assessment Tool of Older Adults

- Katz Index of Independence in Activities of Daily Living (ADL)

- The Mini Mental State Examination (MMSE)

- The Geriatric Depression Scale (GDS)

- Predicting Pressure Ulcer Risk

- The Pittsburgh Sleep Quality Index (PSQI)

- The Epworth Sleepiness Scale

- Assessing Pain in Older Adults

- Fall Risk Assessment

- Assessing Nutrition in Older Adults

- Sexuality Assessment

- Urinary Incontinence Assessment

- Hearing Screening

- Confusion Assessment Method (CAM)

- Caregiver Strain Index (CSI)

- Elder Mistreatment Assessment

- Beers' Criteria for Potentially Inappropriate Medication Use in the Elderly

- Alcohol Use Screening and Assessment

- The Kayser Jones Brief Oral Health Status Examination (BOHSE)

- Horowitz's Impact of Event Scale: An Assessment of Post-Traumatic Stress in Older Adults

- Preventing Aspiration in Older Adults with Dysphagia

- Immunizations for the Older Adult

- Assessing Family Preferences for Participation in Care in Hospitalized Older Adults

- The Lawton Instrumental Activities of Daily Living (IADL) Scale

- The Hospital Admission Risk Profile (HARP)

- Confusion Assessment Method for the Intensive Care Unit (CAM-ICU)

- Avoiding Restraints in Patients with Dementia

- Brief Evaluation of Executive Dysfunction: An Essential Refinement in the Assessment of Cognitive Impairment

- Assessing Pain in Persons with Dementia

- Therapeutic Activity Kits

- Recognition of Dementia in Hospitalized Older Adults

- Wandering in the Hospitalized Older Adult

- Communication Difficulties: Assessment and Interventions

- Assessing and Managing Delirium in Persons with Dementia

- Decision Making and Dementia

- Working with Families of Hospitalized Older Adults with Dementia

- Eating and Feeding Issues in Older Adults with Dementia: Part I: Assessment

- Eating and Feeding Issues in Older Adults with Dementia: Part II: Interventions

summary of the quality assessment tools recommended as best practices by the John A. Hartford Foundation and the Nurse Competence in Aging initiative (see http://www.consultgerirn.org) (**Box 6-11**).

BOX 6-11   Web Exploration

Visit the Hartford Institute's website and browse the tools, videos, and articles available at http://consultgerirn.org/resources/

Summary

Comprehensive assessment of the older adult is an essential component of geriatric nursing care that involves both objective and subjective data collection. Nurses may obtain information about the older adult patient from a variety of sources including the patient, family, friends, caregivers, nursing staff, other team members, charts, and other written documentation. All aspects of the older adult person should be considered, including physical, psychological, socioeconomic, and spiritual. Particular challenges may be encountered when assessing older adults with cognitive impairments. This chapter presented many tools and websites that can assist the nurse in assessing older adults as the initial step in individualizing a plan of care.

Critical Thinking Exercises

1. **In this chapter, we have said that** comprehensive assessment is not a neutral process. Reflect on what that really means and what kinds of things might constitute an unwanted bias to the assessment process.

2. **In this chapter, we have emphasized that** comprehensive assessment makes use of nursing knowledge and understanding of the combined factors of age-related changes, age-associated and other diseases, heredity, and lifestyle choices. Think of an older adult for whom you have provided care and describe that person. Try to outline the factors (age-related changes, age-associated and other diseases, heredity, and lifestyle choices) that are relevant for his or her health assessment.

Personal Reflections

1. In this chapter, we have underlined the importance of the healthcare team and consultation with team members. Reflect on your understanding of the contributions of team members in relation to the assessment of older adults. What are some of your personal qualities in terms of working as a member of the health care team?

2. How would you define "successful aging" in relation to your own aging? What are the implications of your definition in relation to decisions you might make during your lifetime? How might this definition affect the way you view the aging process of others?

References

Adnan, A., Chang, A., Arseven, O. K., & Emanuel, L. L. (2005). Assessment instruments. In L. L. Emanuel (Ed.), *Clinical geriatric medicine* (pp. 121–146). Philadelphia, PA: Saunders.

American Psychiatric Association. (2000). *Diagnostic and statistical manual of mental disorders* (4th ed., text rev.). Washington, DC: Author.

Anderson, M. A. (2003). *Caring for older adults holistically* (3rd ed.). Philadelphia, PA: F. A. Davis.

Annells, M., & Koch, T. (2003). Constipation and the breached trio: Diet, fluid intake, exercise. *International Journal of Nursing Studies, 40,* 843–852.

Anstey, K. J., von Sanden, C., & Sargent-Cox, C. (2007). Prevalence and risk factors for depression in a longitudinal, population-based study including individuals in the community and residential care. *American Journal of Geriatric Psychiatry, 15*(6), 497–505.

Armetta, M., & Molony, C. M. (1999). Topics in endocrine and hematologic care. In S. L. Molony, C. M. Waszynski, & C. H. Lyder (Eds.), *Gerontological nursing: An advanced practice approach* (pp. 359–387). Stamford, CT: Appleton & Lange.

Arterburn, D. E., Crane, P. K., & Sullivan, S. D. (2004). The coming epidemic of obesity in elderly Americans. *Journal of the American Geriatrics Society, 52,* 1007–1012.

Baum, C., Edwards, D. F., & Morrow-Howell, N. (1993). Identification and measurement of productive behaviours in senile dementia of the Alzheimer's type. *The Gerontologist, 33,* 403–408.

Bawden, M. E. (2006). Clean those teeth. *Perspectives, 30*(4), 15.

Beck, C. (1988). Measurement of dressing performance in persons with dementia. *American Journal of Alzheimer's Care and Related Disorders and Research, 3,* 21–25.

Brink, P., & Stones, M. (2007). Examination of the relationship among hearing impairment, linguistic communication, mood and social engagement of residents in complex continuing care facilities. *The Gerontologist, 47*(5), 633–641.

Bruno, L., & Ahrens, J. (2003, November). The importance of screening for depression in home care patients. *Caring,* 54–58.

Bureau of the Census. (1997). *Statistical abstract of the United States 1997* (117th ed.). Washington, DC: U.S. Department of Commerce.

Chan, C. C., & Lee, T. M. (1997). Validity of the Canadian Occupational Performance Measure. *Occupational Therapy International, 4*(3), 229–247.

Crum, R., Anthony, J., Bassett, S., & Folstein, M. (1993). Population-based norms for the Mini-Mental State Examination by age and educational level. *Journal of the American Medical Association, 269*(18), 2386–2391.

Culbertson, D. S., Griggs, M., & Hudson, S. (2004). Ear and hearing status in a multilevel retirement facility. *Geriatric Nursing, 25,* 93–98.

Dawson, P., Wells, D. L., & Kline, K. (1993). *Enhancing the abilities of persons with Alzheimer's disease and related dementias.* New York, NY: Springer.

Dendukuri, N., McCusker, J., & Belzile, E. (2004). The Identification of Seniors at Risk screening tool: Further evidence of concurrent and predictive validity. *Journal of the American Geriatrics Society, 52*, 290–296.

Doerflinger, D. M. C. (2007). The Mini-Cog. *American Journal of Nursing, 107*(12), 62–71.

Dupuis, S. L., Wiersma, E., & Loiselle, L. (2012). Pathologizing behavior: Meanings of behaviors in dementia care. *Journal of Aging Studies, 26*, 162–173.

Ferrini, A., & Ferrini, R. (2012). *Health in the later years.* New York, NY: McGraw-Hill Higher Education.

Fessey, V. (2007). Patients who present with dementia: Exploring the knowledge of hospital nurses. *Nursing Older People, 19*(10), 29–33.

Fields, S. D., & Stano-Paul, L. (2005). Preface: Obesity. *Clinics in Geriatric Medicine, 21*(4), xi–xiii.

Fisher, K. M., & Copenhaver, V. (2006). Assessing the mental health of rural older adults in public housing facilities. *Journal of Gerontological Nursing, 22*(9), 26–33.

Fletcher, A. E., Dickinson, E. J., & Philp, I. (1992). Review: Quality of life instruments for everyday use with elderly patients. *Age and Aging, 21*, 142–150.

Folstein, M. F., Folstein, S. E., & McHugh, P. R. (1975). A practical method for grading the cognitive state of patients for the clinician. *Journal of Psychiatric Research, 12*(3), 189–198.

Forbes, E. J. (1994). Spirituality, aging, and the community-dwelling caregiver and care recipient. *Geriatric Nursing, 15*(6), 297–302.

Gates, G. A., Murphy, M., Rees, T. S., & Fraher, M. A. (2003). Screening for handicapping hearing loss in the elderly. *Journal of Family Practice, 52*(1), 56–62.

Gill, T. M., Williams, C. S., & Tinetti, M. E. (1995). Assessing risk for the onset of functional dependence among older adults: The role of physical performance. *Journal of the American Geriatrics Society, 43*, 604–609.

Guralnik, J. M., Branch, L. G., Cummings, S. R., & Curb, J. D. (1989). Physical performance measures in aging research. *Journal of Gerontology: Medical Sciences, 44*(5), M141–M146.

Guse, L. W., & Masesar, M. (1999). Quality of life and successful aging in long-term care: Perceptions of residents. *Mental Health Nursing, 20*(6), 527–539.

Harrison, T. C., Mackert, M., & Watkins, C. (2010). Health literacy issues among women with visual impairments. *Research in Gerontological Nursing, 3*(1), 49–60.

Institute of Medicine. (2004). *Health Literacy: A Prescription to End Confusion.* Washington, DC: National Academies Press.

Jensen, G. L. (2005). Obesity and functional decline: Epidemiology and geriatric consequence. *Clinics in Geriatric Medicine, 21*(4), 677–687.

Jensen, G. L., & Friedmann, J. M. (2002). Obesity is associated with functional decline in community-dwelling rural older adults. *Journal of the American Geriatrics Society, 50*, 918–923.

Jung, S., Coleman, A., & Weintraub, N. T. (2007). Vision screening in the elderly. *Journal of the American Medical Directors Association, 8*(6), 355–362.

Kahn, R. S. (1964). Comments. In M. P. Lawton & F. G. Lawton (Eds.), *Mental impairment in the aged* (pp. 109–114). Philadelphia, PA: Philadelphia Geriatric Center.

Kane, R., Ouslander, J., & Abrass, J. (1989). *Social assessment: Essentials of geriatrics.* New York, NY: McGraw-Hill.

Kane, R. A. (1995). Comment. In L. Z. Rubenstein, D. Wieland, & R. Bernabei (Eds.), *Geriatric assessment technology: The state of the art* (pp. 99–100). New York, NY: Springer.

Kane, R. L. (1993). The implications of assessment. *Journals of Gerontology, 48*(special issue), 27–31.

Katz, S., Down, T. D., Cash, H. R.. & Grotz, R. C. (1970). Progress in the development of the index of ADL. *The Gerontologist, 10*, 20–30.

Katz, S., Ford, A., Moskowitz, R., Jackson, B., & Jaffee, M. (1963). Studies of illness in the aged: The index of ADL, a standardized measure of biological and psychosocial functioning. *Journal of the American Medical Association, 185*, 94–101.

Kearney, P. M., & Pryor, J. (2004). The international classification of functioning, disability, and health (ICF) and nursing. *Journal of Advanced Nursing, 46*(2), 142–170.

Kitwood, T. (1997). *Dementia reconsidered.* Buckingham, UK: Open University Press.

Kitwood, T., & Bredin, K. (1992). Towards a theory of dementia care: *Personhood and well-being. Ageing and Society, 12*(3), 269–287.

Law, M., Polatajko, H., Pollock, N., McColl, M. A., Carswell, A., & Baptiste, S. (1994). Pilot testing of the Canadian Occupational Performance Measure: Clinical and measurement issues. Canad*ian Journal of Occupational Therapy, 61*(4), 191–197.

Lawton, M. P. (1972). Assessing the competence of older people. In D. Kent & R. Kastenbaum (Eds.), *Research, planning and action for the elderly*. Sherwood, NY: Behavioral Publications.

Lawton, M. P., & Brody, E. M. (1969). Assessment of older people: Self-maintaining and instrumental activities of daily living. *The Gerontologist, 9*(3), 179–186.

Lebowitz, B. D., Pearson, J. L., Schneider, L. S., Reynolds, C. F., Aleropoulos, G. S., Bruce, M. F.,… Parmalee, P. (1997). Diagnosis and treatment of depression in late life: Consensus statement update. *Journal of the American Medical Association, 278*, 1186–1190.

Lee, J. S., Kritchevsky, S. B., Tylavsky, F., Harrie, T. B., Ayonayon, H. N., & Newman, A. B. (2006). Factors associated with well-functioning community-dwelling older adults. *Journal of Nutrition for the Elderly, 26*(1), 27–43.

Luborsky, M. (1997). Attuning assessment to the client: Recent advances in theory and methodology. *Generations, 21*(1), 10–15.

Mahoney, F. I., & Barthel, D. W. (1965). Functional evaluation: The Barthel index. *Maryland State Medical Journal, 14*(2), 61–65.

Mahoney, J., Drinka, T., Abler, R., Gunter-Hunt, G., Matthews, C., Grenstein, S., & Carnes, M. (1994). Screening for depression: Single question versus GDS. *Journal of the American Geriatrics Society, 42*, 1006–1008.

McGuire, K. (2006). Promotion of urinary continence: Management of urinary incontinence in the geriatric setting. *Perspective, 30*(2), 22–23.

Mentes, J.C., &Wang, J. (2011). Measuring risk for dehydration in nursing home residents. *Research in Gerontological Nursing, 4*(2),148–156.

Mesman, G. R., Buchanan, J. A., Husfeldt, J. D., & Berg, T. M. (2011). Identifying preference in persons with dementia: Systematic preference testing vs. caregiver and family member report. *Clinical Gerontologist, 34*, 154–159.

Morley, J. E. (2003). Anorexia and weight loss among older persons. *Journal of Gerontology Biological Sciences, 58*(2), 131–137.

Morris, J. N., & Morris, S. A. (1997). ADL assessment measures for use with frail elders. In J. A. Teresi, M. P. Lawton, D. Holmes, & M. Ory (Eds.), *Measurement in elderly chronic care populations* (pp. 130–156). New York, NY: Springer.

Olenek, K., Skowronski, T., & Schmaltz, D. (2003, August). Geriatric nursing assessment. *Journal of Gerontological Nursing*, 5–10.

Ostbye, T., Tyas, S., McDowell, I., & Koval, J. J. (1997). Reported activities of daily living: Agreement between elderly subjects with and without dementia and their caregivers. *Age and Ageing, 26*, 99–106.

Parker, M. G., & Thorslund, M. (2007). Health trends in the elderly population: Getting better and getting worse. *The Gerontologist, 47*(2), 150–158.

Perry, L., Kendrick, D., Morris, R., Dinan, S., Masud, T., Skelton, D., Iliffe, S. (2012). Completion and return of fall diaries varies with participants' level of education, first language and baseline fall risk. *Journal of Gerontology: Medical Sciences, 67A*(2), 210–214.

Registered Nurses' Association of Ontario. (2003). *Screening for delirium, dementia and depression in older adults*. Toronto, Canada: Author.

Registered Nurses' Association of Ontario. (2004). *Caregiving strategies for older adults with delirium, dementia and depression*. Toronto, Canada: Author.

Reker, G. T., Peacock, E. J., & Wong, P. T. P. (1987). Meaning and purpose in life and well-being: A life span perspective. *Journal of Gerontology, 42*, 44–49.

Reuben, D. B., Herr, K. A., Pacala, J. T., Pollock, B. G., Potter, J. F., & Semla, T. P. (2008). *Geriatrics at your fingertips*. Malden, MA: American Geriatrics Society.

Reuben, D. B., & Sui, A. L. (1990). An objective measure of physical function of elderly outpatients: The physical performance test. *Journal of the American Geriatrics Society, 38*, 1190–1193.

Reuben, D. B., Valle, L. A., Hays, R. D., & Sui, A. L. (1995). Measuring physical function in community-dwelling older persons: A comparison of self-administered, interviewer-administered and performance-based measures. *Journal of the American Geriatrics Society, 43*, 17–23.

Richman, S. M., & Drickamer, M. A. (2007). Gynecologic care of elderly women. *Journal of the American Medical Directors Association, 8*(4), 219–223.

Rowe, J. W., & Kahn, R. L. (1997). Successful aging. *The Gerontologist, 37*, 433–440.

Sabat, S. R., & Collins, M. (1999, January/February). Intact social, cognitive ability and selfhood: A case study of Alzheimer's disease. *American Journal of Alzheimer's Disease*, 112–119.

Seeman, T. E., & Berkman, L. F. (1988). Structural characteristics of social networks and their relationship with social support in the elderly: Who provides support? *Social Science and Medicine, 26*(7), 737–749.

Stewart, S., O'Riley, A., Edelstein, B., & Gould, C. (2012). A preliminary comparison of three cognitive screening instruments in long-term care: The MMSE, SLUMS, and MoCA. *Clinical Gerontologist, 35*, 57–75.

Stolee, P., Patterson, M. L., Wiancko, D. C., Esbaugh, J., Arcese, Z. A., Vinke, A. M., Crilly, R. G. (2003). An enhanced role in comprehensive geriatric assessment for community nurse case managers. *Canadian Journal on Aging, 22*(2), 177–184.

Stoll, R. L. (1979, September). Guidelines for spiritual assessment. *American Journal of Nursing*, 1574–1577.

Stone, L. M., & Lyles, K. W. (2006). Osteoporosis in later life. *Generations, 30*(3), 65–70.

Tappen, R. M. (1994). Development of the refined ADL assessment scale. *Journal of Gerontological Nursing, 20*(6), 36–41.

Tariq, S. H. (2007). Constipation in long-term care. *Journal of the American Medical Directors Association, 8*(4), 209–218.

Tinetti, M. E., Speechley, M., & Ginter, S. F. (1988). Risk factors for falls among elderly persons living in the community. *New England Journal of Medicine, 319*, 1701–1707.

Tomaka, J., Thompson, S., & Palacios, R. (2006). The relation of social isolation, loneliness and social support to disease outcomes among the elderly. *Journal of Aging and Health, 18*(3), 359–384.

Uniform Data System for Medical Rehabilitation (UDSMR). (1996). *Guide for the Uniform Data Set for Medical Rehabilitation (including the FIM instrument)*. Buffalo, NY: Author.

Verbrugge, L. M., & Jette, A. M. (1994). The disablement process. *Social Science and Medicine, 38*, 1–14.

Wilson, K., Mottram, P., & Sexsmith, A. (2007). Depressive symptoms in the very old living alone: Prevalence, incidence and risk factors. *International Journal of Geriatric Psychiatry, 22*, 361–366.

Wallhagen, M. I. (2009). The stigma of hearing loss. *The Gerontologist, 50*(1), 66–75.

Wang, D. S. (2011). Interdisciplinary methods of treatment of depression in older adults: A primer for practitioners. *Activities, Adaptation & Aging, 35*, 298–314.

Woodward, S. (2012). Assessment and management of constipation in older people. *Nursing Older People, 24*(5), 21–26.

World Health Organization [WHO]. (2001). *International classification of function, disability, and health (ICF)*. Geneva, Switzerland: Author.

Yesavage, J. A., Brink, T. L., Rose, T. L., Lum, O., Huang, V., Aday, M., & Leirer, V. O. (1983). Development and validation of a geriatric depression screening scale. *Journal of Psychiatric Research, 17*, 37–49.

For a full suite of assignments and additional learning activities, see the access code at the front of your book.

Unit III
Health Promotion, Risk Reduction, and Disease Prevention

(COMPETENCIES 3–5, 9, 17, 18)

LEARNING OBJECTIVES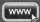

At the end of this chapter, the reader will be able to:

> Discuss the promise and limitations of the Healthy People initiatives.
> Apply the health contract technique and nutritional bull's-eye for behavior change.
> Describe several model health promotion programs.
> Explain the concept of re-engagement and provide examples of it.
> Identify the components of Medicare prevention.
> Explain the importance of life review.
> Recognize the importance of exercise and nutrition for healthy aging.
> Discuss the importance of the Green House project to the future of long-term care.

KEY TERMS

Center for Science in the Public Interest
   (CSPI)
Dependence
Depression
Exercise
Health behavior change
Health contract/calendar
Healthy People initiatives

Life review
Medicare prevention
Mental health
Model health promotion programs
Nutrition
Nutrition bull's-eye
Quality of life
Re-engagement

Chapter 7

(Competencies 4, 5, 9, 17, 18)

Promoting Healthy Aging

David Haber

Health promotion works, no matter what one's age, and even after decades of practicing unhealthy habits. But it does not work for everyone, all the time. So what needs to be done to increase the odds of promoting healthy aging successfully? Certainly the entire burden cannot be placed on the guilt-ridden backs of individuals. The federal and state governments play a significant role, as do religious institutions, businesses, community centers, hospitals, medical clinics, health professionals, educational institutions, families, neighborhoods, and even shopping malls. In this chapter, some of these influences on healthy aging will be explored.

Exercise and *nutrition* are probably the two most widely publicized components of health promotion, and they will be given their due in this chapter as well. We will use a broad definition of health promotion in this chapter, one that includes such diverse topics as self-management through health contracts, promoting mental health through life reviews, promoting *re-engagement* rather than retirement, and promoting the health of frail elders through unique homes rather than through institutions that are merely called (nursing) homes.

One aspect of health promotion lies with the federal government. We'll start by talking about the Healthy People initiatives and Medicare prevention.

Healthy People Initiatives

The federal government has been establishing goals for healthy aging since 1980, when the U.S. Public Health Service published the report *Promoting Health/Preventing Disease: Objectives for the Nation*. This 1980 report outlined 226 objectives for the nation to achieve over the following 10 years. It was referred to by some as Healthy People 1990.

A decade later, in 1990, another 10-year national effort, Healthy People 2000, was initiated by the U.S. Public Health Service to reduce preventable death and disability for Americans. A third effort came with the Healthy People 2010 initiative and 467 objectives distributed over 28 priority areas. Healthy People 2020 sets forth four overarching goals, one of which is to "attain high quality, longer lives free of preventable disease, disability, injury, and premature death" (p. 1).

There are some notable benefits to the *Healthy People initiatives*. On the positive side, these initiatives give recognition to health promotion rather than focusing exclusively on wars on diseases (e.g., tabulating the number of deaths from cancer or heart disease, and then organizing a campaign against them). The Healthy People initiatives are health oriented, and as such they recognize the complexity of the socioeconomic, lifestyle, and other nonmedical influences that impact our ability to attain and maintain health.

A second major benefit of the Healthy People initiatives is that they are focused on documenting baselines, setting objectives, and monitoring progress. For instance, according to the Healthy People 2000 Review, 1998–1999 (National Center for Health Statistics [NCHS], 1999), 15% of the objectives for the year 2000 were met, and 44% demonstrated movement toward the target. However, since the initiative relied mostly on data monitoring and a small amount of publicity—and very little financial support—it is unclear whether Healthy People 2000 contributed directly to this progress. For example, in an area where there was no financial support for encouraging change—being overweight or obese—the trend in America for adults between the ages of 20 and 74 has been in the opposite direction: a steady increase in weight gain for Americans over the decade (NCHS, 1999). There was a similar result with sedentary behavior among Americans. In the absence of financial support for encouraging change in this area, light to moderate physical activity on a near-daily basis between the ages of 18 and 74 had not improved over the decade (NCHS, 1999).

Focusing on those age 65 or over, the Merck Institute on Aging and Health came out with a report card on the Healthy People 2000 initiative (available at http://www.gericareonline.net) that revealed several failing grades. Older Americans did not reach the 2000 target goals, and in fact fell far short of them in the areas of physical activity, being overweight, and eating fruits and vegetables. Additional failing grades were assigned to the target goals of reducing hip fractures for persons age 65 or over and fall-related deaths for persons age 85 or over.

In contrast to the mere monitoring of most Healthy People 2000 target goals, financial assistance was provided to older adults through Medicare during the decade for mammogram coverage, pneumococcal vaccination, and influenza vaccination. With this financial support, the percentage of compliance in these three areas doubled among older adults during the decade (Haber, 2002). Consequently, the Healthy People 2000 target goals were met for mammogram screening and influenza vaccination, and fell just short of being met for pneumococcal vaccination.

This raises the question of whether the federal government should be doing more than monitoring data changes when it comes to promoting healthy aging. A comparable question can be asked of state governments. The Healthy People initiatives were supposed to have had a counterpart initiative at each of the state health departments. In this author's experience with several states, however, the initiatives either have been ignored or the state health department has conducted a modest project that was accomplished several years ago, but did not follow up with additional activity. Financing and leadership are needed to make these programs successful. To find out more about the Healthy People 2020 initiative, go to http://www.healthypeople.gov/2020/Connect/iHealthyPeople2020v25.pdf.

Medicare Prevention

The federal government does more than just establish Healthy People initiatives. It also reimburses Medicare recipients for certain prevention activities (see **Table 7-1**). Some of Medicare's reimbursement policies have emerged from the research evidence reviewed by the U.S. Preventive Services Task Force (USPSTF). USPSTF was launched by the U.S. Public Health Service to systematically review evidence of effectiveness of clinical preventive services. This task force periodically updates its research guidelines on a wide variety of screening and counseling recommendations, such as breast cancer screening, colorectal cancer screening, and counseling to promote physical activity.

These updates have been compiled into a two-volume, loose-leaf notebook and a CD for the period 2001 to 2006. This notebook, and periodic updates after 2006, can be accessed by calling the AHRQ Publications Clearinghouse at (800) 358-9295, by sending an email to ahrqpubs@ahrq.gov, or by visiting the website at http://www.ahrq.gov/clinic/pocketgd.htm.

If you review the USPSTF recommendations, however, you will notice that they are often out of sync with Medicare reimbursement policies. Some reimbursement policies appear to have been influenced more by medical lobbyists advocating for specific segments of the medical industry (e.g., oncology, urology, orthopedics) than by policy derived from evidence-based medicine (Haber, 2001, 2005).

Although the movement into *Medicare prevention*—with substantially expanded coverage in 1998 and 2005—undoubtedly benefits older Americans, there is room for considerable improvement in the way the Medicare program promotes health and prevents disease. Lobbyists have promoted medical screenings that are reimbursed too frequently or over too long a period of time. Some screenings may not be worth the expense (e.g., fecal occult blood test, barium enema, sigmoidoscopy, routine prostate cancer screening, baseline EKG). Conversely, Medicare policy is stingy toward risk reduction counseling, which, not surprisingly, has little if any lobbying effort behind it.

TABLE 7-1   Medicare Prevention

One-time "Welcome to Medicare Physical"
Within 6 months of initial enrollment; no deductible or copayment.
Physician takes history of modifiable risk factors (coverage makes special mention of
depression, functional ability, home safety, falls risk, hearing, vision), height and weight,
blood pressure, EKG.

Cardiovascular screening
Every 5 years; no deductible or copayment.
Ratio between total cholesterol and HDL, triglycerides.

Cervical cancer
Covered every 2 years; no deductible, copayment applies.
Pap smear and pelvic exam.

Colorectal cancer
Covered annually for fecal occult blood test; no deductible or copayment.
Covered every 4 years for sigmoidoscopy or barium enema; deductible and copayment apply.
Covered every 10 years for colonoscopy; deductible and copayment apply.

Densitometry
Covered every 2 years; deductible and copayment apply.

Diabetes screening
Annually (those with prediabetes, every 6 months); no deductible or copayment.
Not covered routinely, but includes most people age 65+ (if overweight, family history, fasting glucose of
100–125 mg/dl [prediabetes], hypertension, dyslipidemia).

Mammogram
Covered annually; no deductible, copayment applies.

Prostate cancer
Covered annually; no deductible or copayment.
Digital rectal examination and PSA test.

Smoking cessation
Two quit attempts annually, each consisting of up to four counseling sessions.
Limited to those with tobacco-related diseases (heart disease, cancer, stroke) or drug regimens that are
adversely affected by smoking (insulin, hypertension, seizure, blood clots, depression). Clinicians are
encouraged to become credentialed in smoking cessation.

Immunization

No deductible or copayment.

Influenza vaccination covered annually; pneumococcal vaccination covered one time, revaccination after 5 years dependent on risk.

Other coverage

Diabetes outpatient self-management training (blood glucose monitors, test strips, lancets; nutrition and exercise education; self-management skills: 9 hours of group training, plus 1 hour of individual training).

Medical nutrition therapy for persons with diabetes or a renal disease:

3 hours of individual training first year, 2 hours subsequent years.

Glaucoma screening annually for those with diabetes, family history, or African American descent.

Persons with cardiovascular disease may be eligible for comprehensive prevention programs by Drs. Dean Ornish and Herbert Benson: coverage 36 sessions within 18 weeks, possible extension to 72 sessions within 36 weeks.

Frequency and duration

These are estimates of what researchers recommend, relying most heavily on the U.S. Preventive Services Task Force recommendations, but not exclusively on them.

Blood pressure: Begin early adulthood, annually, ending around age 80.

Cholesterol: Begin early adulthood, every 2–3 years, ending around age 80.

Colorectal cancer: Begin age 50, every 5–10 years for colonoscopy, ending around age 80.

Mammogram: Begin age 40, every year or two; begin age 50 annually; begin age 65 every 2 years; ending around age 80.

Osteoporosis: Begin early adulthood for women (no frequency recommended); every 2–3 years after age 65 for women, less frequently for men.

Pap test: Begin with female sexual activity, two normal consecutive annual screenings, followed by every 3 years; two normal consecutive annual screenings around age 65, then discontinue.

Prostate cancer: Do not do routinely, except if there is a family history or African American heritage.

Definitions

Hypercholesterolemia: LDL above 160/130/100 (depending on risk factors); HDL below 40; ratio (total/HDL) 4.2 or above.

Diabetes: Fasting glucose 126 mg/dl and above; prediabetes, 100–125 mg/dl.

High blood pressure: Over 140/90; between 120/80 and 140/90 is prehypertensive.

Osteopenia: 1–2.5 standard deviations below young-adult peak bone density.

Osteoporosis: 2.5 standard deviations or more below young-adult peak bone density.

Source: Permission from D. Haber, *Health Promotion and Aging: Practical Applications for Health Professionals.* New York: Springer Publishing Company, 4th edition, 2007, pp. 100–101.

Analysts have argued that prevention resources are limited, and we should re-examine policy that is so heavily focused on medical screenings. Perhaps it would be more effective, and cost-effective, to focus on counseling in the areas of sedentary behavior, inadequate nutrition, smoking and tobacco use, and alcohol abuse (Haber, 2001, 2005).

Medical screenings and immunizations are undeniably important tools for disease prevention, but the data collected by the USPSTF (1996) resulted in a surprising conclusion: "Among the most effective interventions available to clinicians for reducing the incidence and severity of the leading causes of disease and disability in the United States are those that address the personal health practices of patients" (p. xxii). Stated another way "conventional clinical activities (e.g., diagnostic testing) may be of less value to clients than activities once considered outside the traditional role of the clinician," namely, counseling and patient education (USPSTF, 1996, p. xxii).

To end this section on an encouraging note, Medicare prevention is moving in positive directions, providing coverage for:

> Nutrition therapy for persons with diabetes and kidney disease
> An initial physical examination that includes prevention counseling
> Smoking cessation for those who have an illness caused by or complicated by tobacco use
> Comprehensive health promotion programs developed by Drs. Dean Ornish and Herbert Benson, for beneficiaries with heart problems

It is important not only to expand these counseling and health education programs, but also to publicize them. Years after implementation, for instance, only a small percentage of seniors eligible for the newly implemented initial physical examination took advantage of this opportunity (Pfizer, 2007).

Health Behavior Change

Theories help us understand what influences health behaviors and how to plan effective interventions. A theory of *health behavior change* attempts to explain the processes underlying the learning of new health behaviors. The two most widely cited theories of behavior change are social cognitive theory (Bandura, 1977) and stages of change (Prochaska & DiClemente, 1992). Other theories that have marshaled support are health locus of control (Wallston & Wallston, 1982), health belief model (Becker, 1974), reasoned action (Fishbein & Ajzen, 1975), community empowerment (Wallerstein & Bernstein, 1988), and community-oriented primary care (Nutting, 1987).

The author of this chapter is not an advocate of any single theory. Theories are broad and ambitious, attempting to relate a set of concepts systematically to explain and predict events and activities. Concepts, however, are the primary elements of a theory, and each theory has a concept or two that is particularly well developed and helpful in guiding a risk reduction intervention. Borrowing concepts from different theories can help one plan an intervention.

BOX 7-1   Recommended Readings

Birren, J., & Cochran, K. (2001). *Telling the stories of life through guided autobiography groups.* Baltimore, MD: Johns Hopkins University Press.

Freedman, M. (1999). *Prime time: How baby boomers will revolutionize retirement and transform America.* New York, NY: Public Affairs.

Haber, D. (2007). *Health promotion and aging: Practical applications for health professionals* (4th ed.). New York, NY: Springer.

Lorig, K., Ritter, P., Stewart, A., Sobel, D., Brown, B., Bandura, A., et al. (2001). Chronic disease self-management program: 2-year health status and health care utilization outcomes. *Medical Care, 39*(11), 1217–1223.

Rabig, J., Thomas, W., Kane, R., Cutler, L., & McAlilly, S. (2006). Radical redesign of nursing homes: Applying the Green House concept in Tupelo, Mississippi. *The Gerontologist, 46*(4), 533–539.

Thomas, W. (2004). *What are old people for?* Acton, MA: VanderWyk & Burnam.

One behavior-changing tool that borrows concepts from a variety of theories is the *health contract/calendar* (see **Figures 7-1** and **7-2**). The health contract/calendar relies on the self-management capability of a client, after initial assistance is provided by a clinician or health educator. The client is helped to choose an appropriate behavior change goal and to create and implement a plan to accomplish that goal. The statement of the goal and the plan of action are then written into a contract format.

My **health goal** is: _____

My **motivation** for my health goal is:
1. _____
2. _____
3. _____

My Plan of Action

For social or emotional **support** I will…

To **remind** me of new behaviors I will…

Problems that may interfere with reaching my health goal and **solutions**:

My **signature**/   Support person's **signature**

date   date

Figure 7-1 Health contract.

Source: Permission from D. Haber, *Health Promotion and Aging: Practical Applications for Health Professionals.* NY: Springer Publishing Company, 4th edition, 2007, pp. 100–101.

Fill in activities and make an X on each day you complete them.						
Month: _____				Backup plan:		
Sunday	Monday	Tuesday	Wednesday	Thursday	Friday	Saturday
Weekly Success #days completed/ #days contracted						

Figure 7-2 Health calendar.

Source: Permission from D. Haber, *Health Promotion and Aging: Practical Applications for Health Professionals.* NY: Springer Publishing Company, 4th edition, 2007, p. 114.

A health contract is alleged to have several advantages over verbal communication alone, especially when the communication tends to be limited in direction (i.e., mostly from health professional to client). The alleged advantages of a contract, which still need additional empirical testing, are that it is a formal commitment that not only enhances the therapeutic relationship between provider and client, but also requires the active participation of the client. The contract also:

> Identifies and enhances motivation
> Clarifies measurable and modest goals
> Suggests tips to remember new behaviors
> Provides a planned way to involve support persons such as family and friends
> Provides a means to problem-solve around barriers that previously interfered with the achievement of a goal
> Suggests ways to design a supportive environment
> Provides incentives to reinforce behaviors

> Establishes a record-keeping system (i.e., a month-long calendar for the health contract/calendar technique)

The health contract/calendar technique includes a set of instructions (see Haber, 2007b) that help older adults establish a goal, identify motivation, implement a plan of action, identify potential problems, and encourage solutions to overcome these barriers. The contract is signed and dated at the bottom by the older adult and a support person. Progress is typically assessed after one week, and the success of the contract is reviewed at the end of a month. There is also the potential for providing ongoing support.

Health contracts have been applied with varying degrees of success to a wide variety of behaviors, such as drug use, smoking, alcohol abuse, nutrition, and exercise (Berry, Danish, Rinke, & Smiciklas-Wright, 1989; Clark, Keukefeld, & Godlaski, 1999; Cupples & Steslow, 2001; Haber, 2007a; Haber & Looney, 2000; Haber & Rhodes, 2004; Jette et al., 1999; Johnson, Nicklas, Arbeit, Webber, & Berenson, 1992; Leslie & Schuster, 1991; Lorig, Lubeck, Kraines, Seleznickm, Holman, 1996; Lorig et al., 2000; Moore, von Korff, Cherkin, Saunders, & Lorig, 2000; Neale, Singleton, Dupuis, & Hess, 1990; Schlenk & Boehm, 1998; Swinburn, Walter, Arroll, Tilyard, & Fried, 1998).

There are many versions of health contracts ranging from the simple to the complex. Here is an example of a simple weight-loss contract developed by Dr. Joseph Chemplavil, a cardiac endocrinologist in Hampton, Virginia:

I, (patient's name), hereby promise to myself and to Dr. Chemplavil, that I will make every effort to lose my (agreed-upon) weight, and I will pay $1 to Dr. Chemplavil's Dollar for Pound Fund for every pound of weight that I gain, on each visit to the office, by cash. I also understand that I will receive $1 from the same fund for each pound of weight that I lose.

Dr. Chemplavil paid out $1,044 to 118 patients, received $166 from 30 patients, and two patients broke even (Kazel, 2004).

Research on health contracts has been limited and often marred by a lack of random assignment to treatment and control groups, small sample sizes, and lack of replication. In addition, there are several uncertainties about the effectiveness of health contracts in terms of one's ability to identify which components work better than others (e.g., health education, social support, the professional–client relationship, memory enhancement, motivation building, contingency rewards, etc.), whether contracts work better with one type of person than another, and how to determine the content and amount of training that is required for health educators or clinicians to help clients implement health contracts.

Even without a definitive body of research, health contracts are widely used. They are simple to administer, time-efficient, and even cost-effective when medical personnel assign the completion of health contracts to a health educator or trained office worker. The health contract can also be effectively taught to students in the classroom who are interested in health education, risk factor counseling, or program development (Haber, 2007a).

Exercise

The 1996 *Surgeon General's Report on Physical Activity and Health* was an outstanding review of the research on the effects of physical activity on people's health, and it has yet to be improved upon. According to the Surgeon General's report, regular exercise and physical activity improve health in a variety of ways, including a reduction in heart disease, diabetes, high blood pressure, colon cancer, depression, anxiety, excess weight, falling, bone thinning, muscle wasting, and joint pain.

However, 60% of adults did not achieve the recommended amount of physical activity, and 25% of adults were not physically active at all. Inactivity increased with age; by age 75, about one in three men and one in two women engaged in no physical activity. Inactivity was also more common among women and people with lower incomes and less education.

The most significant component of the Surgeon General's report was its advocacy for several tested exercise principles. First, motivation is very important, and to enhance it requires a large degree of modesty in setting goals and at least a small degree of enjoyment—hence, the emphasis on being more physically active rather than a narrow adherence to a rigid exercise regimen.

Second, Americans should get at least 30 minutes of physical activity or exercise most days of the week. This statement provided a major perspective shift from previous recommendations by government and exercise leaders. This new message recommended that Americans become more concerned about total calories expended through exercise than about intensity level or duration of continuous exercise. Regarding intensity level, the report stresses the importance of raising respiratory rate and body warmth—physiological changes that are apparent to the participant—but not to be too concerned about raising intensity level to a target heart rate, particularly if the person is sedentary or has a less than active lifestyle.

Regarding duration of continuous exercise, it is no longer deemed essential to obtain 30 consecutive minutes of exercise. For Americans, the large majority of whom are not too active, accumulating shorter activity spurts throughout the day is effective. Taking a brisk walk in a shopping mall or climbing a few stairs in spare minutes can accumulate the benefits of exercise. A review of the research literature concludes that accumulating several 5- or 10-minute bouts of physical activity over the course of the day provides beneficial health and fitness effects (DeBusk, Stenestrand, Sheehan, & Haskell, 1990; Jakicic, Donnelly, Pronk, Jawad, & Jacobson, 1995; Lee, Sesso, & Paffenbarger, 2000; Murphy, Nevill, Neville, Biddle, & Hardman, 2002; Pate et al., 1995). One study reported that if a person times these bouts of activity correctly they can gain the added benefit of replacing junk food snack breaks (Jakicic et al., 1995).

Regarding exercise itself, it is difficult for adults to go from inactivity to an exercise routine. Thinking about how to accumulate short bouts of activity is a useful way to get started on better health and fitness. For example, nurses can encourage older adults to vacuum the carpet more briskly than normally (even if it means doing it in segments throughout the day), or to put more energy into leaf raking or lawn mowing, gardening with enthusiasm, or dancing to music on the radio. In addition, nurses should not underestimate the ability of older adults to engage in adventurous or unusual sports (see **Figure 7-3**).

Finally, the Surgeon General's report urged Americans to be active most days of the week. We should aim for the habit of everyday physical activity or exercise, but should not allow the occasional lapse to discourage us. Making physical activity or exercise a near-daily routine is more likely to become an enduring habit than the previously recommended three-times-per-week exercise routine.

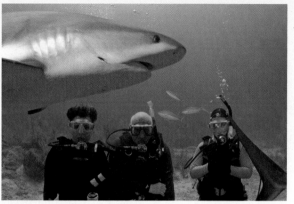

Figure 7-3 Older adults may continue sporting activities well into later life and share them with their grandchildren. These grandparents took their adult grandchild on a shark dive in the Bahamas.

For most older adults, a brisk walking program will provide sufficient intensity for a good aerobics program. An 8-year study of more than 13,000 people indicated that walking briskly for 30 to 60 minutes every day was almost as beneficial in reducing the death rate as jogging up to 40 miles a week (Blair et al., 1989). The authors of a study of 1,645 older adults reported that simply walking 4 hours per week decreased the risk of future hospitalization for cardiovascular disease (LaCroix, Veveille, Hecht, Grothous, & Wagner, 1996).

The National Center for Health Statistics (1985) reported that walking has much greater appeal for older adults than high-intensity exercise. A national survey indicated that a smaller percentage of persons age 65-plus (27%) engaged in vigorous activities, in comparison to 41% of the general adult population; however, people of all age groups (41%) were equally likely to walk for exercise.

Many older adults are concerned about unfavorable weather and may abandon their walking routine as a consequence. Prolonged hot or cold spells may sabotage a good walking program. Rather than discontinue this activity because of the weather, adults may choose to walk indoors at their local shopping malls. Many shopping malls—about 2,500 nationwide—open their doors early, usually between 5:30 and 10:00 a.m., for members of walking clubs.

There is also a relationship between one's neighborhood and one's health. Residents who depend on a car to get to most places and have few sidewalks for safe walking are likely to be more obese and have chronic medical conditions that impact health-related quality of life (Booth, Pinkston, & Boston, 2005; Sturm & Cohen, 2004). For every extra 30 minutes commuters drive each day, they have a 3% greater chance of being obese; in contrast, people who live within walking distance of shops are 7% less likely to be obese (Frank, Andresen, & Schmid, 2004). Older persons who believe their neighborhoods are favorable for walking are up to 100% more physically active (King et al., 2003; Li, Fisher, & Harmer, 2005). People at high risk for inactivity may increase their physical activity when they have access to walking trails (Brownson et al., 2000).

A sedentary person is estimated to walk about 3,500 steps a day, and the average American about 5,130 steps. Many advocates believe Americans should aim for 10,000 steps a day, or about 5 miles. Workplace physical activity, particularly among blue-collar occupations, helps many people reach the 10,000-step target, leaving older adults (and overweight office workers) most likely to be at risk (McCormack, Giles-Corti, & Milligan, 2006).

Pedometers are small devices that count steps, and are typically attached at the waist. They first appeared in Japan in 1965 under the name Manpo-meter—manpo in Japanese means 10,000 steps. Their introduction into America took another few decades, but they have been rapidly increasing in popularity—even McDonald's distributed them for a while as part of an adult Happy Meal called Go Active (salad, bottled water, and a pedometer for $4.99). Studies, though, have been equivocal about the benefits of using a pedometer to motivate individuals.

One study, for instance, reported that pedometers added no additional benefit to a coaching intervention (Engel & Lindner, 2006), whereas another publication noted that it increased the frequency of short walking trips (Stovitz, Van Wormer, Center, & Bremer, 2005). One study reported that cheap pedometers are likely to overestimate the actual number of steps taken (De Cocker, Cardon, & De Bourdeaudhuij, 2006). There are many ways in addition to the use of a pedometer to add steps to a daily routine. For information and guidelines on this topic, contact America on the Move, at http://www.americaonthemove.org.

Another option for older adults is to join a noncompetitive walking or hiking club, or to participate in a nearby walking or hiking event. Two opportunities in this regard are the American Volkssport Association at 800-830-9255 or http://www.ava.org, and the local Sierra Club at http://www.sierraclub.org. If you want to add a mind-body dimension to walking, try ChiWalking, which combines walking with the principles of tai chi (http://www.chiwalking.com).

Traveling to another city can also be an excuse not to exercise, or it can be an opportunity to gather information from the local newspaper or chamber of commerce about a walking tour for an enjoyable way to get exercise and a unique way to learn about offbeat aspects of a city's history. Most if not all big cities have walking tours, and some sound particularly intriguing (such as Oak Park, Illinois's self-guided walking tours of Frank Lloyd Wright homes and the Big Onion walking tours of New York City's ethnic communities and restaurants [http://www.bigonion.com]).

There are many other aspects of exercise besides aerobics that are important for older adults to know about, including strength building, flexibility, and balance. There are also many important topics that need to be considered, such as safety, qualified exercise leaders for older adults, fitness clubs that motivate older adults, and the compatibility of an exercise routine with the medical status of an individual. For a detailed description of a model exercise program and related exercise topics, see Haber (2007b).

Nutrition

Nutrition is only one component in the development and exacerbation of disease (heredity, environment, medical care, social circumstances, and other lifestyle risk factors also play a part), but eating and drinking habits have been implicated in 6 of the 10 leading causes of death—heart disease, cancer, stroke, diabetes, atherosclerosis, and liver disease—as well as in several debilitating disorders like osteoporosis and diverticulosis.

Older adults are in a particularly precarious position because they are more vulnerable to both obesity and malnutrition than other age groups. The highest percentage of obese adults is in the age group 50–69 years, with those ages 70–79 the next most obese (Squires, 2002). Also, older adults are at the highest risk of being malnourished (Beers & Berkow, 2000). Social isolation, dental problems, medical disease, and medication usage are among the risk factors for malnourishment in older adults.

Older adults are more conscientious about nutrition than other age groups, according to one national study (Harris, 1989). In this sample, a higher percentage of those over age 65 (approximately two-thirds) than of those in their 40s (one-half) reported trying "a lot" to limit sodium, fat, and sugar; eat enough fiber; lower cholesterol; and consume enough vitamins and minerals.

If older adults are paying more attention to their nutritional habits, one can only speculate that they may be motivated by more immediate feedback (heartburn, constipation, and so forth), or by feelings of greater vulnerability (higher risk of impairment from disease and of loss of independence). The next cohort of older adults—today's baby boomers—bring more than motivation to the table. They also bring a higher formal education level, including a strong interest in health education.

The federal government provides a modest amount of nutrition education for older adults and the rest of the American public. The 2005 Dieary Guidelines for Americans includes a 70-page blueprint for nutritional policy; a revised Food Guide Pyramid, dubbed MyPyramid; and a website, http://www.mypyramid.gov. The guidelines are redrafted every 5 years by the U.S. Department of Agriculture (USDA) and the Department of Health and Human Services (DHHS). The Food Guide Pyramid, however, had not been updated for 13 years, and the website was a brand new initiative. The entire update was billed as an interactive food guidance system rather than a one-size-fits-all initiative.

The guidelines basically encourage Americans to eat fruits, vegetables, whole grains, and low-fat or fat-free dairy products, and there is much more detail on the consumption of these foods than was provided by previous guidelines. Fruits and vegetables are increased to 5 to 13 servings per day. Salt guidelines are specific for the first time, limiting it to one level teaspoon a day. Trans fat is identified for the first time, and the advice is to keep intake as low as possible. Saturated fat limitations have become specific, keeping it to 10% of calories or less. Cholesterol level is to be less than 300 milligrams. Added sugars or sweeteners are discouraged for the first time, particularly in drinks. Whole grains are differentiated from the broad category of carbohydrates, and the recommendation is that one-half the grain servings should be whole grains.

The website offers people specific dietary recommendations on grains, vegetables, fruit, milk, meat and beans, total fat, saturated fat, cholesterol, sodium, oils, and fats/sugars. Types and duration of physical activity are assessed as well, with specific recommendations. The website is interesting and informative.

Another educational tool is the *nutrition bull's-eye* developed by Covert Bailey (1996). The goal of the bull's-eye is for people to consume the nutritious foods that are listed in the center of it. These foods are low in saturated fat, sugar, and sodium, and high in fiber. They include skim milk, nonfat yogurt, most fruits and vegetables, whole grains, beans and legumes, and water-packed tuna. As you move to the foods listed in the rings farther away from the bull's-eye, you eat more saturated fat, sugar, sodium, and low-fiber foods. In the outer ring of the bull's-eye, therefore, are most cheeses, ice cream, butter, whole milk, beef, cake, cookies, potato chips, and mayonnaise.

Unlike the Food Guide Pyramid, Bailey's bull's-eye is focused on making distinctions within food categories. Whole-wheat products, for instance, are in the bull's-eye, whereas products made from refined white flour and those with added sugar are placed in the outer circles. Fresh fruits and vegetables are in the bull's-eye, but juiced vegetables and fruit that lose fiber and that concentrate sugars are placed in a ring just outside of the bull's-eye. Skim milk, low-fat and nonfat cottage cheese, and part-skim mozzarella are in the center ring, whereas whole milk and most cheeses are in the outer circles of the target.

The author has offered older clients a personalized version of the nutrition bull's-eye. In this version, you begin with a blank bull's-eye, and then add food and drink products that you usually consume to each of the rings. The foods and drinks in the personalized nutrition bull's-eye (see **Figure 7-4**) are clearly superior; the second ring is not quite as nutrient dense; the third ring is neutral, products that are not particularly harmful or helpful; and the outer ring includes the least nutritious foods and drinks that should be consumed sparingly.

In the center and innermost ring of the personalized bull's-eye, patients also add the foods and drinks that they are not currently consuming, but that they

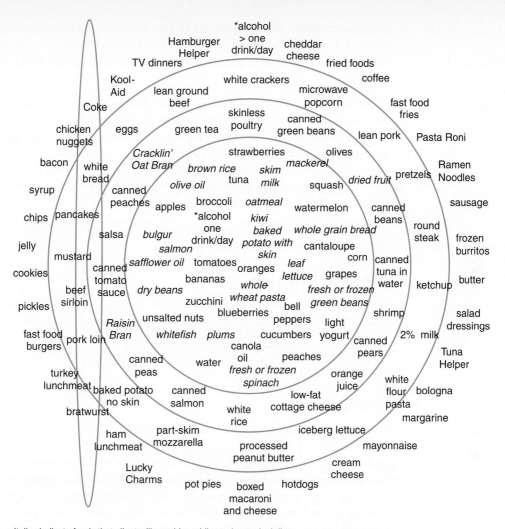

Italics indicate foods that client will consider adding to her typical diet.

Figure 7-4 Personalized nutrition bull's eye.

Source: Permission from D. Haber, *Health Promotion and Aging: Practical Applications for Health Professionals.* NY: Springer Publishing Company, 4th edition, 2007, p. 191.

find sufficiently desirable and are considering adding to their diet (in italics in Figure 7-4). The assignment of food and drink products to each of the rings is likely best done with the aid of a dietitian who can assess their nutritional value. (Darson Rhodes and Mandy Puckett, former nutrition students at Ball State University, identified products for the personalized nutrition bull's-eye in Figure 7-4.)

The *Center for Science in the Public Interest (CSPI)* is the premier educational and advocacy organization for promoting better nutritional habits in the United States. Its educational component consists of the Nutrition Action Healthletter, published monthly, which informs more than 800,000 subscribers, including this author. The organization is best known, however, for its advocacy accomplishments, under the leadership of its executive director and cofounder (in 1971), Michael Jacobson.

Jacobson and CSPI staff, for example, have led the fight for nutrition labels on food items in the supermarket; for exposing the hidden fat in Chinese, Mexican, Italian, and delicatessen food; for pressuring movie theaters to stop cooking popcorn in artery-clogging coconut oil; for warning labels on Procter & Gamble's fake fat, Olean, which may interfere with the absorption of nutrients and cause loose stools and cramping; for more accurate labeling of ground beef in supermarkets; and for the listing of trans fat on nutrition labels.

For more information, contact the Center for Science in the Public Interest at their website, http://www.cspinet.org

Mental Health

Neither the average 50% reduction in income at retirement nor the increases in emotional losses, physical losses, and caregiving responsibilities in later life result in a persistent reduction in life satisfaction among most older adults. As sociologist Linda George (1986) notes, "Older adults are apparently masters of the art of lowering aspirations to meet realities" (p. 7).

Life Review

One tool for preserving or enhancing the *mental health* of older adults is the *life review*, which is an autobiographical effort that can be preserved in print, by tape recording, or on videotape. The review is guided by a series of questions in specific life domains, such as work and family, as well as memories further stimulated through a family photo album, other memorabilia, a genealogy, musical selections from an earlier time, or a trek back to an important place in one's past. It can be conducted by oneself, in a dyad, or as part of a group process. A life review is more likely to be conducted by or with an older adult who is relatively content with his or her life and not seeking therapy than it is to be used therapeutically with an older adult. Nonetheless, life reviews are believed to have therapeutic powers, and they are incorporated into a wide variety of counseling modalities (Haber, 2006).

The psychiatrist Robert Butler first extolled the benefits of the life review process to his colleagues and the public as early as 1961, as a way of incorporating reminiscence in the aged as part of a normal aging process. Dr. Butler described the life review as more comprehensive and systematic than spontaneous reminiscing, and perhaps more important in old age when there may be a need to put one's life in order and to come to an acceptance of present circumstances (Butler, 1995).

The review of positive and negative past life experiences by older adults has enabled them to overcome feelings of depression and despair (Butler, 1974; Butler,

Lewis, & Sunderland, 1991; Watt & Cappeliez, 2000). Another study of the life review process reported positive outcomes in terms of stronger life satisfaction, psychological well-being, self-esteem, and reduced depression (Haight, Michel, & Hendrix, 1998).

Although life reviews are usually helpful for improving the mental health of most older adults who are seeking meaning, resolution, reconciliation, direction, and atonement, physicians, nurses, and other clinic personnel find it is too time-consuming to listen to the reminiscences of older clients in this era of medical care. Health professionals can, however, play a key role in referring older clients to appropriate forums or helping them obtain relevant life review materials.

One book, *Aging and Biography*, by the psychologist James Birren and colleagues (1996), helps guide and provide structure for the life review process by suggesting a focus on several themes, such as love, money, work, and family. Birren also suggests in another book, *Telling the Stories of Life Through Guided Autobiography Groups*, that incorporating life reviews into a small-group format can help in the retrieval as well as with the acceptance of memories (Birren & Cochran, 2001).

With careful monitoring, Birren noted that in his years of experience he has not had a group member report becoming depressed as a result of a life review (Birren & Deutchman, 1991). He warned, however, that persons who are already depressed or otherwise needing therapy should be under the supervision of a qualified professional.

Depression

Whether older adults participate in life reviews or not, they are vulnerable to *depression* due to losses that accompany aging such as widowhood, chronic medical conditions and pain, and functional *dependence* (Lantz, 2002). Not only can these emotional and physical losses lead to depression, but depression in turn can lead to more physical decline (Penninx, Guralnik, Ferruci, et al., 1998).

Although the mechanism is not understood, depression increases the likelihood of mortality from cancer (Penninx, Guralnik, Pahor, et al., 1998) and heart disease (Frasure-Smith, Lesperance, & Talajic, 1995). The mortality rate for depressed patients with cardiovascular disease is twice that of those without depression (Lantz, 2002). Even mild depression can weaken the immune system in older persons if it goes on long enough (McGuire, Kiecolt-Glaser, & Glaser, 2002).

Depression also plays a significant role in suicidal behaviors, and older persons have the highest suicide rate of any age group. Older adults account for 25% of all suicide deaths, though they make up only about 13% of the general population. This elevated suicide rate, however, is largely accounted for by white men age 85 or older. The suicide rate of this age/gender category is six times higher than the overall national rate (Centers for Disease Control and Prevention, 1999).

Depression in older adults often goes undetected until it is too late. Between 63% (Rabins, 1996) and 90% (Katon, von Korff, Lin, Bush, & Ormel, 1992) of depressed older patients go untreated or receive inadequate treatment. One retrospective study of older adults who had committed suicide revealed that 51 of the 97 patients studied had seen their primary care physician within 1 month of their suicide date. Of these 51, only 19 were even offered treatment, and only 2 of the 51 patients studied were provided adequate treatment (Caine, Lyness, & Conwell, 1996).

Barry Lebowitz (1995) of the National Institute of Mental Health estimated that 15% of Americans age 65 or over suffered from serious and persistent symptoms of depression, but only 3% were reported to be suffering from the clinical diagnosis of major depression. In other words, although depressive disorders that fulfill rigorous diagnostic criteria are relatively rare, subthreshold disorders are considerably more common, infrequently diagnosed, or treated with prescribed antidepressants, and because they usually go untreated, are likely to become chronic conditions (Beekman et al., 2002).

Detection of depression is hampered not only by the underreporting of symptoms by older patients, but also by biases on the part of physicians and family members. In one study, 75% of physicians thought that depression was understandable in older persons—that is, a normal facet of old age (Gallo, Ryan, & Ford, 1999). Family members may also view the signs and symptoms of depression as "normal aging," when in fact the persistence of depressive symptoms is not normal.

Dependency

The concepts that best capture the degree of dependency an individual must bear are Activities of Daily Living (ADLs) and Instrumental Activities of Daily Living (IADLs). ADLs measure the individual's ability to perform basic personal care tasks such as eating, bathing, dressing, using the toilet, getting in or out of a bed or chair, caring for a bowel-control device, and walking (the latter being the most common ADL limitation). The average nursing home resident needs help with four or five ADLs.

IADLs measure the individual's ability to perform more complex, multifaceted activities in one's environment, such as home management, managing money, meal preparation, making a phone call, or grocery shopping (the latter being the most common IADL limitation). These limitations typically precede the limitations associated with ADLs.

While ADLs and IADLs can reflect functional impairment on a temporary basis, such as during convalescence from surgery or a temporary disability, with age the limitations are typically chronic. This state of affairs presents not only a physical challenge to the older adults, but a mental health one as well. The primary mental health concern is focused on the quality of one's remaining life, rather than the quantity of years left to live (Haber, 2010). At age 65 we can expect about one-third of our remaining years to be dependent, but by age 85 that increases to two-thirds of our remaining years. With age, dependent living becomes increasingly problematic and is a big contributor to depression (Brenes et al., 2008).

Dependency is often described as frailty when there are three or more ADL deficiencies, combined with weakness and chronic exhaustion. To avoid or slow the descent into frailty, exercise is commonly recommended, even for the very old, but there are many other interventions as well. Smoking cessation, alcohol moderation, nutrition, fall and injury prevention, social support, medical screenings, immunizations, sleep hygiene, and medication management are just a few of the other factors to consider. There is plenty that we can control to lower the probability of a dependent life style or frailty, or at least to shorten this period of dependency as much as possible.

Quality of Life and Wellness

Life is more than the avoidance of dependency, however. We want to promote *quality of life,* which goes beyond mere autonomy in performing ADLs and IADLs. Quality of life may be defined as functional health combined with life satisfaction, a feeling of competency, and a perception of social support. About three-fourths of non-Hispanic Whites and almost two-thirds of African Americans and Hispanic Americans over the age of 65 report a good quality of life, according to the 2004–2006 National Health Interview Survey.

Older adult self-assessments are not always shared by others. Physicians, for instance, often rate the quality of life of older persons lower than do the elders themselves. Physicians are more influenced by objective health factors than are older adults, who tend to adapt to physical deficiencies over time. Even older persons in nursing homes tend to rate their health more positively than others do (Hooyman & Kiyak, 2011).

The broadest perspective on quality of life is reflected in the concept of wellness. Ironically, wellness as a term has not caught on in the medical world, but in both the corporate setting (Jacob, 2002) and the academic one (as evidenced by the name of this author's former employer: The Institute of *Wellness* and Gerontology at Ball State University), the concept finds fertile territory.

The most common conceptualization of wellness divide this term into seven components. These dimensions are:

Physical: Exercise, eat a well-balanced diet, get enough sleep, protect yourself

Emotional: Express a wide range of feelings, acknowledge stress, channel positive energy

Intellectual: Embrace lifelong learning, discover new skills and interests

Vocational: Do something you love, balance responsibilities with satisfying ways to occupy yourself

Social: Laugh often, spend time with family and friends, join a club, respect cultural differences

Environmental: Recycle daily, use energy-efficient products, walk or bike, grow a garden

Spiritual: Seek meaning and purpose, take time to reflect, connect with the universe.

The world of medicine fully embraces the legitimacy of the physical dimension of wellness, but gives much less emphasis to the other six domains. To access the full spectrum of wellness (see **Box 7-2**), you need to seek out the resources that are commonly available in community health. While exercise is the most ubiquitous health program in the community, the other domains of wellness are represented as well. This is the case with many of the model health promotion programs for older adults that are described in the next section.

BOX 7-2   Recommended Electronic Newsletter

Human Values in Aging is edited by Harry (Rick) Moody. It is a free, monthly e-newsletter that contains items of interest about humanistic gerontology, including late-life creativity, spirituality, the humanities, arts and aging, and lifelong learning. For a sample copy or free subscription, email hrmoody@yahoo.com.

Model Health Promotion Programs for Older Adults

Although there is no certain method for determining what constitutes a *model health promotion program*, there has been no shortage of attempts to identify them, develop a catalog that includes a summary of these exemplars, and distribute the catalog around the country in order to encourage their replication. Many of these model health promotion programs have been developed over the years with the aid of federal grants and other funding sources, have gone through multiple program evaluations, and can be helpful to health professionals who are interested in launching or improving their own program.

One of the more recent efforts in this regard has been organized by the Health Promotion Institute (HPI) of the National Council on Aging. The HPI started by summarizing 16 model programs or best practices and compiling them into a loose-leaf directory. The summaries included information on the planning process, implementation of the program, and program evaluations. Each year, new best practices have been added to this directory. If interested in obtaining a copy, contact the National Council on Aging, Health Promotion Institute, 300 D St., SW, #801, Washington, DC 20024; 202-479-1200; or http://www.ncoa.org.

Six model health promotion programs that have focused on older adults and have received national attention are summarized in the following sections. These programs have received federal funding and foundation support to evaluate their effectiveness and to encourage their replication.

Healthwise

The best-known older adult medical self-care program is Healthwise, located in Boise, Idaho. The Healthwise program relies mostly on the Healthwise Handbook, which provides information and prevention tips on 190 common health problems, with information periodically updated. The Healthwise Handbook (Healthwise, 2006) is now in its 17th edition. This handbook includes physician-approved guidelines on when to call a health professional for each of the health problems it covers. Some Healthwise community programs have supplemented the distribution of the handbook with group health education programs or nurse call-in programs. There is a Spanish language edition of the Healthwise Handbook, called La Salud en Casa, and a special self-care guide for older adults called Healthwise for Life.

With the assistance of a $2.1 million grant from the Robert Wood Johnson Foundation, Healthwise distributed its medical self-care guide to 125,000 Idaho households, along with toll-free nurse consultation phone service and self-care workshops. Thirty-nine percent of handbook recipients reported that the handbook helped them avoid a visit to the doctor (Mettler, 1997). Blue Cross of Idaho reported 18% fewer visits to the emergency room by owners of the guide.

Elements of the Healthwise program have been replicated in the United Kingdom, South Africa, New Zealand, Australia, and Canada. In British Columbia, the Healthwise Handbook was distributed to every household, and all 4.3 million residents had potential access to the Healthwise content through a website and a nurse call center. Additional information can be obtained from Donald Kemper or Molly Mettler, at http://www.healthwise.org.

Chronic Disease Self-Management Program

Kate Lorig, a nurse-researcher at the Stanford University School of Medicine, and her medical colleagues have been evaluating community-based, peer-led, chronic disease self-management programs for more than two decades, beginning with the Arthritis Self-Management Program (Lorig et al., 1996). This program has since evolved into a curriculum that is applicable to a wide array of chronic diseases and conditions.

Typically, each program involves about a dozen participants, led by peer leaders who have received 20 hours of training. The peer leaders, like the students, are typically older and have chronic diseases that they contend with. The program consists of six weekly sessions, each about 2.5 hours long, with a content focus on exercise, symptom management, nutrition, fatigue and sleep management, use of medications, managing emotions, community resources, communicating with health professionals, problem solving, and decision making. The program takes place in community settings such as senior centers, churches, and hospitals.

The theoretical basis of the program has been to promote a sense of personal efficacy among participants (Bandura, 1997) by using such techniques as guided mastery of skills, peer modeling, reinterpretation of symptoms, social persuasion through group support, and individual self-management guidance. In addition to improving self-efficacy, Lorig and colleagues (2001) reported reduced emergency room and outpatient visits, and decreased health distress, fatigue, and limitations in role function.

The Chronic Disease Self-Management Program is housed at Stanford University's Patient Education Research Center, 1000 Welch Road, #204, Palo Alto, CA 94304; 650-723-7935; http://patienteducation.stanford.edu/programs/cdsmp.html.

Project Enhance

Senior Services of Seattle/King County began the Senior Wellness Project (later renamed Project Enhance) in 1997 at the North Shore Senior Center in Bothell, Washington. It was a research-based health promotion program that included a component of chronic care self-management that was modeled after Kate Lorig's program (Lorig, Sobel, & Stewart, 1999). The program also included health and functional assessments; individual and group counseling; exercise programs; a personal health action plan with the support of a nurse, social worker, and volunteer health mentor; and support groups. A randomized controlled study of chronically ill seniors reported a reduction in number of hospital stays and average length of stay, a reduction in psychotropic medications, and better functioning in activities of daily living (Leveille et al., 1998).

Project Enhance is a partnership among a university, an area Agency on Aging, local and national foundations, health departments, senior centers, primary care providers, older volunteers, and older participants. Versions of this model program are being replicated at senior wellness sites around the country (80+ sites in the United States) and two sites in Sweden to test its effectiveness in a variety of communities, in an assortment of sites, serving a diversity of clientele. Findings have demonstrated higher levels of physical activity and lower levels of depression among its participants (Dobkin, 2002).

Project Enhance is currently divided into two components: Enhance Fitness and Enhance Wellness. Enhance Fitness is an exercise program that focuses on stretching, flexibility, balance, low impact aerobics, and strength training. Certified instructors have undergone special training in fitness for older adults. Classes last an hour, involve 10 to 25 people, and participants can track their progress through a series of functional evaluations.

Participants who completed 6 months of Enhance Fitness improved significantly in a variety of physical and social functioning measures, as well as reported reduced levels of pain and depression. There was also a reduction in healthcare costs

(Ackerman et al., 2003). The Enhance Fitness program has been replicated in 64 community sites across 6 states.

Enhance Wellness focuses on mental health, with an emphasis on lessening symptoms of depression and other mood problems, developing a sense of greater self-reliance, and lowering the need for drugs that affect thinking or emotions. Enhance Wellness typically consists of a nurse and social worker working with an individual. An analysis of the effectiveness of the program found that it reduced depression 1 year after the program and improved exercise readiness, physical activity levels, and self-reported health (Phelan et al., 2002).

To learn more about Project Enhance, contact Susan Snyder, Program Director at Senior Services of Seattle/King County, at susans@seniorservices.org.

Ornish Program for Reversing Heart Disease

Dr. Dean Ornish, a physician at the University of California at San Francisco and founder of the Preventive Medicine Research Institute, has developed a program for reversing heart disease that has been replicated at several sites around the country. Dr. Ornish (1992) has recommended a vegetarian diet (see **Box 7-3**) with fat intake of 10% or less of total calories, moderate aerobic exercise at least three times a week, yoga and meditation an hour a day, group support sessions, and smoking cessation.

Dr. Ornish and his colleagues have reported that as a result of their program, blockages in arteries have decreased in size and blood flow has improved in as many

---

BOX 7-3   Research Highlight

Aim: The researchers investigated the association between use of the Mediterranean diet and mortality. The effect of a healthy lifestyle on premature death was also examined.

Methods: A cohort of 120,852 men and women ages 55–69 were asked to provide information on their dietary and lifestyle habits. Their mortality was followed for at least 10 years. A combined lifestyle score was given to them based on adhering to four modifiable healthy lifestyle factors: the Mediterranean diet, not smoking, maintaining normal weight, and physical activity. The case-cohort analysis was based on 9,691 deaths using 3,576 members of a subcohort.

Findings: Maintaining a Mediterranean diet showed significantly lower mortality for women, but not for men. However, those with healthier lifestyle scores had a significantly lower rate of mortality.

Application to practice: The data from this study suggested that both men and women who adhere to the four modifiable lifestyle factors can reduce their risk of premature mortality. Nurses can encourage young-old adults to adopt healthy aging practices and these four lifestyle changes that can decrease their risk of premature death.

Source: van den Brandt, P. A. (2011). The impact of a Mediterranean diet and healthy lifestyle on premature mortality in men and women. *American Journal of Clinical Nutrition, 94*, 913–920.

as 82% of their heart patients (Gould et al., 1995). A 5-year follow-up of this program reported an 8% reduction in atherosclerotic plaques, while the control group had a 28% increase. Also during this time, cardiac events were more than doubled in the control group (Ornish et al., 1998).

The applicability of Ornish's program to the average patient is still of uncertain utility. It may take highly motivated individuals (e.g., patients with severe heart disease) and significant medical and health support (requiring significant resources) for the model program to be useful to others. For additional information, contact Dean Ornish at http://www.pmri.org.

Benson's Mind/Body Medical Institute

Dr. Herbert Benson is a physician affiliated with Harvard Medical School and best known for his bestselling books on the relaxation response and for popularizing the term mind/body medicine. For individuals feeling the negative effects of stress, Benson's program teaches them to elicit the relaxation response, a western version of meditation. The Benson–Henry Institute for Mind/Body Medicine's clinical programs treat patients with a combination of relaxation response techniques, proper nutrition and exercise, and the reframing of negative thinking patterns.

Benson's nonprofit scientific and educational institute conducts research; provides outpatient medical services; and trains health professionals, postdoctoral fellows, and medical students. The Benson–Henry Institute for Mind/Body Medicine can be contacted at http://www.massgeneral.org/bhi/.

The research results from Benson's and Ornish's programs attracted the attention of Medicare, which funded a demonstration project to evaluate these programs. As a consequence of the demonstration project, in 2006 Medicare began to reimburse eligible patients for participation in the two cardiac wellness programs, Ornish's Reversing Heart Disease and Benson's Mind/Body Medicine. These two programs have expanded the emphasis in Medicare from acute care medicine, rehabilitative medicine, and prevention to the inclusion of comprehensive wellness.

Strong for Life

The Strong for Life program is a home-based exercise program for disabled and nondisabled older adults. It focuses on strength and balance and provides an exercise video, a trainer's manual, and a user's guide. The program was designed by physical therapists for home use by older adults, and relies on elastic resistive bands for strengthening muscles. The exercise program led to a high rate of exercise adherence among older participants, as well as increased lower extremity strength, improvements in tandem gait, and a reduction in physical disability (Jette et al., 1999).

This program is now housed at Stanford Hospital and clinics at Aging Adult Services 300 Pasteur Drive, HC005Palo Alto, CA 94305-5279; (650) 725-4137; http://stanfordhospital.org/forPatients/patientServices/StrongforLife.html

Re-Engagement Instead of Retirement

In 2011, baby boomers began turning age 65 and started becoming the gerontology boomers. Most of them will not retire, if "retirement" means a type of disengagement. Why will these gerontology boomers be different from the current crop of retirees?

First, the boomers will be the longest-lived cohort of older adults. They may have 25 or 30 years of life to negotiate after giving up their main line of work. How many of them will be comfortable with the idea of a quarter-century without additional earnings? How many will be comfortable letting go of education, exploration, and engagement?

The boomers will be the best-educated cohort of older adults. Between 1950 and 2000, the percentage of Americans age 65 or over with a high school diploma leaped from 18% to 66%; college graduates jumped from 4% to 15%. In 1991, 17% of Americans age 60–64 were involved in adult education; by 1999 that number had jumped to 32%. They say a mind–seventy-six million minds, to be precise–is a terrible thing to waste, not only from the individual's standpoint, but from society's as well.

The boomers will be the healthiest cohort of older adults. Almost 90% of Americans ages 65–74 report that they have no disability, and the disability rate for older Americans continues to decline. An increasing number of older adults are exercising in late life, with brisk walking for exercise becoming commonplace among the old. Not only is a mind a terrible thing to waste, so is a healthy body.

Also, the boomers may become the most-engaged cohort of older adults. Fifty-four percent of boomers say helping others is important to them. A 2002 national survey by Hart Research Associates reported that about 60% of older Americans believe that retirement is a "time to be active and involved, to start new activities and to set new goals." A 2005 survey by Civic Ventures and the MetLife Foundation reported that 58% of leading-edge baby boomers, those between ages 51 and 59, said they want to take jobs that serve their communities.

In addition, the boomers will be the largest cohort of retirees ever. The number of Americans age 65 or older will increase from 35 million in 2000 to more than 70 million in 2030. When these boomers came into the world they revolutionized hospitals and health care just through their sheer size. They did the same thing to public schools, the Vietnam War, and then the housing market, spurring a tremendous growth in building. A cohort this large is unlikely to pass into retirement and leave it unchanged, and boomers are unlikely to accept things as they are.

What might older adults do, if they decide to re-engage rather than retire? Here are two possibilities.

Experience Corps

Experience Corps is a foundation-supported program that has placed 2,000 older adults as tutors and mentors with 20,000 low-income children in urban public elementary schools and afterschool programs in 19 cities. These programs not only boost the academic performance of students, but enhance the well-being of the older volunteers in the process (Fried et al., 2004; Rebok et al., 2004; Tan, Xue, Li, Carlson, & Fried, 2006). Much work remains as two-thirds of the nation's fourth graders in major urban areas are reading below basic levels for their grade. For more information, contact Experience Corps at http://www.experiencecorps.org.

The North Carolina Center for Creative Retirement

The North Carolina Center for Creative Retirement (NCCCR) has implemented a course entitled "Creative Retirement in Uncertain Times." Through lectures, case studies, discussion groups, and community activities, older participants explore their image of retirement, their ability to revitalize themselves, and their plan of action.

With the help of a civic engagement grant from the National Council on Aging, NCCCR created a Leadership Training Program for Older Persons. It enables low-income older adults age 50 or older to gain the skills and confidence necessary to advocate for their peers by becoming effective leaders in community organizations that rarely include representatives from low-income groups.

The North Carolina Center for Creative Retirement can be contacted at http://www.unca.edu/ncccr. For information about demonstration grants awarded to encourage civic engagement, contact the National Council on Aging, 300 D. St., SW, #801, Washington, DC, 20024; 202-479-1200; http://www.ncoa.org.

There are hundreds of courses hosted at institutes of higher education targeted toward older adults, some of which are peer-led by retired older adults. Older adults can find out if there are similar educational offerings in their local area by contacting nearby colleges and universities.

Green House

Nursing homes are not homes—they are institutions. No matter how well run they are, they are not places where most of us want to end up. We are at the beginning of revolutionizing the long-term care industry, and no one has been more innovative and successful at this early stage than William Thomas, MD, founder of the Green House. Dr. Thomas started out his career as a medical director in a nursing home and was saddened by how regimented and joyless the environment was.

In traditional nursing homes, residents are viewed as sick and dependent, which fosters learned helplessness and induced disability. Staff may encourage wheelchair dependency to serve the needs of staff members who are pressed for time. Dressing, feeding, bathing, and toileting need to be routinized and sped up for aides needing to stay on schedule. A staff member is more likely to rely on incontinence briefs than to take the time to develop individualized toileting routines.

Green Houses, in contrast, look like surrounding homes in a residential community. They are homes, not home-like, though they are bigger than the average home. The first ones were constructed in Tupelo, Mississippi, in 2003, and were 6,400 square feet. The rooms in these homes include extra expense, such as ceiling lifts, but these innovations can save costs over the long term by reducing back injuries, employee turnover, and workers' compensation.

Green House workers are paid more and are better trained than the typical nursing assistant, but the extra costs are offset by employee empowerment that reduces staff turnover and additional training expenses. The annual employee turnover rate in the average nursing home is 75%, whereas it was less than 10% in the first Green House in Tupelo. Moreover, not one staff person left during the house's first 3 years of existence.

About 10 people live in a Green House, each having a private room and bath, and access to a central hearth where cooking and socializing are done. There is a surrounding garden for contemplative walks and for growing vegetables and flowers. Doors can be opened to view the garden and hearth from an individual room or closed for privacy. With the circular nature of the individual rooms, both the garden and the central hearth are within 30 feet. There is strategically placed furniture to help with "cruising" to central areas and to help with gains in mobility (see **Case Study 7-1**).

Green Houses promote autonomy. Residents get up, eat, and go to bed when they want. They decide on which foods to eat, and that may even include pizza, wine, or ice cream. Medications are locked in individual rooms, rather than distributed by

---

Case Study 7-1

Dr. Brown is a retired superintendent of a large public school system in the Midwest. He has been widowed for 5 years and just recently retired at the age of 69 after experiencing a fall down a flight of stairs at his home that resulted in a fractured hip, skull fracture, and broken shoulder, for which he has been treated in the hospital and is being discharged soon.
Dr. Brown's two adult children have encouraged him to sell his home and move somewhere where there is help available when he needs it. Dr. Brown hates the thought of a nursing home, especially since his wife spent about a year in one before her death. He is not certain whether an assisted living facility would work for him either. The family asks the hospital nurse for assistance in exploring living options for Dr. Brown.

Questions:

1. What questions should the nurse ask of Dr. Brown to help determine his preferences for living situations?

2. What other factors are essential to know about Dr. Brown in order to assist him with proper choices?

3. Are there any other team members who should be consulted within the hospital that could help with this decision? If so, who?

4. Would a Green House be a better option than assisted or independent living for Dr. Brown? Why or why not? What factors must be considered before answering this question?

a cart that is wheeled from room to room. There are few features that are different from the typical home, and if there are unusual features, they are de-emphasized, like a ceiling lift that is recessed and used only when needed for transfer. Induction cooking in the kitchen prevents residents from burning themselves on a stove. Stoves have shut-off valves, with pot trappers to prevent hot pots from burning residents. A safety gate around the kitchen can be used when necessary.

People in the first 10 Green Houses were selected from nursing homes and represented a typical nursing home population. Of the first 40 selected, 12 had advanced dementia, and all Green House residents had the typical array of physical and cognitive limitations associated with the average nursing home resident.

Decision making is lodged in residents and workers, unless there are safety or budget issues that cannot be handled at that level. Aides are called shahbazim (derived from the mythical Persian royal falcon that protected the king), with the primary job responsibility to protect, nurture, and sustain.

Ideal staff ratio is 1 for every 5 residents; nurse ratio is 1 for every 2 houses (or 1 per 20 people), and administrator ratio (and one assistant) 1 for every 12 houses (or 1 per 120 people). Staff find replacements for themselves if sick, either through a substitute pool or through overtime (which is managed within the allowable budget).

Workers receive 120 hours of additional training in areas such as CPR, first aid, culinary skills, safe food handling, communication, and dementia care. They are better paid than the average long-term care worker ($11 per hour versus $7.50) and are given rotating responsibility (purchasing food and cooking, housekeeping, scheduling, budget, etc.). Unless the nonclinical work teams endanger safety or overspend budget, administrators cannot overrule their decisions.

Every Green House has been fully staffed so far, with never a day understaffed. Wheelchair use has declined, and the strength of residents has increased. Residents have the option to eat in a group or alone, with an individualized menu and pleasant surroundings—referred to as a convivium. A local cookbook is assembled to cater to the tastes of people born in a region. Shahbazim can eat with residents and participate in activities with them, along with family and friends.

Most of these ideas are summarized in William Thomas's book, *What Are Old People For?* and in a journal article titled, "Radical Redesign of Nursing Homes" (Rabig, Thomas, Kane, Cutler, & McAlilly, 2006). In a publication called CNS SeniorCare, Thomas (Rabig et al., 2006) sums up his philosophy:

> Old age, like all the other phases of our lives, should be about life and living. Treating aging as a medical condition that must be managed with the professional distance prescribed by the medical model is wrong and leads to terrible suffering. For decades we have organized the life of the elder or disabled individual in a skilled nursing facility around the needs of the institution, rather than individuals who live there. (p. 14)

The Robert Wood Johnson Foundation provided a $10 million grant (from 2006 to 2010) to establish at least 30 Green Houses around the United States and to allow other long-term care owners and administrators to replicate them through training support and up to $125,000 in predevelopment loans.

Summary

Many exciting changes are taking place in the field of health promotion and aging (see **Box 7-4**). Perhaps it is time to establish a pro-aging movement—in contrast to the commercial and exploitive anti-aging movement. No longer needing to impress employers, in-laws, or peers, older adults are free to be themselves. Aging people have an opportunity to be freer, wiser, more engaged in helping others, and more willing to be an advocate not only for their own health, but for the well-being of society.

BOX 7-4   Web Exploration

Check out current nutrition recommendations at http://www.choosemyplate.gov/.

Critical Thinking Exercises

1. **Are you in favor of the federal government monitoring goals for healthy aging?** If so, how would you improve federal intervention? If not, why?

2. **What do you think is the most important health objective** that should be set for the Healthy People 2020 initiative, and what should federal and state governments do to help?

3. **How familiar are you with the health-promoting resources** in your community? Find one that you are unfamiliar with but believe may be important for older persons. Summarize it sufficiently to answer most questions that older adults might have about it.

4. **What is your opinion** of the existing Medicare prevention coverage? What would you change, and why?

5. **Write a health contract/calendar** for yourself for 1 month. At the end of this time explain your success or lack of such with accomplishing your health goal.

6. **What has been your major barrier** when it comes to engaging in exercise on a regular basis, and have you attempted to overcome it? If so, how?

7. Check out the **nutrition guidelines at Choose My Plate http://www.choosemyplate.gov/,** and see what you can learn about nutrition that is interesting to you. Do you have any suggestions for improving this site?

8. **Research suggests that older adults are more conscious of their nutritional habits** than younger adults. Conduct your own survey of five older adults and five younger adults, asking them to rate how much attention they give to eating what is good for them, using a scale of 1 (not very often) to 10 (all the time). Does your convenience sample corroborate the positive relationship between age and good nutritional habits?

Personal Reflections

1. Create your own nutrition bull's-eye, filling in the foods and drinks that you consume or might consider consuming. Use it for a week to guide your eating choices. Take a list of the food products in the center of your bull's-eye to the supermarket with you. Did you find this technique to be helpful?

2. Have you ever conducted a life review with an older adult? If you have, how satisfying was it for you and for them? If not, why not? How do you feel about not having done one with an older family member?

3. Choose one of the model health promotion programs summarized in this chapter and find out something of interest to you about that program that is not mentioned in this chapter.

4. The author believes that if we become more responsive to the health care needs of older adults, we will probably provide better health care for people of all ages in the United States. What do you think is the logic behind this belief?

5. What does this quotation by Henry Wadsworth Longfellow mean to you? "Age is opportunity no less than youth itself, though in another dress, and as the evening twilight fades away, the sky is filled with stars, invisible by day."

6. Describe a geriatric job, or an aspect of a job, that you would enjoy doing (related to nursing or not) and would be an important service for older adults, but is not currently being done.

References

Ackerman, R. T., Cheadle, A., Sandhu, N., Madsen, L., Wagner, E. H., & LoGerfo, J. P. (2003). Community exercise program use and changes in health care costs for older adults. *American Journal of Preventive Medicine, 25*(3), 232–237.

Bailey, C. (1996). *Smart eating.* Boston, MA: Houghton-Mifflin.

Bandura, A. (1977). *Social learning theory.* Englewood Cliffs, NJ: Prentice Hall.

Bandura, A. (1997). *Self-efficacy: The exercise of control.* New York, NY: W. H. Freeman.

Becker, M. (1974). The health belief model and personal health behavior. *Health Education Monographs, 2*(4), 236.

Beekman, A., Geerlings, S. W., Deeq, D. J., Smit, J. H., Schoevers, R. S., de Beurs, E.,…van Tilburg, W. (2002). The natural history of late-life depression: A 6-year prospective study in the community. *Archives of General Psychiatry, 59*(7), 605–611.

Beers, M., & Berkow, R. (2000). *The Merck manual of geriatrics* (3rd ed.). Whitehouse Station, NJ: Merck Research Laboratories.

Berry, M., Danish, S. J., Rinke, W. J., & Smiciklas-Wright, H. (1989). Work-site health promotion: The effects of a goal-setting program on nutrition-related behaviors. *Journal of the American Dietary Association, 89*(3), 914–920.

Birren, J., & Cochran, K. (2001). *Telling the stories of life through guided autobiography groups.* Baltimore, MD: Johns Hopkins University Press.

Birren, J., & Deutchman, D. (1991). *Guiding autobiography groups for older adults.* Baltimore, MD: Johns Hopkins University Press.

Birren, J., Kenyon, G. M., Ruth, J.-R., Schroots, J. J. F., & Svensson, T. (Eds.). (1996). *Aging and biography: Explorations in adult development.* New York, NY: Springer.

Blair, S., Kohl, H. W. III, Paffenbarger, R. S. Jr., Clark, D. G., Cooper, K. H., & Gibbons, L. W. (1989). Physical fitness and all-cause mortality: A prospective study of healthy men and women. *Journal of the American Medical Association, 262*(17), 2395–2401.

Booth, K., Pinkston, M. M., & Poston, W. S. (2005). Obesity and the built environment. *Journal of the American Dietetic Association, 105*(5 Suppl. 1), S110–S117.

Brenes, G., Penninx, B. W., Judd, P. H., Rockwell, E., Sewell, D. D., & Wetherell, J. L. (2008). Anxiety, depression and disability across the life span. *Aging and Mental Health, 12*, 158–163.

Brownson, R., Housemann, R. A., Brown, D. R., Jackson-Thompson, J., King, A. C., Malone, B. R., & Sallis, J. F. (2000). Promoting physical activity in rural communities: Walking trail access, use, and effects. *American Journal of Preventive Medicine, 18*(3), 235–241.

Butler, R. (1974). Successful aging and the role of the life review. *Journal of the American Geriatrics Society, 22*(12), 529–535.

Butler, R. (1995). Foreword: The life review. In B. Haight & J. Webster (Eds.), *The art and science of reminiscing* (pp. xvii–xxi). Washington, DC: Taylor and Francis.

Butler, R., Lewis, M. I., & Sunderland, T. (1991). Aging and mental health: Positive psychosocial and biomedical approaches. Columbus, OH: Charles E. Merrill.

Caine, E., Lyness, J. M., & Conwell, Y. (1996). Diagnosis of late-life depression: Preliminary studies in primary care settings. *American Journal of Geriatric Psychiatry, 4*(1), S45–S50.

Centers for Disease Control and Prevention. (1999). *Suicide deaths and rates per 100,000.* Retrieved from http://www.aacap.org/galleries/PracticeParameters/Suictabl.pdf

Civic Ventures and MetLife. (2005). *New faces of work survey.* Retrieved from http://civicventures.org/publications/surveys/new_face_of_work/new_face_of_work.pdf

Clark, J., Keukefeld, C., & Godlaski, T. (1999). Case management and behavioral contracting: Components of rural substance abuse treatment. *Journal of Substance Abuse Treatment, 17*(4), 293–304.

Cupples, S., & Steslow, B. (2001). Use of behavioral contingency contracting with heart transplant candidates. *Progress in Transplantation, 11*(2), 137–144.

DeBusk, R., Stenestrand, U., Sheehan, M., & Haskell, W. L. (1990). Training effects of long versus short bouts of exercise in healthy subjects. *American Journal of Cardiology, 65*(15), 1010–1013.

De Cocker, K., Cardon, G., & De Bourdeaudhuij, I. (2006). The validity of the inexpensive "stepping meter" in counting steps in free-living conditions. *British Journal of Sports Medicine, 40*(8), 714–716.

Dobkin, L. (2002). Senior wellness project secures health care dollars. *Innovations, 2*, 16–20.

Engel, L., & Lindner, H. (2006). Impact of using a pedometer on time spent walking in older adults with type 2 diabetes. *Diabetes Education, 32*(5), 98–107.

Fishbein, M., & Ajzen, I. (1975). *Belief, attitude, intention and behavior: An introduction to theory and research.* Reading, MA: Addison-Wesley.

Frank, L., Andresen, M. A., & Schmid, T. L. (2004). Obesity relationships with community design, physical activity, and time spent in cars. *American Journal of Preventive Medicine, 27*(2), 87–96.

Frasure-Smith, N., Lesperance, F., & Talajic, M. (1995). Depression and 18-month prognosis after myocardial infarction. *Circulation, 91*(4), 999–1005.

Fried, L., Carlson, M. C., Freedman, M., Frick, K. D., Glass, T. A., Hill, J., McGill, S.,…Zeger, S. (2004). A social model for health promotion for an aging population: Initial evidence on the Experience Corps model. *Journal of Urban Health, 81*(1), 64–78.

Gallo, J., Ryan, S. D., & Ford, D. E. (1999). Attitudes, knowledge, and behavior of family physicians regarding depression in late life. *Archives of Family Medicine, 8*(3), 249–256.

George, L. (1986, Spring). Life satisfaction in later life. *Generations*, 5–8.

Gould, L., Ornish, D., Scherwitz, L., Brown, S., Edens, R. P., Hess, M. J.,…Billings, J. (1995). Changes in myocardial perfusion abnormalities by positron emission tomography after long-term, intense risk factor modification. *Journal of the American Medical Association, 274*(11), 894–901.

Haber, D. (2001). Medicare prevention: Movement toward research-based policy. *Journal of Aging and Social Policy, 13*(1), 1–14.

Haber, D. (2002). Health promotion and aging: Educational and clinical initiatives by the federal government. *Educational Gerontology, 28*(2), 1–11.

Haber, D. (2005). Medicare prevention update. Journal of Aging and Social Policy, 17(2), 1–6.

Haber, D. (2006). Life review: Implementation, theory, and future direction. *International Journal of Aging and Human Development, 63*(2), 153–171.

Haber, D. (2007a). Health contract in the classroom. *Gerontology and Geriatrics Education, 27*(4), 41–54.

Haber, D. (2007b). *Health promotion and aging: Practical applications for health professionals* (4th ed.). New York, NY: Springer.

Haber, D. (2010). *Health promotion and aging: Practical applications for health professionals* (5th ed.), New York, NY: Springer.

Haber, D., & Looney, C. (2000). Health contract calendars: A tool for health professionals with older adults. *The Gerontologist, 40*(2), 235–239.

Haber, D., & Rhodes, D. (2004). Health contract with sedentary older adults. *The Gerontologist, 44*(6), 827–835.

Haight, B., Michel, Y., & Hendrix, S. (1998). Life review: Preventing despair in newly relocated nursing home residents' short- and long-term effects. *International Journal of Aging and Human Development, 47*(2), 119–142.

Harris, L.. (1989). *The prevention index '89: Summary report.* Emmaus, PA: Rodale Press.

Hart, P. (2002). *The new face of retirement: An ongoing survey of American attitudes on aging.* Retrieved from http://www.experiencecorps.org/images/pdf/new_face_survey_results.pdf

Healthwise. (2006). *Healthwise handbook* (17th ed.). Boise, ID: Author.

Healthy People 2020. (n.d.) *iHealthy People 2020.* Retrieved from http://www.healthypeople.gov/2020/Connect/iHealthyPeople2020v25.pdf

Hooyman, N & Kiyak, H. (2011). *Social gerontology: A multidisciplinary perspective.* Boston, MA: Allyn & Bacon.

Jacob, J. (2002). Wellness programs help companies save on health costs. *American Medical News,* March, 32–33.

Jakicic, J., Donnelly, J. E., Pronk, N. P., Jawad, A. F., & Jacobsen, D. J. (1995). Prescription of exercise intensity for the obese patient: The relationship between heart rate, VO2 and perceived exertion. *International Journal of Obesity, 19*(6), 382–387.

Jette, A., Lachman, M., Giorgetti, M. M., Assmann, S. F., Harris, B. A., Levenson, C.,…Krebs, D. (1999). Exercise—It's never too late: The Strong for Life program. *American Journal of Public Health, 89*(1), 66–72.

Johnson, C. C., Nicklas, T. A., Arbeit, M. L., Webber, L. S., & Berenson, G. S. (1992). Behavioral counseling and contracting as methods for promoting cardiovascular health in families. *Journal of the American Dietetic Association, 92*(4), 479–481.

Katon, W., von Korff, M., Lin, E., Bush, T., & Ormel, J. (1992). Adequacy and duration of antidepressant treatment in primary care. *Medical Care, 30*(11), 67–76.

Kazel, R. (2004, June 28). Dieting for dollars. *American Medical News,* 17–18.

King, W., Brach, J. S., Killingsworth, R., Fenton, M., & Kriska, A. M. (2003). The relationship between convenience of destinations and walking levels in older women. *American Journal of Health Promotion, 18*(1), 74–82.

LaCroix, A., Leveille, S. G., Hecht, J. A., Grothaus, L. C., & Wagner, E. H. (1996). Does walking decrease the risk of cardiovascular disease hospitalization and death in older adults? *Journal of the American Geriatrics Society, 44*(2), 113–120.

Lantz, M. (2002). Depression in the elderly: Recognition and treatment. *Clinical Geriatrics, 10*(2), 18–24.

Lebowitz, B. (1995, Spring). Depression in older adults. *Aging and Vision News, 7,* 2.

Lee, I., Sesso, H. D., & Paffenbarger, R. S. (2000). Physical activity and coronary heart disease risk in men. *Circulation, 102*(4), 981–986.

Leslie, M., & Schuster, P. (1991). The effect of contingency contracting on adherence and knowledge of exercise regimen. *Patient Education and Counseling, 18*(3), 231–241.

Leveille, S., Wagner, E. H., Davis, C., Grothaus, L., Wallace, J., LoGerfo, M., & Kent, D. (1998). Preventing disability and managing chronic illness in frail older adults: A randomized trial of a community-based partnership with primary care. *Journal of the American Geriatrics Society, 46*(10), 1191–1198.

Li, F., Fisher, K. J., & Harmer, P. (2005). Improving physical function and blood pressure in older adults through cobblestone mat walking: A randomized trial. *Journal of the American Geriatrics Society, 53*(8), 1305–1312.

Lorig, K., Lubeck, D., Kraines, R. G., Seleznickm, M., Holman, H. R. (1996). Outcomes of self-help education for patients with arthritis. *Arthritis and Rheumatism, 28*(2), 680–685.

Lorig, K., Ritter, P., Stewart, A.. L., Sobel, D. S., Brown, B. W. J., Bandura, A.,…Holman, H. R. (2001). Chronic disease self-management program. *Medical Care, 39*(11), 1217–1223.

Lorig, K., Sobel, D., Holeman, M. D., Laurent, D., Gonzales, V., & Minor, M. (2000). *Living a healthy life with chronic conditions.* Palo Alto, CA: Bull.

Lorig, K., Sobel, D., & Stewart, A. (1999). Evidence suggesting that a chronic disease self-management program can improve health status while reducing hospitalization: A randomized trial. *Medical Care, 37*(1), 5–14.

Lorig, K., Stewart, A., Ritter, P., Gonzalez, V., Laurent, D., & Lynch, J. (1996). *Outcome measures for health education and other health care interventions.* Thousand Oaks, CA: Sage.

McCormack, G., Giles-Corti, B., & Milligan, R. (2006). Demographic and individual correlates of achieving 10,000 steps/day: Use of pedometers in a population-based study. *Health Promotion Journal of Australia, 17*(1), 43–47.

McGuire, L., Kiecolt-Glaser, J. K., & Glaser, R. (2002). Depressive symptoms and lymphocyte proliferation in older adults. *Journal of Abnormal Psychology, 111*(1), 192–197.

Mettler, M. (1997). *Unpublished update on the Healthwise Handbook program.* Healthwise, Inc., P.O. Box 1989, Boise, ID 83701.

Moore, J., von Korff, M., Cherkin, D., Saunders, K., & Lorig, K. (2000). A randomized trial of a cognitive-behavioral program for enhancing back pain self care in a primary care setting. *Pain, 88*(2), 145–153.

Murphy, M., Nevill, A., Neville, C., Biddle, S., & Hardman, A. (2002). Accumulating brisk walking for fitness, cardiovascular risk, and psychological health. *Medical Science and Sports Exercise, 34*(9), 1468–1474.

National Center for Health Statistics. (1985). *National health interview survey.* Hyattsville, MD: U.S. Public Health Service, Advance Data, 13.

National Center for Health Statistics. (1999). *Healthy People 2000 review, 1998–1999.* Hyattsville, MD: U.S. Department of Health and Human Services.

Neale, A., Singleton, S. P., Dupuis, M. H., & Hess, J. W. (1990). The use of behavioral contracting to increase exercise activity. *American Journal of Health Promotion, 4*(2), 441–447.

Nutting, P. (1987). Community-oriented primary care: From principle to practice. In P. Nutting (Ed.), *Community-oriented primary care.* (pp. xv–xxv). Albuquerque: University of New Mexico Press.

Ornish, D. (1992). *Dr. Dean Ornish's program for reversing heart disease.* New York, NY: Ballantine.

Ornish, D., Scherwitz, L. W., Billings, J. H., Brown, S. E., Gould, K. L., Merritt, T. A.,…Brand, R. J. (1998). Intensive lifestyle changes for reversal of coronary heart disease. *Journal of the American Medical Association, 280*(23), 2001–2007.

Pate, R. R., Pratt, M., Blair, S. N., Haskell, W. L., Macera, C. A., Bouchard, C.,…Wilmore, J. H. (1995). Physical activity and public health. *Journal of the American Medical Association, 273*(5), 402–407.

Penninx, B., Guralnik, J. M., Pahor, M., Ferrucci, L., Cerhan, J. R., Wallace, R. B., & Havlik, R. J. (1998a). Chronically depressed mood and cancer risk in older persons. *Journal of the National Cancer Institute, 90*(24), 1888–1893.

Penninx, B., Guralnik, J. M., Ferucci, L., Simonsick, E. M., Deeq, D. J., & Wallace, R. B. (1998b). Depressive symptoms and physical decline in community-dwelling older persons. *Journal of the American Medical Association, 279*(21), 1720–1726.

Pfizer. (2007). *The health status of older adults.* Retrieved from http://media.pfizer.com/files/products/The_Health_Status_of_Older_Adults_2007.pdf

Phelan, E., Williams, B., Leveille, S., Snyder, S., Wagner, E. H., & LoGerfo, J. P. (2002). Outcomes of a community-based dissemination of the health enhancement program. *Journal of the American Geriatrics Society, 50*(9), 1519–1524.

Prochaska, J., & DiClemente, C. (1992). Stages of change in the modification of problem behaviors. In M. Herson et al. (Eds.), *Progress in behavior modification* (pp. 184–218). CA: Sage.

Rabig, J., Thomas, W., Kane, R., Cutler, L., & McAlilly, S. (2006). Radical redesign of nursing homes: Applying the Green House concept in Tupelo, Mississippi. *The Gerontologist, 46*(4), 533–539.

Rabins, P. (1996). Barriers to diagnosis and treatment of depression in elderly patients. *American Journal of Geriatric Psychiatry, 4*(1), S79–S83.

Rebok, G., Carlson, M. C., Glass, T. A., McGill, S., Hill, J., Wasik, B. A.,...Rasmussen, M. D. (2004). Short-term impact of Experience Corps participation on children and schools. *Journal of Urban Health, 81*(1), 79–83.

Schlenk, E., & Boehm, S. (1998). Behaviors in type II diabetes during contingency contracting. *Applied Nursing Research, 11*(2), 77–83.

Squires, S. (2002, October 14–20). We're fat and getting fatter. *Washington Post National Weekly Edition*, p. 34.

Stovitz, S., VanWormer, J. J., Center, B. A., & Bremer, K. L. (2005). Pedometers as a means to increase ambulatory activity for patients seen at a family medicine clinic. *Journal of the American Board of Family Practice, 18*(5), 335–343.

Sturm, R., & Cohen, D. (2004). Suburban sprawl and physical and mental health. Public Health, 118(7), 488–496.

Swinburn, B., Walter, L. G., Arroll, B., Tilyard, M. W., & Russell, D. G. (1998). The green prescription study: A randomized controlled trial of written exercise advice provided by general practitioners. *American Journal of Public Health, 88*(2), 288–291.

Tan, E., Xue, Q. L., Li, T., Carlson, M. C., & Fried, L. P. (2006). Volunteering: A physical activity intervention for older adults—The Experience Corps program in Baltimore. *Journal of Urban Health, 83*(5), 954–969.

Thomas, W. (2004). *What are old people for?* Acton, MA: VanderWyk & Burnam.

U.S. Preventive Services Task Force. (1996). *Guide to clinical preventive services*. Baltimore, MD: Williams and Wilkins.

Wallerstein, N., & Bernstein, E. (1988). Empowerment education: Freier's ideas adapted to health education. *Health Education Quarterly, 15*(4), 379–394.

Wallston, K., & Wallston, B. (1982). Who is responsible for your health? The construct of health locus of control. In G. Saunders & J. Suls (Eds.), *Social psychology of health and illness*. Hillsdale, NJ: Erlbaum.

Watt, L., & Cappeliez, P. (2000). Integrative and instrumental reminiscence therapies for depression in older adults. *Aging & Mental Health, 4*(2), 166–183.

For a full suite of assignments and additional learning activities, see the access code at the front of your book.

LEARNING OBJECTIVES

At the end of this chapter, the reader will be able to:

> Discuss techniques for assessing and treating factors that lead to functional decline in the elderly.
> Describe recommended screening evaluations for the elderly population.
> Cite the expert recommendations for flu and pneumonia vaccines.
> Identify risk factors and signs of abuse in the elderly.
> Explain the protocol for reporting elder abuse.

KEY TERMS

Activities of daily living (ADLs)
Adult protective services agency
Annoyance
Chronic Disease Self-Management
   Program (CDSMP)
Contracting
Cut down
Dietary Approaches to Stop Hypertension
   (DASH) diet
Eye opener
Framingham Heart Study
Functional decline

Guilt
Health promotion
Health screening
Healthy People 2020
Instrumental activities of daily living
   (IADLs)
Primary prevention
Secondary prevention
Tertiary prevention
U.S. Preventive Services Task Force
   (USPSTF)

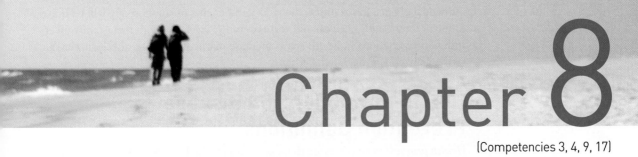

Chapter 8

(Competencies 3, 4, 9, 17)

Identifying and Preventing Common Risk Factors in the Elderly

Joan M. Nelson

Introduction

Health promotion activities can help to prevent functional decline in the elderly. Scientific evidence supports the fact that functional disability is not caused by aging, per se, but results from illnesses and diseases that are related to unhealthy lifestyle decisions. Unhealthy behaviors or lifestyles have been linked to physical decline in later life (Pluijm et al., 2007). This creates an exciting opportunity for nurses to improve the quality of life for the elderly client through evidence-based health promotion activities.

In this chapter, we will review the health promotion and disease prevention guidelines recommended by the following:

> *U.S. Preventive Services Task Force (USPSTF):* The USPSTF was convened by the U.S. Public Health Service to systematically review the evidence of effectiveness of clinical preventive services. The task force is an independent panel of private-sector experts in primary care and prevention whose mission is to evaluate the benefits of individual services and to create age-, gender-, and risk-based recommendations about services that should routinely be incorporated into primary medical care. Its recommendations can be found at http://www.uspreventiveservicestaskforce.org/recommendations.htm.

> *Healthy People 2020:* Healthy People 2020 is an initiative of a Federal Interagency workgroup with input from many governmental and private agencies. It is a set of healthcare objectives designed to improve the health of individuals and communities, eliminate health disparities, and improve access to care. Its recommendations can be found at http://www.healthypeople.gov/2020/about/objectiveDevelopment.aspx.

The recommendations presented in this chapter are guidelines for most patients, most of the time. Clinical judgment must be used in applying these guidelines to individual clients; for example, the risks and benefits of colonoscopy will be quite different for a healthy 75-year-old versus a frail 75- year-old with metastatic cancer. Individual variations in health status increase markedly with age, necessitating an individualized approach to health care.

Health Promotion and Disease Prevention Definitions

Health promotion activities are those activities in which an individual is able to pro-actively engage in order to advance or improve his or her health. *Primary prevention* activities are those designed to completely prevent a disease from occurring, such as immunization against pneumonia or influenza. *Secondary prevention* efforts are directed toward early detection and management of disease, such as the use of colonoscopy to detect small, cancerous polyps. *Tertiary prevention* efforts are used to manage clinical diseases in order to prevent them from progressing or to avoid complications of the disease, as is done when beta-blockers are used to help remodel the heart in congestive heart failure.

Screening

Health screening is a form of secondary prevention and will be a focus of this chapter. In order to endorse screening for a specific disease, the USPSTF considers whether the disease occurs with enough frequency in a population to justify mass screening. The population is more likely to benefit from screening tests for a disease like diabetes, which occurs frequently, than it is to benefit from screening for Addison's disease, which is uncommon. In order to justify the costs and inconvenience of screening, we must be able to detect the condition being screened at a relatively early stage and have effective treatments for the condition. Early detection of the disease has to result in improved clinical outcomes. The screening tests should be relatively noninvasive and acceptable to patients, cost effective and available, and highly sensitive and specific (see **Case Study 8-1**).

Screening recommendations are graded by expert panels according to the strength of the supporting evidence and the net benefit. The USPSTF uses the following rating scale:

> *Level A*: The USPSTF recommends the service. There is high certainty that the net benefit is substantial based on rigorous experimental research with consistent results.
> *Level B*: The USPSTF recommends the service. There is high certainty that the net benefit is moderate or there is moderate certainty that the net benefit is moderate to substantial.

Case Study 8-1

You are working as an RN for a managed care organization. Physicians have complained about their inability to adequately care for their elderly patients given the time constraints imposed by the 20-minute office visit. An innovative strategy—in which RNs meet with all clients over the age of 65 on an annual basis, prior to the physician visit, in order to ensure that recommended screening tests are performed—has been instituted by the HMO.

You are visiting with Hilde M., an 82-year-old woman, who is accompanied by her daughter, Roxanne. Roxanne has called you prior to the visit to inform you about her concerns about her mother's ability to live safely alone at home. She confides that her mother is forgetting many appointments and has fallen at least twice in the

past 3 months. Although Hilde had a minor stroke 3 years ago, she has not been into the office for the past year because she lacks transportation since she gave up driving 2 years ago due to her poor vision. Roxanne has encouraged her mother to move into an assisted-living facility, but Hilde is loathe to sell her home of 50 years and to give up her independence.

Questions:

What screening tests are appropriate for Hilde at this time? Justify your choices. What instruments will you use to perform the appropriate screening tests? What counseling will you provide for Mrs. M. and her daughter, based on the limited information you have been provided?

> *Level C*: Clinicians may provide this service to selected patients depending on individual circumstances. However, for most individuals without signs or symptoms there is likely to be only a small benefit from this service.
> *Level D*: The USPSTF recommends against the service. There is moderate or high certainty that the service has no net benefit or that the harms outweigh the benefits.
> *Level I*: The USPSTF concludes that the current evidence is insufficient to assess the balance of benefits and harms of the service. Evidence is lacking, of poor quality, or conflicting, and the balance of benefits and harms cannot be determined.

The Focus of Health Promotion Efforts

A major focus of health promotion efforts for the elderly is to minimize the loss of independence associated with illness and functional decline. Healthy People 2020 and the USPSTF suggest the following focus areas for nurses in order to promote health and prevent disability in the elderly client:

> Physical activity
> Nutrition
> Tobacco use
> Health screening
> Injury prevention
> Preventive medications and immunizations
> Caregiver support

Many of these foci show considerable overlap with recommendations for younger adults, but some, like injury prevention and hearing and vision screening, are unique to older adults. It is important to consider the impact of health conditions on physical functioning and on quality of life in the older client. This is different from the younger adults' focus on treatment and cure of a single, acute condition. Multiple chronic illnesses are common in the elderly, and cure is often an unrealistic and inappropriate goal. These chronic illnesses can lead to disability and dependency. In fact, almost 15% of Americans over 65 years of age require help with bathing, dressing, meal preparation, or shopping (Centers for Disease Control and Prevention [CDC] and the Merck Company Foundation, 2007). Symptoms that impact functional status should be the focus of interventions with this population. Maintaining independence in *activities of daily living (ADLs)* is an important goal for health promoting activities.

By the time we are 85 years old, one-half of our remaining years of life are expected to be lived dependently, often in a nursing home. About 2.3 million elderly Americans have some functional limitation, and one-half of elderly clients hospitalized for medical illness were found to have some deficiency in ADLs (CDC, 2011d). Some of the preventive strategies that will be discussed in this chapter, like smoking cessation, immunization, physical activity, weight control, blood pressure control, and arthritis and diabetes self-management programs, are known to be effective in lessening disability.

Assessment of functional status requires a multipronged approach. The ADL scale and the *instrumental activities of daily living (IADLs)* scale are valid and reliable self-report tools to assess functional status (Lawton & Brody, 1969). Nurses can use these instruments to identify elderly individuals who are frail and may benefit from an increased level of care or additional in-home support. Fear of being advised to leave their home, however, can cause elderly individuals to deny difficulties. Because the ADL and IADL scales rely on self-reporting, they can fail to detect difficulties when clients are not forthcoming about their limitations.

Performance-based tools, like the Get Up and Go test (Duxbury, 1997), can provide a more objective measurement of functional status and fall risk. This assessment requires clients to rise from a chair, walk 10 feet, turn around, return to the chair, and sit down. These actions are timed and compared with a historic sample of adults without balance problems that were able complete this test in less than 10 seconds. Older adults who are dependent in most activities of daily living and have poor balance and gait may take more than 30 seconds to complete the task. Clients are observed for sitting balance, transfers, gait, and ability to maintain balance while turning. If a gait abnormality is detected, weight-bearing exercise and physical rehabilitation may prevent further decline and lessen the risk of falls.

Frailty is a concept that is often discussed in the literature, but which is difficult to define and is the topic of much debate. Frailty involves visible changes such as weight loss, decreased physical activity, fatigue, weakness, and impaired mobility, as well as the accumulation of health conditions and deficits. There is agreement that frailty is associated with poor health outcomes, increased risk of hospitalization, and limited lifespan (U.S. Preventative Services Task Force [USPSTF], 2012). Several frailty measures exist for use in practice and tool selection should be guided by the skill of the person performing the assessment and the time allocated for the assessment (deVries et al., 2011).

Self-Management

What can nurses do to encourage clients to adopt health-promoting behaviors and manage their chronic illnesses? Kate Lorig, MD, has been instrumental in developing the concept of self-management and outlining the role of the healthcare provider in fostering the client's self-management of his or her chronic condition (Lorig & Holman, 2000). Her research, which was sponsored by the Agency for Healthcare Research and Quality (AHRQ), supported the effectiveness of chronic disease self-management in preventing or delaying disability from chronic diseases. She has described how the self-management concept also may be applied to health promotion activities.

The *Chronic Disease Self-Management Program (CDSMP)* is a 17-hour course for patients with chronic diseases that is taught by trained laypeople (Stanford School of Medicine, 2012). The course goal is to teach patients to improve symptom management, maintain functional ability, and adhere to their medication regimens. The proven effectiveness of the intervention is, at least in part, attributable to the improved self-efficacy of clients who participate in the program. Clients come to believe that they can succeed in managing their illness and preventing disability.

Critical to the concept of self-management is an assessment of the client's goals and concerns, which may be different from the healthcare professional's goals and concerns. The nurse may feel that exercise will help lower her client's blood pressure, which may decrease stroke risk—certainly an important goal. The client's focus, however, may be that he does not want to go shopping for new clothes, needed as a result of his recent weight gain, and his goal is to continue to be able to use his current wardrobe. He will assess the value of his new exercise program in terms of his clothing budget, not in relation to his blood pressure readings.

Lorig & Holman (2000) identified five key elements of self-management programs: problem solving, decision making, resource utilization, forming a healthcare professional–client partnership, and taking action. In the problem-solving phase, a client may identify several barriers to initiating an exercise program and then list strategies for overcoming each barrier, to arrive at a workable strategy. Decision making helps to arm clients with the information needed to make the decisions they need to make on a daily basis. "How do I know when I am exercising too hard?" "Should I exercise when I don't feel well?" The provider plays an important role in providing accurate and sufficient information for clients to make informed decisions. Providers also teach clients to access and evaluate appropriate resources and to create plans that are easily accomplished, limited in scope, and easily evaluated for success. A technique that has proven successful is to ask the client how confident they are on a scale of 1–10 (10 being maximally confident) that they will accomplish their objective. If the score is less than 7, encourage them to set a more realistic goal.

Contracting for health promoting behaviors is another useful strategy. A successful contract for behavior change is very specific. The contract may begin with the overall behavioral goal ("I wish to lose 20 lbs over the next year in order to improve my overall health, strength, and stamina"). The client determines his or her own short-term goal and means of achieving that goal for the next week ("I will exercise for 20 minutes, 3 times this week"). The nurse helps the client to pinpoint exactly how and when that will occur. The client is encouraged to write the exact time that the exercise will occur on his or her calendar, and the exact form the exercise will take ("I will walk around my subdivision, which is 1.25 miles in length, at 10 a.m. on Tuesday, Thursday, and Saturday"). Ideally, the client and nurse will meet at the end of that time period to evaluate and modify the plan for the next week or so. Barriers to implementing the plan are reviewed and taken into consideration in order to rewrite the following week's contract.

Self-management classes and contracting are strategies that can be incorporated through individual sessions or in group meetings, to help implement the health promotion and disease prevention ideas discussed in this chapter.

Physical Activity

Functional decline in the elderly is attributable, at least in part, to physical inactivity. Researchers have correlated physical activity through the lifespan with preservation of cognitive function. See **Box 8-1** for more information about this study. Physical activity can improve quality of life, decrease the risk of death from cardiovascular disease and some cancers, and reduce the risk of bone fractures and falls (CDC, 2011d) (see **Box 8-2**). Despite the well-documented benefits of exercise in reducing blood pressure and cholesterol, improving insulin resistance, reducing weight, strengthening bones, and reducing falls, one-third of adults 65 years of age and older report that they do not engage in any leisure time physical activity (Partnership for Prevention, 2008). In order to receive health benefits from exercise, older adults should engage in 150 minutes of moderate intensity or 75 minutes of vigorous intensity exercise every week (CDC, 2008a).

Physical inactivity causes increased healthcare costs to our nation. In fact, a CDC study has shown that the direct medical costs of inactive Americans are markedly higher than the costs for active Americans. The direct medical costs associated with physical inactivity were nearly $76.6 billion in 2000 (National Center for Chronic Disease Prevention and Health Promotion, 2004).

BOX 8-1   Research Highlight

Aim: This cross-sectional study was designed to determine whether there is a relationship between physical activity at various stages in life and cognitive decline.

Methods: 9,344 women with mean age of 71.6 years completed a questionnaire about their level of physical activity as teenagers, young and middle-aged adults, and older adults. Their cognitive status was assessed, at the time of the study, using the Mini Mental Status Exam. A logistic regression was used to determine the relationship between cognitive function and level of exercise at each phase of life.

Findings: There was a positive relationship between cognitive status and physical activity at any age, but especially during the teen years.

Application to Practice: Nurses should encourage physical activity to help their patients prevent cognitive decline. Lifelong habits related to physical exercise are most effective in preventing dementia, but increasing physical activity at any age is helpful.

Source: Middleton, L. E., Barnes, D. E., Lui, L., & Yaffe, K. (2010). Physical activity over the life course and its association with cognitive performance and impairment in old age. *Journal of the American Geriatrics Society, 58*(7), 1322–1326.

BOX 8-2   Physical Activity Counseling

Level I recommendation: The USPSTF found insufficient evidence to determine whether encouraging or counseling patients to begin an exercise program actually led to improvements in their level of physical activity. There is strong evidence, however, to support the effectiveness of physical activity in reducing morbidity and mortality from chronic illness.

Scientific evidence supports the effectiveness of moderate physical activity in:

> Decreasing overall mortality
> Decreasing coronary heart disease, the leading cause of death in the United States
> Decreasing colon cancer
> Decreasing the incidence and improving the management of diabetes mellitus
> Decreasing the incidence and improving the management of hypertension
> Decreasing obesity
> Improving depression
> Improving quality of life
> Improving functional status
> Decreasing falls and injury

Moderate exercise is defined as 30 or more minutes of brisk walking on 5 or more days per week. Tai chi and yoga are helpful for improving balance and flexibility. Modified exercises, such as armchair exercises, can be helpful for the frail elderly or those with mobility restrictions. Sporadic, vigorous exercise should be discouraged.

Barriers to physical exercise that have been identified by the elderly include lack of access to safe areas to exercise, pain, fatigue, and impairment in sensory function and mobility. These barriers underscore the need to individualize your approach to helping clients develop an exercise regimen tailored to their unique needs and to participate in community efforts to create environments that foster healthy lifestyles. The Partnership for Prevention (2008) developed an excellent community assessment guide with a list of strategies for communities to overcome barriers encountered by older adults to physical activities. This guide, called *Physical Activity Guidelines for Americans*, is accessible on the Web at http://www.health.gov/paguidelines/guidelines/chapter5.aspx.

What can be done to foster participation in physical exercise? Individuals can increase their chances of beginning, and sticking with, an exercise program if they identify activities that can be a regular part of their daily routine and identify individuals who can participate in the exercise with them. Nurses can help clients to assess their current level of activity and barriers that prevent them from exercising. The nurse then can help the client with goal setting, write a prescription for exercise, work with the client to develop an exercise program individually tailored to the client's unique needs, and follow up by telephone at regular intervals to assess progress and barriers. Follow-up phone calls can also be used to assess how well the client has done with accessing community resources.

Nutrition

Four of the 10 leading causes of death in the United States (cancer, diabetes, coronary heart disease, and cerebral vascular accidents) are associated with unhealthy dietary patterns (CDC, 2012a). Most Americans do not eat enough fruits or vegetables and eat too much fat. Healthy People 2020 includes objectives to increase consumption of fruits, vegetables, and whole grains and decrease consumption of solid fats and sugars, as well as increasing the frequency with which healthcare providers counsel patients about nutrition and measure their body mass index (BMI).

Elderly clients may be at increased risk for poor nutrition due to the fact that they have multiple chronic illnesses, may have tooth or mouth problems that can interfere with their ability to eat, may be socially isolated, may have economic hardship, may be taking multiple medications that can cause changes in appetite or gastrointestinal symptoms, and may need assistance with self-care. Weight gain or loss may signal nutritional problems. A BMI of less than 19 can signal undernutrition (Thomas, Ashmen, Morley, & Evans, 2000).

Measurement of body weight over time provides the simplest means of detecting nutritional risk. Unintended weight loss is highly correlated with mortality (Wannamethee, Shaper, & Lennon, 2005). The Mini Nutritional Assessment (MNA) is a tool that can be used by nurses to assess nutritional risk. It is available online at http://www.mna-elderly.com/forms/mini/mna_mini_english.pdf. The MNA is a well-validated, six-item tool that can be quickly administered and used to predict poor health outcomes (Sieber, 2006).

Older adults residing in rehabilitation and long-term care facilities are at very high risk for inadequate nutrition. The Council for Nutritional Clinical Strategies in Long-Term Care developed an evidenced-based guideline for management of adults found to have nutritional compromise (Thomas et al., 2000). This guideline identifies adults with a BMI of less than 21 as potentially at risk and suggests that these adults be targeted for counseling and other interventions. The first step identified in this guideline is to clarify the patient and family's advanced directives. A comprehensive assessment is recommended to identify hydration status, medications, and medical conditions that could contribute to loss of appetite, swallowing difficulties, increased metabolic states, and decreased food intake. Nurses should notify the healthcare provider of the patient's dietary and fluid intake as well as any fevers; fecal impaction; constipation; mood disturbances; nausea, vomiting, or indigestion; signs of pain or infection; or signs of swallowing problems, ill-fitting dentures, or dental problems. Nurses should check the chart for signs of nutritional inadequacy. These would include albumin < 3.4 g/dL, cholesterol < 160 mg/dL, Hgb <12 g/dL, and serum transferrin <180.

Any adult with signs of undernutrition should be instructed to stop any special diets and encouraged to snack and use food supplements, like protein shakes, between meals (not at meal times). Medications should not be administered with meals. Family can be encouraged to provide the older adult with his/her favorite foods and to provide socialization during mealtimes, when possible. A speech therapist can assist with adults who have dysphagia and an occupational therapist is instrumental in identifying adaptive equipment to help older adults with the mechanics of eating. This guideline contains helpful algorithms for nurses and can be accessed at http://www.geroupr.com/nutri.pdf.

Being overweight or obese is also a health risk for older adults due to the associated risks for diabetes, heart disease, and some types of cancer. Adults with BMIs over 25 are considered to be overweight, and those with BMIs over 30 are considered to be obese. Overweight older adults should be counseled to avoid weight gain, whereas those who are in the obese category will benefit from weight loss strategies (see **Box 8-3**).

BOX 8-3   Nutrition Counseling

Level B recommendation: The USPSTF found good evidence to support counseling interventions among adults at risk for diet-related chronic disease. Interventions that have proven to stimulate healthy dietary changes combine nutrition education with behavioral counseling.

General dietary guidelines for older adults include (USDA, 2010):

> Limit alcohol to one drink a day for women, two daily for men.
> Limit fat and cholesterol.
> Maintain a balanced caloric intake.
> Ensure adequate daily calcium, especially for women.
> Older adults should consume foods fortified with vitamins, such as fortified cereals or supplements.
> Older adults who have minimal exposure to sunlight or who have dark skin need supplemental vitamin D. Daily vitamin D intake should be 800–1000 IU and can be derived from fortified foods or supplements (Dawson-Hughes et al., 2010).
> Include adequate whole grains, fruits, and vegetables.
> Drink adequate water.

Tobacco Use

Cigarette smoking is the leading cause of preventable death in the United States. About one-half of the population of people who use tobacco can be expected to die from tobacco-related causes (CDC, 2008b). Elderly Americans are just as likely to benefit from quitting smoking as are younger adults. Quitting smoking can decrease the chance of having a myocardial infarction or dying from lung cancer or heart disease. Nonsmokers have improved wound healing, recovery from illness, and cerebral circulation.

A practice guideline for clinicians to help their patients quit smoking has been developed through the Public Health Service (Tobacco Use and Dependence Guideline Panel, 2008) and is available online at http://www.ncbi.nlm.nih.gov/books/NBK63952/. The task force stresses that the most important step in helping a client to quit smoking is to screen for tobacco use and assess the client's willingness to quit. It outlines the 5 As for clients who are ready to quit smoking and recommends that clinicians use motivational interviewing strategies to increase the likelihood of future quit attempts for those who are not ready to quit. Support to prevent relapse in those who have quit is also recommended.

The 5 As:

Ask about smoking status at each healthcare visit.
Advise client to quit smoking.
Assess client's willingness to quit smoking at this time.
Assist client to quit using counseling and pharmacotherapy.
Arrange for follow-up within one week of scheduled quit date.

Practical tips for the nurse or provider to use in assisting patients who are ready to quit are provided in the guideline. One of the key strategies to use in any behavior change counseling is to encourage the patient to be very specific about what, when, and how he/she plans to make this change. In the case of smoking cessation, the older adult can be encouraged to mark a quit date on his/her calendar and to tell family and friends about plans to quit on that day. All tobacco products should be removed from the home in advance of this quit date. The "Quit Line" (1-800-QUIT-NOW) has additional counseling and support materials. Medications have been shown to increase success with long-term smoking cessation.

BOX 8-4   Tobacco Cessation Counseling

Level A recommendation: The USPSTF found good evidence that screening, brief behavioral counseling, and pharmacotherapy are effective in helping clients to quit smoking and remain smoke-free after 1 year. There are good data to support that smoking cessation lowers the risk for heart disease, stroke, and lung disease.

Safety

Many of the safety recommendations for older adults are similar to those for younger people: use lap and shoulder belts in motor vehicles, avoid driving while intoxicated, use smoke detectors in the home, maintain hot water heaters at or below 120° F. Falls, however, are a safety risk that is relatively unique to the elderly.

Falls are the leading cause of unintentional injury death in older adults in this country. Approximately one-half of elderly adults living in institutions and one-third of community-dwelling elders fall every year (Roman, 2004). Twenty to thirty percent of these falls result in serious injuries, including fractures, traumatic brain injuries, and lacerations (CDC, 2011b). Twenty thousand Americans die as a result of a fall each year. Elderly adults are susceptible to falls as a result of postural instability, decreased muscle strength, gait disturbances and decreased proprioception, visual and/or cognitive impairment, and polypharmacy. Environmental conditions that contribute to falls are slippery surfaces, stairs, irregular surfaces, poor lighting, incorrect footwear, and obstacles in the pathway.

BOX 8-5   Fall Prevention Counseling

Revision of recommendation in progress at this time, but the USPSTF says, "There is strong evidence that several types of primary care applicable falls interventions (i.e., comprehensive multifactorial assessment and management, exercise/physical therapy interventions, and vitamin D supplementation) reduce falls among those selected to be at higher risk for falling. Harms of these interventions appear to be minimal, but future research should confirm this assertion" (Michael et al., 2010, p. iv).

The American Geriatrics Society (2010) and British Geriatrics Society have published a joint guideline on fall prevention for older adults. Nurses should ask all older adults three basic screening questions: "Have you fallen in the past year?"; "If so, what were the circumstances of the fall(s) and how often have you fallen?"; and "Do you have any difficulty with walking or balance?" Patients who have had more than one fall or have had an injury significant enough to require medical care, or who have difficulty with walking or balance, require a full, multifactorial fall risk assessment. An algorithm useful in the assessment and treatment of fall risk can be accessed at http://www.medcats.com/FALLS/frameset.htm. Interventions aimed at reducing the risk of falls include a home safety evaluation with appropriate modifications, discontinuation of high-risk medications, management of postural hypotension, vitamin D supplementation, assessment and treatment of foot problems, and exercise. There are strong data to support the effectiveness of balance and strengthening exercises for fall reduction (Mitty & Flores, 2007), as well as research to support physiologic and environmental risk factor reduction.

Polypharmacy and Medication Errors

Elderly adults are at increased risk of adverse drug effects compared to younger adults, as a result of the fact that they take more medications and the biologic effects of aging and chronic diseases. Medication under- and overutilization by this population has been shown to increase the number of hospitalizations and emergency room visits, to worsen cognitive functioning, and to contribute to falls.

The CDC (2011a) has developed a medication safety program with information for patients about high-risk medications and medication safety strategies. The Food and Drug Administration (2011) is spearheading a multi-agency effort called the "Safe Use Initiative," which aims to coordinate efforts in order to improve the safe use of medications and to prevent harm caused from medication errors, abuse, and misuse. The American Pharmacists Association and the National Association of Chain Drugstores Foundation (2008) created a service model to help with medication management and included a sample format for a personal medication record; it can be accessed at http://www.pharmacist.com/sites/default/files/files/core_elements_of_an_mtm_practice.pdf.

Older adults comprise 12% of the population, but use about one-third of all prescription and over-the-counter drugs sold in the United States. This number is markedly higher for hospitalized patients or those living in nursing homes or assisted-living facilities. Polypharmacy is not always inappropriate in this population of clients who have multiple chronic illnesses, but increased numbers of medications carry increasing risks. Budnitz, Lovegrove, Shehab, and Richards (2011) examined a large national database and discovered that almost 100,000 Americans over the age of 65 were admitted to the emergency department (ED) annually between 2007 and 2009 due to adverse drug events. Over one-half of these admissions were for patients over the age of 80 and four specific classes of medications accounted for over two-thirds of these ED visits: warfarin, insulin, oral hypoglycemic medications, and oral antiplatelet medications.

The American Geriatrics Society (AGS) has recently published an updated version of the Beer's Criteria for Potentially Inappropriate Medications in Older Adults (AGS, 2012). This update came from an extensive review of evidence relating to harm due to these agents and is available as an easy-to use pocket card at http://www.americangeriatrics.org/files/documents/beers/PrintableBeersPocketCard.pdf.

These medications include long-acting benzodiazepines, sedative or hypnotic agents, long-acting oral hypoglycemics, analgesics, antiemetics, and gastrointestinal antispasmodics. Elderly clients who require home care services and are, therefore, among the more disabled, are prescribed these medications even more often than the healthier members of their cohort. See Chapter 11 for a thorough discussion on polypharmacy.

The Screening Tool of Older Persons' Prescriptions (STOPP) and the Screening Tool to Alert to Right Treatment (START) are new, validated tools for identification of inappropriate prescribing in the older adult; these are suggested to be used in conjunction with the Beer's criteria (O'Mahoney et al., 2010). The STOPP and START tools are provided in **Box 8-6**.

BOX 8-6   Screening Tool of Older People's Potentially Inappropriate Prescriptions (STOPP)

The following prescriptions are potentially inappropriate in persons older than 65 years of age

Cardiovascular system

Digoxin at a long-term dose > 125 µg/day with impaired renal function[a] (*increased risk of toxicity*)

Loop diuretic for dependent ankle edema only, i.e., no clinical signs of heart failure (*no evidence of efficacy, compression hosiery usually more appropriate*)

Loop diuretic as first-line monotherapy for hypertension (*safer, more effective alternatives available*)

Thiazide diuretic with a history of gout (*may exacerbate gout*)

Noncardioselective betablocker with chronic obstructive pulmonary disease (COPD) (*risk of bronchospasm*)

Beta-blocker in combination with verapamil (*risk of symptomatic heart block*)

Use of diltiazem or verapamil with NYHA Class III or IV heart failure (*may worsen heart failure*)

Calcium channel blockers with chronic constipation (*may exacerbate constipation*)

Use of aspirin and warfarin in combination without histamine H2 receptor antagonist (except cimetidine because of interaction with warfarin) or proton pump inhibitor (*high risk of gastrointestinal bleeding*)

Dipyridamole as monotherapy for cardiovascular secondary prevention (*no evidence for efficacy*)

(*continues*)

BOX 8-6   Screening Tool of Older People's Potentially Inappropriate Prescriptions (STOPP) (*continued*)

Aspirin with a past history of peptic ulcer disease without histamine H2 receptor antagonist or proton pump inhibitor (*risk of bleeding*)

Aspirin at dose > 150 mg/day (*increased bleeding risk, no evidence for increased efficacy*)

Aspirin with no history of coronary, cerebral, or peripheral arterial symptoms or occlusive arterial event (*not indicated*)

Aspirin to treat dizziness not clearly attributable to cerebrovascular disease (*not indicated*)

Warfarin for first, uncomplicated deep venous thrombosis for longer than 6 months duration (*no proven added benefit*)

Warfarin for first uncomplicated pulmonary embolus for longer than 12 months duration (*no proven benefit*)

Aspirin, clopidogrel, dipyridamole, or warfarin with concurrent bleeding disorder (*high risk of bleeding*)

Central nervous system and psychotropic drugs

Tricyclic antidepressants (TCAs) with dementia (*risk of worsening cognitive impairment*)

TCAs with glaucoma (*likely to exacerbate glaucoma*)

TCAs with cardiac conductive abnormalities (*pro-arrhythmic effects*)

TCAs with constipation (*likely to worsen constipation*)

TCAs with an opiate or calcium channel blocker (*risk of severe constipation*)

TCAs with prostatism or prior history of urinary retention (*risk of urinary retention*)

Long-term (i.e., > 1 month), long-acting benzodiazepines (e.g., chlordiazepoxide, fluazepam, nitrazepam, chlorazepate) and benzodiazepines with long-acting metabolites (e.g., diazepam) (*risk of prolonged sedation, confusion, impaired balance, falls*)

Long-term (i.e., > 1 month) neuroleptics as long-term hypnotics (*risk of confusion, hypotension, extrapyramidal side effects, falls*)

Long-term neuroleptics (> 1 month) in those with parkinsonism (*likely to worsen extrapyramidal symptoms*)

Phenothiazines in patients with epilepsy (*may lower seizure threshold*)

Anticholinergics to treat extrapyramidal side-effects of neuroleptic medications (*risk of anticholinergic toxicity*)

Selective serotonin re-uptake inhibitors (SSRIs) with a history of clinically significant hyponatraemia (*non-iatrogenic hyponatraemia < 130 mmol/l within the previous 2 months*)

Prolonged use (> 1 week) of first generation antihistamines (e.g., diphenydramine, chlorpheniramine, cyclizine, promethazine) (*risk of sedation and anticholinergic side effects*)

Gastrointestinal system

Diphenoxylate, loperamide, or codeine phosphate for treatment of diarrhea of unknown cause (*risk of delayed diagnosis, may exacerbate constipation with overflow diarrhea, may precipitate toxic megacolon in inflammatory bowel disease, may delay recovery in unrecognized gastroenteritis*)

Diphenoxylate, loperamide, or codeine phosphate for treatment of severe infective gastroenteritis, i.e., bloody diarrhoea, high fever, or severe systemic toxicity (*risk of exacerbation or protraction of infection*)

Prochlorperazine (Stemetil) or metoclopramide with parkinsonism (*risk of exacerbating parkinsonism*)

PPI for peptic ulcer disease at full therapeutic dosage for > 8 weeks (*earlier discontinuation or dose reduction for maintenance/prophylactic treatment of peptic ulcer disease, esophagitis or GORD indicated*)

Anticholinergic antispasmodic drugs with chronic constipation (*risk of exacerbation of constipation*)

Respiratory system

Theophylline as monotherapy for COPD (*safer, more effective alternatives; risk of adverse effects due to narrow therapeutic index*)

Systemic corticosteroids instead of inhaled corticosteroids for maintenance therapy in moderate–severe COPD (*unnecessary exposure to long-term side effects of systemic steroids*)

Nebulized ipratropium with glaucoma (*may exacerbate glaucoma*)

Musculoskeletal system

Nonsteroidal anti-inflammatory drug (NSAID) with history of peptic ulcer disease or gastrointestinal bleeding, unless with concurrent histamine H2 receptor antagonist, PPI, or misoprostol (*risk of peptic ulcer relapse*)

NSAID with moderate–severe hypertension (moderate: 160/100– 179/109 mmHg; severe: ≥ 180/110 mmHg) (*risk of exacerbation of hypertension*)

NSAID with heart failure (*risk of exacerbation of heart failure*)

Long-term use of NSAID (> 3 months) for relief of mild joint pain in osteoarthtitis (*simple analgesics preferable and usually as effective for pain relief*)

Warfarin and NSAID together (*risk of gastrointestinal bleeding*)

NSAID with chronic renal failure[b](*risk of deterioration in renal function*)

Long-term corticosteroids (> 3 months) as monotherapy for rheumatoid arthrtitis or osterarthritis (*risk of major systemic corticosteroid side-effects*)

Long-term NSAID or colchicine for chronic treatment of gout where there is no contraindication to allopurinol (*allopurinol first choice prophylactic drug in gout*)

Urogenital system

Bladder antimuscarinic drugs with dementia (*risk of increased confusion, agitation*)

Bladder antimuscarinic drugs with chronic glaucoma (*risk of acute exacerbation of glaucoma*)

Bladder antimuscarinic drugs with chronic constipation (*risk of exacerbation of constipation*)

Bladder antimuscarinic drugs with chronic prostatism (*risk of urinary retention*)

(*continues*)

BOX 8-6 **Screening Tool of Older People's Potentially Inappropriate Prescriptions (STOPP) (*continued*)**

Alpha-blockers in males with frequent incontinence, i.e., one or more episodes of incontinence daily (*risk of urinary frequency and worsening of incontinence*)

Alpha-blockers with long-term urinary catheter in situ (i.e., more than 2 months) (*drug not indicated*)

Endocrine system

Glibenclamide or chlorpropamide with type 2 diabetes mellitus (*risk of prolonged hypoglycaemia*)

Beta-blockers in those with diabetes mellitus and frequent hypoglycaemic episodes (i.e., ≥ 1 episode per month) (*risk of masking hypoglycaemic symptoms*)

Estrogens with a history of breast cancer or venous thromboembolism (*increased risk of recurrence*)

Estrogens without progestogen in patients with intact uterus (*risk of endometrial cancer*)

Drugs that adversely affect those prone to falls (≥ 1 fall in past 3 months)

Benzodiazepines (*sedative, may cause reduced sensorium, impair balance*)

Neuroleptic drugs (*may cause gait dyspraxia, parkinsonism*)

First generation antihistamines (*sedative, may impair sensorium*)

Vasodilator drugs known to cause hypotension in those with persistent postural hypotension (i.e., recurrent > 20 mmHg drop in systolic blood pressure) (*risk of syncope, falls*)

Long-term opiates in those with recurrent falls (*risk of drowsiness, postural hypotension, vertigo*)

Analgesic drugs

Use of long-term powerful opiates (e.g., morphine or fentanyl) as first-line therapy for mild–moderate pain (*WHO analgesic ladder not observed*)

Regular opiates for more than 2 weeks in those with chronic constipation without concurrent use of laxatives (*risk of severe constipation*)

Long-term opiates in those with dementia unless indicted for palliative care or management of moderate/severe chronic pain syndrome (*risk of exacerbation of cognitive impairment*)

Duplicate drug classes

Any regular duplicate drug class prescription (e.g., two concurrent opiates, NSAIDs, SSRIs, loop diuretics, ACE inhibitors) (*optimisation of monotherapy within a single drug class should be observed prior to considering a new class of drug*). This excludes duplicate prescribing of drugs that may be required on a PRN basis, e.g., inhaled beta 2 agonists (long and short-acting) for asthma or COPD, and opiates for management of breakthrough pain

Screening Tool to Alert Doctors to Right Treatments (START)

These medications should be considered for people ≥ 65 years of age with the following conditions, where no contra-indication to prescription exists

Cardiovascular system

Warfarin in the presence of chronic atrial fibrillation

Aspirin in the presence of chronic atrial fibrillation, where warfarin is contraindicated, but not aspirin

Aspirin or clopidogrel with a documented history of atherosclerotic coronary, cerebral, or peripheral vascular disease in patients with sinus rhythm

Antihypertensive therapy where systolic blood pressure consistently > 160 mmHg

Statin therapy with a documented history of coronary, cerebral, or peripheral vascular disease, where the patient's functional status remains independent for activities of daily living and life expectancy is > 5 years

Angiotensin converting enzyme (ACE) inhibitor with chronic heart failure

ACE inhibitor following acute myocardial infarction

[a]Estimated GFR < 50 ml/minute.

[b]Estimated GFR 20–50 ml/minute.

Beta-blocker with chronic stable angina

Respiratory system

Regular inhaled beta 2 agonist or anticholinergic agent for mild to moderate asthma or COPD

Regular inhaled corticosteroid for moderate-severe asthma or COPD, where predicted FEV1 < 50%

Home continuous oxygen with documented chronic type 1 respiratory failure (pO2 < 8.0 kPa, pCO2 < 6.5 kPa) or type 2 respiratory failure (pO2 < 8.0 kPa, pCO2 > 6.5 kPa)

Central nervous system

L-DOPA in idiopathic Parkinson's disease with definite functional impairment and resultant disability

Antidepressant drug in the presence of moderate–severe depressive symptoms lasting at least 3 months

Gastrointestinal system

Proton pump inhibitor with severe gastroesophageal acid reflux disease or peptic stricture requiring dilatation

Fiber supplement for chronic, symptomatic diverticular disease with constipation

Musculoskeletal system

Disease-modifying antirheumatic drug (DMARD) with active moderate–severe rheumatoid disease lasting > 12 weeks

Bisphosphonates in patients taking maintenance oral corticosteroid therapy

Calcium and vitamin D supplement in patients with known osteoporosis (radiological evidence or previous fragility fracture or acquired dorsal kyphosis)

(continues)

BOX 8-6   Screening Tool of Older People's Potentially Inappropriate Prescriptions (STOPP) (*continued*)

Endocrine system

Metformin with type 2 diabetes ± metabolic syndrome (in the absence of renal impairment[a])

ACE inhibitor or angiotensin receptor blocker in diabetes with nephropathy (i.e., overt urinalysis proteinuria or micoralbuminuria > 30 mg/24 hours) ± serum biochemical renal impairment[a]

Antiplatelet therapy in diabetes mellitus if one or more co-existing major cardiovascular risk factors present (hypertension, hypercholesterolaemia, smoking history)

Statin therapy in diabetes mellitus if one or more co-existing major cardiovascular risk factors present

[a]Estimated GFR < 50 ml/minute.

Source: Reprinted with permission from: Gallagher, P., Ryan, C., Byrne, S., Kennedy, J., & O'Mahony, D. STOPP (Screening Tool of Older Person's Prescriptions) and START (Screening Tool to Alert doctors to Right Treatment). Consensus validation. *International Journal of Clinical Pharmacology and Therapeutics, 46*(2), 72–83.

Immunizations

Annual vaccination against influenza is recommended for all adults 65 years of age or older because more than 90% of the deaths from influenza occur in this population. Several studies suggest that flu vaccination is beneficial in preventing illness, hospitalization, and mortality in both community-dwelling and institutionalized elderly individuals (McElhaney, 2011). Due to the decreased immune function that accompanies older age, a new high-dose influenza vaccine is available for older adults. This vaccine contains four times the amount of antigen that is present in other forms of the influenza vaccine (CDC, 2011c) (see **Box 8-7**).

BOX 8-7   Vaccination Recommendations from the CDC for Adults Over Age 65 Years

Annual influenza vaccination—either standard dose trivalent vaccine or high dose (FluZone High Dose)

Amantadine or rimantadine prophylaxis

Older adults, especially those with chronic illnesses or who live in nursing homes, are susceptible to pneumococcal pneumonia, which results in death in over one-third of clients over 65 years of age who acquire the disease. The emergence of drug-resistant strains of pneumococcal pneumonia underscores the importance of acquired immunization against the illness. Pneumococcal vaccine is given once for clients who are 65 years of age or older (see **Box 8-8**). Tetanus and diphtheria are uncommon diseases in the United States, but only 28% of adults age 70 or older are immune to tetanus. It is these adults who account for the majority of tetanus, a disease that results in death in more than one-quarter of cases. The tetanus and diphtheria (Td) vaccine is highly efficacious against tetanus, but immunity may wane after 10 years. Periodic boosters of tetanus vaccine, traditionally given every 10 years in the United States, are recommended for older adults by the USPSTF. The Tdap vaccine, in addition to immunizing against tetanus and diphtheria, also contains pertussis vaccine and is recommended for any older adult who has close contact with infants less than 12 months of age (CDC, 2012b).

BOX 8-8   Vaccination Recommendations

Pneumococcal vaccine once after age 65 years.

Herpes zoster infection can occur at any age, but is far more common in older adults. Over 98% of American adults are believed to have serologic evidence of varicella zoster viral infection and could, at some time in their lives, experience an outbreak of shingles from this infection. An outbreak of herpes zoster causes a painful rash in one or two adjacent dermatomes in the body that lasts for 2 to 4 weeks. The most common complication of this condition is post-herpetic neuralgia (PHN), severe pain that can last for months to years after resolution of the acute rash. It occurs in up to 50% of adults over the age of 60 who have a herpes zoster outbreak (CDC, 2011e). For this reason, the CDC recommends one-time immunization against herpes zoster for adults 60 years of age and older regardless of whether they have had shingles (CDC, 2012b) (see **Box 8-9**).

BOX 8-9   Vaccination Recommendations

Herpes zoster vaccine once after age 60, even if the older adult has had a prior episode of herpes zoster.

Tdap recommended for older adults who have contact with infants < 12 months of age.

Tetanus vaccination—Td or Tdap—every 10 years

Mental Health Screening

Mental health enables individuals to participate in productive activities and relationships and to adjust to change and loss. Mental disorders are characterized by alterations in mood, behaviors, or cognition and are associated with impaired functioning and/or distress. Mental disorders have been associated with complications resulting in disability or death, and they profoundly affect family members as well as patients. Mental disorders are as common in late life as they are during other stages of the life span, but some disorders are relatively unique to elderly clients.

Depression

Although estimates of depression vary widely, up to 37% of community-dwelling older adults are depressed. Depression rates increase markedly among clients who have a chronic illness or disability and have been found to be 12% for hospitalized geriatric clients and over 50% for nursing home residents (Hoover et al., 2010). Elderly men have the highest rates of suicide in the nation.

The diagnostic criteria for depression, according to the *Diagnostic and Statistical Manual of Mental Disorders, 4th ed.* (American Psychiatric Association, 2000) require that five or more of the following symptoms be present almost daily, for a 2-week period, and that they represent a change from baseline functioning and not be directly caused by a medical condition or drug: depressed mood, decreased pleasure or interest in activities, change in appetite or weight that is not a result of dieting, change in sleep pattern, psychomotor retardation or agitation, fatigue or loss of energy, feelings or worthlessness or guilt, recurrent thoughts of death or suicide, or diminished ability to think or concentrate.

There is good evidence to support screening for depression in adults, including older adults. Screening can improve identification of depressed elders and improve outcomes. Screening efforts must be coordinated with effective treatment and follow-up in order to have maximal benefit. Initial screening may be accomplished by asking two questions about mood and anhedonia: "Over the past 2 weeks, have you felt down, depressed, or hopeless?" and "Over the past 2 weeks, have you felt little interest or pleasure in doing things?" A positive response to this initial screen may be followed with the Geriatric Depression Scale (see **Figure 8-1**), which has been found to have 92% sensitivity and 89% specificity for detecting depression in elderly adults (Kurlowicz & Greenberg, 2007). The PHQ-9 is another depression screen that has been validated for use with older adults (Kroenke, Spitzer, & Williams, 2001). The Cornell Scale for Depression in Dementia is a useful tool to use with cognitively impaired older adults (Alexopoulos, Abrams, Young, & Shamoian, 1998). A positive depression screen should be followed with an assessment of suicide risk and substance abuse.

Dementia

Dementia affects almost 50% of elderly Americans 85 years of age or older. Alzheimer's disease (AD) accounts for 60–70% of all cases of dementia and is associated with doubling of the death rate, compared to clients who are free from AD, and markedly increased rates of nursing home admissions. Alzheimer's disease prevalence rates double every 5 years after the age of 65. Multi-infarct dementia accounts for 20–30% of dementias and is the second leading cause of dementia in the United States. Dementia is a chronic and progressive illness characterized by behavioral and cognitive changes that affect memory, problem solving, judgment, and speech and that cause deficits in functional abilities.

Unfortunately, there is insufficient evidence at this time to suggest that population-wide screening of Americans 65 years and older for dementia is beneficial. It is difficult to recognize early AD and though it is difficult to quantify the deficit in dementia diagnosis by primary care providers, a study by Bradford, Kunik, Shultz,

Choose the best answer for how you have felt over the past week:

1. Are you basically satisfied with your life? YES / **NO**
2. Have you dropped many of your activities and interests? **YES** / NO
3. Do you feel that your life is empty? **YES** / NO
4. Do you often get bored? **YES** / NO
5. Are you in good spirits most of the time? YES / **NO**
6. Are you afraid that something bad is going to happen to you? **YES** / NO
7. Do you feel happy most of the time? YES / **NO**
8. Do you often feel helpless? **YES** / NO
9. Do you prefer to stay at home, rather than going out and doing new things? **YES** / NO
10. Do you feel you have more problems with memory than most? **YES** / NO
11. Do you think it is wonderful to be alive now? YES / **NO**
12. Do you feel pretty worthless the way you are now? **YES** / NO
13. Do you feel full of energy? YES / **NO**
14. Do you feel that your situation is hopeless? **YES** / NO
15. Do you think that most people are better off than you are? **YES** / NO

Scoring: One point is given for each depressive symptom answered (these appear in bold). Normal, 0–5; suggests depression, above 5. For additional information on administration and scoring, refer to the following reference.

Figure 8-1 Geriatric Depression Scale (GDS), short form.

Source: Sheikh, J. I., & Yesavage, J. A. (1986). Geriatric Depression Scale (GDS): Recent evidence and development of a shorter version. *Clinical Gerontologist,* 5, 165–172. (Reprinted with permission from Hawthorn Press, Inc.)

Williams, and Singh (2009) verified that missed diagnoses are common. Failure to diagnose early AD may severely compromise client safety as a result of household and motor vehicle accidents. These clients are susceptible to financial losses through errors and scams that prey on the elderly. There is sufficient evidence to support the fact that medication delays the rate of cognitive impairment associated with AD, which can lead to improved quality of life for individuals and families and decreased costs of care for our nation. Experts do recommend thorough screening for clients in whom cognitive impairment is suspected or when concerns are expressed by family members or friends.

Three screening tests are commonly used for all forms of dementia. The Mini Mental State Examination (MMSE) is considered the "gold standard" diagnostic test to detect dementia. It has reasonable sensitivity and specificity, and can be made more sensitive or specific depending on the cutpoint used to diagnose dementia (Folstein, Folstein, & McHugh, 1975). The clock-drawing test, in which the client is asked to draw a clock face and indicate a particular time, is a sensitive but non-specific screening test (Sunderland et al., 1989). The use of informant reporting of an individual's cognitive status has been found to be a useful screening tool, as well.

It is important to distinguish between screening tools and tests used for the differential diagnosis of dementia (see **Box 8-10**). A thorough dementia evaluation involves systematic history and examination, laboratory testing, and brain imaging.

BOX 8-10   Depression and Dementia Screening

Level B recommendation to support screening: The USPSTF found good evidence that screening effectively identifies depressed patients and that treatment of depression improves clinical outcomes as long as there is sufficient staff-assisted depression care to support diagnosis, treatment, and follow-up.

Level I recommendation: The USPSTF found the clinical evidence to be insufficient to recommend screening for all elderly clients in a primary care setting. Most expert panels agree that clients who are suspected of having cognitive impairment or whose families express concern about their cognitive functioning should be screened.

Alcohol Abuse

Two and a half million older Americans have alcohol-related problems (U.S. Department of Health and Human Services, Substance Abuse and Mental Health Services Administration, 2001) that augment problems related to polypharmacy. It is very difficult to diagnose alcohol problems in the elderly for several reasons. Retired people do not have the lifestyle disruptions caused by heavy alcohol use that are commonly encountered in younger adults. They are less likely to be arrested due to disorderly conduct or aggression related to their drinking. Alcoholics over the age of 65 are more likely to be living alone and drinking alone than younger adults. On the other hand, the older drinker is more likely to honestly report his or her drinking to the healthcare provider and is more likely to comply with treatment strategies (see **Box 8-11**).

BOX 8-11   Alcohol Screening

Level B recommendation for screening: The USPSTF found good evidence that screening is beneficial in identifying patients whose alcohol consumption patterns place them at risk for

increased morbidity and mortality, and good evidence that counseling about alcohol reduction can produce sustained benefit over a 6- to 12-month period.

Elderly clients have alcohol-related complications that are not generally seen in younger adults, such as increased rates of hip fractures due to falls and medication reactions due to alcohol's effects on liver enzyme systems.

There is some evidence to suggest that light to moderate alcohol consumption in older adults may reduce the risk of coronary heart disease. The National Institute on Alcohol Abuse and Alcoholism (1998) recommends no more than one drink per day for this purpose. More than 7 drinks per week for women, or 14 drinks per week for men, has been defined as "risky" or "hazardous."

Several screening tools are commonly used to screen for alcohol abuse. The CAGE questionnaire is a self-report screening instrument that is easy and quick to administer (Ewing, 1984). It asks four yes/no questions and requires approximately 1 minute to complete. CAGE is a mnemonic for the four key screening questions:

Cut down: Refers to attempts by the client to cut down on drinking
Annoyance: Related to suggestions by friends or family to cut down on drinking
Guilt: Relates to client guilt about drinking
Eye opener: Relates to the need for a drink in the morning to get going

The CAGE questionnaire has been found to have 75% sensitivity and 96% specificity. The 5 As and 5 Rs strategies, defined under the section on tobacco abuse in this chapter, are also suggested strategies for reducing alcohol consumption.

Another screening tool, the Alcohol Use Disorders Identification Test (AUDIT), is a 10-item screening test developed by the World Health Organization and is sensitive for detecting alcohol dependence and abuse (Babor, Higgins-Biddle, Saunders, & Monteiro, 2001). You can learn more about this screening tool at http://whqlibdoc .who.int/hq/2001/WHO_MSD_MSB_01.6a.pdf

Elder Abuse and Neglect

Unfortunately, it is difficult to estimate the prevalence of elder abuse and neglect in this country due, at least in part, to the lack of appropriate screening instruments and consequent underreporting of abuse and neglect by healthcare professionals. Reporting of elder abuse to the *adult protective services agency* is mandatory in almost all states, but it is estimated that only 1 in 14 cases of elder abuse and neglect is actually reported (National Center on Elder Abuse, 2005). There is a paucity of studies to determine the effectiveness of interventions in decreasing abuse (see **Box 8-12**). Studies directed toward identification of both abuse victims and perpetrators are needed.

Elder abuse may include physical, sexual, psychological, and financial exploitation; neglect; and violation of rights. Physical abuse includes shaking, restraining, hitting, or threatening with objects. Sexual abuse includes unwanted contact with the genitals, anus, or mouth. Clients who are psychologically abused experience threats, insults, or harassment, or are recipients of harsh commands. Financial abuse

---

BOX 8-12　Elder Abuse Screening

Level I evidence: Insufficient evidence to support mass screening based on a lack of research to support the use of any particular screening tool, and lack of evidence to support that identification of risk changes outcomes.

occurs in the form of scams or can be perpetrated by family members who try to misuse a client's money or possessions. Neglect may be intentional or unintentional and occurs when required food, medication, or personal care is not provided. Abandonment is a form of neglect where someone who has agreed to provide care for an elderly client deserts that client. Clients who are denied the right to make their own decisions, even though they are competent to do so, or are not provided privacy or the right to worship are suffering from a violation of their inalienable rights.

Self-neglect, wherein an older adult is unable to provide for his/her own care, is the most common provider-reported form of neglect (Tatara, 1998). Most cases of elder abuse are perpetrated by a family member, and reasons for the abuse include caregiver burnout and stress, financial worries, transgenerational violence, and psychopathology in the abuser. Women and dependent elders tend to be the most vulnerable to abuse.

Assessment of abuse can be very difficult because the victim may be cognitively impaired and unable to describe the abuse. It is not unusual for elderly clients to have multiple bruises due to poor balance and loss of subcutaneous fat. Clues to abuse may include:

> The presence of several injuries in different stages of repair
> Delays in seeking treatment
> Injuries that cannot be explained or that are inconsistent with the client's history
> Contradictory explanations by the caregiver and the patient
> Bruises, burns, welts, lacerations, or restraint marks
> Dehydration, malnutrition, decubitus ulcers, or poor hygiene
> Depression, withdrawal, or agitation
> Signs of medication misuse
> A pattern of missed or cancelled appointments
> Frequent changes in healthcare providers
> Discharge, bleeding, or pain in the rectum or vagina or a sexually transmitted disease
> Missing prosthetic device(s), such as dentures, glasses, or hearing aids

The USPSTF decided that there is insufficient evidence to support mass screening of asymptomatic elderly clients for abuse or for the potential for abuse. Suspected abuse should be evaluated through a thorough history with patients, caregivers, and other significant informants, taken separately. Home visits also can yield important clues to the situation. Physical examination, including mental status and evaluation of mood, is critical. Laboratory and imaging studies can support suspicions of dehydration, malnutrition, medication abuse, and fractures or other injuries.

Several assessment tools may help the nurse to determine whether a client is being abused or is at risk for abuse, although none have been adequately tested for validity, reliability, and generalizability, according to the National Center on Elder Abuse (Wolf, 2007). The Hwalek–Sengstock Elder Abuse Screening Test (H-S/EAST) (Neale, Hwalek, Scott, Sengstock, & Stahl, 1991) and the Vulnerability to

Abuse Screening Scale (Schofield & Mishra, 2003) are commonly used screening instruments that are completed by the older adult. Elder abuse screening tools can be accessed online at http://www.medicine.uiowa.edu/familymedicine/emscreeninginstruments/.

If suspicions are strengthened through this assessment, a collaborative approach to management and prevention is required. Team members include the adult protective services agency, social workers, psychiatrists, lawyers, and law enforcement officials. It is important to ascertain whether the client is in immediate danger, in which case law enforcement will be helpful in removing the client from the dangerous situation. The approach to any abuse case should be coordinated with the adult protective services agency, as mandated by law. Abuse and neglect should be reported within 48 hours of the time that you become aware of the situation. Elder abuse that occurs in nursing homes and assisted-living facilities must be reported to the Long-Term Care Ombudsman Program in most states.

In summary, guidelines for elder abuse treatment recommend that you (1) report abuse and neglect to adult protective services or other state-mandated agencies; (2) ensure that there is a safety plan and assess safety; (3) assess the client's cognitive, emotional, functional, and health status; and (4) assess the frequency, severity, and intent of abuse. It is important that the nurse's involvement does not end with the referral, but includes an ongoing plan of care because elderly persons referred to adult protective services are at increased risk of mortality in the decade following the referral. Chapter 23 provides additional information on the prevention and treatment of elder abuse.

Heart and Vascular Disease

Coronary heart disease (CHD) is the leading cause of death in the United States. Every year over 1 million Americans have a new or recurrent myocardial infarction (MI) or die from coronary heart disease. Almost 50% of patients who suffer MI or sudden death have no prior warning symptoms (Bolooki & Askari, 2010). Most of these unexpected cardiac events and cases of sudden death occur in patients over 65 years of age. For this reason, identification of clients at risk for MI, who may be able to benefit from primary prevention strategies, is desirable. National Health and Nutrition Examination Survey (NHANES) III data (National Center for Health Statistics, 2004) suggest that approximately 25% of U.S. adults may be at high risk for a coronary event and may be potential beneficiaries of primary prevention strategies. The *Framingham Heart Study* has elucidated many of the risk factors associated with coronary heart disease. This study began with over 5,000 male and female subjects about 50 years ago in order to study cardiovascular risk factors. As a result of decades of epidemiologic work, the following risk factors have been identified:

> Age greater than or equal to 50 for men and 60 for women
> Hypertension
> Smoking

> Obesity
> Family history of premature CHD
> Diabetes (considered to be a CHD risk-equivalent, i.e., carries the same risk of a coronary event as known CHD)
> Sedentary lifestyle
> Abnormal lipid levels (Expert Panel on Detection, Evaluation, and Treatment of High Blood Cholesterol in Adults, 2001)

Several emerging risk factors, including homocysteine, lipoprotein(a) [Lp(a)] and infectious agents, are currently under investigation. A risk assessment tool developed as a result of discoveries from the Framingham study can be accessed at http://hin.nhlbi.nih.gov/atpiii/calculator.asp?usertype=prof. The risk factors included in the Framingham calculation of 10-year risk are age, total cholesterol, HDL cholesterol, systolic blood pressure, treatment for hypertension, and cigarette smoking (National Cholesterol Education Program, 2004). Patients who have diabetes or atherosclerotic diseases are known to have a more than 20% chance of a cardiac event in the next 10 years; the tool is not necessary to calculate risk for these patients.

In order to utilize this risk assessment tool, screening for the cardiac risk factors included in the tool must be performed. We will examine these screening guidelines, and the evidence to support these screenings, individually.

Lipids

There is strong evidence to link elevations in total cholesterol (TC) and low-density lipoprotein (LDL-C), and low levels of high-density lipoprotein (HDL-C), with coronary risk. Four large primary prevention trials documented a 30% reduction in cardiac events for clients whose cholesterol was reduced using statin therapy (USPSTF, 2008).

Unfortunately, there were very few subjects older than 65 years of age in primary prevention trials, but there have been studies of older adults with preexisting cardiovascular disease that have shown a reduction in cardiovascular events with the use of statins (USPSTF, 2008). There is no age at which the task force recommends screening be stopped, but cholesterol levels are unlikely to increase after age 65 (see **Box 8-13**). For patients who have been tested and found to have normal levels of cholesterol before the age of 65, testing may not be necessary in later years.

BOX 8-13   Lipid Screening

Level A recommendation for screening: There is strong evidence that correlates lipid abnormalities with cardiac risk. A simple blood test is a valid and reliable method of diagnosing lipid abnormalities, and diet and drug therapies are effective remedies. The USPSTF recommends screening all men over the age of 35 and women over age 45 who are at risk for CHD for lipid disorders.

The ratios of TC to HDL-C or LDL-C to HDL-C are better predictors of risk than TC alone. It is possible to accurately measure TC and HDL-C on nonfasting venous or capillary blood samples, but fasting blood samples are required for accurate LDL-C measurement. Two separate measurements are required for definitive diagnosis. The optimal interval for lipid testing has not been determined, but most expert guidelines support testing every 5 years, with shorter intervals for people who have elevated lipid levels and who may require therapy.

Hypertension

Fifty million Americans have high blood pressure. Older Americans have the highest prevalence of hypertension and are the least effectively treated. Framingham data suggest that clients who have normal blood pressure at age 55 have a 90% chance of developing hypertension at some time in their life. High systolic blood pressure, which is more strongly correlated with CVAs, renal failure, and heart failure than diastolic blood pressure, is the most common form of hypertension in the elderly and is less likely to be well controlled than diastolic blood pressure. The NHANES study found that among subjects 60 years of age or older, isolated systolic hypertension (systolic >140 mmHg with diastolic > 90 mmHg) was present in 65% of cases of high blood pressure.

The Seventh Report of the Joint National Committee on Prevention, Detection, Evaluation, and Treatment of High Blood Pressure (U.S. Department of Health and Human Services, 2004) is a national guideline for blood pressure screening and treatment and can be accessed at www.nhlbi.nih.gov/guidelines/hypertension/. It is important to diagnose and treat hypertension to reduce the incidence of cardiac disease (see **Box 8-14**). The correlation of cardiovascular risk and blood pressure is dramatic: Risk doubles with each increment of 20/10 mmHg after 115/75. Treatment of isolated systolic hypertension in the elderly reduced stroke and coronary heart disease events by 30%, heart failure by 50%, and total mortality by 13% (U.S. Department of Health and Human Services, 2004).

BOX 8-14   Blood Pressure Screening

Level A recommendation: There is strong evidence that blood pressure measurement can identify adults at increased risk for cardiovascular disease due to high blood pressure. Treatment of hypertension substantially decreases the incidence of cardiovascular disease.

Blood pressure readings can be accurately determined by a properly calibrated sphygmomanometer using an appropriately sized cuff. (The cuff's bladder needs to encircle at least 80% of the client's arm.) Clients should have been seated in a chair for at least 5 minutes before blood pressure is measured. The client's feet should be uncrossed on the floor and the arm at heart level. Blood pressure measurements should be validated by measuring pressure in the contralateral arm. It is recommended that hypertension be diagnosed only after two or more elevated readings are obtained on at least two visits over a period of 1 to several weeks.

Lifestyle modifications are effective in preventing hypertension and lowering blood pressure in clients who have hypertension. These lifestyle changes include physical activity, weight loss, reducing dietary sodium, and following the *Dietary Approaches to Stop Hypertension (DASH) diet,* published by the National Institutes of Health (NIH) and downloadable from the Web at http://www.nhlbi.nih.gov/ health/public/heart/hbp/dash/new_dash.pdf. This is a comprehensive plan that can be given to patients and includes a summary of the JNC-7 guidelines on hypertension, the results of studies on the DASH eating plan and its effectiveness in lowering hypertension, a diet journal, a tutorial on reading and understanding food labels, and meal plans using the DASH diet.

Aspirin Therapy

Aspirin therapy has long been known to be effective as a secondary prevention strategy for clients with heart disease, but the risks of gastrointestinal bleeding and hemorrhagic stroke associated with aspirin therapy have delayed recommendations of aspirin as a means of primary prevention. A meta-analysis of five primary prevention trials (USPSTF, 2009a) that showed a 28% reduction of cardiac disease in subjects (most of whom were older than 50) has led experts to recommend aspirin chemoprophylaxis with clients between the ages of 45 and 79 years at high risk for developing CHD (see **Box 8-15**). Gastrointestinal bleeding occurred in about 0.3% of subjects given aspirin for 5 years, causing some concerns about the risk versus benefit of aspirin for primary prevention of heart disease in patients who are at low risk for cardiac illness. The USPSTF states that there is insufficient evidence to recommend for or against aspirin prophylaxis in adults 80 years of age and older (USPSTF, 2009a).

BOX 8-15   Aspirin Therapy

Level A recommendation: There is good evidence that aspirin decreases the incidence of CHD in adults who are at increased risk for heart disease, but aspirin increases the incidence of gastrointestinal bleeding and hemorrhagic strokes. The USPSTF concluded that evidence is strongest to support aspirin therapy in patients at high risk of CHD.

Level I recommendation: There is insufficient evidence to recommend for or against aspirin prophylaxis in men and women 80 years of age and older.

Stroke

Cerebrovascular accidents (CVAs) are the third leading cause of death in the United States, with more than two-thirds of stroke occurring in persons age 65 years or older (American Heart Association, American Stroke Association, 2008).

The physical, psychological, economic, and social costs of CVAs are enormously high, to clients as well as their families. Strokes are a significant cause of dependency among the elderly.

The primary risk factors for ischemic stroke are similar to those described in the previous section on heart disease: increased age, hypertension, smoking, and diabetes. Clients with coronary artery disease are at increased risk for stroke because atherosclerotic vessel disease is a common etiology for the two diseases. Lifestyle factors associated with CVA risk that have been identified by the National Stroke Association are heavy alcohol use, cigarette smoking, sedentary lifestyle, and a high-fat diet. In addition to these risk factors, atrial fibrillation and asymptomatic carotid stenosis place clients at high risk for cerebrovascular disease.

It is estimated that 36% of strokes suffered by clients 80–89 years of age are as a result of nonvalvular atrial fibrillation (National Stroke Association, 1999). Adequate anticoagulation with warfarin therapy in patients with atrial fibrillation has been found to reduce stroke occurrence by 68%, while aspirin therapy was found to reduce CVAs by only 21%. It is based on these data that the National Stroke Association guidelines recommend the use of oral anticoagulation with warfarin for patients older than 75 years of age with nonvalvular atrial fibrillation. Patients 65 to 75 years old with atrial fibrillation, as well as other CVA risks, should be treated with warfarin, and those without additional risk factors may be treated with warfarin or aspirin. The consensus panel of the Stroke Association underscores the importance of weighing the risk of hemorrhage against the benefit of therapy on an individual patient basis.

Carotid stenosis is an important stroke risk factor. However, there is insufficient evidence to recommend screening asymptomatic persons for carotid artery stenosis, using either physical examination or carotid ultrasound. Screening is justified if early treatment can change clinical outcomes and if there are effective, low-risk screening tests. The inability of experts to recommend screening is based on the fact that there is significant debate about the risks and benefits of carotid endarterectomy as a treatment for asymptomatic disease. The American Heart Association (1998) recommends carotid endarterectomy for asymptomatic stenosis when the artery is at least 60% occluded, but the USPSTF does not recommend carotid ultrasound for asymptomatic patients based on remaining questions about the risks and benefits of carotid endarterectomy as a result of varying surgical risks among studies. Physical findings that suggest stenosis, by auscultation of the carotid artery, are a poor predictor of subsequent stroke.

Experts agree that the risk of a stroke can be minimized through treatment of hypertension; using statin therapy after MI for normal and high cholesterol; using warfarin for patients with atrial fibrillation and specific risk factors, and for patients after MI who have atrial fibrillation, left ventricular thrombus, or decreased left ventricular ejection fraction; and modification of lifestyle-related risk factors like smoking, alcohol use, physical activity, and diet.

Thyroid Disease

The USPSTF (2004) has found insufficient evidence to support screening for thyroid disease in adults. Older adults are far more susceptible to thyroid dysfunction than younger adults. Overt disease affects 5% of American adults, but the prevalence of subclinical hypothyroidism (elevated thyroid-stimulating hormone [TSH] with normal levels of thyroid hormone) is 17.4% among women older than age 75 and 6.2% among men over age 65. Approximately 2–5% of these cases of subclinical hypothyroidism will progress to overt hypothyroidism each year (Cooper, 2001). The American Association of Clinical Endocrinologists (AACE Task Force, 2002) has published clinical guidelines for the diagnosis and management of thyroid disease, in which it states that subclinical hypothyroidism may be associated with gastro-intestinal disorders, depression, dementia, lipid disorders, increased likelihood of goiter, and overt thyroid disease.

Subclinical hyperthyroidism is far less common in the population, affecting only a little more than 1% of adults over 60 years of age, but it is present in up to 20% of patients taking levothyroxine for hypothyroidism (AACE Task Force, 2002).

Untreated hyperthyroidism can lead to atrial fibrillation, congestive heart failure, osteoporosis, and neuropsychiatric disorders. Hypothyroidism can cause constipation and ileus, lipid abnormalities, weight gain, decreased cognition, depression, and negative changes in functional status. The goal of screening would be to decrease the negative effects of overt thyroid disease.

The Task Force's inability to recommend for or against screening of asymptomatic persons for thyroid disease results (see **Box 8-16**) from the lack of clarity about the risks of subclinical disease. It is clear that both hypothyroidism and hyperthyroidism cause significant morbidity and need to be treated, but the negative consequences of these diseases appear to be present primarily in patients who present with symptoms of the disease. There are significant costs and risks associated with thyroid replacement, which need to be considered before recommending mass screening. Many patients who receive thyroid hormone replacement develop subclinical hyperthyroidism, which may increase the risk of developing osteoporosis, hip fracture, and atrial fibrillation. The task force recommends that clinicians be cognizant of the signs and symptoms of thyroid disease, and test symptomatic patients; evidence is lacking to justify screening of asymptomatic patients, however. The AACE supports treatment of subclinical hypothyroidism if thyroid antibodies are positive. Thyroid antibodies are elevated in Hashimoto's thyroiditis, the most common cause

---

BOX 8-16   Thyroid Disease Screening

Level I recommendation: There is insufficient evidence to recommend for or against screening based on limited evidence to establish health risks of subclinical disease, and due to the risks of treatment.

of subclinical hypothyroidism. Clients with goiters and positive antibodies are more likely than other patients to progress to overt hypothyroidism.

Osteoporosis

One-half of all postmenopausal women will have a fracture related to osteoporosis at some point in their life. The risk for the development of osteoporosis markedly increases with age, and osteoporosis is responsible for 70% of the fractures that occur in older adults. Women ages 65–69 years have 6 times the risk of osteoporosis than younger postmenopausal women, and that rate increases to 14 times in women ages 75–79 (USPSTF, 2010). Age, low body mass index (BMI), and failure to use estrogen replacement are the strongest risk factors for osteoporosis development (see **Box 8-17**). Other possible risks include White or Asian race, family history of compression or stress fracture, fall risk or history of fracture, low levels of weight-bearing exercise, smoking, excessive alcohol or caffeine use, and low intake of calcium or vitamin D. Certain medications, such as thyroid medication or prednisone, increase the chances of developing osteoporosis.

BOX 8-17   Osteoporosis Screening

Level B recommendation: Osteoporosis is common in the elderly and is correlated with fracture risk. There are good screening tests to diagnose osteoporosis and effective treatments for the disease. Screening is recommended for all women 65 years and older and for women younger than 65 who are at high risk for fractures.

Some men are at increased risk for osteoporosis, and decisions about screening may be made on an individual basis. Men with chronic lung disease, low testosterone levels, and who require steroid medications for extended periods of time are at increased risk of bone loss (National Osteoporosis Foundation [NOF], 2010).

There is a strong association between bone mass and fracture risk, which continues into old age. Multiple studies demonstrate that therapies that slow bone loss are effective in reducing fracture risk, even if they are begun in old age. The USPSTF uses the Frax® tool, developed by the World Health Organization (WHO), which determines an individual's risk for future fractures. Based on the risk factors, screening is recommend for all women over the age of 65 and for women between the ages of 50 and 64 if they meet the 9.3% probability of fracture in the next 10-years based on the Frax® tool (USPSTF, 2011b). Bone density testing at the femoral, neck, and lumbar spine by dual energy X-ray bone densitometry is the gold standard screening tool, and the one most closely correlated with hip fracture risk, though heel measurements using ultrasonography are also predictive of short-term fracture risk. Men make up only 20% of the Americans with osteoporosis. While they are at significantly less risk then women, 1 in 4 men over the age of 50 will incur a fracture due to osteoporosis (NOF, 2010). Despite these statistics, the USPSTF has deemed the available evidence insufficient to recommend osteoporosis screening for males (USPSTF, 2011b).

Vision and Hearing

The prevalence of hearing and visual impairment increases with age and has been correlated with social and emotional isolation, clinical depression, and functional impairment. An objective hearing loss can be identified in 20–40% of adults over the age of 50 and in 80% of adults 80 years of age and older (USPSTF, 2011a). High-frequency loss is the most important contributor to this increase in hearing loss, though up to 30% of cases may be caused or compounded by cerumen impaction or otitis media, which are easily treated (Ivers, Cumming, Mitchell, Simpson, & Peduto, 2003).

About 4% of adults ages 65–74 and 16% of those 80–84 years of age have bilateral visual acuity worse than 20/40. Macular degeneration is the most common cause of visual loss in elderly Whites, whereas African Americans are more likely to lose vision as a result of cataracts, glaucoma, and diabetes. Visual impairment has been correlated with falls and hip fractures in the elderly (Ivers et al., 2003).

The Snellen eye chart is a useful tool for detecting refraction errors but is, unfortunately, ineffective at detecting early macular degeneration. The USPSTF (2009b) has also found insufficient evidence to suggest that screening and treatment to improve visual acuity also improve functional outcomes in older adults. Ophthalmology referral may be useful for clients whose corrected vision is worse than 20/40, or who report visual problems that limit activities such as reading or driving. Many expert panels, including the American Academy of Ophthalmology, the American Optometric Association, and Prevent Blindness America, recommend regular ophthalmologic exams for adults over 65 years of age (40 years of age for African Americans) based on the fact that effective glaucoma screening should be performed by eye specialists with specialized equipment to evaluate the optic disc and measure visual fields. The optimal frequency for glaucoma screening has not yet been determined.

The USPSTF (2011a) found insufficient evidence for screening for hearing impairment for older adults (see **Box 8-18**), based on a lack of demonstrated improvement in quality of life after improvement of hearing with hearing aids. Simple testing for hearing loss using a whisper voice test from a distance of 2 feet

---

BOX 8-18   Hearing and Vision Screening

Level I recommendation: More research is needed to understand the benefits of hearing screening.

Level I recommendation: There is insufficient evidence to recommend for or against screening for visual acuity changes or for glaucoma in adults.

and asking the older adult about his or her perceived hearing loss were effective at detecting hearing loss (see **Figure 8-2**).

Prostate Cancer

Prostate cancer is both the second most-common form of cancer and the second most-common cause of cancer death among U.S. men. The risk of developing prostate cancer increases with age and is the second leading cause of death overall in American men (American Cancer Society, 2012c). The disease is most prevalent in African Americans and least prevalent among Asian Americans.

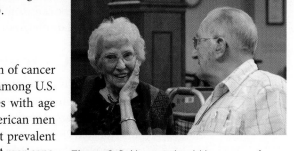

Figure 8-2 Nurses should be aware of the many sensory changes that come with advancing age.

Two tests are commonly used in prostate cancer screening: the digital rectal exam (DRE) and the prostate-specific antigen (PSA) blood test. "The pooled sensitivity, specificity, and positive predictive value for PSA were 72.1%, 93.2% and 25.1%, respectively; and for DRE were 53.2%, 83.6% and 17.8%, respectively" (Mistry & Cable, 2003, p. 95). Benign prostatic hypertrophy is common in older men, and the presence of this disease increases the likelihood of false-positive testing with the PSA. Most prostate cancers are slow-growing and unlikely to be a cause of significant morbidity and mortality in older men. The greatest controversy regarding screening for prostate cancer is the inability to accurately predict which cancers will be aggressive and require treatment, and which are unlikely to metastasize.

The USPSTF recommends against screening for prostate cancer in men over the age of 75, due to their limited life expectancy. Discussion of this complex issue, including the pros and cons of screening, is recommended for men younger than age 75 (see **Box 8-19**). The CDC has a set of patient education materials designed to help guide this discussion, which can be found at http://www.cdc.gov/cancer/dcpc/publications/prostate.htm.

BOX 8-19   Prostate Cancer Screening

Level I recommendation: There is insufficient evidence to recommend screening based on inconclusive evidence that screening with DRE and PSA improves health outcomes.

Level D recommendation: The USPSTF recommends against screening for men 75 years of age and older. Men with a life expectancy of less than 10 years are unlikely to benefit from prostate screening.

A large clinical trial sponsored by the National Cancer Institute called "The Prostate, Lung, Colon and Ovarian (PLCO) Cancer Screening Trial" was designed to determine whether prostate screening, and early detection of prostate cancer, improved patient outcomes (National Cancer Institute, 2012). In a report from this PLCO screening trial, a 7-year, controlled, multicenter trial of over 75,000 men who were randomized to receive either usual care or DRE and PSA testing was described.

Men in the experimental group received more frequent prostate cancer screening than those in the control group but were not found to have any difference in prostate cancer-related death (Andriole et al., 2009).

Breast Cancer

Breast cancer is the most common cancer among U.S. women, and the prevalence of the disease increases with age. According to the CDC (2010), 3–4% of women who are 60 years old today will get breast cancer by the age of 70. In 2011 there were an estimated 20,050 new in situ cases and 98,080 invasive cases of breast cancer in women over the age of 65, with 22,660 deaths (American Cancer Society 2012a). Other risk factors for the disease include family history of breast cancer, atypical hyperplasia in breast tissue, obesity, use of postmenopausal hormones, and birth of a first child when a woman is over 30 years of age. The USPSTF recommends biennial breast cancer screening for women between the ages of 50 and 75 years; however, the Task Forces finds the evidence to be insufficient to rationalize screening by mammography for women over the age of 75 (USPSTF, 2009c). This is despite the fact that women between the ages of 75 and 79 have the highest rate of breast cancer (American Cancer Society, 2012a). Although disease prevalence is high in this population, the Task Force wondered whether early detection of disease would improve health outcomes in a population that also has a higher incidence of other chronic illnesses. They wondered if there was an upper age limit at which breast cancer screening would no longer be beneficial (see **Box 8-20**).

BOX 8-20   Breast Cancer Screening

Screening with mammography (with or without clinical breast exam): Level B evidence: There is fair evidence to support benefit from breast cancer screening for women between the ages of 50 and 74 by mammogram every 2 years. Level I recommendation for screening of women 75 years and older.

Clinical breast exam screening: Level I evidence.

Self breast exam screening: Level D evidence. The task force recommends against teaching women to do self-breast examination.

Screening tests used to detect breast cancer include mammography, clinical breast exam by a healthcare provider, and both mammography and magnetic resonance imaging (MRI) for women at very high risk for development of breast cancer (Saslow et al., 2007). The sensitivity of mammography to detect breast cancer varies widely, depending on a woman's age, whether she takes hormonal replacement, the technical quality of the testing equipment, and the skill of the radiologist. Overall, the test is more sensitive for older women than for younger women. Unfortunately, there are many false-positive tests, and up to one-quarter of women who have annual mammograms may need to undergo unnecessary, invasive follow-up testing as a result of false-positive tests from mammography at some point in their lives. No studies have looked at the effectiveness of clinical breast exam without concurrent mammography to detect breast cancer. The USPSTF recommends against teaching the self-breast exam, concluding that the harms likely outweigh derived benefits and has found insufficient evidence for clinical breast exams by healthcare providers or for diagnostic MRIs (USPSTF, 2009c).

Colorectal Cancer Screening

Colorectal cancer is both the third most-common cancer in the United States and the third leading cause of cancer death in the United States (American Cancer Society 2012b). The prevalence of the disease increases with age, and over 90% of colorectal cancer is diagnosed in clients over the age of 50 (American Cancer Society, 2011). The American Cancer Society released screening guidelines in 2008 that emphasize the importance of detecting precancerous growths as opposed to cancer itself. There are several good screening methodologies available to detect these precancerous lesions: annual fecal immunochemical test (FIT), stool DNA test (sDNA), annual fecal occult blood testing (FOBT), double-contrast barium enema, CT colonography every 5 years, flexible sigmoidoscopy every 5 years, or colonoscopy every 10 years. Choice of screening test is determined based on client risk factors and preference. Patients who are at an average risk for developing colorectal cancer should be screened regularly from the ages of 50 through 75 using one of these testing methods (USPSTF, 2008). The best methodology for FOBT is the three consecutive stool samples that are collected at home by the patient on an annual basis. These tests should be examined without rehydration due to the decreased specificity of the test that is associated with rehydration of the samples. A single guiaic test, performed in the office with DRE, is not recommended as an adequate screening test (National Guideline Clearinghouse, 2009).

Patients who have a history of adenomatous polyps or inflammatory bowel disease, or a family history of colorectal cancer or adenomatous polyps, should receive colonoscopy. Screening for these high-risk clients is begun before age 50.

Colonoscopy is the most sensitive of the screening methodologies but is associated with the highest costs and risks. These risks include a small risk of perforation and bleeding and the risks associated with sedation, which is required for the procedure.

There is strong evidence to support colorectal screening for men and women age 50 or older, but insufficient evidence to determine which of the various screening options is the preferred method for screening (see **Box 8-21**). As of 2011, only 50% of patients over the age of 50, for whom screening is recommended, report compliance with the American Cancer Society colorectal screening guidelines (American Cancer Society 2012b).

BOX 8-21   Colorectal Screening

Level A recommendation: The task force strongly recommends colorectal screening by FOBT, sigmoidoscopy, or colonoscopy for adults between the ages of 50 and 75.

Level C recommendation: For adults between the ages of 76 and 85.

Level D recommendation: For adults over age 85.

Summary

In summary, there are many effective screenings for various diseases common to the elderly population. Nurses should utilize the appropriate resources to obtain and put into practice screening of aged patients according to the USPSTF guidelines. (**Table 8-1** contains a summary of guidelines.) Proper screening of older adults can save lives.

TABLE 8-1   Summary of USPSTF Screening Recommendations for Older Adults

Screening Test	Recommendation	Level of Evidence
Physical activity	Physical activity has a positive impact on health but we don't know whether counseling about exercise is effective in helping people to begin exercising.	Level I
Nutrition	Counseling clients with hyperlipidemia or cardiovascular disease risk factors about nutrition is beneficial.	Level B
Tobacco use	Screening is helpful in identifying tobacco use, and counseling is effective in helping people quit smoking.	Level A
Depression	Screening is effective in identifying depression and treatments are effective if adequate staff support is available.	Level B
Dementia	Insufficient evidence to support mass screening of elders for dementia, but good evidence to suggest screening to follow up on family or client's concerns about memory loss.	Level I
Alcohol abuse	Screening is beneficial and treatment is effective.	Level B

Elder abuse and neglect	No evidence that either screening or interventions are effective.	Level I
Lipids	Good evidence to support that treatment and screening are effective.	Level A
Hypertension	Good evidence to support that treatment and screening are effective.	Level A
Aspirin therapy for men over 45 years and women over 55 years of age	Good evidence to support aspirin therapy in clients at high risk for CV disease.	Level A; Level I for adults over 80 years of age
Cerebrovascular disease	Insufficient evidence for use of carotid ultrasound to screen for carotid stenosis as a CVA risk factor.	Level I
Thyroid disease	Insufficient evidence to support screening for thyroid disease.	Level I
Osteoporosis	Screening is recommended for all women over 65 years of age.	Level B
Vision and hearing	Insufficient evidence that hearing screening and treatment actually improves function; Glaucoma testing by an ophthalmologist is recommended for adults at risk of developing glaucoma.	Level I
Prostate cancer	Insufficient evidence to recommend screening.	Level I for adults less than 75 years of age; Level D for adults greater than 75 years of age
Breast cancer	Mammography is recommended every 2 to 3 years as a screening for breast cancer for older women.	Level B for women between the ages of 50 and 74; Level I for women age 75 and over
Colorectal cancer	Screening for colorectal cancer by FOBT, FIT, sigmoidoscopy, sDNA, double contrast barium enema, or colonoscopy is recommended.	Level A for adults less than 76 years of age; Level C for those aged 76–85; Level D for those over age 85

Critical Thinking Exercises

1. Iola R., a 72-year-old, overweight woman, tells you that she wishes that she could exercise, but that she can never bring herself to begin an exercise program. She knows that her hypertension, diabetes, and high cholesterol would benefit from regular exercise. She is caring for her grandchildren 3 days per week and can't find the time to engage in regular exercise. She is not sure if it is safe to walk alone around her neighborhood, anyway. Explain how you could use the concepts of self-management of chronic illness and contracting to help Iola begin an exercise program. What benefits might she obtain through regular exercise? How frequently should she plan to exercise?

2. Mr. Gottlieb complains that he has been falling a lot recently. He can remember at least three falls in the past 6 months, but luckily, none have resulted in injury yet. His friend is living in a nursing home as a result of complications and debility that followed a hip fracture, and Mr. Gottlieb does not want the same fate for himself. Describe how you will assess and manage Mr. Gottlieb's fall risk.

3. Mrs. Hall is a 94-year-old woman with Alzheimer's disease. Her daughter is her primary caregiver and calls to report that caring for her mother has become intolerable. "I can't make her eat, drink, or stop her incessant whining." You notice that Mrs. Hall has not been in to see her primary care doctor in over 3 years, but that she has been in to the emergency department four times in the past year for dehydration, urinary tract infections, and behavior management. You want to assess the home situation for safety and provide caregiver support to the patient's daughter. What signs of abuse and neglect might you look for through a chart review? Through a clinic visit and evaluation of the client? Through laboratory testing? How could you get a better assessment of the actual home situation? If your suspicions are strengthened, how will you proceed to intervene with this case of suspected elder abuse and neglect?

Personal Reflections

1. In the case described in #3 of the Critical Thinking Exercises, which of the two clients described, Mrs. Hall or her daughter who initially called you, is your primary patient? Do you have loyalties to both? How could you address the care needs of Mrs. Hall's daughter?

2. Do you feel that you can counsel a client about health promotion if you do not adopt these behaviors yourself?

3. Mr. J., an 88-year-old gentleman, had a colonoscopy 6 years ago in which an adenomatous polyp was removed. His gastroenterologist has asked for your help in bringing Mr. J. back for follow-up testing. You call the patient who tells you that, although he recognizes the risk, he is not willing to undergo the procedure again. He believes his life expectancy is limited anyway and would prefer not to know if he has another polyp because he would not want to undergo surgery anyway. What do you do?

References

Alexopoulos, G. S., Abrams, R. C., Young, R. C., & Shamoian, C. A. (1988). Cornell Scale for Depression in Dementia. *Biological Psychiatry, 23*, (3), 271–284.

American Association of Clinical Endocrinologists [AACE] Task Force. (2002). American Association of Clinical Endocrinologists medical guidelines for clinical practice for the evaluation and treatment of hyperthyroidism and hypothyroidism. *Endocrine Practice, 8*(6), 457–467.

American Cancer Society [ACS]. (2011) *Colorectal cancer facts and figures 2011–2013*. Atlanta, GA: Author. Retrieved from http://www.cancer.org/acs/groups/content/@epidemiologysurveilance/documents/document/acspc-028323.pdf

American Cancer Society [ACS]. (2012a). Breast cancer facts and figures 2011–2012. Atlanta, GA: Author. Retrieved from http://www.cancer.org/acs/groups/content/@epidemiologysurveilance/documents/document/acspc-030975.pdf

American Cancer Society [ACS]. (2012b). *Colorectal cancer early detection*. Retrieved from http://www.cancer.org/Cancer/ColonandRectumCancer/MoreInformation/ColonandRectumCancerEarlyDetection/colorectal-cancer-early-detection-acs-recommendations

American Cancer Society [ACS]. (2012c). *Prostate cancer*. Retrieved from http://www.cancer.org/Cancer/ProstateCancer/DetailedGuide/prostate-cancer-key-statistics

American Geriatrics Society [AGS]. (2010). *AGS/BGS clinical practice guideline: Prevention of falls in older persons*. Retrieved from http://www.americangeriatrics.org/health_care_professionals/clinical_practice/clinical_guidelines_recommendations/prevention_of_falls_summary_of_recommendations

American Geriatrics Society [AGS] 2012 Beers Criteria Update Expert Panel. (2012). American Geriatrics Society updated Beers criteria for potentially inappropriate medication use in older adults. *Journal of the American Geriatrics Society, 60*(4), 616–631. doi: 10.1111/j.1532-5415.2012.03923.x

American Heart Association. (1998). Guidelines for carotid endarterectomy. A statement for healthcare professionals from a special writing group of the Stroke Council, American Heart Association. *Circulation, 97*, 501–509.

American Heart Association, American Stroke Association. (2008). *Heart disease and stroke statistics*. Retrieved from http://www.americanheart.org/downloadable/heart/1200082005246HS_Stats%202008.final.pdf

American Pharmacists Association and National Association of Chain Drug Stores Foundation. (2008). *Medication therapy management in pharmacy practice: Core elements of an MTM service model*. Retrieved from http://www.pharmacist.com/sites/default/files/files/core_elements_of_an_mtm_practice.pdf

American Psychiatric Association [APA]. (2000). Diagnosis and statistical manual of mental disorders, (4th ed.). Washington, DC: Author.

Andriole, G. L., Crawford, E. D., Grubb, R. L. III, Buys, S. S., Chia, D., Church, T. R., …Berg, C. D, (2009). Mortality results from a randomized prostate cancer screening trial. *New England Journal of Medicine, 360*, 1310–1319.

Babor, T. F., Higgins-Biddle, J. C., Saunders, J. B., & Monteiro, M. G. (2001). The alcohol use disorders identification test (2nd ed.). *World Health Organization*. Retrieved from http://whqlibdoc.who.int/hq/2001/WHO_MSD_MSB_01.6a.pdf

Bolooki, H. M., & Askari, A. (2010). Acute myocardial infarction. Cleveland Clinic Publications: Disease Management Project. Retrieved from http://www.clevelandclinicmeded.com/medicalpubs/diseasemanagement/cardiology/acute-myocardial-infarction/#s0015

Bradford, A., Kunik, M. E., Schultz, P., Williams, S. P., & Singh, H. (2009). Missed and delayed diagnosis of dementia in primary care: prevalence and contributing factors. *Alzheimer's Disease & Associated Disorders, 23*(4), 306–314.

Budnitz, D. S., Lovegrove, M. C., Shehab, N., & Richards, C. L. (2011). Emergency hospitalizations for adverse drug events in older adults. *New England Journal of Medicine, 365*, 2002–2012.

Centers for Disease Control and Prevention [CDC]. (2008a). *Fact sheet for health professionals on physical activity guidelines for older adults*. Retrieved from http://www.cdc.gov/nccdphp/dnpa/physical/pdf/PA_Fact_Sheet_OlderAdults.pdf

Centers for Disease Control and Prevention [CDC]. (2008b). *Smoking-attributable mortality, years of potential life lost and productivity losses—United States, 2000–2004.* Retrieved from http://www.cdc.gov/mmwr/preview/mmwrhtml/mm5745a3.htm

Centers for Disease Control and Prevention [CDC]. (2010). Risk of breast cancer by age. Retrieved from http://www.cdc.gov/cancer/breast/statistics/age.htm

Centers for Disease Control and Prevention [CDC]. (2011a). *Adults and older adult adverse drug events.* Retrieved from http://www.cdc.gov/MedicationSafety/Adult_AdverseDrugEvents.html

Centers for Disease Control and Prevention [CDC]. (2011b). *Falls among older adults: An overview.* Retrieved from http://www.cdc.gov/homeandrecreationalsafety/falls/adultfalls.html

Centers for Disease Control and Prevention [CDC]. (2011c). *Fluzone high-dose seasonal influenza vaccine.* Retrieved from http://www.cdc.gov/flu/protect/vaccine/qa_fluzone.htm

Centers for Disease Control and Prevention [CDC]. (2011d). Phys*ical activity for everyone.* Retrieved from http://www.cdc.gov/physicalactivity/everyone/health/index.html

Centers for Disease Control and Prevention [CDC]. (2011e). Shingles (Herpes zoster). Retrieved from http://www.cdc.gov/shingles/hcp/clinical-overview.html

Centers for Disease Control and Prevention [CDC]. (2012a). Fast stats. Leading causes of death. Retrieved from http://www.cdc.gov/nchs/fastats/lcod.htm.

Centers for Disease Control and Prevention [CDC]. (2012b). *Recommended adult immunization schedule—United States.* Retrieved from http://www.cdc.gov/vaccines/recs/schedules/downloads/adult/mmwr-adult-schedule.pdf

Centers for Disease Control and Prevention [CDC] & the Merck Company Foundation. (2007). *The state of aging and health in America, 2007.* Whitehouse Station, NJ: The Merck Company Foundation.

Cooper, D. S. (2001). Subclinical hypothyroidism. *The New England Journal of Medicine, 345,* 260–265.

Dawson-Hughes, B., Mithal, A., Bonjour, J. P., Boonen, S., Burckhardt, P., Fuleihan, G. E. H., … Yoshimura, N. (2010). IOF position paper: Vitamin D recommendations for older adults. *Osteoporosis International, 21,* 1151–1154.

deVries, N. M., Staal, J. B., van Ravensberg, C. D., Hobbelen, J. S. M, Olde Rikkert, M. G. M, & Nijhuis-van der Sanden, M. W. G. (2011). Outcome instruments to measure frailty: A systematic review. *Ageing Research Reviews, 10,* 104–114.

Duxbury, A. S. (1997). Gait disorders in the elderly: Commonly overlooked diagnostic clues. *Consultant, 37,* 2337–2351.

Ewing, J. A. (1984). Detecting alcoholism. The CAGE questionnaire. *Journal of the American Medical Association, 252,* 1905–1907.

Expert Panel on Detection, Evaluation, and Treatment of High Blood Cholesterol in Adults. (2001). Executive summary of the third report of the National Cholesterol Education Program (NCEP) Expert Panel on Detection, Evaluation, and Treatment of High Blood Cholesterol in Adults (Adult Treatment Panel III). *Journal of the American Medical Association, 285*(19), 2486–2497.

Folstein, M. F., Folstein, S. E., & McHugh, P. R. (1975). "Mini-mental state." A practical method for grading the cognitive state of patients for the clinician. *Journal of Psychiatric Research, 12,* 189–198.

Food and Drug Administration [FDA]. (2011). Safe use initiative. Retrieved from http://www.fda.gov/Drugs/DrugSafety/SafeUseInitiative/default.htm

Hoover, D. R., Siegel, M., Lucas, J., Kalay, E., Gaboda, D., Devanand, D. P., & Crystal, S. (2010). Depression in the first year of stay for elderly long-term nursing home residents in the USA. *International Psychogeriatrics, 22,*(7), 11, 1161–1171.

Ivers, R. Q., Cumming, R. G., Mitchell, P., Simpson, J. M., & Peduto, A. J. (2003). Visual risk factors for hip fracture in older people. *Journal of the American Geriatric Society, 51,* 356–363.

Kroenke, K., Spitzer, R. L., & Williams, J. B. (2001). The PHQ-9: Validity of a brief depression severity measure. *Journal of General Internal Medicine, 16,* (9), 606–613.

Kurlowicz, L., & Greenberg, S. (2007). *The geriatric depression scale (GDS).* Hartford Institute for Geriatric Nursing, 4. Retrieved from http://www.consultgerirn.org/uploads/File/trythis/issue04.pdf

Lawton, M. P., & Brody, E. M. (1969). Assessment of older people: Self-maintaining and instrumental activities of daily living. *Gerontologist, 9,* 179–186.

Lorig, K., & Holman, H. (2000). Self management education: Context, definition and outcomes and mechanisms. Australian Government Department of Health and Ageing. Retrieved from http://www.chronicdisease.health.gov.au/pdfs/lorig.pdf

McElhaney, J. (2011). Influenza vaccine responses in older adults. *Ageing Research Reviews, 10*(3), 379–388.

Michael, Y. L., Lin, J. S., Whitlock, E. P., Gold, R., Fu, R., O'Connor, E. A., Zuber, S. P.,…Lutz, K. W. (2010). Interventions to prevent falls in older adults: An updated systematic review. Rockville, MD: Agency for Healthcare Research and Quality.

Middleton, L. E., Barnes, D. E., Lui, L., & Yaffe, K. (2010). Physical activity over the life course and its association with cognitive performance and impairment in old age. *Journal of the American Geriatrics Society, 58,* (7), 1322–1326.

Mistry, K., & Cable, G. (2003). Meta-analysis of prostate-specific antigen and digital rectal examination as screening tests for prostrate carcinoma. *Journal of the American Board of Family Practice, 16,* 95–101.

Mitty, E., & Flores, S. (2007). Fall prevention in assisted living: Assessment and strategies. *Geriatric Nursing, 28*(6), 349–357.

National Cancer Institute. (2012). Screening for prostate cancer in older patients (PLCO screening trial). Retrieved from http://clinicaltrials.gov/show/NCT00002540

National Center for Chronic Disease Prevention and Health Promotion. (2004). *Improving nutrition and increasing physical activity.* Centers for Disease Control and Prevention. Retrieved from http://www.cdc.gov/nccdphp/publications/factsheets/Prevention/pdf/obesity.pdf

National Center for Health Statistics. (2004). *Third National Health and Nutrition Examination Survey (NHANES III) public-use data files.* Retrieved from http://www.cdc.gov/nchs/products/elec_prods/subject/nhanes3.htm

National Center on Elder Abuse. (2005). Fact sheet. Elder abuse prevalence and incidence. Retrieved from http://www.ncea.aoa.gov/ncearoot/Main_Site/pdf/publication/FinalStatistics050331.pdf

National Cholesterol Education Program. (2004). *Risk assessment tool for estimating 10-year risk of developing hard CHD (myocardial infarction and coronary death).* Retrieved from http://hin.nhlbi.nih.gov/atpiii/calculator.asp?usertype=prof

National Guideline Clearinghouse. (2009). *Guideline synthesis: Screening for colorectal cancer.* Retrieved from http://http://www.guideline.gov/syntheses/synthesis.aspx?id=16435

National Institute on Alcohol Abuse and Alcoholism. (1998). *Alcohol and aging, alcohol alert #40.* Retrieved from http://pubs.niaaa.nih.gov/publications/aa40.htm

National Osteoporosis Foundation [NOF]. (2010). *The clinician's guide to the prevention and treatment of osteoporosis.* Retrieved from http://www.nof.org/professionals/clinical-guidelines.

National Stroke Association. (1999). Stroke prevention. Retrieved from http://www.stroke.org/site/PageServer?pagename=prevent

Neale, A. V., Hwalek, M. A., Scott, R. O., Sengstock, M. C., & Stahl, C. (1991). Validation of the Hwalek-Sengstock elder abuse screening test. *Journal of Applied Gerontology, 10*(4), 406–418.

O'Mahoney, D., Gallagher, P., Ryan, C., Byrne, S., Hamilton, H., Barry, P.,…Kennedy, J. (2010). STOPP and START criteria: A new approach to detecting potentially inappropriate prescribing in old age. *European Geriatric Medicine, 1*(1), 45–51.

Partnership for Prevention. (2008). *Physical activity guidelines for Americans, Chapter 5.* Retrieved from http://www.health.gov/paguidelines/guidelines/chapter5.aspx

Pluijm, S. M., Vasser, M., Puts, M. T., Dik, M. G., Schalk, B. W., van Schoor, N. M., … Deeq, DJ. (2007). Unhealthy life styles during the life course: Association with physical decline in late life. *Aging Clinical and Experimental Research, 19*(1), 75–83.

Roman, M. (2004). Falls in older adults. *AACN ViewPoint, 26*(2), 1–7.

Saslow, D., Boetes, C., Burke, W., Harms, S., Leach, M. O., Lehman, C. D., …American Cancer Society Breast Cancer Advisory Group. (2007). American Cancer Society guidelines for breast screening with MRI as an adjunct to mammography. *CA: A Cancer Journal for Clinicians, 57*(2), 75–89.

Schofield, M. J., & Mishra, G. D. (2003). Validity of self-report screening scale for elder abuse: Women's Health Australia Study. *The Gerontologist, 43*(1), 110–120, Table 1.

Sieber, C. C. (2006). *Nutritional screening tools—How does the MNA compare?* Proceedings of the session held in Chicago, May 2–3, 2006 (15 years of mini-nutritional assessment). *Journal of Nutrition Health and Aging, 10*(6), 488.

Stanford School of Medicine. (2012). Chronic disease self-management program. Retrieved from http://patienteducation.stanford.edu/programs/cdsmp.html

Sunderland, T., Hill, J. L., Mellow, A. M., Lawlor, B. A., Gundersheimer, J., Newhouse, P. A., & Grafman, J. H. (1989). Clock drawing in Alzheimer's disease. A novel measure of dementia severity. *Journal of the American Geriatric Society, 7*(8), 725–729.

Tatara, T. (1998). *The national elder abuse incidence study.* The National Center on Elder Abuse. Retrieved from www.ncea.aoa.gov/ncearoot/Main_Site/Library/Statistics_Research/National_Incident.aspx

Thomas, D. R., Ashmen, W., Morley, J. E., & Evans, W.J. (2000). *Nutritional management in long-term care: Development of a clinical guideline. Council for Nutritional Strategies in Long Term Care. The Journals of Gerontology. Series A, Biological Sciences and Medical Sciences, 55A*(12), M725–M734.

Tobacco Use and Dependence Guideline Panel. (2008). *Treating tobacco use and dependence: 2008 update.* Rockville, MD: U.S. Department of Health and Human Services. Public Health Service.

U.S. Department of Agriculture [USDA]. (2010). *Dietary guidelines for Americans, 2010.* Retrieved from http://www.health.gov/dietaryguidelines/dga2010/dietaryguidelines2010.pdf

U.S. Department of Health and Human Services, National Institutes of Health, & National Heart, Lung, and Blood Institute. (2004). *The seventh report of the Joint National Commission on the prevention, detection, evaluation, and treatment of high blood pressure.* Retrieved from http://www.nhlbi.nih.gov/guidelines/hypertension/jnc7full.pdf

U.S. Department of Health and Human Services, National Institutes of Health, & National Heart, Lung, and Blood Institute. (2006). *DASH eating plan: Lower your blood pressure.* Retrieved from http://www.nhlbi.nih.gov/health/public/heart/hbp/dash/new_dash.pdf

U.S. Department of Health and Human Services, Substance Abuse and Mental Health Services Administration. (2001). *Alcohol use among older adults. Pocket screening instruments for health care and social service providers.* Retrieved from http://www.kap.samhsa.gov/products/brochures/pdfs/Pocket_2.pdf

U.S. Preventive Services Task Force [USPSTF]. (2008). *Screening for lipid disorders in adults.* Retrieved from http://www.uspreventiveservicestaskforce.org/uspstf08/lipid/lipidrs.htm

U.S. Preventive Services Task Force [USPSTF]. (2009a). *Aspirin for the primary prevention of cardiovascular events.* Retrieved from http://www.uspreventiveservicestaskforce.org/uspstf/uspsasmi.htm

U. S. Preventive Services Task Force [USPSTF]. (2009b). *Screening for impaired visual acuity in older adults.* Retrieved from http://www.uspreventiveservicestaskforce.org/uspstf09/visualscr/viseldrs.htm#rationale

U.S. Preventive Services Task Force [USPSTF]. (2009c). Screening for breast cancer. Retrieved from http://www.uspreventiveservicestaskforce.org/uspstf/uspsbrca.htm

U.S. Preventive Services Task Force [USPSTF]. (2010). *Screening for osteoporosis: Recommendations and rationale.* Retrieved from http://www.uspreventiveservicestaskforce.org/3rduspstf/osteoporosis/osteorr.htm

U.S. Preventive Services Task Force [USPSTF]. (2011a). *Screening adults aged 50 years and older for hearing loss.* Retrieved from http://www.uspreventiveservicestaskforce.org/uspstf11/adulthearing/adulthearart.htm

U.S. Preventive Services Task Force [USPSTF]. (2011b). *Screening for osteoporosis.* Retrieved from http://www.uspreventiveservicestaskforce.org/uspstf10/osteoporosis/osteors.htm

U.S. Preventive Services Task Force http://www.uspreventiveservicestaskforce.org/uspstf10/osteoporosis/osteors.htm. (2012). *Focus on older adults.* Retrieved from http://www.uspreventiveservicestaskforce.org/tfolderfocus.htm

Wannamethee, S. G., Shaper, A. G., & Lennon, L. (2005). Reasons for intentional weight loss, unintentional weight loss and mortality in older men. *Archives of Internal Medicine, 165*(9), 1035–1040.

Wolf, R. (2007). *Risk assessment instruments*. NCEA. Retrieved from http://www.ncea.aoa.gov/main_site/library/Statistics_Research/Research_Reviews/risk_assessment.aspx

For a full suite of assignments and additional learning activities, see the access code at the front of your book.

Unit IV

Illness and Disease Management

(COMPETENCIES 9, 15–18)

At the end of this chapter, the reader will be able to:

> Name the major risk factors associated with cardiovascular disease (CVD).
> Discuss the impact of the major CVDs seen in older adults on the health of the U.S. population.
> Recognize signs of myocardial infarction that may be unique to the older adult.
> Utilize resources and research to promote heart-healthy lifestyles in older adults.
> State the warning signs of stroke.
> Apply the Mauk model for poststroke recovery to the care of stroke survivors.
> Identify common treatments for pneumonia, tuberculosis (TB), and chronic obstructive pulmonary disease (COPD).
> Discuss how to minimize risk factors for common gastrointestinal problems in the elderly.
> Describe nursing interventions for patients dealing with gastroesophageal reflux disease (GERD).
> Discuss ways to prevent catheter-associated urinary tract infection (CAUTI).
> Identify signs, symptoms, and treatments for benign prostatic hyperplasia (BPH) and vaginitis.
> Recognize common treatments for several cancers in older adults: bladder, prostate, colorectal, cervical, and breast.
> List several medications that can contribute to male impotence.
> Recognize the clinical treatments for persons with Parkinson's disease (PD).
> Devise a nursing care plan for someone with Alzheimer's disease (AD).
> Discuss possible causes and solutions for dizziness in the elderly.
> List the modifiable risk factors for osteoporosis.
> Distinguish between osteoarthritis and rheumatoid arthritis in relation to typical presentation, treatment, and long-term implications.
> Contrast rehabilitative care for older adults with hip and knee replacement surgery.
> Describe the most effective way to condition a stump to promote use of a prosthesis.
> Distinguish the signs and symptoms of cataracts, glaucoma, macular degeneration, and diabetic retinopathy.
> Contrast management of the four most common eye disorders seen in the elderly.
> Distinguish among the three major types of skin cancer.

> Identify signs and symptoms of herpes zoster appearing in the elderly.
> Review prevention of the most common complications of diabetes in older adults.
> Devise a plan for good foot care for older adults with diabetes.
> Synthesize knowledge about hypothyroidism into general care of the older adult.

KEY TERMS

Activities of daily living (ADLs)
Age-related macular degeneration (ARMD)
Alzheimer's disease (AD)
Angina
Atherosclerosis
Benign paroxysmal positional vertigo (BPPV)
Benign prostatic hyperplasia (BPH)
Bone mineral density (BMD)
Cardiovascular disease (CVD)
Cataracts
Catheter-associated urinary tract infection (CAUTI)
Cerebrovascular accident (CVA)
Chronic bronchitis
Chronic obstructive pulmonary disease (COPD)
Congestive heart failure (CHF)
Continuous bladder irrigation (CBI)
Corneal ulcer
Coronary artery disease (CAD)
Coronary heart disease (CHD)
Cystectomy
Diabetic retinopathy
Diverticulitis
Dysphagia
Emphysema
Erectile dysfunction (ED)
Gastroesophageal reflux disease (GERD)
Glaucoma
Gonioscopy
Helicobacter pylori (*H. pylori*)
Hemiparesis
Hemiplegia

Herpes zoster
Histamine 2 (H2) blockers
Hypertension (HTN)
Incontinence
Instrumental activities of daily living (IADLs)
Intraocular pressure (IOP)
Mauk model for poststroke recovery
Meniere's syndrome
Myocardial infarction (MI)
Osteoporosis
Otoconia
Parkinson's disease (PD)
Peripheral artery disease (PAD)
Peripheral vascular disease (PVD)
Phantom limb pain
Proliferative retinopathy
Prostate-specific antigen (PSA)
Proton pump inhibitors (PPIs)
Radical prostatectomy
Retinal detachment
Scatter laser treatment
Stroke
Tinnitus
Tonometer
t-PA (tissue plasminogen activator)
Transient ischemic attack (TIA)
Transurethral resection of the prostate (TURP)
Tuberculosis (TB)
Urinary tract infection (UTI)
Urostomy
Vitrectomy

Chapter 9

(Competencies 9, 15, 17,18)

Management of Common Illnesses, Diseases, and Health Conditions

Kristen L. Mauk
Patricia Hanson
Debra Hain

The purpose of this chapter is to present basic information related to common diseases and disorders experienced by older adults. It is assumed that the reader of this text has fundamental nursing knowledge and will study disease processes more in depth in other courses. Extensive discussion of the nursing care and treatment of each disease is beyond the scope of this text, but nurses are encouraged to refer to traditional medical–surgical textbooks for further reading. The discussion in this chapter will use a systems approach to provide a "snapshot" of essential information regarding background, risk factors, signs and symptoms, diagnosis, and usual treatment, while emphasizing any important aspects unique to care of the elderly with each disorder. Unit 5 provides a thorough discussion of some additional common problems and geriatric syndromes.

Cardiovascular Problems

Several conditions and diseases related to the cardiovascular system are common in older adults. The specific conditions discussed in this section include *myocardial infarction (MI)*, *hypertension*, *angina*, *congestive heart failure (CHF)*, *coronary artery disease (CAD)*, *stroke*, and *peripheral vascular disease*.

By 2030, 40.5% of the U.S. population is projected to have some form of *cardiovascular disease (CVD)* (Heidenreich et al., 2011). In Canada, 28% of all male deaths and 29.76% of all female deaths in 2000 were due to heart disease and stroke (Heart and Stroke Foundation of Canada, 2008). The American Heart Association (AHA, 2012b) lists the following as the major cardiovascular diseases: hypertension (HTN), *coronary heart disease (CHD*; includes myocardial infarction and angina), congestive heart failure (CHF), and stroke. These will be discussed in the following sections.

Hypertension

Background/Significance

In 2008, 64% of men and 59.3% of women ages 65–74 were diagnosed with HTN; of those age 75 years or older, 66.7% of men and 78.5% of women had HTN. African Americans continue to have a 1.6 times greater risk than Whites of having a fatal stroke, and a 4.2 times greater chance of developing end stage renal disease (Centers for Disease Control and Prevention [CDC], 2011).

Risk Factors/Warning Signs

Risk factors for hypertension include family history, ethnicity, poor diet, being overweight, excessive alcohol intake, a sedentary lifestyle, and certain medications (see **Table 9-1**). A blood pressure consistently under 120/80 is desirable. As persons age, the systolic blood pressure (the measure of the heart at work) tends to rise, but because of the significant risk of stroke associated with hypertension, older adults are being treated earlier and more aggressively than in years past. Although some clinicians used to consider HTN in the elderly as a blood pressure greater than 160/90, because of the rise in systolic blood pressure with age, those with isolated systolic HTN (i.e., a systolic BP over 140 and a diastolic BP less than 90) should be aggressively treated (Reuben et al., 2004). Complete information about the Joint National Committee's seventh report (JNC 7) for control of high blood pressure can be found at http://www.nhlbi.nih.gov/guidelines/hypertension/.

Assessment/Diagnosis

Blood pressure is determined by many factors, some of which, such as the condition of the heart and blood vessels, are influenced by age. Over 95% of hypertension is called "essential" hypertension; that is, it has no known cause (Mayo Clinic, 2011). High blood pressure may also result from disease processes. Additionally, those with prehypertension, a systolic blood pressure between 120 and 139 or a diastolic blood pressure between 80 and 89 on multiple readings, should receive a recommendation

TABLE 9-1 Risk Factors for Hypertension
Heredity
Race (African American)
Increased age
Lack of physical activity
Male gender
High sodium intake
Diabetes or renal disease
Heavy alcohol consumption
Obesity
Some medications

Source: AHA, 2012e.

to make lifestyle changes, because they often develop hypertension. Diagnosis of hypertension should be based on several readings at different times or visits to the primary healthcare provider.

Interventions

Lifestyle modifications may help older adults to control blood pressure. **Table 9- 2** lists recommended strategies for older adults. In addition, several medications may be used to treat hypertension in the elderly (see **Table 9-3**). The goal of medical treatment in older adults is to lower the blood pressure to 120/80 or below.

TABLE 9-2   Strategies to Help Older Adults Control High Blood Pressure
Limit alcohol intake to one drink per day.
Limit sodium intake.
Stop smoking.
Maintain a low-fat diet that still contains adequate vitamins and minerals by adding leafy green vegetables and fruits.
Do some type of aerobic activity nearly every day of the week.
Lose weight. (Even 10 pounds may make a significant difference.)
Have blood pressure checked regularly. Report any significant rise in blood pressure to the physician.
Take medications as ordered. Do not skip doses.

TABLE 9-3 Some Types of Medications Used to Treat Cardiovascular Disease		
Classification	**Action**	**Example**
+Diuretics	Decrease water and salt retention	Furosemide (Lasix)
+Beta-blockers	Lower cardiac output and heart rate	Atenolol (Tenormin)
+ACE inhibitors	Block hormone that causes artery constriction	Captopril (Capoten)
+Central alpha agonists	Block constriction of vessels	Clonidine (Catapres)
+Calcium channel blockers	Relax blood vessels to the heart	Amlodipine (Norvasc)
+Angiotensin II receptor blockers	Relax blood vessels by blocking angiotensin II	Irbesartan (Avapro)
+Vasodilators	Relax the walls of the arteries	Hydralazine (Apresoline)
*Digitalis	Strengthens and slows the heart	Digoxin (Lanoxin)
*Potassium	Helps control heart rhythm	K-Dur, K-Tab
*Blood thinners	Prevent clots	Warfarin (Coumadin); Heparin

+Medications used for both CHF and HTN
*Medications used for CHF

Thiazide diuretics or beta-blockers are often used as drugs of choice for those elderly who do not have other coexisting medical conditions. It is not uncommon for older adults to require more than one and even up to several medications to achieve adequate control. In fact, combination therapy for older adults allows for smaller doses of each drug and may help avoid side effects. The most common combinations are a thiazide diuretic with either a potassium-sparing diuretic, a beta-blocker, a calcium channel blocker, angiotensin-converting enzyme inhibitors (ACEIs), or angiotensin receptor blockers (ARBs) (National Institutes of Health [NIH], 2008).

Older adults should work with their physicians and nurses to achieve good control of their blood pressure, because it is a risk factor and contributor to many other serious health conditions including heart disease, stroke, and renal disease. Nurses may need to do extensive teaching about lifestyle modifications to assist older adults with smoking cessation and appropriate dietary choices. Remember that in addition to promoting nutrition, nurses should teach patients to read labels, avoid processed foods, prepare foods appropriately, and drink adequate amounts of fluids to stay hydrated.

Coronary Heart Disease

Coronary heart disease (CHD), also called coronary artery disease (CAD) or ischemic heart disease, affects millions of people each year in many countries. This condition is caused by hardening and narrowing of the blood vessels of the heart (*atherosclerosis*), resulting in an impaired blood supply to the myocardium. Thirteen million Americans are affected each year. The rates for older females after menopause are more than twice that of older females prior to menopause. Over 82% of people who die with CHD are age 65 years or over (AHA, 2012c). Angina and myocardial infarction are two results of CHD that will be discussed here.

Angina

Background/Significance

Angina pectoris is chest pain that results from lack of oxygen to the heart muscle. A small number of deaths are attributed to this cause each year, but mortality statistics related to angina are often included with CHD reports. Only about 20% of heart attacks are preceded by diagnosed angina.

Risk Factors/Warning Signs

Among Americans ages 40–74, the prevalence of angina is slightly higher for females, significantly higher for Mexican American males and females, and slightly higher, though not significantly so, for African American females (AHA, 2012b). According to the AHA, the incidence of angina per 1,000 people aged 65–74 is highest for non-Black males (28.3), followed by Black males (22.4), Black females (15.5), and non-Black females (14.1) (AHA, 2012a, 2012b).

Angina is usually the first symptom of CAD in the older adult. Older adults with angina may first complain of dyspnea, dizziness, or confusion versus classic chest pain (O'Donnell et al., 2012).

Assessment/Diagnosis

Angina is classified as stable or unstable. Although the symptoms of angina may be similar to myocardial infarction, there are several notable differences. Angina often occurs related to exercise or stress and is relieved by rest and/or nitroglycerin. The associated chest pain is generally shorter (less than 5 minutes) than MI, though the classic presentation is squeezing pain or pressure in the sternal area. In addition to a thorough history and checking vital signs, a 12-lead EKG and lab tests will help rule out or confirm an MI.

Intervention/Strategies for Care

Treatment is ongoing for angina. Unstable angina may require hospitalization, whereas stable angina can be managed with medication and lifestyle modifications aimed at reducing the workload on the heart and the accompanying oxygen demand. Teaching of patients and families will include weight management, stress management, limiting caffeine, smoking cessation, an exercise regimen that considers the person's myocardial capacity, control of hypertension, and medical management of any coexisting endocrine disorder (such as hyperthyroidism). Beta-blockers and calcium channel blockers are often prescribed to decrease the oxygen demand on the heart. Patients should be alerted to side effects from these medications, such as fatigue, drowsiness, dizziness, and slow heart rate.

Myocardial Infarction

Background/Significance

Since 2000 there has been a decrease in the incidence of myocardial infarction, from 224 per 1,000 to 208 per 1,000 (Yen et al., 2010) The risk of MI increases with age; men have the highest incidence of MI until approximately age 70, when the incidences of MI converge and the rate of MI for men and women equalizes (Zafari & Yang, 2012).

Risk Factors/Warning Signs

Risk factors for MI include hypertension, race (especially African American males with HTN), high-fat diet, sedentary lifestyle, diabetes, obesity, high cholesterol, family history, cigarette smoking, excessive alcohol intake, and stressful environment. Many of these risk factors are modifiable or controllable. Warning signs of MI are listed in **Table 9-4**. It is important to note that the warning signs are often very different for women than they are for men (see **Case Study 9-1**). Women often do not have the substernal chest pain, but more often experience sharp pain, fatigue, weakness, and other nonspecific symptoms (Garas & Zafari, 2006). Symptoms may occur as much as 1 month prior to the occurrence of a myocardial infarction. These symptoms include unusual fatigue (70%), sleep disturbance (48%), shortness of breath (42%), indigestion (39%), and anxiety (35%) (Health Education Solutions, 2012).

TABLE 9-4   Warning Signs of Heart Attack
Chest pain appearing as tightness, fullness, or pressure
Pain radiating to arms
Unexplained numbness in arms, neck, or back
Shortness of breath with or without activity
Sweating
Nausea
Pallor
Dizziness
*Unexplained jaw pain
*Indigestion or epigastric discomfort, especially when not relieved with antacids

*Of particular significance in the elderly

Case Study 9-1

Mr. Jones is a 62-year-old man who lives next door to you. He comes over while you are out in your yard and says, "You're a nurse, so I have this question for you. I have had this annoying heartburn all day that just doesn't go away no matter what I do." He points to his epigastric area. "It just feels like this pressure right here and makes me a little sick to my stomach." Mr. Jones looks pale and a bit diaphoretic.

Questions:

1. What is your best response to this situation?

2. What could these signs and symptoms indicate?

3. What would you expect Mr. Jones to do at this point?

4. Are there any other questions you could ask that would provide additional information about the potential seriousness of his complaint?

Assessment/Diagnosis

Diagnosis may include a variety of tests, including electrocardiogram (ECG) and angiogram or cardiac catheterization to visualize any areas of blockage. **Figure 9-1** shows the results of an angiogram with some degree of blockage in a major heart vessel. Such procedures are generally done in a special catheterization lab within a heart center or hospital by a cardiologist. Important nursing interventions after these procedures include keeping the leg straight with pressure on the femoral artery entry site per the facility's protocol. Instruction of the patient and family after this outpatient procedure should include emphasis on the importance of monitoring the entry site. Patients should be taught that bleeding at the site is considered an emergency and that firm, direct pressure must be applied to the site immediately. It is common for bruising to occur, and limits to lifting and driving should be strictly followed after the procedure to prevent complications.

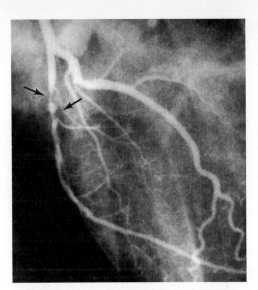

Figure 9-1 Coronary angiogram illustrating segmental narrowing (arrows).

Source: Leonard Crowley, *An Introduction to Human Disease: Pathology and Pathophysiology Correlations* (9th Edition). Burlington, MA: Jones & Bartlett Learning, 2013.

Interventions

Thrombolytic therapy, if administered early in the course of MI, significantly reduces the morbidity and mortality associated with MI (Kulick, 2012). The following steps are recommended, if possible, while awaiting emergency treatment:

1. Have the patient rest.
2. Provide supplemental oxygen.
3. Give nitroglycerin sublingually every 5 minutes times three and monitor vital signs.
4. Give aspirin if not contraindicated.

Some nurses use the mnemonic MONA (morphine, oxygen, nitroglycerin, aspirin) to remember the steps in acute care treatment of MI. If neither oxygen nor nitroglycerin is available, proceed with giving aspirin.

Usual medical treatment of MI includes several options, depending on the results of the diagnostic tests and extent of damage and blockage. Angioplasty (see **Figure 9-2**) is a common procedure that uses a balloon, stent, or other device to open the blocked vessel. Coronary artery bypass graft (CABG), commonly known as open-heart surgery, is often used for those with blockages in several major arteries in order to restore blood flow (see **Figure 9-3**). Pharmacological treatment may include beta-blockers, angiotensin-converting enzyme (ACE) inhibitors, and antihypertensives, to name a few. The recovery period will include careful monitoring in cardiac intensive care, then progression to cardiac rehabilitation, where patients will be closely monitored after discharge and assisted by specialized nurses to make lifestyle modifications to promote maximal recovery and return to function. Patients are discharged from the hospital as early as possible; therefore, the

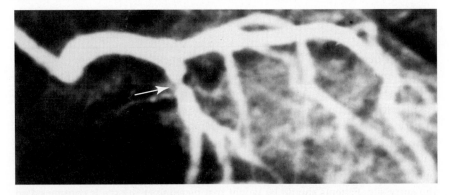

Figure 9-2a Coronary angioplasty. A severely narrowed coronary artery (arrow) shown by angiogram.

Source: Leonard Crowley, *Introduction to Human Disease* (6th ed.). Sudbury, MA: Jones & Bartlett Publishers, 2005.

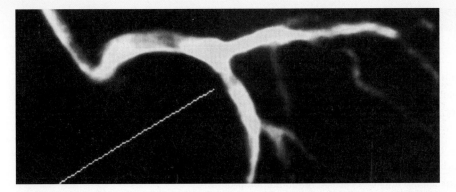

Figure 9-2b B, Same artery after successful dilation by angioplasty.

Source: Leonard Crowley, *Introduction to Human Disease* (6th ed.). Sudbury, MA: Jones & Bartlett Publishers, 2005.

cardiac rehabilitation will likely occur on an outpatient basis. It is important to encourage patients to follow through with cardiac rehabilitation even though they may be feeling well.

Persons surviving a heart attack should be dedicated to reducing risk factors associated with heart disease. **Table 9-5** lists several strategies for older adults to prevent a first or recurring heart attack. Nurses should encourage patients to attend cardiac rehabilitation programs during the posthospitalization period. The American Heart Association website has information about cardiac rehabilitation, its necessity in recovery from MI, and its ongoing importance for achieving optimal wellness. (AHA, 2012a). Support groups for survivors and families may also be helpful. Family members, particularly spouses, should be included in the rehabilitation process.

Congestive Heart Failure

Background/Significance

The incidence of congestive heart failure (CHF) varies among races and across age groups. For example, White men have an incidence of 15.2 per 1,000 between the ages of 65 and 74, 31.7 per 1,000 between the ages of 75 and 84, and 65.2 per 1,000 when greater than 85 years of age. Considering these same age ranges, the incidence of heart failure for White women is 8.2, 19.8, and 45.6, respectively; for Black men 16.9, 25.5, and 50.6, respectively; and for Black women, 14.2, 25.5, and 44.0, respectively (AHA, 2012d). The lifetime risk for someone to have CHF is 1 in 5. The risk of CHF in older adults doubles for those with blood pressures over 160/90. Seventy-five percent of those with CHF also have hypertension (AHA, 2012e). The major risk factors for CHF are diabetes and MI. Congestive heart failure often occurs within 6 years after a heart attack.

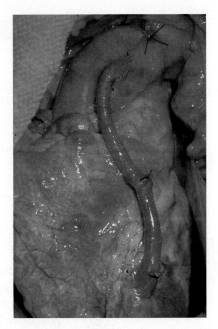

Figure 9-3 Vein graft extending from aorta above the origin of the coronary arteries to the anterior interventricular (descending) coronary artery distal to the site of arterial narrowing.

Source: Leonard Crowley, *An Introduction to Human Disease: Pathology and Pathophysiology Correlations* (9th Edition). Burlington, MA: Jones & Bartlett Learning, 2013.

TABLE 9-5   Strategies for Older Adults to Reduce Risk of Heart Attack
Exercise regularly.
Do not smoke.
Eat a balanced diet with plenty of fruits and vegetables; avoid foods high in saturated fats.
Maintain a healthy weight.
Manage stress appropriately.
Control existing diabetes by maintaining healthy blood sugars and take medications as prescribed.
Limit alcohol intake to one drink per day for women and two drinks per day (or less) for men.
Visit the doctor regularly.
After a heart attack, participate fully in a cardiac rehabilitation program.
Involve the entire family in heart-healthy lifestyle modifications.
Report any signs of chest pain immediately.

TABLE 9-6   Signs and Symptoms of Chronic Heart Failure
Shortness of breath
Swelling of the legs, ankles, and feet
Coughing or wheezing
Fatigue
Lack of appetite or nausea
Confusion
Increased heart rate
Sudden weight gain
Decreased tolerance for physical activity

Source: Mayo Clinic, 2012b

Risk Factors/Warning Signs

Signs and symptoms of heart failure are many; these appear in **Table 9-6**. It is essential that older adults diagnosed with CHF recognize signs of a worsening condition and report them promptly to their healthcare provider. Older adults may present with atypical symptoms such as decreased appetite, weight gain of a few pounds, or insomnia (Amella, 2004).

Assessment/Diagnosis

For in-home monitoring, daily weights at the same time of day with the same clothes on the same scale are essential. The physician or primary care provider will give guidelines for the patient to call if the weight exceeds his or her threshold for weight gain. This is usually between 1 and 3 pounds. The decision regarding when to call the primary care provider is made based upon the severity of the HF and the relative stability/frailty of the patient. In the office or long-term care setting, O_2 saturation levels can be easily monitored. An O_2 saturation of less than 90% in an older person is cause for concern and further investigation.

Intervention/Strategies for Care

Treatment for CHF involves the usual lifestyle modifications discussed for promoting a healthy heart (see Table 9-5), as well as several possible types of medications. These include ACE inhibitors, diuretics, vasodilators, beta-blockers, blood thinners, angiotensin II blockers, calcium channel blockers, and potassium. Digoxin, once a mainstay in the treatment of CHF, is rarely used now, although it may be seen on occasion. Most CHF is managed with lifestyle modifications and medications; however, in extreme cases, surgery may be a treatment option if valvular repair/replacement or heart transplant becomes necessary.

In addition, nurses should teach older adults about lifestyle modifications that can decrease and/or help manage the workload on the heart (see **Box 9-1**). To minimize exacerbations, patient and family counseling should include teaching about the use of medications to control symptoms and the importance of regular monitoring with a health care provider (Agency for Healthcare Research and Quality [AHRQ], 2012; Hunt et al., 2009). These teaching points appear in **Table 9-7.** With the proper

---

BOX 9-1   Resources About Cardiovascular Disease

American Heart Association
  1-800-AHA-USA1
  http://www.americanheart.org

American Society of Hypertension (ASH)
  http://www.ash-us.org

American Stroke Association
  1-888-4-STROKE
  http://www.strokeassociation.org

Heart and Stroke Foundation of Canada
  http://www.heartandstroke.ca

Heart and Stroke Foundation of Alberta, Canada
  http://www.heartandstroke.ab.ca

National Emergency Medicine Association
  http://www.nemahealth.org

National Institute of Neurological Disorders and Stroke
  http://www.ninds.nih.gov

National Stroke Association
  http://www.stroke.org

South African Heart Association
  http://www.saheart.org

TABLE 9-7   Lifestyle Modifications to Teach Older Adults with Heart Failure

Limit or eliminate alcohol use (no more than 1 oz. ethanol per day = one mixed drink, one 12-oz. beer, or one 5-oz. glass of wine).

Maintain a healthy weight. Extra pounds put added stress and workload on the heart. Weigh daily and report weight gains of 5 pounds or more to healthcare provider.

Stop smoking (no tobacco use in any form).

Limit sodium intake to 2–3 g per day—read the labels: avoid canned and processed foods. Take care with how foods are cooked or prepared at home (e.g., limit oils and butters).

Take medications as ordered—do not skip doses. Report any side effects to the physician.

Exercise to tolerance level—this will differ for each person. Remain active without overdoing it.

Alternate rest and activity. Learn energy conservation techniques.

combination of treatments such as lifestyle changes and medications, many older persons can still live happy and productive lives with a diagnosis of heart failure and minimize their risk of complications related to this disease.

Stroke

Stroke, also known as *cerebrovascular accident (CVA)* or brain attack, is an interruption of the blood supply to the brain that may result in devastating neurological damage, disability, or death. Approximately 795,000 people in the United States have a new or recurrent stroke each year (American Stroke Association [ASA], 2012a).

Background/Significance

Stroke accounts for 1 in 18 deaths, making it the fourth leading cause of death in the United States. A death from stroke occurs every 4 minutes and the cost of stroke treatment and disability was over $73 billion in 2010. Death from stroke is generally higher among females, with higher rates in Black males (67.7/100,000) and females (57.0/100,000) than in Caucasians (ASA, 2012a). In Canada, stroke is the fourth leading cause of death, affecting 50,000 people each year (Heart and Stroke Foundation of Canada, 2009).

There are two major types of stroke: ischemic and hemorrhagic. The vast majority of strokes are caused by ischemia (87%), usually from a thrombus or embolus (ASA, 2012a). The symptoms and damage seen depend on which vessels in the brain are blocked. Carotid artery occlusion is also a common cause of stroke related to stenosis (see **Figure 9-4**).

Risk Factors/Warning Signs

Some risk factors for stroke are controllable and others are not; risk factors appear in **Table 9-8**. The most significant risk factor for stroke is hypertension. Controlling high blood pressure is an important way to reduce stroke risk. Those with a blood pressure of less than 120/80 have half the lifetime risk of stroke as those with hypertension (ASA, 2012a). Smoking 40 or more cigarettes per day (heavy smoking) increases the stroke risk to twice that of light smokers. If a person quits smoking, their risk after 5 years mirrors that of a nonsmoker, so older adults should be particularly encouraged to stop smoking.

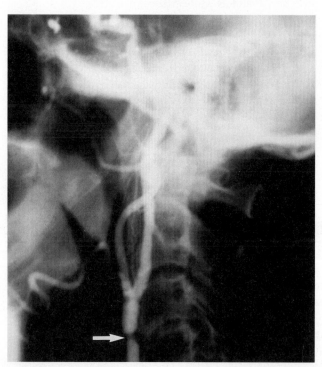

Figure 9-4 Angiogram showing narrowed carotid artery.

Source: Leonard Crowley, *An Introduction to Human Disease: Pathology and Pathophysiology Correlations* (9th Edition). Burlington, MA: Jones & Bartlett Learning, 2013.

TABLE 9-8 Risk Factors for Stroke	
Controllable	**Uncontrollable**
Hypertension	Advanced age
High cholesterol	Gender (males more than females until menopause)
Heart disease	
Smoking	
Obesity	Race (African Americans more than Whites)
Stress	
Diabetes	
Depression	Heredity
Atrial fibrillation	

TABLE 9-9   Warning Signs of Stroke
• Sudden numbness or weakness of face, arm, or leg, especially on one side of the body
• Sudden confusion; trouble speaking or understanding
• Sudden trouble seeing in one or both eyes
• Sudden trouble walking, dizziness, or loss of balance or coordination
• Sudden severe headache with no known cause

Source: American Stroke Association, 2012b

Several warning signs are common with stroke (see **Table 9-9**). Thromboembolic strokes are more likely to show classic signs than hemorrhagic strokes, which may appear as severe headaches but with few other prior warning signs. A quick initial evaluation for stroke can be performed by assessing for three easy signs: facial droop, motor weakness, and language difficulties.

Other warning signs of stroke include a temporary loss of consciousness or the appearance of the classic warning signs that go away quickly (see **Case Study 9-2**). *Transient ischemic attacks (TIAs)* are defined as those symptoms similar to stroke that go away within 24 hours (and usually within minutes) and leave no residual effects. Most TIAs in Whites are from atherothrombotic disease, with another 20% from cardiac emboli and 25% from occlusion of smaller vessels (Warlow, Sudlow, Martin, Wardlaw, & Sandercock, 2003). Those having a TIA are 10 times more likely to have a stroke than those who have not had a TIA (ASA, 2012b, 2012c).

Assessment and Diagnosis

There are several tools for assessing for signs and symptoms of stroke; one easy acronym is FAST:

F stands for facial droop. Ask the person to smile and see if drooping is present.
A stands for arm. Have the person lift both arms straight out in front of him. If one is arm is drifting lower than the other, it is a sign that weakness is present.

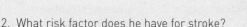

Case Study 9–2

Your grandfather is 85 years old and tells you at a family gathering that yesterday he had some blurred vision and numbness down his right arm. He didn't tell his wife or anyone else because the symptoms went away within 10 minutes, but he wanted to tell you just in case he should have it checked out.

Questions:

1. What should you tell your grandfather? What do his symptoms possibly indicate?

2. What risk factor does he have for stroke?

3. What other questions should you ask to gain more information?

4. What is the next step of action that your grandfather should take?

5. Should anything be discussed with his wife? If so, what?

6. At this point, are there specific topics that should be taught to your grandfather?

S stands for speech. Ask the person to say a short phrase such as "light, tight, dynamite" and check for slurring or other abnormal speech.

T stands for time. If the first F-A-S checks are not normal, then one is to remember F-A-S-T that time is important and the emergency medical system should be activated (National Stroke Association, 2012).

Older adults experiencing the warning signs of stroke should note the time on the clock and seek immediate treatment by calling 911 (ASA, 2012b). Transport to an emergency medical facility for evaluation is essential for the best array of treatment options. A history and neurological exam, vital signs, as well as diagnostic tests including electrocardiogram (ECG), chest X-ray, platelets, prothrombin time (PT), partial thromboplastin time (PTT), electrolytes, and glucose are routinely ordered. Diagnostic imaging may include computed tomography (CT) without contrast, magnetic resonance imaging (MRI), arteriography, or ultrasonography to determine the type and location of the stroke. The CT or MRI should ideally be done within 90 minutes so that appropriate emergency measures may be initiated to prevent further brain damage.

Interventions

The first step in treatment is to determine the cause or type of stroke. A CT scan or MRI must first be done to rule out hemorrhagic stroke (see **Figure 9-5**). Hemorrhagic stroke treatment often requires surgery to evacuate blood and stop the bleeding.

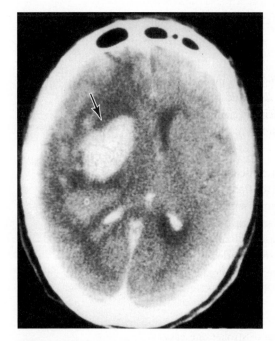

Figure 9-5 CT scan showing cerebral hemorrhage.

Source: Leonard Crowley, *An Introduction to Human Disease: Pathology and Pathophysiology Correlations* (9th Edition). Burlington, MA: Jones & Bartlett Learning, 2013.

Acute Management

The American Heart/American Stroke Association has published numerous guidelines for the treatment of various types of stroke. These can be accessed through the ASA's website at http://www.strokeassociation.org/STROKEORG/Professionals/Professionals_UCM_308581_SubHomePage.jsp. On this homepage for professionals, nurses can find stroke statements and guidelines that provide the best up-to-date information based on evidence. Those hospitals that have been certified as Primary or Comprehensive Stroke Centers by the Joint Commission have met strict criteria for the treatment of stroke and may be preferred places for care.

The gold standard at present for treatment of ischemic stroke is *t-PA (tissue plasminogen activator)*. At this time, t-PA must be given within 3 hours after the onset of stroke symptoms. This is why it is essential that older adults seek treatment immediately when symptoms begin. Only about 3–5% of people reach the hospital in time to be considered for this treatment (ASA, 2012d). t-PA may be effective for a select group of patients after the 3-hour window (up to 4.5 hours), and this treatment window has been approved in Canada (Heart and Stroke Foundation of Canada, 2009). New treatments are being explored to extend the treatment window, including the use of a synthetic compound derived from bat saliva that contains an anticoagulant-type property. The major side effect of t-PA is bleeding. t-PA is not effective for all patients, but may reduce or eliminate symptoms in over 40% of those who receive it at the appropriate time (Higashida, 2005). Other, much less common procedures such as angioplasty, laser emulsification, and mechanical clot retrieval may be options for treatment of acute ischemic stroke.

Additionally, the use of cooling helmets to decrease the metabolism of the brain is thought to preserve function and reduce ischemic damage. The roles of hyperthermia, hyperglycemia, and hypertension are all being further explored, as these are known to be associated with mortality and other poor outcomes related to ischemic stroke.

To prevent recurrence of thromboembolic stroke, medications such as aspirin, ticlopidine (Ticlid), clopidogrel (Plavix), dipyridamole (Persantine), heparin, warfarin (Coumadin), and enoxaparin (Lovenox) may be used to prevent clot formation. Once the stroke survivor has stabilized, the long process of rehabilitation begins. Each stroke is different depending on location and severity, so persons may recover with little or no residual deficits or an entire array of devastating consequences.

The effects of stroke vary, but may include *hemiplegia, hemiparesis*, visual and perceptual deficits, language deficits, emotional changes, swallowing dysfunction, and bowel and bladder problems. Ninety percent of all *dysphagia* results from stroke (White, O'Rourke, Ong, Cordato, & Chan, 2008). Although the deficits that present themselves depend on the area of brain damage, it is sometimes helpful to picture most strokes as involving one side of the body or the other. A person with left-brain injury presents with right-sided weakness or paralysis, and a person with right-sided stroke presents with left-sided weakness or paralysis. **Table 9-10** lists common deficits caused by stroke, seen in varying degrees, and some common problems associated with strokes on one side of the brain versus the other.

Poststroke Rehabilitation

Rehabilitation after a stroke focuses on several key principles. These include maximizing functional ability, preventing complications, promoting quality of life, encouraging adaptation, and enhancing independence. Rehabilitation emphasizes the survivor's abilities, not disabilities, and helps him or her to work with what he or she has while acknowledging what was lost.

If significant functional impairments are present, evaluation for transfer to an intensive acute inpatient rehabilitation program is recommended. Inpatient rehabilitation units offer the survivor the best opportunity to maximize recovery, including functional return. An interdisciplinary team of experienced experts, including nurses, therapists, physicians, social workers, and psychologists, will

TABLE 9-10 Common Deficits Caused by Stroke		
Common Characteristics Associated with Stroke of Either Side	**Right Hemisphere Stroke**	**Left Hemisphere Stroke**
Weakness/paralysis	Left hemiparesis or hemiplegia	Right hemiparesis or hemiplegia
Fatigue	Left homonymous hemianopsia	Right homonymous hemianopsia
Depression	Difficulty with cognitive tasks such as spatial-perceptual tasks, sequencing, following multistep instructions, and writing	Aphasia (especially expressive type)
Emotional lability		Reading/writing problems
Some memory impairment		Dysarthria
Sensory changes		Dysphagia
Social isolation	Memory deficits related to performance	Anxiety when trying new tasks
Altered sleep patterns	May not recognize or accept limitations or deficits	Tendency to worry and be easily frustrated
	Overestimating abilities	Slow, cautious
	Impulsive	Memory deficits related to language
	Quick movements	
	Anosognosia or other forms of left-sided neglect	
	Impaired judgment	
	Inappropriately low anxiety	
	Higher risk for falls due to lack of safety awareness	
	Deficits less easily recognized by others	

help the survivor and the family to adapt to the changes resulting from the stroke. Although the goal of rehabilitation will usually be discharge back to the previous home environment, this is not always possible. Advanced age and functional capacity, particularly ambulatory ability, may be predictors of discharge to a nursing home (Lutz, 2004).

The *Mauk model for poststroke recovery* (Easton, 2001; Mauk, 2006) (see **Box 9-2**) can help guide nursing practice by suggesting focused interventions for each of the six phases of stroke recovery. **Tables 9-11** and **9-12** list the major

---

BOX 9-2 Research Highlight

Aim: To test the accuracy of nursing students in assessing the phases of a stroke model.

Methods: A sample of 30 nursing student volunteers was provided a 15-minute overview and diagram of the Mauk model for poststroke recovery. Then they were asked to read five case studies and use the Mauk model to assess the phase of stroke being described.

Findings: The six phases of poststroke recovery emerging from the data were labeled in a model: agonizing, fantasizing, realizing, blending, framing, and owning. The majority of respondents (57%) were able to rate the correct phase of stroke recovery with 100% accuracy. Areas of the model that needed clarification were identified as the blending and owning phases.

Application to practice: Nursing students were able to quickly learn and correctly identify the phases of the Mauk model. Parts of the model can benefit with more clarification and increased testing. By using the Mauk model for poststroke recovery, nurses can more efficiently target their care by focusing nursing interventions unique to the phase of recovery in which survivors are. Nurses should assess the phase of recovery and focus on care interventions related to the essential tasks for each phase.

Source: Mauk, K. L., Lemley, C., Pierce, J., & Schmidt, N. A. (2011). The Mauk model for poststroke recovery: Assessing the phases. *Rehabilitation Nursing, 36*(6), 241–247.

TABLE 9-11 The Six Phases (Concepts) of the Poststroke Journey with Characteristics

Phase/Concept	Characteristics/Subconcepts
Agonizing	Fear, shock/surprise, loss, questioning, denial
Fantasizing	Mirage of recovery, unreality
Realizing	Reality, depression, anger, fatigue
Blending	Hope, learning, frustration, dealing with changes
Framing	Answering why, reflection
Owning	Control, acceptance, determination, self-help

Source: Easton, K. L. (2001). *The poststroke journey: From agonizing to owning.* Doctoral dissertation. Wayne State University. Detroit, MI: Author

TABLE 9-12 Summary of Major Survivor and Nursing Tasks for Each Phase of the Poststroke Journey		
Phase	**Survivor Task**	**Nursing Task**
Agonizing	Survival	Protection and physical care
Fantasizing	Ego protection	Reality orientation and emotional support
Realizing	Facing reality	Emotional and psychosocial support
Blending	Adaptation	Teaching
Framing	Reflection	Listening; providing reason for the stroke
Owning	Moving on	Enhancing inner and community resources

Source: Easton, K. L. (2001). *The poststroke journey: From agonizing to owning.* Doctoral dissertation. Wayne State University. Detroit, MI: Author.

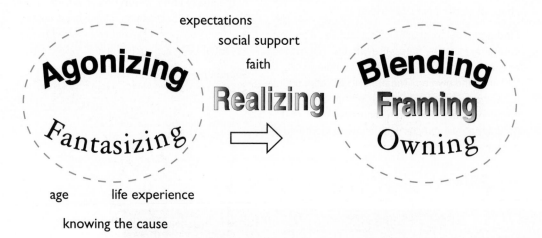

Figure 9-6 The Mauk model of poststroke recovery.

concepts and subconcepts of the model (see **Figure 9-6**) and the major tasks for survivors and nurses. Nursing diagnoses common to stroke rehabilitation appear in **Table 9-13.**

Stroke survivors maintained high expectations for recovery during the first 3 months (Anderson & Marlett, 2004; Rochette, Korner-Bitensky, & Lavasseur, 2006; Wiles, Ashburn, Payne, & Murphy, 2002, 2004). A study on motor stroke

TABLE 9-13 Common Problems Related to Stroke

Common Potential Nursing Diagnoses Related to Stroke	Common Medical Complications After Stroke
Activity intolerance	Depression
Aspiration, risk for	Deep vein thrombosis
Body image, disturbed	Dysphagia (sometimes resulting in aspiration)
Communication, impaired verbal	Pressure ulcers
Constipation, risk for	Neurogenic bowel
Coping, ineffective	Neurogenic bladder
Disuse syndrome, risk for	Shoulder subluxation
Fall, risk for	Spasticity
Fatigue	
Fear	
Grieving	
Hopelessness	
Injury, risk for	
Knowledge, deficiency	
Mobility: physical, impaired	
Nutrition, imbalanced: less than body requirements	
Self-care deficit: bathing/hygiene	
Self-care deficit: dressing/grooming	
Self-care deficit: feeding	
Self-care deficit: toileting	
Sensory perception, disturbed (tactile,visual)	
Sexual dysfunction	
Skin integrity, risk for impaired	
Social isolation	
Spiritual distress, risk for	
Tissue integrity, risk for impaired	
Tissue perfusion, ineffective, cerebral	
Unilateral neglect	
Urinary elimination, impaired	
Walking, impaired	

recovery showed that 3 years after motor stroke, function was stable, psychological outcomes were improved, and there was a low mortality rate (Hinkle, 2010). Rehabilitation was found to be helpful in stroke recovery. Realistic expectations should be based on current evidence (see **Box 9-3**) and can be reinforced by therapists and nurses. It is important to remember with less than optimal outcomes in the immediate months after stroke survival not to destroy hope of an increased quality of life.

Patient and Family Education

A large amount of teaching is often done by stroke rehabilitation nurses who work with older survivors. Training informal caregivers has been shown to improve quality of life for stroke survivors and their caregivers, and to decrease costs over time (Kalra et al., 2004). Many topics may need to be covered, depending on the extent of brain damage that has occurred. Some topics should be addressed with all survivors and their families. These include knowing the warning signs of stroke and how to activate the emergency response system in their neighborhood, managing high blood pressure, understanding what medications are ordered as well as how often to take them and why, the importance of regular doctor visits, preventing falls and making the home environment safe, available community education and support groups, and the necessity of maintaining a therapeutic regimen and lifestyle to decrease the risk of complications and recurrent stroke. All survivors will need assistance in re-integrating into the community. This is generally begun in the rehabilitation setting.

Family caregivers of stroke survivors must also deal with many issues. A classic study by Mumma (1986) revealed that stroke patients and their spouses perceived losses in such areas as mobility, traveling, the ability to do certain desired activities,

---

BOX 9-3 Evidence-Based Practice Highlight

The author implemented a research utilization project with 35 female stroke survivors in a free-standing rehabilitation facility. A control group of 35 patients discharged from the same facility and not receiving the educational intervention were used as a control group. The interdisciplinary team at the rehabilitation facility agreed to implement the following four interventions that were shown in the literature to provide best evidence for practice: (1) enhanced bladder history, (2) timed and prompted voiding, (3) bathroom training programs, and (4) pelvic floor exercises. The outcomes of the project showed the women who received the interventions showed a significantly higher mean FIM change in bladder FIM score than the control group. Consistent implementation of evidence-based practice in the area of bladder management with female stroke survivors resulted in better bladder management for patients.

Source: Cournan, M. (2012). Bladder management in female stroke survivors: Translating research into practice. *Rehabilitation Nursing, 37*(5), 220–230.

and independence. A study by Pierce, Gordon, and Steiner (2004) revealed that families dealing with stroke survivors identified five top self-care needs that they wished to have information about: preventing falls, maintaining adequate nutrition, staying active, managing stress, and dealing with emotional and mood changes. Conversely, nurses chose topics such as understanding the disease process, preventing pressure ulcers, demonstrating safe transfer technique, preventing aspiration, and dealing with communication and social interaction problems as being more important. These differing results demonstrate a need for teaching that goes beyond what is taught in the traditional hospital setting. Pierce, Steiner, and associates (2004) also found that using an Internet-based support group for rural caregivers produced positive responses and suggested common problems that caregivers face. These include such things as changing roles, problem solving, feeling connected with the family and survivor, using spirituality to cope, and balancing feelings of success in adapting with losses that have occurred. Other studies have supported the need for family caregivers to have extensive support as the stroke victim and his or her family members transition from the acute care setting to home (Cameron & Gignac, 2008; Lefebure, Levert, Pelchat, & Lepage, 2008; Steiner et al., 2008). Lutz and Young (2010) suggested that a systematic, comprehensive assessment be done of the family, patient, and caregiver, including examining resources and implementing case management across the continuum of care that also considers the needs and preferences of the caregiver in addition to the stroke survivor.

Outcomes for geriatric stroke survivors are enhanced by intensive rehabilitation programs, whether offered in rehabilitation units or in skilled nursing facilities (Duraski, Denby, Danzy & Sullivan, 2012; Jett, Warren, & Wirtalla, 2005). **Table 9-14** presents general approaches to care for stroke survivors. Generally, advanced age is considered to be a negative factor in recovery from stroke, but factors such as motivation and hope must also be considered in the rehabilitation process. In addition, much of the research literature regarding functional level of recovery after stroke suggests that return of function peaked and did not significantly progress much after the 3- to 6-month mark poststroke. However, emerging research suggests that survivors can and do continue to make improvements in daily function even years after a stroke (Duraski et al., 2012; Easton, 2001; Hinkle, 2010). Much of this improvement may be in the area of *instrumental activities of daily living (IADLs)*, or home activities that the survivor wished to resume after the stroke. New research out of the Cincinnati College of Medicine in Ohio suggests that even mental practice of upper arm mobility may have a significant and positive impact on a stroke survivor's ability to use the affected upper limb (Morris, 2006; Page, Levine, & Leonard, 2005). Many survivors will continue to benefit from outpatient therapies in occupational therapy, physical therapy, and/or speech therapy. Some will need referral to vocational counseling if they wish to return to work. Others may need to follow up with an orthotist for splints or other orthotic devices.

TABLE 9-14   General Approaches to Traditional Nursing of the Stroke Survivor

Common Characteristics Associated with Stroke of Either Side	Right Hemisphere Stroke	Left Hemisphere Stroke
When working with the patient, encourage use of the affected side to reduce neglect.	Foster a calm and unhurried care environment.	Speak slowly and distinctly. Use simple sentences for those with aphasia.
When the person is alone, place items (such as the call light, tissues, and other personal items) on the unaffected side to promote self-care and safety and to avoid isolation.	Break tasks into simple steps.	Encourage all forms of communication.
Use a variety of teaching modalities during educational sessions to promote learning.	Be especially attentive to safety issues that may arise from poor judgment and lack of safety awareness. Protect the patient from injury.	Use a variety of communication techniques: gesturing, cues, pointing, writing, communication boards, yes/no questions (if appropriate). Find what is most effective for each person.
Minimize distractions during educational sessions. Keep these teaching items short and relevant.	Be alert for possible deficits that may not be overt. Avoid overstimulation.	Allow time for the person to respond to questions.
Use terms such as affected/unaffected side or weak/strong side instead of good/bad.		Provide teaching in a quiet, structured environment. Monitor the patient for swallowing difficulties.
Use critical pathways or care plans to promote consistency of care, but remember that each survivor is unique and be sure to adapt nursing care accordingly.		Promote a positive self-image by attention to good grooming, personal hygiene, and positive reinforcement.
Alternate rest and activity.		
Build endurance slowly. Remember that a stroke is exhausting to the entire body.		
Include the person and family in the plan of care.		
Assist the patient and family in setting reasonable goals.		

Common Characteristics Associated with Stroke of Either Side	Right Hemisphere Stroke	Left Hemisphere Stroke
Make early referrals to stroke services or the specialized stroke team.		
Connect the family with a stroke support group or club.		
Use a discharge follow-up plan.		

Source: Adapted from Easton, 1999, p. 196, with permission of author.

Peripheral Artery Disease (PAD)

Background/Significance

Peripheral artery disease (PAD), the most common type of peripheral vascular disease (PVD), affects 8–12 million Americans, 12–20% of those over the age of 65, and could reach as many as 9.6 million Americans by the year 2050 (Cleveland Clinic, 2013).

Risk Factors/Warning Signs

The risk factors for PAD are the same as those for CHD, with diabetes and smoking being the greatest risk factors (AHA, 2011). According to the American Heart Association, only 25% of those older adults with PAD get treatment.

Assessment/Diagnosis

The most common symptoms of PAD are leg cramps that worsen when climbing stairs or walking, but dissipate with rest, commonly called intermittent claudication (IC). The majority of persons with PAD have no symptoms (AHA, 2005). PAD is a predictor of CHD and makes a person more at risk for heart attack and stroke. Left untreated, PAD may eventually lead to impaired function and decreased quality of life, even when no leg symptoms are present. In the most serious cases, PAD can lead to gangrene and amputation of a lower extremity.

Interventions

Most cases of PAD can be managed with lifestyle modifications such as those discussed previously for heart-healthy living. Nurses should also encourage patients with PAD to discuss their symptoms with both their healthcare provider and a physical therapist, because some patients find symptom relief through a combination of medical and therapy treatments (Aronow, 2007; Cleveland Clinic, 2013).

Respiratory Problems

Respiratory problems are common among older adults and a leading contributor to mortality and morbidity. This section will present information on pneumonia, chronic obstructive pulmonary diseases (COPDs), and tuberculosis. There are many nursing interventions to enhance quality of life for older adults with breathing problems. These will also be reviewed.

Pneumonia

Background

According to the CDC (2010), chronic lower respiratory disease and pneumonia with influenza are the third and ninth leading causes of death, respectively, among older adults. Adults 65 years and older were disproportionately affected by these disorders as compared to younger adults; the risk of mortality increases with age. A study using data from the National Hospital Discharge Survey concluded that the rates of hospitalization between 1988 and 2002 for pneumonia in older adults ≥85 years increased to about 1 in 20 patients (Fry et al., 2005). In 2005 there were 651,000 hospital discharges of males diagnosed with pneumonia and 717,000 discharges of females, with greater than 62,000 deaths attributed to pneumonia (American Lung Association [ALA], 2008). The majority of these cases occurred in those age 65 and older, with this population having 5–10 times the risk of death from pneumonia as younger adults (Kennedy-Malone, Fletcher, & Plank, 2004).

Pneumonia is infection of the lung parenchyma that can be caused by a variety of organisms including bacteria, viruses, and mycoplasmas (Weinberger, 2004; ALA, 2012b). The two most common pathways through which microorganisms invade the lung are inhalation of droplet particles carrying infectious pathogens and aspiration of oropharyngeal secretions (Weinberger et al., 2004). Older adults are considered at particularly high risk for pneumonia with a significantly increased risk for serious infection when they have comorbidities such as chronic obstructive lung disease, heart failure, immunosuppression, cerebrovascular disease, and poor mobility (ALA, 2012a; Weinberger, 2004). The incidence of community-acquired pneumonia (CAP) among older adults (≥65 years) is about 221.3 per 10,000 (ALA, 2008). When bacteria are the cause, the most common pathogen is *Streptococcus* with about 50% of people with CAP requiring hospitalization (ALA, 2012b; Weinberger, 2004). When hospitalized this population is at risk for poor health outcomes including respiratory failure requiring ventilator support; sepsis; and longer length of hospitalization, duration of antibiotic therapy, and other supportive treatment (ALA, 2012b).

Risk Factors/Warning Signs

The onset of bacterial pneumonia can be sudden or gradual; however, older adults may not present with typical symptoms of chills, fever, chest pain, sweating, productive cough, or dyspnea and instead they may have acute alerted mental status (confusion/delirium). Cases of viral pneumonia account for about half of all types of pneumonia and tend to be less severe than bacterial pneumonia. Symptoms of viral pneumonia include fever, nonproductive hacking cough, muscle pain, weakness, and shortness of breath.

Assessment and Diagnosis

Diagnosis is made through chest X-ray, complete blood count, and/or sputum culture to determine the type and causal agents (if bacterial). A thorough history and physical that includes assessment of dentition, swallowing ability, and eating (watch for coughing while eating) to evaluate for aspiration risk should be done. Crackles may be heard in the lungs through auscultation, and chest pain with shortness of breath may be present.

Interventions

Bacterial pneumonia can often be treated successfully when detected early, and viral pneumonia generally heals on its own (antibiotics are not effective if pneumonia is caused by a virus), though older adults may experience a greater risk of complications than younger adults. Oral antibiotics will significantly help most patients with bacterial pneumonia, and even though many older persons may require hospitalization, intravenous (IV) antibiotics have not been shown to be necessarily more effective than oral types, with IV treatment resulting in longer hospital stays and more hospital-acquired problems (Loeb, 2002).

Aspiration pneumonia is caused by inhalation of a foreign material, such as fluids or food, into the lungs. This occurs more often in persons with impaired swallowing (see Chapter 17 for a discussion on dysphagia), those who have esophageal reflux disease, or who are unconscious. One particular danger to which nurses should be alert is those older adults receiving tube feedings. Care must be taken to avoid having the person in a laying position during and immediately after tube feeding because aspiration can occur; it is important to note that tube feedings do not reduce the risk of aspiration. Having the head of the bed elevated or, even better, the person in a sitting position when eating or receiving enteral nutrition helps to avoid the potential complication of pneumonia related to aspiration.

When recovering from pneumonia, the older adult should be encouraged to get plenty of rest and take adequate fluids to help loosen secretions (with accommodations made to support the added need to urinate due to the increased fluid intake, a common reason why older adults may not drink adequate fluids). Tylenol or aspirin (if not contraindicated by other conditions) can be taken to manage fever as well as aches and pains. Exposure to others with contagious respiratory conditions should be avoided. Respiratory complications are often what lead to death in the older adults, so they should be cautioned to report any changes in respiratory status such as increased shortness of breath, high fever, or any other symptoms that do not improve. Symptoms typically resolve before radiographic resolution of the infiltrate (what would be seen on the chest X-ray), so it is important to follow up with a chest X-ray to assure resolution of the pneumonia.

Prevention of pneumonia is always best. Adults over the age of 65 are advised to get a pneumonia vaccine (pneumococcal polysaccharide vaccine, or PPV), although its effectiveness may be somewhat diminished in higher risk groups than in healthy adults (ALA, 2008). This vaccine is generally given one time, though sometimes a revaccination is recommended after about 6 years for older adults with higher risk. A yearly flu vaccine is also recommended for older adults, because pneumonia is a common complication of influenza in this age group. Medicare will cover these vaccines for older persons, so cost should not be a prohibiting factor in prevention.

Chronic Obstructive Pulmonary Disease

Background

Chronic obstructive pulmonary disease (COPD) refers to a group of diseases resulting in airflow obstruction due to smoking, environmental exposures, and genetics. However, smoking is clearly the most common cause of COPD. The two disorders most commonly included under the umbrella of COPD are *emphysema* and *chronic bronchitis*. Although the pathophysiological mechanisms contributing to airflow obstruction is different in these two disorders, most patients demonstrate features of both emphysema and chronic bronchitis.

In 2008, the CDC released a report naming COPD as the third leading cause of death in the United States (Minino, Xu, and Kochanek, 2008). There are more than 12 million people in the United States diagnosed with COPD. However, due to the underdiagnosis of the disease, only estimations of the prevalence of COPD are available, which suggest that approximately 24 million people are living with COPD (ALA, 2012). Slightly more females than males are affected, with female smokers having a 13 times greater chance of death from COPD than nonsmoking females (ALA, 2004).

Chronic Bronchitis

Chronic bronchitis is a common COPD among older adults. It results from recurrent inflammation and mucus production in the bronchial tubes. Repeated infections produce blockage from mucus and eventual scarring that restricts airflow. The American Lung Association (2012a) stated that about 8.5 million Americans had been diagnosed with chronic bronchitis as of 2005. Females are twice as likely as males to have this problem.

Emphysema

Emphysema results when the alveoli in the lungs are irreversibly destroyed. As the lungs lose elasticity, air becomes trapped in the alveolar sacs, resulting in carbon dioxide retention and impaired gas exchange. More males than females are affected with emphysema, and most (91%) of the 3.8 million Americans with this disease are over the age of 45 (ALA, 2004).

Risk Factors/Warning Signs

The major risk factor for COPD is smoking, which causes 80–90% of COPD deaths. Other risk factors appear in **Table 9-15**. Alpha-1-antitrypsin deficiency is a rare cause of COPD, but can be ruled out through blood tests. Although "COPD is almost 100% preventable by avoidance of smoking" (Kennedy-Malone et al., 2003), environmental factors play a strong role in the incidence of COPD. Approximately 19.2% of people with COPD can link the cause to work exposure, and 31.7% have never smoked (ALA, 2008).

The signs and symptoms of chronic bronchitis include increased mucus production, shortness of breath, wheezing, decreased breath sounds, and chronic productive cough. Chronic bronchitis can lead to emphysema. Signs and symptoms of emphysema include shortness of breath, decreased exercise tolerance, and cough.

TABLE 9-15   Risk Factors for COPD
Smoking
Air pollution
Second-hand smoke
Heredity
History of respiratory infections
Industrial pollutants
Environmental pollutants
Excessive alcohol consumption
Genetic component (alpha-1-antitrypsin deficiency)

Assessment and Diagnosis

Persons with COPD often experience a decrease in quality of life as the disease progresses. The shortness of breath so characteristic of these diseases impairs the ability to work and do usual activities. According to a survey by the American Lung Association (2004), "half of all COPD patients (51%) say their condition limits their ability to work [and] limits them in normal physical exertion (70%), household chores (56%), social activities (53%), sleeping (50%), and family activities (46%)" (p. 3). Diagnosis is made through pulmonary function and other tests, a thorough history, and a physical.

Interventions

Although there are no easy cures for COPD, older adults can take several measures to improve their quality of life by controlling symptoms and minimizing complications. These include lifestyle modifications such as smoking cessation, medications (see below), oxygen therapy, and pulmonary rehabilitation (see **Table 9-16**). Older adults should have influenza and pneumonia vaccinations (National Heart Lung and Blood Institute, [NHLBI], 2010). Oxygen therapy is required in those individuals demonstrating hypoxemia based on resting, nocturnal, and ambulatory oximetry readings.

Medications are used to help control symptoms, but they do not change the downward trajectory of COPD that occurs over time as lung function worsens. Typical medications given regularly include bronchodilators through oral or inhaled routes. Antibiotics may be given to fight infections and systemic steroids for acute exacerbations.

In extreme cases, lung transplantation or lung volume reduction surgery may be indicated. Older persons with severely impaired lung function related to emphysema may be at higher risk of death from these procedures and have poorer outcomes.

Nurses working with older adults with COPD will find it challenging to assist them with a home maintenance program that addresses their unique needs with this chronic disease. Teaching should involve the patient and family and should plan for the long term. Reducing factors that contribute to symptoms, medication usage, alternating rest and activity, energy conservation, stress management, relaxation, and the

TABLE 9-16 Strategies for Symptom Management for Older Adults with COPD

Do not smoke.
Avoid second-hand smoke.
Avoid air pollutants and other lung irritants.
Exercise regularly as tolerated or prescribed.
Maintain proper nutrition.
Maintain adequate hydration—especially water intake.
Take medications as ordered: bronchodilators (antibiotics and steroids for exacerbations).
Use energy conservation techniques.
Alternate activities and rest.
Learn and regularly use breathing exercises.
Learn stress management and relaxation techniques.
Recognize the role of supplemental oxygen.
Receive yearly pneumonia and influenza vaccines to avoid serious infections.
Investigate pulmonary rehabilitation programs.
Join a support group for those with breathing problems and their families.
Explore any possible surgical options with the physician.

role of supplemental oxygen should all be addressed. Many older adults with COPD find it helpful to join a support group for those who are living with similar problems.

Tuberculosis

Background

Tuberculosis (TB), caused by *Mycobacterium tuberculosis*, is a contagious infection that involves the lungs but can attack any part of the body. Primary TB is caused by inhalation of air droplets from an infected person through coughing, sneezing, laughing, or other activities in which particles become airborne (NCBI, 2011). Older adults and immuno-compromised persons are at the greatest risks. According to the CDC's Morbidity and Mortality Weekly Report [MMWR] (2012b), the incidence of TB in 2011 has declined by 6.4% since 2010. There are a reported 3.4 cases per 100,000 populations in the United States, which translates to about 10,521 new TB cases in 2011. However, data continue to point to a trend of foreign-born or racial/ethnic minorities being disproportionately affected by TB compared to U.S.-born persons. This gap is continuing to widen despite an overall decreased number of cases in both groups (CDC, 2012b). The AIDS epidemic has contributed to the spread of TB, particularly in less developed countries; this may be due to the suppression of the immune system that is associated with AIDS.

Risk Factors/Warning Signs

Nursing home residents are considered an at-risk group due to the typically higher rates found in this population. General guidelines from the Advisory Committee for

Elimination of Tuberculosis (Centers for Disease Control and Prevention [CDC], 1990) set a concrete strategy for prevention and management of TB in nursing homes to decrease the spread among this institutionalized and vulnerable population. Thus, older adults who may be discharged from acute care facilities to a nursing home will generally undergo TB skin testing prior to discharge.

Screening for TB is simple and can be done at the local health department, clinic, or doctor's office. A Mantoux test is an intradermal injection that is read for results 48–72 hours after administration. A result of 11 mm or greater of induration (not redness, but swelling) is considered a positive result. It is recommended that older adults undergo a two-step screening wherein the test is given again, because there are many false results in the older adults. A positive TB skin test should be followed up with a chest X-ray to rule out active disease.

It must be noted that persons who received a vaccine for TB may have a positive reaction. A TB vaccine is commonly given in many countries outside the United States.

A person can be infected with TB and have no symptoms; this means they may have a positive skin test, but cannot spread the disease. Such a person can develop TB later if left untreated. Those with active TB can spread the disease to others and should be treated by a physician or other healthcare provider. The signs and symptoms of TB appear in **Table 9-17**.

Assessment and Diagnosis

For older adults born in the United States, a positive skin test may prompt the healthcare provider to initiate preventative treatment. The medication isoniazid (INH) is generally given to kill the TB bacteria. Treatment with INH often lasts at least 6 months. Few adults have side effects from the medication, but those that are possible include nausea, vomiting, jaundice, fever, abdominal pain, and decreased appetite. Patients taking INH should be cautioned not to drink alcohol while on the medication.

TABLE 9-17   Signs and Symptoms of Tuberculosis
A severe cough that lasts more than 2 weeks
Chest pain
Bloody sputum
Weakness
Fatigue
Weight loss
*Chills
*Fever
*Night sweats

*May not be present in the elderly.
Source: CDC, 2008.

Interventions

Patients with active TB can be cured, but the medication regimen is complex, with several different drugs taken in combination. Caution should be taken to avoid spread of the disease. This generally means isolation for patients in the hospital with active TB. In 1998, the FDA approved a new medication, rifapentine (Priftin), to be used with other drugs for TB. Medications should be strictly taken for the entire period of time (many months) to kill all of the bacteria. Older adults may need assistance with keeping track of these medications; evaluation of medication management should be included in the assessment. The use of a medication box set up by another competent and informed family member to ensure compliance with the medication regimen may be helpful, because it can be overwhelming for some persons. Adequate rest, nutrition, and hydration, as well as breathing exercises, may help with combating the effects of TB. Since over half of all patients with actively diagnosed TB have come to the United States from other countries, language may be a barrier. Education requires understanding and may necessitate an interpreter to ensure understanding of the complex regimens required to eradicate the bacteria.

Gastrointestinal Disorders

Gastrointestinal problems are among the most frequent complaints of older adults. Several common disorders will be discussed here, including gastroesophageal reflux, peptic ulcer, *diverticulitis*, constipation, and several types of cancers.

Gastroesophageal Reflux Disease

Background/Significance

Although *gastroesophageal reflux disease (GERD)* is common among older adults, the true prevalence is not known, as many patients with GERD-related symptoms never discuss their problems with their primary care provider. GERD is thought to occur in 5–7% of the world's population, with 21 million Americans affected (International Foundations for Functional Gastrointestinal Disorders, 2008), and is found in both men and women.

Risk Factors/Warning Signs

Pathophysiological changes that occur in the esophagus (reduced lower esophageal pressure and length, impaired motility of the esophagus, and reduced salivary secretion), hiatus hernia, and certain medications and foods increase the risk for GERD. Obesity and activities that increase intra-abdominal pressure such as wearing tight clothes, bending over, or heavy lifting have also been linked to GERD (MedlinePlus, 2005). The cardinal symptom of GERD is heartburn; however, older adults may not present with this, but rather complain of atypical symptoms such as pulmonary conditions (bronchial asthma, chronic cough, or chronic bronchitis), otorhinolaryngeal problems (hoarseness, pain when swallowing foods, or chronic laryngitis), or noncardiac chest pain (Pilotto & Franceschi, 2009). GERD can result in chronic mucosal inflammation with erosive esophagitis and ulceration, which can be further complicated by strictures and bleeding (Pilotto & Franceschi, 2009). The chronic backflow of acid into the esophagus can lead to abnormal cell development (Barrett esophagus) that increases the risk for esophageal adenocarcinoma. Therefore, it is essential that nurses consider atypical presentations of GERD when caring for older adults.

Assessment and Diagnosis

Older adults often present with atypical symptoms, making the diagnosis of GERD very challenging. As people age the severity of heartburn can diminish, while the complications, such as erosive esophagitis, become more frequent. Therefore, endoscopy should be considered as one of the initial diagnostic tests in older adults who are suspected of having GERD (Pilotto & Franceschi, 2009). Examination of the esophagus, stomach, and duodenum through a fiber-optic scope (endoscopy) while the person receives conscious sedation allows the gastroenterologist to visualize the entire area, identify suspicious areas, and obtain biopsies as needed. *Helicobacter pylori*, a chronic bacterial infection in humans, is a common cause of GERD, affecting about 30% to 40% of the U.S. population. Testing for *H. pylori* can be done during the endoscopy or by urea breath testing or stool antigen testing (Ferri, 2011).

Interventions

The objectives of treatment include: (1) relief of symptoms, (2) healing of esophagitis, (3) prevention of further occurrences, and (4) prevention of complications (Pilotto & Francheschi, 2009). Lifestyle and dietary modifications are important aspects of care. The nurse should recommend smoking cessation; limiting or avoiding alcohol; and limiting chocolate, coffee, and fatty or citrus foods. Medications should be reviewed and offending medications modified, as certain medications decrease the lower esophageal sphincter (LES), allowing acid to backflow into the esophagus. These include anticholinergic drugs, some hormones, calcium channel blockers, and theophylline. Avoidance of food or beverages 3–4 hours prior to bedtime, weight loss, and elevation of the head of the bed on 6-to-8 inch blocks are some other interventions that may help alleviate symptoms. Pharmacological treatments with antacids in conjunction with *histamine 2 (H2) blockers* (Tagmet, Zantac, Axid, and Pepcid) are used for mild GERD. If these are ineffective in controlling symptoms, then the *proton pump inhibitors (PPIs)* are the next drugs of choice, which include

---

BOX 9-4   Resources for Those with GERD

American College of Gastroenterology (ACG)
   4900-B South 31st Street
   Arlington, VA 22206-1656
   703-820-7400
   http://www.acg.gi.org

American Gastroenterological Association (AGA)
   4930 Del Ray Avenue
   Bethesda, MD 20814
   301-654-2055
   http://www.gastro.org

omeprazole, lansoprazole, rabeprazole, pantoprazole, and esomeprazole. The H2 blockers are often prescribed twice a day and the PPIs once a day; however, sometimes these may be ordered twice daily. These medications should be taken on an empty stomach. Laparoscopic fundoplication surgery, although controversial, may be indicated in adults who fail treatments and have severe complications.

Peptic Ulcer Disease

Background/Significance

Each year, about 5 million people in the United States are affected by peptic ulcer disease (PUD), with about 12% occurrence in those over age 75 years and 9.6% in people ages 65–74. The overall trend for incidence of PUD has been declining in young men; however, the opposite is true for older women (Anand, 2013). Early identification and treatment is important, because about 25% of people with PUD have serious complications such hemorrhage, perforation, or gastric outlet obstruction (Ramakrishnam & Salinas, 2007). Ulcers are a common cause for hospitalizations for upper gastrointestinal (GI) bleeding in the United States (Laine & Jensen, 2012). Upper GI bleeds occur in about 15 to 20% of adults, with about 20% of episodes in older adults occurring with no symptoms of the disease. Although a small percentage of people experience perforation the risk of death is high in older adults when it does occur (Martinez & Mattu, 2006).

Risks/Warning Signs

The most common causes of PUD are *H. pylori* infection and use of nonsteriodal anti-inflammatory drugs (NSAIDS). Other risk factors include smoking, drinking alcohol, caffeine, and stress. In hospitalized adults, critical illness, surgery, or hyporvolemia contribute to development of an ulcer (Ramakrishnam & Salinas, 2007). The most common symptom is dyspepsia (indigestion), which can classified as ulcer-like or food-provoked. Ulcer-like is the most common and is manifested by burning pain and epigastric, hunger-like pain that is relieved with food, antacids, and/or medications classified as antisecretory agents. Patients with food-provoked dyspepsia may present with epigastric discomfort and fullness after eating a meal, belching, early satiety, nausea, and occasional vomiting. These symptoms can overlap (Soll, 2011). Older adults may experience "silent" PUD, which makes it difficult to identify before complications occur (Barkun & Leontiadis, 2010).

Assessment and Diagnosis

The diagnosis is made through the history and physical. The typical symptoms are episodic gnawing or burning epigastric pain, often occurring 2 to 5 hours after meals. The older adult should be evaluated for anemia, hematemesis, melena, or heme-positive stool suggesting a GI bleed. Vomiting is suggestive of an obstruction, weight loss and anorexia of cancer, and persistent upper abdominal pain radiating to the back may indicate perforation. Adults 55 years and older presenting with any of these symptoms should promptly be referred to a gastroenterologist for further evaluation. Patients should be tested for *H. pylori* with a urea breath test, stool antigen test, or endoscopic biopsy. When there are acute problems, such as a GI bleed, older adults may have an atypical presentation of acute confusion, restlessness, abdominal distention, and falls (Ramakrishnam & Salinas, 2007).

Interventions

The treatment depends on the cause. If *H. pylori* is present, then eradication with antibiotics and antisecretory therapy for about 10 to 14 days is indicated. Administration of proton pump inhibitors (PPIs), bismuth, many antibiotics, and an upper GI bleed can lead to false-negatives. It is essential to address risk factors, as stated above (Ramakrishnam & Salinas, 2007). If the person is taking NSAIDs for pain, discuss alternatives such as acetaminophen and nonpharmacological treatments. Lifestyle modifications such as avoidance of late meals, elevation of head of bed, weight loss in overweight or obese people, smoking cessation, and avoidance of recumbency for 2 to 3 hours after meals (American Gastroenterology Association [AGA], 2008) should be taught. Medications, such as PPIs or histamine H2-receptor blockers, are used to heal an ulcer. If for some reason aspirin or NSAID cannot be discontinued, use of a PPI is more effective. Prevention should always be reinforced; it is important to identify those at risk (previous ulcer, use of NSAIDS, anticoagulant therapy, over 70 years of age, *H. pylori* infection, and use of oral corticosteroids) and then use PPIs and educate the person about prevention measures (Lockrey & Lim, 2011).

Diverticulitis

Background/Significance

Diverticulitis is an inflammation or infection of the pouches of the intestinal mucosa (see **Figure 9-7**). Diverticular disease is more common among older adults than younger people (Tursi, 2007). Sixty-five percent of older adults will develop diverticulosis ("pouches of the intestinal mucosa in the weakened muscle wall of the large bowel" [Eliopoulos, 2005, p. 321]) by 85, with some going on to develop diverticulitis (Kennedy-Malone et al., 2004). The exact cause of diverticulosis is not known, but it is speculated that a diet low in fiber and high in refined foods causes the stool bulk to decrease, leading to increased colon transit time. Retention of undigested foods and bacteria results in a hard mass that can disrupt blood flow and lead to abscess formation. The earlier the diagnosis and treatment, the better the outcomes will be; however, complications such as bleeding increase the risk of less-than-optimal outcomes.

Risks/Warning Signs

Risk factors for diverticulosis include obesity, chronic constipation, straining, irregular and uncoordinated bowel contractions, and weakness of bowel muscle due to aging. Other risk factors are directly related to the suspected cause of the condition; these include older than 40 years of age, low-fiber diet, and the number of diverticula in the colon (Thomas, 2011). Diverticulosis can present with pain in the left lower quadrant (LLQ), can get worse after eating, and may improve after a bowel movement. Warning signs of diverticulitis include fever, increased white blood cell count, bleeding that is not associated with pain, tachycardia, nausea, and vomiting.

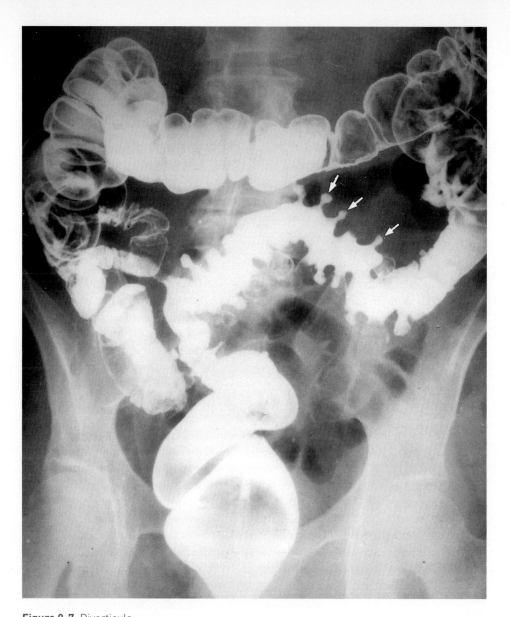

Figure 9-7 Diverticula.

Source: Leonard Crowley, *Introduction to Human Disease* (6th ed.). Sudbury, MA: Jones & Bartlett Publishers, 2005.

Assessment and Diagnosis

Evaluation of the abdomen may reveal tenderness in the LLQ and there may be rebound tenderness with involuntary guarding and rigidity. Bowel sounds may be initially hypoactive and can be hyperactive if the obstruction has passed. Stool may be heme-positive. The initial evaluation is abdominal X-ray films, followed by a barium enema, though a CT scan with oral contrast is more accurate in diagnosing (Thomas, 2011). A complete blood count should be obtained to assess for infection and anemia.

Interventions

Diverticulosis is managed with a high-fiber diet or daily fiber supplementation with psyllium. Diverticulitis is treated with antibiotics, but in acute illness the person may require hospitalization for IV hydration, analgesics, bowel rest, and possible NG tube placement. Morphine sulfate should be avoided because it increases the intraluminal pressures within the colon, causing the symptoms to get worse (Thomas, 2011). In some cases, either where the person has complications that do not resolve with medical management or has several repeated episodes, a colon resection may be needed. Patient education should include information about diet, avoidance of constipation and straining during bowel movements, and when to seek medical care. The diet should include fresh fruits, vegetables, whole grains, and increased fluid intake, unless contraindicated.

Constipation

Background/Significance

Constipation is the most common bowel problem in older adults. The definition varies by patients and healthcare providers, but the ROME III criteria for chronic constipation provide a definition based on symptoms. Constipation is a preventable and treatable problem that requires identification of the risk factors (see **Table 9-18**) to reduce the occurrence of complications. Some of the complications that can occur include fecal incontinence, fecal impaction, urinary retention, rectal prolapse, diverticular disease, and impaired quality of life (Harari, 2009).

Risks/Warning Signs

Constipation is often multifactorial, with causes that can include a combination of systemic or local conditions. Some of the risk factors include impaired mobility, medications (anticholinergics, analgesics, iron supplements, and calcium supplements), depression, neurological conditions (dementia, Parkinson's disease, stroke, diabetes mellitus, and spinal cord injury), dehydration, low dietary fiber, metabolic disturbances (hypothyroidism, hypercalcemia, hypokalemia, and uremia), undergoing dialysis, mechanical obstruction, and decreased access to toilet (Harari, 2009). Warning signs include constipation with a family history of colon cancer, rectal bleeding, unexplained anemia, weight loss, or narrowed caliber of stool (Ham, Sloane, Warshaw, Bernard, & Flaherty, 2007).

TABLE 9-18   Factors to Consider in Bowel Management

Uncontrollable Factors	Controllable Factors
Family history	Diet
Presence of neurogenic bowel	Fiber
	Fluids
Existence of prior bowel disease	Timing
	Activity
	Positioning
	Medications

Assessment and Diagnosis

Nurses should include assessment of bowel elimination that focuses on predisposing causes. History should include all over-the-counter medications, diet and fluid intake, and physical activity. Other assessments include psychosocial, mental health (mood), cognitive, and laboratory studies (CBC, electrolytes, glucose, and thyroid profile). The diagnosis is based on clinical presentation and physical examination. It is important to determine the onset and duration of the constipation, along with functional and nutritional status. Abdominal assessment and rectal exam should include checking stool for occult blood.

Interventions

Initial interventions should focus on lifestyle and dietary modifications (see **Table 9-19**). Bulk agents (e.g., psyllium, methylcellulose) should be considered for those who do not respond to lifestyle changes, and for those who do not respond to bulking agents, osmotic laxatives (e.g., lactulose, sorbitol) should be considered. Residents of nursing homes appear to respond to stimulant laxatives (e.g., senna, bisacodyl). Enemas should not be used on a regular basis and should be reserved for those who do not respond to treatments or who have evidence of fecal impaction. Nonpharmacological interventions include regular exercise, establishment of a regular routine for toileting (assure privacy), and encouragement of a high-fiber diet with adequate fluid intake (unless contraindicated).

TABLE 9-19 Principles of Bowel Programs to Prevent Constipation
• Start with a clean bowel. (Administer needed medications or enemas to cleanse the bowel prior to initiating a program or protocol.)
• Try all-natural means first: fiber, fluids, activity, timing, positioning.
• Be sure the person is taking adequate fiber and fluids before adding medications.
• Change only one item at a time in the program. Allow several days to pass before evaluating the effectiveness of the change. If needed, add another intervention.
• Stool softeners are given for hardened stool, and the person must drink at least a liter of fluid per day for them to be effective.
• Peristaltic stimulators are useful when the person is unable to move the stool down into the rectum.
• Use the least caustic type of suppository that is effective for the older person.
• Avoid the use of bedpans—have the person sit upright on the toilet or commode.
• Avoid the regular use of enemas.

Cancers

Aging is a major risk factor for cancer. Cancer is the second-leading cause of death after heart disease. Esophageal, stomach, colorectal, and pancreatic cancers will be discussed here, but a more thorough discussion of care of the older adult with cancer is provided in Chapter 30.

Colorectal

Background/Significance

Colorectal (CRC) cancer is the second most commonly diagnosed cancer and the second leading cause of mortality in the United States (Richardson, Tai & Rim, 2011) yet the most curable form of cancer if the disease is localized to the bowel (National Cancer Institute, 2008). The vast majority of this type of cancer is adenocarcinoma arising from colonic polyps. Although most polyps do not become malignant, the risk of cancer increases as the polyp size increases (Edwards, 2002). Strong evidence supports that screening for CRC can reduce the incidence and the risk of mortality (Richardson et al., 2011).

Risks/Warning Signs

Risk factors include a first-degree relative with colorectal cancer, age 50 or older, hereditary disease such familial polyposis, and a history of ulcerative colitis or Crohn's disease. Other risk factors are high-fat diet, alcohol consumption, cigarette smoking, sedentary lifestyle, and exposure to environmental toxins. Warning signs such as abdominal pain, palpable mass in lower right quadrant, anemia, and dark red or mahogany-colored blood mixed in the stools are indicative of tumors of right colon. Manifestations of tumors on the left include progressive abdominal distention, pain, vomiting, constipation, and bright red blood on the surface of the stool (McCance, Huether, Brashers, & Rote, 2010).

Assessment and Diagnosis

The nurse should evaluate bowel elimination patterns when obtaining the history to determine if there has been a change. According to the American Cancer Society, screening recommendations are based on the level of risk. Those with an average risk should begin screening at age 50 years with an annual fecal occult blood test and flexible signmoidoscopy every 5 years or colonoscopy every 10 years. People at a high risk should have a colonoscopy every 3–5 years starting at age 40.

Interventions

Educate older adults about the risks of colorectal cancer and recommend screening as appropriate. Teach them how to lower their risks by maintaining a diet that is high in grains, fruits, and vegetables, and low in processed red meats; replacing

Vitamin D when deficient; adding calcium and folic acid supplements; avoiding excessive alcohol; and increasing their physical activity.

Gastric (Stomach)

Background/Significance

Despite a decline in the incidence of stomach cancer, this condition comprises about 2% (21,230) of all new cancers and causes about 10,540 deaths each year (American Cancer Society, 2012e). The average age of diagnosis is 70 years; approximately two-thirds of people with stomach cancer are age 65 or older. There is a greater incidence among men than in women, as well as in Hispanics, African Americans, and Asian/Pacific Islanders as compared to Caucasians (American Cancer Society, 2005). If detected early, there is a good prognosis, but once a tumor has advanced, patients may quickly deteriorate.

Risks/Warning Signs

There are several risk factors for stomach cancer. *H. pylori* appears to be the major cause, especially in the distal aspect of the stomach. People who have been treated for mucosa-associated lymphoid tissue (MALT) lymphoma have an increased risk, which may be related to *H. pylori* bacteria. Consumption of large amounts of smoked foods, salted fish and meat, and picked vegetables; smoking cigarettes (particularly of the upper portion of the stomach); obesity (not strong link); previous gastric surgeries; pernicious anemia; blood type A; and family history of gastric adenocarcinoma are other risk factors (American Cancer Society, 2012e). Patients may not have signs of the cancer until later in the disease, when the prognosis is poor.

Assessment and Diagnosis

Early in the disease patients may be asymptomatic or experience vague symptoms such as loss of appetite (especially for meat), malaise, and "indigestion." As the disease progresses, they may have unintentional weight loss, upper abdominal pain, vomiting, change in bowel habits, and anemia due to occult bleeding (McCance et al., 2010). Diagnostic tests will depend on the symptoms the person is experiencing. The best way to diagnose is by performing an EGD so there is direct visualization and the ability to obtain a biopsy.

Interventions

Surgery is the standard treatment for gastric cancers. Nurses can help with primary prevention of stomach cancer by educating older adults about how to reduce risks and identify early symptoms. Dietary changes are a significant way to reduce risks; a diet lower in red meats and higher in antioxidants has a protective effect (American Cancer Society, 2012e). In addition, weight loss and smoking cessation may also be beneficial. Encourage regular physical exams and reporting of suspicious symptoms, as early testing can help decrease the risk of mortality.

Esophagus

Background/Significance

The risk of cancer of the esophagus increases as a person ages; in 2005–2009, the median age at diagnosis was 68 years of age, while 69 years was the average age of death (Howlader et al., 2009). The two most common types of cancers of the esophagus are adenocarcinoma, followed by squamous cell carcinoma. Early detection is key because the prognosis for either type is relatively poor.

Risks/Warning Signs

Squamous cell carcinoma is associated with malnutrition. This can be related to lower socioeconomic status, poor dietary habits, alcoholism, tobacco use, obesity, radiation exposures, and chronic GERD (American Gastroenterology Association, 2008). Adenocarcinoma is related to reflux esophagitis and hiatal hernia; these both can cause erosive esophagitis and ulcerations, which can lead to Barrett esophagus and cancer (McCance et al., 2010). The most common warning sign is heartburn initiated by spicy or highly seasoned foods.

Assessment and Diagnosis

The nurse should assess for heartburn after eating spicy foods and when lying down. Dysphagia that can present as pressure-like and may radiate to the back between the scapulae is another common symptom. In older adults, symptoms may not appear until the cancer advanced, when the cancer has most likely metastasized. Older adults with dysphagia should undergo an EGD.

Interventions

Nurses can initiate primary prevention by encouraging smoking cessation and limitation of alcohol intake (a maximum of one drink per day for females and two for males). Older adults should be educated about risk factors and when to notify healthcare professionals of symptoms that may warrant further evaluation.

Pancreas

Background/Significance

The incidence of pancreatic cancer has increased over the past few years to the point where the lifetime risk of developing it is 1.47% (American Cancer Society, 2013). Pancreatic cancer is found more often in older adults and is a leading cause of death in this age group. It is estimated that about 44,000 people will be diagnosed with and about 37,390 will die of pancreatic cancer in 2012 (Howlader et al., 2008). The prognosis is poor because there are often suboptimal responses to treatment.

Risks/Warning Signs

Risk factors include tobacco smoking and smokeless tobacco use (about twice as high for cigarette smokers as compared to nonsmokers), family history, diabetes mellitus, obesity, and possibly high levels of alcohol consumption. Unfortunately, early warning signs often are absent. Symptoms that require further evaluation are weight loss, pain in upper abdomen that radiates to the back, and high blood glucose levels. Sometimes tumors develop near the common bile duct, causing an obstruction that leads to jaundice; this may allow for earlier diagnosis.

Assessment and Diagnosis

Patients may present with vague, diffuse pain that is located in the epigastric area of the left upper quadrant. Diarrhea can be an early symptom, and weight loss can be a late finding. At the present time there are no early diagnostic methods. A CT scan can be done to identify pancreatic cancer; however, endoscopic ultrasonography is more sensitive in detecting the cancer (McPhee, Papadakis, & Rabow, 2012).

Interventions

Surgery, radiation therapy, and chemotherapy are all treatment options, but these are done with the hopes of extending survival or as part of palliative care. Less than 20% of people diagnosed with pancreatic cancer are candidates for surgery because the cancer often has metastasized by the time of diagnosis. For those people for whom the disease is localized and who have small cancers (<2 cm) with no lymph node metastases and no extension outside the capsule of the pancreas, the 5-year survival rate for surgical treatment is about 18 to 24%. Hospice should be considered as early as possible when the prognosis is terminal. (see **Box 9-5**)

BOX 9-5   Resources for Those with Common Cancers

American Cancer Society (all forms of cancer)
    I Can Cope (community support groups)
    1599 Clifton Road, N.E.
    Atlanta, GA 30329
    1-800-ACS-2345
    http://www.cancer.org

American Urological Association
    Online patient information resource http:// www.urologyhealth.org

Bladder Health Council
    c/o American Foundation for Urologic Disease
    1000 Corporate Boulevard, Suite 410
    Linthicum, MD 21090
    800-828-7866

National Breast Cancer Foundation
    http://www.nationalbreastcancer.org

Genitourinary Problems

The elderly may experience several major problems related to the reproductive and urinary systems. This section will discuss some common problems, including urinary tract infection, bladder cancer, atrophic vaginitis, breast cancer, *benign prostatic hyperplasia (BPH)*, prostate cancer, and erectile dysfunction. Urinary incontinence, which is common in older adults, is addressed in its own chapter (Chapter 15) under a section on geriatric syndromes. Although just a brief synopsis of specific cancers are given here, Chapter 30 is devoted to the discussion of care of the older adult with cancer, so the reader may find additional resources in that chapter.

Urinary Tract Infection

Background/Significance

Urinary tract infections (UTIs), also called cystitis (inflammation of the bladder), are common among older adults and are more frequent in women. They are a primary cause of urinary incontinence and delirium. *Catheter-associated urinary tract infections (CAUTIs)* are more common among older adults (Fakih et al., 2012) and are mainly attributed to the use of indwelling urinary catheters. Many indwelling catheters are thought to be unnecessary (Cochran, 2007) and one study noted that physicians were often not aware of the purpose for which their patients had a catheter inserted (Saint, Meddings, Calfee, Kowlaski, & Krein, 2009). UTIs have been show to increase morbidity and mortality, length of hospital stay, and cost of hospitalization (Kleinpell, Munro, & Giuliano, 2008). CAUTI is considered preventable and is not reimbursed by Medicare, so hospitals will largely assume the financial costs for preventable infections of this type. Since nurses play a key role in inserting, maintaining, and decision making regarding catheter use, it is essential that those working with older adults be alert to current guidelines for catheter use.

Risk Factors/Warning Signs

Several risk factors are associated with UTIs. These include being female, having an indwelling urinary catheter, the presence of urological diseases, and hormonal changes associated with menopause in women. Signs and symptoms of UTIs include urinary frequency and burning or stinging felt during voiding. Pain may be felt above the pubic bone, and a strong urge to void but with small amounts of urine expelled are also symptoms. The most significant risk factor for CAUTI is prolonged use of an indwelling catheter. In hospital-acquired UTIs, 75% are associated with the use of an indwelling catheter (CDC, 2012). In women, signs and symptoms of CAUTI may be more severe than those reported by patients in the community who do not have an indwelling catheter. Lethargy, malaise, onset or worsened fever, flank pain, and altered mental status have been associated with CAUTI (Hooton et al., 2010).

Assessment/Diagnosis

Nurses should thoroughly assess and document patients' urinary output, including amounts, color, odor, appearance, frequency of voiding, urgency, and episodes of incontinence. A urine specimen should be obtained if UTI is suspected. Laboratory results will show the type of organism causing the infection, and the sensitivity will tell what medication the organism is susceptible to. These results should be reported promptly to the physician or nurse practitioner caring for the patient so that a diagnosis and treatment plan can be made.

Interventions

Prevention of UTIs is considered a primary nursing strategy. Elderly female patients can be instructed to make lifestyle modifications such as increasing their fluid intake; emptying the bladder after sexual intercourse; practicing good perineal hygiene, including wiping front to back after toileting; getting enough sleep; and avoiding stress (PubMed Health, 2011). Although many of these common-sense strategies are recommended by primary care providers, there is a lack of scientific evidence to support many of them. Many UTIs will clear up on their own, particularly if the person increases oral fluid intake during early symptoms. However, with many older adults, antibiotic treatment may be needed. In general, a course of 3 days for healthy adults is thought to be sufficient, but for more resistant bacteria, a longer course more than 5 days may be needed (PubMed Health, 2011). For those with repeated or chronic UTIs, a low dose of antibiotics taken for 6–12 months may be indicated (Hooton et al., 2010). Monitor the patient's temperature at least every 24 hours (Carpenito, 2013). Encourage fluids. If an indwelling catheter is in place, evaluate if continued use is necessary.

If the underlying cause is CAUTI, treatment will be more aggressive. To prevent CAUTI, nurses should thoroughly assess and document a patient's urinary output as with a suspected standard UTI. Appropriate uses of indwelling catheters may include those with acute urinary retention, the acutely ill who need more accurate monitoring of urinary output, perioperative patients having certain surgeries, those with sacral or coccygeal wounds and incontinence, those with prolonged immobility such as spinal injury, and persons at end of life (Health Care Infection Control Practices Advisory Committee [HICPAC], 2009). Alternatives to indwelling catheters should be considered for appropriate patients. Intermittent catheterization, if appropriate, is preferred over indwelling catheter use, especially for long-term maintenance of bladder management (Hooton et al., 2010). Condom catheters may be an appropriate choice for some males. If an indwelling urinary catheter is necessary, sterile technique on insertion should be strictly observed and asepsis maintained afterwards. The catheter should be removed as soon as possible to reduce the risk of CAUTI. Clear removal guidelines for catheters should be established and in place for all patients (Romito, Beaudoin, & Stein, 2011). Some suggested strategies to include in hospital protocols are electronic medical record reminders to the nurse or physician and automatic stop dates (Hooton et al., 2010). There are many resources for nurses and patients that can help prevent CAUTI: A simple FAQ page for patients and families can be found at http://www.cdc.gov/hai/pdfs/uti/CA-UTI_tagged.pdf and the HICPAC clinical practice guideline for professionals can be found at http://www.cdc.gov/hicpac/pdf/CAUTI/CAUTIguideline2009final.pdf.

Bladder Cancer

Background/Significance

Bladder cancer occurs mainly in older adults, with an average age at diagnosis of 73 years, with 9 out of 10 cases of bladder cancer diagnosed in persons over age 55. The ACS (2012c) reported that over 73,000 cases were diagnosed in 2012 and that this diagnosis rate has been relatively stable over the last 20 years. Men are three times as likely to get cancer of the bladder as women (American Foundation for Urologic Disease, 2008) and the incidence increases with age.

Risk Factors/Warning Signs

Risk factors include chronic bladder irritation and cigarette smoking, the latter contributing to over half of cases (see **Case Study 9-3**). Male gender and age are also risk factors. The classic symptom of bladder cancer is painless hematuria, which may be a reason that older adults sometimes do not seek treatment right away.

Assessment/Diagnosis

Assessment begins with a thorough history and physical. Be sure to ask the patient if he/she has experienced any bleeding or observed blood with voiding; older adults may attribute the bleeding to hemorrhoids or other causes and feel that because there is no pain, it could not be serious. Diagnosis may involve several tests including an intravenous pyelogram (IVP), urinalysis, and cystoscopy (in which the physician visualizes the bladder structures through a flexible fiber-optic scope). This is a highly treatable type of cancer when caught early. In fact, the ACS (2012c) estimates that there were more than 500,000 survivors of this cancer in 2012.

Interventions

Once diagnosed, treatment depends on the invasiveness of the cancer. Treatments for bladder cancer include surgery, radiation therapy, immunotherapy, and chemotherapy (ACS, 2012c). Specifically, a transurethral resection (TUR) may

---

Case Study 9-3

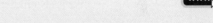

Dr. Johnson is a 62-year-old dentist who runs a busy practice in a large suburb of Chicago. He had been a smoker for over 30 years but recently quit. For some time he has noted little spots of blood in his urine, but he did not have pain, so he attributed it to some prostate problems he has had in the past. Dr. Johnson hears a couple of his patients discussing a mutual friend with bladder cancer who has similar symptoms, and this prompts him to visit his family physician for a checkup. After several tests and a cystoscopy, Dr. Johnson is diagnosed with early stage bladder cancer.

Questions:

1. What risk factors did Dr. Johnson have for bladder cancer?

2. What primary sign did he exhibit?

3. Since his cancer was detected early, what treatments might be options in his case?

4. If Dr. Johnson's cancer becomes invasive, what other options are available for treatment?

5. Describe the nursing implications and care required if Dr. Johnson needed to have a cystectomy.

6. How would you explain a cystectomy to his family?

involve burning superficial lesions through a scope. Bladder cancer may be slow to spread, and less invasive treatments may continue for years before the cancer becomes metastatic, if ever.

Immune/biological therapy includes Bacillus Calmette-Guérin (BCG) wash, an immune stimulant that triggers the body to inhibit tumor growth. BCG treatment can also be done after TUR to inhibit cancer cells from re-growing. Treatments are administered by a physician directly into the bladder through a catheter for 2 hours once per week for 6 or more weeks (Mayo Clinic, 2012a). The patient may be asked to lie on his/her stomach, back, or side throughout the procedure. The nurse should instruct the patient to drink plenty of fluids after the procedure and to be sure to empty the bladder frequently. In addition, because the BCG contains live bacteria, the patient should be taught that any urine passed in the first 6 hours after treatment needs to be treated with bleach: One cup of undiluted bleach should be placed into the toilet with the urine and allowed to sit for 15 minutes before flushing (Mayo Clinic, 2012a).

If the cancer begins to invade the bladder muscle, then removal of the bladder (*cystectomy*) is indicated to prevent metastasis. Additional diagnostic tests will be performed if this is suspected, including CT scan or MRI. Chemotherapy and/or radiation may be used in combination with surgery. When the cancerous bladder is removed, the person will have a *urostomy*, a stoma from which urine drains into a collection bag on the outside of the body, much like a colostomy. Bleeding and infection are two major complications after surgery, regardless of type. Nursing care includes assessment and care of the stoma, emptying and changing collection bags as needed, monitoring output, and assessing for bleeding and infection. Significant education of the patient related to intake/output, ostomy care, appliances, and the like is also indicated.

Female Reproductive System

Two major problems common among older females will be discussed here. These include atrophic vaginitis and and breast cancer. Additional information related to cancer care appears in Chapter 30.

Atrophic Vaginitis

Background/Significance

Normal aging changes in the female reproductive system (see Chapter 29) make elderly women more at risk for infection: Less vaginal lubrication and more alkaline pH due to lower estrogen levels put elderly women at increased risk of vaginitis, and the vaginal canal also becomes more fragile with age due to atrophy. Vaginitis, or inflammation of the vaginal canal and the external genitalia (vulva), may have several causes, including bacteria, yeast, viruses, organisms passed between sexual partners, chemical irritants (such a douches), or even clothing. Atrophic vaginitis (AV) is one of the most common problems, affecting

10–50% of postmenopausal women (Reimer & Johnson, 2010). Often, the symptoms are mistaken for a normal part of aging and women may not report them to their primary care provider.

Risk Factors/Warning Signs

Atrophic vaginitis is caused by low estrogen levels. It may be progressive in relationship to the time after the onset of menopause because of sustained low levels of estrogen. Signs and symptoms of AV include abnormal vaginal discharge, burning, itching, tenderness, dryness, soreness, sparse labial hair, and pain with sexual intercourse (WebMD, 2012).

Assessment/Diagnosis

Because there are many major causes of vaginitis, and more than one can be present at the same time, the underlying cause of vaginitis can be difficult to diagnos. Older women with the above symptoms should be referred to their primary care provider or gynecologist for appropriate treatment. However, since AV is relatively common among postmenopausal women, the nurse practitioner or physician examining the patient will largely rely on the patient's description of symptoms and a thorough history and physical examination for diagnosis. This includes inspection of the vaginal and cervical areas (with speculum use). No laboratory tests are generally needed to diagnose AV in the postmenopausal woman.

Interventions

Treatment for AV is prescribed on an individual basis. The Society of Obstetricians and Gynecologists of Canada (SOGC) and the North American Menopause Society (NAMS) "recommend the use of nonhormonal lubricants or moisturizers and maintenance of sexual activity as first-line treatment" (Reimer & Johnson, 2010, p. 26). If the patient does not respond to this, then hormone-based therapy is considered.

There are several different types of hormonal therapy to treat AV. Vaginal estrogen therapy comes in the form of creams, vaginal rings, or tablets. Treatments with creams may be messier than the rings or tablets, and may be prescribed daily or twice weekly depending on the medication used (Reimer & Johnson, 2010). The use of local estrogen therapy can significantly improve symptoms of vaginal dryness, and it promotes sexual and urogenital health (North American Menopause Society, 2012).

For general vaginal health, women should be instructed to avoid douching and the use of feminine deodorant sprays or perfumes. Wearing cotton undergarments may also help. A water-soluble lubricant, such as K-Y gel, should be used during intercourse if vaginal dryness is a problem; the use of other lubricants such as Vaseline contributes to cases of vaginitis other than atrophic. In addition, cigarette smoking can increase the potential for AV, so smoking cessation is encouraged.

Breast Cancer

Background/Significance

Breast cancer is the second leading cancer diagnosis for women after skin cancer. The ACS estimated 226,870 new cases of invasive breast cancer in 2012, as well as 62,300 cases of new in situ cancer in women and about 2,190 cases of breast cancer in men. It was also estimated that 39,920 women would die from breast cancer in 2012 (ACS, 2012a). The incidence of breast cancer in women over 50 has declined since the year 2000, and this is attributed largely to the decrease in use of menopausal hormone therapy (MHT), previously known as hormone replacement therapy (HRT) (ACS, 2012a; BreastCancer.org, 2012; McEneaney, 2012). Most breast cancers are diagnosed in women over the age of 65 (National Breast Cancer Foundation, 2012). White women have a higher incidence of breast cancer after age 45, while African American women have a higher incidence rate prior to age 45 years and a higher likelihood of dying from breast cancer at any age (ACS, 2012a; BreastCancer.org, 2012). Men may also develop breast cancer, though this is much less frequent, and they should not be excluded from education about the disease.

Risk Factors/Warning Signs

There are several risk factors for breast cancer, some controllable, some not. These include family history, late menopause, having the first child after age 30, obesity, high fat intake, and alcohol consumption. Of course, primary nursing care focuses on those factors that can be modified. Geriatric nurses should be particularly aware of the importance of early detection among those older women who are at higher risk.

Signs and symptoms of breast cancer include a breast mass or lump, breast asymmetry, dimpling of the skin or "orange peel" appearance, discharge, and nipple changes (Kennedy-Malone et al., 2004; ACS, 2012d). Early detection by screening is important since there may not be any pain or other symptoms associated with early stages of breast cancer.

Assessment and Diagnosis

An abnormality, such as a lump felt upon examination of the breasts either by the patient or primary care provider, may be the first indication of a problem. In general, however, most breast lumps are benign and could be due to factors other than cancer, such as fibrocystic disease.

A breast exam performed by a clinician, mammography, and biopsy, in addition to lab tests, chest X-ray, and bone scans, are indicated for diagnosis (see **Case Study 9-4**). Stage I breast cancer has a 98% survival rate at 5 years (National Breast Cancer Foundation, 2012), so early diagnosis and treatment is essential.

Interventions

Screening is an important intervention for prevention and early detection. Screening guidelines for older women have changed significantly in recent years, based on current evidence. Starting at age 40, women should have clinical breast exam CBE

Case Study 9-4

Mrs. Valdez is a 65-year-old woman who comes to the physician's office after experiencing enlargement of her right breast upon self-exam. The nurse observes during the physician's physical examination that Mrs. Valdez's right breast is twice as large as the left one and has a puckered appearance. The physician tells Mrs. Valdez that she will need to have some tests and a biopsy and then he leaves the room. Mrs. Valdez looks at the nurse and asks, "What does he mean? What is wrong with me?"

Questions:

1. What should the nurse explain to Mrs. Valdez at this point? What educational materials might she need?

2. What tests would the nurse expect the physician to order?

3. Are there possible risk factors for breast cancer that Mrs. Valdez might have? If so, what are they?

4. Given the physical observations, what would the nurse expect to see done for this patient?

and mammography yearly "as long as a woman is in good health" (ACS, 2012d, p. 1). The CDC guidelines (2012a) state that women aged 50–74 years should have a screening mammography every 2 years. Current evidence is insufficient to support screening for breast cancer in women over 75 (U.S. Preventive Services Task Force, 2009).

Nursing care is important at all levels of prevention. Nurses working with older adults should encourage appropriate screening according to recommended guidelines, and the elderly should be encouraged to have regular checkups with their physician. Although controversy exists over the use of mammography, it remains an effective means to detect many cancerous tumors at an earlier stage with minimal risk to the person, but screening should begin in middle adulthood.

Treatment for breast cancer depends on stage, but includes any combination of radiation, chemotherapy, or surgery. Depending on the type of tumor, hormone therapy may also be effective. Older women undergoing mastectomy as treatment for breast cancer may require more time for recovery. Promotion of the return of full range of motion to the arm on the operative side is essential. This may require physical therapy in addition to the psychosocial and emotional support involved in rehabilitation.

Male Reproductive System

The most common disorders related to the reproductive system among older men include benign prostatic hyperplasia (BPH), cancer of the prostate, and *erectile dysfunction (ED)*.

Benign Prostatic Hyperplasia

Background

BPH, also known as prostatism, results from noncancerous enlargement of the prostate gland that is associated with advanced age. This condition affects 50% of men ages 51–60 and up to 90% of men over 80 years (American Urological Association, 2010). Although the enlargement is benign, it is sometimes associated with prostate cancer, so men with this condition should be carefully monitored.

Risk Factors/Warning Signs

Reasons for why the prostate tends to enlarge as a man ages are unclear. Known risk factors for BPH are few, but include advanced age and family history; in fact, BPH is so common with advanced age that nearly all men would have some prostate enlargement if they lived long enough. BPH occurs when the enlarged prostate squeezes and compresses the urethra, causing symptoms such as a decreased urinary stream, increased frequency, increased urgency, nocturia, incomplete emptying, dribbling, a weak urine stream, and urinary *incontinence* (see **Table 9-20**). The urge to void may be so frequent in men with BPH (as often as every 2 hours) that it can interfere with sleep and activities of daily living.

Assessment and Diagnosis

Diagnosis is made using any number or combination of tests and studies including digital rectal exam (DRE), urinalysis, postvoiding residual, *prostate-specific antigen (PSA)*, urodynamic studies, ultrasound, and cystoscopy. The DRE and PSA are used to help rule out prostate cancer as a cause of the symptoms.

Interventions

Medical treatment generally includes medications and surgery. The two most frequently used types of medications are alpha-blockers and 5-alpha-reductase inhibitors. Alpha-blockers, such as alfuzosin, doxazosin (Cardura), terazosin (Hytrin BPH), and tamsulosin (Flomax MR), work to relieve symptoms of BPH by relaxing the smooth muscle of the prostate and bladder neck to allow urine to flow more easily. None of the four medications listed has been convincingly shown to be more effective than the other (American Urological Association, 2010). A 5-alpha-reductase inhibitor such as finasteride (Proscar) works differently, by shrinking the prostate to promote urine

TABLE 9-20 Signs and Symptoms of BPH
Decreased urinary stream
Urinary frequency
Urinary urgency
Nocturia
Urinary incontinence
Incomplete bladder emptying
Urinary dribbling
Feelings of urge to void but difficulty starting urine stream
Decreased quality of life related to symptoms
Altered sleep patterns related to nocturia

flow, but has sexual side effects such as impotence (American Urological Association, 2010; Mead, 2005; U.S. Department of Health and Human Services, National Kidney and Urological Diseases Information Clearing House [NKUDIC], 2012).

There are several surgical procedures that can be used to treat BPH. One of the most common surgical interventions for BPH is a *transurethral resection of the prostate (TURP)*. During this procedure, the urologist resects the enlarged prostate gland through a cystoscope (see **Figure 9-8**). Older men sometimes call this the "Rotor Rooter" surgery. Nursing care after this procedure is essential to avoid complications related to the heavy bleeding that may occur. The patient will have an indwelling urinary catheter with three ports. Postoperatively, *continuous bladder irrigation (CBI)* must be maintained to prevent dangerous clotting of the blood. The nurse is responsible for assessing the color of the urine draining from the catheter. The urine in the tube should be charted with specific terms such as bright red, brick red, tea colored, amber, yellow, or clear. The number and size of clots draining from the catheter should be described. The goal of the CBI is to flush the bladder, so the nurse must regulate the rate of the fluid to keep the urine yellow

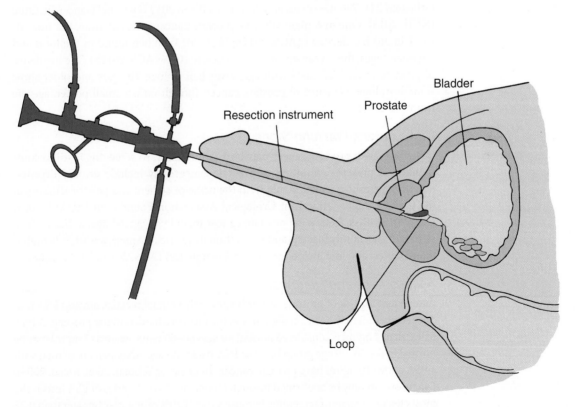

Figure 9-8 TURP.

Source: Leonard Crowley, *Introduction to Human Disease* (6th ed.). Sudbury, MA: Jones & Bartlett Publishers, 2005.

or as clear as possible. CBI will continue postoperatively until the bleeding stops. Bleeding complications may result if the CBI is allowed to go dry or the catheter is removed too soon after surgery. In the event that the patient is unable to void after removal of the catheter post-TURP, the catheter may need to be reinserted. If the nurse is unable to reinsert the catheter, the physician may need to be called in to do this. Nurses should be particularly alert to the potential for complications in older men after this procedure.

A newer procedure that has shown promising results is holmium laser enucleation of the prostate (HoLEP). Although the HoLEP procedure generally takes longer than the TURP, it has some added benefits, such as a low incidence of needing further surgery and the ability to take a larger and better tissue sample for examination than with TURP. However, most residents are still being taught TURP as the gold standard of treatment for treatment of BPH (Bhojani & Lingeman, 2011).

Prostate Cancer

Background

Prostate cancer is the second leading cause of cancer death in U.S. males, with an estimated 241, 740 new cases and 28,170 deaths in 2012 (National Cancer Institute [NCI], 2013). One in 6 men will have prostate cancer in his lifetime, but mortality (1 in 36) has declined (ACS, 2012b; NCI, 2013). When found in the local and regional stages, the 5-year survival rate is nearly 100% (ACS, 2012b). The incidence of prostate cancer increases with age. Over half of men 70 years and older show some histologic evidence of prostate cancer, though only a small percentage die from this disease.

Risk Factors/Warning Signs

Older men with prostate cancer may be asymptomatic, so screening is still recommended. If present, symptoms of prostate cancer may include urinary urgency, nocturia, painful ejaculation, blood in the urine or semen, and pain or stiffness in the back or thighs (American Urological Association Foundation [AUAF], 2008; NCI, 2013). Risk factors for prostate cancer include advanced age, a diet high in saturated fats, family history, and race/ethnicity (African Americans slightly higher than Whites, and low incidence among Asian males) (ACS, 2013); AUAF, 2008).

Assessment and Diagnosis

Assessment for risk of prostate cancer begins with a digital rectal exam and PSA test. The rectal exam may detect malignancy in the form of a hard, nodular prostate. A PSA of less than 4 ng/ml is considered normal for ages 60–69 years, whereas 7 ng/ml may be normal in the 70–79 age group because PSA rises with age. Sixty percent of men with a PSA above 10 ng/ml have prostate cancer (Bradway & Yetman, 2002; Mead, 2005). Diagnosis can only be confirmed through biopsy, however. A series of PSA tests is the most effective means of screening, because a rise of 20% over a year (greater than 0.75 ng/ml per year) generally indicates cancer (Mead, 2005).

Interventions

If a biopsy of the prostate is needed, the nurse can educate the patient on what to expect. The biopsy is often done in the urologist's office. Usually, local anesthetic is used. The physician will use a special needle to take samples of the prostate, which is accessed through the rectal wall. Several samples will be taken. The procedure generally takes around 10 minutes, and the patient may be ordered some antibiotics to take afterwards to prevent possible infection after the procedure (ACS, 2012b). The biopsy samples will be sent to a lab where the pathologist will examine them. If found to be cancerous, the tumor will be graded and discussion of treatment will be done with the physician and patient.

Treatment depends on the stage of cancer growth, but for more localized cancers it generally includes three major options: *radical prostatectomy*, radiation therapy, and active surveillance. The "decision to proceed to prostate biopsy should be based primarily on PSA and Digital Rectal Examination (DRE) results, but should take into account multiple factors including free and total PSA, patient age, PSA velocity, PSA density, family history, ethnicity, prior biopsy history, and comorbidities" (AUAF, 2009, p. 5–6). The patient's age, health condition, and life expectancy should be considered when planning treatment.

Because a radical prostatectomy is major surgery and carries some inherent risks, all options should be considered with the older patient. The major problems after surgery to remove the prostate include urinary *incontinence* (which is often temporary) and impotence. The skill and experience of the surgeon can decrease the risk of urinary incontinence after surgery.

A holistic approach to care may include dietary changes such as a low-fat diet and the addition of vitamin E, selenium, and soy protein (Bradway & Yetman, 2002). It is important that a patient not adopt complementary medicine treatments without talking with his doctor.

Nursing care surrounding treatment for prostate cancer will involve helping families to explore their options, linking them to community resources, and providing education related to managing postoperative complications if surgery is indicated. Geriatric nurses should be informed as to the various options available for treatment of impotence that accompanies this type of surgery. Couples should be provided with support group information as well as information on penile implants and other devices that patients may wish to consider after recovery.

Erectile Dysfunction

Background

Erectile dysfunction (ED), also known as impotence, is defined as the inability to achieve and sustain a sufficient erection for intercourse. Erectile dysfunction is found in approximately 17% of men over age 60 and 47% of men age 75 years or older (NKUDIC, 2012). About 30 million American men are affected by ED

(NKUDIC, 2012). The incidence of ED increases with age, but it is not inevitable and is highly treatable in many cases.

Risk Factors/Warning Signs

The causes of ED may be many, including diabetes, hypertension, multiple sclerosis, spinal cord injury, thyroid disorders, alcoholism, renal failure, hypogonadism, other diseases, some medications (see **Table 9-21**), and psychological factors (such as fear, guilt, or depression). Smoking, alcoholism, and obesity may also contribute to ED. In men over age 75, ED has a positive correlation with prostate and urinary problems as well as advanced age (Shabsigh, Perleman, Lockhart, Lue & Broderick, 2005).

Assessment and Diagnosis

Assessment of ED should include a thorough patient history, physical and psychological exam, and lab tests. Interviewing the man's sexual partner may also provide clues as to the cause of ED. Determining whether the cause is physical, psychological, or a combination of both is a good place to start. It is important for nurses to note that ED can also be an important predictor of overall health in older men (Shabsigh et al., 2005).

Interventions

Treatment for ED usually begins with the least invasive strategies. This could include lifestyle modifications such as smoking cessation, monitoring alcohol intake, dietary changes for weight control, and increasing exercise. If the problem seems more psychological than physical (after testing), referral to a qualified counselor or psychiatrist may be ordered. Medications should be examined for those contributing to ED, and adjustments or alternatives to those medications should be explored with the primary care provider.

Other treatment options for ED fall into several categories, including oral medications, vacuum pump devices, penile implants, and drugs injected into the penis. Sildenafil (Viagra) is an oral medication that is taken 1 hour prior to sexual activity. It is contraindicated in those with heart disease and may result in some cardiovascular-related side effects including headache, flushing, and nasal

TABLE 9-21 Medications That May Affect Sexual Function
Anticholinergics
Antidepressants
Antihypertensives
Digoxin
Hypnotics
Sedatives
Sleeping medications
Tranquilizers

congestion. Other oral products on the market (Cialis, Levitra) are based on similar principles. A complaint about Viagra is the possibility of irreversible visual impairment in some men, but screenings for those at increased risk for this complication (those with certain characteristics in the inner eye being at higher risk) can be done by most primary care physicians or ophthalmologists.

Vacuum devices have a good acceptance in the elderly population, with a 70–90% success rate (Reuben et al., 2008). These devices work in various ways to pump or draw blood into the penis and use another mechanism, such as a ring around the base of the penis, to help sustain the erection for intercourse. Risks from use of this device would include bruising or bleeding (in extreme cases). Nursing instruction to couples on the use of such a device is essential to prevent harm. Other treatments for ED include medications that may be injected directly into the penis to cause temporary erection, and some persons may opt for having surgery to insert a penile implant. There are two types of penile implants: one that results in permanent erection and one that may be pumped to cause erection and then released. All options should be explored with persons wishing information on treatment of ED.

Neurological Disorders

Several neurological disorders are common to the elderly, including diseases and conditions that are often secondary to common diseases. Two of the most frequently occurring neurological diseases in the elderly will be discussed here: *Parkinson's disease (PD)* and *Alzheimer's disease (AD)*. Chapter 10 is devoted to nursing management of dementia, so the reader is referred there for a more thorough discussion.

Stroke may also be considered a neurological disorder, but was discussed previously in the section on circulation problems. Complications that affect the neurological system as a result of a variety of causes may include seizures, tremor (see discussion on PD), peripheral neuropathy (see discussion on diabetes), and dizziness.

Alzheimer's Disease

Background

Alzheimer's disease (AD) is the most common type of dementia seen in older adults. Other forms of dementia include vascular dementia, dementia with Lewy bodies, and Parkinson's dementia. Care of the person with AD provides an example of nursing interventions for all persons with dementia. One is eight older adults has AD, and it is the sixth leading cause of death in the United States (Alzheimer's Association, 2012b).

An estimated 5.4 million Americans of all ages have Alzheimer's disease in 2012. This figure includes 5.2 million people age 65 years and over, along with 200,000 individuals under age 65 who have younger-onset Alzheimer's (Alzheimer's

Notable Quotes

"My father started growing very quiet as Alzheimer's started claiming more of him. The early stages of Alzheimer's are the hardest because that person is aware that they're losing awareness. And I think that that's why my father started growing more and more quiet."

—Patti Davis regarding her father, President Ronald Reagan

Association, 2012b). By 2050, the number of individuals age 65 and over with Alzheimer's could range from 11 million to 16 million unless science finds a way to prevent or effectively treat the disease. (Alzheimer's Association, 2012b).

Those affected with AD may live from 3–20 years or more after diagnosis, making the life span with this disease highly variable. Eight percent of people with AD are cared for in their home by unpaid family members (Alzheimer's Association, 2012b). The annual estimated cost of AD in healthcare services was about $200 billion in 2012 (Alzheimer's Association, 2012b). Alzheimer's disease results in lost productivity and strain on family; considering the increasing number of people expected to develop AD, these costs are expected to exceed $163 billion per year by 2050 (National Conference of Gerontological Nurse Practitioners & National Gerontological Nursing Association, 2008a). These statistics reveal that AD has and will continue to have a great impact on our society.

Risk Factors/Warning Signs

Advanced age is the single most significant risk factor for AD (Alzheimer's Association, 2012a). Nearly half (45%) of people over the age of 85 have AD. More women than men have AD, but this is because women live longer than men, not because gender is a risk factor. Family history and heredity are also identified risk factors for AD, as are head trauma and poor cardiac health.

Assessment and Diagnosis

Alzheimer's disease is characterized by progressive memory loss. The person affected by AD is gradually less able to remember new information and memory lapses begin to affect daily function. It is a terminal disease that over its course will eventually leave a person completely dependent upon others for care. Initially, the clinical progression of the disease is slow with mild decline; however, deterioration increases the longer the person lives, with an average life span of 8 years after diagnosis (Cotter, 2002; Fletcher, Rapp, & Reichman, 2007). The underlying pathology is not clear, but a growth of plaques and fibrillary tangles, loss of synapses, and neuronal cell loss are key hallmarks of AD that interfere with normal cell growth and the ability of the brain to function. Absolutely definitive diagnosis is still through autopsy, although clinical guidelines make diagnosis easier than decades ago when less was known about the disease. Primary care physicians generally make the diagnosis through a thorough history, physical exam, cognitive testing, and labs. New criteria for diagnosis include staging the disorder and biomarkers (beta amyloid and tau in the cerebrospinal fluid and blood) (Alzheimer's Association, 2012b). A MRI of the brain may be ordered to rule out other causes of symptoms.

The clinical course of AD is divided into several stages, depending on the source consulted. For the purposes of this text, early, middle, and late phases will be described; however, it should be noted that the Alzheimer's Association lists seven stages for AD, ranging from no symptoms to very severe decline (Alzheimer's Association, 2012a).

In the early course of AD, the person may demonstrate a loss of short-term memory. This involves more than common memory loss, such as where the keys were put, and may involve safety concerns such as forgetting where one is going while driving. The inability to perform math calculations and to think abstractly may also be evident. In the middle or moderate phase, many bodily systems begin to decline. The person may become confused as to date, time, and place. Communication skills become impaired and personality changes may occur. As cognitive decline worsens, the person may forget the names of loved ones, even their spouse. Wandering behavior as well as emotional changes, screaming, delusions, hallucinations, suspiciousness, and depression are common. The person with AD is less able to care for her- or himself and personal hygiene suffers. In the most severe and final phase, the person becomes completely dependent upon others, experiences a severe decline in physical and functional health, loses communication skills, and is unable to control voluntary functions. Death eventually results from body systems shutting down and may be accompanied by an infectious process.

Although there is no single test, and the diagnosis may be one of exclusion, early diagnosis is important to maximize function and quality of life for as long as possible. Persons experiencing recurring and progressing memory problems or difficulties with daily activities should seek professional assistance from their physician. Warning signs of Alzheimer's are listed in **Table 9-22**.

Interventions

Treatment for AD is difficult. There are several medications (such as Aricept, Namenda, Razadyne, and Exelon) that may help symptoms (such as memory), but they do not slow the course of the disease. There is currently no cure; however, research continues to occur in pharmacology, nonpharmacology, and the use of stem cells to manage symptoms and perhaps one day eradicate the disease.

TABLE 9-22   Ten Warning Signs of Alzheimer's Disease
Memory loss that interferes with daily life
Challenges in problem solving
Difficulty performing familiar tasks
Confusion related to time and place
Visual problems
Problems with language (new problems with talking or writing)
Misplacing things in unusual places and not being able to find them
Poor or decreased judgment
Withdrawal from usual activities
Changes in mood or personality

Source: Alzheimer's Association, 2012c.

Nursing care will focus on symptom management, particularly in the areas of behavior, safety, nutrition, and hygiene. Behavioral issues such as wandering and outbursts pose a constant challenge. Many long-term care facilities have instituted special units to care for Alzheimer's patients from the early to late stages of the disease. These units provide great benefits such as consistent and educated caregivers with whom the patient or resident will be familiar, a safe and controlled environment, modified surroundings to accommodate wandering behaviors, and nursing care 24 hours a day. Additionally, nurses are present to manage medications and document outcomes of therapies. However, many family members wish to care for their loved ones at home for as long as possible.

Thus, another important aspect of care in AD is care for the caregivers. Howcroft (2004) suggested that "support from carers is a key factor in the community care of people with dementia, but the role of the caregiver can be detrimental to the physical, mental, and financial health of a carer" (p. 31). She goes on to say that the caregivers of persons with AD would benefit from training in how to cope with behaviors that arise in these patients and how to cope with practical and legal issues that may occur.

Research from Paun, Farran, Perraud, and Loukissa (2004; see also Mannion, 2008a, 2008b) showed that ongoing skills were needed by family caregivers to deal with the progressive decline caused by AD. In fact, "a 63% greater risk of mortality was found among unpaid caregivers who characterized themselves as being emotionally or mentally strained by their role versus noncaregivers" (National Conference of Gerontological Nursing Practitioners & National Gerontological Nursing Association, 2008b, p. 4). Adapting to stress, working on time management, maximizing resources, and managing changing behavior were all skills caregivers needed to develop in order to successfully manage home care of their loved ones. When interventions and resources were not used by caregivers in the early stages of the care recipient's AD, the risk of a healthy patient being institutionalized due to caregiver burden was higher (Miller, Rosenheck & Schneider, 2012). Caregivers needed not only to acquire knowledge and skills, but also to make emotional adjustments themselves to the ever-changing situation. Such findings suggest that nurses should focus a good deal of time on educating caregivers of persons with AD to cope with, as Nancy Reagan put it, "the long good-bye."

Scientists continue to explore the causes of AD and hope in the near future to be able to isolate the gene that causes it. In the meantime, results from a fascinating longitudinal study (called the Nun study) on aging and AD, which used a group of nuns who donated their brains to be examined and autopsied after death, has suggested that there is a connection between early "idea density" and the emergence of AD in later life. That is, essays the nuns wrote upon entry to the convent were analyzed and correlated with those who developed AD. It was found that those with lower idea density (verbal and linguistic skills) in early life had a significantly greater chance of developing AD (Grossi, Buscema, Snowdon, & Antuono, 2007; Snowdon, 2004). The nun study has allowed researchers to examine hundreds of brains so far in nuns who died between 75 and 107 years of age and discover other important facts such as a relationship between stroke and the development of AD in certain individuals, and the role of folic acid in protecting against development of AD (Snowdon, 2004). Scientists from a number of fields continue to research the causes and possible treatments for AD and the Nun study project is continuing at the University of Minnesota. Snowdon's research suggests that early education, particularly in verbal and cognitive skills, may protect persons from AD in later life.

Parkinson's Disease

Background

Parkinson's disease is one of the most common neurological diseases, affecting at least 4 million people in the United States (National Parkinson Foundation, 2013). Parkinson's disease usually affects people over the age of 50, and the likelihood of developing PD increases with age (National Institute of Neurological Disorders and Stroke, 2008); the average age of onset is about 59 years of age (APDA, 2013). It affects both men and women, particularly those over the age of 60 years (National Parkinson Foundation, 2013). Parkinson's disease was first described by Dr. James Parkinson as the "shaking palsy," so named to describe the motor tremors witnessed in those experiencing this condition.

Parkinson's disease is a degenerative, chronic disorder of the central nervous system in which nerve cells in the basal ganglia degenerate. A loss of neurons in the substantia nigra of the brainstem causes a reduction in the production of the neurotransmitter dopamine, which is responsible for fine motor movement. Dopamine is needed for smooth movement and also plays a role in feelings and emotions. One specific pathological marker is called the Lewy body, which under a microscope appears as a round, dying neuron.

Risk Factors/Warning Signs

Parkinson's disease has no known etiology, though several causes are suspected. There is a family history in 15% of cases. Some believe a virus or environmental factors play a significant role in the development of the disease. A higher risk of PD has been noted in teachers, medical workers, loggers, and miners, suggesting the possibility of a respiratory virus being to blame. More recent theories blame herbicides or pesticides. An emerging theory discusses PD as an injury related to an event or exposure to a toxin versus a disease. Interestingly, coffee drinking and cigarettes are thought to have a protective effect in the development of PD (Films for the Humanities and Sciences, 2004).

The signs and symptoms of PD are many; however, there are four cardinal signs: bradykinesia (slowness of movement), rigidity, tremor, and gait changes such as imbalance or uncoordination. A typical patient with PD symptoms will have some distinctive movement characteristics with the components of stiffness, shuffling gait, arms at the side when walking, incoordination, and a tendency to fall backward. Not all patients exhibit resting tremor, but most have problems with movement, such as difficulty starting movement, increased stiffness with passive resistance, and rigidity, as well as freezing during motion (NINDS, 2012). Additional signs, symptoms, and associated characteristics of PD appear in **Table 9-23**. Advanced PD may result in Parkinson's dementia.

TABLE 9-23 Signs, Symptoms, and Associated Problems Seen in Persons with Parkinson's Disease
Bradykinesia
Rigidity
Tremor
Pill rolling
Incoordination
Shuffling gait, arms at side
Freezing of movements
Balance problems (tendency to fall backward)
Vocal changes; stuttering
Swallowing problems
Drooling
Visual disturbances
Bowel and bladder dysfunction
Sexual dysfunction
Dizziness
Sweating
Dyskinesias
Sleep pattern disturbances
Dementia
Memory loss
Emotional changes
Confusion
Nightmares
Twitching
Handwriting changes
Depression
Anxiety
Panic attacks
Hallucinations
Psychosis

Assessment and Diagnosis

Diagnosis of PD is made primarily on the clinician's physical examination and thorough history taken from the patient and/or family. Nurses should note that several other conditions may cause symptoms similar to PD, such as the neurological effects of tremor and movement disorders. These may be attributed to the effects of drugs or toxins, Alzheimer's disease, vascular diseases, or normal pressure hydrocephalus, and not be true PD. There is no one specific test to diagnose PD, and labs or X-rays rarely help with diagnosis.

Interventions

Management of PD is generally done through medications. Levodopa, a synthetic dopamine, is an amino acid that converts to dopamine when it crosses the blood–brain barrier. Levodopa helps lessen most of the serious signs and symptoms of PD. The drug helps at least 75% of persons with PD, mainly with the symptoms of bradykinesia and rigidity (NINDS, 2008). One important side effect to note is hallucinations. A more common treatment, and generally the drug of choice, involves a medication that combines levodopa and carbidopa (Sinemet), resulting in a decrease in the side effect of nausea seen with Levodopa therapy alone, but with the same positive control of symptoms, particularly with relation to movement. Patients should not be taken off of Sinemet precipitously, so it is important to check all of a patient's medications if they are admitted to either acute or long-term care. Dopamine agnoists trick the brain into thinking it is getting dopamine. This class of medications is less effective than Sinemet, but may be beneficial for certain patients. The most commonly prescribed dopamine agonists are pramipexole (Mirapex) and ropinirole (Requip) (Parkinson's Disease Foundation, 2012). Medications such as Sinemet show a wearing-off effect, generally over a 2-year period. During this time, the person must take larger doses of the medication to achieve the same relief of symptoms that a smaller dose used to bring. For an unknown reason, if the medication is stopped for about a week to 10 days, the body will reset itself and the person will be able to restart the medication at the lower dose again until tolerance is again reached. This time off from the medication is called a "drug holiday" and is a time when the person and family need extra support, because the person's symptoms will be greatly exacerbated without the medication. The earliest drugs used for PD symptom management were anticholinergics such as Artane and Cogentin, and these medications are still used for tremors and dystonias associated with wearing-off and peak dose effects (Parkinson's Disease Foundation, 2012).

There are many other treatments for Parkinson's disease being explored. These include deep brain stimulation (DBS), with electrode-like implants that act much like a pacemaker to control PD tremors and other movement problems. The person using this therapy will still have the disease and generally uses medications in combination with this treatment, but may require lower doses of medication (NINDS, 2012). Thalamotomy, or surgical removal of a group of cells in the thalamus, is used in severe cases of tremor. This will manage the tremors for a period of time, but is a symptomatic treatment, not a cure. Similarly, pallidotomy involves destruction of a group of cells in the internal globus pallidus, an area where information leaves the basal ganglia. In this procedure, nerve cells in the brain are permanently destroyed.

Fetal tissue transplants have been done experimentally in Sweden with mild success in older adults and more success among patients whose PD symptoms were a result of toxins. Stem cell transplant uses primitive nerve cells harvested from a surplus of embryos and fetuses from fertility clinics. This practice, of course, poses an ethical dilemma and has been the source of much controversy and political discussion.

A more recent development includes the use of adult stem cells, a theory that is promising but not yet well researched. Cells may be taken from the back of the eyes of organ donors. These epithelial cells from the retina are micro-carriers of gelatin that may have enough cells in a single retina to treat 10,000 patients (Films for the Humanities and Sciences, 2004). In addition, cells modified from the skin of patients with PD can be engineered to behave like stem cells (NINDS, 2012). Both of these alternatives present a more practical and ethically pleasing source of stem cells than embryos.

Other research includes areas in which nurses may advocate for evidence-based practice in their facilities or organization. For example, Tai Chi has been shown to be effective in improving balance and reducing falls for PD patients (NINDS, 2012). Rehabilitation units have been using Tai Chi for similar benefits in other patients with neurological deficits. Simple interventions such as using Wii games to promote activity and exercise may be explored. The role of caffeine in PD is also being examined. In a small randomized control study of 61 patients with PD, caffeine equivalent to 2–3 cups of coffee per day was given to subjects and compared with a control group of those taking a placebo. Those patients receiving the caffeine intervention showed little improvement in daytime sleepiness, but modest improvement in PD severity scores related to speed of movement and stiffness (Postuma et al., 2012). Further study with larger groups was recommended by the researchers.

Much of the nursing care in PD is related to education. Because PD is a generally chronic and slowly progressing disorder, patients and family members will need much instruction regarding the course of the disease and what to anticipate. Instruction in the areas of medications, safety promotion, prevention of falls, disease progression, mobility, bowel and bladder, potential swallowing problems, sleep promotion, and communication is important. Most of the problems seen as complications of PD are handled via the physician as an outpatient, but certainly complications such as swallowing disorders as the disease progresses may require periods of hospitalization. When persons suffer related dementia in the final phases of the disease, they are often cared for in long-term care facilities that are equipped to handle the challenges and safety issues related to PD dementia. Areas for teaching appear in **Table 9-24**. In addition, access to resources and support groups is essential. A list of helpful resources and agencies is provided in **Box 9-6**.

fluid in the inner ear, which is the cause of
of being unsteady or dizzy may last for as
episode (Mayo Clinic, 2012).

As mentioned previously, BPPV is the
older age group, accounting for as much a
incidence with age (Hain, 2003, 2012). BF
("rocks in the ears") become dislodged from
elsewhere in the vestibular system. Althou;
BPPV is not known, the degeneration of th
occurs with normal aging is thought to pl
do not respond to traditional medication
should be suspected. A key to diagnosis of
the patient is laid down quickly from a sitti
side and hung over the back of the exam
nystagmus if the cause is BPPV.

Interventions

Treatment for dizziness depends on the un
body position, behavioral modification is ir
ziness, medication may be helpful. For dizzi
may be used over a 3-week period to impro
ease, meclizine may help with acute sympto:
therapy might be initiated to decrease vasc

BPPV can be treated in the office by tl
or even a physical therapist with knowledg
maneuver is a technique by which the pati
tions and head turns to promote return of t
ear. After this treatment, the patient must st
sleep in a recliner chair at 45 degrees for tl
be instructed to avoid head positions that
(Hain, 2003). Other maneuvers and even s
rare variations of BPPV; these would be rec
by-case basis.

Dizziness, whatever the cause, can be par
can interfere with activities of daily living, tl
of independence. Elders may decrease activ
to the fear of dizzy spells or of falling. It is a l
tinuing driving, which may be depressing tc
other cases the fear of having to stop driving
attention. Early diagnosis of the cause of diz
starting treatment sooner and avoiding com
syncope or vertigo.

TABLE 9-24 Client/Family Teaching Regarding Parkinson's Disease Key Areas

Medication therapy (side effects, wearing off, drug holidays, role of diet in absorption)
Safety promotion/fall prevention
Disease progression
Effects of disease on bowel and bladder, sleep, nutrition, attention, self-care, communication, sexuality, and mobility
Swallowing problems
Promoting sleep and relaxation
Communication
Role changes
Caregiver stress/burden—need for respite
Community resources

BOX 9-6 Resources for Those with Parkinson's Disease

American Parkinson Disease Association
800-223-2732
http://www.apdaparkinson.org

Michael J. Fox Foundation for Parkinson's Research
212-509-0995
http://www.michaeljfox.org

National Institute of Neurological Disorders and
Stroke (NINDS)
800-352-9424
http://www.ninds.nih.gov

National Parkinson Foundation
800-327-4545
http://www.parkinson.org

Parkinson's Disease Foundation
800-457-6676
http://www.pdf.org

Dizziness

Background

Dizziness is quite common in older adults, affecting about 30% of those over age 65. It represents about 2% of the consultations in primary health care (Hansson, Mansson, & Hakanson, 2005) and is the most common complaint in those over 75 who are seen by office physicians (Hill-O'Neill & Shaughnessy, 2002). There are four major types of dizziness according to Hill-O'Neill and Shaughnessy: vertigo, presyncope (light-headedness), disequilibrium (related to balance), and ill-defined (i.e., it does not fit in any other categories). These are further explained under assessment and diagnosis.

Risk Fac~

Risk factors
problems, o
cervical spo
symptoms c
lasting for
medications

Signs an
ance, and na
something a

Assessm

Vertigo—a
brought on
the wrong p
ear; *Menier*
motion; or
sclerosis.

Presynco
is associated
suddenly ch
the heart. It
hypovolemi

Disequili
Causes of d
muscle prob

The four
included in
as other inn
side effects c
and benign

Dizziness
such as dizzi

Otologica
Ramaswamy
The most co
syndrome is
attributed tc
decrease in h
tinnitus (rin
O'Neill & Sh

Nurses should encourage older adults with complaints of dizziness to seek medical help. Treatment may be with medication, simple maneuvers, or lifestyle changes. Emotional support during diagnosis and testing, and reassurance that most causes of dizziness are treatable, can be a comfort to the older adult with this problem.

Seizures

Background

Once thought to be mainly a disorder of children, recurrent seizures or epilepsy is thought to be present in about 7% of older adults (Spitz, 2005) and is usually related to one of the common comorbidities found in older adults (Bergey, 2004; Rowan & Tuchman, 2003). Epilepsy affects up to 3 million Americans of all ages (Velez & Selwa, 2003). Davidson & Davidson (2012) summarized findings of most studies on epilepsy in older adults with these main points:

1. the elderly succumb to seizures and epilepsy more than any other age group;
2. the largest identifiable cause of seizures and epilepsy in the elderly is cerebrovascular disease;
3. the symptoms of seizures and epilepsy in the elderly are more vague than in younger adults;
4. finding an appropriate treatment for the elderly is complicated by adverse drug reactions, drug interactions, polypharmacy, absorption rates, and other challenging health issues; and
5. approximately 100 in every 100,000 patients over the age of 65 experience a seizure or epilepsy. (p. 11)

Seizures can be caused by a variety of conditions in older persons, but "the most common cause of new-onset epilepsy in an elderly person is arteriosclerosis and the associated cerebrovascular disease" (Spitz, 2005, p. 1), accounting for 40–50% of seizures in this age group (Rowan & Tuchman, 2003). Seizures are associated with stroke in 5–14% of survivors (Spitz, 2005; Velez & Selwa, 2003). Other common causes of epilepsy in the elderly include Alzheimer's disease and brain tumor. A list of potential causes of seizures in older adults appears in **Table 9-25**.

TABLE 9-25   Possible Causes of Seizures in the Elderly
Stroke or other cerebrovascular disease
Arteriosclerosis
Alzheimer's disease
Brain tumor
Head trauma
Intracranial infection
Drug abuse or withdrawal
Withdrawal from antiepileptic drug

TABLE 9-24 Client/Family Teaching Regarding Parkinson's Disease Key Areas

Medication therapy (side effects, wearing off, drug holidays, role of diet in absorption)

Safety promotion/fall prevention

Disease progression

Effects of disease on bowel and bladder, sleep, nutrition, attention, self-care, communication, sexuality, and mobility

Swallowing problems

Promoting sleep and relaxation

Communication

Role changes

Caregiver stress/burden—need for respite

Community resources

BOX 9-6 Resources for Those with Parkinson's Disease

American Parkinson Disease Association
800-223-2732
http://www.apdaparkinson.org

Michael J. Fox Foundation for Parkinson's Research
212-509-0995
http://www.michaeljfox.org

National Institute of Neurological Disorders and Stroke (NINDS)
800-352-9424
http://www.ninds.nih.gov

National Parkinson Foundation
800-327-4545
http://www.parkinson.org

Parkinson's Disease Foundation
800-457-6676
http://www.pdf.org

Dizziness

Background

Dizziness is quite common in older adults, affecting about 30% of those over age 65. It represents about 2% of the consultations in primary health care (Hansson, Mansson, & Hakanson, 2005) and is the most common complaint in those over 75 who are seen by office physicians (Hill-O'Neill & Shaughnessy, 2002). There are four major types of dizziness according to Hill-O'Neill and Shaughnessy: vertigo, presyncope (light-headedness), disequilibrium (related to balance), and ill-defined (i.e., it does not fit in any other categories). These are further explained under assessment and diagnosis.

Risk Factors/Warning Signs

Risk factors for dizziness include advanced age, sudden change in position, inner ear problems, orthostatic hypotension, cerebrovascular disease, cardiovascular disease, cervical spondylosis, vestibular diseases, Meniere's disease, and TIAs. The signs and symptoms of dizziness can vary from lightheadedness lasting seconds to dizziness lasting for days (as in *benign paroxysmal positional vertigo (BPPV)*). Certain medications can also cause dizziness.

Signs and symptoms of BPPV include dizziness, presyncope, feelings of imbalance, and nausea. The symptoms begin when the person changes head position, even something as usual as tipping the head back or turning the head in bed.

Assessment and Diagnosis

Vertigo—a false sense of motion or spinning—may be caused by BPPV, which is brought on by normal calcium carbonate crystals breaking loose and falling into the wrong part of the inner ear. It can also be caused by inflammation in the inner ear; *Meniere's syndrome*; vestibular migraine; acoustic neuroma; rapid changes in motion; or more serious problems such as stroke, brain hemorrhage, or multiple sclerosis.

Presyncope is when the older person complains of feeling faint or light-headed. It is associated with a drop in blood pressure such as occurs when the person sits up or suddenly changes to a standing position, or with an inadequate output of blood from the heart. It can also be caused by medications that induce orthostatic hypotension, hypovolemia, low blood sugar, or some other cause of lack of blood flow to the brain.

Disequilibrium is a loss of balance or the feeling of being unsteady when walking. Causes of disequilibrium include vestibular problems, sensory disorders, joint or muscle problems, or medications.

The fourth category is really a "catch all" for possible causes of dizziness not included in the first three categories. Problems in this category include such things as other inner ear disorders, anxiety disorders, hyperventilation, cerebral ischemia, side effects of medications, Parkinsonian symptoms, hypotension, low blood sugar, and benign positional vertigo.

Dizziness is generally treatable by addressing the cause. However, in some cases, such as dizziness associated with poststroke, it can be a permanent impairment.

Otological dizziness (a major classification in the elderly, according to Hain and Ramaswamy [2005]) refers to vertigo caused by changes in the vestibular system. The most common types in the elderly are Meniere's syndrome and BPPV. Meniere's syndrome is common in those over age 50. The cause is unknown, though it is often attributed to a virus or bacterial infection. Signs and symptoms include a rapid decrease in hearing; a sense of pressure or fullness in one ear, accompanied by loud *tinnitus* (ringing in the ears); and then vertigo (Hain & Ramaswamy, 2005; Hill-O'Neill & Shaughnessy, 2002; Hain, 2012). It may involve the excessive buildup of fluid in the inner ear, which is the cause of the feeling of fullness in the ear. A feeling of being unsteady or dizzy may last for as little as 30 minutes or for days after the episode (Mayo Clinic, 2012).

As mentioned previously, BPPV is the most common cause of dizziness in the older age group, accounting for as much as 50% of all dizziness, with an increasing incidence with age (Hain, 2003, 2012). BPPV occurs when debris called *otoconia* ("rocks in the ears") become dislodged from their usual place in the ear and get stuck elsewhere in the vestibular system. Although in most cases the underlying cause of BPPV is not known, the degeneration of the vestibular system in the inner ear that occurs with normal aging is thought to play a major role. In cases of vertigo that do not respond to traditional medication for dizziness (such as Antivert), BPPV should be suspected. A key to diagnosis of BPPV is Hallpike's maneuver, in which the patient is laid down quickly from a sitting position, with the head turned to the side and hung over the back of the exam table. This will produce a characteristic nystagmus if the cause is BPPV.

Interventions

Treatment for dizziness depends on the underlying cause. For dizziness caused by body position, behavioral modification is indicated. Depending on the cause of dizziness, medication may be helpful. For dizziness of acute onset, methylprednisolone may be used over a 3-week period to improve vestibular function. In Meniere's disease, meclizine may help with acute symptom relief. If the cause is TIAs, then aspirin therapy might be initiated to decrease vascular risk factors (Reuben et al., 2008).

BPPV can be treated in the office by the physician, advanced practice nurse, or even a physical therapist with knowledge of the proper maneuvers. The Epley maneuver is a technique by which the patient is put into a series of specific positions and head turns to promote return of the otoconia to their proper place in the ear. After this treatment, the patient must stay in the office for 10 minutes and then sleep in a recliner chair at 45 degrees for the following 2 nights. They should also be instructed to avoid head positions that cause BPPV for at least another week (Hain, 2003). Other maneuvers and even surgical treatment may be necessary in rare variations of BPPV; these would be recommended by the physician on a case-by-case basis.

Dizziness, whatever the cause, can be particularly distressing to the older adult. It can interfere with activities of daily living, the ability to drive, and the maintenance of independence. Elders may decrease activities and spend more time at home due to the fear of dizzy spells or of falling. It is a leading cause of elderly persons discontinuing driving, which may be depressing to them and limit their social activity. In other cases the fear of having to stop driving will keep a person from seeking medical attention. Early diagnosis of the cause of dizziness can result in better outcomes by starting treatment sooner and avoiding complications that can result from bouts of syncope or vertigo.

Nurses should encourage older adults with complaints of dizziness to seek medical help. Treatment may be with medication, simple maneuvers, or lifestyle changes. Emotional support during diagnosis and testing, and reassurance that most causes of dizziness are treatable, can be a comfort to the older adult with this problem.

Seizures

Background

Once thought to be mainly a disorder of children, recurrent seizures or epilepsy is thought to be present in about 7% of older adults (Spitz, 2005) and is usually related to one of the common comorbidities found in older adults (Bergey, 2004; Rowan & Tuchman, 2003). Epilepsy affects up to 3 million Americans of all ages (Velez & Selwa, 2003). Davidson & Davidson (2012) summarized findings of most studies on epilepsy in older adults with these main points:

1. the elderly succumb to seizures and epilepsy more than any other age group;
2. the largest identifiable cause of seizures and epilepsy in the elderly is cerebrovascular disease;
3. the symptoms of seizures and epilepsy in the elderly are more vague than in younger adults;
4. finding an appropriate treatment for the elderly is complicated by adverse drug reactions, drug interactions, polypharmacy, absorption rates, and other challenging health issues; and
5. approximately 100 in every 100,000 patients over the age of 65 experience a seizure or epilepsy. (p. 11)

Seizures can be caused by a variety of conditions in older persons, but "the most common cause of new-onset epilepsy in an elderly person is arteriosclerosis and the associated cerebrovascular disease" (Spitz, 2005, p. 1), accounting for 40–50% of seizures in this age group (Rowan & Tuchman, 2003). Seizures are associated with stroke in 5–14% of survivors (Spitz, 2005; Velez & Selwa, 2003). Other common causes of epilepsy in the elderly include Alzheimer's disease and brain tumor. A list of potential causes of seizures in older adults appears in **Table 9-25**.

TABLE 9-25   Possible Causes of Seizures in the Elderly
Stroke or other cerebrovascular disease
Arteriosclerosis
Alzheimer's disease
Brain tumor
Head trauma
Intracranial infection
Drug abuse or withdrawal
Withdrawal from antiepileptic drug

There are three major classifications of epilepsies, although there are many additional types. Generalized types are more common in young people and associated with grand mal or tonic-clonic seizures. A number of cases have an undetermined origin and may be associated with certain situations such as high fever, exposure to toxins, or rare metabolic events. In older adults, localized (partial or focal) epilepsies are more common, particularly complex partial seizures (Luggen, 2009). In contrast to young adults, Rowan and Tuchman (2003) cite other differences in seizures in the elderly: low frequency of seizure activity, easier to control, high potential for injury, a prolonged postictal period, and better tolerance with newer antiepileptic drugs (AEDs). Additionally, older adults may have coexisting medical problems and take many medications to treat these problems.

Risk Factors/Warning Signs

Risk factors for seizures in older adults include cerebrovascular disease (especially stroke), age, and head trauma. The most obvious signs and symptoms of epilepsy are seizures, although changes in behavior, cognition, and level of consciousness may be other signs. Also, note that exposure to toxins can cause seizures that are not epilepsy. Complex partial seizures in older adults may include symptoms such as "confusion, memory loss, dizziness, and shortness of breath" (Davidson & Davidson, 2012, p. 16). Automatism (repetitive movements), facial twitching with following confusion, and coughing are also signs of the more-common complex partial seizure (Luggen, 2009).

Assessment and Diagnosis

Diagnosis is made by careful description of the seizure event, a thorough history, and physical. Eyewitness accounts of the seizure incident can be quite helpful, although many community-dwelling older adults go undiagnosed because their seizures are never witnessed. In addition, complete blood work, neuroimaging, chest X-ray, electrocardiogram (ECG), and electroencephalogram (EEG) help determine the cause and type of seizure (National Institute for Health and Clinical Excellence [NICE], 2012).

Interventions

Treatment for epilepsy is aimed at the causal factor. The standard treatment for recurrent seizures is antiepilepsy drugs (AEDs). The rule of thumb, "start low and go slow," for medication dosing in older adults particularly applies to AEDs. The elderly tend to have more side effects, adverse drug interactions, and problems with toxicity levels than younger people.

Research has suggested that older adults may have better results with fewer side effects with the newer AEDs than the traditional ones, though about 10% of nursing home residents are still medicated with the first-generation AEDs (Mauk, 2004). The most common older medications used to treat seizures include barbiturates (such as phenobarbital), benzodiazepines (such as diazepam/Valium), hydantoins (such as phenytoin/Dilantin), and valproates (such as valproic acid/Depakene) (Deglin & Vallerand, 2005; Resnick, 2008).

Several newer drugs are also used, depending on the type of seizure. Second-generation AEDs, including gabapentin (Neurontin), lamotrigine (Lamictal), oxcarbazepine (Trileptal), levetiracetam (Keppra), pregabalin (Lyrica), tiagabine (Gabitril), and topiramate (Topamax), are generally recommended over the older AEDs; however, older AEDS such as phenytoin (Dilantin), valproate (Depakote), and carbamazepine (Tegretol) are the most commonly prescribed treatment options (Resnick, 2008). Each of these medications has specific precautions for use in patients with certain types of medical problems or for those taking certain other medications. When assessing for side effects in older patients, be sure to be alert to potential GI, renal, neurological (ataxia), and hepatic side effects. Additionally, some newer extended-release AEDs are thought to be better tolerated and have a lower incidence of systemic side effects (such as tremors) (Uthman, 2004).

Musculoskeletal Disorders

Among older adults, there are several significant musculoskeletal problems that can significantly impact quality of life. Osteoporosis can lead to fractures. Arthritis is a major source of pain among older adults, and those who experience related decreased range of motion may have joint replacement surgery. Some of these common disorders will be discussed in this section.

Osteoporosis

Background/Significance

Osteoporosis is a bone disorder characterized by low bone density or porous bones. Over 44 million Americans, including 55% of adults age 50 or over, have this disease. Although often thought of as a woman's disease, by age 90 17% of men have osteoporosis as do 32% of women (Khosla, 2010; Cawthon, 2010). Older persons of all ethnic backgrounds may experience osteoporosis, though it is more common among Whites and Asians. The risk factors for this disorder are many and appear in **Table 9-26**.

Risk Factors/Warning Signs

A major complication of osteoporosis is fractures. These are especially common in the vertebral spine, hips, and wrists. The cumulative cost for treatment of osteoporosis and associated fractures and pain is expected to rise to $204 billion during the period of 2006–2015 and to exceed $228 billion during 2016–2025 (USPSTF, 2011). Because there are sometimes no signs or symptoms during the early course of bone deterioration, osteoporosis is often undiagnosed and untreated until fracture occurs.

Assessment/Diagnosis

Osteoporosis-related fractures may lead to pain, immobility, and other complications. If signs and symptoms are present besides fractures, they may take the form of pain and kyphosis (see **Figure 9-9**). Diagnostic testing would reveal decreased bone density and any pathological fractures present via X-ray. On occasion, hairline fractures do not manifest themselves with the initial X-ray, but appear 5–10 days after the initial assault.

TABLE 9-26 **Risk Factors for Osteoporosis**
Personal history of fracture after age 50
Current low bone mass
History of fracture in a first-degree relative
Being female
Being thin and/or having a small frame
Advanced age
A family history of osteoporosis
Estrogen deficiency as a result of menopause, especially early or surgically induced
Abnormal absence of menstrual periods (amenorrhea)
Anorexia nervosa
Low lifetime calcium intake
Vitamin D deficiency
Use of certain medications, such as corticosteroids and anticonvulsants
Presence of certain chronic medical conditions
Low testosterone levels in men
An inactive lifestyle
Current cigarette smoking
Excessive use of alcohol
Being White or Asian, although African Americans and Hispanic Americans are at significant risk as well

Source: From the National Osteoporosis Foundation, 2008, p. 1.

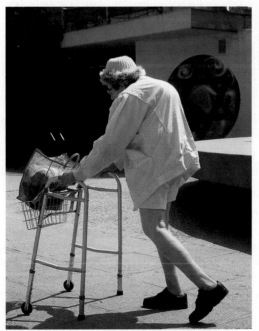

© Bill Aron/PhotoEdit

Figure 9-9 Kyphosis.

Interventions

Because this is a highly treatable and often preventable disease when detected early, all women over the age of 65 years should have *bone mineral density (BMD)* or bone mass measurement done, while women with risk factors for osteoporosis should have BMD at age 60 (AHRQ, 2013). Steps can be taken to prevent osteoporosis by habits that help build strong bones before the age of 20, when bones are fully developed. Preventing osteoporosis in adolescent years would include eating a well-balanced diet with plenty of calcium and vitamin D, no smoking or excessive alcohol intake, plenty of weight-bearing exercise, and discussing any needed treatments with the physician to minimize the risk of the disease. It should be noted that most of the calcium in the diet of American children comes from milk, though yogurt, broccoli, and certain enriched cereals may provide additional sources. Nurses can be active in primary prevention of osteoporosis through educating children in schools about the effects of this disease in later life and how to prevent it.

Treatment of existing osteoporosis takes many forms. Postmenopausal women are often prescribed biphosphonates (such as Fosamax), calcitonin (Miacalcin), or estrogen/hormone replacement medications (such as Estratab or Premarin). Some of these medications are aimed at promoting adequate amounts of calcium in the bones, whereas the hormone replacement therapies replace the estrogen not being produced after menopause, which helps create more of a balance between the delicate hormones that guide bone reabsorption and demineralization. The use of estrogen replacement therapy was once used to decrease the incidence of serious fractures in postmenopausal women, but now only selective estrogen receptor modulators are approved for this use (Gallagher & Levine, 2011) due to the associated side effects. Weight-bearing exercises and getting enough calcium in the diet or through supplementation are other treatments to consider. If vitamin supplementation is used, it is essential that the patient take not only calcium but also vitamin D to promote the absorption of the calcium. Nurses should encourage patients to discuss all treatment options with their physicians. Nutritional counseling and the role of sunlight (a source of vitamin D) and exercise should also be addressed. One potential exercise that is being explored for its benefit for both balance and promoting bone health is Tai Chi, a form of Eastern martial arts—one randomized controlled trial demonstrated that the Tai Chi group should increased balance (Shan et al., 2008).

Arthritis

Arthritis, or inflammation of the joint, is the number one chronic complaint and cause of disability in the United States (Arthritis Foundation, 2012), affecting nearly 46 million people (1 in 5 adults, or 20% of the U.S. population) at a cost of $128 billion per year (Arthritis Foundation, 2012; CDC, 2011). There are over 100 types of arthritis, with the two most common being osteoarthritis (OA) and rheumatoid arthritis (RA). These will be discussed here in relationship to their impact on the lives of older adults. Rheumatic diseases affect approximately 21% of the US population, 1.3 million with RA (Helmick et al., 2008).

Osteoarthritis

Background/Significance

Osteoarthritis (OA) is also called degenerative joint disease, osteoarthrosis, hypertrophic arthritis, and degenerative arthritis (Arthritis Foundation, 2012). It affects about 13.9% of the U.S. population age 25 or older and 33.6% of those 65 or older, which equals an estimated 26 million adults (Arthritis Foundation, 2012; CDC, 2011). Bitton (2009) estimated that the cost of osteoarthritis to be approximately $89.1 billion, including both direct and indirect costs as well as lost wages due to time off from work.

Risk Factors/Warning Signs

The cause of OA is unknown, but it affects females more often than males, and risk increases with certain factors. Modifiable risks include obesity, joint injury, occupation, structural alignment, and muscle weakness. Nonmodifiable risks include gender (women are more at risk), age, race (White and Asian people are at higher risk), and genetic predisposition (CDC, 2011). At this point, it is unknown whether smoking increases risk.

Assessment and Diagnosis

This disease is characterized by chronic deterioration of the cartilage at the ends of the bones; eventually, the bones at the joint become inflamed due to cartilage breakdown, which released cytokines (inflammation proteins) and enzymes that further damage the cartilage. This results in a change in the shape and make-up of the joint so that it will not function smoothly. Bone fragments and cartilage may float in what joint fluid there is, causing irritation and pain, and often resulting in bone spurs (osteophytes) forming near the end of the bone (Arthritis Foundation, 2012).

Signs and symptoms of OA include pain, stiffness (especially in the morning), aching, some joint swelling, and inflammation. Osteoarthritis targets joints such as the fingers, feet, knees, hips, and spine (Yurkow & Yudin, 2002). Heberden's nodes (bony enlargements at the end joints of the fingers) and Bouchard's nodes (bony enlargements at the middle joints of the fingers) are common (see **Figure 9-10**). Radiographs would show increased heat at the site of inflammation as well as bone deterioration. As OA progresses, the individual may experience crepitus, limping, limited range of motion, increased pain, and even fractures. Diagnosis is made through various lab tests, X-rays, MRIs, or CT scans to visualize areas of damage.

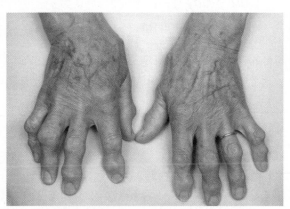

© Visuals Unlimited

Figure 9-10 Bouchard's and Herberden's nodes.

Interventions

The most common associated complication of OA is pain. Although there is no cure for OA, treatment is generally aimed at symptom reduction through lifestyle modifications, nonpharmacological therapies, and medication. For example, risk factors that can be modified, such as excessive stress to the joint (perhaps caused by sports or obesity), should be addressed with exercise programs for strengthening muscles and weight loss (see **Case Study 9-5**). Exercise programs that are holistic and interdisciplinary, particularly those offered in rehabilitation units, may help individuals cope with pain and increase functional levels. In addition, many persons use alternative methods of pain control in combination with medications. **Table 9-27** provides a summary of common treatments for pain for those with OA.

Medications used for treatment of OA include acetaminophen (Tylenol), aspirin, nonsteroidal anti-inflammatory drugs (NSAIDs) such as ibuprofen and naproxen, COX-2 inhibitors (such as celecoxib/Celebrex), tramadol (Ultram), and antidepressants. Other therapies include injection of steroids into the joint to decrease inflammation or injection of synthetic material (such as Synvisc) that acts as a lubricant in the absence of synovial fluid to provide comfort. Other therapies to preserve motion and decrease pain include heat or cold, splints, adaptive equipment, aquatic therapy, and nutrition. In cases of severe dysfunction and pain, surgery with joint replacement may be an option.

Important for any nurse caring for older persons taking NSAIDs is the awareness of common side effects. The most common adverse effects of NSAIDs include gastrointestinal symptoms such as stomach upset, nausea, vomiting, and more seriously, gastric ulcers. COX-2 drugs were thought to minimize these effects. Currently all COX-2 medications except Celebrex have been pulled from the market due to associated cardiac risk (Frisco, 2013).

Case Study 9-5

Mrs. Chiu is a small, 100-pound, 90-year-old Chinese woman with fractures of the vertebral spine. Because of kyphosis and pain associated with osteoporosis, Mrs. Chiu has been bedbound in a nursing home for several months. Her family visits regularly and has many questions about her condition, especially if it is something that her teenage granddaughters might develop.

Questions:

1. What are Mrs. Chiu's known risk factors for osteoporosis and resulting fractures?

2. How should you answer the family's questions?

3. Are the granddaughters at risk because Mrs. Chiu has osteoporosis? If so, what can they do to prevent it?

4. What teaching should be done with this family?

TABLE 9-27   Treatments for Pain Associated with Osteoarthritis

Pharmacological	Nonpharmacological
Acetaminophen	Moist heat
Aspirin	Warm paraffin wraps
NSAIDs	Stretch gloves or stockings
Capsaicin (topically, with other therapies)	Range of motion exercises
Nabumetone	Upper extremity activities (such as piano playing, typing, card-playing)
	Swimming
	Adaptive equipment
	Heat/cold applications
	Warm bath (limit to 20 minutes)
	Good posture
	Supportive shoes
	Well-balanced diet
	Maintenance of appropriate weight

Rheumatoid Arthritis

Background/Significance

Rheumatoid arthritis is characterized by remissions and exacerbations of inflammation within the joint. It affects the fingers, wrists, knees, and spine. In contrast to OA, RA is caused by chronic inflammation that can cause severe joint deformities and loss of function over time (see **Figure 9-11**).

Rheumatoid arthritis affects over 2 million Americans and is more common in women than men. It is generally diagnosed between the ages of 40 and 50 and can cause significant disability for adults who live into old age with this disorder (Mayo Clinic, 2012c). Although the cause is unknown, researchers believe RA may be due to a virus or hormonal factors. In 1987, Peter Gregersen identified the relationship between five specific amino acids and RA, hypothesizing that the area of the genome known as the major histocompatibility complex was critical to RA susceptibility. Twenty years later the ability to fine-map the MHC was discovered. With this technique it is expected that scientists will be able to identify the specific area of the MHC and the triggering mechanism in the HLA proteins responsible for RA. Knowing the cause of the antigens that initiate RA will be the first step towards better treatment for the disease (Von Radowitz, 2012).

Risk Factors/Warning Signs

Risk factors for RA include being female, having a certain predisposing gene, and exposure to an infection. Advanced age is a risk factor until age 70, after which incidence decreases. Cigarette smoking over a period of years is another risk factor.

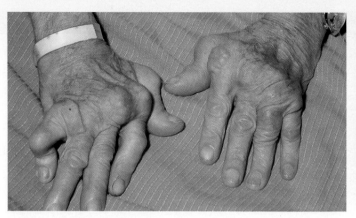
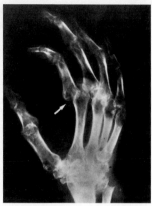

Figure 9-11 Rheumatoid arthritis.

Source: Leonard Crowley, *An Introduction to Human Disease: Pathology and Pathophysiology Correlations* (9th Edition). Burlington, MA: Jones & Bartlett Learning, 2013.

There are numerous potential complications with RA, including lung disease (Antin-Ozerkis et al., 2010), increased risk of diabetes (Solomon et al., 2010), and cardiac arrhythmias, specifically atrial fibrillation (Gabriel & Crowson, 2012). Patients with RA need to be educated and cautioned to pay attention to any signs and symptoms of these potential diseases and to seek medical attention, and not "write them off" to an RA exacerbation.

Assessment and Diagnosis

Signs and symptoms of RA are systemic and include malaise, fatigue, symmetrical patterns of joint inflammation, pain, stiffness, swelling, gelling (joints stiff after rest), elevated sedimentation rate, presence of serum rheumatoid factor, and elevated white blood cell count (WBC) in the synovial fluid of the inflamed joint. Radiographs will show erosion of the bone. Pain is more prevalent in RA, and joint deformities can cause more debilitation than is generally seen with OA. In addition, RA often strikes in young to middle adulthood, with more degeneration seen over time than with OA.

Interventions

The treatment for RA is similar to OA with the exception that anti-inflammatory and immune-suppressing drugs may play a more important role. DMARDs (disease-modifying anti-rheumatic drugs) are also used in RA. Historically these drugs were not used until all other medications had been tried; now, however, the DMARDs are often used within 3 months of diagnosis, the intention being to modify the disease process and prevent the deformities and pain associated with the disease. These medications may not show results for several months, and nurses should teach patients to recognize signs of infections such as chills, pain, and fever.

Nurses should expect to see many complications associated with arthritis. Some potential nursing diagnoses are pain, impaired physical mobility, fatigue, decreased endurance, powerlessness, self-care deficits, sleep pattern disturbance, depression, impaired coping, social isolation, fear, anxiety, and body-image disturbance. Goals for care include promoting independence within limitations, pain management, and education.

Educational programs for persons with arthritis should include exercise and mobility, education, counseling, individual physical and occupational therapy, and a focus of independence in *activities of daily living (ADLs)* with self-care. These types of programs help decrease disability, pain, and the need for assistance, as well as reduce joint tenderness. Pain coping and exercise training may also enhance pain control.

Joint Replacement

Joint replacement is used for several different diagnoses, including fracture, immobility, and intractable pain. The two most commonly performed joint replacement surgeries are total hip arthroplasty and total knee arthroplasty. Knee replacements are mainly related to advanced arthritis that causes severe pain and decreased function. Hip replacements may also be done related to arthritis or due to fracture, usually from falling.

Steel, Clark, Lang, Wallace, and Melzer (2008) and Constantinescu, Goucher, Weinstein, and Fraenkel (2009) reported significantly fewer joint replacements done on Hispanics and Blacks than Whites, due to reasons beyond access and financial resources. The researchers suggested that cultural differences, values, and attitudes might also play a role in seeking joint replacement.

Total Hip Arthroplasty/Replacement
Background/Significance

Hip replacement surgery may be indicated when an older person demonstrates lack of function, trouble with ADLs, and continued pain that is not sufficiently addressed with traditional medical therapy. Certainly, those with certain types of hip fractures will be candidates for this surgery also. In women, body weight and older age have been found to be risk factors for needing hip replacement due to OA (National Institute of Arthritis and Musculoskeletal and Skin Diseases, 2003).

Interventions

During hip replacement, a prosthetic device made of metal, plastic, ceramic, or various other substances is substituted for the worn-out, damaged, or fractured portions of the hip. The implant is made of a ball-type device on a stem that fits into the femur. The socket of the pelvis helps hold the ball that is articulated onto the joint (see **Figure 9-12**). During surgery, physicians may choose to cement the prosthesis into the femur or not. Staples are generally used to close the wound, with

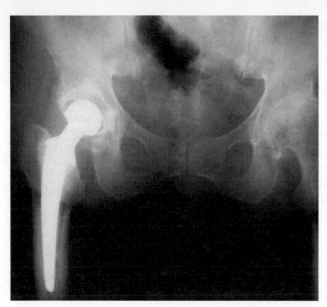

Figure 9-12 Total hip prosthesis.

Source: Leonard Crowley, *Introduction to Human Disease* (6th ed.). Sudbury, MA: Jones & Bartlett Publishers 2005.

a nonstick dressing applied. Staples are usually removed 7–10 days after surgery, depending on healing of the wound. Sometimes physicians will order half of the staples removed initially and the other half later. Steri strips may be applied to assist with wound edge approximation.

Postoperatively, the person will remain in acute care for several days to a week, and then many older adults may need rehabilitation services as inpatients or outpatients, depending on comorbidities, physical condition, and family support. Weight bearing is progressive and depends upon the physician's orders based on the condition of the bones observed during surgery. It is essential that the nurse and other team members strictly observe weight-bearing instructions (such as toe-touch, partial, or full) to avoid injury to the healing hip. Dislocation of the traditional prosthesis can also result from not following routine hip precautions after surgery. Routine hip precautions include not crossing the legs at the knees or ankles, not bending in a chair more than 90 degrees, keeping a pillow between the knees (to maintain abduction) until determined by the physician, and avoiding lying on the operative side until the physician gives permission to do so. Surgical procedures for total hip arthroplasty continue to advance. Minimally invasive surgery may require the same precautions as traditional surgery depending upon the approach of the surgeon. Single incision using a frontal approach is being done in select hospitals across the United States and has the advantage of not requiring mobility limitations immediately after surgery (Alcelik et al., 2012; Wong et al., 2011; Neville, Dvorkin, Chittenden, & Fromm, 2008).

Nursing instruction to patients and family members should include watching for signs and symptoms of wound infection. Patients should report any redness, swelling, drainage, or odor from the operative site. A small amount of brownish drainage from the site a few days postoperatively is normal. Fever or malaise could also be signs of infection and should be promptly reported to the physician. These nursing implications apply to all surgical procedures.

Additionally, reminders about routine hip precautions (as indicated by the procedure performed), exercises, and ambulation as indicated by the physical therapist, as well as traveling implications, should be given. Some prostheses will cause the alarm at airport security to go off. Teach patients to inform security personnel of their hip prosthesis prior to entering the security gate.

Dr. Robert Zann, an orthopedic specialist, stated that recovery from hip replacement surgery generally takes longer than many patients think: "It is interesting that patients undergoing hip replacement surgery will uniformly reach their maximum improvement between 1–2 years" (2005, p. 1). Physicians attribute this to the need for tissue healing (of which 90% occurs in the first 3 months) and return of muscles to normal function and strength, which takes longer.

Total Knee Arthroplasty/Replacement

Background/Significance

Similar to hip replacement, knee replacement is done when a person is experiencing decreased range of motion, trouble walking or climbing stairs, and increased degeneration of the joint so as to impair quality of life. This most often occurs as a result of arthritis (either osteo- or rheumatoid arthritis).

Interventions

Total knee replacement (TKR) surgery involves resurfacing or removing the distal portion of the femur that articulates with the end of the shin bone. The prosthesis consists of metal and plastic or similar materials that are cemented onto the newly resurfaced areas of the articulating bones. Although often done under general anesthetic, this surgery can also be performed under spinal anesthesia. Sometimes blood loss is significant, so patients may be asked to donate their own blood ahead of time to be given back to them in the event it is needed. In addition, a growing trend is toward bilateral knee replacement in those persons requiring both knees to be surgically repaired. The benefits of this are the one-time operative anesthetic and room costs, and many physicians feel recovery from bilateral replacement is similar to single replacement. However, the pain and lack of mobility, as well as the significant increase in the assistance needed after surgery when a bilateral replacement is done, may make this less than ideal for most older patients. Surgical procedures for TKR have not evolved quite as rapidly as total hip arthroplasy; however, additional procedures include partial knee replacement, which might be performed in lieu of TKR. Despite the procedure, nursing care remains constant.

Discomfort after knee surgery is generally severe in the first few days. Nurses should encourage patients to use cold packs on the operative area for the first day and take pain and sleeping medications as ordered. In addition, alternative therapies such as guided imagery have been shown to help with pain management (Posadzi & Ernst, 2011). Many joint replacement patients feel a loss of control and independence. Nurses can help the recovery process by maintaining a professional therapeutic relationship with patients. This has been shown to assist older persons in regaining their sense of independence (Heikkinen et al., 2008).

Therapy will begin immediately in the acute care hospital. Although weight bearing does not usually occur until 24 hours after surgery, sitting in a chair and using a continuous passive motion machine (CPM), if ordered, will ease recovery. The use of a CPM is generally based on the surgeon's preference. There is research to support it, as well as studies indicating that walking soon after surgery has an equal effect and makes the CPM unnecessary. However, in cases of an older person who may not have the mobility skills initially after surgery that a younger person would, a CPM may be beneficial to keep the joint flexible and decrease pain.

Dr. Zann (2005) indicated that "patients undergoing total knee replacement do not achieve their maximum improvement until 2–4 years" (p. 1). This is attributed to the lack of muscular structures that surround and protect the knee and the need for the ligaments and tendons to adapt to the indwelling prosthesis. Recovery times vary and depend upon a number of variables, including the patient's overall health, age, comorbidities, and motivation. Patients report that the new knee joint never feels normal even years after the surgery, but they do experience an increase in function and generally much less pain than before.

Nursing implications include teaching the patient about signs and symptoms of infection, care of the surgical site (if staples are still present), pain management, and expectations for recovery. A range of motion from 0–90 degrees is the minimum needed for normal functioning. Most prostheses will allow up to about 120 degrees of flexion, though 110 degrees is considered good range of motion after knee replacement. After discharge, a walker is usually used in the first few weeks, followed by light activities 6 weeks after surgery. In addition, the patient's spouse may experience feelings of being overwhelmed due to role transitions that occur after surgery and during the recovery period. Nurses can help facilitate this transition by providing education and discussing realistic expectations (Walker, 2012).

Amputation

Background/Significance

Amputation is an acquired condition that results in the loss of a limb, typically from disease, injury, and/or associated surgery. There are approximately 278,000 new amputees each year in the United States (Amputation Statistics, 2012). Seventy-seven percent of these cases are from circulatory problems, particularly PVD related to diabetes, while most of the rest are attributed to trauma.

Risk Factors/Warning Signs

Most amputations involve the lower extremities, above or below the knee. The greatest risk factor for amputation is diabetes with accompanying peripheral vascular disease, with African American men having a 2.3 times greater rate of amputation than Whites with diabetes. Advanced age and the incidence of diabetes in the elderly make this a potential problem in the older age group. Additionally, a recent study showed that HgbA1c level was a significant predictor of foot amputation (Palmer et al., 2004).

Assessment/Diagnosis

In the acute phase of recovery after surgery, it is important to prevent contractures of the knee joint (if present) and attempt to maintain normal muscle power and range of motion in remaining joints. The limb should not be hung over the bedside or placed in a dependent position. Both in acute care and rehabilitation, the stump should be conditioned to prepare for the wearing of a prosthesis. In certain circumstances, an older person may choose, in consultation with the physician, not to wear a prosthesis. This generally occurs when there are other health issues, such as poor balance from another disease or disorder that would make falling and injury more likely with prosthetic use.

Interventions

Initially, there may be drainage from the surgical site, and a sterile dressing will be kept in place and changed at least daily. Eventually, the staples or sutures will be removed and a thick, black eschar will form at the amputation site and gradually come off. An Ace wrap or stump shrinker sock (elastic) is used to help prepare the stump for wearing the prosthesis. Several factors should be considered when preparing the stump to wear a prosthesis. These include a movable scar, lack of tenderness/sensitivity, a conical shape, firm skin, and lack of edema. All of these can be achieved by proper wrapping of the stump to maximize shrinkage and minimize swelling. The prone position, if tolerable, is an excellent way to promote full extension of the residual limb.

It is also important for the person to begin therapy right away. Chin and colleagues (2003) state that the higher/more proximal the amputation, the higher the energy expenditure to walk: Transfemoral amputation requires at least a 65% increase, traumatic amputation at least a 60% increase. The elderly generally have a 40% decrease in speed and 80% more energy expenditure. When using the prosthesis at first, an older adult may tire easily. Be sure to take into account any coexisting problems, such as cardiopulmonary disease, when considering energy expenditure. The newest technologies allow prosthetics to be light, durable, and more comfortable.

Nurses will need to teach patients and families about stump care, mobility, adaptation, coping, and self-care. Home maintenance, dealing with complications and/or additional health problems, wear and tear on non-weight-bearing joints, adapting to the environment, accessibility, stigma, depression, role changes, decreased energy, and chronic pain are all issues to be aware of related to amputation. It is likely that the person with lower extremity amputation will experience some shoulder problems over time due to the additional stress on this non-weight-bearing joint. Remember that alteration in body image is a significant hurdle to overcome for some individuals. *Phantom limb pain*, or pain sensations in the nonexistent limb, is more common after traumatic amputations and may last for weeks after amputation. Massage and medications may help with this type of pain control (Beers, 2005). Additionally, proper wrapping of the stump (in a figure-eight wrap) may help decrease the chance of phantom limb pain later (Kalapatapu, 2012).

In general, older persons with amputation may return to a normal quality of life with some adaptations. The care provided by nurses and physicians in rehabilitation after amputation may make the difference in the person's ability to cope with the changes that result after surgery. Geriatric nurses can facilitate the transition back into the community after amputation by educating patients and families about resources to assist with adaptation.

Sensory Impairments

Although many normal aging changes occur in the sensory system, most of the common abnormalities seen in the elderly are related to vision. According to Lighthouse International (2005), a leading resource on vision impairment and visual rehabilitation, the most common age-related vision problems are cataracts, glaucoma, macular degeneration, and diabetic neuropathy. This section will discuss these impairments and others. As diseases related to the senses of touch, hearing, and taste are rare, these will not be discussed here. The other most common sensory problem in older adults is chronic sinusitis, which will also be discussed.

Cataracts

Background

Cataracts are responsible for 51% of world blindness, representing about 20 million people (World Health Organization [WHO], 2010). More than 90% of cataracts are age-related. Cataracts are so common in older adults that some almost consider them an inevitable consequence of old age and often fail to report during the history and physical. According to the University of Washington, Department of Ophthalmology (2008), 400,000 new cases of cataract development are diagnosed each year, 1,350,000 cataract extractions are currently performed each year, 3,700,000 visits to a doctor related to cataracts occur each year, and 5,500,000 people have visual obstruction due to cataracts.

Risk Factors/Warning Signs

Advancing age is the biggest risk factor for the development of cataracts. Other risk factors include diabetes, uveitis, intraocular tumor, long-term use of medications such as corticosteroids, excessive exposure to sunlight, blunt or penetrating trauma, and excessive exposure to heat or radiation. Tobacco use, family history of cataracts, high alcohol intake, and lack of dietary antioxidants also puts the person at risk for cataract development (Gerzevitz, Porter, & Dunphy, 2011). The etiology is thought to be from oxidative damage to lens protein that occurs with aging. Although about half of people between 65 and 75 years of age have cataracts, they are most common in those over age 75 (70%), and there are no ethnic or gender variations (Trudo & Stark, 1998).

Assessment and Diagnosis

Cataracts cause no pain or discomfort and may be manifested by gradual opacity of the lens, which affects the ability to see clearly. This causes decreased visual acuity, sensitivity to glare, and altered color perception. Older adults may not be aware of the problem until visual changes occur. They may report blurred or distorted vision or complain of glare when driving at night. The person may present with a fall due to visual changes. Some older adults will disclose that their reading vision has improved and they no longer need reading glasses, something called "second sight." Eventually the pupil changes color to a cloudy white (see **Figure 9-13**). Generally, the most common objective finding is decreased visual acuity, such as that measured with a Snellen eye chart. The patient should be referred to an ophthalmologist for further evaluation and consideration of surgery.

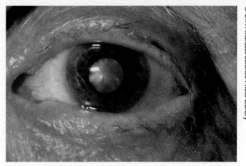

Figure 9-13 A cataract.

Interventions

Although changes in eyeglasses are the first option, when quality of life becomes affected, the most effective treatment for cataracts is surgery. Surgery is relatively safe and usually is done as an outpatient procedure. The opaque lens is removed and replaced with an artificial intraocular lens. This is the most common operation among older adults, and more than 95% of them have better vision after surgery (Trudo & Stark, 1998). The benefits of surgery include improved visual acuity, depth perception, and peripheral vision, leading to better outcomes related to ADLs, quality of life, and reduced risk of falls. Complications associated with surgery are rare but include retinal detachment, infection, and macular edema. The lens is removed through an incision in the eye and an intraocular lens is inserted. The surgical incision is either closed with sutures or can heal itself. After surgery, patients will need to avoid bright sunlight; wear wrap-around sunglasses for a short time; and avoid straining, lifting, or bending. Cataract surgery today offers a safe and effective treatment to maintain independence and improve quality of life for older adults.

Glaucoma

Background

Glaucoma is a group of degenerative eye diseases with various causes that leads to progressive optic neuropathy, in which the optic nerve is damaged by high *intraocular pressure (IOP)*, resulting in blindness (Podolsky, 1998). Glaucoma is a leading cause of visual impairment and the second leading cause of blindness in the United States, and occurs more often in those over 40, with an increased incidence with age (3% to 4% in those over age 70) (Fingeret, 2010; Kennedy-Malone et al., 2004; Podolsky, 1998).

Risk Factors/Warning Signs

Unlike cataracts, there are some ethnic distinctions with the development of glaucoma. African Americans tend to develop it earlier than Caucasians, and females more often than males. Glaucoma is more common in African Americans, Asian Americans, and Alaska Natives. Other contributing factors include eye trauma, small cornea, small anterior chamber, family history, cataracts, and some medications (Eliopoulos, 2005; Kennedy-Malone et al., 2004).

Assessment and Diagnosis

Although the cause is unknown, glaucoma results from pupillary blockage that limits flow of aqueous humor, causing a rise in intraocular pressure. Two major types are noted here: acute and chronic. Acute glaucoma is also called closed angle or narrow angle. Signs and symptoms include severe eye pain in one eye, blurred vision, seeing colored halos around lights, red eye, headache, nausea, and vomiting. Symptoms may be associated with emotional stress. Acute glaucoma is a medical emergency and the patient should seek emergency help immediately. Blindness can occur from prolonged narrow angle glaucoma.

Chronic glaucoma, also called open angle or primary open angle, is more common than acute (90% of cases are this type), affecting over 2 million people in the United States. One million people probably have glaucoma and don not know it, and 10 million people have above normal intraocular pressure that may lead to glaucoma if not treated (University of Washington, Department of Ophthalmology, 2008). This type of glaucoma occurs gradually. Peripheral vision is slowly impaired. Signs and symptoms include tired eyes, headaches, misty vision, seeing halos around lights, and worse symptoms in the morning. Glaucoma often involves only one eye, but may occur in both.

Interventions

Since there is no scientific evidence of preventative strategies, early detection in those at risk is important. Treatment is essential to prevent loss of vision, because once vision has been lost to glaucoma, it cannot be restored. Diagnosis is made using a *tonometer* to measure IOP; normal IOP is 10–21 mmHg. Ophthalmologic examination will reveal changes in the color and contour of the optic nerve when glaucoma is present. *Gonioscopy* (direct exam), which is performed by an optometrist or ophthalmologist, provides another means of evaluation.

Treatment is aimed at reducing IOP. Medications to decrease pressure may be given, and surgical iridectomy to lower the IOP may prevent future episodes of acute glaucoma. In chronic glaucoma, there is no cure, so treatment is aimed at managing IOP through medication and eyedrops. Nurses should regularly evaluate if the person is consistently using the eyedrops as prescribed and, if not, determine why and develop strategies to improve medication adherence. In some cases it may be appropriate to have patients demonstrate how they administer the eyedrops. In addition, older adults should be assessed for safety related to visual changes and also reminded to schedule and attend regular visits with their ophthalmologist.

Macular Degeneration

Background

Age-related macular degeneration (ARMD) is the most common cause of blindness for those over age 60, affecting about 12 million Americans over the age of 40 and more than 1 out of every 3 people over age 75 (Seftel, 2005; Starr, Guyer, & Yannuzzi, 1998). Macular degeneration occurs in approximately 10% of long-term care residents age 66–74 years and increases to 30% for those residents age 75–85 (Stefanacci, 2007). About 11 million people in the United States have some from of ARMD and this number is expected to increase to approximately 22 million by 2050.

Risk Factors/Warning Signs

Age is a major risk factor; 3.8% of Americans between the ages of 50 and 59 years have some form of ARMD, with about 14.4% of older adults ages 70–79 having the disease (American Health Assistance Foundation [AHAF], 2012). Other risk factors include smoking, hypertension, diabetes mellitus, family history of macular degeneration, female gender, obesity, Caucasian, prolonged exposure to ultraviolet light, and diet high in fat and/or low in nutrients and antioxidants. Inactivity has also been linked to ARMD, which is most likely related to the increased risk for cardiovascular disease.

Assessment and Diagnosis

Macular degeneration results from damage or breakdown of the macula and subsequent loss of central vision. Generally associated with the aging process, it can also result from injury or infection. Two types are noted: dry (nonexudative) and wet (exudative). Dry macular degeneration affects 90% of those with the disease (Lighthouse International, 2005) and has a better prognosis. The dry type progresses slowly, with more subtle changes in vision than the wet type, which comes on suddenly and may cause more severe loss in vision. The signs and symptoms of ARMD are decreased central vision, seeing images as distorted, decreased color vision, and sometimes a central scotoma (a large, dark spot in the center of vision).

Interventions

Although there is no cure for macular degeneration, some new therapies show promise (see **Case Study 9-6**). Photodynamic therapy uses a special laser to seal leaking blood vessels in the eye. Antioxidant vitamins (C, D, E, and beta-carotene) and zinc also seem to slow the progress of the disease (Age-Related Eye Disease Study Authors [AREDS], 2001). Retinal cell transplantation or regeneration works by harvesting cells from the body and injecting them into diseased macular sites in the hope that new and healthy cells will grow, thus reversing the damage caused by ARMD (Macular Degeneration Foundation, 2005).

New medications have been approved for the treatment of macular degeneration. Ranibizumab (Lucentis) was approved in 2006, and not only has it shown promise in stopping the progression of macular degeneration, but approximately 50% of the patients taking the medication have shown an improvement in their vision to 20/40. It is given by injection into the eye by an ophthalmologist every 4 weeks for 2 years. Bevacizumab (Avastin) has been used in the treatment of wet macular degeneration and was widely used prior to the advent of ranibizumab. In 2011 Eylea (afibercept

Case Study 9–6

Mrs. Booker has recently been diagnosed with ARMD. She is distressed to feel she is going blind and there is nothing she can do about it. She expresses these frustrations to the nurse and asks for help.

Questions:

1. What should the nurse's response be?

2. What initial adaptations need to be made early in the disease process?

3. Are there any things that Mrs. Booker can do now to help modify her environment for this progressive vision loss? What would those things be?

4. To which resources should the nurse refer Mrs. Booker for further information and support?

injection) was approved by the FDA to treat the wet form of ARMD. Pegaptanib (Macugen) was approved in 2004 for the treatment of neovascular macular degeneration. It is also injected directly into the eye and targets endothelial growth factor (Stefanacci, 2007).

Chances are that most gerontological nurses will care for older adults with ARMD. Initially, small changes in the environment should be encouraged, such as better lighting in hallways, minimizing glare from lamps or shiny floors, and decorating living spaces in contrasting colors (McGrory & Remington, 2004). Visual adaptive devices such as magnifying glasses and reading lamps may provide temporary help as vision worsens. Auditory devices such as books on tape and adaptation of the environment to the visual impairment may help maintain independence. Nurses should be aware of the treatments being researched (see **Box 9-8**) and can assure patients that although there is no cure at present, there is hope for the future (see **Box 9-7**). Encourage patients to exercise; avoid overexposure to the sun; wear sunglasses and a hat; maintain a healthy weight; eat a nutritious diet that includes leafy green vegetables, fruit, fish, and foods containing vitamins D, E, and C, beta-carotene, and omega 3-fatty acids. It is also important that blood pressure and blood sugar are controlled.

It is crucial to remind patients not to just assume that visual changes are "due to aging," but that they may be treatable. Many people avoid seeking treatment for fear that nothing can be done and that they could lose their driver's license.

Diabetic Retinopathy

Background

Diabetes has become an epidemic in the United States. *Diabetic retinopathy*, a complication of diabetes mellitus, is a leading cause of blindness among adults age 25 to 74. Approximately 700,000 have proliferative diabetic retinopathy with an

BOX 9-7   Resources for Those with Visual Impairments

American Academy of Ophthalmology
   P.O. Box 7424
   San Francisco, CA 94120-7424
   415-561-8500
   http://www.aao.org

American Council of the Blind
   1155 15th Street, NW, Suite 720
   Washington, DC 20005
   http://www.acb.org

American Printing House for the Blind
   P.O. Box 6985
   1839 Franklin Avenue
   Louisville, KY 40206
   http://www.aph.org

EyeCare America
   A Public Service Foundation of the American
   Academy of Ophthalmology
   1-877-887-6327
   1-800-222-3937
   http://www.eyecareamerica.org

Lighthouse International
   111 East 59th Street
   New York, NY 10022-1202
   1-800-334-5497
   1-800-829-0500
   http://www.lighthouse.org

Macular Degeneration Foundation
   http://www.eyesight.org

National Eye Institute
   31 Center Drive MSC 2510
   Bethesda, MD 20892-2510
   301-496-5248
   http://www.nei.nih.gov

BOX 9-8   Web Exploration

Visit Lighthouse International at http://www.lighthouse.org and read about new software that may assist persons with visual problems.

annual incidence of about 65,000 (Klein, Knudtson, Lee, Gangnan, & Klein, 2009). Blindness results from the breakage of tiny vessels in the retina as a complication of diabetes and generally affects both eyes. The exact mechanism is not known, but the longer a person has diabetes, the more likely he or she is to suffer visual impairment (Eyecare America, 2005). Currently approximately 7 million diabetics suffer from diabetic retinopathy, 700,000 are at risk for blindness, and 16 million are prime targets for blinding disorders (University of Washington, Department of Ophthalmology, 2008).

Risk Factors/Warning Signs

There are no early warning signs of diabetic retinopathy, so it is essential that older adults with diabetes have a dilated eye exam each year. Early diagnosis and treatment can prevent much of the blindness that occurs from this disorder.

Assessment and Diagnosis

During the eye exam the eye care professional will do a visual acuity test, a dilated eye exam, and tonometry. If a person complains of seeing spots floating in the visual field, bleeding may be occurring and the person should see an eye doctor as soon as possible.

There are four stages of diabetic retinopathy. These appear in **Table 9-28**. Of the four stages, *proliferative retinopathy* is the most severe and accounts for 64% of vitreous hemorrhage in non-type 1 diabetic patients and for 89% of vitreous hemorrhage in type 1 diabetics (Manuchehri & Kirkby, 2003). As new, fragile, and abnormal blood vessels grow to compensate for the blocked vessels in the retina, these vessels may leak blood into the eye, causing swelling of the macula and blurred vision. This is what causes much of the blindness seen with diabetic retinopathy.

Interventions

The first three stages of diabetic retinopathy are not treated. The first priority in treating proliferative retinopathy is to treat the cause of the vitreous hemorrhage itself. This is followed by a procedure called *scatter laser treatment* that helps shrink the abnormal vessels (Manuchehri & Kirkby, 2003). This procedure may require at least two visits, because multiple areas away from the retina are burned with a laser in order to shrink abnormal vessels. Although patients may note some loss of peripheral sight and/or color vision with this procedure, it is the standard for preserving the majority of central and essential vision.

For more severe cases of bleeding in the eye, a *vitrectomy* may be needed. When blood collects in the center of the eye, a vitrectomy allows removal of the vitreous gel that has blood in it through a small incision in the eye. The blood-contaminated vitreous gel is replaced with a saline-type solution. This is often done as an outpatient procedure. The patient will need to wear an eye patch for days to weeks and use medicated eyedrops to prevent infection. After a vitrectomy, the person's eye may be red and sensitive for some time.

TABLE 9-28 Four Stages of Diabetic Retinopathy		
Stage	**Description**	**Pathophysiology**
Stage 1	Mild nonproliferative retinopathy	Microaneurysms in retina
Stage 2	Moderate nonproliferative retinopathy	Blockage of some blood vessels supplying retina
Stage 3	Severe nonproliferative retinopathy	Blockage of many blood vessels supplying retina; retina is deprived of needed circulation
Stage 4	Proliferative retinopathy	Advanced stage; new blood vessels that are abnormal and easily breakable form to compensate for blockage of circulation to retina; these vessels may break and leak to cause macular edema and blurred vision

Source: National Eye Institute, 2005.

The most important nursing consideration in caring for older persons who may be at risk for diabetic retinopathy is to emphasize prevention of this complication. Treatment becomes necessary with more severe cases, so the best treatment is prevention through regular eye exams, good control of blood sugars, monitoring hypertension, and controlling cholesterol levels. The nurse should encourage the older adult with diabetes to develop a good working relationship with a trusted eye care professional.

Retinal Detachment

Although not as common as the other visual problems discussed, *retinal detachment* may occur in the older adult. It can be the result of trauma to the eye. Symptoms may be gradual or sudden and may look like spots moving across the eye, blurred vision, light flashes, or a curtain drawing. If an older person presents with such symptoms, he or she should seek immediate medical help. Keep the person quiet to minimize further detachment. Surgery may be required to save vision.

Corneal Ulcer

Corneal ulcers are more common in the elderly than in younger age groups due to decreased tearing that occurs with normal aging. Also, many elderly patients have worn contact lenses, either for a very long time or as a result of cataract surgery; improper cleaning or accidents can occur when placing the lenses, which can cause corneal abrasions. The ulcers may also result from inflammation of the cornea related to stroke, fever, irritation, dehydration, or a poor diet. Corneal ulcers are difficult to treat and may leave scars that affect vision. Signs of corneal ulcer may include bloodshot eye, photophobia, and complaint of irritation. The nurse should encourage the older person to seek prompt assistance from an eye care professional.

Chronic Sinusitis

Background

One of the common health complaints of the elderly is chronic sinusitis. About 14.1% of Americans 65 and older report suffering from chronic sinusitis; for those 75 years and older, the rate is slightly lower at 13.5% (American Academy of Otolaryngology, 2012). Age-related physiological and functional changes that occur can cause restrictions to the airflow. This results from irritants blocking drainage of the sinus cavities, leading to infection.

Risk Factors/Warning Signs

Symptoms include a severe cold, sneezing, cough (that is often worse at night), hoarseness, diminished sense of smell, discolored nasal discharge, postnasal drip, headache, facial pain, fatigue, malaise, and fever (Kelley, 2002).

Assessment and Diagnosis

Upon physical examination, the person may complain of pain on palpation of the sinus areas, and edema and redness of the nasal mucosa may be evident. Allergies, common cold, and dental problems should be ruled out for differential diagnosis. When symptoms continue over a period of weeks and up to 3 months and are often recurring, chronic sinusitis should be suspected. A CT scan of the sinuses will show areas of inflammation.

Interventions

Treatment for chronic sinusitis is with antibiotics, decongestants, and analgesics for pain. Inhaled corticosteroids may be needed to reduce swelling and ease breathing. Irrigation with over-the-counter normal saline nose spray is often helpful and may be done two to three times per day. The person with chronic sinusitis should drink plenty of fluids to maintain adequate hydration and avoid any environmental pollutants such as cigarette smoke or other toxins. Chronic sinusitis is a condition that many older adults wrestle with their entire life. Avoidance of precipitating factors for each individual should be encouraged.

Integumentary Problems

Many changes occur in the integumentary system with normal aging. These are discussed in Chapter 29. One of the most common problems in the elderly is a skin breakdown due to pressure ulcers. The treatment of pressure ulcers is discussed at length in Chapter 20. Skin cancer and herpes zoster infection (shingles) are also common ailments. These two disorders will be briefly addressed here.

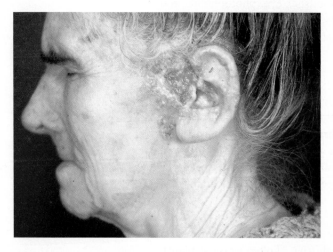

Figure 9-14 Basal cell carcinoma.

Source: Leonard Crowley, *Introduction to Human Disease* (6th ed.). Sudbury, MA: Jones & Bartlett Publishers, 2005.

Skin Cancers

Background

There are three major types of skin cancer: basal cell, squamous cell, and malignant melanoma (MM).

Basal cell carcinoma (see **Figure 9-14**) is the most common skin cancer, accounting for 65–85% of cases (Kennedy-Malone et al., 2000). According to the American Cancer Society (2008a), this means that about 800,000–900,000 cases of basal cell carcinoma are diagnosed each year. Squamous cell carcinoma is more common in African Americans and is also less serious than malignant melanoma. It accounts for approximately 200,000–300,000 new cases yearly. Malignant melanoma accounts for only 3% of all skin cancers, but it is responsible for the majority of deaths from skin cancer. Older adults are 10 times more likely to get MM than adults under age 40 (Johnson & Taylor, 2012). About 8,420 people were estimated to die from malignant melanoma in 2008. The American Cancer Society (2008a) estimated that in 2008 there would be 62,480 new cases of malignant melanoma in the United States.

Risk Factors/Warning Signs

Older adults are more susceptible to skin cancers because of a variety of factors. These include exposure to carcinogens over time (such as UV radiation) and immunosenescence, or a decline in immune function. The major risk factor for all types of skin cancer is sun exposure.

Assessment and Diagnosis

Annual physical examinations should include inspection of the skin for lesions. Older adults should be taught to report any suspicious areas on their skin to the physician. Persons should particularly look for changes in shape, color, and whether a lesion is raised or bleeds.

Basal Cell Carcinoma

Basal cell carcinoma (BCC) is the most common kind of skin cancer. It is often found on the head or face, or other areas exposed to the sun. Although there are different forms of BCC, the nodular type is most common, and appears as a raised, firm, papule that is pearly or shiny with a rolled edge (Johnson & Taylor, 2012). Patients often complain that these lesions bleed and scab easily. When treated early, it is easily removed through surgery and is not life threatening, though it is often recurring.

Squamous Cell Carcinoma

Squamous cell carcinoma (SCC) also appears as lesion on areas of the body exposed to the sun, or from other trauma such as radiation. HPV is a risk factor of SCC, and metastasis is more common than with BCC. The lesions of SCC appear scaly, pink, and thicker than BCC. Their borders may be more irregular and the lesions may look more like an ulceration.

Malignant Melanoma

Malignant melanoma has a more distinctive appearance than other types of skin cancer. The areas appear asymmetric with irregular borders, a variety of colors (including black, purplish, and pink), and size greater than 6 mm. Malignant melanoma is often identified with the ABCDE method (see **Figure 9-15**) and accounts for the vast majority of deaths from skin cancer.

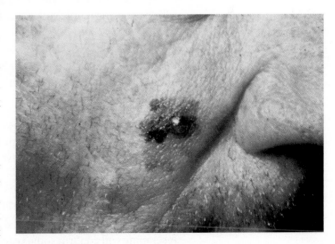

Figure 9-15 Malignant melanoma.

Source: Leonard Crowley, *Introduction to Human Disease* (6th ed.). Sudbury, MA: Jones & Bartlett Publishers 2005.

Interventions

The best treatment for skin cancer in the elderly is prevention. All older persons, especially those with fair skin who are prone to sunburn, should wear sunblock and protective clothing. Most skin cancers, when treated early, have a good prognosis.

All skin lesions larger than 6 mm, or those with any of the ABCDE signs, should be referred for biopsy. There are many nonsurgical interventions. These include cryotherapy, radiotherapy (for superficial BCC or SCC) electrodessication and curettage, and topical treatments. Topical treatments are generally not as effective as more aggressive interventions, but research is ongoing in this area.

The prognosis for MM depends on the extent and staging of the tumor, but when caught very early, the cure rate is nearly 100%. Malignant melanoma presenting in older adults is often more advanced and aggressive. Malignant melanoma metastases sites are typically the lymph nodes, liver, lung, and brain (Johnson & Taylor, 2012). Surgical treatment is required in malignant melanoma, with chemotherapy and radiation. Adjuvant treatments for MM are also often used.

Herpes Zoster (Shingles)

Background

Commonly known as shingles, *herpes zoster* is the reactivation of the virus that causes chicken pox. Older persons may be infected with this latent varicella virus after initial exposure to it in the form of chicken pox. The virus then lays dormant in the neurons until it is reactivated, often due to immunosuppression, when it appears in the form of painful vesicles along the sensory nerves. This reactivation tends to occur only once in a lifetime, with repeat attacks occurring about 5% of the time (Flossos & Kostakou, 2006). Herpes zoster occurs in both men and women equally, with no specific ethnic variations, but is more common in the elderly.

Risk Factors/Warning Signs

Risk factors for developing shingles are age over 55 years, stress, and a suppressed immune system. For many older women particularly, emotional or psychological stress can trigger reactivations.

Signs and symptoms of herpes zoster include painful lesions that erupt on the sensory nerve path, usually beginning on the chest or face. These weepy vesicles get pustular and crusty over several days, with healing occurring in 2–4 weeks (Kennedy-Malone et al., 2004).

Assessment and Diagnosis

Diagnosis can be made by clinical appearance of the lesions and a history of onset. A scraping will confirm some type of herpes virus. The most common complaint of those with herpes zoster is severe pain that usually subsides in 3–5 weeks (NINDS, 2013). Postherpetic neuralgia, a complication of herpes zoster, may last 6–12 months after the lesions disappear and may involve the dermatome, thermal sensory deficits, allodynia (the perception of pain where pain should not be), and/or severe sensory loss, all of which can be very distressing for the patient (Flossos & Kostakou, 2006).

Interventions

Anitviral medications such as acyclovir are used to treat shingles, but must be given within 48 hours of the eruption of the lesion. Topical ointments may help with pain and itching. Pain medications, particularly acetaminophen, are appropriate for pain management in older adults. Persons with pain that lasts past 6 weeks after the skin lesions are gone and that is described as sharp, burning, or constant require reevaluation by a physician. Postherpetic neuralgia usually disappears within a year (NINDS, 2005). As of March 2011, a preventive vaccine was approved for persons over age 50 (NINDS, 2013) that cuts risk of acquiring shingles in half.

Nursing interventions for the older adult with shingles are largely to recommend rest and comfort. The patient should be advised to seek medical attention as soon as he or she suspects shingles, in order to receive the best results from acyclovir. The virus will run its course, but the person is contagious while vesicles are weepy. Persons should not have direct contact (even clothing) with pregnant women, people who have not had chicken pox, other elderly persons, or those with suppressed immune systems. The older person with shingles may experience concerns with pain management and feel a sense of isolation, particularly if they live alone. Arranging for a family member or friend who does not have a high risk of infection to check on the older person at home is advisable. Zostavax, a vaccine for shingles, has become available, and it is recommended for all persons age 60 or older. At this time it is covered by Medicare (see **Case Study 9-7**).

Case Study 9-7

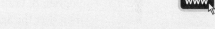

Eloise Mitchell is a 90-year-old female who lives alone in a senior living apartment. She has three children, none of whom live nearby. Although she has been in good health, Ms. Mitchell has recently experienced weight loss and frequent "colds." She was recently diagnosed with shingles and comes to you, the nurse for the senior living complex, for some help. How would you respond to the following questions from Ms. Mitchell?

Questions:

1. What caused the shingles?

2. The doctor says it's like chicken pox, but I wasn't exposed to that, so how did I get it?

3. Why is there so much pain with this problem? Is there anything I can do to get relief? The medication doesn't help that much.

4. Can I really have sores on the bottom of my feet and in my mouth?

5. How long am I contagious?

6. When will I start to feel better? I had a friend who was under the weather for months! Is that usual?

7. Can I ever get this again? If so, how can I prevent it? It's awful!

Endocrine/Metabolic Disorders

Two of the most common disorders in this category among older adults are diabetes and hypothyroidism. These will be discussed in this section.

Diabetes Mellitus

Background

Diabetes mellitus is a common metabolic disorder that affects carbohydrate, lipid, and protein metabolism. It is estimated that about 8.3% (25.8 million) of persons in the United States have diabetes mellitus (American Diabetes Association, 2013). There are two major types of diabetes, type 1 (T1DM) and type 2 (T2DM). T1DM is characterized by autoimmune destruction of the insulin-producing beta cells of the pancreas, leading to a deficiency of insulin. New-onset of adult T1DM in older adults rarely happens; however, due to better treatment of T1DM, older adults who have been diagnosed at an earlier age are living longer. About 90% of older adults with diabetes have T2DM, which is often related to obesity. T2DM is characterized by hyperglycemia and insulin resistance; however, impaired insulin secretion may also be present. Diabetes mellitus is a major cause of disability and death in the United States, and is the seventh leading cause of death among older adults.

Risk Factors/Warning Signs

The risk of diabetes increases with age (45 years and older). Other risk factors include family history, obesity, race (African Americans, Hispanics, Native Americans, Asian Americans, Pacific Islanders), hypertension (blood pressure greater than or equal to 140/90 mmHg), less "good" cholesterol (less than 35 mg/dl), lack of exercise, polycystic ovary syndrome, having a history of delivering large babies (≥9 pounds), personal history of gestational diabetes, and prediabetes (Laberge, Edgren, & Frey, 2011). It is estimated that 11.5 million women and 12.0 million men over the age of 60 have diabetes, but many do not know it. Type 2 is the most common type in older women (CDC, 2007). The Indian Health Service reported via the National Diabetes Survey of 2007 that of the 1.4 million Native Americans and Alaska Natives in the United States, 14.2% age 20 years or older have diagnosed diabetes. Rates vary by region, from 6.0% of Alaska Natives to 29.3% of Native Americans in southern Arizona (CDC, 2007). The risk of death from DM is significantly higher among older Mexican American, African American, and Native American women when compared to Whites. The CDC (2005) names obesity, weight gain, and physical inactivity as the major risk factors for DM among women.

Assessment and Diagnosis

The most common presentation for older adults with T1DM is hyperglycemia. Older adults may not have the classical symptoms such as polydipsia, polyuria, polyphagia, and weight loss; instead, they may have an atypical presentation (Chang & Halter, 2009). They may first present with falls, urinary incontinence, fatigue, or confusion. Because older adults may have T2DM for years before it is diagnosed, they often have macroscualar and microvascular complications at the time of diagnosis, so evaluation of these should be considered at this time.

Interventions

Prevention is the best approach to care, which involves identifying those at risk and encouraging lifestyle change. Older adults with diabetes mellitus have a high risk for complications related to macrovascular disease, microvascular disease, and neuropathy. Macrovascular diseases include coronary heart disease, stroke, and peripheral vascular disease, which can lead to amputation. Microvascular diseases are chronic kidney disease, which is the most common cause of end-stage renal disease, and diabetic retinopathy, which can lead to blindness. Peripheral neuropathy presents as uncomfortable, painful sensations in the legs and feet that are difficult to treat. A lack of sensation may also be present and contribute to the risk of falls. There is no cure for peripheral neuropathy, and it tends to be a complication for which patients experience daily challenges trying to manage the symptoms. A combination of medication to address pain and interventions by a physical therapist seems to be the best current treatment. Most of the complications of DM seen in the elderly have been discussed elsewhere in this chapter.

Treatment is aimed at helping patients to achieve and maintain glycemic control to decrease risk of complications. The initial treatment approach is to work with the older adult to establish treatment goals aimed at reducing long-term complications. This often requires working within an interprofessional team. Aggressive treatment may be appropriate for most older adults; however, the risk of hypoglycemia is higher in older adults. Older adults with hypoglycemia may have an atypical presentation with acute onset of confusion, dizziness, and weakness instead of tremors or sweating. The best measure of good blood glucose management and controlled blood sugars is HgbA1c levels (glycosylated hemoglobin). This measure of hemoglobin provides insight into the previous 3 months of blood sugar control. If HgbA1c is elevated, it indicates that the blood sugar has been high over time. For most people, HgbA1c ≤7% indicates optimal glycemic control; however, due to poor health outcomes, for frail older adults or those with a life expectancy ≤5 years this may not be the best, and HgbA1c of 8% might be more appropriate.

Management is successful when a balance is achieved among exercise, diet, and medications. Medications may be oral hypoglycemics or insulin injection. Insulin injection is used in T1DM and may be prescribed for T2DM because as the person ages, beta-cell function declines. If insulin is needed, it is important to consider if there are visual problems or hand arthritis that limits the dexterity necessary to prepare and inject the medication. For some, a simple regimen such as premeasured doses and easier injection systems (e.g., insulin pens with easy-to-set dosages) is the best. Nurses will need to do a significant amount of teaching (see **Tables 9-29** and **9-30**) regarding the signs and symptoms of hyper- and hypoglycemia and the role of medications in managing blood sugar.

TABLE 9-29	The National Diabetes Education Program's Seven Principles for Management
Principle 1: Find out what type of diabetes you have.	
Principle 2: Get regular care for your diabetes.	
Principle 3: Learn how to control your diabetes.	
Principle 4: Treat high blood sugar.	
Principle 5: Monitor your blood sugar level.	
Principle 6: Prevent and diagnose long-term diabetes problems.	
Principle 7: Get checked for long-term problems and treat them.	

Source: National Diabetes Education Program, 2005, p. 1.

TABLE 9-30	Key Areas for Nursing Teaching of Older Persons with Diabetes
Proper nutrition	
Exercise	
Medications	
Signs and symptoms of hyper- and hypoglycemia	
Meaning of lab tests: FBS, blood glucose, HgbA1c	
Use of a glucometer	
Foot care	
Importance of adherence to therapeutic regimen	
Possible long-term complications	
Prevention of complications	
Develop a plan of action for when illness occurs	

Although much of the teaching done with older adults is usually in the acute care hospital or rehabilitation setting, telephone follow-up calls have been shown to improve patient adherence to diet. Additionally, a significant finding of Kim and Oh's (2003) research was that patients receiving phone calls from the nurse about adherence to the prescribed regimen for diabetes management showed improved HgbA1c over those who did not have follow-up phone calls.

Thorough evaluation of readiness to learn and of the ability of an older person to manage his or her medications must be done. Older adults who need to give themselves insulin injections may experience anxiety about learning this task. Demonstration, repetition, and practice are good techniques for the older age group. Adaptive devices such as magnifiers may help if the syringes are hard to read. A family member should also be taught to give the insulin to provide support and encouragement, although the older adult should be encouraged to remain independent in this skill if possible. Williams and Bond (2002) suggested that programs that promote confidence in self-care abilities are likely to be effective for those with diabetes. A plan for times of sickness and the use of a glucometer to monitor blood sugars will also need to be addressed. Additionally, the dietician may be consulted to provide education for the patient and family on meal planning, calorie counting, carbohydrate counting, and nutrition. Many patients benefit from weight loss, so the nutritionist can assist with dietary planning in this regard also.

Due to the increased risk of infection and slow healing that result from diabetes, foot care is an essential component in teaching older adults to manage DM. Some experts believe that good preventive foot care would significantly reduce the incidence of amputation in the elderly. Older persons with DM should never go barefoot outside. Extremes in temperature should be avoided. Shoes should be well fitting and not rub. Socks should be changed regularly. Elders should be taught to inspect their feet daily, with a mirror if needed. Corns and ingrown toenails should be inspected and treated by a podiatrist, not by the patient. Older persons should see their podiatrist for a foot inspection at least yearly. Patients should be cautioned that even the smallest foot injury, such as a thorn or blister, can go unnoticed and unfelt—and often results in partial amputations that lead to a cascade of lower extremity problems.

Hypothyroidism

Background

Hypothyroidism results from lack of sufficient thyroid hormone being produced by the thyroid gland. Older adults may have subclinical hypothyroidism, in which the TSH (thyroid-stimulating hormone) is elevated and the T4 (thyroxine or thyroid hormone) is normal; 4.3–9.5% of the general population has this problem (Woolever & Beutler, 2007). In this condition, the body is trying to stimulate production of more thyroid hormone. Some older adults with this condition will progress to have primary or overt hypothyroidism, which is when the TSH is elevated and T4 is decreased. Hashimoto's disease is the most common cause and represents 90% of all patients with hypothyroidism (American Association of Clinical Endocrinologists [AACE], 2005; Woolever & Beutler, 2007), though certain pituitary disorders, medications, and other hormonal imbalances may be causal factors.

Risk Factors/Warning Signs

Older adults may present an atypical picture, but the most common presenting complaints are fatigue and weakness. **Table 9-31** provides additional classic signs and symptoms.

Assessment and Diagnosis

Diagnosis should include a thorough history and physical; bradycardia and heart failure are often associated factors. Lab tests should include thyroid and thyroid antibody levels (common to Hashimoto's), and lipids, because hyperlipidemia is also associated with this disorder.

TABLE 9-31 Signs and Symptoms of Hypothyroidism
*Weakness
*Fatigue
Dry skin
Brittle hair
Hair loss
Weight gain (7–20 pounds)
Cold sensitivity
Puffy face
Headache
Difficulty sleeping
Goiter
Trouble breathing or swallowing
Constipation
Ataxia
Depression
Bradycardia
Anorexia

*Primary signs in the elderly; others may or may not be present.
Source: AACE, 2005; Freil & Cotter, 2002; Reuben et al., 2008.

Interventions

Treatment centers on returning the thyroid hormone level to normal. This is done through oral thyroid replacement medication, usually L-thyroxine. In older adults with coexisting cardiovascular disease, starting with the usual doses may exacerbate angina and worsen the underlying heart disease, so it is important to start low and go slow. Titration should be done cautiously, with close monitoring of the older adult's response to the medication. The does should be adjusted on 6-week intervals until euthyroid (normal levels of thyroid hormone) is achieved. Once the TSH is within normal limits, checking the TSH should be done every 6 to 12 months to monitor effectiveness and blood levels, because hyperthyroidism is a side effect of this therapy and can have serious implications on the older person's health.

Nurses should teach patients about the importance of taking thyroid medication at the same time each day without missing doses. Sometimes older adults have other problems associated with hypothyroidism, such as bowel dysfunction and depression. Any signs of complicating factors should be reported to the physician, and doctors' appointments for monitoring should be religiously kept. Strategies for managing fatigue and weakness should also be addressed, because some lifestyle modifications may need to be made as treatment is initiated.

Summary

This chapter provided brief and concise snapshots of illnesses, diseases, and health conditions common to older adults. Students and health professionals may learn additional information about these problems in greater detail from other courses or sources. This chapter focused on a review of basic knowledge but added specific information related to older adults who may require interventions related to certain common conditions.

There are several notable conditions commonly seen in older adults that may be the result of a variety of factors, not just one physical problem or disease. These include depression, anxiety, delirium, dementia, and insomnia. Common geriatric syndromes are discussed in separate chapters in this text and readers are encouraged to refer to these for more specific information on these conditions.

Critical Thinking Exercises

1. This chapter discusses a great deal of content. Choose one health condition or disease that interests you most and search the Internet site of the organization dedicated to that cause. What resources are available for persons with this problem?

2. Volunteer through your local hospital to help with stroke and/or blood pressure screenings of older adults. Note any common risk factors you observe among the persons that are being screened.

3. Visit a support group related to one of the long-term conditions discussed in this chapter. It might be a stroke survivor's meeting, the breather's club, or a Parkinson's disease group. Listen to the participants and their family members. Write down anything new you learned about how people live with and manage this condition. Talk personally with a family who is living with the condition that you are further investigating. Talk to participants and their family members. Write down anything new you learned about how people live with and manage this condition.

4. Go to your local mall, church, shopping center, restaurant, or other place where seniors living in the community might gather. Listen to casual conversations between older adults. What types of health problems and concerns do they express?

5. Talk to a nurse who works in the emergency room, or to a local cardiologist. Ask what symptoms they have seen in older adult patients who were diagnosed with myocardial infarction. How are these symptoms different from or similar to a classic presentation?

Personal Reflections

1. Of the disorders presented in this chapter, which are the most familiar to you? Which do you feel you need to do more reading about? Have you ever cared for an older patient with any of these problems? Did the information in the text present what you saw as signs and symptoms in this patient?

2. Which of the diseases in this chapter do you feel are most common in the people you take care of? Have you noticed any ethnic or cultural differences in the geographic area where you work?

3. If an older person came to you and wanted to know about one of the diseases in this chapter, what would you tell the person? How is your comfort level with what needs to be taught for each of the disorders in this chapter?

4. Make a list of three diseases that you are least knowledgeable about and re-read that section of this chapter. Memorize the signs and symptoms, and think about the nursing interventions you should use.

References

Agency for Healthcare Research and Quality [AHRQ]. (2012). *Management of chronic heart failure. A national guideline.* Retrieved from http://guideline.gov/content.aspx?id=10587

Agency for Healthcare Research and Quality [AHRQ]. (2013). Routine osteoporosis screening recommended for all women over age 65. Retrieved from http://www.ahrq.gov/news/press/pr2011/tfosteopr.htm

Age-Related Eye Disease Study Authors. (2001). A randomized, placebo-controlled, clinical trial of high-dose supplementation with vitamins C and E, beta carotene, and zinc for age-related macular degeneration and vision loss. *Archives of Ophthalmology, 119,* 1417–1436.

Alcelik, I., Sukeik, M., Pollock, R., Misra, A., Naguib, A., & Haddad, F. S. (2012). Comparing the midvastus and medial parapatellar approaches in total knee arthroplasty: A meta-analysis of short term outcomes. *Knee, 19*(4), 229–236.

Alzheimer's Association. (2012a). *What is Alzheimer's?* Retrieved from http://www.alz.org/alzheimers_disease_what_is_alzheimers.asp

Alzheimer's Association (2012b). *2012 Alzheimer's disease facts and figures.* Retrieved from m http://www.alz.org/downloads/facts_figures_2012.pdf

Alzheimer's Association (2012c). *Ten early signs and symptoms of Alzheimer's.* Retrieved from http://www.alz.org/alzheimers_disease_10_signs_of_alzheimers.asp

Amella, G. J. (2004). Presentation of illness in older adults. *American Journal of Nursing, 104*(10), 40–51.

American Academy of Otolaryngology. (2012). Head and Neck. Retrieved from http://www.entnet.org/

American Association of Clinical Endocrinologists. (2005). *Hypothyroidism.* Retrieved from http://www.aace.com/publications/guidelines

American Cancer Society [ACS]. (2005). *Stomach cancer.* Retrieved from http://www.cancer.org/cancer/stomachcancer/index

American Cancer Society [ACS]. (2008). *Basal cell carcinoma statistics.* Retrieved from http://www.cancer.org/cancer/skincancer-basalandsquamouscell/detailedguide/skin-cancer-basal-and-squamous-cell-key-statistics

American Cancer Society. (2013). Pancreatic Cancer. Retrieved from http://www.cancer.org/acs/groups/cid/documents/webcontent/003131-pdf.pdf

American Cancer Society [ACS]. (2012a). *Cancer facts and figures.* Retrieved from http://www.cancer.org/acs/groups/content/@epidemiologysurveilance/documents/document/acspc-031941.pdf

American Cancer Society [ACS]. (2012b). *Prostate cancer.* Retrieved from http://www.cancer.org/Cancer/ProstateCancer/DetailedGuide/prostate-cancer-diagnosis

American Cancer Society [ACS]. (2012c). Bladder cancer. Retrieved from http://www.cancer.org/Cancer/BladderCancer/DetailedGuide/bladder-cancer-key-statistics

American Cancer Society [ACS]. (2012d). American Cancer Society recommendations for early breast cancer detection in women without breast symptoms. Retrieved from http://www.cancer.org/cancer/breastcancer/moreinformation/breastcancerearlydetection/breast-cancer-early-detection-acs-recs

American Diabetes Association. (2013). Diabetes statistics. Retrieved from http://www.diabetes.org/diabetes-basics/diabetes-statistics/

American Cancer Society. (2013). Prostate Cancer. Retrieved from http://www.cancer.org/cancer/prostatecancer/detailedguide/prostate-cancer-risk-factors

American Foundation for Urologic Disease [AFUD]. (2008). *Bladder cancer.* Retrieved from http://www.urologyhealth.org/urology/index.cfm?article=100

American Urological Association Foundation. (2008). The management of localized prostate cancer. Retrieved from http://www.auanet.org/content/media/pc08.pdf

American Gastroenterology Association. (2008). *Gastroesophageal reflux disease.* Retrieved from http://www.gastro.org/wmspage.cfm?parm1=848#GERD?

American Health Assistance Foundation [AHAF]. (2012). About glaucoma. Retrieved from http://www.ahaf.org/glaucoma/

American Heart Association (2011). About peripheral artery disease. Retrieved from http://www.heart.org/HEARTORG/Conditions/More/PeripheralArteryDisease/About-Peripheral-Artery-Disease-PAD_UCM_301301_Article.jsp

American Heart Association [AHA]. (2012a). *Cardiac rehabilitation.* Retrieved from http://www.heart
.org/HEARTORG/Conditions/More/CardiacRehab/Cardiac-Rehab_UCM_002079_SubHomePage.jsp

American Heart Association [AHA]. (2012b). *Heart disease and stroke statistics. 2012 update.* Retrieved
from http://my.americanheart.org/professional/General/Heart-Stroke-2012-Statistical-Update_
UCM_434526_Article.jsp

American Heart Association [AHA]. (2012c). *Statistical fact sheet 2012 update: African Americans and
cardiovascular diseases.* Available at http://www.heart.org/idc/groups/heart-public/@wcm/@sop/
@smd/documents/downloadable/ucm_319568.pdf

American Heart Association [AHA]. (2012d). *Understand your risk for high blood pressure.* Retrieved
from http://www.heart.org/HEARTORG/Conditions/HighBloodPressure/UnderstandYour
RiskforHighBloodPressure/Understand-Your-Risk-for-High-Blood-Pressure_UCM_002052_
Article.jsp

American Heart Association (AHA). (2012e). High Blood Pressure. Retrieved from http://www.heart
.org/idc/groups/heart-public/@wcm/@sop/@smd/documents/downloadable/ucm_319587.pdf

American Lung Association [ALA]. (2004). *Chronic obstructive pulmonary disease (COPD) fact sheet.*
Retrieved from http://www.lung.org/lung-disease/copd/resources/facts-figures/COPD-Fact-Sheet
.html

American Lung Association [ALA]. (2008). *Pneumonia fact sheet.* Retrieved from http://www.lung.org/
lung-disease/influenza/in-depth-resources/pneumonia-fact-sheet.html

American Lung Association [ALA]. (2012a). Understanding COPD. Retrieved from http://www.lung.org/
lung-disease/copd/about-copd/understanding-copd.html

American Lung Association [ALA]. (2012b). Understanding Pneumonia. Retrieved from http://www.
lung.org/lung-disease/pneumonia/understanding-pneumonia.html

American Parkinson Disease Foundation. (2013). Basic information about PD. Retrieved from http://
www.apdaparkinson.org/publications-information/basic-info-about-pd/

American Stroke Association [ASA]. (2012a). *Impact of stroke.* Retrieved from http://www
.strokeassociation.org/STROKEORG/AboutStroke/Impact-of-Stroke_UCM_310728_Article.jsp

American Stroke Association [ASA]. (2012b). *Stroke risk factors.* Retrieved from http://www
.strokeassociation.org/STROKEORG/AboutStroke/UnderstandingRisk/Understanding-Stroke-
Risk_UCM_308539_SubHomePage.jsp

American Stroke Association [ASA]. (2012c). *Stroke treatments.* Retrieved from http://
www.strokeassociation.org/STROKEORG/AboutStroke/Treatment/Treatment_UCM_310892_
Article.jsp

American Stroke Association [ASA]. (2012d). *Warning signs.* Retrieved from http://
www.strokeassociation.org/STROKEORG/WarningSigns/Warning-Signs_UCM_308528_
SubHomePage.jsp

American Urological Association. (2010). *Guidelines for management of benign prostatic hyperplasia.*
Retrieved from http://www.auanet.org/content/clinical-practice-guidelines/clinical-guidelines/
main-reports/bph-management/chap_1_GuidelineManagementof(BPH).pdf

American Urological Association Foundation. (2009). *Prostate specific antigen best practice statement: 2009 update.* Retrieved from http://www.auanet.org/content/guidelines-and-quality-care/
clinical-guidelines/main-reports/psa09.pdf

Amputation Statistics. (2012). Retrieved from http://www.statisticbrain.com/amputee-statistics/

Anand, B. S. (2013). Peptic ulcer disease. Retrieved from http://emedicine.medscape.com/article/
181753-medication

Anderson, S., & Marlett, S. (2004). The language of recovery: How effective communication of information is crucial to restructuring post-stroke life. *Topics in Stroke Rehabilitation, 11*(4), 55–67.

Antin-Ozerkis, D, Evans, J, Rubinowitz, A., Homer, RJ & Matthay, RA. (2010). Pulmonary manifestations
of rheumatoid arthritis. *Clinics in Chest Medicine* 3(3): 451–78.

Aronow, W. S. (2007). Recognition of aortic stenosis in the elderly. *Geriatrics, 62*(12), 23–32.

Arthritis Foundation. (2012). *Osteoarthritis.* Retrieved from http://www.arthritis.org/what-is-
osteoarthritis.php

Beers, M. H. (Ed.). (2005). *Merck manual of geriatrics*. Whitehouse Station, NJ: Merck Research Laboratories.

Bergey, G. E. (2004). Initial treatment of epilepsy: Special issues in treating the elderly. *Neurology, 63*(10), S40–S48.

Bhojani, N. & Lingeman, J. E. (2011). Surgery for BPH/LUTS: Is TURP still the gold standard? *Urology Times, 39*(13), 38–39.

Bitton, R. (2009). The economic burden of osteoarthritis. American Journal of Managed Care, 15(8 Suppl), S230–5.

Bradway, C. W., & Yetman, G. (2002). Genitourinary problems. In V. T. Cotter & N. E. Strumpf (Eds.), *Advanced practice nursing with older adults: Clinical guidelines* (pp. 83–102). New York, NY: McGraw-Hill.

BreastCancer.org. (2012). *U.S. breast cancer statistics*. Retrieved from http://www.breastcancer.org/symptoms/understand_bc/statistics.jsp

Cameron, J., & Gignac, M. A. M. (2008). "Timing it right": A conceptual framework for addressing the support needs of family caregivers to stroke survivors from the hospital to home. *Patient Education and Counseling, 70*(3), 305–314.

Carpenito, L. J. (2013). *Nursing Diagnosis: Application to Clinical Practice*. Philadelphia, PA: Walters Kluwer/Lippincott Williams & Wilkins.

Cawthon, P. (2011). Gender differences in osteoporosis and fractures. *Clinical Orthopaedics & Related Research, 469*(7), 1900–1905. doi: 10/1007s11999-011-1780-7

Centers for Disease Control and Prevention [CDC]. (1990). *Prevention and control of tuberculosis in facilities providing long-term care to the elderly: Recommendations of the Advisory Committee for Elimination of Tuberculosis*. Retrieved from http://www.cdc.gov/niosh/topics/tb/

Centers for Disease Control and Prevention [CDC]. (2005). *Diabetes and women's health across the life stages: A public health perspective*. Retrieved from http://www.cdc.gov/diabetes/pubs/pdf/women.pdf

Centers for Disease Control and Prevention [CDC]. (2007). *National diabetes fact sheet 2007*. Retrieved from http://www.cdc.gov/diabetes/pubs/pdf/ndfs_2007.pdf

Centers for Disease Control and Prevention. (2010). *Pneumococcal vaccination*. Retrieved from http://www.cdc.gov/vaccines/vpd-vac/pneumo/default.htm

Centers for Disease Control and Prevention [CDC]. (2011a). National diabetes fact sheet: National Estimates and general information on diabetes and prediabetes in the United States.

Centers for Disease Control and Prevention [CDC]. (2011b). *Summary health statistics for US Adults, 2010, Table 2*. Retrieved from http://www.cdc.gov/nchs/data/series/rs_10/sr10_252.pdf

Centers for Disease Control and Prevention [CDC]. (2012a). *Screening*. Retrieved from http://www.cdc.gov/cancer/breast/basic_info/screening.htm

Centers for Disease Control and Prevention [CDC]. (2012b). Trends in Tuberculosis – United States, 2011. *Morbidity and Mortality Weekly Report, 61*(11), 181–185.

Chang, A.M. & Halter, J.B. (2009). Diabetes mellitus. In Halter, J. B., Ouslander, J. G., Tinetti, M. E., Studenski, S., High, K. P., & Asthana, S. *Hazzard's Geriatric Medicine and Gerontology* (6th ed., pp.1308–1332.) New York, NY: McGraw-Hill.

Chin, T., Sawamura, S., Shiba, R., Oyabu, H., Nagakura, Y., Takase, I., Machida, K., & Nakagawa, A. (2003). Effect of an intelligent prosthesis (IP) on the waling ability of young transfemoral amputees: Comparison of IP users with able-bodied people. *American Journal of Physical Medicine & Rehabilitation, 82*(6), 447–451.

Cleveland Clinic. (2013). Peripheral artery disease. Retrieved from http://my.clevelandclinic.org/heart/disorders/vascular/default.aspx

Cochran, S. (2007). Care of the indwelling cather: Is it evidence-based? *Journal of Wound, Ostomy, Continence Nursing, 34*(3), 282–288.

Constantinescu, F., Goucher, S., Weinstein, A., & Fraenkel, L. (2009). Racial disparities in treatment preferences for rheumatoid arthritis. *Medical Care, 47*(3), 350–355. doi: 10.1002/rnj.054

Cournan, M. (2012). Bladder management in female stroke survivors: Translating research into practice. *Rehabilitation Nursing, 37*(5), 220–230.

Cotter, V. T. (2002). Dementia. In V. T. Cotter & N. G. Strumpf (Eds.), *Advanced practice nursing with older adults: Clinical guidelines* (pp. 183–200). New York, NY: McGraw-Hill.

Davidson, P. & Davidson, K. (2012). Electroencephalography in the elderly. *Neurodiagnostic Journal, 52*(1), 3–19.

Deglin, J. H., & Vallerand, A. H. (2005). *Davis's drug guide for nurses*. Philadelphia, PA: F. A. Davis.

Duraski, S. A., Denby, F. A., Danzy, L. V., & Sullivan, S. (2012). Stroke. In K. L. Mauk (Ed.) *Rehabilitation nursing: A contemporary approach to practice*. (pp. 215–254). Sudbury, MA: Jones & Bartlett Learning.

Easton, K. L. (2001). *The post-stroke journey: From agonizing to owning*. Doctoral dissertation. Wayne State University.

Edwards, W. (2002). Gastrointestinal problems. In V. T. Cotter & N. E. Strumpf (Eds.), *Advanced practice nursing with older adults: Clinical guidelines* (pp. 201–216). New York, NY: McGraw-Hill.

Eliopoulos, C. (2005). *Gerontological nursing*. Philadelphia, PA: Lippincott.

Eyecare America. (2005). *Diabetes: An eye exam can save your life*. Brochure: Author.

Fakih, M. G., Greene, M. T., Kennedy, E. H., Meddings, J. A., Krein, S. L., Olmsted, R. N., & Saint, S. (2012). Introducing a population-based outcome measure to evaluate the effect of interventions to reduce catheter-associated urinary tract infection. *American Journal of Infection Control, 40*(4), 359–364.

Ferri, F. F. (Ed.). (2011). *Ferri's Clinical Advisor, 2011*. Philadelphia: Elsevier Mosby.

Films for the Humanities and Sciences. (2004). *The Parkinson's enigma* (DVD). Princeton, NJ: Author.

Fingeret, M. (2009). The Management of Glaucoma. *Chilton's review of optometry, 113*, 7.

Fletcher, K., Rapp, M. P., & Reichman, W. R. (2007). Optimal management of Alzheimer's disease: A multimodal approach. Special report published by *Geriatrics*.

Flossos, A., & Kastakou, C. (2006). A review of postherpetic neuralgia. *Internet Journal of Pain Symptom Control & Palliative Care, 4*(2). Retrieved from http://web.ebscohost.com/ehost/delivery? vid=7&hid=112&sid=8ba80619-4e14-896e

Freil, M. A., & Cotter, V. T. (2002). Thyroid disorder. In V. T. Cotter & N. E. Strumpf (Eds.), *Advanced practice nursing with older adults: Clinical guidelines* (pp. 127–139). New York, NY: McGraw-Hill.

Frisco, D. J. (2013). About Celebrex (celecoxib) COX-2 inhibitor. Retrieved from http://www.spine-health.com/treatment/pain-medication/about-celebrex-celecoxib-cox-2-inhibitor

Fry, A. M, Shay, D. K., Holman, R. C., Curns, A. T., & Anderson, L. J. (2005). Trends in Hospitalization for Pneumonia Among Persons Aged 65 Years or Older in the United States, 1988–2002. *Journal of the American Medical Association, 294*(21), 2712–2719.

Gabriel, S. E. & Crowson, C. S. (2012). Risk factors for cardiovascular disease in rheumatoid arthritis. *Current Opinion in Rheumatology, 24*(2), 171–176.

Gallagher, J. C. & Levine J. P. (2011). Preventing osteoporosis in symptomatic postmenopausal women. *Menopause, 18*(1), 109–118.

Garas, S., & Zafari, A. M. (2006). Mycardial infarction. eMedicine. Retrieved from http://www.emedicine.com/MED/topic1567.htm

Gerzevitz, D., Porter, B. O., Dunphy, L.M. (2011). Eyes, ears, nose and throat. In Dunphy, L. M., Winland-Brown, J. E., Portor, B. O., Thomas, D. J. *Primary Care: The Art and Science of Advanced Practice Nursing* (3rd ed., pp. 245–330). Philadelphia, PA: Davis.

Grossi, E., Buscema, M. P., Snowdon, D. & Antuono, P. (2007). Neuropathophysiological findings processed by artificial neural networks (ANNs) can perfectly distinguish Alzheimer's patients from controls in the Nun study. *BioMed Central Neurology online*. doi: 10.1186/1471-2377-7-15.

Hain, T. C. (2003). *Benign paroxysmal positional vertigo*. Retrieved from http://www.tchain.com

Hain, T. (2012). Dizziness in older people. Retrieved from http://www.dizziness-and-balance.com/disorders/age/Dizziness%20in%20the%20Elderly.htm

Hain, T. C., & Ramaswamy, T. (2005). Dizziness in the elderly. Retrieved from http://www.galter.north-western.edu/geriatrics/chapters/dizziness.cfm

Ham, R. J., Sloane, P.D., Warshaw, G.A., Bernard, M.A., & Flaherty, E (2007). *Primary care geriatrics: a case-based approach* (5th ed.). Philadelphia, PA: Elsevier Mosby.

Hansson, E. E., Mansson, N.-O., & Hakansson, A. (2005). Balance performance and self-perceived handicap among dizzy patients in primary healthcare. *Scandinavian Journal of Primary Health Care, 23*, 215–220.

Harari, D. (2009). Constipation. In Halter J. B., Ouslander, J. G., Tinetti, M. E., (Eds.), *Hazzard's Geriatric Medicine and Gerontology*. (6th ed., pp. 1103–1122). New York, NY: McGraw-Hill.

Health Care Infection Control Practices Advisory Committee. (2009). *Guideline for prevention of catheter-associated urinary tract infection*. Retrieved from http://www.cdc.gov/hicpac/pdf/CAUTI/CAUTIguideline2009final.pdf

Health Education Solutions. (2012). Symptoms of heart attack may present differently in men and women. Retrieved from http://www.healthedsolutions.com/articles/signs-and-symptoms-heart-attack

Heart and Stroke Foundation of Canada. (2009). *Stroke treatments*. Retrieved http://www.heartandstroke .com/site/c.ikIQLcMWJtE/b.3483943/k.DA86/Stroke___Treatment.htm

Heidenreich, P. A., Trogdon, J. G., Khavjou, O. A., Butler, J., Dracup, K., Ezekowitz, M. D., Finkelstein, E. A., … Woo, J. (2011). Forecasting the future of cardiovascular disease in the United States: A policy statement from the American Heart Association. *Circulation, 123*, 993–944.

Helmick, C. G., Felson, D. T., Lawrence, R. C., Gabriel, S., Hirsch, R., Kwoh, C. K,…Stone, J. H. (2008). Estimates of the prevalence of arthritis and other rheumatic conditions in the United States. *Arthritis & Rheumatism 58*(1), 15–25.

Heikkinen, K., Helena, L., Taina, N., Anne, K., & Sanna, S. (2008). A comparison of two educational interventions for the cognitive empowerment of ambulatory orthopaedic surgery patients. *Patient Education and Counseling, 73*(2), 272–279.

Higashida, R. (2005). *Nonpharmacologic therapy for acute stroke*. Paper presented at the American Stroke Association International Stroke Conference 2005, State-of-the-Art Stroke Nursing Symposium, New Orleans, Louisiana.

Hill-O'Neill, K. A., & Shaughnessy, M. (2002). Dizziness and stroke. In V. T. Cotter & N. E. Strumpf (Eds.), *Advanced practice nursing with older adults: Clinical guidelines* (pp. 163–182). New York, NY: McGraw-Hill.

Hinkle, J. (2010). Outcomes three years after motor stroke. *Rehabilitation Nursing Journal, 35*(1), 23–30.

Hooton, T. M., Bradley, S. F., Cardenas, D. D., Colgan, R., Geerlings, S. E., Rice, J. C., Saint, S.,….Nicolle, L. E. (2010). Diagnosis, prevention, and treatment of catheter-associated urinary tract infection in adults. *Clinical Infectious Diseases, 50*(5), 625–663.

Howcroft, D. (2004). Caring for persons with Alzheimer's disease. *Mental Health Practice Journal, 7*(8), 31–37.

Howlader, N., Noone, A. M., Krapcho, M., Neyman, N., Aminou, R., Waldron, W., … Edwards, B. K. (2011). SEER cancer statistics review, 1975–2008. *Bethesda, MD: National Cancer Institute, 19*.

Hunt, A. H., Abraham, W. T., Chin, M. H., Feldman, A. M., Francis, G. S., Ganiats, T. G., Jessup, M., … Yancy, C. W. (2009). 2009 focused update incorporated into the ACC/AHA 2005 Guidelines for the diagnosis and management of heart failure in adults. *Journal of the American College of Cardiology*. Retrieved from http://content.onlinejacc.org/article.aspx?articleid=1139601

International Foundations for Functional Gastrointestinal Disorders. (2008). *About GERD*. Retrieved from http://www.aboutgerd.org/

Jett, D. U., Warren, R. L., & Wirtalla, C. (2005). The relation between therapy intensity and outcomes of rehabilitation in skilled nursing facilities. *Archives of Physical Medicine and Rehabilitation, 86*(3), 373–379.

Johnson, S. R. & Taylor, M. A. (2012). Identification and management of malignant skin lesions among older adults. *The Journal for Nurse Practitioners, 8*(8), 610–161.

Kalapatapu, V. (2012). *Lower extremity amputation*. Retrieved from http://www.uptodate.com/contents/lower-extremity-amputation

Kalra, L., Evans, A., Perez, I., Melbourne, A., Patel, A., Knapp, M., & Donaldson, N. (2004). Training carers of stroke patients: Randomized controlled trial. *British Medical Journal, 328*, 1099–1103.

Kelley, M. F. (2002). Respiratory problems in older adults. In V. T. Cotter & N. E. Strumpf (Eds.), *Advanced practice nursing with older adults: Clinical guidelines* (pp. 67–82). New York, NY: McGraw-Hill.

Kennedy-Malone, L. D., Fletcher, K. R., & Plank, L. M. (2004). *Management guidelines for nurse practitioners working with older adults.* Philadelphia, PA: F. A. Davis.

Kim, H., & Oh, J. (2003). Adherence to diabetes control recommendations: Impact of nurse telephone calls. *Journal of Advanced Nursing, 44*(3), 256–261.

Khosla, S. (2010). *Update in male osteoporosis. Journal of Clinical Endocrinology and Metabolism, 95*(1), 3–10.

Kleinpell, R. M., Munro, C., & Guiliano, K. K. (2008). Targeting health care-associated infection: Evidence-based strategies. In R. G. Hughes (Ed.), *Patient safety and quality: An evidence-based handbook for nurses* (AHRQ Publication No. 08-0043). Retrieved from www.ahrq.gov/qual/nurseshdbk/

Klein, R., Knudtson, M. D., Lee, K. E., Gangnon, R., & Klein, B. E. (2009). The Wisconsin Epidemiologic Study of Diabetic Retinopathy XXIII. The Twenty-Five-Year Incidence of Macular Edema in Persons with Type 1 Diabetes. *Ophthalmology, 116*(3), 497.

Kulick, D. L. (2012). Heart attack treatment. Retrieved from http://www.medicineNet.com

Laberge, M., Edgren, A. R. & Frey, R. J. (2009). Diabetes mellitus, Type 1. *The Gale Encyclopedia of Medicine* (3rd ed.). Jacqueline L. Longe, Ed. Detroit, MI: Gale.

Laine, L., & Jensen, D. M. (2012). Management of patient with ulcer bleeding. *American Journal of Gastroenterology* doi: 10.1038/ajg.2011.480

Lefebure, H., Levert, M., Pelchat, D., & Lepage, J. (2008). Nature, sources and impact of information or the adjustment of family caregivers: A pilot project. *Canadian Journal of Nursing Research, 40*(1), 143–160.

Lighthouse International. (2005). *The four most common causes of age-related vision loss.* Retrieved from http://www.lighthouse.org

Lockrey, G., & Lim, L. (2011). Peptic ulcer disease in older people. *Journal of Pharmacy Practice and Research, 41*(1), 58.

Loeb, M. (2002). Community-acquired pneumonia. *American Family Physician.* Retrieved from http://www.aafp.org/afp/2011/0715/p218.html

Luggen, A. (2009). Epilepsy in the elderly. *The Clinical Advisor.* Retrieved from http://www.clinicaladvisor.com/epilepsy-in-the-elderly/article/129590/3/

Lutz, B. J. (2004). Determinants of discharge destination for stroke patients. *Rehabilitation Nursing, 29*(5), 154–163.

Lutz, B., & Young, M. E. (2010). Rethinking intervention strategies in stroke family caregiving. *Rehabilitation Nursing, 35*(4), 152–160.

Macular Degeneration Foundation. (2005). *As therapy for macular degeneration, regenerating retinal cells moves several steps closer to reality.* Retrieved from http://www.eyesight.org

Mannion, E. (2008a). Alzheimer's disease: The psychological and physical effects of the caregivers' role. Part 1. *Nursing Older People, 20*(4), 27–32.

Mannion, E. (2008b). Alzheimer's disease: The psychological and physical effects of the caregivers' role. Part 2. *Nursing Older People, 20*(4), 33–38.

Manuchehri, K., & Kirby, G. R. (2003). Vitreous haemorrhage in elderly patients: Prevention and management. *Drugs & Aging, 20*(9), 655–661.

Martinez, J. P., & Marttu, A. (2006). Abdominal pain in the elderly. *Emergency Medicine Clinics of North America, 24,* 371–388.

Mauk, K. L. (2004). Pharmacology update: Antiepileptic drugs. *ARN Network,* 20 (5), 3, 11.

Mauk, K. L. (2006). Nursing interventions within the Mauk model for poststroke recovery. *Rehabilitation Nursing, 31*(6), 257–263.

Mauk, K. L., Lemley, C., Pierce, J., & Schmidt, N. A. (2011). The Mauk model for poststroke recovery: Assessing the phases. *Rehabilitation Nursing, 36*(6), 241–247.

Mayo Clinic (2011). *Essential hypertension.* Retrieved from http://www.Mayoclinic.com/health=high=blood=pressure/ds00100/DSECTION=causes

Mayo Clinic (2012a). *Bacilllus of Calmette and Guerin Vaccine Live (intravesical route).* Retrieved from http://www.mayoclinic.com/health/drug-information/DR600215/DSECTION=proper-use

Mayo Clinic (2012b). *Heart failure symptoms.* Retrieved from http://www.mayoclinic.com/health/heart-failure/DS00061/DSECTION=symptoms

Mayo Clinic (2012c). *Rheumatoid arthritis.* Retrieved from http://www.mayoclinic.com/health/rheumatoid-arthritis/DS00020/tab=InDepth

Mayo Clinic. (2013). Benign paroxysmal positional vertigo (BPPV). Retrieved from http://www.mayoclinic.com/health/vertigo/DS00534

McCance, K. L., Huether, S. E., Brashers, V. L., & Rote, N. S. (2010). *Pathophysiology: The Biologic Basis for Disease in Adults and Children* (6th ed.). Maryland Heights, MD: Mosby Elsevier.

McEneaney, M. J. (2012). Individualizing management for common concerns of postmenopausal women. *The Journal for Nurse Practitioners, 8*(6), 470–474.

McGrory, A., & Remington, R. (2004). Optimizing the functionality of clients with age-related macular degeneration. *Rehabilitation Nursing, 29*(3), 90–94.

McPhee, S. J., Papadakis, M. A., & Rabow, M. W. (2012). Current Medical Diagnosis & Treatment 2012. *LANGE McGraw-Hill Medical, 50.*

Mead, M. (2005). Assessing men with prostate problems: A practical guide. *Practice Nurse, 29*(6), 45–50.

MedlinePlus. (2005). *GERD.* Retrieved from http://www.nlm.nih.gov/medlineplus/gerd.html

Miller, E. A., Rosenheck, R. A., & Schneider, L. S. (2012). Caregiver burden, health utilities, and institutional service use in Alzheimer's disease. *International Journal of Geriatric Psychiatry, 27*(4), 382–393.

Miniño, A.M., Xu, J., Kochanek, K.D. (2010). Deaths: Preliminary Data for 2008. *National Vital Statistics Reports, 59*(2), 1–52. Retrieved from http://www.cdc.gov/nchs/data/nvsr/nvsr59/nvsr59_02.pdf

Morris, H. (2006). Dysphagia in the elderly—A management challenge for nurses. *British Journal of Nursing, 15*(15), 558–562.

Mumma, C. (1986). Perceived losses following stroke. *Rehabilitation Nursing, 11*(3), 19–24.

National Heart Lung and Blood Institute [NHLBI]. (2010). How Is COPD Treated? Retrieved from http://www.nhlbi.nih.gov/health/health-topics/topics/copd/treatment.html

National Breast Cancer Foundation. (2012). *Breast cancer.* Retrieved from http://www.nationalbreastcancer.org/edp/

National Cancer Institute [NCI]. (2008). *Cancer fact sheet. Colon and rectal cancer.* Retrieved from http://www.cancer.gov/cancertopics/types/colon-and-rectal

National Cancer Institute [NCI]. (2013). *Prostate cancer.* Retrieved from http://www.cancer.gov/cancertopics/types/prostate

National Center for Biotechnology Information. (2011). Pulmonary Tuberculosis. Retrieved from http://www.ncbi.nlm.nih.gov/pubmedhealth/PMH0001141/

National Conference of Gerontological Nurse Practitioners & National Gerontological Nursing Association. (2008a). Current treatment options and management strategies in Alzheimer's disease and related dementias. *Counseling Points, 1*(1), 4–13.

National Conference of Gerontological Nurse Practitioners & National Gerontological Nursing Association. (2008b). Current treatment options and management strategies in Alzheimer's disease and related dementias. *Counseling Points, 1*(3), 4–12.

National Diabetes Education Program. (2005). *Guiding principles for diabetes care: For healthcare providers.* Retrieved from http://www.ndep.nih.gov/diabetes/pubs/GuidPrin_HC_Eng.pdf

National Diabetes Survey. (2007). *National diabetes.* fact sheet. Retrieved from http://www.cdc.gov/diabetes/pubs/pdf/ndfs_2007.pdf. Retrieved from http://www.nationaldiabetessurvey.org

National Eye Institute, U.S. National Institutes of Health. (2005). *Diabetic retinopathy: What you should know.* Retrieved from http://www.nei.nih.gov/health/diabetic/retinopathy.asp#1

National Institute of Arthritis and Musculoskeletal and Skin Diseases. (2003). *Scientists identify two key risk factors for hip replacement in women.* Retrieved from http://www.niams.nih.gov

National Institute of Neurological Disorders and Stroke [NINDS]. (2005). *NINDS shingles information page.* Retrieved from http://www.ninds.nih.gov

National Institute of Neurological Disorders and Stroke [NINDS]. (2008). *Parkinson's disease.* Retrieved from http://www.ninds.nih.gov

National Institute of Neurological Disorders and Stroke [NINDS]. (2012). Parkinson's Disease information page. Retrieved from http://www.ninds.nih.gov/disorders/parkinsons_disease/parkinsons_disease.htm

National Institute of Health and Clinical Excellence [NICE]. (2012). *The epilepsies: The diagnosis and management of the epilepsies in adults and children in primary and secondary care. Clinical guideline no. 137.* London: Author.

National Institutes of Health [NIH]. (2008). *The seventh report of the Joint National Committee on Prevention, Detection, Evaluation, and Treatment of High Blood Pressure (JNC 7).* Retrieved from http://www .nhlbi.nih.gov/guidelines/hypertension/

National Osteoporosis Foundation. (2008). *Fast facts on osteoporosis.* Retrieved from http://www .nof.org/professionals/Fast_Facts_Osteoporosis.pdf

National Parkinson Disease Foundation. (2013). Parkinson Disease. Retrieved from http://www.parkinson .org/parkinson-s-disease.aspx

National Stroke Association [NSA]. (2012). *Warning signs of stroke.* Retrieved from http://www.stroke .org/site/PageServer?pagename=symp

Neville, D. A., Dvorkin, M., Chittenden, M. E., & Fromm, L. (2008). The new era of total hip replacement *OR Nurse 2008*, 18–25.

North American Menopause Society. (2012). Menopause. *The Journal of The North American Menopause Society, 19*(3), 257–271. DOI: 10.1097/gme.0b013e31824b970a

O'Donnell, S., McKee, G.; O'Brien, F., Mooney, M. & Moser, DK (2012). Gendered symptom presentation in acute coronary syndrome: A cross sectional analysis. *International Journal of Nursing Studies, 49*(11), 1325–1332.

Palmer, A. J, Rose, W. J., Minshallbm, M. E., Hayesm, C., Ogelsby, A. & Spinnas, A. (2004) Impact of HgA1c, lipids, and blood pressure on long term outcomes: An analysis using the CORE diabetes model. *Current Medical Research and Opinion, 20*(s1), 953–958.

Page, S. J., Levine, P., & Leonard, A. C. (2005). Effects of mental practice on affected limb use and function in chronic stroke. *Archives of Physical Medicine and Rehabilitation, 86*(3), 399–402.

Parkinson's Disease Foundation. (2012). *Prescription medications.* Retrieved from http://www.pdf.org/ parkinson_prescription_meds

Paun, O., Farran, C. J., Perraud, S., & Loukissa, D. A. (2004). Successful caregiving of persons with Alzheimer's disease: Skill development over time. *Alzheimer's Care Quarterly, 5*(3), 241–251.

Pierce, L. L., Gordon, M., & Steiner, V. (2004). Families dealing with stroke desire information about self-care needs. *Rehabilitation Nursing, 29*(1), 14–17.

Pierce, L. L., Steiner, V., Govoni, A. L., Hicks, B., Cervantez Thompson, T. L., & Friedemann, M. L. (2004). Internet-based support for rural caregivers of persons with stroke shows promise. *Rehabilitation Nursing, 29*(3), 95–99.

Pilotto, A., & Franceschi, M. (2009). Upper gastrointestinal disorders. In Halter, J.B., Ouslander, J. G., Tinetti, M.E., Studenski, S., High, K. P., & Asthana, S. *Hazzard's Geriatric Medicine and Gerontology* (6th ed., pp. 1075–1090). New York, NY: McGraw-Hill.

Podolsky, M. M. (1998). Exposing glaucoma. *Postgraduate Medicine, 103*(5), 131–152.

Posadzi, P., & Ernst, E (2011). Guided imagery for musculosketetal pain: A systematic review. *Clinical Journal of Pain, 27*(7), 645–653.

Postuma, R. B., Lang, A. E., Munhoz, R. P., Charland, K., Pelletier, A., Moscovich, M., Filla, L., … Shah, B. (2012). Caffeine for treatment of Parkinson Disease. *Neurology.* Retrieved from http://www.neurology .org/content/early/2012/08/01/WNL.0b013e318263570d.short#cited-by

PubMed Health. (2011). *Fact sheet: Cystitis in women.* Retrieved from http://www.ncbi.nlm.nih.gov/ pubmedhealth/PMH0005174/

Ramakrishnam, K. & Salinas, R. C. (2007). Peptic ulcer disease. *American Family Physician, 76*, 1005–1012.

Reimer, A. & Johnson, L. (2010). Atrophic vaginitis: Signs, symptoms, and better outcomes. *The Nurse Practitioner, 36*(1), 22–28.

Resnick, B. (2008). Treatment options for seizures in older adults. *Assisted Living Consult.* Retrieved from http://www.assistedlivingconsult.com/issues/04-01/alc12-Seizure-121.pdf

Reuben, D. B., Herr, K. A., Pacala, J. T., Pollock, B. G., Potter, J. F., & Semla, T. P. (2004). *Geriatrics at your fingertips* (7th ed.). Malden, MA: American Geriatrics Society.

Reuben, D. B., Herr, K. A., Pacala, J. T., Pollock, B. G., Potter, J. F., & Semla, T. P. (2008). *Geriatrics at your fingertips* (10th ed.). Malden, MA: American Geriatrics Society.

Richardson, L. C., Tai, E., & Rim, M. P. H. (2011). Vital Signs: Colorectal Cancer Screening, Incidence, and Mortality- United States, 2002–2010. *Morbidity and Mortality Weekly Report, 60*(26).

Rochette, A., Korner-Bitensky, N., & Lavasseur, M. (2006). Optimal participation: A reflective look. *Disability and Rehabilitation, 28*(19), 1231–1235.

Romito, D., Beaudoin, J. M., & Stein, P. (2011). Urinary tract infections in patients admitted to rehabilitation from acute care settings: A descriptive research study. *Rehabilitation, 36*(5), 216–222.

Rowan, J., & Tuchman, L. (2003). Management of seizures in the elderly. *Seizure Management, 2*(4), 10–16.

Saint, S., Meddings, J., Calfee, D., Kowlaski, C., & Krein, S. (2009). Catheter-associated urinary tract infection and the Medicare rule changes. *Annals of Internal Medicine, 150*, 877–884.

Seftel, D. (2005). *Adult macular degeneration.* Retrieved from http://www.eyesight.org/Macular_Degeneration/Adult_MD/adult_md.html

Shabsigh, R., Perleman, M. A., Lockhart, D. C., Lue, T. F. & Broderick, G. A. (2005). Health issues of men: Prevalence and correlates of erectile dysfunction. *The Journal of Urology, 174*(2), 662–667.

Shan, C. L, James, C. R., Chyu, M. C., Brismee, J. M., Zumualti, M. A., & Paklikuha, W. (2008). *Effects of tai chi on gait kinetic, physical function and pain in elderly with knee.* Retrieved from http://www.medicinenet.com/osteoporosis/article.htm

Snowdon, D. (2004). *Testimony of Dr. David Snowdon.* Presented to the Subcommittee on Labor, Health, and Human Services, and Education and Related Agencies Committee on Appropriations. March, 2004.

Schneeweiss, S. (2010). Risk of diabetes among patients with rheumatoid arthritis, psoriatic arthritis and psoriasis. *Annals of the Rheumatic Diseases, 69*(12), 2114–2117.

Soll, A. H. (2011). Overview of the natural history and treatment of peptic ulcer disease. Retrieved from http://www.uptodate.com/contents/overview-of-the-natural-history-and-treatment-of-peptic-ulcer-disease

Spitz, M. (2005). Epilepsy in the elderly. *Epilepsy/Professionals Spotlight, 2*(2), 1–2.

Starr, C. E., Guyer, D. R., & Yannuzzi, L. A. (1998). Age-related macular degeneration. *Postgraduate Medicine, 103*(5), 153–166.

Steel, N., Clark, A., Lang, W., Wallace, R. B., & Melzer, D. (2008). Racial disparities in the receipt of hip and knee joint replacements are not explained by need: The health & retirement study 1996–2004. *Journal of Gerontology Series A: Biological Sciences and Medical Sciences, 63*(6), 629–634.

Stefanacci, R. G. (2007, March/April). Let's not lose sight of residents' visual health. *Assisted Living Consult*, 23–26.

Steiner, V., Pierce, L., Drahuschak, S., Nofziger, E., Buchanan, D., & Szirony, T. (2008). Emotional support, physical help and health of caregivers of stroke survivors. *Journal of Neuroscience Nursing, 40*(1), 48–54.

Thomas, D.J. (2011). Abdominal problems. In Dunphy, L.M., Winland-Brown, J. E., Portor, B. O., Thomas, D. J. *Primary Care: The Art and Science of Advanced Practice Nursing* (3rd ed., pp. 492–581). Philadelphia, PA: Davis.

Trudo, E. W., & Stark, W. J. (1998). Cataracts. *Postgraduate Medicine, 103*(5), 114–130.

Tursi, A. (2012). Advances in the management of colonic diverticulitis. *Canadian Medical Association Journal, 184*, 14770–14776.

United States Preventive Services Task Force [USPSTF]. (2009). *Screening for breast cancer.* Retrieved from http://www.uspreventiveservicestaskforce.org/uspstf/uspsbrca.htm

United States Preventive Services Task Force [USPSTF]. (2011). *Osteoporosis.* Retrieved from http://uspreventiveservicestaskforce.org/3rduspstf/osteoporosis/osteoor.htm.

University of Washington, Department of Ophthalmology. (2008). *Cataract statistics.* Retrieved from http://www.universityofwashington/ophthalmology.org

U.S. Department of Health and Human Services, National Kidney and Urological Diseases Information Clearing House [NKUDIC]. (2012). *Prostate enlargement: Benign prostatic hyperplasia.* Retrieved from http://kidney.niddk.nih.gov/kudiseases/pubs/prostateenlargement/#common

Uthman, B. M. (2004). *Successfully using antiepileptic drugs in the elderly.* Paper presented at the 6th annual U.S. Geriatric and Long Term Care Congress, Orlando, FL.

Velez, I., & Selwa, L. M. (2003). Seizure disorders in the elderly. *American Family Physician, 67*(2), 325–332.

Von Radowitz, J. (5 March 2012). New research claims rheumatoid arthritis breakthrough. *The Independent.* Retrieved Jan 21, 2013 from http://www.independent.co.uk/life-style/health-and-families/health-news/new-research-claims-rheumatoid-arthritis-breakthrough-7537207.html

Walker, J. (2012). Care of patients undergoing joint replacement. *Nursing Older People 24*(1), 14–20.

Warlow, C., Sudlow, C., Martin, D., Wardlaw, J., & Sandercock, P. (2003). Stroke. *Lancet, 362*(9391), 1.

WebMD. (2012). *Women's health.* Retrieved from http://women.webmd.com/guide/sexual-health-vaginal-infections

Weinberger, S.E. (2004). Principles of Pulmonary Medicine (4th ed.). Philadelphia, PA: Saunders.

White, N. G., O'Rourke, F., Ong, B. S., Cordato, D. J., & Chan, D. K. Y. (2008). Dysphagia: Causes, assessment, treatment and management. *Geriatrics, 63*(5), 15–18.

Wiles, R., Ashburn, A., Payne, S., & Murphy, C. (2002). Patients' expectations of recovery following stroke: A qualitative study. *Disability and Rehabilitation, 24*(16), 841–850.

Wiles, R., Ashburn, A., Payne, S., & Murphy, C. (2004). Discharge from physiotherapy following stroke: The management of disappointment. *Social Science & Medicine, 59*(6), 1263–1273.

Williams, K. E., & Bond, M. J. (2002). The roles of self-efficacy, outcome expectancies and social support in the self-care behaviours of diabetics. *Psychology, Health & Medicine, 7*(2), 127–141.

Wong, J. M., Khan, W. S., Chimutengwende-Gordon, M., & Dowd, G. S. E. (2011). Recent advances in designs, approaches and materials in total knee replacement: Literature review and evidence today. *Journal of Perioperative Practice, 21*(5), 165–171.

World Health Organization [WHO]. (2010). Prevention of blindness and visual impairment. Retrieved from http://www.who.int/blindness/causes/priority/en/index1.html

Woolever, D. R., & Beutler, A. I. (2007). Hypothyroidism: A review of the evaluation and management. *Family Practice Recertification, 29*(4), 45–52.

Yen, R. W., Sidney, M. S., Chanra, M., Sorel, M. M., Selby, J. V., & Go, A. S. (2010). Myocardial infarction. *American Journal of Medicine, 363*, 2155–2165.

Yurkow, J., & Yudin, J. (2002). Musculoskeletal problems. In V. T. Cotter and N. E. Strumpf (Eds.), *Advanced practice nursing with older adults: Clinical guidelines* (pp. 229–242). New York, NY: McGraw-Hill.

Zann, R. B. (2005). *Joint replacement in normal joints.* Retrieved from http://www.ortho-spine.com

Zafari, A. M., & Yang, R. H. (2012). Myocardial infarction. http://emedicine.medscape.com/article/155919-overview

For a full suite of assignments and additional learning activities, see the access code at the front of your book.

LEARNING OBJECTIVES

www

At the end of this chapter, the reader will be able to:

> Differentiate among dementia, depression, and delirium.
> Identify the stages and clinical features of dementia.
> Describe procedures for diagnosing dementia.
> Recognize and address the common causes of delirium.
> Discuss the theoretical foundations of nursing care for persons with dementia.
> Contrast pharmacological and nonpharmacological interventions for dementia, delirium, and depression.
> Apply basic principles to provide safe and effective care for persons with dementia.
> List specific nursing interventions for behavioral and psychological symptoms of dementia.
> Recognize the role of adult day services in the care of persons with dementia.
> Identify the role that palliative care/hospice care plays for individuals with dementia and their families.

KEY TERMS

www

Acetylcholine

Agnosia

Alzheimer's disease (AD)

Anticholinergic

Aphasia

Apolipoprotein E-e4 (APOE-e4)

Apraxia

Beta-amyloid plaques

Cholinesterase

Cholinesterase inhibitor (CEI)

Delirium

Dementia

Depression

Executive function

Hallucinations

Hospice

Palliative Care

Neurofibrillary tangles

Neurotransmitter

Paranoia

Chapter 10

Nursing Management of Dementia

Christine E. Schwartzkopf
Prudence Twigg

The purpose of this chapter is to present basic information about dementia, delirium, and depression. These conditions are sometimes referred to as the "3 Ds" of geriatrics because they are fairly common in older adults and their signs and symptoms often overlap. Additionally, this chapter includes information on pharmacological and nonpharmacological treatments and care approaches to improve care for older adults with dementia (see **Box 10-1**).

BOX 10-1   Web Exploration

Review the following resources about dementia, delirium, and depression:

Alzheimer's Association: http://www.alz.org

American Association for Geriatric Psychiatry: http://www.aagpgpa.org

National Institute of Mental Health: http://www.nimh.nih.gov

National Institute of Neurological Disorders and Stroke: http://www.ninds.nih.gov

National Institute on Aging: http://www.nia.nih.gov

Dementia

Dementia is a general term that refers to progressive, degenerative brain dysfunction, including deterioration in memory, concentration, language skills, visuospatial skills, and reasoning, that interferes with a person's daily functioning. Although dementia is much more common in older adults than in younger persons, dementia is not considered a normal part of aging. The most common type of dementia (see **Box 10-2**) is *Alzheimer's disease (AD)*, named after Dr. Alois Alzheimer, who first described the condition about 100 years ago. Alzheimer's disease did not begin to be commonly diagnosed and systemically studied until the 1970s (National Institute on Aging, 2007).

BOX 10-2   Most Common Types of Dementia in Older Adults

Alzheimer's disease (most common)

Vascular dementia (considered the second most-common form of dementia, after Alzheimer's)

Mixed Alzheimer's/vascular dementia

Parkinson's dementia

Lewy body dementia

Frontotemporal lobe dementia

Notable Quotes

"The journey into dementia has its disappointments to be endured as well as its triumphs to be cherished. In all of the ambiguities and confusion there may also be signs of hope, for this is a journey with intersecting signposts; reminders of the past and pointers to the future. There are always fresh opportunities for a new walk on a new day."

—Rosalie Hudson. (2006). Spirited walking. In M. Marshall & K. Allan (Eds.), *Dementia: Walking not wandering* (p. 113). London, UK: Hawker.

Currently, about 5.4 million people in the United States have Alzheimer's disease. With the changing demographics of the U.S. population leading to a higher percentage of older adults, the number of Americans with AD is projected to rise to about 11 to 16 million by the year 2050. Dramatic increases in the number of "oldest-old" (those whose age is >85 years) across all racial and ethnic groups contributes to this increased prevalence. As will be discussed throughout this chapter, the needs of persons with dementia are complex and costly, both financially and psychologically, with families providing most of the care. There are no specific interventions for the prevention of AD, and the current treatments offer only modest benefits (Alzheimer's Association, 2012).

Although the aging brain undergoes many developmental changes, mild cognitive impairment (MCI), an intermediate state between normal aging and dementia, is characterized by acquired cognitive deficits; these changes *do not* significantly interfere with the daily functioning of most older adults. Studies conducted on MCI have introduced new concepts regarding the possible distinctions between normal and pathologic aging of the brain. The hippocampus, a region of the brain important to learning and memory, gradually loses volume as part of the normal aging process. This loss is significantly accelerated in older people with Alzheimer's disease, especially if they have vascular problems or diabetes. An international team of researchers has identified four genes that may play a role in the age-related decline of hippocampal volume, a finding that may provide insight to risk for cognitive decline and Alzheimer's disease (Bis et al., 2012).

Persons with AD, however, have numerous pathological brain changes that contribute to their symptoms. The pathological hallmarks of AD are beta-amyloid plaques and neurofibrillary tangles. The plaques are dense deposits around neurons. The tangles build up inside nerve cells. Together, the plaques and tangles interfere with normal nerve cell function and lead to neuronal death (National Institute on Aging, 2007). Plaques made up of abnormal deposits of beta-amyloid protein are a hallmark of Alzheimer's disease. The toxic buildup begins when the beta-secretase enzyme (BACE), working in concert with a partner enzyme, snips a small fragment of amyloid precursor protein (APP) and releases beta-amyloid from the cell membrane of neurons. The beta-amyloid can then gradually clump together to form the well-known plaques that may cause damage to brain cells (Obregon et al., 2012). See the section on the nervous system in Chapter 5 for more specific information about brain changes with aging and Alzheimer's disease.

Alzheimer's dementia is the most common type of dementia, accounting for an estimated 60–80% of cases, although several other types of dementia are also commonly seen in older adults. Vascular dementia (previously known as multi-infarct or poststroke dementia) is the second most-common type of dementia, and combinations of Alzheimer's and vascular dementia are also quite common (called "mixed dementia"). Vascular dementia may occur rather acutely after a cerebrovascular accident (CVA, or stroke) or more insidiously due to chronic atherosclerosis of cerebral arteries. Much like the coronary arteries, cerebral arteries are negatively affected by factors such as hyperlipidemia, smoking, and hypertension, causing decreased blood flow to the brain and neuronal death (Alzheimer's Association, 2012). The clinical signs and symptoms of dementia due to Alzheimer's and vascular causes are similar, and generally, the assessment of and interventions for these dementias are similar.

Parkinson's disease (PD) is a chronic neurodegenerative disease characterized by motor symptoms in the early stages, but cognitive symptoms and dementia may develop in the later stages of PD. Lewy body dementia (LBD) is a variant of dementia with a specific pathological finding in the brain (abnormal deposits of a protein, alpha-synuclein). Clinically, LBD can be distinguished from AD by:

> Motor symptoms in the early stage of LBD (which occur in the late stage of AD)
> Visual hallucinations in early LBD (which occur in the middle stage of AD, if at all)
> Fluctuating mental status as a feature of LBD (which usually occurs only due to delirium in AD)

It is not uncommon for persons with LBD to initially be suspected of having PD, due to their motor symptoms (e.g., decreased range of motion and gait instability), although their motor symptoms do not respond to dopaminergic agents given for PD.

Frontotemporal dementia or frontal lobe dementia (FLD) affects the frontal and temporal lobes of the brain and is often characterized by early deficiencies in *executive functioning* (e.g., planning and making decisions), while memory may initially remain fairly intact. There are three types of FLD:

> **Progressive behavior/personality decline**—characterized by changes in personality, behavior, emotions, and judgment (e.g., behavioral variant frontotemporal dementia).
> **Progressive language decline**—marked by early changes in language ability, including speaking, understanding, reading, and writing (e.g., primary progressive aphasia).
> **Progressive motor decline**—characterized by various difficulties with physical movement, including shaking, difficulty walking, frequent falls, and poor coordination.

Persons with FLD often experience personality changes and disinhibition (saying and doing inappropriate things) much earlier than persons with AD (Alzheimer's Association, 2012).

Normal pressure hydrocephalus (NPH) is a relatively rare type of dementia, but an important subtype, primarily because, if identified early, it may be partially reversible with surgical intervention. The symptoms of NPH are related to an abnormal accumulation of cerebrospinal fluid and are clinically distinguishable from other dementias by a triad of symptoms: slowed cognitive processes, gait disturbances, and urinary incontinence with a relatively acute onset (Alzheimer's Association, 2012).

Other, less common dementias include Huntington's disease (hereditary), Wernicke–Korsakoff's syndrome (most commonly caused by chronic alcoholism), and Creutzfeldt–Jakob disease (a very rare, rapidly progressing fatal dementia related to "mad cow disease"). Down's syndrome is also associated with the eventual development of dementia. About 65% of persons with Down's syndrome who are over 60 years old will have dementia. Although there are many types of dementia, the majority of cases are attributable to Alzheimer's and/or vascular dementia (Alzheimer's Association, 2012).

Risk Factors for Dementia

The main risk factor for developing Alzheimer's-type dementia is age, but AD is not a normal part of aging. The risk for AD doubles every 5 years after age 65 years. By age 85, about one-half of people will have symptoms of Alzheimer's. Family history also plays a role in the risk for developing dementia. Having a first-degree relative (parent, sibling, or child) with Alzheimer's increases the risk, and the risk increases even more if more than one first-degree relative has had the disease. Some of the increased risk is heredity (genetics), while some risk is related to shared environmental/lifestyle factors (see **Box 10-3**), though both may play a role in the increased risk within families (Alzheimer's Association, 2012). Neuroimaging and genetic testing have aided in the identification of individuals at increased risk for dementia.

One gene that increases the risk for Alzheimer's in the general population is the presence of *apolipoprotein E-e4 (APOE-e4)*. The other common forms of the APOE gene (e2 and e3) are not associated with Alzheimer's. Each person inherits two APOE genes, so some people will have no APOE-e4, some may have one APOE-e4 (higher risk for AD), and a few may have two copies of APOE-e4 (highest risk for AD). The APOE-e4 gene has varying penetrance, however, so even persons at the highest risk may never develop the disease. The APOE gene codes for proteins associated with cholesterol transport in the body. There are rarer genes that are associated with the risk for Alzheimer's, but these genes tend to be concentrated within a few hundred well-identified families (Alzheimer's Association, 2012). Although many people

BOX 10-3 Risk Factors for Dementia	
Age	History of head trauma
Family history	Vascular disease
Genetic factors	Certain types of infections

worry about having the APOE-e4 gene, routine genetic screening is not recommended. The value of having such knowledge is questionable because of the varying predictive ability and lack of treatment for the presence of the gene.

On the other hand, there are several modifiable risk factors that can lower one's risk for developing Alzheimer's and/or vascular dementia. Persons with a history of head injury, head trauma, and traumatic brain injury are associated with increased risk for developing dementia later in life. Groups that routinely experience head injuries, such as boxers, football players, and combat veterans, may be at risk of dementia, late-life cognitive impairments, and evidence of tau tangles (a hallmark of AD) at autopsy. Protecting the head from injury by using seatbelts and bicycle/motorcycle helmets throughout the life span is one way to lower the risk for dementia. Vascular disease contributes to the risk for dementia, so taking care of one's brain, in much the same way that one can prevent heart disease, is another good way to lower the risk for dementia. Some data indicate that cardiovascular disease risk factors such as physical inactivity, high cholesterol, diabetes, smoking, and obesity are associated with a higher risk of developing dementia. Unlike genetic risks, cardiovascular risk factors are modifiable. Therefore, maintenance of ideal body weight, exercising, avoiding smoking, and controlling hyperlipidemia and hypertension may all help to lower the risk of dementia. Finally, exercising the brain with lifelong cognitive activity, along with consuming a diet low in saturated fats and rich in vegetables, may support brain health (Alzheimer's Association, 2012).

Medical Diagnosis of Alzheimer's Disease/Dementia

When an older adult and/or their family members suspect memory problems and possibly dementia (see **Box 10-4**), the first step is a visit to the primary care provider (PCP). It is not uncommon for family members and friends to notice changes and request an evaluation even though the older adult may not think there are any problems. Conversely, some older adults without significant cognitive problems may be overly concerned about mild memory lapses and request evaluations. Whenever the cognitive function of an older adult is in question, the best course of action is to seek a medical evaluation. More and more PCPs are routinely screening for cognitive impairment in older adults using short questionnaires at office visits for

BOX 10-4 Possible Warning Signs of Dementia	
Frequent forgetfulness, especially of recent events	Poor judgment, especially with finances
Difficulty with common tasks (e.g., cooking)	Misplacing objects in unusual places (e.g., puts clothes in bathtub, puts purse in oven)
Forgetting common words	Changes in mood, behavior, or personality
Becoming lost in familiar areas	Lack of interest/involvement in life activities

other medical problems. The goal of this practice is to identify and treat dementia in the early stage, before the symptoms are more apparent and when interventions tend to be more successful.

Alzheimer's disease has several clinical features including, but not limited to, memory impairment (see **Box 10-5**). Memory impairment alone does not indicate AD; rather, the cognitive deficits and memory impairment must significantly interfere with functioning. Additionally, the diagnostic criteria require that one of the following features also be present: impaired executive function, aphasia, apraxia, or agnosia. Executive function refers to higher level functions such as the ability to think abstractly, plan, organize, complete sequences of action, and make decisions. Impaired executive function significantly affects a person's ability to complete day-to-day tasks. Even an activity as simple as getting dressed in the morning requires planning, decision making, and sequencing. *Aphasia* refers to language deficits, typically a lack of complex language (e.g., less vocabulary) and word finding difficulties (e.g., can't think of the right word to speak) early in AD. *Apraxia* is the inability to carry out motor activities, even though there are no motor deficits (e.g., unable to comb one's hair even though the arms have full range of motion). *Agnosia* refers to the failure to recognize sensory stimuli (e.g., cannot look at a wristwatch and name what it is). In AD, the history of the cognitive deficits is that they have occurred gradually over a relatively long period of time (months to a few years).

In addition to having the preceding deficits, to make a diagnosis of AD, the clinician must ensure that nothing else but AD accounts for the deficits observed. Therefore, a significant part of diagnosing AD is ruling out other possible causes of cognitive deficits such as delirium, depression, other central nervous system disorders, medication side effects, and numerous medical conditions that impact cognitive function.

The primary care provider (PCP) evaluating cognitive problems in an older adult will conduct a history and physical examination. The medical history, particularly

---

BOX 10-5 Diagnostic Criteria for Alzheimer's Disease

- Multiple cognitive deficits/impairment
  1. Impaired short- or long-term memory AND
  2. At least one of the following:
     - Impaired executive function (abstraction, planning, organizing, sequencing)
     - Aphasia (language disturbance)
     - Apraxia (impaired purposeful movements)
     - Agnosia (inability to recognize sensory stimuli)
- The changes significantly interfere with social and/or occupational function and represent a decline from previous level of function.
- The course has been a gradual onset and continuing decline.
- The changes do not occur exclusively during delirium.
- The changes are not better accounted for by another condition (systemic disorders, central nervous system disorders, substances, other psychiatric conditions).

the onset, type, and duration of symptoms, may help distinguish chronic from acute cognitive changes. A thorough physical examination, including laboratory tests, may help identify possible reversible causes of the cognitive changes. Several medical disorders that can be identified with laboratory tests can contribute to cognitive problems in older adults, including severe liver disease, hypothyroidism, vitamin B_{12} deficiency, hypercalcemia, and latent syphilis. The patient's medication list should be carefully reviewed to determine any current medications that may be causing or worsening cognitive impairment. (A pharmacist may be enlisted to help with this review.) **Box 10-6** lists common medications that may cause or worsen cognitive impairment. Many of these medications appear on a list that is famous, or perhaps infamous, in the world of geriatrics: Beers's criteria for potentially inappropriate drugs in older adults (Fick et al., 2003). Medication issues will be discussed in more detail later in this chapter.

Usually, imaging of the head/brain will be conducted. Although Alzheimer's disease cannot be directly diagnosed by a computed tomography (CT) scan of the head or magnetic resonance imaging (MRI) of the brain, these studies may identify or rule out other possible causes of cognitive decline (such as the presence of a tumor, or evidence of a stroke) and may confirm the presence of vascular disease

BOX 10-6　Common Medications That Can Cause or Worsen Confusion

Any anticholinergic agents or those with significant anticholinergic effects

Analgesics

　Propoxyphene (found in Darvon and Darvocet)

　Meperidine (Demerol)

　Opiates in excessive doses

Antiemetics

Promethazine (Phenergan)—anticholinergic

Antihistamines

Diphenhydramine (Benadryl)—anticholinergic

Antihypertensives

Clonodine (Catapres)

Antipruritics

Hydroxyzine (Atarax)—anticholinergic

Antiseizure medications (most, to some degree)

Phenobarbital

Anxiolytics

　Meprobamate (Equanil)

　Benzodiazepines (Ativan, Xanax, Valium)

Bladder relaxants

Oxybutynin (Ditropan)—anticholinergic

Gastrointestinal antispasmodics

　Dicyclomine (Bentyl)—anticholinergic

　Hyoscyamine (Levsin)—anticholinergic

H2 antagonists

Cimetidine (Tagamet)—anticholinergic

Muscle relaxants

Cyclobenzaprine (Flexeril)—anticholinergic

Tricyclic antidepressants

Amitriptyline (Elavil)—anticholinergic

(Alzheimer's Association, 2012). The American Association for Geriatric Psychiatry (AAGP) has recommended that a CT or MRI be conducted as part of a dementia workup and that positron emission tomography (PET) scans not be used routinely to diagnose dementia (AAGP, 2004b). PET scans of the brain are more commonly used in dementia research than in clinical practice.

Any possible medical problems contributing to cognitive changes will usually be treated before concluding that the older adult has dementia. Notably, delirium should be excluded and depression should be excluded or diagnosed and treated before a diagnosis of dementia can be firmly established.

The PCP may do simple "paper and pencil" screening tests to determine the presence and degree of cognitive impairment. If the screening tests are suspicious for cognitive impairment, the PCP may refer the older adult to a psychologist and/or psychiatrist for further testing, although many PCPs are comfortable making the diagnosis of dementia without referral to a specialist. The AAGP, however, recommends that the diagnosis of dementia be made by physicians with experience in geriatrics: geriatric internists, geriatric psychiatrists, neurologists with training in the area of cognitive disorders, or family practitioners with expertise in geriatrics (AAGP, 2004b).

There are several common neuropsychological screening tests that can be administered to older adults. In the past, the most popular screening test was the Mini Mental State Examination (MMSE), which is scored from 0–30; 30 is considered normal (Folstein, Folstein, & McHugh, 1975). The MMSE, however, is no longer available in the public domain and so is not as commonly used, though you may still hear clinicians refer to it. Alternatives to the MMSE include the Mini-Cog (Borson, Scanlan, Brush, Vitallano, & Dokmak, 2000) and the St. Louis University Mental Status (SLUMS) examination (Tariq, Tumosa, Chibnall, Perry, & Morley, 2006). (See **Box 10-7** to access these and other assessment tests referred to in this chapter.) Psychologists and/or psychiatrists administering neuropsychological tests for cognitive impairment may administer much more complicated and time-intensive tests to determine the exact nature of the cognitive deficits.

BOX 10-7   Resources for Assessment Available on the Internet

Assessing and Managing Delirium in Older Adults with Dementia:

http://www.consultgerirn.org/uploads/File/trythis/try_this_d8.pdf

Assessing Pain in Persons with Dementia:

http://consultgerirn.org/uploads/File/trythis/try_this_d2.pdf

Avoiding Restraints in Patients with Dementia:

http://www.nursingcenter.com/prodev/ce_article.asp?tid=776342

Beers Criteria for Potentially Inappropriate Medication Use in Older Adults: Parts I and II:

http://consultgerirn.org/uploads/File/trythis/issue16_1.pdf

http://consultgerirn.org/uploads/File/trythis/issue16_2.pdf

Brief Evaluation of Executive Dysfunction:

http://consultgerirn.org/uploads/File/trythis/try_this_d3.pdf

Communication Difficulties: Assessment and Interventions in Hospitalized Older Adults with Dementia:

http://www.nursingcenter.com/prodev/ce_article.asp?tid=776481

Confusion Assessment Method (CAM):

http://www.nursingcenter.com/prodev/ce_article.asp?tid=756744

Decision Making and Dementia:

http://consultgerirn.org/uploads/File/trythis/issue_d9.pdf

Eating and Feeding Issues in Older Adults with Dementia: Parts I and II:

http://consultgerirn.org/uploads/File/trythis/try_this_d11_1.pdf

http://consultgerirn.org/uploads/File/trythis/try_this_d11_2.pdf

Geriatric Depression Scale (GDS):

http://www.nursingcenter.com/prodev/ce_article.asp?tid=743421

Mental Status Assessment of Older Adults: The Mini-Cog:

http://www.nursingcenter.com/prodev/ce_article.asp?tid=756614

National Alzheimer's Project Act

http://www.nia.nih.gov/newsroom/2012/02/we-cant-wait-administration-announces-new-steps-fight-alzheimers-disease

Nursing Standard of Practice Protocol: Recognition and Management of Dementia:

http://consultgerirn.org/topics/dementia/want_to_know_more

St. Louis University Mental Status Examination (SLUMS):

http://medschool.slu.edu/agingsuccessfully/pdfsurveys/slumsexam_05.pdf

---

BOX 10-8   Diagnosis of Dementia

History and physical examination

Review of medications

Laboratory tests: complete blood count (CBC), complete metabolic panel (CMP), thyroid-stimulating hormone (TSH), vitamin B_{12} level, syphilis serology

Neuropsychological testing

Imaging studies: CT scan and/or MRI, PET scan (not routinely)

Many persons with a new diagnosis of (see **Box 10-8**) dementia and/or their families may believe that the diagnosis is incorrect. Receiving a diagnosis of dementia is almost uniformly devastating to the client and/or family, and initially, denial is a common psychological coping mechanism. When the previously mentioned diagnostic steps are completed, however, the diagnostic certainty for the diagnosis of "probable dementia" is quite high (about 90%), higher than for many other medical illnesses (National Institute on Aging, 2007). Clients and families who remain uncertain about the diagnosis should be counseled to seek a second opinion from a physician specializing in the diagnosis and treatment of dementia. From a medical, psychosocial, and financial planning perspective, acceptance of the diagnosis by the client and family and subsequent steps to act on the knowledge can positively influence care outcomes. Prolonged denial of the diagnosis tends to worsen the situation for both the client and family and delay necessary treatment. Older adults with dementia and their families should be referred to the Alzheimer's Association (http://www.alz.org), a national organization with local chapters, for support services.

Stages of Alzheimer's Disease

Alzheimer's disease is commonly divided into three stages for the purpose of clinical management: mild, moderate, and severe (National Institute on Aging, 2007) (see **Box 10-9**). During the mild stage of AD, symptoms are often subtle and may go unnoticed by the person and his or her family and friends or may be attributed to "just getting older," resulting in a delay in diagnosis and appropriate treatment. Behavioral and psychological symptoms of dementia (BPSD) are most commonly exhibited during the moderate stage (see **Figure 10-1**) and often lead

---

BOX 10-9 Characteristics of Alzheimer's Disease by Stage

Mild Stage

- Memory loss
- Getting lost in familiar places
- Having more difficulty doing normal daily tasks
- Difficulty with managing finances
- Making bad decisions
- Not being as talkative or verbally fluent
- Being more moody or anxious

Moderate Stage

- Increased memory loss and confusion
- Short attention span
- Difficulty with language, numbers
- Difficulty with reasoning
- Inability to learn new things or to adapt to new situations
- Restlessness, agitation, anxiety, tearfulness, wandering—especially in the late afternoon or at night ("sundowner syndrome")

- Repetitive statements, questions, or movements
- Hallucinations, delusions, paranoia, irritability
- Impulsivity (saying or doing things he or she normally would not)
- Perceptual-motor problems (interfering with activities of daily living)

Severe Stage

- Weight loss
- Seizures in some patients
- Dysphagia (difficulty swallowing)
- Vocalizations, but speech usually unintelligible
- Increased time spent sleeping
- Bowel and bladder incontinence
- Loss of recognition of family
- Pressure ulcers
- Neuromuscular symptoms (contractures)

to institutionalization due to the need for 24-hour supervision. BPSD will be discussed in more detail later in this chapter. The person with severe AD requires total care for all needs and will most often die of complications (aspiration pneumonia) related to dysphagia, unless another medical condition causes death sooner.

Reisberg and colleagues (2002) have identified seven stages of AD (ranging from Stage 1: "no impairment" to Stage 7: "very severe cognitive decline"). Regardless of the staging system employed, persons with AD may pass through the stages of the disease at varying rates, but generally die within 4 to 6 years of diagnosis, although most have had the disease for some time before diagnosis. However, the course of AD is quite variable and can range from 3 to 20 years (Alzheimer's Association, 2012).

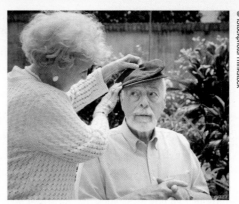

Figure 10-1 Family members may be the first to notice signs of cognitive decline.

Pharmacological Intervention for Dementia

The American Association for Geriatric Psychiatry (AAGP, 2006) has published principles for care for persons with Alzheimer's disease, including principles of pharmacological management. Ideally, pharmacological therapy for AD would prevent *beta-amyloid plaques* and/or ameliorate the neuronal damage caused by the plaques and *neurofibrillary tangles*. Unfortunately, currently no medications are available that have this mechanism of action, although many new promising agents are being studied. Two classes of medications currently are approved for the treatment of Alzheimer's dementia: *cholinesterase inhibitors (CEIs)* and N-methyl-D-aspartate (NMDA) receptor antagonists. Both classes provide their therapeutic effect by acting on neurotransmitters. Several neurotransmitters in the brain are affected by the pathological changes associated with Alzheimer's disease.

Acetylcholine is a *neurotransmitter* in the brain, known to be important for memory. Medications or diseases that inhibit acetylcholine interfere with memory. Early in the course of AD, neuronal loss causes a decrease in the acetylcholine available for normal neurotransmission. Direct supplementation with acetylcholine is not currently feasible. Acetylcholine is naturally degraded in the brain by an enzyme, acetylcholinesterase. Cholinesterase inhibitors (CEIs) exert their therapeutic effect by blocking the enzyme, resulting in a net increase in acetylcholine.

Four drugs are currently approved for treatment of AD (see **Box 10-10**). The first CEI developed was tacrine (Cognex); however, this agent is no longer commonly used due to its dosing schedule (four times a day) and potential liver complications. The three remaining CEIs that commonly are prescribed for AD are donepezil (Aricept), rivastigmine (Exelon), and galantamine (Razadyne). The CEIs are generally started as early as possible in AD and continued throughout the

BOX 10-10   Medication Treatment for Alzheimer's Disease

Medication	Target Dose
Cholinesterase inhibitors (CEIs)	
Donepezil (Aricept)	10 mg po q. daily
Galantamine (Razadyne ER)	24 mg po q. daily
Rivastigmine (Exelon)	6 mg po bid or 9.5 mg patch daily
N-methyl-D-aspartate (NMDA) receptor antagonists	
Memantine (Namenda)	10 mg po bid

Refer to a pharmacology text for more specific information about medications for dementia.

disease course until no longer effective based on clinical judgment, although only donepezil is approved by the FDA for use in severe AD. The CEIs are generally well tolerated, although, when initiated, clients may complain of gastrointestinal (GI) side effects (nausea, diarrhea), due to the cholinergic effects of the medication on the GI tract. For this reason, the CEIs are usually started at low doses and then gradually titrated up (usually over a period of about 6 weeks) to the target dose in order to lessen side effects. Rivastigmine is also approved for use in mild to moderate Parkinson's dementia. All of the CEIs, however, are often prescribed off-label for dementias other than AD.

Glutamate is the main excitatory neurotransmitter in the brain. Glutamate excitotoxicity (due to excess glutamate) has been implicated in the pathogenesis of AD. When neurons die due to plaques and tangles, glutamate is released in large amounts into the extracellular fluid, increasing NMDA receptor activation and intracellular calcium influx into adjacent neurons. Excess intracellular calcium kills the remaining healthy neurons. Although excess glutamate is not the cause of AD per se, the cascading effect of neuronal death, excess glutamate, and further neuronal loss is believed to play a role in the progression of the disease.

Memantine (Namenda) is an NMDA noncompetitive receptor antagonist, currently the only medication in this class, and helps to protect neurons from glutamate excitotoxicity without completely eliminating the glutamate necessary for normal neurological function (see **Box 10-11**). Memantine is generally well tolerated, can be safely administered with donepezil or other *cholinesterase* inhibitors, and the combination has been found to be more effective than cholinesterase inhibitors alone. Memantine is currently approved for moderate to severe stage AD, although some clinicians may prescribe the medication for early stage AD or other dementias (off-label use). Memantine, like the CEIs, is generally started at a low dose and gradually titrated up to the target dose (usually over a period of about 4–6 weeks) to lessen side effects.

BOX 10-11   Research Highlight

Aim: This review study evaluated the evidence for the effectiveness of cholinesterase inhibitors and memantine in achieving clinically relevant outcomes for patients with Alzheimer's disease.

Methods: A literature search for all published English-language randomized controlled clinical trials that evaluated the pharmacologic agents for adults with AD yielded 96 publications of 59 unique studies eligible for review.

Findings: Both cholinesterase inhibitors and memantine demonstrated consistent clinical effects in the areas of cognition and global assessment; however, the effect sizes were small. Most of the studies were short (6 months), limiting the ability to make conclusions about the effects of the medications on the progression of dementia. Other limitations included inclusion of only patients with mild or moderate AD, poor reporting of adverse effects of the medications, and limited evaluation of behavior and quality of life as possible outcome indicators.

Application to practice: Cholinesterase inhibitors and memantine for the treatment of AD show statistically significant results but only marginal clinical improvement in cognition and global (overall) assessment measures. Nurses should use this knowledge when teaching patients and families about the benefits of medication therapy in AD.

Source: Raina, P., Santaguida, P., Ismaila, A., Patterson, C., Cowan, D., Levine, M., Booker, L., & Oremus, M. (2008). Effectiveness of cholinesterase inhibitors and memantine for treating dementia: Evidence review for a clinical practice guideline. *Annals of Internal Medicine, 148*, 379–397.

The cholinesterase inhibitors and memantine slow the progression of dementia, but do not stop the decline. After several months or years of treatment, however, the person receiving treatment may have significantly higher function than if he or she had not been treated at all. For this reason, once the medications are started, they are usually not discontinued unless significant side effects develop (rare after continuous use). Suddenly discontinuing the medications may result in a significant observable decline that may not be reversed by restarting the medications. If the medications are stopped for some reason for a period of days or weeks, and then restarted, the lowest dose is restarted and then titration proceeds back up to the target dose. Eventually, when the client is in the most advanced stage of AD and is clearly no longer benefiting from the medications (nonambulatory, mute, unable to recognize family members), the medications are usually weaned off.

Indirectly, good treatment for other medical conditions, particularly the management of vascular disease and associated conditions such as hypertension, hyperlipidemia, hyperglycemia, and elevated homocysteine levels, may help slow the progression of dementia. Vitamin E supplementation, as an antioxidant, is available over the counter and may be recommended for AD by some clinicians, although the daily dose should not exceed 400 IU due to concerns about toxicity and cardiovascular side effects. Medications not currently recommended for the treatment of Alzheimer's disease include estrogen replacement, anti-inflammatory agents (e.g., ibuprofen), and gingko biloba, although estrogen and ibuprofen may be appropriate for other uses (AAGP, 2006).

Numerous new medications for Alzheimer's disease are being investigated in drug trials. The next generation of drugs is designed to prevent and/or destroy deposits of beta-amyloid plaque that kill the brain's nerve cells, which leads to the devastating loss of cognition and function that characterizes Alzheimer's. Some trials are exploring the strong correlation between heart disease and diabetes as Alzheimer's risk factors. Cholesterol-lowering drugs (statins) and the diabetes drug rosiglitazone (Avandia) are being trialed for Alzheimer's disease.

Medications That Can Cause or Worsen Confusion

With an understanding of some of the neurotransmitters affected by Alzheimer's disease and the medications used to treat dementia, one can imagine that some medications could worsen confusion in persons with dementia. This is, indeed, the case. Particularly problematic are agents that block acetylcholine. Medications classified as *anticholinergic* or medications otherwise classified but with significant anticholinergic effects can be expected to worsen cognitive function in persons with dementia (see Box 10-6). Additionally, any medications that have central nervous system effects have the potential to negatively affect cognitive functioning.

Delirium

Delirium is a syndrome (group of symptoms) that occurs relatively acutely and is often called acute confusion—unlike dementia, which is characterized as chronic confusion. Delirium typically develops over a period of hours or days and is caused by some other underlying medical problem. Delirium can present with a hyperalert state (in which the person attends to all environmental stimuli simultaneously), hypoactive state (in which the patient seemingly retreats into inner thoughts and experiences that are abnormal), or mixed presentation. Delirium is considered to have a clinical presentation that is "characteristic" (Burns, Gallagley, & Byrne, 2004). A person of any age, when acutely ill, may experience delirium or acute confusion; however, older adults are at higher risk than younger adults, and older adults with preexisting dementia are at highest risk for developing delirium when acutely ill or injured. Not surprisingly, there is a high incidence of delirium among older adults in acute care hospitals, estimated to be as high as 80% (Foreman, Wakefield, Culp, & Milisen, 2001). Causes of delirium may include but are not limited to: medication side effects, chronic alcoholism, tumors or infections in the brain, blood clots in the brain, vitamin B12 deficiency, and/or some thyroid, kidney, or liver disorders (see **Box 10-12**).

Inouye and colleagues (1990) developed an instrument, the Confusion Assessment Method (CAM), to assist nurses and others to identify delirium quickly and accurately using the four basic features of delirium: (1) acute onset or fluctuating course, (2) inattention, (3) disorganized thinking, and (4) altered level of consciousness.

BOX 10-12 Common Causes of Delirium in Older Adults

Inadequate or inappropriate pain control	Hypo/hyperglycemia
Fecal impaction	Fluid/electrolyte imbalance
Medications (see also Box 10-7)	Hypoxia
Infections (urinary, respiratory, skin)	Head trauma

A diagnosis of delirium is made if both features 1 and 2 are present along with either of features 3 or 4. The CAM can be accessed online (see Box 10-7).

The nurse plays a critical role in identifying whether an older adult has experienced an acute change in mental status that could be delirium, assessing for delirium (using an instrument like the CAM), reporting the change to the physician or nurse practitioner, implementing appropriate interventions, and continuing to evaluate the client for signs and symptoms of further decline or improvement.

The primary treatment for delirium is to discover and treat the etiology or cause. The typical medical workup for the possible causes of delirium includes physical examination, laboratory tests (complete blood count, basic metabolic panel, and urinalysis), and imaging of the head/brain if trauma is suspected (e.g., delirium occurring after a recent fall). The medication list should be scrutinized for agents that are known to cause or worsen confusion (see Box 10-6). Particular attention should be paid to medications that have recently been started or increased. A pharmacist may be enlisted to assist with the review of medications.

Secondary interventions for delirium include keeping the patient comfortable, treating symptoms (e.g., with pain medication, oxygen, or intravenous fluids), and ensuring the safety of the client. Some persons with delirium may be quite lethargic (hypoactive delirium) whereas others may be very agitated (hyperactive delirium). Either situation presents a nursing challenge. For the lethargic client, oral intake may be compromised and the client is at risk for dehydration and aspiration pneumonia; impaired mobility increases the risk for pressure ulcers. The client with agitated delirium may be at risk for harming self and/or others and may require the judicious use of medications (e.g., benzodiazepines, antipsychotics). Physical restraints should be avoided if at all possible because they tend to cause more panic and agitation in older adults with delirium and can result in serious injury.

Other nursing interventions include moving the older adult to a room nearer the nursing station (for closer observation), implementing risk-for-falls protocols, providing one-to-one care and supervision, eliminating "tethers" when medically feasible (e.g., indwelling catheters, oxygen tubing), and eliminating confusing external stimuli (e.g., television). Generally, a calm, quiet environment is the most beneficial for a client with delirium. With appropriate medical care, delirium will eventually clear. One of the main goals of nursing care for delirium is to prevent further complications from developing during this acute syndrome. Delirium is further discussed in Chapter 13.

Depression

The risk for depression increases in older adults with chronic illnesses, including dementia. Content in Chapters 11 and 12 also discussed delirium and depression. *Depression* in the older adult is often not as obvious or as easily diagnosed as in young or middle-aged adults. Older adults may deny depression due to the stigma that this cohort often attaches to mental illness. Older adults, their families, and/ or healthcare providers may incorrectly attribute depressive symptoms to normal aging. Many older adults do not meet the strict criteria for a diagnosis of major depression (see **Box 10-13**), and yet have significant depressive symptoms. Although the prevalence of major depression in older adults is actually lower than that of younger and middle-aged adults, about 8–20% of older adults living in the community and 25–40% of older adult nursing home residents have significant depressive symptoms (AAGP, 2004a).

The nurse can play an important role in recognizing possible symptoms of depression and reporting them to the primary care provider, screening for

---

BOX 10-13   Diagnostic Criteria for Major Depression (DSM-IV and ICD-10 Criteria)

At least five of the following symptoms for at least 2 weeks:

- Depressed mood*
- Diminished interest or pleasure*
- Significant involuntary weight loss/gain or appetite change
- Insomnia/hypersomnia
- Psychomotor agitation/retardation
- Fatigue/loss of energy
- Feelings of worthlessness/guilt
- Impaired concentration
- Recurrent thoughts of death or suicide

*Must have one of these symptoms

The symptoms must cause significant distress or impaired function and cannot be better accounted for by other medical conditions, substances, or bereavement.

Source: Modified from American Psychiatric Association (2000). *Diagnostic and statistical manual of mental disorders* (4th ed., text revision). Washington, DC: Author.

depression, and educating older adult clients and their families about depression. The most commonly used screening tool for depression in older adults is the Geriatric Depression Scale (GDS), a 30-item yes–no questionnaire developed by Yesavage and colleagues (1983), and subsequently shortened to a 15-item scale (Sheikh & Yesavage, 1986). See Box 10-7 to access the GDS online. The GDS and other screening tools, however, do not replace the need for a clinical examination to diagnose the condition. Many clinicians are qualified to diagnose and treat geriatric depression including primary care providers, psychiatrists, and psychiatric clinical nurse specialists.

Symptoms of depression may overlap with symptoms of dementia. For example, persons with depression frequently have poor concentration that may worsen performance on cognitive tests. Ordinarily, older adults with cognitive symptoms will be evaluated for both dementia and depression. If depressive symptoms are present, treatment with antidepressants and/or psychotherapy will be initiated. Mild cognitive symptoms in older adults often improve with the treatment of depression; however, some older adults will eventually be diagnosed with both dementia and depression.

BOX 10-14　Important Points About Depression in Older Adults

Prevalent condition	Symptoms may overlap with dementia
Often under recognized	Common cause of excess disability
Often undertreated	Potentially life-threatening
May not meet strict diagnostic criteria	Treatable
May present with anxiety, agitation, or insomnia	

Depression in older adults (with or without dementia) often includes symptoms of anxiety (see Chapter 14), agitation, and insomnia. Therefore, an important step in evaluating these symptoms in older adults is to screen for depression. Unfortunately, some older adults with depression are inappropriately treated for months or years with sedating medications to control these symptoms without ever being treated for the primary cause of their symptoms, depression. A complete discussion of geriatric depression is beyond the scope of this text; the reader is referred to mental health nursing texts for more information on the evaluation for and treatment of depression. The symptoms of dementia, delirium, and depression often overlap. See **Table 10-1** for a summary of some of the key similarities and differences.

TABLE 10-1 Comparison of Signs and Symptoms of Dementia, Depression, and Delirium

	Dementia	Depression	Delirium
Onset	Gradual over months to years.	Usually gradual.	Acute over hours to days.
Course	Slowly progressive, irreversible, minimally treatable.	Chronic, but sometimes abrupt with psychosocial stressors. Treatable.	Fluctuating. Reversible with identification and treatment of cause.
Level of Consciousness	Alert.	Alert.	Altered, cloudy, fluctuating.
Memory	Impaired. Initially short-term memory loss, eventually long-term memory loss.	Intact, but my exhibit poor effort on memory tests.	Short-term memory loss.
Orientation	Impaired to time, then place, and eventually person, including self.	Intact.	Impaired, fluctuating.
Psychomotor Speed	Normal. Slowed in advanced stages.	May be normal, hypoactive, or hyperactive.	Hypoactive, hyperactive, or mixed.
Language	Word-finding difficulties. Impairment increases with disease progression.	Normal. May not initiate much conversation.	Often incoherent.
Hallucinations	Usually visual if present. Most common in middle stage.	None less psychotic depression.	Common, tend to be tactile and visual.

Caring for the Person with Dementia
Theories of Dementia Care

Several theories of dementia care have been developed and tested. The Progressively Lowered Stress Threshold (PLST) model of Hall and Buckwalter (1987) focuses on the relationship between environmental stimuli and the lowered stress threshold of the person with dementia, identifying common stressors that may lead to behavioral and psychological symptoms—for example, misleading or inappropriate stimuli; excessive external demands; physical stressors; and changes in the environment, routine, or caregiver (Hall, 1994). Using this model, nurses focus on supporting the personal resources of the person with dementia (e.g., providing rest periods) and controlling that person's environment (e.g., assigning the same nursing assistant to care for the person when possible).

The Enablement Model of dementia care (Dawson, Wells, & Kline, 1993) focuses on supporting the remaining abilities of the person with dementia in order to avoid excess disability (i.e., functional impairment above and beyond what should be expected based on degree of dementia). Using this model, when abilities are still present (e.g., self-feeding), nurses focus on promoting the use of the retained abilities (e.g., setting up the meal tray for the client). When abilities have been lost due to progressive dementia (e.g., drinking from a glass without spilling), nurses focus on assisting the client and manipulating the environment to support the client (e.g., providing a "sippy" cup with a lid).

The Need-Driven Dementia-Compromised Behavior (NDB) model has conceptualized behavioral and psychological symptoms of dementia as resulting from background and proximal factors (Algase et al., 1996; Kolanowski, 1999). Background factors are person-related and more enduring; these include neurological factors, cognitive abilities, health status, and psychosocial history. Proximal factors are more amenable to change and include physiological and psychological need states, and the physical and social environment. The background and proximal factors interact to produce need-driven behaviors. The nurse considers the background factors in providing care and intervenes to change proximal factors that may be contributing to behavioral symptoms.

The antecedent-behavior-consequence (ABC) model can be used to analyze and understand the behavioral symptoms of persons with dementia (Smith, Buckwalter, & Mitchell, 1993). Using the ABC model, the nurse would first observe and describe the behavior. Next, the nurse would identify the antecedents or "triggers" that occurred before the behavior. Common triggers for behavioral symptoms in persons with dementia include, but are not limited to, personal care discomfort or embarrassment (e.g., bathing, toileting), the person with dementia misinterpreting environmental cues (e.g., a misplaced personal item must have been stolen), and caregiver approaches (e.g., rushing tasks). Finally, the nurse considers the consequences or reactions that may have worsened the behavior (e.g., yelling at the person with dementia who is resisting a bath). After analyzing the behavior using the ABC model, the nurse can plan changes to the antecedents and consequences to help prevent the behavioral symptom from recurring.

Retrogenesis theory, sometimes referred to as "reverse Piaget theory," describes the decline in cognition and function of persons with dementia in terms of reverse development (Reisberg et al., 2002). Retrogenesis theory posits that persons with dementia tend to lose cognition and function in the reverse order of acquisition. Using this theory, the nurse would understand why a person with severe dementia may put nonfood items in the mouth (analogous to Piaget's sensorimotor stage of infant development). The nurse would focus on providing an environment and activities consistent with the client's cognitive developmental stage. An important caveat to the use of this theory is that we do not want to fall into the habit of treating persons with dementia like children or referring to them as "babies." Persons with dementia should always be treated as adults, but knowledge of their cognitive stage of development can enhance understanding and promote more appropriate interventions.

Lawton's person–environment (P–E) fit theory (1982) can be used as a theoretical basis for providing care to persons with dementia. (See the discussion of this theory in Chapter 3.) The environmental docility hypothesis, formulated by Lawton, posits that persons with a disability, including dementia, will be more dependent upon the physical and social environment. An appropriate environment will support higher functioning. "Environmental press" is the degree to which the environment challenges the individual. If the environment is too complex, a person with dementia may become frustrated and withdraw from activity; conversely, if the environment is too trivial, the person with dementia will not be challenged to maintain cognitive and functional abilities. Using the P–E fit theory, the nurse can formulate plans of care that adjust the environmental conditions to challenge, without frustrating, the person with dementia.

Person-centered care, based on the work of Kitwood (1997), is not a true theory, but an approach to dementia care that incorporates several principles: (1) learning about the history and preferences of the person with dementia, (2) developing genuine relationships between persons with dementia and caregivers, (3) promoting physical and emotional comfort, and (4) respecting the choices of persons with dementia and their families (Talerico, O'Brien, & Swafford, 2003).

Behavioral and Psychological Symptoms of Dementia

In the past, persons with Alzheimer's disease and other dementias were often labeled as having "problem behaviors" or "behavioral disturbances." You may still hear some clinicians using these terms. A consensus group of the International Psychogeriatric Association (IPA, 2002), however, has recommended that the term *behavioral and psychological symptoms of dementia*, or BPSD (see Box 10-11), be used instead,

BOX 10-15   Behavioral and Psychological Symptoms of Dementia (BPSD)

Behavioral Symptoms

Physical aggression (hitting, kicking, biting)

Verbal agitation (screaming, meaningless vocalizations)

Physical agitation (restlessness, purposeless movements)

Wandering (continuous walking around aimlessly)

Sexual disinhibition (exposing genitals, masturbating in public)

Hoarding (keeping/hiding unusually large amounts of what are often useless items)

Verbal aggression (swearing at, threatening others)

Shadowing (following another person around closely for long periods of time)

Psychological Symptoms

Anxiety

Depressive symptoms (feeling sad, poor sleep and/or appetite, lack of interest in life)

Hallucinations (seeing or hearing things that others do not)

Delusions (holding false beliefs)

Paranoia (having unreasonable fears)

emphasizing the understanding that such symptoms are disease-related. BPSD includes symptoms of disturbed perception, thought content, mood, or behavior. Behavioral symptoms can typically be assessed objectively by observing the person with dementia. Psychological symptoms are usually assessed by talking to the person with dementia and/or their families and caregivers.

The estimated frequency of BPSD varies considerably. Anywhere from 20–73% of persons with dementia may experience delusions, 15–29% have *hallucinations,* up to 20% show aggression and hostility, and as many as 80% have depressive symptoms (Finkel, 1998). If left untreated, BPSD contributes to premature institutionalization, increased financial costs, increased caregiver stress, excess disability for the person with dementia, and decreased quality of life for the person with dementia and their caregivers (IPA, 2002). The frequency of BPSD tends to peak in the middle stages of dementia and wane in the later stages.

Some types of BPSD are more common in certain types of dementia. For example, visual hallucinations and sexual disinhibition are more common in Lewy body dementia and frontotemporal lobe dementia, respectively. Common delusions in dementia include the belief that others are stealing things, that one's spouse is having an affair, that one's spouse or other loved one is an imposter, or that one has been abandoned. One of the more difficult situations nurses employed in nursing homes often encounter is trying to find out if a particular item really was stolen from an older adult (a crime) or if the belief is falsely held by the older adult (a delusion). Visual hallucinations are more common than auditory hallucinations in persons with dementia and are more common in persons with visual deficits, who are presumably misinterpreting visual stimuli. Close attention to lighting, eliminating confusing visual stimuli, and providing visual aids may decrease visual hallucinations. When a person with dementia has ongoing disturbing hallucinations, delusions, and/or *paranoia,* a diagnosis of "psychosis of Alzheimer's disease" may be made, and the condition may be treated with antipsychotic medication.

Agitation is a nonspecific term often applied to the behavior of persons with dementia. Cohen-Mansfield (1996) studied agitation extensively and identified four subtypes of agitation: physically nonaggressive behaviors (e.g., restlessness, pacing), verbally nonaggressive behaviors (e.g., complaining, interrupting), verbally aggressive behaviors (e.g., screaming, swearing), and physically aggressive behaviors (e.g., hitting, kicking, biting). When a person with dementia becomes agitated, the possibility of delirium should be considered.

Pharmacological Treatment for Behavioral and Psychological Symptoms of Dementia

Generally, nonpharmacological treatments for BPSD are initiated first and preferred due to potential medication side effects in older adults. When symptoms are uncomfortable for the person with dementia or the behaviors endanger self or others, and have not responded to nonpharmacological treatments, then medications are prescribed. See **Box 10-16** for a list of medications commonly prescribed for BPSD.

Older antidepressants, such as amitriptyline (Elavil), are generally avoided in older adults with dementia due to their adverse side effect profiles (anticholinergic). Generally, the selective serotonin reuptake inhibitors (SSRIs) and serotonin norepinephrine reuptake inhibitors (SNRIs) are safe and effective with minimal side effects. The most common side effect of these classes is gastrointestinal upset when the medications are started, so starting doses are usually low and gradually titrated upward. Paroxetine (Paxil) is often avoided because this agent has the most anticholinergic side effects in its class. Although gradual dose reductions, unless contraindicated, of all psychotropic medications are mandated in the nursing home setting, many clinicians continue antidepressants indefinitely due to the high rate of recurrence of geriatric depressive symptoms when medications are withdrawn (AAGP, 2004b).

Antipsychotics are generally reserved for psychotic or serious behaviors endangering self or others. Antipsychotics are not considered effective for dementia per se. The atypical antipsychotics carry a "black box warning" concerning the increased risk for adverse cardiovascular events (AAGP, 2004b). Generally, the atypical antipsychotics are preferred over the conventional antipsychotics due to the side effect profiles, although haloperidol (Haldol) is commonly used in acute care for delirium. Benzodiazepines are used cautiously in older adults due to their side effect profile, particularly increased risk for falls. Psychotropic drug

BOX 10-16 Common Medications Prescribed for BPSD

Class/Medications	Common Uses

Selective serotonin reuptake inhibitors
    Fluoxetine (Prozac)
    Sertraline (Zoloft)
    Paroxetine (Paxil)
    Citalopram (Celexa)
	Depression, agitation, and/or anxiety attributed to depression

Serotonin norepinephrine reuptake inhibitors
    Venlafaxine (Effexor)
    Duloxetine (Cymbalta)
	Depression, agitation, and/or anxiety attributed to depression

Other antidepressants
    Mirtazapine (Remeron)
    Trazadone (Desyrel)
	Depression, used at lower doses for insomnia and appetite stimulation

Mood stabilizers
    Divalproex (Depakote)
    Benzodiazepines*
	Low doses for insomnia,
	Bipolar-type depression, agitation
	Anxiety, agitation

Antipsychotics
    Risperidone (Risperdal)
    Olanzapine (Zyprexa)
    Quetiapine (Seroquel)
    Aripiprazole (Abilify)
    Ziprasidone (Geodon)
	Psychotic symptoms, mania, adjunct therapy for depression, violent behavior

Conventional/typical antipsychotics Haloperidol (Haldol)	Delirium, violent behavior

*Check the Beer's list for cautions in older adults.

use in the nursing home setting is highly regulated. Regular review of the risks and benefits along with trials of periodic gradual dose reductions are mandated unless clinically contraindicated.

A more complete discussion of pharmacological therapy for persons with dementia is beyond the scope of this chapter. For more information, please consult psychiatric nursing and pharmacology texts.

Nonpharmacological Treatment for Dementia

Nurses, as an interdependent intervention, administer medications prescribed for persons with dementia. The largest role for nurses in dementia care, however, is applying the nursing process to promote comfort, function, and dignity for persons with dementia. The nurse uses theories about dementia care to guide assessment, nursing diagnosis, planning, intervention, and ongoing evaluation. The role of the nurse is particularly important in assessing and treating BPSD. When evaluating any acute changes in the cognition, behavior, and mood of persons with dementia, recall that delirium is a common cause of these changes.

General Interventions

Reality orientation is a technique that presents information to persons with dementia about themselves and their orientation in time and place. Nurses using reality orientation frequently remind the person with words and other cues (e.g., clocks, calendars). A systematic review of studies of reality orientation found that the technique could improve both cognitive and behavioral outcomes (Spector, Orrell, Davies, & Woods, 2008). Reality orientation, however, may actually increase distress in some persons with dementia, who may be convinced of some other reality and resent being "corrected."

BOX 10-17   General Approaches to Managing Behavioral and Psychological Symptoms of Dementia (BPSD)

Try nonpharmacological before pharmacological interventions.

Maintain a calm, familiar environment and routine.

For specific BPSD:

Identify and describe the behavior in as much detail as possible.

Identify the antecedents (triggers) and consequences of the behavior (per the ABC model).

Identify the desired behavioral outcome.

Implement interventions.

Evaluate the effectiveness of interventions.

Validation therapy (VT), which was developed by Naomi Feil (1993), is a systematic method for communicating with and caring for persons with dementia in an empathic and individualized manner. Validation therapy recognizes that older adults with dementia are unique, valuable individuals who should be accepted nonjudgmentally. Within the VT framework, the behavior of persons with dementia is viewed as having meaning and is not just caused by physical and functional changes in the brain (the medical model of dementia). Furthermore, VT posits that older adults with impaired memory are often trying to resolve uncompleted developmental tasks from earlier in life, thus accounting for their tendency to dwell more on remote rather than recent memories. Feil developed her own classification of chronic confusion in older adults called the four stages of resolution: malorientation, time confusion, repetitive motion, and vegetation. Communication and care are based on the stage of resolution. The goals of VT are to reduce anxiety, restore a sense of self-worth, and improve function for the person with dementia. A systematic review of VT for persons with dementia concluded that there were too few good studies and relatively small numbers of subjects to draw any conclusions about the effectiveness of VT (Neal & Barton Wright, 2008).

Validation therapy and reminiscence therapy (RT) share several principles and approaches, though validation therapy relies less on cognitive ability and thus can theoretically be used into much later stages of dementia. Reminiscence therapy was developed for use with older adults by Norris (1986), based on Butler's (1963) work on life review. The purpose of RT is to promote adjustment and integrity for older adults through structured remembering and reflecting on the past. Reminiscence therapy may be conducted individually, but is frequently a group activity for persons with dementia living in institutions, often incorporating refreshments. A systematic review of RT for persons with dementia concluded that there were too few good studies and too many variations in treatment protocols to evaluate the effectiveness of RT (Woods, Spector, Jones, Orrell, & Davies, 2008).

Environmental Interventions

Managing the environment of the person with dementia is a component of most theories of dementia care. The acute care environment, with its multiple and competing stimuli, can be very stressful for persons with dementia, who have decreased ability to adapt to change. Nurses should assess and modify the environment to control the information the patient is receiving (see **Box 10-18**).

BOX 10-18 Examples of Environmental Interventions

Physical Environment

Areas for safe wandering.

Alarms on exits and/or the person to detect elopement.

Adequate, but not harsh, lighting during the day.

Low lighting at night.

Soft background music.

Appropriate, nonconfusing sensory stimuli.

Comfortable room temperature.

Temporal Environment

Establish a meaningful routine.

Alternate activity and rest periods.

The impact the environment has on patient behavior may fluctuate, depending on the degree of activity occurring at any given time. Behavioral symptoms are more likely to occur during periods of high activity: 7 to 10 a.m., noon to 2 p.m., and 4 to 7 p.m. In an acute care environment, these times represent periods of high activity: shift changes, meal times, sending and receiving patients from operating rooms, doctor rounds, and visiting hours. Carefully planning activities to minimize additional procedures and demands during peak periods may prevent unnecessary stress and behavioral outbursts (Gitlin, Liebman, & Winter, 2003).

Physical Comfort Interventions

Interventions to promote elimination, comfort, sensory function, and adequate sleep and nutrition (discussed in other areas of this text) will contribute to overall well-being for persons with dementia and reduce the risk for BPSD.

Pain Management and Alzheimer's Disease

Many people with Alzheimer's disease are unable to report their pain. In such cases, nurses must rely on observation to assess for pain behaviors. Each person might have a "pain signature," which means that one person's pain may cause him or her to become agitated and combative, whereas another may withdraw. Failure to recognize and treat pain can lead to sleep disturbances, malnutrition, depression, decreased mobility, needless suffering, and inappropriate psychotropic medication use (American Geriatrics Society [AGS], 2002).

One of the most important steps in evaluating any patient, especially for those with Alzheimer's disease, is to obtain a baseline pain assessment. Changes in baseline are then used to determine the need for adjustments in the treatment plan, such as the addition of an analgesic or dose adjustment. Because self-report is the single most reliable indicator of pain, those who are able to communicate verbally should be asked about their pain level. A pain assessment, such as a 0–10 scale or a faces pain rating scale, should be used to determine pain intensity. For more impaired clients, the nurse should assess for crying, moaning, groaning, and other verbalizations that may be indicative of pain, along with possible nonverbal expressions of pain (see **Box 10-19**). It is important to assess pain at rest and during activity. Pain behaviors are often more obvious during activities such as repositioning and bathing. See Box 10-7 for more information on how to assess for pain in persons with dementia.

The principles of good pain management for adults with Alzheimer's apply universally to those with the disease. Nonpharmacological interventions (see **Box 10-20**) should be tried first for mild pain and used along with pharmacological interventions in moderate to severe pain. Nonopioid analgesics should be considered for mild to moderate pain. Opioid analgesics are added to the treatment plan for more severe pain. If neuropathic pain is suspected, adjuvant analgesics such as local anesthetics, anticonvulsants, and antidepressants may be indicated. Opioid analgesics are generally

---

BOX 10-19   Possible Nonverbal Expressions of Pain

Agitation	Restlessness
Increased confusion	Changes in eating and sleeping habits
Decreased mobility	Withdrawal
Combativeness	Aggression
Resistance to care	Rubbing/holding a particular area of the body
Guarding	Rapid breathing
Grimacing	

BOX 10-20 Nonpharmacological Interventions for Pain

Distraction

Massage

Heat/cold application

Gentle movement/repositioning

Participation in normal activities as able

BOX 10-21 Key Points for Pain Control

Persons with dementia may not be as able to report pain.

Always consider pain as a possible cause of behavioral symptoms.

Assess for possible objective indicators of pain.

Administer analgesics routinely for painful conditions when the person cannot ask.

---

started at very low doses and titrated upward based on continuing evaluation. When opioids are administered, it is particularly important to assess bowel function, because the person with dementia may not be able to report constipation (AGS, 2002).

Activity Interventions

Persons with dementia need a balance between stimulating and calming activities. Too much or too little activity may lead to behavioral and psychological symptoms. When evaluating behavioral symptoms, note the time of day and the level of activity at the time the symptoms occurred.

Interdisciplinary teamwork (see **Figure 10-2**) between nursing and the activities service is needed to assess the person's normal schedule of activities, looking for prolonged periods of activity or inactivity. Adjustments can be made to increase or decrease activity. In addition to the quantity of activity, the quality of activity is important. Generally, persons with dementia respond most positively to meaningful activities that are connected to their personal history and preferences. Lifelong personality characteristics may also be used to help choose appropriate activities (Kolanowski & Buettner, 2008). More extroverted individuals may prefer small group activities; more introverted individuals may prefer one-on-one or individual activities. Group physical activity can help meet both exercise and socialization needs (Netz, Axelrad, & Argov, 2007).

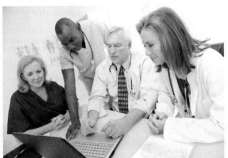

© iStockphoto.com/asiseeit

Figure 10-2 Interdisciplinary teamwork is important in providing quality care for older adults with dementia.

Communication Interventions

Language and speech become progressively impaired in dementia, but maintaining communication is critical to effective care for persons with dementia. Keep in mind that behavior is a form of communication, and as dementia progresses it becomes more and more important for the nurse to analyze and interpret the behavior of a person with dementia in that context. For example, a person with dementia who is exhibiting a behavioral symptom may just need food, fluids, or to be toileted, but be unable to express that need. Nurses who routinely care for persons with dementia in long-term care become experts at interpreting the meaning of particular behaviors. See **Box 10-22** for suggested communication techniques.

BOX 10-22   Suggested Communication Techniques

Speak to the person distinctly and in simple phrases/sentences.

Speak as one adult to another.

Smile.

Avoid "elderspeak" (sing-song baby talk).

Keep the pace of the conversation slow.

Listen.

Allow sufficient time for responses.

Be calm, remain patient, and speak softly.

Maintain eye contact.

Use nonverbal cues: Point or demonstrate what you want done.

Repeat instructions as often as necessary.

Lower voice to accommodate age-related hearing changes.

For persons with limited speech, try using yes–no questions.

Observe carefully for a person's nonverbal cues.

Interventions for Particular Behaviors

Nurses caring for persons with dementia are often challenged to address particular behaviors. Keeping in mind that these behaviors are most often symptoms of the disease process, the nurse can analyze the behaviors using the ABC model. An important step in this process is examining the possible antecedents, causes, or triggers for the behavior (see **Box 10-23**). When the antecedents of the behavior have been identified, the nurse can plan care to help prevent that behavior in the future. For example, if a person with dementia becomes agitated every time he or she has to void, scheduled toileting could be implemented to avoid this behavior. Nursing care for the behavioral symptoms of

---

BOX 10-23   Common Behavioral Triggers

Hunger

Thirst

Toileting needs

Feeling too hot/too cold

Pain

Boredom

Overstimulation

Certain people

Certain activities (meals, baths)

dementia is quite individualized because the cause of and approach to the behavior are very much dependent on the personal and contextual factors. There are, however, some general approaches to particular behaviors (see **Boxes 10-24** through **10-28**).

BOX 10-24   Suggested Interventions for Agitation/Aggression

Avoid provoking situations.

Intervene early, before the behavior escalates.

Remain calm; speak in a soft voice.

Approach slowly from the front.

Avoid startling the person.

Stay at the eye level of the person.

Avoid touching initially; wait until the person is calmer.

Distract the person.

Avoid rational arguments.

Avoid physical restraint if at all possible.

Identify and address unmet needs (food, fluid, toileting).

BOX 10-25   Suggested Interventions for Resistance to Bathing

Remain calm.

Use a soft voice.

Choose a time when the person is most rested and least confused.

Consider the person's lifelong preferences:

   Shower vs. bath

   Morning vs. evening

Maintain a leisurely pace. Avoid rushing the person.

Premedicate with analgesics if pain with movement is an issue.

Allow the person to wear underwear or a patient gown, if desired.

Avoid spraying water directly on the head or face.

Pantomime the desired hygiene activities.

Use distraction: conversation, snacks, or music.

When complete, give praise for clean appearance.

BOX 10-26   Suggested Interventions for Wandering

Assess for unmet needs.

Reassure the person that he or she is in the right place.

Use identification bracelets (in case he or she gets lost).

Place alarms on the person and/or doors to detect elopement.

Provide a safe wandering "path."

Provide alternative activities.

Minimize medication use (to reduce risk for falls).

Visually disguise exits.

Provide daily exercise.

Provide simple snack foods to be eaten "on the run."

BOX 10-27   Suggested Interventions for Delusions/Paranoia

Assist the person to keep track of personal items.

Avoid defensiveness if accused.

Do not argue with the person.

Maintain a simple, noncluttered environment.

Avoid whispering in front of the person.

Note: Antipsychotic medications are often required.

BOX 10-28   Suggested Interventions for Inappropriate Sexual Behavior

If disrobed, offer clothing.

If masturbating:

   Avoid laughing, scolding, or confrontation.

   Guide to a private place.

   Distract the person.

Activities of Daily Living

As the disease progresses, persons with dementia become more dependent upon caregivers for assistance with activities of daily living (ADLs). See **Boxes 10-29** and **10-30** for suggested interventions in these areas.

BOX 10-29   Suggested Interventions for Eating/Feeding Issues

Thoroughly prepare meal trays (open cartons, cut food).

Offer small, frequent meals and snacks.

At meals, provide one food and one utensil at a time.

Provide nutritious finger foods.

Provide nutritional supplements, if indicated.

Offer fluids in containers that can be self-managed ("sippy" cups, sports bottles).

Request speech therapy (ST) and occupational therapy (OT) services, if needed.

Provide adaptive utensils, if indicated. (OT will order.)

Assist the client to feed self, rather than feeding, whenever possible.

Use "hand-over-hand" feeding (your hand guides theirs).

Gently cue the person to continue eating, chewing, and swallowing.

Avoid making comments about manners or messiness.

Provide the person with dignified protection for clothing.

If agitation develops during feeding, stop and retry a little later.

Avoid force feeding.

Reassure the person that his or her food has been paid for (a common concern).

Monitor body weight to detect gains or losses.

BOX 10-30 Suggested Interventions to Promote Continence/Toileting

Ensure that toilets are visible.

Keep bathroom doors open.

Place signs/pictures as visual cues.

Keep paths to the bathroom clear.

Systematically assess voiding and bowel patterns.

Offer toileting frequently.

Use incontinence pads/briefs, as needed.

For persons who can still toilet, use "pull-up"-type protective products.

Provide adequate fluids during the day.

Limit fluids at bedtime.

Avoid beverages with caffeine.

Ensure adequate fiber in diet.

Settings for Care: Focus on Adult Day Services

Adult day services are the cornerstone of community-based, long-term care alternatives. These services are designed to meet the needs of cognitively and functionally impaired adults through individualized plans of care (National Adult Day Services Association [NADSA], n.d.). Most frequently referred to as adult day care (ADC), these services offer consumers the opportunity to continue living at home while receiving needed services in a safe, structured environment. They offer a comprehensive program that provides a variety of health, social, and related services in a protective setting during the daytime hours: midday meals, structured recreational activities, socialization opportunities, and appropriate cognitive stimulation (see **Box 10-31**). Over the past 10 years, the number of adult day services has increased to about 3,400 nationwide, serving about 150,000 older adults each day (NADSA, n.d.). Consumers of adult day care increasingly have more healthcare and functional needs. Over 50% of ADC consumers have dementia.

BOX 10-31 Typical Adult Day Services

Recreational therapy/activities

Meals

Social services

Transportation

Personal care: bathing, hair and nail care

Nursing services

Rehabilitation services (less commonly offered)

Medical services (less commonly offered)

As the older adult population increases, adult day services will undoubtedly become more appealing to consumers. Caregivers using ADC for older adults with dementia have more time to rest, run errands, and do other business. Adult day services assist persons with dementia to function at their highest level, strengthen caregivers' abilities and coping skills, and delay institutionalization.

Hospice/Palliative Care

End-of-life care is often fragmented among providers and provider settings, leading to a lack of continuity of care, which impedes the ability to provide high-quality, interdisciplinary care.

Dementia and cognitive impairment are on the rise. Alzheimer's disease is the sixth-leading cause of death in the United States overall and the fifth-leading cause of death in Americans age >65 years. Alzheimer's disease is becoming a more common cause of death as the population of the United States and other countries age. Although deaths from other major causes continue to experience significant declines, those from AD have continued to rise by 66% between 2000 and 2008. (Alzheimer's Association, 2012)

A blurred distinction exists between death *with* dementia and death *from* dementia. The different ways in which dementia eventually ends in death can create ambiguity about the underlying cause of death. Severe dementia frequently causes symptoms and complications of chronic disease and terminal illness, as immobility, bedsores, swallowing disorders, malnutrition, and delirium affect many people at the end of life. These can lead to the risk of pneumonia, which has been found as the most common cause of death among the elderly with dementia.

Realizing there is no "right" place to die, where we die is not usually something we get to decide. But, if given the choice, each person and/or his or her family should consider which type of care makes the most sense, where that kind of care can be provided, and whether family/friends are available to help. Enhanced communication among patients, families, and providers is crucial to high quality end-of-life care.

Recently, the term *palliative care* has come to mean more than just treating symptoms. In the United States, palliative care refers to a comprehensive approach to improving the quality of life for people who are living with potentially fatal diseases. It provides support for family members, very similar to the more familiar concept of hospice care.

In a palliative care program, a multidisciplinary healthcare team works with both the patient and family to provide any support—medical, social, or emotional—needed to live with a chronic illness. Palliative care can be provided in hospitals, nursing homes, outpatient palliative care clinics, certain other specialized clinics, or at home. Medicare covers some of the treatments and medicine, and veterans may be eligible for palliative care through the Department of Veterans Affairs.

Who Can Benefit?

Palliative care is a resource for anyone with a long-term disease that will, in time, probably cause their death, not just for people who might die soon. Those suffering from medical diseases, such as heart failure, chronic obstructive pulmonary disease, or chronic renal failure; individuals with disabilities such as Parkinson's disease; or patients with dementia can benefit through palliative care (see **Case Study 10-1**).

Case Study 10-1

Sam was retired from the U.S. Air Force. He was diagnosed with dementia at age 78. As the disease progressed and ADLs became more difficult, Sam's family wanted to explore more treatment options to slow the disease. Through palliative care provided by the Veterans Health Administration, Sam was able to receive the comfort care and emotional support he and his family needed to cope with his health problems. As Sam stabilized, he was discharged home. The program provided help around the house and other support for Sam's wife, making it easier for her to care for him at home.

In time, if a doctor believes the patient is not responding to treatment and is likely to die within 6 months, there are two possibilities:

> palliative care could transition to hospice care, or
> palliative care could continue, with increasing emphasis on comfort care and less focus on medical treatment (See **Box 10-32**).

BOX 10-32　Some Differences Between Palliative Care and Hospice

	Palliative Care	Hospice
Who can be treated?	Anyone with a serious illness	Anyone with a serious illness whom doctors think has only a short time to live, often less than 6 months
Will my symptoms be relieved?	Yes, as much as possible	Yes, as much as possible
Can I continue to receive treatments to cure my illness?	Yes, if you wish	No, only symptom relief will be provided
Will Medicare pay?	It depends on your benefits and treatment plan	Yes, it pays all hospice charges
Does private insurance pay?	It depends on the plan	It depends on the plan
How long will I be cared for?	This depends on what care you need and your insurance plan	As long as you meet the hospice's criteria of an illness with a life expectancy of months, not years
Where will I receive this care?	Home Assisted living facility Nursing home Hospital	Home Assisted living facility Nursing home Hospice facility Hospital

See the section on end-of-life care in Chapter 24 for more specific information about hospice and palliative care.

At this point, providing comprehensive comfort care to the dying person as well as support to his or her family make more sense. *Hospice* is designed for this situation. The patient beginning hospice care understands that his or her illness is not responding to medical attempts to cure or to slow the disease's progress. Hospice care is beneficial, yet underutilized in advanced dementia. Patients dying with dementia who receive hospice care have better symptom management (Kiely, Givens, Shaffer, Teno, & Mitchell, 2010), fewer hospitalizations, and greater family satisfaction with care than those not receiving hospice care. Trends indicate that hospice enrollment is increasing.

Advance Directives

Although advance directives and advance care planning can be important tools to assist those facing end of life, the evidence suggests that end-of-life decision making in the United States is often poorly implemented (U.S. Department of Health and Human Services, 2008).

Preparing an advance directive prior to the onset of cognitive impairment or conditions such as Alzheimer's disease is very important. A person in the early stages of these conditions will likely still have the capacity to express their preferences and complete an advance directive if they had not already done so.

People with Alzheimer's have the legal right to limit or forgo medical or life-sustaining treatment, including the use of mechanical ventilators, cardiopulmonary resuscitation, antibiotics, and artificial nutrition and hydration. These wishes can be expressed through their advance directives.

Nurses should:

> Urge preparation of advance directives early in adulthood
> Help families to continue supporting the advance care wishes of their loved ones, especially when their cognitive health is declining
> Encourage review of prepared documents on an annual basis

Legislative Action

Reducing the burden of Alzheimer's disease on patients and their families (see **Box 10-33**) is an urgent national priority. The National Alzheimer's Project Act was signed into law in January 2011, calling for the expansion and coordination of research and health service delivery across federal agencies for Alzheimer's disease and related dementias.

The top priorities of the Act are to place significant focus on the millions of persons in the United States in the advanced stage of the disease, for whom there is a great need and opportunity to improve patient outcomes, contain healthcare expenditures, reduce disparities, and better coordinate care. It stresses the need for initiatives aimed at the prevention and early detection of dementia. These new efforts to fight Alzheimer's disease included making an additional $50 million available for cutting-edge Alzheimer's research. Together, the fiscal years 2012 and 2013 investments total $130 million in new Alzheimer's research funding—over 25% more than the current annual Alzheimer's research investment.

The additional NIH research funding will support both basic and clinical research. Investments will include research to identify genes that increase the risk of Alzheimer's disease and testing therapies in individuals at the highest risk for the disease. On the clinical side, the funds may be used to expand efforts to move new therapeutic approaches into clinical trials and to develop better databases to assess the nation's burden of cognitive impairment and dementia.

This announcement also includes an additional $26 million earmarked for support for caregivers in the community, improving healthcare provider training, and raising public awareness. The preliminary framework for the National Alzheimer's Disease Plan identifies key goals, including preventing and treating Alzheimer's disease by 2025 (National Institute on Aging, 2012).

Summary

There are many challenges that face the gerontological nurse who is working with patients with dementia. As the population continues to age, the number of persons with dementia will also grow, so nurses need to be well informed about dementia care. There are reliable assessment tools to assist nurses in recognizing dementia in earlier stages. The content of this chapter presented many suggestions of interventions for the common behaviors encountered among persons with dementia and for their caregivers.

Notable Quotes

"The intuitive mind is a sacred gift, and the rational mind its faithful servant. We have created a society that honors the servant and has forgotten the gift."

—Albert Einstein

BOX 10-33 Research Highlight

Aim: To understand how spouses experience dementia in their loved one.

Method: Transcripts were analyzed of 19 90-minute support group meetings for spouses of those with dementia. Spouses were ages 67–82, caring for their partner with dementia within about the same age group. Participants in the support group were all White, non-Hispanic with an N of 11 and mostly female.

Results: Fourteen metaphors used by the participants were identified. These included the following: Journey, machine or circuit, basic orientation, harm or abuse, game metaphor, hand, child, container (caregiver feels trapped), image, struggle, weight, loss, story/performance, and honeymoon/dream.

Application to practice: Nurses can use this data to inform their conversations with spouses of those experiencing dementia. Listening for metaphoric conversation and understanding this as a way of relating experiences and emotions can better inform the support health professionals provide for caregiving spouses.

Source: Golden, M. A., Whaley, B. B. & Stone, A. M. (2012). "The system is beginning to shut down": Utilizing caregivers' metaphors for dementia, persons with dementia, and caregiving. *Applied Nursing Research, 25*, 146–151.

Critical Thinking Exercises

1. Delirium may present as hypoactive or hyperactive. Which type of delirium do you think is more likely to be identified by nurses in the clinical setting, and why?

2. Why do individuals with delirium tend to be unable to communicate appropriately? What are the characteristic features associated with delirium? What are the primary risk factors for the development of delirium? Is delirium a reversible disorder?

3. Evaluate the medication list of one of your clinical clients with dementia or delirium in relation to the Beer's criteria for potentially inappropriate medications for older adults.

4. Given the modest benefits of cholinesterase inhibitors and memantine in the treatment of dementia, debate the pros and cons of administering these medications for persons with dementia.

5. Choose a client in your clinical setting who has dementia. Practice communication strategies.

Personal Reflections

1. Have you ever cared for a patient or family member with dementia? How did you feel about this experience? What did you find most frustrating? How did you handle specific symptoms that caused changes in behavior?

2. What risk factors do you personally have for AD? Are there any activities that you can do to decrease your personal risk?

3. What do you consider the difference between chronic and acute illness?

4. This chapter focused on the nurse's role, but what challenges do you think family members face in caring for loved ones with AD?

References

Algase, D. L., Beck, C., Kolanowski, A., Whall, A., Berent, S., Richards, K., & Beattie, E. (1996). Need-driven dementia-compromised behavior: An alternative view of disruptive behavior. *American Journal of Alzheimer's Disease, 11*(6), 10–19.

Alzheimer's Association. (2012). Alzheimer's disease facts and figures. *Alzheimer's and Dementia, 8,* 131–168.

American Association for Geriatric Psychiatry [AAGP]. (2004a). *Geriatrics and mental health: The facts.* Retrieved from http://www.gmhfonline.org/prof/facts_mh.asp

American Association for Geriatric Psychiatry [AAGP]. (2004b). *PET scans for the diagnosis of Alzheimer's disease.* Retrieved from http://www.gmhfonline.org/prof/facts_PETscans2004.asp

American Association for Geriatric Psychiatry [AAGP]. (2006). *Position statement: Principles of care for patients with dementia resulting from Alzheimer disease.* Retrieved from http://www.gmhfonline.org/prof/position_caredmnalz.asp

American Geriatrics Society, Panel on Persistent Pain in Older Persons. (2002). The management of persistent pain in older persons. *Journal of the American Geriatrics Society, 50*(6 Suppl.), S205–S224. Retrieved from http://onlinelibrary.wiley.com/doi/10.1046/j.1532-5415.50.6s.1.x/abstract

American Psychiatric Association [APA]. (2000). *Diagnostic and statistical manual of mental disorders* (4th ed., text rev.). Washington, DC: Author.

Bis, J. C., DeCarli, C., Smith, A. V., van der Lijn, F., Crivello, F., Fornage, M.,…Cohorts for Heart and Aging Research in Genomic Epidemiology Consortium. (2012). Common variants at 12q14 and 12q24 are associated with hippocampal volume. *Nature Genetics, 44*(5), 545–551. doi:10.1038/ng.2237

Borson, S., Scanlan, J. M., Brush, M., Vitallano, P., & Dokmak, A. (2000). The Mini-Cog: A cognitive "vital signs" measure for dementia screening in multi-lingual elderly. *International Journal of Geriatric Psychiatry, 15*(11), 1021–1027.

Burns, A., Gallagley, A., & Byrne, J. (2004). Delirium. *Journal of Neurology, Neurosurgery, and Psychiatry, 75*, 362–367.

Butler, R. N. (1963). *The life review: An interpretation of reminiscence in the aged.* Psychiatry, 26, 65–68.

Cohen-Mansfield, J. (1996). Conceptualization of agitation results based on the Cohen-Mansfield Agitation Inventory and the Agitation Behavior Mapping Instrument. *International Psychogeriatrics, 8*(3 Suppl.), 309–315.

Dawson, P., Wells, D. L., & Kline, K. (1993). *Enhancing the abilities of persons with Alzheimer's and related dementias: A nursing perspective.* New York, NY: Springer.

Feil, N. (1993). The validation breakthrough: *Simple techniques for communicating with people with Alzheimer's-type dementia.* Baltimore, MD: Health Professions Press.

Fick, D. M., Cooper, J. W., Wade, W. E., Waller, J. L., Maclean, J. R., & Beers, M. H. (2003). Updating the Beers criteria for potentially inappropriate medication use in older adults. *Archives of Internal Medicine, 163*, 2716–2725.

Finkel, S. I. (1998). The signs of the behavioural and psychological symptoms of dementia. *Clinician, 16*(1), 33–42.

Folstein, M., Folstein, S. E., & McHugh, P. R. (1975). "Mini-Mental State": A practical method for grading the cognitive state of patients for the clinician. *Journal of Psychiatric Research, 12*(3), 189–198.

Foreman, M. D., Wakefield, B., Culp, K., & Milisen, K. (2001). Delirium in elderly patients: An overview of the state of the science. *Journal of Gerontological Nursing, 27*(4), 12–20.

Gitlin, L. N., Liebman, J., & Winter, L. (2003). Are environmental interventions effective in the management of Alzheimer's disease and related disorders?: A synthesis of the evidence. *Alzheimer's Care Quarterly, 4*(2), 85–107.

Golden, M. A., Whaley, B. B. & Stone, A. M. (2012). "The system is beginning to shut down": Utilizing caregivers' metaphors for dementia, persons with dementia, and caregiving. *Applied Nursing Research, 25*, 146–151.

Hall, G. R. (1994). Caring for people with Alzheimer's disease using the conceptual model of Progressively Lowered Stress Threshold in the clinical setting. *Nursing Clinics of North America, 29*(1), 129–141.

Hall, G. R., & Buckwalter, K. C. (1987). Progressively lowered stress threshold: A conceptual model for the care of adults with Alzheimer's disease. *Archives of Psychiatric Nursing, 1*, 399–406.

Inouye, S., van Dyck, C., Alessi, C., Balkin, S., Siegal, A., & Horwitz, R. (1990). Clarifying confusion: The confusion assessment method. *Annals of Internal Medicine, 113*(12), 941–948.

International Psychogeriatric Association [IPA]. (2002). *Behavioral and psychological symptoms of dementia (BPSD).* Retrieved from http://www.ipa-online.net/pdfs/1BPSDfinal.pdf

Kiely, D. K., Givens, J. L., Shaffer, M. I., Teno, J. M., & Mitchell, S. L. (2010). Hospice use and outcomes in nursing home residents with advanced dementia. *Journal of the American Geriatric Society, 58*, 2284–2291.

Kitwood, T. (1997). *Dementia reconsidered: The person comes first.* Buckingham, UK: Open University Press.

Kolanowski, A., & Buettner, L. (2008). Prescribing activities that engage passive residents: An innovative method. *Journal of Gerontological Nursing, 34*(1), 13–18.

Kolanowski, A. M. (1999). An overview of the need-driven, dementia-compromised behavior model. *Journal of Gerontological Nursing, 25*(9), 7–9.

Lawton, M. P. (1982). Competence, environmental press, and the adaptation of older people. In M. P. Lawton, P. G. Windley, & T. O. Byerts (Eds.), *Aging and the environment: Theoretical approaches* (pp. 33–59). New York, NY: Springer.

National Adult Day Services Association [NADSA]. (n.d.). *Adult day services: The facts.* Retrieved from http://www.nadsa.org

National Institute on Aging. (2007). *Alzheimer's disease: Unraveling the mystery.* Retrieved from http://www.nia.nih.gov/Alzheimers/Publications/alzheimers-disease-unraveling-mystery

National Institute on Aging. (2012). We can't wait: Administration announces new steps to fight Alzheimer's disease. Retrieved from http://www.nia.nih.gov/newsroom/2012/02/we-cant-wait-administration-announces-new-steps-fight-alzheimers-disease

Neal, M., & Barton Wright, P. (2008). Validation therapy for dementia. [Systematic Review]. *Cochrane Dementia and Cognitive Improvement Group Cochrane Database of Systematic Reviews, 2.*

Netz, Y., Axelrad, S., & Argov, E. (2007). Group physical activity for demented older adults: Feasibility and effectiveness. *Clinical Rehabilitation, 21*(11), 977–986.

Norris, A. D. (1986). *Reminiscence with elderly people.* London, UK: Winslow.

Obregon, D., Hou, H., Deng, J., Giunta, B., Tian, J., Darlington, D.,...Tan, J. (2012). Soluble amyloid precursor protein-α modulates β-secretase activity and amyloid-β generation. *Nature Communications, 3, 777.* doi: 10.1038/ncomms1781

Raina, P., Pasqualina, S., Ismaila, A., Patterson, C., Cowan, D., Levine, M.,...Oremus, M. (2008). Effectiveness of cholinesterase inhibitors and memantine for treating dementia: Evidence review for a clinical practice guideline. *Annals of Internal Medicine, 148,* 379–397.

Reisberg, B., Franssen, E. H., Souren, L. E. M., Auer, S. R., Akram, I., & Kenowsky, S. (2002). Evidence and mechanisms of retrogenesis in Alzheimer's and other dementias. American *Journal of Alzheimer's Disease and Other Dementias, 17*(4), 202–212.

Sheikh, J. I., & Yesavage, J. A. (1986). Geriatric Depression Scale (GDS). Recent evidence and development of a shorter version. In T. L. Brink (Ed.), *Clinical gerontology: A guide to assessment and intervention* (pp. 165–173). New York, NY: Haworth Press.

Smith, M., Buckwalter, K., & Mitchell, S. (1993). Acting up and acting out: Assessment and management of aggressive and acting out behaviors. In M. Smith, K. Buckwalter, & C. M. Mitchell (Eds.), *The geriatric mental health training series.* New York, NY: Springer.

Spector, A., Orrell, M., Davies, S., & Woods, B. (2008). Reality orientation for dementia. [Systematic Review]. *Cochrane Dementia and Cognitive Improvement Group Cochrane Database of Systematic Reviews, 2.*

Talerico, K. A., O'Brien, J. A., & Swafford, K. L. (2003). Person-centered care: An important approach for 21st century health care. *Journal of Psychosocial Nursing and Mental Health Services, 41*(11), 12–16.

Tariq, S. H., Tumosa, N., Chibnall, J. T., Perry, M. H., & Morley, J. E. (2006). Comparison of the Saint Louis University Mental Status Examination and the Mini-Mental State Examination for detecting dementia and mild neurocognitive disorder: A pilot study. *American Journal of Geriatric Psychiatry, 14,* 900–910.

U.S. Department of Health and Human Services. (2008). *Advance Directives and Advance Care Planning: Report to Congress.* Retrieved from http://aspe.hhs.gov/daltcp/reports/2008/adcongrpt.htm

Woods, B., Spector, A., Jones, C., Orrell,, M., & Davies, S. (2008). Reminiscence therapy for dementia. [Systematic Review]. *Cochrane Dementia and Cognitive Improvement Group Cochrane Database of Systematic Reviews, 2.*

Yesavage, J. A., Brink, T. L., Rose, T. L., Lum, O., Huang, V., Adey, M. B., & Leirer, V. O. (1983). Development and validation of a geriatric depression screening scale: A preliminary report. *Journal of Psychiatric Research, 17,* 37–49.

For a full suite of assignments and additional learning activities, see the access code at the front of your book.

Unit V
Management of Geriatric Syndromes

LEARNING OBJECTIVES www

At the end of this chapter, the reader will be able to:

> Evaluate the patient's medication list to formulate a plan to address medication-related problems before they occur.
> Identify evidence and references in medical literature that demonstrate polypharmacy's impact on patient outcomes.
> Recognize the symptoms of the syndrome of polypharmacy in elderly patients, acknowledging that the symptoms may be quite distant from the cause.
> Understand how goals of care influence appropriateness of medication choice.
> Identify drugs that are being used to treat side effects of other drugs.
> Explain how medications are tested for safety and efficacy with relationship to the elderly.
> Develop a personal system of addressing polypharmacy and medication-related problems in the clinical setting.
> Discuss how increasing medication burden can pose a hazard to the cognitively impaired elder.
> Describe why nurses have a unique perspective and role in the healthcare team when it comes to medication use and outcomes.

KEY TERMS www

Activity of daily living (ADL)
Adverse drug reaction (ADR)
Beers criteria
Brown bag assessment
Delirium
Dementia
Depression
Falls
Geriatric syndrome
Iatrogenic harm/iatrogenesis
Instrumental activity of daily living (IADL)
Isolation

Medication administration record (MAR)
Medication-related problem (MRP)
Morbidity
Mortality
Pharmacodynamics
Pharmacokinetics
Pharmacogenomics
Polypharmacy
Prescribing cascade
START criteria
STOPP criteria

Polypharmacy

Demetra Antimisiaris
Dennis J. Cheek

Background

Polypharmacy, or the concurrent use of multiple medications, fits the definition of a *geriatric syndrome* in that it is a common health condition in older adults that does not fit into the category of a discrete disease. Geriatric syndromes are highly prevalent within the older age group, multifactorial in etiology, and are associated with substantial morbidity and mortality (Inouye, Stuenksi, Tinetti, & Kuchel, 2007). There are four shared characteristics associated with an increased risk of living with geriatric syndromes: older age, baseline cognitive impairment, baseline functional impairment, and impaired mobility. These are markers of frailty, and generally the more frail a person is, the higher the chance that the person will experience multiple geriatric syndromes, including poor outcomes with medication use. An understanding of the relationship between frailty and medication misadventure will help clinicians identify and intervene to prevent potential polypharmacy-caused *morbidity* and *mortality*. Frailty alters *pharmacokinetics* (how drugs are absorbed, metabolized, and eliminated), *pharmacodynamics* (how drugs work in the body), and a person's ability to manage medications. Age is not necessarily a direct indication of frailty. Persons living with chronic disease who are under 65 years of age can be frail and face some of the same risks as an older frail person with respect to medication outcomes. Conversely, older people who are relatively healthy can tolerate and manage medications as well as a younger adult. A person's physiologic reserve is a strong determinant of one's ability to tolerate medications and resist medication harm. We will discuss polypharmacy as a geriatric syndrome; however, the principles presented are applicable to anyone utilizing medications, especially the chronically ill and frail.

Statistics on the number of medications utilized per person in the United States are slow to appear in the literature. The Agency for Healthcare Research and Quality, a federally funded agency, in their May 2009 statistical brief noted that as of 2006, the average senior used approximately six prescriptions, which is up from five noted in the past decade. This report also documents that the number of prescriptions per person increases with age (Stagnitti, 2009). The Kaiser Foundation Annual report on State Health Facts reveals that adults aged 19–64 filled an average of 11.3 prescriptions per person in 2010, while the elderly (65 years and older) filled an average of 31.1 prescriptions per person in 2010. Intuitively, this trend is likely to keep increasing over time. From the time period of year 2000–2008, the number of people using one, two and, five prescription medications within the past month increased from 4% to 48%, 25% to 31% and 6% to 11% respectively (Gu, Dillon, & Burt, 2010). The total number of prescriptions per capita in the United States, including all age groups, is increasing over time; the number of scripts per capita as of 2010 was standing at 12, an increase from the 1997 level of 8.9 (Kaiser Foundation, 2010). There are many factors driving the trend towards increased medication use in the population-at-large. The most obvious is that there are just more medications available than ever before. The Physicians' Desk Reference (PDR) in 1969 consisted of 1,415 pages of monographs for every prescription and over-the-counter product available in the United States. By 2012, the PDR consisted of 3,151 pages for just the prescription products alone, with a separate book approximately 800 pages in length to cover the over-the-counter (OTC) products (PDR, 2008). Additionally, an average of 27 products are approved by the Food and Drug Administration (FDA) annually with very few taken off the market during the same time period (Vandegrift & Datta, 2006).

The risks associated with multiple medication use are present at any age, but in the elderly who are frail and living with increasing multiple chronic diseases, that risk is more prevalent. Polypharmacy, like any other geriatric syndrome, can look on the surface like a specific disease state, while in actuality the symptoms observed are due to multiple and distant causes. A common example is when an elder is taking OTC NSAID (non-steroidal anti-inflammatory) pain medications and their blood pressure is mysteriously and suddenly elevated. Typically, the patient will be diagnosed as having worsening hypertension and a new hypertension medication will be prescribed, when the real cause is an OTC NSAID. This is usually not reported to the physician by the patient because the patient perceives OTC products as insignificant and is not aware of the connection between blood pressure and NSAID use.

How many medications used at the same time are enough to be labeled polypharmacy? As you can see in the above example, it only takes one when viewing polypharmacy as a harmful syndrome. Although the word polypharmacy is derived from the Greek words "poly," meaning many, and "pharmakon," which means drug, polypharmacy as a syndrome can involve any one medication or multiple medications that in combination cause harm, are unnecessary, or used inappropriately (Masoodi, 2008). Most medical literature commonly defines polypharmacy as the concomitant use of five medications; however, a particular number of drugs utilized at the same time do not always predict medication harm. Polypharmacy is seen among all age groups, but the combination of multiple chronic diseases, multiple doctors, multiple pharmacies, *isolation*, and advanced age increases the risk of medication harm. Consider polypharmacy in light of the following polypharmacy syndrome risk factors: 30% of elders live alone (which increases to 47% for women over 75), 41% of seniors reported taking five or more prescription medications, more than 50% have two or more physicians, and an estimated 64% of older individuals without *dementia* have some cognitive impairment (Caracciolo, Gatz, Xu, Perdersen, & Fratiglioni, 2012; Wilson, Schoen, & Neuman, 2007).

Polypharmacy poses a greater hazard for the elderly patient because of a diminished ability to eliminate medications as well as diminished physiological reserves. These issues, in combination with impairment in cognition, cause problems with an elder's ability to manage medications and report when adverse events occur.

Significance of the Problem
Morbidity, Mortality, and Costs

Inadvertent harm caused by the syndrome of polypharmacy accounts for numerous unnecessary costs to the healthcare system and patients (Budnitz, Lovegrove, & Shehab, 2011). It has been estimated that of hospitalized patients, 2,216,000 experience serious *adverse drug reactions (ADRs)*, and of these patients 106,000 die annually from an ADR (Lazarou, Pormeranz, & Corey, 1998). To place this statistic in perspective: Deaths from ADRs, if included in Centers for Disease Control and Prevention (CDC) rankings of causes of death, would place ADRs as the fifth leading cause of death annually, ahead of Alzheimer's disease, diabetes and kidney disease (CDC, 2012). However, statistics on ADRs are only as accurate as one's ability to recognize when an ADR is the cause. Most reported ADRs are incidents where a medication was given and the person died shortly thereafter or a person is hospitalized for an ADR specifically and the result was death. The number of deaths attributed to organic causes such as kidney failure, which were actually caused by organ damage due to chronic or acute medication use, is still not well quantified. It is important to be aware that current statistics on the deaths or harm due to ADRs all come mostly, if not all, from hospital records or institutional records such as nursing homes (where ADRs are often underreported due to lack of recognition of medication side effects). Therefore, the magnitude of ADR-related morbidity and mortality occurring in the ambulatory population-at-large is overlooked. The reported statistics on ADRs thus are a potential underestimate of the true overall harm resulting from medication use.

In older patients (those over 65 years of age), up to 30% of the persons admitted to the hospital are admitted for medication-related problems (Marcum et al., 2012). In the nursing home setting, for every $1.00 spent on drugs, $1.33 in healthcare resources are consumed to treat drug-related problems (Bootman, Harrison, & Cox, 1997). Overall, the economic impact of *medication-related problems (MRPs)* would result in MRPs being the fifth-highest cost of disease (if MRPs were considered a disease) impacting people over 65 years of age in the United States. That means that MRPs would cost less than diabetes, Alzheimer's disease, cancer, and cardiovascular disease, but would cost more than osteoarthritis, stroke, osteoporosis, and Parkinson's disease. The risk of ADRs rises exponentially with the addition of each new medication to a person's drug regimen. Despite this, as a society, we are increasing our concomitant use of medication more each year (Denham, 1990).

An Important Historical Perspective

The stunning statistics on individual medication burden and medication-related harm associated with polypharmacy seems to have silently developed as our society rapidly increases the use of medications over a relatively short period of time. We are at an unprecedented time in history where people are taking medications in a way as never before. Consider that our knowledge and ability to design drugs to fight disease is a relatively recent phenomenon. This means that an understanding of what happens when multiple medications are combined is in its infancy.

It wasn't until the mid-to-late 1800s that ether was determined to be a safer anesthetic than chloroform. Little discussion of specific dosing for specific patient types circulated in those days: It was one physician-scientist learning through trial and error and keeping notes in his corner of the world, in contrast to the way we derive and disseminate medical data and knowledge today. The first medication in the era of modern medicine use was in the early 1900s when aspirin was discovered to be a universal pain reliever. After that, in the 1930s and 1940s, penicillin and the first semi-synthetic antibiotic, tetracycline, were developed. The field of pharmaco-kinetics was discovered in the 1960s and 1970s, and we started to understand that drugs are absorbed into the body, distributed, and eliminated primarily through the kidneys and liver.

In the late 1990s, with the mapping of the human genome for the first time, we then discovered that we all have a genetic, set-at-birth capacity to metabolize medications through numerous different pathways, each one working at a different rate in different people (*pharmacogenomics*). Yet for most medications we still have standard recommended doses for all adults regardless of individual pharmacogenomics. Today, knowledge of the physiology of aging is expanding, and even starting in our late 20s it is suggested that persons slowly move towards becoming frail. As we lose muscle mass and our percentage of body fat increases, we become increasingly frail and our organs become more impaired. Medications can behave differently than they did in the fairly healthy, carefully selected individuals the drugs were tested in for safety, efficacy, and FDA approval. In addition to new knowledge of the physiology of aging, the first clinical studies of polypharmacy and its relationship to morbidity, impaired function, and outcomes started to emerge just after the turn of this century.

Guidelines and Medical Literature on Polypharmacy

The guidance on recommended medication use to treat chronic disease and medical problems is designed to demonstrate efficacy and rarely designed to tell how drugs will perform in the frail elder. Drugs are brought to market through an FDA-guided safety and efficacy trial process, which does not often include the older patient or the patient who has multiple problems and takes multiple combinations of medications. For example, a medication being tested to treat Alzheimer's dementia (AD), which didn't make it to market, had the following exclusion criteria: the patient would not qualify for the drug trial if they had "neurodegenerative disease and/or dementias other than AD, are a frequent smoker and/or frequent consumer of caffeine, have hypothyroidism, or folic acid deficiency or B12 deficiency, a history or presence of stroke or epilepsy, a history of an MI [myocardial infarction] within 5 years, severe hypotension or hypertension requiring therapy, uncontrolled atrial fibrillation or AV block higher than 1st degree" (Sunovion Pharmaceuticals, 2006). Most of the patients ineligible for this drug trial possessed many of the characteristics found in patients with dementia who will ultimately use the medication, but the medication would be brought to market having been tried in a very different, and much healthier, group of patients. Additionally, how many patients are not going to smoke or consume coffee and soft drinks with caffeine? The take-home point is that most drugs studied in drug trials, including safety and efficacy trials for FDA approval and those aimed at proving drug efficacy in various disease states, do not include subjects who are likely to have poor or dangerous outcomes. Because the studies are designed mainly to look for efficacy, they are designed for success in proving efficacy, as opposed to looking for toxicity in the frailest patients. This means that most of the frail elders, the older old, or the people with multiple chronic disease and end organ damage will not be represented in our evidence-based guidance. It is easy to see why the elderly suffer poor outcomes caused by polypharmacy, given the way medications are tested for efficacy. Elders have multiple comorbidities, use more medication than younger patients, and are not included in drug studies unless they are fairly healthy.

Another discrepancy between the literature on medication and the actual elderly medication user is that OTC drug and supplement use is not accounted for in the medical literature except on a case by case basis. It has been documented that 30% of elders take an analgesic medication and more than 60% of those individuals cannot identify the active ingredient in their brand of pain reliever. Overall, 40% of Americans believe that OTC medications are too weak to cause any real harm (Zagaria, 2009). These are alarming facts in light of the record number of medications that are going from prescription to over-the-counter status.

The elder-at-large is not as carefully followed as the study subjects are by the study investigator physicians and the team of clinical trial professionals. Older adult patients are faced with the challenges of aging and poor health such as multiple doctors, pharmacies, transitions of care, psychosocial isolation, and challenges performing their *activities of daily living (ADLs)* and *instrumental activities of daily living (IADLs)*, all of which impact the ability to safely use medications but are not necessarily accounted for in the guidance. So the assumption that what worked well in the medical literature, which produced guidelines or brought new drugs to market, will work well in the elderly patient is a false assumption under the current healthcare system.

We should assume that in elders, guidelines on disease state management are guidelines and not absolute benchmarks to reach in order to reap good outcomes. This is an important point since healthcare systems are increasingly moving towards rewards for meeting chronic disease management guidelines, and it is important to consider that those guidelines were not tested in the very old and very frail. An example would be the CMS PQRI (now called PQRS) program, which offers incentives to prescribers for meeting criteria for disease management; one example would be that a person with documented cardiovascular disease is prescribed a statin (PQRI, n.d). Additionally, there is the literature that makes sweeping health policy suggestions, like a piece suggesting that statins should be served at fast food outlets in the condiments (Ferenczi, Asaria, Hughes, Chaturvedi, & Francis, 2010). Statins have not been tested in many older patients and there are very few study subjects above the age of 72 in the studies from which the guidelines for statin use were derived. Even the JUPITER trial (Justification for the Use of Statins in Prevention: an Intervention Trial Evaluating Rosuvastatin), which was aimed at studying primary prevention in men over 50 and women over 60 years of age with elevated C-reactive protein, did not include any subjects over 71 years of age despite being conducted at 1,315 sites in 26 countries (Ridker et al., 2008).

An individualistic approach to each elder is necessary for safe medication use. This is not to suggest that guidance on adult disease management is not important, but to emphasize that guidance needs to be individualized for the frail elder until such time that more specific guidelines for elders becomes available. As we age, we become more physiologically diverse from one another through different environmental exposures, disease states, and genetic influences (see **Figure 11-1**).

Unfortunately, the individual approach takes time, which the office visit typically does not allow for. The average office visit consists of 15 minutes, of which 7 minutes

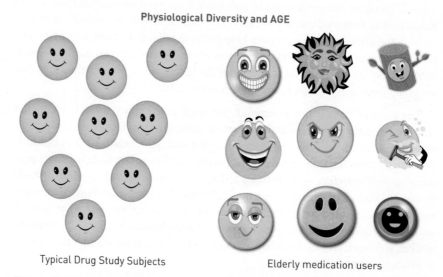

Physiological Diversity and AGE

Typical Drug Study Subjects   Elderly medication users

Figure 11-1 Cohort on the left represents the homogeneity of the typical study subject. Much of our study data and guidelines are built upon the study design seen on the left, but applied to the group on the right—the elderly, who are individually quite diverse.

are dedicated to greeting and social discussion, leaving a little over 7 minutes to address a patient's problems. According to one study, the result is an average of 3 minutes dedicated to discussion of medications per typical office visit (Tai-Seale, McGuire, & Zhang, 2007). If you are a frail elder on 20 medications, no one may be assessing the overall regimen for appropriateness, adherence, and side effects beyond the obvious such as bleeds or abnormal lab values, which may cue the prescriber that something may be wrong with the medication regimen.

The healthcare community is beginning to study the impact of higher overall drug burden on elder function and well-being. From 1986 to 2011, there have been 19 studies using rigorous observational or interventional designs examining the relationship between medication use and functional status decline in the elderly. Of these, three studies found an increased risk in functional decline among elders living with polypharmacy overall. Benzodiazepine use and functional decline were associated in four studies. As for antidepressants, one study found no relationship between antidepressant use and functional status, and another randomized trial found amitriptyline to impair some measures of gait. Anticholinergic burden was associated with worsening functional status in two studies. Several studies looked at multiple central nervous system drugs and found links to greater declines in self-reported mobility, with one study reporting hospitalized rehabilitation patients who used hypnotics/anxiolytics having a lower functional independence measure in motor gains than nonusers. Antihypertensive medications have been linked to impairment in functional status in two studies (Peron, Gray, & Hanlon, 2011).

Risk Factors

Multiple Medications: The Prescribing Cascade—Is It The Medication Or The Disease?

As mentioned earlier, the more medications a person takes concurrently, the higher the risk of experiencing an MRP. Any one medication possesses multiple inherent risks (see **Figure 11-2**). There is the immediate risk of any medication causing anaphylaxis, and then there are the typical known side effects, the atypical side effects, the counterintuitive side effects, the dose limitations, the long-term use side effects, and the user error side effects. Take hydrochlorothiazide (HCTZ), a common "water" pill. Usually people think about monitoring for low potassium, but HCTZ requires ongoing monitoring not only of potassium, but also chloride, sodium, magnesium, lipids (can contribute to hyperlipidemia), uric acid (can lead to gout), complete blood counts (can cause hemolytic anemia, thrombocytopenia), and glucose (can increase glucose resistance). HCTZ is a medication that patients sometimes take more than recommended because they diagnose themselves as needing to lose water,

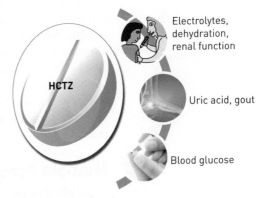

Electrolytes, dehydration, renal function

HCTZ

Uric acid, gout

Blood glucose

Figure 11-2 Illustration of the multiple monitoring issues that have to be addressed even in commonly utilized medications such as hydrochlorothizide (HCTZ).

so adherence assessment is important in determining if side effects are relevant to regular use or hidden misuse of medication.

When medication side effects are treated with other medications, it is called the *prescribing cascade*. Usually, the practice of treating medication side effects with other medications is not intentional and is due to the mistaken identification of a medication side effect as organic in origin (caused by a disease or condition). Occasionally, in patients who necessitate extreme doses of a medication to control a condition for which there are no alternative treatments, side effects are anticipated and purposefully treated with other medications because the risk of discontinuation of the first medication outweighs the benefit. An example might be a patient who demonstrates extreme agitation and aggression without high-dose antipsychotic therapy and would be unable to live successfully in the community or be part of an institutional setting appropriate for their well-being without the risky antipsychotic use. Under such circumstances, the expected side effects of extrapyramidal syndrome (movement disorder) and metabolic syndrome might be treated with benztropine (a strong anticholinergic, used to address the drug-induced movement disorder) and glyburide. Benztropine can cause serious side effects itself, such as cardiac problems, impaired cognition, urinary retention, ocular issues, and temperature deregulation, as can glyburide, which can cause hypoglycemia and requires constant glucose monitoring. With the intentional use of medications to treat the side effects of another medication, the clinician should document the rationale for doing so, including the risks versus benefits, and the monitoring parameters along with the recommended intervals of monitoring.

More times than not, the use of medications to treat the side effects of other medications is not intentional and, as a consequence, unnecessary and inappropriate use of medications occurs. The following prescribing cascade case illustrates a common polypharmacy scenario (see **Case Study 11-1**).

This was an actual case in which a patient had been diagnosed with and treated for Parkinson's disease, despite the real cause of her movement disorder being the combination of drugs that are known (or not-so-well known) to induce movement disorders as a side effect (Mellor, Ahme, & Thomson, 2009; Alvarez & Evidente, 2008). The diagnosis of Parkinson's disease was made by her primary care doctor. She had moderate to severe dementia and lacked the verbal ability to describe the history of the onset of her movement disorder, which contributed to the inappropriate diagnosis that masked the true underlying cause of symptoms related to medication use.

Multiple Prescribers and Iatrogenic Harm

Today's healthcare system is very complex and patients are handled by multiple physicians, facilities, healthcare agencies, and pharmacies. A well-known book entitled *To Err is Human* published statistics from a Harvard medical practice for the year 1984 and found that adverse events were responsible for 13.6% of all deaths and that 2.6% of errors resulted in permanent, disabling injury. It was determined

Case Study 11–1: Is it the Drug or the Disease?

J.C. is an 84 year old female who presented to an assisted living home for assistance with her IADLs. Upon review of her admit medication orders, it was noted that she had some medications that are known to be inappropriate to use in the elderly, such as fluoxetine and metoclopramide (per the Beers Criteria). She had a significant amount of aphasia, tremor, and periods of agitation and aggression reportedly due to her dementia.

PMH

Hypertension	Vascular dementia
Parkinson's disease	Depression
Chronic atrial fibrillation	Osteoarthritis

Medications Upon Admission

Warfarin 4mg daily	Memantine 10mg twice daily
Fluoxetine 20mg daily	Tramadol 25mg up to four times daily
Carbidopa-levodopa 25/100mg three times daily	Metoprolol 25mg XL daily
Metoclopramide 10mg 30 minutes before meals	Hydrochlorothiazide 25mg daily
Donepezil 10mg daily	Quetiapine 25mg twice daily
Acetaminophen 325mg two tablets every 8 hours	

Medication Adjustments:

When the attending physician reviewed her case, she immediately recognized that the fluoxetine was too long-acting for use in elders and discontinued it (American Geriatrics Society Beers Criteria Update Expert Panel, 2012). The half-life of fluoxetine is about 48–70 hours with an active metabolite that can remain in the body for another 15 days; in an elder, this can be longer. This long half-life elevates the risk that elders will build up too much fluoxetine due to impaired clearance. Most psychoactive medications cannot be abruptly stopped, but fluoxetine's half-life is so long that it self-tapers as it takes its time eliminating and is one of the only psychoactive medications that can be stopped immediately. The doctor's plan was to start citalopram in a few weeks instead of fluoxetine. She also immediately discontinued the metoclopramide, recognizing that its antidopaminergic effect is not safe to use in patients with movement disorders. She discontinued the tramadol due to its risk of not clearing efficiently in renally impaired patients, and J.C.'s estimated creatinine clearance was calculated at less than 30ml/min. She instead prescribed routine acetaminophen for J.C.'s arthritis pain.

When the tramadol, fluoxetine and metoclopramide were removed, her tremor went away and therefore she didn't need to take carbidopa-levodopa anymore. Her quality of life improved dramatically. J.C. was better able to walk and participate in activities and self-care. The elimination of the offending medications also revealed that her dementia-related behaviors of aggression and agitation were actually akathisia related to the use of fluoxetine, tramadol, and metoclopramide. Her orders for an antipsychotic agent twice daily were eliminated as a result. The patient lived the rest of her life pleasantly with dementia as her primary problem and was much more comfortable than when first presented.

by expert opinion that 56% of these adverse outcomes were preventable (Kohn, Corrigan, & Donaldson, 1999). This is known as *iatrogenic harm* or *iatrogenesis,* meaning doctor- or healthcare-created harm. Decades ago this complex dynamic in the healthcare system was less prevalent because there were fewer medications, interventions, and specialists. Elders are unfamiliar with how to safely negotiate their way through today's complicated healthcare system. When today's elders were younger, the medical system left the coordination of a person's health care to the physician's office. Generally, a person would see one doctor for all their problems, and that doctor would spend a great deal of time with them, knew all of their history, came to the hospital when they were admitted, and knew their family and medications because that one doctor treated the whole family over their lifetime and was the sole prescriber. The average number of physicians that a patient over 65 years old today sees is 7. It would not be self-evident to an elder (or perhaps anyone) that bringing *all* of their medications to all seven doctor visits and the hospital is a necessary precaution to foster safer medication assessment. For seniors living with 5 or more chronic conditions (approximately 20% of seniors) this number goes up to 14 different doctors at different addresses. This group also averages over 40 office visits in one year (Berenson, 2010).

Medication reconciliation by healthcare professionals is a serious challenge for numerous reasons. One of the most significant threats to sound medication reconciliation is the systemic problem of transitions of care. This leaves the patient as the healthcare provider's only witness to all of the medication changes. The patients themselves are perplexed by having to navigate a healthcare system that is very complex, difficult to understand, and hard to follow. Another threat to medication reconciliation is having to follow multiple providers' instructions and order changes, especially for elderly patients who are too ill to absorb so much constantly changing information. Serious medication-related problems can occur as a result of lack of coordination of care, lack of patient advocacy, and poor communication between providers. Today, the elder is faced with multiple physicians, multiple prescribers, and the obligation to coordinate their own care. The more an elder is exposed to the healthcare system, the higher the risk for iatrogenic harm (Permpongkosol, 2011).

Despite the multiple exposures to physicians' offices and hospitals and the seemingly multiple missed opportunities to catch medication errors, most adverse drug events are rooted in the encounter with the prescriber, with a lesser part of the cause attributed to adherence. A study of the incidence and preventability of adverse drug events in community-dwelling elders found that 58.4% started at the prescribing stage, with 60.8% of these events caused by poor drug monitoring and 21% attributed to problems with patient adherence to the prescribed regimen. (The percentages do not add up to 100% because of overlap of causes per adverse drug event studied.) (Gurwitz et al., 1995). Healthcare providers such as nurses and clinical pharmacists can make a large impact by ensuring that the correct monitoring occurs and not assuming that the prescribers have that aspect covered. Monitoring for medication safety can include laboratory tests, drug interaction checks, physical assessment, and psychological assessment. Appropriate medication monitoring will be discussed in subsequent sections.

Multiple Pharmacies

With the advent of mail-order pharmacies and multiple chain stores at every corner, people are filling prescriptions at multiple pharmacies instead of filling all of their prescriptions at one pharmacy. The practice of using one pharmacy for all of a person's prescription, over-the-counter, vitamin, and supplement purchases was an additional check of the overall medication regimen's safety. The old-style, single pharmacy relationship was also another point of accessibility for the patient to gain consultation on how to correctly take their medications. The virtual elimination of the single pharmacy model, in addition to studies demonstrating that patients are no longer receiving oral or written instructions from their physicians and pharmacists, leaves the prescription bottle label as the most important guide to medication use (Metlay et al., 2005; Morris, Tabak, & Gondek, 1997). The barriers to safe and effective medication use are both systemic and patient-centered. Health literacy is increasingly becoming recognized as a significant factor at any age. Ideally, the pharmacy would be an excellent point for patient education and counseling to help overcome literacy challenges. One study looked at nearly 400 English-speaking adults in 3 primary care clinics to study the patient's understanding of instructions on 5 prescription container labels. The investigators also assessed whether the subjects could actually demonstrate one of the label's dosing instructions using actual pills. The ability to correctly understand the 5 labels ranged from 67.1% to 91.1%, with people reading at or below 6th grade level less likely to understand all 5 labels. Although 70.7% of the patients with low literacy correctly stated the instructions reading "take two tablets by mouth twice daily," only 34.7% could demonstrate the number of pills to be taken daily. In this study, as with many others, the greater the number of prescription medications, the greater the likelihood of misunderstanding (Davis et al., 2006). In elderly patients, literacy may be added to other challenges such as cognitive, sensory, and functional impairment.

Older Age: Frailty, Chronic Disease, Cognitive Impairment, and Altered Pharmacokinetics

There is irony in the fact that the population most likely to utilize a higher medication burden is the one facing increasing challenges to successful medication management: the elderly. Management of medications is not so different from other IADLs such as balancing a checkbook, planning to cook a meal and going to the grocery store, or doing the laundry. These activities require *intact* executive function, logical memory, verbal memory, attention, linguistic capacity, and other domains of cognitive function. To complete the ancillary tasks associated with medication management, such as shopping (procuring medication), finances (paying for medications), arranging transportation or driving (doctor's appointments), and using a telephone (calling pharmacies and physicians' offices), various domains of cognition in addition to intact executive function have to work well together (Hall, Hoa, Johnson, Barber, & O'Bryant, 2011).

Medications are additionally dangerous in the elderly because of frailty and the physiological changes that occur with age and impact pharmacokinetics and pharmacodynamics. When we age, muscle turns to fat, altering the distribution of fat- and water-soluble drugs: The volume of distribution of fat-soluble drugs becomes larger and that of water-soluble drugs becomes smaller. This means, for example, that many medications that are psychoactive or target pain will take longer to work upon *initial* dosing because the volume of distribution is larger. However, once distribution is accomplished, the frail elderly patient will be more sensitive to the drug's effects. Conversely, water-soluble drugs will become active in the plasma faster due to smaller volumes of distribution in the elderly. Along with frailty comes protein wasting and typically lower albumen and protein levels. The medications that are highly protein- and albumin-bound in the plasma will be less bound in an older person, resulting in a high fraction of active drug or "free drug" floating around in the blood. What this means clinically is that when a subtherapeutic drug level result comes from the lab for a highly protein-bound drug, there may be no need to increase the dose since the percentage of unbound or free (active) drug is still high (see **Figure 11-3**).

Frailty is also accompanied by changes in the physiological function of the organs and tissues. Medications that are designed to work on various receptors may not find enough receptors to work on because they have diminished in number. One example of a common physiological change with age is altered baroreceptor activity. Orthostatic hypotension is common in elders, even without diuretic therapy or beta-blocker use, because baroreceptors become less sensitive to changes in posture and the other compensatory systems that react to postural changes cannot respond because they are altered by frailty. Another example is the blood–brain barrier, an important structure that drugs are commonly designed around. Psychoactive medications are designed to be lipid- or fat-soluble because the brain is primarily made of lipids and the blood–brain barrier readily allows lipid-soluble compounds to enter the brain. Just as oil mixes with oil and not water, lipid-soluble drugs readily pass into the central nervous system and brain due to their fat-soluble properties, while water-soluble drugs do not. The blood–brain barrier works to let fat-soluble drugs into the brain and keep water-soluble (or polar) substances out. With age this mechanism breaks down due to frailty, so, for example, some urinary

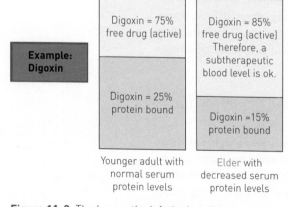

Example: Digoxin

Digoxin = 75% free drug (active)

Digoxin = 25% protein bound

Younger adult with normal serum protein levels

Digoxin = 85% free drug (active) Therefore, a subtherapeutic blood level is ok.

Digoxin =15% protein bound

Elder with decreased serum protein levels

Figure 11-3 The box on the left depicts digoxin protein binding in a younger adult; the box on the right depicts digoxin binding in an older adult with lower protein and albumin stores. Adapted from: Bateman, D. N. (2004). "Digoxin-speci" c antibody fragments: how much and when? *Toxicology Review, 23*, 135–143.

incontinence (UI) medications (such as oxybutynin), which traditionally are well-known to cause confusion and memory impairment due to anticholinergic effects, have been redesigned to not cross into the brain by the addition of a polar entity, making them water soluble. Theoretically, this allows the newer UI medication to do its anticholinergic work in the periphery and not affect the brain. Unfortunately, these strongly anticholinergic drugs can cross into the frail brain through the compromised blood–brain barrier (Chancellor et al., 2012). Although newer UI medications are marketed to be safer and cause less confusion in the frail elder, the safety profile is not reliable because of age-related changes in the blood–brain barrier.

Transitions of Care

Earlier we discussed the increased risk of MRPs related to the increasing numbers of physicians and pharmacists that a patient utilizes. Transitions of care are another glaring source of medication misadventure. Increased transitions of care from one setting to another lead to a higher risk for MRPs. It has been estimated that up to 67% of medication histories taken in the healthcare setting have one or more errors in them, and that 46% of medication errors are made at admission or discharge with new prescriptions (Sullivan, Gleason, & Rooney, 2005; National Audit Office [NAO], 2005). It is easy to see how there can be a detrimental snowballing effect in elders transitioning frequently from one care setting to another, trying to rely upon the healthcare system to keep the medication list current and correct. **Case Study 11-2** illustrates the common scenario of a patient entering the hospital and being discharged on additional inappropriate and unnecessary medications.

Case Study 11–2: Go to the Hospital and Come Back With Four More Medications

www.

K.L. is an 84-year-old male who was sent to the hospital for treatment of possible urinary tract infection (UTI) and dizziness with fever. He has lived in assisted living at SHV assisted living facility (ALF) for the past 4 years. K.L.'s hospital course was complicated by aggressive antibiotic treatment resulting in a *C. difficile* infection and diarrhea. Geriatric Nurse Practitioner B.G. came in to round on K.L. the first day after he returned from the hospital. B.G. compared her chart records to the new posthospital discharge records and found several discrepancies and inappropriate medication changes:

Ht = 6 ft 1 in, Wt = 178 #, BP = 125/65, RR = 18, HR = 72

PMH: DM2, HTN, OsteoArthritis, CAD, Afib, chronic UTI (colonization)

Labs: CMP within normal limits (WNL) except for Creatinine 1.8, BUN = 32, glucose 72; K = 3.0

CBC WNL; Lipid Panel TC = 70, LDL = 127, HDL = 65

(continues)

Case Study 11–2: Go to the Hospital and Come Back With Four More Medications (continued)

From ALF to ED	Hospital DC summary	Current in ALF chart	Assessment and de-prescribing by GNP
Metoprolol XL 25 mg daily	Metoprolol XL 25 mg daily	Metoprolol XL 25 mg daily	
Digoxin 0.125 mg every other day	Amiodarone 200 mg twice daily	Amiodarone 200 mg twice daily	*Cardio consult placed him on amiodarone, purposefully avoided in the past, will switch back to digoxin every other day (Bahr, Lackner, & Pacala, 2008)* **DC amidarone.**
Warfarin 3 mg daily	Warfarin 3 mg daily	Warfarin 3 mg daily	
Lisinopril 20 mg daily	Lisinopril 20 mg daily	Lisinopril 20 mg daily	
Amlodipine 5 mg daily	Amlodipine 10 mg daily	Amlodipine 10 mg daily	*Amlodipine dose increased by hospitalist targeting BP = 120/80; too low for K.L. due to orthostasis and age.* **Decrease to 5 mg.**
Metformin 500 mg BID	Metformin 500 mg BID	Metformin 500 mg BID	
	Glyburide 5 mg daily	Glyburide 5 mg daily	*Hypoglycemic and on glyburide. Glipizide a better choice in renal impairment (dose adjustment). Glyburide should be avoided in CrCl, 50ml/min. His est. CrCl = 33.3m/min. (American Geriatric Society Beers Criteria.)* **DC (discontinue, his BG likely went up due to acute infection)**
	Simvastatin 40 mg daily	Simvastatin 40 mg daily	*His lipid panel indicates that he does not need statin therapy, and amlodipine when given with simvastatin per FDA warning requires simvastatin dose of not more than 20 mg daily.* **DC**
	Nitrofurantoin 100 mg daily	Nitrofurantoin 100 mg daily	*Contraindicated in patients with CrCl < 60ml/min. (nitrofurantoin package insert)* **DC—patient known to have UT bacterial colonization.**
Cranberry supplement	Vancomycin oral 250 mg every 8 hours for 10 days	Vancomycin oral 250 mg every 8 hours for 10 days	*Not clear when vancomycin started, need to clarify how many days remain, then re-culture.*
	Pantoprozole 20 mg daily prn	Pantoprozole 20 mg daily	*This was a prn AST order (routine in hospital) carried forward to discharge which was* **mistranscribed to be routine. DC**
	Diclofenac 75 mg twice daily prn	Diclofenac 75 mg twice daily	*NSAIDS are contraindicated in patients on warfarin, and high risk for CV events in elders. (American Geriatrics Society Beers Criteria).* **DC.**
Routine APAP	Same	Same	*Same*

Isolation

Isolation is a growing problem amongst the elderly, especially with the aging of the baby boomer generation. With the Boomers, there was a marked increase in the number of women not having children or families. Also, more than ever, families are geographically spread out as opposed to living and working in the same town in which they were born. The typical factors leading to isolation are gender (women more than men), health status, death of a spouse, disability, and loss of social network. These risk factors are additive (Holmen, Ericsson, & Winblad, 2000). When an elder is isolated, it is difficult to assess their ability to self-care, their level of well-being, worsening health, and multiple other aspects of their lives. The absence of a social group makes medication side effects difficult to differentiate from new medical problems because no one is present to witness the onset of a problem, nor is anyone able to bear witness to the elder's ability to adhere to the prescribed regimen.

Warning Signs

Nonspecific Complaints

The typical medication-related problem presents itself as a nonspecific complaint as opposed to an obvious reaction to a medication. In the case of anaphylaxis, it is easy to attribute the cause to the medication; however, many medication side effects reveal themselves insidiously, presenting over time as problems like an upset stomach, headache, dry mouth, decreased mental sharpness, agitation or edginess, a sudden change in appetite, insomnia, or hypersomnolence. This is one of the reasons that polypharmacy occurs so easily. A patient goes into the 15-minute doctor's visit with a nonspecific complaint and it typically does not get recognized as a medication side effect, instead becoming another diagnosed condition, leading to another prescription (see **Figure 11-4**).

It is important to always remember that symptoms caused by medication side effects can seem quite unrelated to the actual medication. For example, the headache caused by a cardiac medication (due to vasodilation) is directly caused by the drug's intended action, while another symptom, such as gout, is an indirect outcome of using diuretics, particularly thiazide diuretics. The separation between the actual presenting problem and the origin of the problem as side effect of a drug leads to many misdiagnoses. More prescribing to "chase" the problem rather than fix it at the level of the cause occurs because of the lack

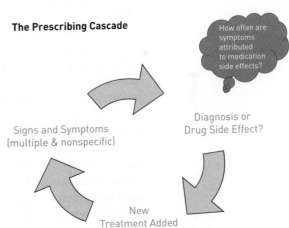

The Prescribing Cascade

How often are symptoms attributed to medication side effects?

Diagnosis or Drug Side Effect?

Signs and Symptoms (multiple & nonspecific)

New Treatment Added

Figure 11-4 The Prescribing Cascade illustrated as a never ending cycle of treating medication side effects that are inaccurately assessed as medical (or organic) problems rather than medication side effects, leading to more medications being prescribed, leading to more side effects.

of connection between drug use and new problems. Tracing a patient's problem back to the offending drug is a challenge because it requires a high level of technical skill and time. One way to ensure that a medication cause is not overlooked is to approach each problem a patient presents with as a possible medication-caused problem and do the research to see if any of their medications have some connection, direct or indirect, to the presenting problem.

Timeline

Being aware of the emergence of a new problem (drug side effect) and the timing of the start of a new drug therapy is the most obvious method of detecting MRPs. The challenge comes with patients who are poor historians (and even cognitively intact elders can get mixed up about what they take and when if the number of medications they take is high). Another challenge, which is often overlooked, is the hidden use of OTCs, supplements, and herbal products. The presenting problem could be caused by unreported use of these products or sporadic use, which may cause a direct effect or compete with an existing stable regimen to destabilize the routine medications. An example of this could be warfarin users who occasionally utilize acetaminophen-containing products. It could be OTC cough and cold preparations, plain acetaminophen, or as-needed prescription opioid combination products that can raise their INR unexpectedly. It usually has to be a high dose of acetaminophen for about one week to make an impact on INR. In this example, there is no direct toxicity from the acetaminophen, but the indirect change in INR can occur and be in effect even after the acetaminophen is discontinued. The clinician may not connect the two as the cause of the MRP because the OTC product is not in use anymore.

Falls

Falls are always of concern in the elderly in the community and in hospital settings. The drugs usually associated with falls are the benzodiazepines, muscle relaxants, first generation antihistamines, and opioids. As with most aspects of MRP assessment, the importance of suspecting the unsuspecting cannot be emphasized enough. In elders, especially with dementia, falls occur in the absence of benzodiazepines and other medications typically associated with falls. The reasons are numerous, including neurological changes effecting gait and balance, weakness due to frailty, and environmental factors. Some patients are fallers, regardless of what medications they are using. However, in a thorough assessment of medication-induced falls, all medications must be considered. Unsuspected medications such as diuretics and cholinesterase inhibitors (donepezil, galantamine, or rivastigmine) can lead to falls, although they typically are not considered drugs that lead to falls. If you think carefully, you can trace the connection between a drug's effects and its potential for causing falls. Consider diuretics: Diuretics cause increased urine output, urge to rush to the restroom, orthostasis, and dehydration. Cholinesterase inhibitors are actually documented in the medical literature as increasing risk of falls, which would be predictable when you know that these medications increase levels of acetylcholine, which in turn can cause bradycardia, increased gastrointestinal motility, and urinary

BOX 11-1 Evidence-Based Practice Example

This meta-analysis aimed to examine the effectiveness of "cholinesterase inhibitors (ChEIs) and Memantine on the risk of falls, syncope, and related events, defined as fracture and accidental injury" (p. 1019). A meta-analysis of randomized controlled trials was conducted from numerous databases through 2009. The settings were the community and nursing homes. Participants yielded from the search included those from 54 placebo-controlled randomized trials that reported data on the factors of interest. ChEI use was associated with greater risk of syncope than placebo, but not fractures, falls, or accidental injury. Memantine was not associated with falls, syncope, or accidental injury, but was correlated with fewer fractures. Gerontological nurses should realize that ChEIs may increase the risk of syncope in older adults, and Memantine may have a favorable effect on fracture. The authors suggested that more research is needed to confirm and explain the observation of the reduction in number of fractures for those taking Memantine.

Source: Kim, D. H., Brown, R. A., Ding, E. L., Kiel, D. P., & Berry, S. D. (2011). Dementia Medications and Risk of Falls, Syncope, and Related Adverse Events: Meta-Analysis of Randomized Controlled Trials. *Journal of the American Geriatrics Society, 59,* 1019–1031.

incontinence, all of which can play a part in falls (Gill et al., 2009). Many cardio-vascular medications can contribute to falls in elders by dropping blood pressure too low, causing orthostatic hypotension, or crossing into the brain and causing confusion. Beta-blockers are an example of this; if the blood pressure therapy drops blood pressure too low, beta-blockers can blunt the baroreceptor and cardiovascular response to postural changes and can cross into the brain to cause confusion. Even some lipophilic statins can cause confusion and contribute to falls, especially in a frail elder whose blood–brain barrier is no longer intact. One prospective cohort study demonstrated that withdrawing (meaning discontinuation of or decreasing in dose) medications that increase fall risk is an effective intervention for lowering the incidence of falls. Their list of target drugs included a majority of psychoactive medications and some cardiovascular medications, plus oral hypoglycemic agents. They found that this decrease in falls effect is more highly correlated with the withdrawal of cardiovascular drugs than the other classes studied (van der Velde, Stricker, Pols, & van der Cammen, 2007). Falls are common in elders and are "never events" per Medicare in hospitals. Medications increase the risk of falls. Awareness that other drugs in addition to the common list of fall-causing drugs, which mostly includes medications that cause drowsiness, better leads the clinician to connect the falls to unsuspecting medications causing falls (see **Box 11-1**).

Sudden Change in IADLs or ADLs

A global sign in the elderly that a problem or problems are developing is when their ability to carry out ADLs and IADLs change, especially if there is an abrupt change. It was not until the mid-2000s that studies have shown a clear relationship among drug burden and functional impairment, increased hospitalization, and even death.

Dry Brain — confusion*
Dry Mouth — can't eat
Dry Eyes — blurry vision
Dries up urine — urinary retention
Dries up bowels — constipation

*Note that medications used for dementia, such as donepezil or Aricept, are procholinergic (opposite of anticholinergic) and anticholinergic medications can impair cognition.
(Campbell et al., 2009)

Figure 11-5 Anticholinergic side effects.

In particular, anticholinergic medications cause significant impairment in function and can accelerate progression of dementia, which results in less and less ability to participate in IADLs and ADLs (see **Figure 11-5**).

One study demonstrated that as anticholinergic medications are added, each additional unit of drug burden had a negative effect on physical function similar to that of three additional physical comorbidities, and a greater effect than anxiety, *depression*, or cognitive impairment. In the same study, each additional unit of anticholinergic drug burden had a negative effect on cognitive task performance similar to that of four additional physical comorbidities and half the effect of anxiety, depression, or cognitive impairment (Hilmer et al., 2007). Another study demonstrated that chronic exposure to anticholinergic medications in patients who were taking cholinesterase inhibitors to treat Alzheimer's disease experienced an acceleration of the worsening of the disease, which was double the rate of those who did not take anticholinergic medications (Lu & Tune, 2003). Lastly, a study looking at the most frail cohort of elders (nursing home patients) where they "de-prescribed" or discontinued an average of 2.8 medications per patient in the intervention arm versus the usual care arm, found that the mortality rate in the intervention arm was 21% versus 45% in the usual care group. The intervention group's rate of referral to the emergency department was 11.8% while the usual care group was sent to the emergency room at a rate of 30%. The 2.8 medications that the investigators chose to discontinue were conservative choices with the aim of selecting just the most unnecessary medications, such as extra laxatives or nitrates for a patient without documented angina at rest (Garfinkel, Zur-Gil, & Ben-Israel, 2007). This and other studies have demonstrated that high medication burden, despite being used to improve health, can actually result in unnecessary functional impairment and even death, while decreasing drug burden can improve functionality significantly.

Assessment

Nurses have an exclusive place in the healthcare team when it comes to medications. They are the only member of the healthcare team that actually witnesses the patient's use and outcome of medications, at least in the institutional setting. One of the cornerstones of nursing education is patient assessment and the increased amount of time spent involved in face-to-face patient care, relative to other healthcare professionals. Nurses have extensive knowledge of the pharmacological aspects of the medication, including intended effect, side effects, administration, and monitoring parameters. Nurses have been administering, monitoring, educating, and documenting all components of medication use for decades. This is why nurses are in a position to make a significant contribution to combating the harms of medication misadventures. Many of the principles of medication and polypharmacy assessment are intuitive to nurses, and the following specific assessment skills can add to nursing's important role in minimizing polypharmacy harm.

Brown Bag Assessment

Many people have heard of the term brown bag medication assessment, which means that patients bring in all of the medications that they are currently taking, including OTCs, supplements, and herbals, to their clinic visits or hospitalizations for assessment. This method is far superior to relying on patient self-report, internal medical records, or transferred medical records from other providers. The only consistent factor throughout the healthcare system is the patient, and having the patient bring in what they are taking at that specific point in time is the most revealing way to assess medication use. The reliability of any one medical chart's drug list is unknown as changes happen between visits to various specialists, hospitals, and the primary physician, which are not always reflected in a transferred list. Sometimes, comparing various chart lists and physician consult summaries leads to even more confusion. Also, the chart medication lists omit quite a bit of over-the-counter use documentation.

The benefit of the *brown bag assessment*, other than being superior to self report, is that the clinician can see how many tablets or capsules are present versus the last time the medications were filled (date on label) to probe for adherence. If time permits, it is helpful to contact the patient's pharmacy (or pharmacies) and ask for a faxed drug list to compare to the medications brought in for the brown bag assessment. The patient can also be queried on how they take the medication and their knowledge of what the medications are for while viewing the medication, which is superior to asking about their medication use by name due to common memory and literacy challenges.

Gait and Frailty

Whenever possible, observation of the patient's functional ability is helpful in detecting potential MRPs. As discussed earlier, the physiological changes that occur with advanced age lead to changes in the way medications are metabolized, distributed, and take effect, and these changes can increase the risk of toxicity. Where an elder is on the spectrum of frailty is important to recognize when assessing for risk of poor medication outcomes. Observing ambulation is one of the most telling assessment tools in determination of frailty (Cesari et al., 2006). Geriatricians routinely use a test called the "get up and go" test, which has an elder seated in a chair with arms get out of the chair, walk several paces, and return to the chair. The clinician observes for ability to support themselves sitting, if they can stand without too much arm assistance, gait and balance, and ability to pivot and turn easily. Failure to perform any or all of these steps indicates possible sarcopenia and frailty.

Medication Adherence Rating Scales and Tests

There are numerous clinical tests for assessment of medication adherence, which may be useful in identifying physical and cognitive barriers to successful medication management; however, each one has limits in terms of validation in the literature for universal applicability and clinical practicality. For example, there are instruments that utilize the patient's own medications and there are some that utilize simulated medications, but there are no studies comparing these different types head-to-head to determine which type is more universally valid. Some instruments take up to 30 minutes or longer to perform, while some take 15 minutes, and whether these time requirements are clinically useful or not have not been studied. The instruments are measuring only cognitive and physical capacity to perform medication adherence; however, medication management and adherence is a very complex task that involves motivation and beliefs about each medication, perception of self-efficacy, ability to access medications, relationships with healthcare providers, and cultural and lifestyle factors. As such, the assessment instruments found in the literature currently could be utilized as a screen for physical and cognitive barriers to medication adherence and management but not necessarily as predictive of poor medication outcomes. The brown bag assessment, in addition to assessment of cognitive status utilizing common standard clinical tests such as the MMSE (Mini-Mental Status Exam) or CLOX (an executive clock-drawing task) (Folstein, Folstein, & McHugh, 1975; Royal, Cordes, & Polk, 1998), are more comprehensive than the medication screens currently found in the literature. The ultimate assessment is the in-home visit and assessment.

Take-Home Medical Administration Record

Occasionally, you will be faced with a patient for whom the brown bag assessment does not work. This might be a patient that brings you all of the medications they ever had from 20 years ago to date and cannot tell you what they are currently taking or not; or a patient who, in the middle of the assessment, starts to describe the "pink" pill that they forgot to bring in; or you are unable to get a list of prescribed medications from other healthcare provider due to HIPAA concerns, so you cannot complete the medication reconciliation. Is there an alternative method of medication reconciliation? There is: You can give the patient a homework assignment in the form of a take-home *medication administration record (MAR)*. This exercise can provide you with a few important bits of data with respect to ability to complete the assignment. It will either tell you that the patient has challenges with medication management (perhaps due to literacy, or cognition, or just complexity of regimen), or, hopefully, clarify what the patient is actually taking. Firstly, it forces the patient (or family) to list the medications taken daily and track days 1–31 regarding what was taken at what time of day. Instruct the patient or caregiver on how to fill it out, including how to document missed doses, and what efficacy and side effect items should be recorded, such as blood pressure, nocturia, sleeping patterns, or glucose levels. The patient and/or caregiver's ability to complete this record will give you some idea of their understanding of what the patient is taking, any problems with understanding the regimen, and how the medications are being used.

Literacy Screen

To successfully utilize today's healthcare system, the patient is required to understand, seek, and actively obtain health information, which can be rather complex at times. Add to that the heretofore described lack of one-on-one explanation and counseling about how to use medications, and the patient is left relying on one primary skill to follow instructions on how to safely use medications: reading. Reading labels and

Risk Factors **437**

information provided from the pharmacy about medications (OTC or prescription) is the main source of guidance on medication use. Medication information presented on an OTC package or patient information handout accompanying a prescription is quite complex. Therefore, even if a patient is well-educated, being able to digest the complex information provided in print about medications and act upon that information is quite a challenge; for the patient who has limited reading capacity, the challenge is even more formidable. Health literacy is composed of many contexts: the ability to extract, understand, and use health-related information (Ishikawa, Takeuchi, & Yano, 2008). There are numerous health literacy assessments that are validated but not used in the practical clinical setting because they take too much time to administer. If time allows, the 3-level HL Scale and the 3-brief SQs are the most comprehensive instruments to measure health literacy (Sayah, Williams, & Johnson, 2012). A brief screen that focuses on the reading component of health literacy is the SILS, or Single Item Literacy Screener, which consists of one question: *"How often do you need to have someone help you when you read instructions, pamphlets, or other written material from your doctor or pharmacy?"* Possible responses are *1-Never, 2-Rarely, 3-Sometimes, 4-Often, and 5-Always.* Scores greater than 2 are considered positive for some difficulty reading health-related material (Morris, MacLean, & Chew, 2006).

Swallowing Status

Swallowing status is a commonly overlooked aspect of assessment for MRPs. Screening for patients with swallowing difficulty should be a routine part of the assessment. The link between difficulty swallowing and medication crushing should be assessed. Patients often alter dosage forms at home by crushing and do not report it to their physicians. One study showed that 1 in every 4 doses administered in the nursing home setting contains an error (Haw, Stubbs, & Dickens, 2007), and the most common error was crushing medication inappropriately. How many patients crush or alter their medications at home is not well quantified, but it is likely that patients are less aware of the dangers of altering dosage forms than healthcare professionals. When a patient is experiencing toxicity or inefficacy relative to their medications, it could be simply because they are altering their tablets and capsules to be able to swallow them or other reasons. It is well-known to nurses that crushing a tablet, cutting a nonscored tablet in half, or breaking the seal of a capsule of long-acting products can result in a very high dose designed to be released over 12 to 24 hours being released all at once, resulting in toxicity. The difficulty comes in knowing what is alterable and what is not. In general, long-acting products that are given once daily or have an SR, XR, CR, or LA designation should not be crushed or split. Also, products that are toxic to the caregiver or patient upon contact should not be altered, such as chemotherapeutic agents (such as tamoxifen), hormonally active agents (such as finasteride), or an irritant (such as hydroxyurea). The following case illustrates two principles in assessment of MRPs: the importance of taking medication dosage form alterations into account and how the signs of medication harm can seem very disconnected from the causative medication (see **Case Study 11-3**).

Case Study 11-3: She Nearly Died From One Medication

M.C. was admitted to an skilled nursing facility for rehabilitation post-partial glossectomy for a recurrent carcinoma of the tongue. Her past medical history was significant for osteoarthritis, lupus, dizziness, syncope, falls, hypertension, osteoporosis, and hypothyroidism. Her medications were: Levothyroxine 75 mcg daily, Oyster-CalD 500 mg BID, Senna-S daily, Alendronate 70 mg weekly, Oxycodone/ Acetaminophen prn, Acetaminophen prn, and Milk of Magnesia. On 11/03/08, the nursing staff notified M.C.'s physicians of her complaints of a burning tongue and refusing food, resulting in weight loss and general decline. The team PharmD visited on 11/11/08 and when presented with the patient's complaint, noted the patient was refusing medication and food due to "bad taste" and "burning." Otherwise, she was cognitively intact with excellent postsurgical wound healing and absence of inflammation or exudates. Other common causes of glossitis had been excluded. Following a review of the nursing notes and medication record, a pattern of food refusal emerged. It appeared to be a weekly occurrence, coinciding with the scheduled dosing of alendronate, which can be caustic to the gastric and esophageal mucosa (Gonzalez-Moles & Bagan-Sebastian, 1999). The nursing staff confirmed adherence to appropriate alendronate administration, i.e., before breakfast with 8 oz. of water and remaining upright for 30 minutes. But, then the staff admitted that all tablets on two shifts were being crushed, despite lack of documentation of crushing in the MAR. The weekly dose of alendronate at 10 pm after dinner but right before going to bed was directly irritating the patient's buccal and esophageal mucosa. The nursing staffs were unaware and lacked training about crushing sustained release tablets, which was done routinely, and the dispensing pharmacy failed to provide any "Do Not Crush" labels. This is not surprising considering that one in every four doses administered in the nursing home setting contains an error, and the most common error was crushing medications inappropriately (Haw, Stubbs, & Dickens, 2007). Given the frequency with which patients in the long-term care setting have swallowing difficulties, coupled with the frequency of bisphosphonate use, this case is presented to alert others to this potentially life threatening scenario.

The challenge, even for healthcare professionals, is knowing which medications outside the obviously labeled SR, XR, SA, or CR are safe to crush. One place to look for information is the Institute for Safe Medication Practices (ISMP) at http://www.ismp.org. This website is an excellent resource for safe medication use and includes information on medication administration timeliness, high alert medications, and many other medication use tools. Specifically, they have a frequently updated "Do Not Crush" medication list, which lists medications not to be crushed and the reasons why. Another place to seek information on which medications are crushable and which are not is to consult references pertaining to tube feedings, as you will find lists of liquid alternatives as well as reviews of which tablets and capsules are safe to alter. Lastly, you can put a request in to your pharmacist and have them find the information for you if it is not already clearly labeled on the medication itself.

Collateral History: Adult Child or Caregiver

When taking a medication history with an elderly patient, it is not always easy to determine the influence of possible cognitive impairment. Whenever possible, try to get a caregiver or family member to corroborate the patient's report of medication use and side effects. It is not uncommon for elders who are experiencing functional decline with or without cognitive impairment to report that they are having no problems out of fear that they may lose autonomy and independence. Falls are perceived as a sign that they are growing old and dependent therefore elders hesitate to report falls to their family and physicians (Biderman, Cwikel, Fried, & Galinsky, 2002). Impaired ability to drive is another topic that can be medication-related that requires caregiver verification, as the elderly sometimes are unaware of their driving impairment or unwilling to report it. It may be necessary to ask the elderly patient's caregiver to keep an MAR or a log of symptoms, OTC use, and other medication-related data if they or the patient cannot accurately report this information.

Beers Criteria and START and STOPP Criteria

Some explicit criteria that provide information on potentially inappropriate medications (PIMs) for use in the elderly are available. The most popular of these are the *Beers criteria*, the *START criteria* (Screening Tool to Alert doctors to the Right Treatment) and the *STOPP criteria* (Screening Tool of Older People's potentially inappropriate Prescriptions). The Beers criteria was updated in 2012, and the new version includes 53 medications/drug classes divided into 3 categories: potentially inappropriate drugs in all older people, potentially inappropriate drugs in those with certain disease states, and drugs to be used with caution in older people (American Geriatric Society, 2012). The START and STOPP screening tools also address PIMs in the elderly and features a rather practical organizational structure that includes identification of excessive prescribing and prescribing oversight, categorized by physiological system, and recognizes high-risk groups such as patients with dementia or patients who fall (Barry, Gallagher, Ryan, & O'Mahony, 2007; Gallagher & O'Mahony, 2008). These are useful, educational references and each brings a different perspective on various mechanisms of medication harm in elders. While they do not list every single medication that can place an elder at risk, they cover the major categories and by referring them often, the clinician will eventually become familiar with the thought process behind identification of potentially inappropriate medication use in the elderly.

Diagnosis

Polypharmacy-induced harm and MRPs are typically diagnosed through deductive means. When presented with a patient experiencing a problem and trying to ascertain whether that problem is caused by medications, there are several items that are important to rule out. These items should be a routine part of the medication differential diagnosis. Firstly, patient adherence to the medication regimen documented and corrections to the patient medication list should be made. A common source of drug toxicity in the elderly—impaired renal drug clearance—should be assessed by calculating current estimated kidney function. Laboratory tests recommended in drug monographs should be performed routinely; however, due to the complexity of our healthcare system, the routine monitoring of labs is often overlooked. If obvious causes of MRPs cannot be detected and the problem persists, then a trial drug discontinuation, if possible, may reveal the source of the problem.

Laboratory Results

The following are some of the common diagnostic lab parameters that are assessed in working up a case of MRPs.

Complete Metabolic Panel and Basic Metabolic Panel. The complete metabolic panel (CMP) and basic metabolic panel (BMP) are essential tests used to monitor therapy when taking just about any medication. The CMP monitors kidney and liver function, glucose, calcium, protein levels, and electrolyte and fluid balance, while the BMP monitors kidney function, glucose, calcium, and electrolyte and fluid balance. When medications known to cause electrolyte imbalances, such as diuretics, are being used, BMPs should be performed weekly for 2–3 weeks when starting therapy and periodically once stable on the new diuretic. Most recommendations on how often to monitor BMP while taking diuretics state "periodically" after the initial weeks of use (where monitoring occurs frequently). This nonspecific time interval is confusing to clinicians and leaves the time period in between electrolyte, fluid, and kidney function assessment open to individual clinician interpretation. In elderly and frail patients, the most conservative course of action is best because in the elderly, dangerous changes in electrolyte levels can occur abruptly, because elders have less homeostatic reserve, and because they are subjected to numerous new medications added to their daily regimen and sometimes have inconsistent food and fluid intake. So, "periodically" in a relatively healthy younger adult taking a diuretic could safely be interpreted as every 6 months to 1 year after stable on the diuretic therapy, but in an elder could mean every 2–3 months depending on how many other comorbidities and medications are involved.

There are instances when an abnormality may show up on the BMP or CMP that seems very unrelated and distant from the medications the patient is taking. For example, you might expect that patients taking vitamin D do not need a CMP because the only lab monitoring necessary would be vitamin D levels, but a CMP still needs to be monitored because aggressive vitamin D supplementation can result in sudden changes in calcium.

Various laboratory tests are mandated per the FDA drug monograph for each particular medication. Some common medications requiring lab monitoring are listed in **Table 11-1**.

Medication	Tests	Reason
Amiodarone	TSH, LFT, Serum Creatinine & Creatinine Kinase (CPK)	Hypo- or hyperthyroid levels. Hepatotoxicity (fatal at times), Rhabdomyolysis
Valproic acid	CMP, CBC, Serum Drug Levels (albumin, serum protein)	Hyponatremia, SIADH, pancytopenia, thrombocytopenia, hepatotoxicity
Phenytoin	Serum Creatinine (initiation of therapy), CBC, LFTs, Serum Drug Levels (albumin, serum protein)	Hepatotoxicity, leukopenia, agranlucytosis, pancytopenia, megaloblastic anemia, no loading dose with renal impairment
ASA, Naproxen, Celecoxib,	Serum Creatinine, CBC, gFOBT (fecal occult blood test)	Renal impairment, GI bleeds
Warfarin	PT/INR, CBC, gFBOT	Monitor INR target, GI bleeds
Statin Therapy	CPK, lipid panel, baseline LFTs	Rhabdomyolysis, LFT at baseline, monitor need for statin and efficacy

TABLE 11-1   Commonly Utilized Medications That Should be Monitored Closely in Elders

Source: See FDA drug monograph (package insert) under prescribing information for detailed explanation.

Lastly, one of the most common polypharmacy-related complaints is memory or cognitive impairment. If a patient presents with these complaints, in addition to assessment for the obvious medication-induced causes such as strongly anticholinergic medications, it is important to rule out common organic causes such as hypothyroidism and vitamin deficiencies. Elders should have their TSH, B12, and folate level assessed when working up the complaint of cognitive impairment.

Cockroft and Gault Creatinine Clearance

Many medications have an FDA drug monograph recommendation for renal adjustment, even some that would not be suspected such as medications that are perceived to be only of concern for hepatic clearance like lovastatin, rosuvastatin, or simvastatin. On lab reports, the renal function is reported in glomerular filtration rate, or GFR. Creatinine clearance is a way of approximating GFR, but it is important to recognize that the GFR reported on most hospital and outpatient lab reports is not the same as the renal function estimation that the FDA uses for drug dose adjustments. The FDA has adopted the Cockroft and Gault method as the standard upon which dose recommendations are based. Creatinine clearance can be calculated by several methods: the Modification of Diet in Renal Disease (MDRD) formula, which has been considered a very accurate estimate of GFR although it underestimates GFR in obese patients while overestimates GFR in underweight patients; the Salazar method, which is validated to be more accurate in obese patients; and many others. The important point when determining dose adjustments for medication is to use the Cockroft and Gault method because that is the basis for the FDA dose adjustment recommendations (U.S. Department of Health and Human Services [U.S. DHHS], 2012). It makes little sense to use other GFR estimations when they are irrelevant to the Cockroft and Gault values reported in the FDA recommendations (see **Figure 11-6**).

Cockroft and Gault Method

A method of estimating renal function

[creatinine clearance ml/min]

$$CrCl_{men} = \frac{(140 - Age) \times LBW^*}{Scr \times 72}$$

$(CrCl_{women} = CrCl_{men} \times 0.85)$

Always use Cockroft and Gault equation because all FDA drug monographs are standardized to C&G.

*Use Lean Body Weight (Ideal Body Weight), especially in elders with poor muscle mass

LBW: Lean Body Weight in Kg

CrCl: Creatinine Clearance in mL/min

SCr: Serum creatinine in mg/dL

Figure 11-6 Cockroft and Gault equation.

Abbreviated Morisky Scale

(A Screen for Medication Behaviors & Adherence)

1. Do you ever forget to take your medicine?
2. Are you careless at time about taking your medicine?
3. When you feel better, do you sometimes stop taking your medicine?
4. Sometimes if you feel worse when you take the medicine, do you stop taking it?

Scoring: high to low; yes=0, no=1
The lower the score, the more likely further medication use assessment is warranted.

Figure 11-7 The abbreviated Morisky scale to assess medication use behavior. It consists of four questions and a higher score estimate is correlated with better adherence.

Source: Morisky, Green, Levine, 1986.

Diagnosing Problems with Medication-Taking Behavior

Medication adherence and behavior assessment is a key part of detecting MRPs and polypharmacy-related potential harm. Medication adherence is the degree to which the patient is actually taking the total prescribed medication regimen, while medication-taking behavior involves the decisions a patient makes and acts upon related to the use of their medication regimen. Medication-taking behavior is influenced by patient beliefs, attitudes, preferences, experiences, and goals related to drug therapy.

The brown bag method is a thorough and time-consuming method of assessment, but should be performed at least annually, with results documented in the patient's chart, because it is for now the gold standard for office assessment of medication use (though in-home visits are the ultimate medication assessment setting). For brief patient encounters, a widely accepted medication-taking behavior screen that can be a means of assessing adherence is a four-item question sequence called the Abbreviated Morisky Scale (an eight-item scale exists as well) (Morisky, Green, & Levine, 1986) (see **Figure 11-7**).

Trial Discontinuations

A carefully considered trial discontinuation of a medication is one of the best ways to diagnose an MRP. For example, if a patient is experiencing generalized muscle pain or memory impairment while taking a statin, it would be of no harm to discontinue the medication for a few days and see if the muscle pain or cognition improves. A study showed that atorvastatin can be discontinued in patients who have stable cardiovascular status for up to 6 weeks and it does not appear to increase the risk of cardiac events (McGowan, 2004). The type of medication considered is of most importance. For example, warfarin trial discontinuation would not be performed without very careful consideration of the risks versus benefit in light of the INR and side effects such as bleeding, and a maintenance psychoactive medication requires careful tapering to avoid precipitation of seizures. But there are some instances in which a trial discontinuation would be easy to implement safely. If a patient were utilizing OTC products that seem to correlate with possible side effect symptoms, then a trial discontinuation would be in order. The discontinuation of multiple medications at the same time is not a good practice and ordinarily reserved for emergency situations such as life-threatening *delirium* in a frail elder, and then medications are typically cut down to a minimal number.

Interventions and Strategies for Care

Polypharmacy is one of the few reversible and preventable causes of iatrogenic harm. The challenge is that reversing and preventing medication-related problems requires careful monitoring, medication use, and prescribing. This ongoing process requires provider and patient awareness, education, and accountability; tracking and reconciliation of the processes of medication use; follow up; information transfer; and patient and family education and engagement. There is a striking similarity to the challenge of coordinating transitions of care and the silent harm that lack of thoughtful transitions of care causes (National Transitions of Care Coalition [NTOCC], 2008). Strategies for intervention should include addressing psychological functioning, physiological functioning, cultural factors, health literacy and linguistic factors, financial factors, spiritual and religious functioning, physical and environmental safety, and family and community support. All of the above factors impact a person's relationship to medications and how utilization occurs.

The following strategies for intervention can help lower the risk of polypharmacy and medication misadventures.

Decrease the Number of Unnecessary or Harmful Medications

To decrease polypharmacy, start with matching each medication to one or more of the patient's diagnoses and do your best to verify the right medication is being used for a valid purpose. There can be more than one medication for a particular diagnosis or more than one diagnosis for a particular medication (i.e., lisinopril for hypertension and renal protection in diabetic patients); however, there should not be any medications being used without good reason (see **Figure 11-8**). Any leftover or unmatched medication that the patient is taking should be considered for discontinuation after verification that it is not necessary. For example, patients often get started

> **Notable Quotes**
>
> "Any symptom in an elderly patient should be considered a drug side effect until proven otherwise."
>
> —J. Gurwitz, Brown University Long-Term Care Quality Letter, 1995.

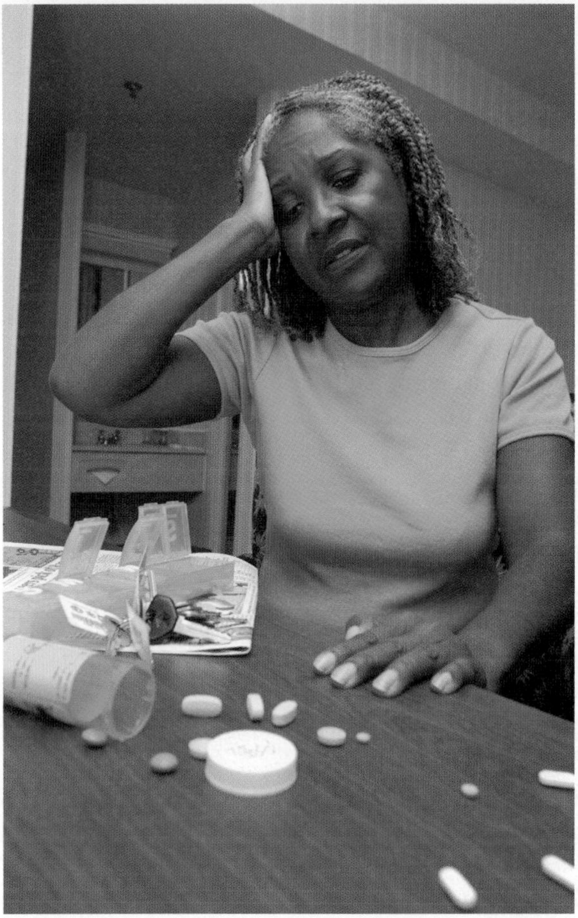

Figure 11-8 Failure to take medications or attend to other health needs can be a sign that an older adult lacks motivation to adhere to the medication regimen.

on stomach acid suppression therapy (AST) in the hospital as a precaution against stress ulcers; the AST often gets carried forward after hospitalization without a specific diagnosis such as peptic ulcer disease, gastroesophageal reflux, or esophagitis that necessitates AST use. Occasionally, a diagnosis will get attached to the discharge AST just because clinic staff or a provider makes the assumption that it must be used for gastroesophageal reflux. The challenging facet of this exercise is to verify diagnosis, which as described in Case Study 11-1 of this chapter, can be inaccurate.

Another common "diagnosis" which is often not accurate is a patient's allergy list. Sometimes people are listed as being allergic to a medication when they actually perceived a bad experience or got a transient upset stomach (or coincidental nausea) with a particular medication; they are not truly allergic in the sense of anaphylaxis, rashes, and hives. Just as medications have to be matched to a diagnosis, allergies should be matched as closely as possible to a verifiable contraindication to taking a particular medication. The reason this practice helps fight polypharmacy is that occasionally you will get a patient who has a list of 10 allergies, which means they have to take a dangerous alternative medication or multiple suboptimal medications when, in fact, one of the safer medications on the allergy list might actually be tolerable.

Another method for decreasing the number of medications a patient needs to manage and be exposed to is to review the medications and question what is wanted versus needed. There are clearly medications that serve a necessary purpose and are needed for the well-being of the patient. For example, a patient with atrial fibrillation who is taking warfarin to prevent a stroke, despite being a patient who falls frequently and is not at higher risk of bleeds from the warfarin than usual (the oldest old patients and most frail patients), still has a better benefit-to-risk ratio on warfarin than off. Sometimes, however, patients are taking medications that are not so necessary because their *family* wants them to take it or they harbor a false belief that the medication is necessary and/or safe. These drugs are more wanted than needed for patient well-being and the clinician trying to lower MRP risk should evaluate, document, and address this issue. **Case Study 11-4** illustrates a situation where, despite many compelling reasons to discontinue medications that the family wanted for the patient, ultimately the family would keep the questionable medications. This

Case Study 11–4: When Drugs That Are a "Want" Are Used Over Drugs That Are a "Need"

K.L. is an 88-year-old female living at home with her daughter, who is a single mother and works full time. K.L.'s daughter, L.C., is not ready to place her mother in a care home and says that she can handle her mother's rising need for hospitalization and increased care burden. K.L. was recently hospitalized for confusion and suffering a severe fall, which did not result in any broken bones. Her fall was due to multifactorial causes including dehydration, overmedication for hypertension (inappropriate blood pressure goals), and the psychoactive medications she was taking. L.C. has come to take her mother home from the hospital. K.L.'s confusion has improved, and her fluid status has been addressed. L.C. was not accepting of the medication changes made by the medical team.

L.C. stated that she would not take her mother home without the quetiapine and lorazepam

because she cannot sleep at night due to her mother's behaviors, which included wandering. The medical team explained that quetiapine and lorazepam were discontinued due to their likely contribution to K.L.'s fall and the inappropriateness of indication. They explained that the use of antipsychotics, in particular in the elderly, for behaviors related to dementia is an off-label use and reserved for severe agitation, restlessness, and behaviors leading to potential harm of the patient. The increased mortality risk inherent with the use of antipsychotic agents in the elderly was explained, especially in light of her mother's compromised cardiac status due to age and lifelong history of cardiovascular disease. The team also explained that mirtazapine and trazodone would function to calm her mother in addition to starting donepezil, which may decrease her episodes of confusion.

Ultimately, L.C. stood by her desire to keep her mother on quetiapine and lorazepam because she felt that without those medications, she couldn't manage to keep her mother at home and still work herself. She also stated that K.L. had been taking them for 2 years already without incident, and that they left their new PCP because he tried to discontinue the same medications 2 months ago. The team had L.C. sign a consent form for the quetiapine discharge prescription (since it is an off-label use) and documented in the discharge summary that L.C. had been advised about the risks of using lorazepam despite K.L.'s fall risk and that L.C. stated she was going to get lorazepam anyway from her physician in the community if they didn't provide it at discharge. The team then discontinued the trazodone and mirtazepine discharge orders.

Medications upon admission	Medications upon discharge
Lisinopril 20 mg daily	Lisinopril 20 mg daily
Hydrochlorothiazide 25 mg daily	Metoprolol XL 25 mg daily
Atenolol 100 mg daily	Donepezil 5 mg (follow up in office next week)
Quietiapine 25 mg BID	Mirtazapine 7.5 mg at HS
Lorazepam 1 mg at HS	Trazodone 50 mg prn at HS
Amlodipine 10 mg daily	
Atorvastatin 40 mg daily	

case also illustrates the limitations of managing medication use in the outpatient setting and the role of the clinician in attempting to implement ethical practices that are not always accepted by the patient or his/her caregiver. The clinician's role in this scenario is to take the effort to explain the risks and try to change the riskier medications to less risky medications. If that fails, it is important to document the attempt and outcome in the medical record. The use of consent forms for high-risk medications is a practice that is gaining in use, although it is not common, though it is used more frequently in the nursing home setting, where lawsuits are increasingly targeting the use of antipsychotics and high-risk medications.

The decision about which medications are necessary and which are not is a complex one. To help you understand more about appropriateness and risks of medications in the elderly, it is useful to make use of point-of-care apps on your smart phone or computer (such as Epocrates, Lexicomp, or Micromedex) or use online databases such as Drugs.com, or RxList. At first, it will be tedious to look up medications, but over time, you will become familiar with the common medications utilized by the elderly and how risks apply to their age group.

Appropriate Choices and Doses

How do clinicians know what are appropriate medications and doses for use in elders? Some medications are widely known as being high risk in the elderly. For example, medications new to market are notorious for bringing harm to the elderly and most geriatricians recommend waiting 5–7 years post-marketing of a new drug before using in the elderly. This allows the FDA to gather postmarketing data, which includes more elders than the safety and efficacy trials. Checking for appropriate dose in the elderly is another way to catch medications at high-risk for inappropriate dosing use before it is too late. Do not forget the saying "start low and go slow" when increasing doses in elders. The point-of-care apps and medication databases will often specifically state what doses are considered appropriate in the elderly in addition to listing monitoring parameters of particular importance in elders.

As described earlier, matching the diagnosis list to the medications taken helps sort out unnecessary from necessary medication. The next thing to do is scan for medications that are known to cause problems in the elderly. Are any of the medications discussed in the Beers criteria or START and STOPP assessment tools? Are there any medications that commonly cause electrolyte imbalances, such as diuretics? Any that can cause confusion, such as motion sickness treatments or sedating antihistamines? Many medication reference databases will at least note which medications, when used in the elderly, require caution. The recommendations are not very specific, because medications are not specifically tested in elders very often, but when cautions are listed under the category "geriatric patients," as clinicians we should look further at specific monitoring parameters and both common and uncommon side effects to extrapolate the reasons why cautions are issued with respect to the use in elders. The START, STOPP, and Beers assessment references are more specific with regard to dose, type of medication, and which clinical scenario is appropriate.

Periodic assessment of the goals of care should be performed for the elderly. The goals of care in the elderly may be quite different than the goals of care in a middle-aged adult. Also, goals of care in an elderly patient can change from decade to decade or even year to year, so consideration of goals of care should be a part of all medication assessments. Commonly, elders are subjected to unnecessary medication risks because their prescribers have not taken into consideration that the goals of care for an elder may be quite different than that of a younger patient and that the risk-versus-benefit ratio may be unfavorable for an elder who is frail and taking a heavy medication burden. A example illustrating this point was the surprising outcome of the Action to Control Cardiovascular Risk in Diabetes (ACCORD) trial (Dluhy, 2008). The ACCORD trial looked at blood pressure, lipids, and glucose control in diabetics aged 40 to 79 who had been diagnosed with type 2 diabetes mellitus for an average of 10 years. One of the clinical questions they were trying to answer was: Would very tight control of blood glucose, HA1c < 6%, result in reduced cardiovascular events in patients with established cardiovascular (CV) disease or additional CV risk factors? The intensive glucose control group had a higher mortality rate than the standard care group, particularly the arm over 65 years of age. The higher mortality rate in the over-65 years intensive therapy group resulted in a halting of the study in the over 65 age group intensive therapy arm of the study. It is thought that the drug side effects and combinations were major contributors to the poor outcomes in this study arm. The ACCORD study outcome illustrates the risk of any type of extreme therapy due to the untested nature of combinations of doses and drugs in older patients with varying degrees of disease and physiological compromise. Also as a result of this and other studies, the American Diabetes Association and American Geriatrics Society (AGS) have recommended that HA1c targets be "individualized," while the AGS also recommends a HA1c target of 8 for older, frailer patients with a life expectancy of less than 5 years, the reason being that the goals of preventing end organ damage due to diabetes mellitus (hyperglycemia) is not as important as protecting people in that group from hypoglycemia, which can lead to dementia, worsening of cognition, and other serious neurological impairments. In considering interventions for polypharmacy, for each medication the questions of what the long-term goal of the medication use is versus the person's life expectancy, balanced with quality of life and potential risk of side effects, should be considered.

Foster Medication Literacy

During the assessment of your patient's understanding of medication purpose, dosing, and side effects, it may become evident that a medication literacy challenge exists. The traditional method of verbally reviewing the medication regimen before discharging the patient from care may or may not work. A few additional steps and repetition of information may provide improved medication understanding for success in home medication management. Patients who track their medication by color and pill size should be redirected towards the medication name and purpose, which should be repeatedly explained if necessary (and presented in written form) (see **Box 11-2**). The problem with identification of medications by size, shape, and color is that at any time a generic substitution could occur and the same medication may look totally different with the next refill. If size, shape, and color are the only means by which a patient can track medication, it would be advisable to set the patient up with routine medication checks in which they bring in all of their medications monthly and are coached on which one to take at the appropriate time and in the appropriate manner.

Creating a medication administration sheet that lists what should be taken when and any precautions, such as with or without food, is a useful tool to help patients increase their medication literacy. Having clear and simple written material is an especially important cue for patients with cognitive impairment. One place to find free downloadable medication record sheet templates is the Microsoft Office website: http://office.microsoft.com/en-us/templates/medication-log-TC102826189.aspx

For patients who have very limited reading ability, it is advisable to use the simpler forms and draw symbols in wherever possible instead of words (i.e., instead of P.M., draw the moon, instead of A.M., draw the sun).

A patient's feelings of self-efficacy and beliefs about medication use have a profound impact on their success or failure in using medications. Medication prioritization, which is when patients adhere to the medications that they perceive work as opposed to those that seem to have no effect, can occur. Medications which are easily perceived as effective by patients include pain medications

---

BOX 11-2   Research Highlight

Aim: The aim of this study was to examine the impact of a self-administration of medication program (SAMP) on the competence of elderly hospital inpatients to manage medications.

Methods: The SAMP was made up of three stages: education, progressing to supervised self-administration, and then to independent self-administration. The Drug Regimen Unassisted Grading Scale (DRUGS) was used by the nursing staff and pharmacist to assess patients' ability to successfully manage medications. Adherence behaviors related to medications were also measured.

Findings: The sample was rather small (a pilot study) consisting of 24 patients, mainly female,

high functioning, and with a mean age of about 77 years. They had 9 medications to manage. Twenty-two of the 24 participants were successful in completing the SAMP.

Application to practice: An inpatient SAMP did improve the ability of older adult patients to competently manage and adhere to their medication regimen.

Source: Lam, P., Elliott, R. E., & George, J. (2011). Impact of a self-administration of medications programme on elderly inpatients' competence to manage medications: a pilot study. *Journal of Clinical Pharmacy and Therapeutics, 36*, 80–86.

or sleep aids, which, when taken, result in a noticeable effect of somnolence or relief from pain. A hypoglycemic agent used by a patient who measures their blood glucose routinely can be seen as efficacious if their blood glucose measurements are on target when taking the medication and not when the medication dose is missed. Theses sorts of medication experiences will result in the most adherence and be prioritized by the patient because they perceive that taking the medication is providing a positive outcome. Medications that do not provide a measurable obvious effect are more challenging when it comes to adherence (Rifkin et al., 2010).

Patients who take blood pressure medications but do not track their blood pressure, or who take statins for lipid level control, may skip doses because they usually feel the same whether they take these medications or not. As healthcare providers, health literacy can be promoted regarding patient medications in terms of expected effects, monitoring for efficacy, and side effects of the medication, which in turn will foster adherence and more effective medication use.

Access to Medications

You might discover that patients alter their medication regimen because they cannot afford their medications. This occurs often during the Medicare D "doughnut hole" time of the year (typically July until the end of the year), when Medicare D beneficiaries hit a maximum prescription coverage spending limit that stops their coverage but then picks up above a much higher amount. The patient has to cover the costs of medications on their own for a few months and sometimes until the beginning of the new year, when the benefit cycle starts again. The "doughnut hole" coverage gap is supposed to be eliminated by the year 2020.

One cause of poor Medicare D coverage and a shorter time to reaching the "doughnut hole" is if an elder enrolled in Medicare D misses the opportunity every year from October 15th to December 7th for open enrollment. During open enrollment, it is prudent for community-dwelling seniors enrolled in Medicare D to go online with their current medication list at hand, at the following website: http://plancompare.medicare.gov/pfdn/FormularyFinder/LocationSearch.

This website allows seniors or caregivers to compare plan coverage for their specific medications to find the plan that offers the best coverage. The coverage changes frequently (usually annually), which is why it is important to review coverage and make use of open enrollment to switch into a better plan if possible. Elders residing in long-term care facilities can switch plans on a monthly basis, as opposed to community dwellers who may only switch during open enrollment. (Note: Not all seniors have Medicare D, especially if their retirement benefits offer better coverage.)

There are other options to aid coverage of medications. The first is to make use of the pharmacies that offer a $4 or discount formulary. These formularies differ from pharmacy to pharmacy, but the lists for each pharmacy should be online. Some offer a 30-day supply of some generics for $4, 90 days for $10, and there are even some pharmacies who offer a free 10-day supply of select antibiotics. Typically, mail order pharmacies offer a 90-day supply for a 1-month copay. For medications that are not on most formularies and are very expensive, there are patient assistance programs available through the pharmaceutical companies. There are also copay assistance programs and low-income subsidy programs that patients can apply for and are easily located by searching the Internet. Patients and providers can go to http://www.partnersind.com (an outreach and education program led by California pharmacy schools), to learn more about Medicare Part D resources.

Summary

In elderly patients, the likelihood that a medication will cause some harm or impairment is heightened by impaired physiology, heavy medication burden, and increased inappropriate medication use by both the healthcare system and the patient. The complex considerations involved in fostering the appropriate use of each medication are often overlooked by all. Nurses are in a special place to make a positive impact by assessing for MRPs and intervening to improve medication outcomes. This chapter covers many aspects of medication misadventure, and it may seem overwhelming, but with application of even a few interventions to identify and fight MRPs, patient outcomes can be markedly improved. The healthcare system needs to take on the problem of MRPs, but until it does, individual clinicians can help by developing some interventions that work in their practice setting and by teaching others about how to assess and impact MRPs using the techniques found in this chapter.

Critical Thinking Exercises

1. **You are working in a nursing home** and caring for two women with the same initials. They look alike and both have middle-stage dementia, so they are not reliable with giving their names. The nursing home does not allow name bands. How will you identify each resident when you go to deliever medications? What strategies could help prevent a medication error from occurring in this situation?

2. **You observe the morning labs from one of your 89-year-old patients** who is being assessed for renal failure. The serum creatinine is only slightly off normal. What is a better and more accurate way to estimate the patient's renal function prior to giving medications that are renally cleared and why?

3. **What are the most likely times** that an older person will experience side effects from a medication? Why are these times that the nurse should be extra vigilant?

Personal Reflection

1. Think about the American Nurses Association Code of Ethics. According to the *Code of Ethics for Nurses*, what is your obligation if you know that a medication error has been made? What principles are upheld in the daily work of administering medications?

2. Have you ever made a medication error? What did you do about it? What effect did it have on the patient or resident? On you as the care provider? Can you identify what you would have done differently to prevent the error?

3. How will you use the information in this chapter to provide better care related to medications and older adults? What helpful piece(s) of information can you immediately apply to your clinical practice?

References

Alvarez, M., & Evidente, V. (2008). Understanding drug-induced Parkinsonism: Separating pearls from oysters. *Neurology, 70*(8), e32–34.

American Geriatrics Society [AGS] 2012 Beers Criteria Update Expert Panel. (2012). American Geriatrics Society updated Beers criteria for inappropriate medication use in older adults. *Journal of American Geriatric Society, 60*(4), 616–631.

Bahr, J., Lackner, T., & Pacala, J. T. (2008) Amiodarone-induced central nervous system toxicity in the frail geriatric patient: A case report and review of the literature. *Annals of Long Term Care, 16*(8), 37–40.

Barry, P. J., Gallagher, P., Ryan, C., & O'Mahony, D. (2007). START (screening tool to alert doctors to the right treatment)—An evidence-based screening tool detect prescribing omissions in elderly patients. *Age and Ageing, 36*(6), 632–638.

Bateman, D. N. (2004). Digoxin-specific antibody fragments: how much and when? *Toxicology Review, 23*, 135–143.

Berenson, R. (2010). *The Medicare chronic care improvement program*. Retrieved from http://www.urban .org/publications/900714.html#n1

Biderman, A., Cwikel, J., Fried, A.V., & Galinsky, D. (2002). Depression and falls among community dwelling elderly people: A search for common risk factors. *Journal of Epidemiology Community Health, 56*, 631–636.

Bootman, J. L., Harrison, D. L., & Cox, E. (1997). The health care cost of drug-related morbidity and mortality in nursing facilities. *Archive of Internal Medicine, 157*, 2089–2096.

Budnitz, D. S., Lovegrove, M. C., & Shehab, N. (2011). Emergency hospitalizations for adverse drug events in older Americans. *New England Journal of Medicine, 365*(21), 2002–2012.

Campbell, N., Boustani, M., Limbil, T., Ott, C., Fox, C., Maidment, I.,…Gulati, R. (2009). The cognitive impact of anticholinergics: A clinical review. *Clinical Interventions in Aging, 4*, 225–233.

Caracciolo, B., Gatz, M., Xu, W., Pedersen, N. L., & Fratiglioni, L. (2012). Differential distribution of subjective and objective cognitive impairment in the population: A nationwide twin-study. *Journal of Alzheimer's Disease, 29*(2), 393–403. doi: 10.3233/JAD-2011-111904.

Centers for Disease Control and Prevention [CDC]. (2012). *Centers for Disease Control leading cause of death 2010*. Retrieved from http://www.cdc.gov/nchs/fastats/lcod.htm

Cesari, M., Leeuwenburgh, C., Lauretani, F., Onder, G., Bandinelli, S., Maraldi, C., & Guralnik, J. M. (2006). Frailty syndrome and skeletal muscle: Results from the invecciare in chianti study. *American Journal of Clinical Nutrition, 83*(5), 1142–1148.

Chancellor, M. B., Staskin, D. R., Kay, G. G., Sandage, B. W., Oefelein, M. G., & Tsao, J. W. (2012). Blood–brain barrier permeation and efflux exclusion of anticholinergics used in the treatment of overactive bladder. *Drugs & Aging, 29*(4), 259–273.

Davis, T. C., Wolf, M. S., Bass, P. F, 3rd, Thompson, J. A., Tilson, H. H., Neuberger, M., & Parker, R.M. (2006). Literacy and misunderstanding prescription drug labels. *Annal of InternalMedicine, 145,* 887–894.

Denham, M .J. (1990). Adverse drug reactions. *British Medical Bulletin, 46,* 53–62.

Dluhy, R. G., & McMahon, G. T. (2008). Intensive glycemic control in the ACCORD and ADVANCE trials. *New England Journal of Medicine, 358,* 2545–2559.

Ferenczi, E. A., Asaria, P., Hughes, A. D., Chaturvedi, N., & Francis, D. P. (2010). Can a statin neurtralize the cardiovascular risk of unhealthy dietary choices? *American Journal of Cardiology, 106*(4), 587–592.

Folstein, M. F., Folstein, S. E., & McHugh, P.R. (1975) "Mini-Mental State:" A practical method for grading the cognitive state of patients for the clinician. *Journal of Psychiatric Research, 12,* 189–198.

Gallagher, P., & O'Mahony, D. (2008). STOPP (screening tool of older persons' potentially inappropriate prescriptions): Application to acutely ill elderly patients and comparison with Beers' criteria. *Age and Ageing, 37*(6), 673–679.

Garfinkel, D., Zur-Gil, S., & Ben-Israel, J. (2007). The war against polypharmacy: A new cost-effective geriatric-palliative approach for improving drug therapy in disabled elderly people. *Israel Medical Association Journal, 9,* 430–434.

Gill, S. S., Anderson, G. M., Fischer, H. D., Bell, C. M., Li, P., Normand, S. L., & Rochon, P. A. (2009). Syncope and its consequences in patients with dementia receiving cholinesterase inhibitors: A population-based cohort study. *Archive of Internal Medicine, 169*(9), 867– 873.

Gonzalez-Moles M. A., & Bagan-Sebastian J. V. (1999). Alendronate-related oral mucosa ulcerations. *Journal of Oral Pathology and Medicine, 29*(10), 514–518.

Gu, Q., Dillon, C. F., & Burt, V. L. (2010). Prescription drug use continues to increase: U.S. prescription drug data for 2007–2008. *NCHS Data Brief, 42,* 1–8.

Gurwitz, J. H. (1995). Investigating polypharmacy presents numerous opportunities for problem solving. *Brown University Long-Term Care Quality Letter, 7*(9), 1.

Hall, J. R., Hoa, V. T., Johnson, L. A., Barber, R. C., & O'Bryant, S. E. O. (2011). The link between cognitive measures and ADLs and IADL functioning in mild Alzheimer's: What has gender got to do with it? *International Journal of Alzheimer Disease.* Advance online publication. doi:10.4061/2011/276734.

Haw, C., Stubbs, J., & Dickens, G. (2007). An observational study of medication administration errors in old-age psychiatric inpatients. *International Journal of Qualitative Health Care, 4*(19), 210–216.

Hilmer, S. N., Mager, D. E., Simonsick, E. M., Cao, Y., Ling, S. M., Windham, B. G., ... Abernethy, D. R. (2007). A drug burden index to define the functional burden of medications in older people. *Archive of Internal Medicine, Volume, 167*(8), 781–787.

Holmen, K., Ericsson, K., & Winblad, B. (2000). Social and emotional loneliness among nondemented and demented elderly people. *Archives of Gerontology and Geriatrics, 31*(3), 177–192.

Inouye, S. K., Stuenski S., Tinetti, M. E., & Kuchel, G. A. (2007). Geriatric syndromes: Clinical, research and policy implications of a core geriatric concept. *Journal of the American Geriatric Society, 55*(5), 780–791.

Ishikawa, H., Takeuchi, T., & Yano, E. (2008). Measuring functional, communicative, and communicative, and critical health literacy among diabetic patients. *Diabetes Care, 31,* 874–879.

Kaiser Foundation. (2010). *Retail prescription drugs filled by pharmacies (annual capita per age) 2010.* Retrieved from http://www.statehealthfacts.org/comparemapdetail.jsp?ind=268&cat=5&sub=66&yr=138&typ=1

Kim, D. H., Brown, R. A., Ding, E. L., Kiel, D. P., & Berry, S. D. (2011). Dementia medications and risk of falls, syncope, and related adverse events: Meta-analysis of randomized controlled trials. *Journal of the American Geriatrics Society, 59,* 1019–1031.

Kohn, L., Corrigan, J., & Donaldson, M. (1999). *To err is human: Building a safer health system.* Washington, DC: National Academies Press.

Lam, P., Elliott, R. E., & George, J. (2011). Impact of a self-administration of medications programme on elderly inpatients' competence to manage medications: A pilot study. *Journal of Clinical Pharmacy and Therapeutics, 36,* 80–86.

Lazarou, J., Pomeranz, B. H., & Corey, P. N. (1998). Incidence of adverse drug reactions in hospitalized patients. *Journal of the American Medical Association, 279,* 1200–1205.

Lu, C. J., & Tune, L. (2003). Chronic exposure to anticholinergic medications adversely affects the course of Alzheimer's Disease. *American Journal of Geriatric Psychiatry, 11*, 458–461.

Marcum, Z. A., Amuan, M. E., Hanlon, J. T., Aspinall, S. L., Handler, S. M., Ruby, C. M., & Pugh, M. J. (2012). Prevalence of unplanned hospitalizations caused by adverse drug reactions in older veterans. *Journal of the American Geriatric Society, 60*(1), 34–41.

Masoodi, N. A. (2008). Polypharmacy: To err is human, to correct divine. *British Journal of Medical Practioners, 1*(1), 6–9.

McGowan, M. P. (2004). There is no evidence for an increase in acute coronary syndromes after short-term abrupt discontinuation of statins in stable cardiac patients. *Circulation, 110*, 2333–2335.

Mellor, K., Ahme, D., & Thomson, A. (2009). Tramadol hydrocholirde use and acute deterioration in Parkinson's disease tremor. *Movement Disorders, 24*(4), 622–623.

Metlay, J. P., Cohen, A., Polsky, D., Kimmel, S. E., Koppel, R., & Hennessy, S. (2005). Medication safety in older adults: home-based practice patterns. *Journal of the American Geriatric Society, 53*(6), 976–982.

Morisky, D. E., Green, L. W., & Levine, D. M. (1986). Concurrent and predictive validity of a self-reported measure of medication adherence. *Medical Care, 24*(1), 67–74.

Morris, L. A., Tabak, E. R., & Gondek, K. (1997). Counseling patients about prescribed medication: 12-year trends. *Medical Care, 35*, 996–1007.

Morris, N. S., MacLean, C. D., & Chew, L. D. (2006) The single item literacy screener: Evaluation of a brief instrument to identify limited reading ability. *British Medical Council Family Practice, 7*, 21. doi: 10.1186/1471-2296-7-21.

National Audit Office [NAO]. (2005). *A safer place for patients: Learning to improve patient safety.* Retrieved from http://www.nao.org.uk/publications/0506/a_safer_place_for_patients.aspx

National Transitions of Care Coalition. (2008). *Transitions of care measures 2008.* Retrieved from http://www.ntocc.org/Portals/0/PDF/Resources/TransitionsOfCare_Measures.pdf

Permpongkosol, S. (2011). Iatrogenic disease in the elderly: Risk factors, consequences and prevention. *Clinical Interventions in Aging, 6*, 77–82.

Peron, E. P., Gray, S. L., & Hanlon, J. T. (2011). Medication use and functional status decline in older adults: A narrative review. *The American Journal of Geriatric Pharmacotherapy, 9* (6), 378–391.

Physicians' Desk Reference. (1969). *PDR* (32nd edition). Montvale, NJ: Thomson.

Physicians' Desk Reference. (2008). *PDR* (62nd edition). Montvale, NJ: Thomson.

PQRI. (n.d.). Retrieved from https://www.cms.gov/Regulations-and-guidance/Legislation/EHRIncentivePrograms/downloads//MU_Stage1_ReqOverview.pdf

Ridker, P. M., Danielson, E., Fonseca, F. A., Genest, J., Gotto, A. M., Jr, Kastelein, J. J., …JUPITER Study Group. (2008). Rosuvastatin to prevent vascular events in men and women with elevated C-reactive protein. *New England Journal of Medicine, 359*(21), 2195–2207.

Rifkin, D. E., Laws, M. B., Rao, M., Balakrishnan, V. S., Sarnak, M. J., & Wilson, I. B. (2010). Medication adherence behavior and priorities among older adults with CKD: A semistructured interview study. *American Journal of Kidney Diseases, 56*(3), 439–446.

Royal, D. R., Cordes, J. A., & Polk. M. (1998). CLOX: An executive clock drawing task. *Journal of Neurology, Neurosurgery and Psychiatry, 64*, 588–594.

Sayah, F. A., Williams, B., & Johnson, J, A. (2012). Measuring health literacy in individuals with diabetes: A systematic review and evaluation of available measures. *Health Education & Behavior.* Advance online publication. doi: 10.1177/1090198111436341.

Stagnitti, M. N. (2009). *Average number of total (including refills) and unique prescriptions by select person characteristics, 2006.* Retrieved from http://www.meps.ahrq.gov/mepsweb/data-files/publications/st245/stat245.pdf

Sullivan, C., Gleason, K., & Rooney, D. (2005). Medication reconciliation in the acute care setting: Opportunity and challenge for nursing. *Journal of Nursing Care Quality, 20*(2), 95–98.

Sunovion Pharmaceuticals. (2006). Safety and efficacy study of AC-3933 in adults with mild to moderate Alzheimer's disease. In ClinicalTrials.gov [Internet]. Bethesda, MD: National Library of Medicine. Retrieved from http://www.clinicaltrials.gov/ct2/show/NCT00359944

Tai-Seale, M., McGuire, T. G., & Zhang, W. (2007). Time allocation in primary care office visits. *Health Services Research, 42*(5), 1871–1894.

U.S. Department of Health and Human Services [U. S. DHHS], Food and Drug Administration [FDA]. (2012). *Guidance for industry pharmacokinetics in patients with impaired renal function—Study design, data analysis, and impact on dosing and labeling.* Retrieved from http://www.fda.gov/downloads/Drugs/GuidanceComplianceRegulatoryInformation/Guidances/ucm072127.pdf

van der Velde, N., Stricker, B., Pols, H., & van der Cammen T. J. (2007) Risk of falls after withdrawal of falls-risk-increasing drugs: A prospective cohort study. *British Journal of Clinical Pharmacology, 63*(2), 232–237.

Vandegrift, D., & Datta, A. (2006). Prescription drug expenditures in the U.S.: The effects of obesity, demographics and new pharmaceutical products. *Southern Economic Journal, 73*(2), 515–529.

Wilson, I. B., Schoen, C., & Neuman, P. (2007). Physician–patient communication about prescription medication nonadherence: A 50-state study of America's seniors. *Journal of General Internal Medicine, 22*(1), 6–12.

Zagaria, M. A. (2009). OTCs & seniors: risks and safeguards. *US Pharmacopedia, 4*(34) (OTC trends suppl), 12–15.

For a full suite of assignments and additional learning activities, see the access code at the front of your book.

LEARNING OBJECTIVES

At the end of this chapter, the reader will:

> Acknowledge the complex health and cost issues related to falls for older adults.
> Describe older adults with a predisposition for falls and falls with injury.
> Identify intrinsic and extrinsic risk factors for falls in older adults.
> Incorporate a patient-specific fall risk assessment into an individualized plan of care.
> Recognize medications associated with falls in older adults.
> Identify patients at risk for restraints.
> Discuss nonrestraint interventions to prevent falls.

KEY TERMS

Chemical restraint
Environmental hazards
Extrinsic risk factors
Fall injury risk factors
Fall risk assessment

Intrinsic risk factors
Nonrestraint fall prevention
   interventions
Physical restraint
Safety promotion

Falls in Older Adults

Marge Dean
Barbara Harrison
DeAnne Zwicker

Introduction

Falls are one of the most common adverse events that threaten the quality of life of older adults. According to the Centers for Disease Control and Prevention (CDC), one in three adults over the age of 65 fall annually. Falls are preventable injuries, yet in 2009, falls resulted in 2.2 million emergency room visits with almost 600,000 resulting in hospitalizations (CDC, 2012). Falls can result in no injury, minor injury, or life-changing injuries. Almost 30% of those who fall experience moderate to severe injuries including hip fracture, head trauma, and lacerations (CDC, 2012). In 2009, almost 40,000 older adults died from unintentional injuries, most resulting from falls (CDC, 2012). Direct medical costs of falls totaled a little over $19 billion, with $179 million for fatal falls and $19 billion for nonfatal fall injuries in 2000 (Stevens, Corso, Finkelstein, & Miller, 2006), which is equal to $28.2 billion in 2010 dollars. Fall prevention by nurses will not only save lives, but reduce healthcare costs as well.

Falls among older adults are *not* a normal consequence of aging; they are considered a geriatric syndrome most often due to multiple predisposing factors and intrinsic and extrinsic risks. The frequency of falls increases with age and frailty. "A fall may be the first indicator of an acute problem (infection, postural hypotension, cardiac arrhythmia), may stem from a chronic disease (Parkinson's, dementia, diabetic neuropathy), or may be a marker for the progression of age-related changes in vision, gait, and strength" (Rubenstein & Josephson, 2006, p. 807). Although there is no universal consensus on the definition of a fall (World Health Organization [WHO], 2010), a fall has been defined as "an event which results in a person unintentionally coming to rest on the ground or another lower level; not as a result of a major intrinsic event (such as a stroke) or overwhelming hazard" (Tinetti, Speechley, & Ginter, 1988, p. 1703). Older adults are more likely to fall in all settings, but are at higher risk in hospital settings (Tinetti & Kumar, 2010).

Falls in the Hospital Setting

Falls are a common problem for hospitalized older adults. Up to 50% of the hospitalized patients in the United States are at risk for falls, and almost half of those who fall suffer an injury (CDC, 2012). Falls are also the most common adverse incident in hospitals, with reported rates of between 3 and 5 falls per 1,000 bed-days, which roughly equals one million inpatient falls occurring in the United States each year (Oliver, Healey, & Haines, 2010). The 2011 Institute of Medicine report, *The Future of Nursing: Leading Change, Advancing Health* reported evidence linking nursing to high quality care for patients, including protecting their safety. When caring for hospitalized older adults, one of nurses' primary responsibilities is maintaining patient safety and preventing iatrogenic events, which include falls.

The complex hospital environment plays a role in older adult falls. Alarms, medical equipment, lack of personal assistance, assistive devices, furniture, and partial side rails have all proven to be environmental hazards associated with falls (Hendrich, 2006; Letts et al., 2010). Older adults in the hospital may have health conditions that place them at risk for falls; for example, delirium may develop due to an infection and cause older adults to be confused or inattentive, which has been linked to hospital falls (Harrision, Ferrari, Campbell, Maddens, & Whall, 2010).

Older adults who experience a fall while hospitalized may experience physical and functional impairments, loss of independence, disability, and death (Hughes et al., 2008). Besides physical injuries, there are psychological consequences, such as increased fear of falling, anxiety, helplessness, or depression (Boyd & Stevens, 2009; Nordell, Andreasson, Gall, & Thorngren, 2009). These psychological consequences, particularly fear of falling (fallophobia), can lead older adults to walk less, lose strength, and then curtail activities that that provide quality in their lives. Thus, fall prevention for hospitalized older adults is critically important to nurses as they develop interventions that promote safety, quality care, and satisfaction for patients who must be hospitalized.

Falls occurring in the hospital are an important concern for nurses because they represent a national measure of quality and safety in the National Database of Nursing Quality Indicators (NDNQI). The American Nurses Association has included patient falls as one of the top 10 nurse-sensitive quality indicators (Montalvo, 2007) and The Joint Commission on Accreditation of Healthcare Organizations has designated patient falls as one of its National Patient Safety Goals (The Joint Commission, 2011). The WHO has described falls and fall related injuries as "major public health challenges that call for global attention. This problem will increase in magnitude as the numbers of older adults increase in many nations throughout the world" (WHO, 2010, p. 30).

Aside from the impact falls have on patients; outcomes of falls also affect hospitals' cost per admission and length of stay. Older adults who sustain a fall while hospitalized utilize more healthcare resources than persons who do not fall. Reimbursement policies set by the Centers for Medicare and Medicaid Services (CMS) have also established limits on hospital reimbursement for care related to fall-related injury (Inouye, Brown, & Tinetti, 2009). Avoidance of the adverse outcomes associated with falls is especially important for judicious use of healthcare resources. Thus, evidence-based fall prevention programs in inpatient settings will not only save lives, but reduce healthcare costs as well.

Implications of Falls

Fractures are the second-most-serious health consequence of falls. Of those who fall, 20–30% suffer moderate to severe injuries and 10–20% experience a fracture (Alexander, Rivara, & Wolf, 1992; CDC, 2012). The most common fractures are of the vertebrae, hip, forearm, leg, ankle, pelvis, upper arm, and hand (Scott, 1990). The incidence of hip fracture is greater in older women but death (mortality) from hip fracture is higher among older men (Fransen et al., 2002). At least 50% of elderly persons who were ambulatory before fracturing a hip do not recover their pre-fracture level of mobility (Beers & Berkow, 2005). About 5% of older adults with hip fractures die while hospitalized; overall mortality in the 12 months after a hip fracture ranges from 12% to 67% (Beers & Berkow, 2005). Excess mortality after hip fracture (adjusting for race and age) was 9% in women and 24% in men in the year after fracture, and at 5 years postfracture was 24% in women and 26% in men (Robbins, Biggs, & Cauley, 2006).

In addition to fractures, over 50% of falls result in at least some minor injury such as lacerations and bruises (Beers & Berkow, 2005). Falls that do not result in injury may still have serious consequences such as a fear of falling again. With fallaphobia, older adults often reduce mobility. This reduction in mobility can lead to a decline in functional capacity, dependence on others, and an increased risk of falls. Further complications resulting for decreased mobility include decline in muscle strength and range of motion, and joint stiffness further compromising mobility. Quality of life may also deteriorate drastically after a fall.

Older adults who fall, particularly those who fall repeatedly, tend to have deficits in activities of daily living and are at high risk for subsequent hospitalization, further disability, institutionalization, and death. Falls are reported to be a contributing factor in 40% of nursing home admissions (Beers & Berkow, 2005). In 2003, the CDC reported that more than 13,700 people age 65 or older died from fall-related injuries The total cost of all fall injuries for people age 65 or older in 2000 was $19 billion; by 2020, the cost of fall injuries is expected to reach $54.9 billion (CDC, 2012).

Risk Factors

In older adults, falls rarely have one cause. Falls are often due to complex interactions of age-related decline, acute illness, chronic disease, postural control, and other factors such as intrinsic behaviors and mobility capacity (Flaherty & Resnick, 2011). Nurses routinely assess patients and their environment and are instrumental in implementing interventions to prevent falls. In order to accurately assess risk for falls, a comprehensive knowledge of factors that contribute to a fall is essential. Risk factors for falls can be categorized into intrinsic and extrinsic factors. *Intrinsic risk factors* are related to the patient's physiology and physical changes associated with aging, such as decreased vision, and disorders affecting the physical function needed to maintain balance. These functions include vestibular, proprioceptive, and visual function, as well as cognition and musculoskeletal function (see **Table 12-1**).

Illnesses and disease states are also intrinsic risk factors for falls. Cognitive impairment—specifically impairment of executive function—is a risk factor for falls in older adults (Muir, Gopaul, & Montero Odasso, 2012). In a systematic review of research involving falls in the elderly, Rubenstein and Josephson (2006) found that muscle weakness increased fall risk up to four times. Balance deficits, cognitive impairment, age greater than 80 years, and visual impairment all increased fall risk three-fold. Older adults with diabetes, low body mass index (BMI), depression, and foot problems are at higher risk for falls according to the World Health Organization (2010). While there are many intrinsic risk factors that usually contribute to the majority of falls in older adults, physical and/or cognitive impairments contribute most to falls and fall-related injuries.

Extrinsic risk factors are related to the physical environment such as lack of grab bars, poor condition of floor surfaces, inadequate lighting, and inadequate or

---

TABLE 12-1   Intrinsic Risk Factors for Falls in the Hospital Setting

Advancing age
Cardiac arrhythmias
Cognitive impairment (slow thinking, poor planning, memory loss)
Delirium (acute cognitive impairment)
Frailty
Use of pain or sleep medications
Use of alcohol
Impaired mobility and balance
History of a fall in past year
Illnesses affecting oxygen saturation (pneumonia, COPD)
Illnesses affecting musculoskeletal system (such as stroke, MS, Parkinson's disease)
Urinary or bowel problems (infection, incontinence, urgency)
Sensory defects such as peripheral neuropathy, poor vision, depth perception, peripheral vision

improper use of assistive devices. In the institutional care environments, extrinsic hazards include IV poles, oxygen tubing, height of beds or stretchers, and side rails. Use of restraints and bed rails increases the risk of falls because patients attempt to free themselves from these constraints. Assessing individual patient's intrinsic and extrinsic risk factors will aid in developing the appropriate interventions and plan of care to prevent falls.

Fall Risk Assessment

Older adults admitted to acute care, rehabilitation, or long-term care settings should have an initial *fall risk assessment* on admission, after any change in condition, and at regular intervals throughout their stay (Nicklin, 2006). A number of fall assessment tools are available to assess inpatient risk of falls, but no single tool has been adopted universally. Most tools contain a fall history, an examination of mental and mobility status, a checklist for the presence of sensory deficits, a list of medications the client is taking, and a list of primary and secondary diagnoses. Two examples are the Tinetti Performance-Oriented Mobility Assessment (see **Table 12-2** and

TABLE 12-2 Nursing Assessment to Identify Intrinsic Risk Factors for Falls	
Physical Assessment	**Problem**
Pulse	Arrhythmias, bradycardia
Blood pressure	Postural hypotension
	Orthostatic blood pressure
Respiratory	Low oxygen saturation leads to confusion
Vision screening	Deficits in acuity, depth perception, peripheral vision and use of glasses
Muscle strength	Weakness in one or both sides
ROM in neck, spine, and extremities	Limitation in range of motion
Gait and balance	Deficits in postural control, balance, coordination, station, and gait
Pain	Limits normal function
Mental status/Level of consciousness (LOC)	Changes in thinking, attention, planning
Memory	Unable to remember safety instructions

*LOC= Alert, confused, drowsy, unresponsive

Box 12-1) and the Timed Get Up and Go Test, which have high sensitivity and specificity in identifying fallers from nonfallers (Shumway-Cook, Brauer, & Woollacott, 2000). The Morse Fall Scale is depicted in **Table 12-3**. Another evidence-based fall-risk assessment tool for older adults is the Hendrich II Fall Risk Model (Hendrich, Bender, & Nyhuis, 2003), available at http://consultgerirn.org/uploads/File/trythis/try_this_8.pdf. These and other fall risk assessment tools (see **Box 12-2**) for both community and institutional care can be found at Minnesota Falls Prevention at http://www.mnfallsprevention.org. While there are several independent experimental studies to support the reliability of fall risk assessment instruments, a systematic review found that further research is recommended to study the sensitivity and specificity of screening tools to accurately predict fall risk, particularly in the community setting (Gates, Smith, Fisher, & Lamb, 2008).

BOX 12-1   Performance-Oriented Mobility Assessment (Tinetti, 1986)

Tinetti Performance-Oriented Mobility Assessment (POMA) The Tinetti assessment tool is an easily administered task-oriented test that measures an older adult's gait and balance abilities.	Date	Date	Date	Date
Balance Tests: Subject is seated on hard, armless chair				
SITTING BALANCE Leans or slides in chair = 0, Steady, safe = 1				
ARISES Unable without help = 0; Able, uses arms = 1, Able without using arms = 2				
ATTEMPTS TO RISE: Unable w/o help = 0; Able, requires > 1 attempt = 1; Able in 1 attempt = 2				
IMMEDIATE STANDING BALANCE (first 5 seconds) Unsteady (sway/stagger/feet move) = 0; Steady, w/ support = 1; Steady w/o support = 2				
STANDING BALANCE Unsteady = 0; Steady, stance > 4-inch BOS & requires support = 1;Narrow stance, w/o support = 2				
STERNAL NUDGE (feet close together) Begins to fall = 0; Staggers, grabs, catches self = 1; Steady = 2				

Tinetti Performance-Oriented Mobility Assessment (POMA) The Tinetti assessment tool is an easily administered task-oriented test that measures an older adult's gait and balance abilities.	Date	Date	Date	Date
EYES CLOSED (feet close together) Unsteady = 0; Steady = 1				
TURNING 360 DEGREES Discontinuous steps = 0; Continuous steps = 1				
TURNING 360 DEGREES Unsteady (staggers, grabs) = 0;Steady = 1				
SITTING DOWN Unsafe (misjudges distance, falls) = 0;Uses arms, or not a smooth motion = 1; Safe, smooth motion = 2				
BALANCE SCORE TOTAL	/16	/16	/16	/16
GAIT INITATION (immediate after told "go") Any hesitancy, multiple attempts to start = 0; No hesitancy = 1				
STEP LENGTH R swing foot passes L stance leg = 1; L swing foot passes R = 1				
FOOT CLEARANCE R foot completely clears floor = 1; L foot completely clears floor = 1				
STEP SYMMETRY R and L step length unequal = 0; R and L step length equal= 1				
STEP CONTINUITY Stop/discontinuity between steps = 0; Steps appear continuous = 1				
PATH (excursion) Marked deviation = 0; Mild/moderate deviation or use of aid = 1; Straight without device = 2				
TRUNK Marked sway or uses device = 0; No sway but knee or trunk flexion or spread arms while walking = 1; None of the above deviations = 2				
BASE OF SUPPORT Heels apart = 0; Heels close while walking = 1				

(*continues*)

BOX 12-1   Performance-Oriented Mobility Assessment (Tinetti, 1986) (continued)

Tinetti Performance-Oriented Mobility Assessment (POMA) The Tinetti assessment tool is an easily administered task-oriented test that measures an older adult's gait and balance abilities.	Date	Date	Date	Date
GAIT SCORE TOTAL	/12	/12	/12	/12
ASSISTIVE DEVICE				
TOTAL SCORE (BALANCE + GAIT)	/28	/28	/28	/28
FALL RISK (minimal >23, Mod. 19–23, High <19)				
Nurse's initials				

Scoring/interpretation: Scored on a three point ordinal scale which ranges from 0 to 2. "2" indicates the highest level of independence, and "0" indicates the highest level of impairment. The two part scale includes a total balance score of 16 and total gait score of 12, for a total possible score of 28. Scores of 25–28 indicate low fall risk, 19–24 medium fall risk, and <19 high fall risk.

BOX 12-2   Research Highlight

Aim: This study was done to test the sensitivity, specificity and feasibility of four fall risk assessment tools.

Method: The four fall risk assessment tools were tested simultaneously in May–June 2006. All 4 assessment tools were completed on a total of 1,546 patients.

Findings: The use of tools was moderately consistent among registered nurses, but the education provided did not entirely eliminate problems with accuracy. The sensitivity of the instruments ranged from 57.1–100% and specificity ranged from 24.9–69.3%.

Application to practice: Sensitivity and specificity of tools are important factors to consider when nurses choose to implement one—specifically, knowing if a tool accurately predicts fall risk. Educating nursing staff on assessment and interventions is also important to reduce the risk of falls. Nurses need to test fall risk assessment tools in their own organizations and with specific populations.

Source: Chapman, J., Bachand, D., & Hyrkas, K. (2011). Testing the sensitivity, specificity and feasibility of four falls risk assessment tools in a clinical setting. *Journal of Nursing Management, 19*, 133–142.

There are several fall assessment tools that are used to predict the risk of falls. To be effective, a fall assessment tool must be short, individualized to the patient, applicable to the setting, readily available to the staff, and have demonstrated validity and reliability. Fall-risk tools have different cut-off points concerning the patients' fall-risk level. Some tools have two fall-risk categories (low/no risk and high risk)

TABLE 12-3	Morse Fall Scale		
Variables		**Numeric Values**	**Score**
1.	History of falling	No 0 Yes 25	_____
2.	Secondary diagnosis	No 0 Yes 15	_____
3.	Ambulatory aid None/bed rest/nurse assist Crutches/cane/walker Furniture	0 15 30	_____
4.	IV or IV Access	No 0 Yes 20	_____
5.	Gait Normal/bed rest/wheelchair Weak Impaired	0 10 20	_____
6.	Mental status Oriented to own ability Overestimates or forgets limitations	0 15	_____
Morse Fall Scale Score = Total _____			

To obtain total score, add up score column.
High risk: Score of 45 or higher
Moderate risk: Score of 25–44
Low risk: Score of 0–24

based on one cut-off point (Hendrich Falls Risk Scale), while other tools have three fall risk categories (no risk, low risk, and high risk) based on two cut-off points/scores (The Morse Fall Scale; Chapman, Bachand, & Hyrkas, 2011). Fall-risk assessment tools also need to be tested for specificity and sensitivity within the population in which it is being used. The specificity and sensitivity of the fall risk tool may be significantly different from one community/population to another patient population. (Chapman et al., 2011).

Nurses must also assess older adults for risk of injury if a fall was to occur. All falls should be carefully evaluated for the underlying contributing factors, but the incidence of recurrent falls is a significant risk factor for serious injury. The older adult should be asked to describe the sensations or events that preceded the fall; circumstances surrounding the fall, such as what activity they were engaged in; the location of the fall; witnesses to the fall; and injuries sustained. The nurse should perform a thorough assessment to determine injuries from the fall and contributing intrinsic health factors such as bradycardia or orthostatic hypotension (see Table 12-3).

Risk factors for serious injury include diagnoses of osteoporosis, previous joint replacement, and spinal abnormalities. Other *fall injury risk factors* for include current use of anticoagulants such as warfarin or aspirin and labs such as low platelet count, elevated INR, or other clotting factors. Most hospitals now have a post-fall protocol that includes assessment for signs or symptoms of fracture or potential for spinal injury before the patient is moved, and neurological observations for all patients where head injury has occurred, to improve outcomes. Some hospitals utilize a rapid response team to assess patients who have fallen due to risk for serious injury and death. After a fall has occurred, it is important that a thorough medical assessment be done to identify any potential hidden injuries. A multidisciplinary-team assessment of the patient who has fallen is another intervention that nurses can initiate to identify potential risk factors not previously found to prevent further falls and/or injuries.

Fall Prevention and Safety Promotion Strategies

Surveillance is one of the primary *safety promotion* interventions used by hospital nurses. The Institute of Medicine (IOM) report, *Keeping Patients Safe*, defined surveillance as "observing changes in patient conditions that may signal a decline in condition along with taking an action to prevent complications" (IOM, 2003, p 12.). Surveillance interventions include frequent rounding, moving patients closer to the nurses' station, assignment of sitters, and observation devices. Surveillance is sometimes supported by technological devices such as alarms, pressure mats, video monitoring, and portable trigger alarms. The evidence for technological devices to reduce falls is limited in part because few studies have documented their effectiveness.

Fall prevention strategies are likely to be more effective if they include an interdisciplinary approach to the process. The most important factor in developing a fall prevention plan is to individualize the interventions that are specific to the patient's risk factors. General fall interventions for all patients in the acute care setting include orienting older adults to their environment with an emphasis on safety and educating them and their family members of their risk of falling and the strategies needed to prevent falls. Other *nonrestraint fall prevention interventions* include providing patients with nonskid slippers or shoes; removal of obstacles and clutter in the room; having the commode close to the bed for independently functioning older adults; and having the call light, bedside table, and other needs within easy reach. Glasses and hearing aids should be worn, although caution is warranted with multifocal lenses during ambulation. *Physical restraints* and raised side rails should be avoided as they increase the risk of falls, particularly falls with serious injury: Patients injure themselves when climbing over or around side rails, and patients who attempt to climb over the rails fall from a greater height, which results in the more serious injury (O'Keefe, Jack, & Lye, 1996). Maintaining the bed in the lowest position will also reduce the severity of injury if a fall occurs. The Institute for Clinical Systems Improvement (ICSI) has developed evidence-based interventions to reduce falls in acute care settings (Degelau et al., 2012). The urgent priority in all settings, particularly acute care, is not only to reduce number of falls, but to eliminate falls with injury entirely. Individually tailored use of the fall prevention interventions discussed here will help to reduce serious injuries, particularly avoidance of physical restraints, which includes side rails.

Another form of restraint that places older adults at risk for falls is *chemical restraints*, which includes any medication that can cause a patient to be drowsy or less alert. Psychotropic medications classes such as benzodiazepines, antipsychotics, pain medications, or other sedating medications are a form of chemical restraint and can lead to falls and hip fracture (Flaherty & Resnick, 2011). Although pain and other sedating medications may be required to treat a patient's condition, nurses need to evaluate the patient's response to these medications and suggest dose adjustment when physical or cognitive impairment increases due to medications. Surveillance for changes in patient conditions that may signal a decline in condition is a primary nursing responsibility. Other surveillance interventions, including making hourly rounds and checking on patients with altered cognition more frequently, may also help to reduce falls (Murphy, Labonte, Klock, & Houser, 2008).

Fall prevention interventions include those that reduce the impact of intrinsic risk factors. Ambulating persons with cognitive impairment helps to maintain their mobility and strength, thus preventing functional decline. Providing interesting activities (books, memory games, newspapers) can maintain orientation to the environment and reduce the risk of delirium, which significantly increases fall risk. Older adults with cognitive impairment are one of the highest fall-risk groups of patients when in the hospital setting and are also at highest risk for overmedication. A program that aides in reducing falls in cognitively impaired older adults is the Hospital Elder Life Program (HELP; Inouye, 2000). This program employs volunteers to aide in walking patients with cognitive changes to help maintain both physical and cognitive function. The reader can find out more about this program at www.hospitalelderlifeprogram.org/public/public-main.php

In summary, nurses caring for older adults in an acute care setting (hospital, rehabilitation, skilled nursing facility) must provide frequent and ongoing assessment of fall risk; implement fall prevention strategies; and educate staff, families, and patients about fall prevention. Fall prevention is a major indicator of quality nursing care and is also essential to nursing care that is safe and cost effective for older adults.

Falls in the Community Setting

Falls in the community are all too common and often cause a change in the person's ability to live life independently, particularly when it results in a fracture, especially in those with a hip fractures. After a fall, many older adults develop a fear of falling; this can result in reduced mobility, which often leads to a decline in muscle strength and flexibility and can actually increase the risk of future falls due to poorer musculoskeletal functioning. Both a history of falls and prior nursing home placement are a significant predictor of future nursing home placement for older adults (Spoelstra, Given, You, & Given, 2012).

The cost of a fall is not only high for the older adult but also for the healthcare system. The (CDC, 2012) estimates that in 2010, $28.2 billion was spent for care of injuries from falls of older adults. The cost estimates come from a variety of sources, including the initial emergency room work up of the fall injury, followed by the hospitalization, and often a transfer for rehabilitation to yet another institution before being released to home care. The cost also includes healthcare personnel, drugs, durable medical supplies, and any surgery costs. The need for ongoing nursing care at home or in an assisted living or long-term care setting may be required, increasing the costs to older adults and the system substantially. Some older adults never return to home after a fall, particularly the frail and those with cognitive impairment.

Risk Factors

Tinetti, Speechly, and Ginter (1988) were the first to identify fall risk factors in the community setting for persons over the age of 65 years. They identified the following risk factors: postural hypotension, use of benzodiazepines or sedatives and hypnotics, use of four or more medications, impairment in muscle strength or range of motions, and *environmental hazards*. Since that time, other researchers have identified the following community risk factors: (1) comorbid conditions including diabetes, stroke, syncope, anemia, Alzheimer's, Parkinson's, and vitamin D deficiency; (2) patient characteristics including gait problems, postural hypotension, difficulty to getting out of chair, impaired activities of daily living (ADLs) performance, difficulty following instructions, impulsivity, fear of falling, and use of psychotropic medications; and (3) community conditions including uneven surfaces, poorly lit environments, lack of support rails, and other environmental hazards. See **Table 12-4** for fall-risk factors identified in the community and **Table 12-5** for preventive actions for specific risk factors for older adults in the community setting (Gillespie et al., 2009).

TABLE 12-4 Risk Factors for Falls, Injuries, and Fall-Related Deaths in the Community			
Intrinsic Risk Factors	**Fall Risk**	**Injury Risk**	**Mortality Risk**
Demographics			
Age: Older Age (especially >70yrs)	Yes	Yes	Yes
Gender	Female	Female	Male >85
Race	Caucasian	Caucasian	Caucasian
Cognitive Function			
Cognitive impairment	Yes	No data	No data
Fallophobia (fear of falling)	Yes	Yes	No data
Inability to follow instructions	Yes	No data	No data

Intrinsic Risk Factors	Fall Risk	Injury Risk	Mortality Risk
Physical Function			
Gait problems	Yes	No data	No data
Impaired ability to perform ADLs	Yes	Yes	No data
Impaired muscle strength or range of motion	Yes	Yes	No data
Poor/fair self-reported health	Yes	Yes	No data
Vision problems	Yes	No data	No data
Physical Status			
BMI less than 22.8 kg/m²	No data	Yes	Yes
Frailty	No data	Yes	Yes
Low body weight	Yes	Yes	No data
Disease States			
Alzheimer's disease	Yes	No data	No data
Anemia (including mild anemia)	Yes	No data	No data
Diabetes	Yes	No data	No data
Diabetic foot ulcer	Yes	No data	No data
Fall in the past 12 months	Yes	Yes	No data
Parkinson's disease	Yes	No data	No data
Postural hypotension	Yes	No data	No data
Previous fracture	No data	Yes	No data
Stroke	Yes	Yes	No data
Subdural hematoma (chronic)	Yes	Yes	No data
Syncope	Yes	No data	No data
Vitamin D deficiency	Yes	Yes	No data

(continues)

TABLE 12-4   Risk Factors for Falls, Injuries, and Fall-Related Deaths in the Community (*continued*)

Intrinsic Risk Factors	Fall Risk	Injury Risk	Mortality Risk
Medications			
Use of four or more medications	Yes	No data	No data
Anti-epileptics	No data	Yes	No data
Antihypertensives	Yes	No data	No data
Antiplatelet therapy	No data	No data	Yes
Psychotropics	Yes	No data	No data
Sedatives and hypnotics	Yes	No data	No data
Extrinsic Risk Factors			
Environmental hazards	Yes	No data	No data
Footwear, nonsupportive (e.g., slippers)	Yes	No data	No data
Hospitalization, recent	Yes	No data	No data
Wheelchair use, reckless wheelchair use	Yes	No data	No data

Source: Currie, L. Fall and injury prevention. (2008). In R.G. Hughes (Ed.). *Patient safety and quality: An evidence-based handbook for nurses* (pp. 1–56). Rockville, MD: Agency for Healthcare Research and Quality.

Who is more at risk for a fall? Age and gender are associated with falls and morbidity and mortality due to falls (CDC, 2006). Fall rates increase with age. In those 65 to 85 years old, females in the community were more likely to fall and males were more likely to die from fall injuries (Hughes et al., 2008). The oldest-old (those 85 years and older) are at the highest risk for falls, with the fall risk escalating in those over age 85 to four times greater than the 65–74 age group. Older adults over age 75 and older are four to five times more likely to be hospitalized for a fall (CDC, 2006).

Falls are the leading cause of death due to injury among older adults, with 87% of all fractures in the elderly due to falls. Risk factors for injury in the community are better characterized by research. Risk factors for fall-related fractures in women over

TABLE 12-5 Risk Factors in the Community and Preventive Interventions

Risk	Preventive Action
Balance disorder	Exercise program: improve strength, balance, flexibility, or endurance
	Teach use of assistive device for ambulation as needed
Dementia	Test memory, vitamin D, maintain social and mental skills
Poor vision	Regular eye check ups to monitor/treat cataracts, glaucoma, macular degeneration
Low lighting in home	More lights, increase wattage, night light
Polypharmacy	Have primary care provider and pharmacist review meds
	Discontinue those that cause dizziness & are known to contribute to falls
Home environment	Home health referral to evaluate home for safety concerns
Cardiac Issues	Check blood pressure for orthostatic hypotension and low heart rate that might require pacemaker insertion
Footwear	Shoes need to be in good condition, with nonslip soles and good fit

Source: Gillespie. L. D. LD, Gillespie, W. J. WJ, Robertson, M. C. MC, Lamb, S. E. SE, Cumming, R. G. RG, & Rowe, B. H BH. (2003). Interventions for preventing falls in elderly people. *Cochrane Database of Systematic Reviews,* Issue 4.

age 70 years included: (1) a fall in the past 12 months, (2) increasing age, (3) prior factors, and (4) low body weight (Porthouse et al., 2004). A study in the community identified nine characteristics that were predictors of fractures, including being female over age 75; Caucasian race; BMI less than 22.8 kg/m^2; cognitive impairment; stroke history; impairment in one or more ADLs; taking antiepileptic drugs; and difficulty performing heavy work, walking a mile, or climbing stairs (Colon-Emeric, Pieper, & Artz, 2002).

Ethnic and gender differences also define who is more at risk for a fall. Caucasian populations had a 2.5 times greater chance of death from fall than Blacks. Men were 46% more likely to die from a fall than older women, and women were 58% more likely to have a nonfatal fall than older men. However, women, especially White women, were found to have more hip fractures than older males and Black and Asian women (WHO, 2010). Fall-related injuries account for up to 15% of rehospitalizations in the first month after discharge from hospital (Mahoney et al., 2000). Based on data from 2000, total annual estimated costs were between $16 billion and $19 billion for nonfatal, fall-related injuries and approximately $170 million dollars for fall-related deaths across care settings in the community. Many of the falls with injury risk factors are consistent with fall risk factors, thus indicating a need for quality screening in the community-dwelling older adult.

Fall Prevention and Safety Promotion Strategies

The American Geriatrics Society (AGS) and British Geriatrics Society (BGS) (2010) Panel on Prevention of Falls in Older Persons agrees that the prevention of falls is an important responsibility of healthcare professionals. The panel looked at 2010 fall prevention guidelines that can reduce the risk of injury from a fall for the older adult in the community. The AGS/BGS panel of experts recommended that older adults be asked at least once a year by health professionals if they have fallen because older adults often will not volunteer this information unless queried. If the older adult has fallen or if they have gait or balance problems, a multifactorial fall risk assessment is recommended. The healthcare provider/nurse should look for under-lying factors that may have contributed to falls, such as medications, exacerbation of a chronic medical problem, or development of a new acute problem. A fall or a change in functional status is often the first sign of a health problem in older adults, thus community nurses must promptly notify the primary provider for follow-up.

The community fall risk assessment includes evaluation of functional status such as ability to perform ADLs, appropriate use of adaptive equipment such as canes or walkers, and fear of falling. In the community setting, physical therapists can assess the older adult for the appropriate assistive device as well as for proper footwear. In general, footwear should have low heels with a large amount of surface contact. Physical and/or occupational therapy assessments provide some insight into older adults' risk for a future fall as well. A home safety evaluation may be done to assess the safety of the living environment and to identify hazards and fall risks that can be modified to improve the safety of the home. Falls can be prevented by remov-ing loose cords and throw rugs or improving lighting in bathrooms. Occupational therapists typically perform home evaluations, so community or home health nurses may request an order from the primary provider for an occupational therapy consult to perform a home safety evaluation.

Exercise programs are recommended for community-dwelling older adults at risk for falling. Evidence has shown that Tai Chi and physical therapy can reduce falls by increasing balance and strength, thus improving function and gait in the older adult (Chang et al., 2004; Li et al., 2005). The National Institute on Aging has published a guide for older adults that can assist them in finding an exercise program for daily use that is adapted to their current abilities and strength (www.nia.nih.gov/health/publication/falls-and-fractures). Community nurses can access and provide this information to at-risk older adults and their family.

Like the ICSI in acute care, the AGS/BGS (2012) panel also recommends a mul-tifactorial intervention that is tailored to the individual older adult's level of cogni-tion and physical ability. Education of the older adult and his or her family support system helps to sustain the interventions. The AGS/BGS panel also suggests that healthcare providers who assess the needs must also follow-up to ensure the fall prevention strategies are implemented. Home health nurses, physical therapists, and occupational therapists are in an optimal position to follow up on the fall prevention plan, evaluate its effectiveness, reinforce its use, and ensure safety in the home setting (see **Boxes 12-3, 12-4**, and **12-5**).

Another fall prevention strategy is a regularly scheduled eye exam to identify problems that are correctable, such as cataracts, and improve the older adult's vision. Correction of the cataracts using surgery significantly reduced the relative risk of falls; however, second surgeries showed no additional benefit. While regular eye exams are regarded as good practice, correction of this deficit alone has not yet demonstrated an effect on reducing falls. If included with multifactorial interventions, though, falls are reduced (Flaherty & Resnick, 2011).

BOX 12-3 Evidence-Based Practice Highlight

Multifactorial, multidisciplinary, health and environmental risk factor screening and intervention programs in community-dwelling older adults with a history of falling have shown to be beneficial in reducing falls. (Gillespie et al., 2003), Systematic Review (Level I evidence).

BOX 12-4 Categories of Falls

Incident reports in the acute care setting use the following ANA–NDNQI fall-related injuries categories:

1. *None* indicates that the patient did not sustain an injury secondary to the fall.

2. *Minor* indicates those injuries requiring a simple intervention.

3. *Moderate* indicates injuries requiring sutures or splints.

4. *Major* injuries are those that require surgery, casting, further examination (e.g., for a neurological injury).

5. *Deaths* refers to those that result from injuries sustained from the fall.

BOX 12-5 Nursing Quality Indicators

Nursing-sensitive quality indicators for acute care settings and Montalvo (2007) indicates that patient falls are one of the American Nurses Association's 10 nurse-sensitive quality indicators and the Joint Commission on Accreditation of Healthcare Organizations has also designated patient falls as one of its National Patient Safety Goals (The Joint Commission, 2011). The World Health Organization (WHO) has described falls and fall-related injuries as "major public health challenges that call for global attention. This problem will increase in magnitude as the numbers of older adults increase in many nations throughout the world " (WHO, 2010, p. 30).

Cardiovascular conditions and/or medications can be associated with falls. Postural hypotension (blood pressure that drops as one moves from lying to sitting and from sitting to standing) is a common problem caused by aging and is a fall-risk factor for older adults. Checking the older adult for postural hypotension can be done during clinic and/or home health visits. Nurses can educate patients about slowly changing positions and notify primary care providers of the identified problem for possible treatment. Assessing for postural hypotension is particularly important in older adults taking cardiac medications such as antihypertensives, beta blockers, and diuretics. Nurses may also find arrhythmias or slow heart rate (bradycardia) when assessing the older adult and will need to report these findings to the primary care provider for follow up.

Calcium and vitamin D (800 IU) supplementation are recommended to maintain healthy bones and assist in prevention or slowing of osteoporosis, particularly in those shown to be deficient in vitamin D. There is evidence that vitamin D supplementation also decreases the risk of falling in older adults deficient in vitamin D3 (Kavlani et al., 2010).

The use of some medications is associated with falls. In 2012 the AGS released the updated Beer's Criteria, which identifies medications and doses of medication that may be harmful to adults age 65 and older. Judicious use of medications, avoiding inappropriate medications, and following the Beer's guidelines may reduce falls and/or fall injuries in older adults. Two key principles in prescribing for older adults are "less is more" and "start low and go slow," which refers to starting doses at lowest levels to reduce potential overdose of medications. Cautious prescribing practices can lessen problems such as delirium, gastrointestinal bleeding, falls, and fractures in the older adult. The Beer's Criteria supports the CDC recommendations for medication reduction or withdrawal, especially for those taking four or more medications (American Geriatrics Society, 2012; CDC, 2012). Regular medication review and discontinuing unnecessary therapy decreases the risk of adverse drug events (Rochon, 2006). Nurses give and monitor patient medications on a regular basis. Becoming familiar with high-risk medications and notifying the primary provider can help in reducing adverse drug events and falls (Zwicker & Fulmer, 2012). Medications implicated in falls include benzodiazepines, sedatives and hypnotics, antidepressants, antipsychotics (neuroleptics), antiarrhythmics, digoxin, diuretics, and alcohol (Gray-Miceli & Quigley, 2012).

Community Resources for Fall Prevention

Fall prevention resources in the community are often available. One example of a community-based program is the Los Angeles Falls Prevention Coalition, which developed programs to specifically assist community-dwelling older adults (http://www.stopfalls.org). To reach the diverse community, this program provides

Evidence-Based Practice Point

"Start low and go slow" with new medications. When starting pharmacological treatment in older adults, the initial dose may need to be lower than the dose listed. Dosing is usually based on research performed in younger adults. If after a predetermined amount of time this dose is not adequate to produce the desired effect, the dose then should be increased slowly until the therapeutic effect is achieved, monitoring closely for side effects.

information on the website in multiple languages to assist the public and health-care providers on fall prevention. This program, which can be replicated, is also connected to the StopFalls Network California and offers a Fall Prevention Advocacy Toolkit.

The CDC provides information on fall prevention in the home, especially the bathroom, which is the number one location of older adult falls with injury. The CDC recommends nonslip surfaces in bathtubs and showers and the use of grab bars in and out of the tub and shower to lessen the chance of a fall. Likewise, a home health nurse can alert a social worker to find resources or request a physical or occupational therapy consult in order to correct the safety issues. The Age Page of the National Institute on Health and Aging also provides community-dwelling older adults and their caregivers with home-based fall prevention and safety strategies at http://www.nia.nih.gov/health/publication/falls-and-fractures.

The Hartford Institute for Geriatric Nursing provides excellent guidelines for nurses caring for the older adult. An evidence-based fall prevention protocol pro-vides a guideline for nurses caring for older adults in the community or in acute care (Gray-Miceli & Quigley, 2012). An outline format of the protocol is available at http://www.consultgerirn.org. The Hendrich II Fall Risk Model may be used to assess the risk of falls in older adults and is also provided at the Hartford Institute website under "Falls." The Get Up & Go Test (Applegate, Blass, & Franklin, 1990) is also provided at the Hartford Institute website and can be administered during routine nursing care to assess risk of falls. To complete the Get Up & Go, the patient is asked to rise from a sitting position and take a few steps. A normal exam shows no loss of balance, pushing up from seated position with one attempt, and an ability to take steps without swaying or need for support (Gray-Miceli & Quigley, 2012; Podsiadlo, 1991).

Summary

Nurses hold a pivotal position in community and acute care settings in assessing older adults for fall risk, developing and implement-ing patient-specific interventions, and providing education to the patient/family that will reduce older adult falls, disability from frac-tures, head trauma, or even death. National healthcare organizations such as the CDC, Hartford Institute, National Institutes of Health, AGS, and other programs provide valuable tools and resources (see **Box 12-6** and **Case Study 12-1**) that can be utilized by the nurse providing health care to older adults. By spending a few minutes to assess the older adult's risk for falls during routine care, the nurse can provide fall risk interventions and education that may help the older adult maintain functional status and ultimately improve quality of

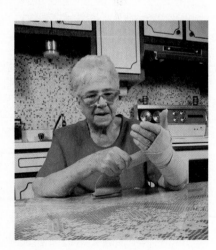

Figure 12-1 Falls can results in serious injury to older adults.

life. Interventions that reduce falls in older adults will also reduce the cost to the healthcare system by limiting the number of older adults who visit the emergency room or are hospitalized as the result of a fall that may have been prevented. Environmental and multifactorial assessments and interventions can make the difference between safety and falling. Nursing actions are key in preventing falls for older adults.

BOX 12-6   Resources

Agency for Healthcare Research and Quality

http://guideline.gov/content.aspx?id=12265&search=falls

American Geriatric Society Clinical Practice Guideline: Prevention of Falls in Older Persons Summary of Recommendations

http://www.americangeriatrics.org/health_care_professionals/clinical_practice/clinical_guidelines_recommendations/prevention_of_falls_summary_of_recommendations

Center for Disease Control and Prevention Compendium of Effective Fall Interventions: What Works for Community-Dwelling Older Adults, 2nd Edition

http://www.cdc.gov/homeandrecreationalsafety/Falls/compendium/0.0_toc.html

Cochrane Summaries

http://summaries.cochrane.org/CD007146/interventions-for-preventing-falls-in-older-people-living-in-the-community

Fall Prevention Center of Excellence: This website identifies best practices in fall prevention and helps communities offer fall prevention programs to older people who are at risk of falling

http://www.stopfalls.org

University of Iowa, Fall Prevention Toolkit

http://www.healthcare.uiowa.edu/igec/falls-prevention-toolkit/demographic.asp

Hartford Institute for Geriatric Nursing. Nursing Standard of Practice Protocol: Fall Prevention

http://consultgerirn.org/topics/falls/want_to_know_more

Joint Commission Safety Standards

http://www.jointcommission.org/standards_information/npsgs.aspx

National Council on Aging

http://www.ncoa.org/improve-health/center-for-healthy-aging/

US Department of Veteran's Affairs. Patient Safety Standards

http://www.patientsafety.gov/CogAids/FallPrevention/index.html#topofpage

World Health Organization Fall Fact Sheet

http://www.who.int/mediacentre/factsheets/fs344/en/index.html

Case Study 12–1

Mrs. Jones is 72-year-old Caucasian female who lives alone and was found on the floor by her neighbor, who comes for coffee each morning. The patient reported "I think I slipped on something," although the neighbor reported no obstacles or wet floor. Mrs. Jones also commented she had been feeling a little dizzy since yesterday. Mrs. Jones has a history of heart disease, high blood pressure, and diabetes. She had her blood pressure medicine, "the diuretic," increased two days ago.

Questions:

1. What are the potential fall risk factors for Mrs. Jones?

2. What assessment would you perform?

3. What are the likely findings?

4. What interventions might you discuss with Mrs. Jones?

5. What educational information would you provide?

Critical Thinking Exercises

1. Read the *Fall Prevention Center of Excellence* website at http://www.stopfalls.org. Discuss your findings with another student nurse in one of your clinical groups.

2. Evaluate one fall-risk assessment tool and discuss its strengths and weaknesses. You can review fall-risk assessment tools at www.consultgerirn.org, under "Falls," see

Box 12-6, review the research of Scott, Votova, Scanlan, & Close (2007).

3. Read Table 12-3 on fall assessment. Describe how you would assess an 86-year-man with atrial fibrillation who has fallen at home. Describe how you would assess an 84-year-old woman with osteoporosis who has fallen getting out of bed in the hospital.

Personal Reflections

1. Have you ever cared for an older adult patient who fell in the hospital? How did it happen? How did the patient feel about that experience? What injuries occurred? Did the fall change how you think about the nursing role in surveillance or safety?

2. Have you ever cared for an older adult who fell at home? How did the patient feel about that experience? What injuries occurred? Did the patient experience a fear of falling after that? Did the fall change how you think about the nursing role in the home/community?

References

Alexander, B. H., Rivara, F. P., & Wolf, M. E. (1992). The cost and frequency of hospitalization for fall-related injuries in older adults. *American Journal of Public Health, 82*(7), 1020–1023.

American Geriatrics Society. (2012) American Geriatrics Society updated Beers criteria for potentially inappropriate medication use in older adults. *Journal of the American Geriatrics Society, 60*(4), 616–631.

American Geriatrics Society & British Geriatrics Society. (2010). *Clinical Practice Guideline: Prevention of Falls in Older Adults.* Retrieved from http://www.americangeriatrics.org/files/documents/health_care_pros/Falls.Summary.Guide.pdf

Applegate, W. B., Blass, J., & Franklin, T. 1990). Instruments for the functional assessment of older patients. *New England Journal of Medicine, 322,* 1207–1214.

Beers, M. & Berkow, R. (2005). The Merck manual of geriatrics (5th Ed.). Whitehouse Station, NJ: Merck.

Boyd, R., & Stevens, J. A. (2009). Falls and fear of falling: Burden, beliefs and behaviours. *Age and Ageing, 38*(4), 423–428.

Centers for Disease Control and Prevention [CDC]. (2006). Annual rate of nonfatal, medically attended fall injuries among adults aged >65 years—United States, 2001–2003. *Morbidity and Mortality Weekly Report, 55*(31), 857.

Centers for Disease Control and Prevention. (2012). Costs of falls among older adults. Retrieved from http://www.cdc.gov/HomeandRecreationalSafety/Falls/fallcost.html

Centers for Disease Control and Prevention. (2012). Fall among older adults: An overview. Retrieved from http://www.cdc.gov/HomeandRecreationalSafety/Falls/adultfalls.html

Chang, J. T., Morton, S. C., Rubenstein, L. Z., Mojica, W. A., Maglione, M., Suttorp, M. J....Shekelle, P. G. (2004). Interventions for the prevention of alls in older adults: Systematic review and metal-analysis of randomized clinical trials. *British Medical Journal, 328*(7441), 680.

Chapman, J., Bachand, D., & Hyrkas, K. (2011) Testing the sensitivity, specificity and feasibility of four falls risk assessment tools in a clinical setting. *Journal of Nursing Management, 19,* 133–142.

Colon-Emeric, C. S., Pieper, C. F., & Artz, M. B. (2002). Can historical and functional risk factors be used to predict fractures in community dwelling older adults. *Osteoporosis International, 13*(12), 955–961.

Currie, L. (2008). Fall and injury prevention. In R.G. Hughes (Ed.). *Patient safety and quality: An evidence-based handbook for nurses* (pp. 1–56). Rockville, MD: Agency for Healthcare Research and Quality.

Degelau, J., Belz, M., Bungum, M., Flavin, P. L., Harper, C., Leys, K....Webb, B. (2012). *Prevention of falls (Acute care).* Institute for Clinical Systems Improvement. Retrieved from www.icsi.org/falls__acute_care___prevention_of__protocol_/falls__acute_care___prevention_of__protocol__24255.html

Flaherty, E. & Resnick, B. (Eds). (2011). *Geriatric nursing review syllabus: A core curriculum in advanced practice geriatric nursing* (3rd ed.). New York, NY: American Geriatrics Society.

Fransen, M., Woodward, M., Norton, R., Robinson, E., Butler, M., & Campbell, A. J. (2002). Excess mortality or institutionalization after hip fracture: men are at greater risk than women. *Journal of American Geriatric Society, 50,* 685–690.

Gates, S., Smith, L. A., Fisher, J. D. & Lamb, S. E. (2008). Systematic review of accuracy of screening instruments for predicting fall risk among independently living older adults. *Journal of Rehabilitation Research & Development, 45*(8), 1105–1116.

Gray-Miceli, D. & Quigley, P.A. (2007). Fall prevention: Assessment, diagnoses, and intervention strategies. In M. Boltz, E. Capezuti, T. Fulmer, & D. Zwicker (Eds.). *Evidence based geriatric nursing protocols for best practice* (4th ed.). New York, NY: Springer.

Gillespie, L. D., Gillespie, W. J., Robertson, M. C., Lamb, S. E., Cumming, R. G., & Rowe, B. H. (2003). Interventions for preventing falls in elderly people. *Cochrane Database of Systematic Reviews,* Issue 4.

Harrison, B. E., Ferrari, M., Campbell, C., Maddens, M., & **Whall, A**. (2010). Evaluating the relationship between inattention, impulsivity related falls in hospitalized older adults. *Geriatric Nursing, 31*(1), 8–16.

Hendrich, A. L., Bender, P. S., & Nyhuis, A. (2003). Validation of the Hendrich II fall risk model: A large concurrent case control study of hospitalized patients. *Applied Nursing Research, 16*(1), 9–21.

Hendrich, A. L. (2006). Inpatient falls: lessons from the field. Retrieved from http://www.psqh.com/mayjun06/falls.html

Hughes, K., van Beurden, E., Eakin, E. G., Barnett, L. M., Patterson, E., Backhouse, J....Newman, B. (2008). Older persons' perception of risk of falling: implications for fall-prevention campaigns. *American Journal of Public Health, 98*(2), 351–357.

Inouye, S. (2000). *The hospital elder life program (HELP).* Yale University School of Medicine. Retrieved from http://www.hospitalelderlifeprogram.org/public/public-main.php

Institute of Medicine. (2011). *The future of nursing: Leading change, advancing health.* Washington, DC: National Academies Press.

Institute of Medicine. (2003). *Keeping Patients Safe: Transforming the Work Environment of Nurses.* Washington, DC: National Academies Press.

Inouye, S., Brown, C., and Tinetti, M. (2009). Medicare Nonpayment, Hospital Falls, and Unintended Consequences, *New England Journal of Medicine,* 360, 2390–2393.

The Joint Commission. (2011). *National Patient Safety Goals.* Retrieved from http://www.health.uab.edu/13428/

Kavlani, R. R., Stein, B., Valiyil, R., Manno, R, Maynard, R. W. & Crews, D. C. (2010). Vitamin D treatment for the prevention of falls in older adults: Systematic review and analysis. *Journal of the American Geriatrics Society, 58*(7), 1299–1210.

Letts, L., Moreland, J., Richardson, J., Coman, L., Edwards, M., Ginis, K....Wishart, L. (2010). The physical environment as a fall risk factor in older adults: Systematic review and meta-analysis of cross-sectional and cohort studies. *Australian Occupational Therapy Journal, 57*(1), 51–64.

Li, F., Harmer, P., Fisher, K. J., McAuley, E., Chaumeton, N., Eckstrom, E., & Wilson, N. L. (2005). Tai chi and fall reductions in older adults: A randomized controlled trial. *Journal of Gerontology, 60*(2), 187–194.

Mahoney, J. E., Palta, M., Johnson, J., Jalaluddin, M., Gray, S., Park, S., & Sager, M. (2000). Temporal association between hospitalization and rate of falls after discharge. *Archives of Internal Medicine, 160*(18), 2788–2795.

Montalvo, I., (September 30, 2007). The National Database of Nursing Quality Indicators™ (NDNQI®) *OJIN: The Online Journal of Issues in Nursing.* Vol. 12 No. 3, Manuscript 2

Muir, S. W., Gopaul, K., & Montero, Odasso, M. M. (2012). The role of cognitive impairment in fall risk among older adults: A systematic review and meta-analysis. *Age and Ageing, 41*(3), 299–308. doi:10.1093/ageing/afs012

Murphy, T., Labonte, P., Klock, M., & Houser, L. (2008). Falls prevention for elders in acute care: An evidence-based nursing practice initiative. *Critical Care Nursing Quarterly, 31*(1), 33–39.

Nicklin, D. (2006). Physical assessment. In J. J. Gallo, H. K. Bogner, T. Fulmer, & G. H. Paveza (Eds.), *Handbook of geriatric assessment* (4th ed., pp. 273–317). Sudbury, MA: Jones & Bartlett.

Nordell, E., Andreasson, M., Gall, K., & Thorngren, K. (2009). Evaluating the Swedish version of the Falls Efficacy Scale-International (FES-I). *Advances in Physiotherapy, 11*(2), 81–87.

O'Keefe, S., Jack, I., & Lye, M. (1996). Use of restraints and bedrails in a British hospital. *Journal of the American Geriatrics, 44,* 1086–1088.

Oliver, D., Healey, F., & Haines, T. P. (2010). Preventing falls and fall-related injuries in hospitals. *Clinics in Geriatric Medicine, 26,* 645–692.

Podsiadlo, D., & Richardson, S. (1991). The timed "up & go": A test of basic functional mobility for frail elderly persons. *Journal of the American Geriatrics Society, 39,* 142–148.

Porthouse, J., Birrks, Y. F., Torgerson, D. J., Cockayne, S., Puffer, S., & Watt, I. (2004). Risk factor for fracture in a UK population: A prospective cohort study. *QJM, 97*(9), 569–574.

Robbins, J. A., Biggs, M. L., & Cauley, J. (2006). Adjusted mortality after hip fracture: From the cardiovascular health study. *Journal of the American Geriatric Society, 54,* 1885–1891.

Rochon, P. A. (2006). *Drug prescribing for older adults.* Retrieved from http://www.uptodate.com/contents/drug-prescribing-for-older-adults

Rubenstein, L. Z. & Josephson, K. R. (2006). Falls and their prevention in elderly people: What does the evidence show? *Medical Clinics of North America. 90*(5), 807–824.

Scott, J. C. (1990). Osteoporosis and hip fractures. *Rheumatic Disease Clinics of North America, 16*(3), 717–740.

Scott, V., Votova, K., Scanlan, A., & Close, J. (2007). Multifactorial and functional mobiity assessment tools for fall risk among older adults in community, home-support, long-term, and acute care settings. *Age and Ageing, 36*, 130–139. Retrieved from http://knowledgetranslation.ca/sysrev/articles/project51/Scott2007.pdf

Shumway-Cook, A., Brauer, S., & Woollacott, M. (2000). Predicting the probability for falls in community-dwelling older adults using the Timed Up & Go Test. *Physical Therapy, 80*(9), 896–930.

Spoelstra, S. L., Given, B., You, M., & Given, C. W. (2012). The contribution falls have to increasing risk of nursing home placement in community-dwelling older adults. *Clinical Nursing Research, 21*(1), 24–42.

Stevens, J. A., Corso, P. S., Finkelstein, E. A., & Miller, T. R. (2006). The costs of fatal and nonfatal falls among older adults. *Injury Prevention, 12*, 290–295.

Tinetti, M. E. (1986). Performance-oriented assessment of mobility problems in elderly patients. *Journal of the American Geriatric Society, 34*(2),119–126.

Tinetti, M.E., & Kumar C. (2010). The patient who falls: It's always a trade-off. *Journal of the American Medical Association. 303*(3), 258–266.

Tinetti, M. E., Speechley, M. & Ginter, S. F. (1988). Risk factors for falls among elderly persons living in the community. *New England Journal of Medicine, 319*(26), 1701–1707.

World Health Organization [WHO]. (2010). *A global report on falls prevention: Epidemiology of falls.* Retrieved from http://www.who.int/ageing/projects/1.Epidemiology%20of%20falls%20in%20older%20age.pdf

Zwicker, D. & Fulmer, T. (2012). Reducing adverse drug events. In M. Boltz, E. Capezuti, T. Fulmer, & D. Zwicker (Eds.). *Evidence-based geriatric nursing protocols for best practice* (4th ed.). New York, NY: Springer.

For a full suite of assignments and additional learning activities, see the access code at the front of your book.

LEARNING OBJECTIVES

At the end of this chapter, the reader will be able to:

> Define delirium.
> Explain common causes of delirium in older adults.
> Describe signs and symptoms of delirium.
> Distinguish between delirium and dementia.
> Discuss appropriate treatment of delirium in a variety of settings.

KEY TERMS

Agitation

Attention

Combativeness

Delirium

Hyperactive form

Hypoactive form

Language

Memory

Mixed form

Orientation

Precipitating factors

Predisposing factors

Reasoning

Thought process and content

Wandering

Chapter 13

Delirium

Susan Saboe Rose

Definition and Etiology

Delirium is one of the most common psychiatric conditions in frail older adults, and one of the leading causes of preventable injury in older patients (Rothschild & Leape, 2000). Derived from the Latin term meaning "off the track," delirium refers to a transient global cognitive disorder or group of symptoms associated with complex medical comorbidities. The definition of delirium, as determined by the Diagnostic and Statistical Manual of Mental Disorders, Fourth Edition (DSM-IV) includes four main criteria, as described in **Table 13-1** (American Psychiatric Association, 2000).

Delirium is an acute disorder of attention and cognitive functioning, and a psychiatric manifestation of a medical or surgical diagnosis (Wiesenfeld, 2008). Nursing care for the individual with delirium is targeted toward identification and removal or treatment of underlying causes; promotion of safety; reorientation to baseline level of cognition; and promotion of adequate hydration, nutrition, elimination, and sleep.

TABLE 13-1 DSM-IV Criteria for Delirium

- Disturbance of consciousness (i.e., reduced clarity of awareness of the environment) with reduced ability to focus, sustain, or shift attention.

- A change in cognition or the development of a perceptual disturbance that is not better accounted for by a preexisting, established, or evolving dementia.

- The disturbance develops over a short period of time (usually hours to days) and tends to fluctuate during the course of the day.

- There is evidence from the history, physical examination, or laboratory findings that the disturbance is caused by the direct physiological consequences of a general medical condition.

Delirium may present in various stages of arousal, which complicates the assessment process, and may lead to an inaccurate or missed diagnosis (Waszynski, 2007; Wiesenfeld, 2008). Three forms of delirium are described in the literature: hyperactive, hypoactive, and mixed.

The *hyperactive form* of delirium often presents with psychomotor agitation and a plethora of psychiatric symptoms, such as confusion, hallucinations, or delusions. The hyperactive form is the most recognized form of delirium and is associated with perceptual disturbances and delusions in more than 70% of sufferers (Boettger & Breitbart, 2011). Manifestations of the hyperactive form of delirium could include *agitation*, such as pulling at tubes or catheters; restlessness; attempts to climb out of bed or elope; physical aggression; or *combativeness*.

The *hypoactive form* of delirium may mimic a stupor or coma and occurs more commonly than the hyperactive form. Hypoactive delirium has a higher mortality rate than hyperactive delirium, largely due to the effects of immobility (O'Keeffe & Lavan, 1999). Often called "quiet" delirium because it is characterized by a flat affect or apathy and often present in otherwise calm and seemingly alert patients (Truman & Ely, 2003), this type of brain dysfunction carries a more grim prognosis than hyperactive delirium and is the most commonly missed subtype of delirium (Camus et al., 2000; Meagher, Hanlon, Mahony, Casey, & Trzepacz, 2000; Peterson et al., 2003). Manifestations may include lethargy, inattention, or severe somnolence. The prevalence of perceptual disturbances or delusions affects roughly one-half of patients with hypoactive delirium (Boettger & Breitbart, 2011).

The *mixed form* of delirium is the most frequent subtype of delirium. The mixed form presents with both hyperactive and hypoactive features. It is not uncommon for delirious individuals to have daytime somnolence accompanied by nocturnal agitation and insomnia. Alternatively, individuals may fluctuate between the hyper- and hypoactive forms during the course of a few hours.

Symptoms of delirium include disturbance of consciousness and perceptual disturbances that develop over a short period of time and fluctuate during the course of the day. Disturbance of consciousness may be manifested as reduced awareness of the environment, inability to stay focused on a topic, disorganized speech, inattention, becoming easily distracted, or withdrawing from others, with very little response to the environment. Cognitive and perceptual disturbances may include poor memory for recent events, disorientation, rambling or nonsensical speech, restlessness, agitation, irritability, combative behavior, and disrupted sleep habits. Emotional disturbances, such as depression, anxiety, fear, and hopelessness, are common. Delirium-related psychoses often include frightening visual hallucinations and persecutory delusions (Trzepacz, 1996).

Although delirium may mimic a dementia, delirium is a separate syndrome and differs from dementia in key areas. One of the most important differences between delirium and dementia has to do with the onset of symptoms. In delirium, the onset of confusion and disordered thinking occurs fairly abruptly, within a short period of

TABLE 13-2 Differentiating Delirium from Dementia	
Delirium	**Dementia**
• Acute confusional state	• Chronic confusional state
• Abrupt onset (hours to days)	• Gradual decline (months to years)
• Impaired attention and focus	• Attention fairly preserved
• Fluctuating mentation and cognition	• Mentation is generally constant
• Potentially reversible	• Irreversible

time, such as a few hours, days, or weeks. In contrast, dementia typically begins with minor symptoms that gradually progress over time, such as months to years. The ability to maintain attention or stay focused is also different. In delirium, attention is significantly impaired, while individuals with dementia are generally able to remain alert until latter stages of the disease. Finally, delirium is characterized by fluctuation in mentation and thinking throughout the day. While individuals with dementia can have "good and bad periods" during the day, their memory and thinking skills tend to stay at a fairly constant level. Characteristics that differentiate delirium from dementia are described in **Table 13-2**.

The most important distinction between delirium and dementia is the potentially reversible attribute of delirium. Unlike dementia, which is a chronic, progressive, and ultimately fatal trajectory, delirium is an abrupt onset of confusion with an optimistic rate of reversibility. With aggressive treatment of underlying causes, it is possible to return the individual to his or her predelirium baseline.

That said, the nature of delirium accelerates the pace of cognitive decline; therefore, the longer the delirium persists, the less robustly the individual will recover. Persistent delirium syndromes are associated with poorer outcomes (Cole, Ciampi, Belzile, & Zhong, 2009), and delirium-related symptoms of inattention, disorientation, and impaired memory may persist up to 12 months after diagnosis (McCusker, 2003). Kiely and associates examined 412 patients with delirium and found that nearly one-third remained delirious 6 months after hospitalization, and those with persistent delirium were 2.9 times as likely to die during the next year than those patients in whom delirium had resolved (Kiely et al., 2009). In fact, the duration of delirium is one of the strongest risk factors for death, length of stay in the hospital, cost of care, and long-term cognitive impairment. As Ely (2002) points out, there are few developments in the course of critical illness that portend a grimmer prognosis than the development of delirium that does not readily resolve.

Background

The mechanism of delirium is not fully understood. There are numerous etiologies involved, and efforts to clarify the complexities often result in oversimplified explanations. One of the most predominant hypotheses describes delirium as a reversible impairment of cerebral oxidative metabolism plus multiple neurotransmitter abnormalities. Numerous neurotransmitters have been linked to delirium, such as acetylcholine, dopamine, serotonin, GABA, and melatonin (Alagiakrishnan & Blanchette, 2012; Alagiakrishnan & Wiens, 2004; Trzepacz, 1994).

Acetylcholine plays a key role in delirium, explaining why anticholinergic medications can cause delirium even in healthy individuals. Delirium is theorized to decrease acetylcholine synthesis in the central nervous system (CNS), and serum anticholinergic activity correlates with the severity of delirium (Campbell et al., 2009; Mach, Dysken, & Kuskowski, 1995). The role of acetylcholine also explains the difficulty differentiating delirium from dementia: Alzheimer's disease is characterized by a loss of cholinergic neurons, illuminating why delirious individuals may exhibit similar symptoms as individuals with dementia.

Of particular importance to the treatment of delirium is a reciprocal relationship between cholinergic and dopaminergic activities, explaining why dopamine blockers such as haloperidol are useful in treating delirium-related psychosis (Alagiakrishnan & Blanchette, 2012; Alagiakrishnan & Wiens, 2004; Flacker & Lipsitz, 1999).

Physiological conditions, such as constipation and urinary retention, can also contribute to delirium. Delirium that results from urinary retention is referred to as "cystocerebral syndrome," and hypothesized by Waardenburg (2008) as a catecholamine surge that occurs as a result of increased bladder-wall tension causing increased sympathetic tone.

Significance of the Problem

Delirium is a medical emergency associated with increased morbidity and mortality. The prevalence of delirium has been widely examined, and a variety of prevalence rates are available in the literature. The wide variation in the numbers underscores the difficulty recognizing delirium due to the fluctuating nature of the condition.

Siddiqui, House, and Holmes (2006) found the prevalence of delirium at admission ranged from 10% to 31%, with an occurrence rate per admission that varied between 11% and 42%. The prevalence of delirium has been reported to be from 10% to as high as 80% in hospitalized medically ill patients to terminally ill patients (Brown & Boyle, 2002; Uguz et al., 2010). Delirium after cardiac surgery has a reported incidence of 3% to 73% (Sockalingam et al., 2005). Other rates in the literature range around from 14% to 56% of hospitalized individuals, as many as 80% of patients in intensive care, and 40% of individuals in long-term care facilities (Foreman, Wakefield, Culp & Milisen, 2001; Inouye, 1994, 2006; Kurlowicz, 2001; Waszynski, 2007).

Patients undergoing surgery have higher risk of developing delirium, with a peak in severity generally occurring on the second postoperative day. The incidence of postoperative delirium varies from 10% to 50% (Dyer, Ashton, & Teasdale, 1995), and individuals undergoing orthopedic surgery are particularly vulnerable (Bitsch, Foss, Kristensen, & Kehlet, 2004).

Up to 70% of older adults in the intensive care unit may suffer from an episode of delirium (McNicoll et al., 2003), with an additional 30% of patients having a milder form of delirium called subsyndromal delirium, in which core diagnostic symptoms are present but the severity is less than a formal diagnosis of delirium (Ouimet et al., 2007). Despite high prevalence rates in the intensive care unit (ICU), delirium often goes unrecognized by clinicians (Ely et al., 2004) or the symptoms are incorrectly attributed to dementia, depression, or incorrectly considered an expected and inconsequential complication of critical illness (Girard, Pandharipande, & Ely, 2008).

Delirium is commonly superimposed on underlying dementia, compounding both its symptoms and severity. Fick, Agostini, and Inouye (2002) found that the prevalence of delirium superimposed on dementia ranged from 22% to 89% and was associated with increased mortality. The presence of a superimposed delirium increases both the severity and the intensity of underlying dementia-related cognitive and perceptual disturbances, and poses an additional layer of complexity to symptom management.

Delirium is an independent predictor of death in older medical patients, and vigilant attention to identification and treatment is vital. Mortality rates for delirium are very high, particularly in hospitalized elders. In patients who are admitted with a delirium, mortality rates range from 10% to 26% (Pompei et al., 1994); however, patients who develop delirium during their hospitalization have a mortality rate of 22% to 76%, as well as a high rate of death in the months following discharge (American Psychiatric Association, 1999). These high mortality rates underscore the emergent nature of delirium.

Mortality rates aside, delirium in elders is also associated with prolonged hospital stays, increased complications, increased cost, and long-term disability (Edlund et al., 2006; Pompei et al., 1994; Tullmann, Fletcher, & Foreman, 2012). Delirium is associated with increased use of physical restraints (Micek, Anand, Laible, Shannon, & Kollef, 2005), and is also a predictor of long-term cognitive and functional decline (Fick et al., 2002). Lakatos and colleagues (2009) studied 252 hospitalized patients and found an association between delirium and prevalence of falls. Similarly, DeCrane, Culp, and Wakefield (2011) studied 320 patients for a 12-month period and found that delirium increased the risk of falling.

In 2007, the Centers for Medicare and Medicaid Services proposed inclusion of delirium to a list of "never" events—a list of hospital-acquired conditions for which a hospital would receive no payment. Although the verdict is still out at the time of this publication, the proposal of this inclusion underscores the preventive nature of delirium and behooves clinicians to aggressively target early recognition and treatment of delirium.

Risk Factors

Risk factors for delirium are best understood as predisposing and precipitating factors. *Predisposing factors* are those baseline vulnerabilities that are possessed by the patient prior to hospitalization. Predisposing factors include brain diseases or cognitive impairments such as dementia, stroke, or Parkinson's disease. Other common predisposing factors include polypharmacy, sensory impairment such as vision or hearing loss, functional impairment, medical comorbidities, or history of alcohol abuse. Age is also a predisposing factor, as elderly patients are at the highest risk for delirium. Additional predisposing factors include infection, metabolic disturbances, dehydration, immobility, malnutrition, or advanced cancer. Both undertreated pain and pain medications can predispose the patient to delirium. Inouye, Viscoli, Horowitz, Hurst, and Tinetti (1993) identified salient predisposing factors for development of delirium in hospitalized patients as (1) sensory impairment; (2) history of cognitive impairment; (3) sleep deprivation; (4) immobility; and (5) dehydration.

Precipitating factors are those events or conditions that occur during hospitalization to trigger a delirium. Precipitating factors include acute cardiac or pulmonary events, bed rest, drug withdrawal, fecal impaction, fluid or electrolyte disturbances, and indwelling devices such as urinary catheters. Additional precipitating factors include infections, medications, restraints, severe anemia, uncontrolled pain, and urinary retention. An increased number of room changes, absence of a clock or watch, absence of reading glasses or hearing aids, and sleep deprivation can also precipitate delirium.

Delirium can be conceptualized as a tangle of strings. Each string is either a predisposing factor (a vulnerability possessed by the patient prior to hospitalization) or a precipitating factor (an event or condition occurring during hospitalization.) The treatment of delirium is comparable to teasing out the strings of a tangle, removing strings, or managing them to reduce risk of harm (George, 2007).

Inouye (2006) found that delirium is rarely caused by a single factor; rather, it represents an intrinsically multifactorial syndrome. The effects of baseline and precipitating factors on the development of delirium are cumulative. Individuals who are highly vulnerable to delirium at baseline may develop delirium with any precipitating factor, whereas patients with low vulnerability could be resistant to development of delirium, even with noxious insults.

Medications are commonly implicated in delirium and can serve as both predisposing and precipitating factors. The etiology of delirium is multifactorial; therefore, it is difficult to firmly establish a causal role for any individual medication (Moore & O'Keeffe, 1999). The cumulative effect of anticholinergic medications may determine development of delirium rather than any single agent. Although not an inclusive list, **Table 13-3** includes medications that can contribute to delirium.

BOX 13-1 Predisposing and Precipitating Factors in Delirium

Predisposing Factors (Baseline Vulnerability)

- Advanced cancer
- Alcoholism
- Anemia
- Cognitive impairment
- Certain medications or polypharmacy
- Chronic pain
- Dehydration
- Fluid and electrolyte imbalances
- Hypoxia
- Impaired cardiac or respiratory function
- Infection; usually urinary tract or pneumonia
- Malnutrition
- Medical comorbidities
- Metabolic disturbances, electrolyte imbalance
- Sensory impairment, vision or hearing loss
- Unfamiliar surroundings

Precipitating Factors (Triggers)

- Absence of a clock or watch
- Absence of reading glasses or hearing aids
- Acute cardiac or pulmonary events
- Bedrest, immobility
- Drug withdrawal
- Fecal impaction
- Fluid or electrolyte disturbances
- Increased number of room changes
- Indwelling devices, such as urinary catheters
- Medications
- Nosocomial or hospital-acquired infections
- Restraints
- Severe anemia
- Sleep deprivation
- Uncontrolled pain
- Urinary retention

TABLE 13-3 Common Anticholinergic Medications (With Examples) That Can Cause or Worsen Confusion

Analgesics: propoxyphene, meperidine, excess doses of opiates
Antiemetics: promethazine
Antihistamines: diphenhydramine, chlorpheniramine, promethazine
Antihypertensives: clonidine, beta-blockers
Antipruitics: hydroxyzine
Anticonvulsants: phenobarbital, carbamazepine
Antivertigo: meclizine, scopolamine
Anxiolytics: meprobamate or paroxetine
Benzodiazepines: alprazolam, diazepam, lorazepam
Bladder relaxants: oxybutynin propantheline, solifenacin, tolterodine
Gastrointestinal antispasmotics: dicyclomine, hyoscyamine
H2 antagonists: cimetidine, ranitidine
Muscle relaxants: cyclobenzaprine, baclofen
Sedatives-hypnotics: chloral hydrate
Tricyclic antidepressants: amitriptyline, desipramine

In particular, anticholinergic medications are associated with confusion and cognitive impairment in older adults. Cholinergic disturbance is theorized as the central lesion in delirium (Tune, 2001). Anticholinergic drugs act by blocking acetylcholine receptors in the central and peripheral nervous system. Impaired cholinergic neurotransmission has been implicated in the pathogenesis of delirium, and anticholinergic medications are well-known causes of acute and chronic confusional states.

Anticholinergic medications contribute to delirium in several ways. The accumulation of medications, both those that are prescribed as well as those purchased over-the-counter (OTC), can increase the overall anticholinergic burden and contribute to anticholinergic toxicity. Additionally, anticholinergic effects on the peripheral nervous system include urinary retention and constipation, both of which are directly linked to delirium. Adding insult to injury, urinary retention and constipation are also linked to urinary tract infections, which further increases risk of delirium, cumulating in a "vicious cycle" of treatment and side effects (Tune, 2001).

Updated frequently, the "Beers list" refers to a list of potentially inappropriate medications. Originally developed and published by Beers and colleagues in 1991 (Beers et al., 1991), the list was subsequently revised in 1997, 2003, and 2012 (Beers, 1997; Fick et al., 2003; American Geriatrics Society, 2012). This list contains potentially inappropriate medications and classes of medications to avoid in older adults, medications that can exacerbate certain conditions and diseases, and medications that should be used with caution in older adults. The Beers list is available on a pocket card from the American Geriatrics Society, and can be downloaded at http://www.americangeriatrics.org

It is important to note that many deliriogenic medications can be purchased without a prescription. Several OTC medications, such as antihistamines and cold formulas, are fairly anticholinergic and can contribute to delirium. Many OTC sleeping medications contain diphenhydramine or other antihistamines; these medications cause sedation, but also contribute to constipation, urinary retention, and confusion. It is important to inquire if patients are using any OTC medications and caution them on potentially unsafe side effects.

Warning Signs

Agitation is a common delirium prodromal feature and a common warning sign of impending delirium. Prodromal symptoms often occur 1 to 3 days prior to the development of delirium, and include restlessness, anxiety, irritability, distractibility, and disruption of sleep that may progress to daytime somnolence and nighttime wakefulness (Schulte, 2003).

Duppils & Wikblad (2004) studied 103 patients after hip surgery to examine behavior changes during the prodromal stage of delirium. Of those patients who met criteria for delirium, 62% exhibited a change in behavior before the onset of delirium. The most commonly observed behavioral changes were anxiety, disorientation, and urgent calls for attention, and the most evident symptoms occurred roughly 6 hours prior to the onset of delirium. De Jonghe et al. (2007) also studied prodromal delirium symptoms in elderly patients undergoing hip surgery and found that early symptoms of memory impairment, incoherence, disorientation, and underlying somatic illness predicted delirium.

Any sudden change in cognition or increase in agitation should be investigated. A person of any age, when acutely ill, may experience delirium; however, older adults with preexisting dementia are at highest risk for developing delirium when acutely ill or injured.

Assessment

Assessment of the frail elderly patient is complicated, particularly when advanced age is combined with comorbid conditions. Geriatric syndromes, such as confusion, weakness, lethargy, falls, and urinary incontinence are generally more common manifestations of illness in older adults than the common symptoms of fever or abnormal lab values that are typically seen with younger patients (Weber, 2010). In fact, it is not uncommon for an older adult with a urinary tract infection to present with altered mental status (AMS) as the sole symptom, and with an absence of fever or any change in blood chemistry.

Arguably, the single most important factor in assessment is knowledge of the patient's baseline level of physical and cognitive functioning. The establishment of a baseline against which to compare assessment data is critical. If the patient is too confused to respond, then data should be elicited from the patient's family or caregivers. All components of the patient's prior level of function, including basic activities of daily living (ADLs) such as bathing, dressing, toileting, and ambulation should be compared to current levels of functioning. The patient's baseline functional status for instrumental ADLs, such as food preparation, management of medications, housekeeping, bill-paying, and transportation, should also be queried.

Mental Status Examination

Nursing assessment is a key factor in recognition of delirium. Since the nature of delirium involves fluctuation of altered levels of consciousness throughout the day, nurses are in the best position to observe this fluctuation over the course of a shift. The mental status examination is the most crucial portion of the nursing assessment, as a thorough evaluation of cognition is required to determine whether the patient meets criteria for delirium. Assessment of mental status generally includes evaluation of basic domains of cognitive functioning: attention, orientation, language, memory, and reasoning, as well as thought process and content. A brief format for assessing domains of cognitive functioning in delirium is described in **Figure 13-1**.

FIGURE 13-1 Brief Mental Status Examination for Delirium (Rose, 2010)

Components	Characteristics	How to Assess	Changes in Delirium
Attention	Sustained focus Vigilance	"I'd like you to start at December, and say the months backwards."	Acute decline and impairment in attention
Orientation	Awareness of person, place, and time	"How old are you? What is the name of this building? What is today's date? What day of the week is this? About what time is it?"	Disorientation to time is a common finding. Disorientation to place may also occur.
Language	Object recognition and naming Verbal fluency Comprehension	Show the patient an object, such as a watch, and then less common parts of the watch. "What do you call this? And what do you call this part of the watch?" (Wristband, clasp or buckle, face or dial, stem or winder). "I'm going to give you one minute, and I'd like you to name as many of the United States as you can. Ok? Start."	Naming may be impaired. Verbal fluency may be diminished. Comprehension will fluctuate.
Memory	Registration and recall of recently presented information, remote memory for historical events	"I'm going to give you three words to remember. Say these words: Apple, penny, green. Say them again. Now I am going to distract you, and will ask you those words in a few minutes." "A few minutes ago, you memorized three words. What were they?" "Now I'm going to test your memory for things in the past. Do you remember when President Kennedy died? How did he die? Where did that happen? Who took his place as president?"	Registration and recall are likely to be grossly impaired in delirium. Recognition from a list may also be impaired. Remote memory is likely to be impaired in delirium.
Reasoning	Abstract concept formation, complex problem-solving	"Have you ever heard the phrase, 'People that live in glass houses shouldn't throw stones?' What does that mean?" "What would you do if you saw a small child in the middle of the road?" "I'd like you to draw the face of a clock, and place the hands at 10 minutes past 11:00."	Reasoning is likely to fluctuate, in accordance with waxing/waning of delirium.

Components	Characteristics	How to Assess	Changes in Delirium
Thought Process	Quality and coherence of thought	"Do you feel like your thoughts are jumbled, or moving at a different speed than normal?"	Thought process is disordered in delirium. Racing thoughts are common in hyperactive delirium, and cognitive slowing is common in hypoactive delirium.
Thought Content	Subject matter of thought	"Do you ever feel like your mind is playing tricks on you?" "Do you find that you've been having odd thoughts recently?" "Have you been having any unusual sensations or visions that just started in the past few days?"	Visual and tactile hallucinations are common in delirium. Auditory hallucinations are less common, and gustatory hallucinations are uncommon. Delusions are very common.

Attention centers around the ability to disengage, reengage, and sustain focus and vigilance. This can be tested with exercises such as reverse weekdays, reverse month order, or subtraction. One of the most common tests of attention is to ask the patient to start at December, and say the months of the year in reverse. Report as the number of correct months: for example, "The patient scored 9/12 on reverse month order." Other tests of attention include asking the patient to perform serial subtractions, such as starting at 20 and subtracting by threes, or starting with 100 and subtracting by sevens. Attention is almost always impaired in delirium, and provides a good benchmark for determination of improvement or decline.

Orientation is a function of memory and involves awareness of the dimensions of person, place, and time. Orientation to person is generally not impaired with delirium. From an existential perspective, awareness of self may be the last cognitive process to develop and the earliest to decline; however, from a cognitive perspective, one's name is among the earliest cognitive representations to develop and usually the last to be lost. Therefore, it is very unusual for a delirious individual to not recall their own name, and such a finding would most likely represent an amnestic condition other than delirium.

Orientation to place can be assessed by asking the patient to state the name of the hospital or care facility. Orientation to time can be assessed by asking the patient to state their current age, and other indications of time, such as the month, year, and approximate time of day. Report as correct, followed by incorrect responses: for example, "The patient was correct on location, month, year, but incorrect on age, date, and weekday." Unlike orientation to the dimension of person, disorientation to place and time are very common in delirium.

Language refers to the capacity for acquiring and using systems of communication. The cognitive domain of language generally refers to primary linguistic functions, such as object recognition and naming, verbal fluency, and comprehension. Object recognition and naming can be tested by asking the patient to identify a common object, such as a watch, followed by familiar, but less common objects, such as the watchband, clasp, face, and stem. Report as correct, then incorrect responses: for example, "The patient was able to correctly identify a watch, band, and clasp, but was unable to come up with the name for the face or stem." Word recognition, grammar, and naming are generally preserved, despite aging or disease, and are less likely to be affected by delirium.

Verbal generative fluency refers to the ability to initiate and sustain communication. This can be tested by asking the patient to name as many animals or specific items as they can in a minute. Generation of 12 to 20 unique responses in a 60-second period is considered a normal response for younger adults; however, verbal generative fluency decreases with age, so an abnormal finding is not necessarily indicative of delirium. Report as the number of items in a time period: for example, "The patient was able to list 14 of the United States in a 60-second period."

Comprehension refers to a level of understanding. Comprehension can be assessed by asking the individual to repeat salient points of a conversation, or by asking questions to determine understanding. Report in terms of description: for example, "The patient did not appear to understand how to use a call light, and was observed speaking to it like a telephone." Comprehension is frequently impaired in delirium. In fact, the nature of delirium is characterized by fluctuating levels of cognition, so comprehension is likely to fluctuate accordingly. This is important to remember, as the patient will have periods of lucidity, which will alternate with periods of confusion and inattention. Patient teaching will need to be maximized during periods of lucidity.

Memory includes primary, secondary, and tertiary memory. Primary or working memory refers to *registration*, and can be tested by giving a patient several words or a phrase to remember: "I am going to give you three words to remember: apple, penny, green. Say those words back to me." Registration is reported as the number of correctly registered words: for example, "The patient scored 3/3 on registration." It is important to make sure the patient can repeat the words back to you. Recall cannot be tested if the patient is unable to register the words in the first place.

Secondary memory refers to *recall*, and can be tested by asking the patient to recall the three words after a few minutes. "A few minutes ago, you were given three words to remember. Repeat those words now." *Cued recall* refers to the use of a category prompt or hint. "Was one of those words a piece of fruit? A coin?

A color?" It is important to note that cued recall is a normal finding in older adults; requirement of a category prompt does not necessarily indicate impairment. If cued recall is impaired, then move on to *recognition*. "Was the fruit an apple, a pear, or a banana? Was the coin a penny, nickel, or quarter? Was the color red, green, or yellow?" Report as the number of correct responses, always including the prior score on registration; for example, "The patient scored 3/3 on registration, 0/3 on recall, 1/3 on cued recall, and was able to recognize 1 of the 2 remaining words when presented with a list." As previously mentioned, impairment in spontaneous recall and requirement of a category prompt is a normal finding in older adults. That said, impairment in cued recall or recognition from a list is considered abnormal, and likely to be impaired in delirium.

Tertiary or remote memory refers to recall of public events throughout history, or facts learned long ago. Remote memory is tested by asking the patient questions about salient events that occurred during their lifetime, such as the death of President Kennedy or the events of September 11, 2001. Report as the number of correct responses followed by incorrect responses: for example, "The patient was able to correctly account for 1/4 airplanes on 9/11/2001, and had an incorrect recollection of events surrounding New York City." Remote memory is also likely to be affected by delirium.

Reasoning refers to abstract concept formation and executive functioning. Reasoning can be tested by asking the patient to interpret a proverb or aphorism, define an abstract concept, or solve a problem. Test by asking the patient to interpret an aphorism, such as "A stitch in time saves nine." Alternatively, you could ask the patient to solve a problem that requires formulation of a strategy: for example, "What would you do if you were stranded on vacation with no money? How would you get home?" Reasoning is frequently impaired, and may fluctuate in accordance with the waxing and waning of mentation that is characteristic of a delirium.

One of the most common ways to assess reasoning is with the Clock Drawing Test (CDT). The CDT assesses capacity for planning, organizing, sequencing, and abstraction, and is a very common test of executive functioning. The following instructions are given: "Draw the face of a clock, place numbers on the clock, and put the hands at 10 minutes past 11 o'clock." There are numerous ways to score the CDT, but the most beneficial is to simply describe what was correct and what was not. Report in terms of planning (circle size), organizing (placement of numbers), sequencing (inclusion of all numbers in the correct order), and abstraction (hand placement and length). For example, "The patient was able to adequately plan a circle large enough to accommodate all of the numbers. Organization and sequencing were impaired, and numbers were placed in incorrect positions. Abstraction was grossly impaired, as the patient was unable to determine any semblance of hand placement."

Other than tests of attention, the CDT is one of the most commonly used determinants of improvement or decline in delirium. As portrayed in **Figure 13-2**, the CDT provides a stark visual illustration of the disorganized cognition that accompanies delirium. This particular CDT also provides an example of the potential for cognitive improvement with aggressive treatment of delirium.

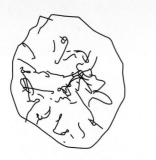
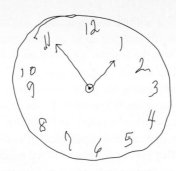

Figure 13-2 Clock drawing test during and after an episode of delirium.

Source: Newton, Kuebrich, & Rose, 2012; used with permission.

Thought process and content refer to the quality, coherence, and content of thought. Thought process includes such features as tempo, perseveration, and organization. Thought content may include delusions, visual hallucinations or misrepresentations, obsessions, or preoccupations. Thought process and content are assessed by observation of the patient during an interview. Speed of processing can be observed by paying attention to latencies in response, or asking the patient if they feel like their thoughts are moving faster or slower than usual. Grossly disordered thinking can be fairly evident, but less obvious presentations may take time to become noticeable. It is important to perform this portion of the assessment in a supportive and matter-of-fact way, as delirious patients may be frightened by their internal thought processes and become suspicious or guarded with interview. Report thought process and content together: for example, "Thought process is disordered, and content includes persecutory delusions, such as believing that she is being poisoned."

Standardized Tests for Delirium

Scales help us understand the level of symptomology of our patients, aid diagnosis, and help gauge treatment efficacy (Nash & Rose, 2012). The nurse plays a critical role in identifying whether an older adult has experienced an acute change in mental status that could be delirium.

Inouye and colleagues (1990) developed the Confusion Assessment Method (CAM) to assist nurses and others to identify delirium quickly and accurately using the four basic features of delirium: (1) acute onset or fluctuating course, (2) inattention, (3) disorganized thinking, and (4) altered level of consciousness. A diagnosis of delirium is made if both features 1 and 2 are present, along with either features 3 or 4. The CAM is commonly used by both nursing and medical staff, and considered by many to be the "gold standard" for recognition of delirium. Report as whether or not the criteria are met: for example, "The patient meets CAM criteria for delirium." CAM criteria is listed in **Table 13-4**.

Although the CAM is sensitive for recognition of delirium, it does not provide a measure of severity. The Delirium Rating Scale-revised-98 is a 16-item clinician-administered scale that provides a measure of delirium severity that can be used to monitor change over time (Trzepacz et al., 2001).

Two common tools for assessing delirium in patients in the ICU are the Confusion Assessment Method for the ICU (CAM-ICU) (Ely, 2002) and the Intensive Care Delirium Screening Checklist (ICDSC) (Bergeron, Dubois, Dumont, Dial, & Skrobik, 2001). The CAM-ICU was adapted from the original CAM, and is comprised of a

TABLE 13-4 Confusion Assessment Method Criteria
Confusion Assessment Method (CAM) Algorithm
1. Acute onset and fluctuating course
2. Inattention
3. Disorganized thinking
4. Altered level of consciousness
Diagnosis by CAM requires 1 and 2, and either 3 or 4.

serial assessment tool for use by bedside clinicians that has been adapted for the critical care setting. The ICDSC is an eight-item delirium checklist, based on data from the previous 24 hours. All of the above instruments require training prior to use.

Diagnosis

The most important objective in a delirium workup is to diagnose the cause of the confusion. Any acute episode of confusion warrants a clinical evaluation by a physician or nurse practitioner. Once the determination of delirium has been obtained, the assessment shifts to a focus on investigating possible causes of delirium.

Nursing diagnostics include monitoring of vital signs. Oxygen saturation is important, as hypoxia or carbon dioxide retention can contribute to delirium. Bladder scans are also important, as urinary retention is both a predictor and an outcome of delirium.

Nursing assessment skills are particularly needed to monitor for signs of infection. The two most common sources of infection in older adults are urinary tract infections (UTI) and pneumonia. Assess for symptoms of UTI, such as a new onset of urinary incontinence, urinary retention, foul or odorous urine, frequency, or dysuria. Monitor for symptoms of pneumonia by auscultating lung sounds and notifying the medical staff of aberrancies.

Undertreated pain is a common contributor to delirium. Pain is particularly difficult to assess in older adults who also have cognitive impairment. Frequent vocalizations and repeated phrases such as "Help me, help me" are commonly associated with pain. Resistance to care, rubbing a particular body part, or combativeness when being bathed can also serve as indicators of pain.

Standard "Delirium labs" include a complete blood count (CBC), comprehensive metabolic panel, and urinalysis. Additional labs generally include a vitamin B12 level; folate, magnesium, and phosphate levels; toxicology; and blood glucose levels to search for potential contributors to delirium. If indicated, a rapid plasma reagin (RPR) is included.

Delirium is a medical emergency, and neuroimaging is generally indicated. A head CT will help determine the presence of a stroke or if trauma related to a recent fall is suspected. Abdominal series are frequently performed to rule out medical culprits, such as constipation. Chest X-ray is indicated if there is a suspicion of pneumonia. An electrocardiogram (EKG) is important, especially if the patient requires treatment with neuroleptic medications, as they can contribute to cardiac arrhythmias.

Other consultations include speech pathology for swallowing evaluations to assess risk of aspiration, as it relates to fluctuating mentation and levels of consciousness. Aspiration precautions are particularly important in the hypoactive or mixed forms of delirium.

Medication review by a clinical pharmacist is commonly requested, as polypharmacy can contribute to delirium. Particular attention should be paid to medications that have recently been started or increased. As described earlier, it is not uncommon for antihistamines to contribute to a delirium because of their anticholinergic properties. In fact, most over-the-counter sleep aids tend to contain antihistamines and are particularly deliriogenic. Additionally, the abrupt discontinuation of some medications, such as benzodiazepines, opioids, or select serotonin reuptake inhibitors (SSRIs), are associated with severe withdrawal syndromes, which can contribute to delirium.

"I WATCH DEATH" is a commonly used mnemonic to evaluate for the presence of contributing factors for delirium (Wise, 1986). The reference to death in the mnemonic is a sobering reminder of the high mortality risks of delirium and the need for timely diagnosis and intervention (see **Table 13-5**).

TABLE 13-5 *"I WATCH DEATH"* **Mnemonic (Wise, 1986)**	
Infection	HIV, sepsis, pneumonia
Withdrawal	Alcohol, barbiturate, sedative/hypnotic
Acute metabolic	Acidosis, alkalosis, electrolyte disturbance, hepatic failure, renal failure
Trauma	Closed-head injury, heat stroke, postoperative, severe burns
CNS pathology	Abscess, hemorrhage, hydrocephalus, subdural hematoma, infection, seizures, stroke, tumors, metastases, vasculitis, encephalitis, meningitis, syphilis
Hypoxia	Anemia, carbon monoxide poisoning, hypotension, pulmonary or cardiac failure
Deficiencies	Vitamin B12, folate, niacin, thiamine
Endocrinopathies	Hyper/hypoadrenocorticism, hyper/hypoglycemia, myxedema, hyperparathyroidism
Acute vascular	Hypertensive encephalopathy, stroke, arrhythmia, shock
Toxins or drugs	Prescription drugs, illicit drugs, pesticides, solvents
Heavy Metals	Lead, manganese, mercury

Nursing assessment is a key factor and frontline concept, both for identification and reduction of delirium risk factors. Salient nursing diagnoses are included under the Cognitive-Perceptual functional health pattern (Carpenito-Moyet, 2008), and may include confusion, disturbed sensory perception, impaired thought processes, and impaired comfort. Other common nursing diagnoses in the setting of delirium include constipation, urinary retention, anxiety, risk of aspiration, and risk for injury (Gordon, 1982).

Given the emergent nature of delirium, early identification of nursing diagnoses is important. It is necessary to be proactive and notify appropriate medical staff of any concerns about potential risks factors, immediately implement a plan of care, and continue close supervision.

Interventions

Treatment of delirium occurs in tandem with treatment of the underlying cause. For example, if the delirium is a result of a urinary tract infection, the combination of antibiotics as well as antipsychotics may be necessary.

Treatment requires an almost obsessional attention to the patient. The nature of delirium is one of waxing and waning, and vigilance is required to recognize the overall pattern of delirium. Some fluctuations may be subtle, while others may have more of a circadian pattern, with nocturnal agitation. As a general rule, suspect that a delirium may be at play when your cognitive assessment differs from that performed by a nurse colleague at a different time of day.

Wiesenfeld (2008) suggests the ADVISE model, as outlined in **Table 13-6**. Advocacy includes standing up for the delirious patient who is unable to speak for themselves. Diligence is necessary to explore potential deliriogenic contributors, rather than attributing confusion as an expected complication in older adults. Vigilance is vital to ensure that predisposing risk factors are explored and

TABLE 13-6 **ADVISE Model for Delirium Intervention (Wiesnefeld, 2008)**	
Advocacy	Advocacy for the delirious patient
Diligence	Diligence in exploring potential deliriogenic contributors
Vigilance	Vigilance to removal of contributing factors
Integration	Integration of a multidisciplinary approach
Support	Support of patient and family distress
Education	Education of delirium triggers

precipitating risk factors are removed. Integration of all disciplines on the healthcare team is essential to ensure that all clinical providers understand the presence of a delirium and support the plan of care. Support of patient and family distress is critical, as delirium can be a frightening ordeal. Education of patient and family is important to control risk factors and prevent further episodes of delirium.

One of the primary goals of treatment is management of delirium-related behaviors so that treatment of the underlying condition can be achieved. Behavioral and psychological symptoms occur in 90% of patients with cognitive impairment. Behavioral disorders in delirium tend to be more severe than those seen in dementia, but of shorter duration. The remainder of this chapter will focus on nursing interventions for specific behavioral challenges.

Pain

Management of pain is crucial, as undertreated pain is a precipitating factor for delirium. While postoperative pain may be a more recognizable condition, pain can occur from a variety of sources. Fundamentally, one of the most common sources of pain in hospitalized older adults is musculoskeletal pain related to immobility. Complicating things further, many clinicians incorrectly assume opioids are the cause of delirium in patients with pain, leading to a reduction in dosage or discontinuation of pain medications altogether. In fact, undertreated pain may be a stronger risk factor for delirium than pain medications (Robinson & Vollmer, 2010). Pain management regimens that involve scheduled analgesia are associated with lower incidence of delirium.

One of the more circuitous pathways in which pain contributes to delirium has to do with inappropriate and continued secretion and/or action of antidiuretic hormone (ADH). Undertreated pain contributes to the syndrome of inappropriate ADH secretion (SIADH), which in turn contributes to hyponatremia, which in turn contributes to delirium. In older adults, even the mildest dip in sodium can result in delirium. Hyponatremia-related deliriums also have a fairly pronounced anxiety component. Additionally, hyponatremia-related deliriums tend to take a long time to resolve, and symptoms often persist long after the sodium normalizes. Therefore, thorough and vigilant monitoring for pain can go a long way toward reduction of delirium risk factors.

Agitation

One of the most common precipitants of delirium-related agitation is excess stimulation. The hospital environment is filled with extraneous noises, such as alarms, telephones, and pagers that emit hundreds, if not thousands, of audible sounds each day. The cumulative effect of the overabundance of auditory and visual stimulation can be overwhelming to the individual with delirium. Delirium can be thought of as a "conceptual fog" in which every fragment of visual, auditory, tactile, and gustatory stimulation must be processed and interpreted by a fragile, delirious brain. Now think of the average hospital room, with all of the various sounds, shapes, colors, and smells. One of the best ways to reduce agitation is simply to remove excess stimulation. Eliminating extraneous noises, such as overhead paging; removing clutter from the patient's line of sight; removing excess equipment; turning off the television; and trying to limit as much stimulation as possible can go a long way toward reducing delirium-related agitation. Nicknamed "Feng Shui for the Frontal Lobe" (Rose, 2010), basic nursing interventions to reduce stimulation can significantly reduce agitation in individuals with cognitive impairment. Given that some forms of delirium may have a mortality rate of up to 76%, these basic nursing interventions can literally be lifesaving.

One of the most common precipitating factors in agitation is a result of an adverse reaction to medication. Psychotropic medications are often used to treat delirium-related psychosis. Akathisia is a sense of internal restlessness that drives agitation, and it is a common side effect of neuroleptic medication. Paradoxically, higher doses of medications can cause worsening of the symptoms that they are designed to treat. The geriatric mantra of "Start Low, Go Slow" is of particular importance when giving psychotropic medications for delirium-related psychosis and agitation.

One of the best strategies for agitated and restless individuals is to help them out of bed and assist them with ambulation to burn off pent-up energy. Scheduled ambulation can go a long way toward reducing agitation, and the benefits of ambulation on sleep and well-being are well known. If the patient is unable to ambulate, consider having them rise to standing at the bedside, with their feet on the floor and eyes on the horizon. This type of spatial reorientation can help burn off energy and improve endurance in individuals who lack the strength to ambulate.

One common behavioral challenge is preventing delirious individuals from pulling out tubes and lines, posing a safety issue. Camouflaging medical equipment can help discourage delirious patients from pulling out tubes. Consider extra tape on the IV site, or wrap it with gauze. Consider double-gowning a patient with a telemetry box between layers to discourage removal. Abdominal binders are useful for discouraging self-removal of surgical tubes, and long pants are useful to help protect urinary catheters.

Combativeness

One of the strongest predictors of combativeness in cognitively impaired elders is constipation (Leonard, Tinetti, Allore, & Drickamer, 2006). Constipation is commonly seen in delirium. Delirious patients are particularly at risk of dehydration, as they may be confused and pull out intravenous tubes or may harbor delusions about food and drink. Patients with delirium are also prone to immobility, as they are less likely to ambulate independently. Prevention and treatment of constipation can go a long way toward reducing agitation and aggression.

It is important to monitor bowel status and aim for a daily bowel movement in the delirious patient. Provide stimulus to defecation, such as coffee or prune juice. Assist the patient to the bathroom to allow for suitable positioning instead of using a bedpan. Check for bowel impaction if no bowel movement is noted within 48 hours in the delirious patient.

Urinary retention is also a contributor to combativeness. Urinary retention is both a predictor and an outcome of delirium; it is also a precipitating factor that may trigger a delirium, due to a catecholamine surge from increased bladder-wall tension. At the same time, the role of acetylcholine in delirium increases the risk of urinary retention. This vicious cycle results in retention as both a risk factor for delirium and a common outcome of delirium. Although it may be tempting to try to avoid performing a bladder scan on a combative patient, vigorous monitoring for urinary retention is important—both for early detection of delirium as well as for prevention of further delirium-related aggression. Additionally, a scheduled protocol of bladder scan and intermittent straight catheterization is preferable to the use of an indwelling urinary catheter.

Avoiding fatigue and sleep deprivation can also significantly reduce combativeness. Prevention is vital; it is important to avoid overstimulation, hunger, thirst, and frustration. Cluster activities at night in order to allow for maximum hours of sleep at night. Allow adequate rest periods during the day, and provide a calm and quiet environment when the delirious individual begins to show symptoms of aggression. A small snack can go a long way toward redirecting frustration and providing a calming distraction.

Inattentiveness

Inattentiveness is a key component of delirium and one of the defining characteristics. Inattentiveness may range from grossly disordered thinking to mildly disorganized thought processes. Inattentiveness may be attributed to normal aging, contributing to underrecognition of delirium. It is not unusual to see notations in the medical record describing an individual as "pleasantly confused" without any further evidence that delirium may be present.

Inattentive behaviors may pose safety risks to delirious patients. For example, they may not remember to ask for help before getting out of bed, or may not recognize that they are tethered to a cardiac monitor or oxygen regulator. They may have difficulty remembering patient instructions, such as how to use a call light. Frequent observation is necessary.

Nursing interventions to help with inattentiveness are geared toward increasing sustained focus. For individuals with severe inattention, short exercises such as listing the days of the week forward and backwards are useful. As the patient's confusion improves, increase the complexity of the exercises to forward and back month order or mathematical problems. Giving a delirious patient some simple arithmetic problems to work on helps with sustained attention and focus, and also provides cognitive stimulation. Sorting cards or folding laundry is a good activity for individuals with inattention, as it helps with sustaining focus over time. Family members can assist in this process; for example, ask the family of a delirious patient to bring in familiar photographs of family members and help the patient to organize the photos into family groups.

Wandering and Exit-Seeking

Wandering is a common symptom in individuals suffering from cognitive impairment, including delirium. It is not uncommon for delirious patients to misjudge their level of wellness, believe they are ready for discharge, and decide to try to leave the hospital setting while they are still fairly confused and disoriented.

There are numerous causes for wandering, including distorted memories of once-familiar surroundings or difficulty adapting to new surroundings. Delirium-related mental changes and disorientation can cause worsening of perceptual distortions that can prompt wandering and exit-seeking.

Wandering that occurs at the same time every day may be linked to a lifelong routine, such as going to work. It is not uncommon for patients to become restless in the late afternoon, or try to elope at the change of shift as they see individuals leaving the unit.

Issues around toileting are common precipitators for wandering behaviors. Looking for a restroom is a frequent impetus for wandering in delirious individuals. Frequent toileting is a good way to prevent wandering, as is the use of signs and arrows to identify restrooms.

Excess stimulation is another culprit in wandering. It is not uncommon for delirious patients to flee rooms with excess clutter. The overstimulating environment of the busy hospital unit can contribute to a desire to elope to a quieter setting.

Wandering patients often head directly to their only exit: public transportation. A well-publicized episode of wandering in a delirious patient was illustrated in the case of a 78-year-old individual who wandered away from a hospital in Denver, Colorado, eventually found his way onto a public bus, then a Greyhound station, and was eventually discovered 3 days later in San Diego (Fong, 2007). The visual appeal of a bus stop for a wandering individual is such a common stimuli that the Benrath Senior Center in Dusseldorf, Germany built a fake bus stop in front of the hospital. It has been a very successful program; wandering patients often settle there, and the bus stop offers a neutral ground to wait until the nursing staff can soothe them back inside (Miller, 2011).

Sleep

Disruption of the sleep–wake cycle is common in delirium, as is nocturnal agitation. Even in the absence of delirium, sleep in older adults is problematic. In the seventh and eighth decade of life, the circadian rhythms tend to flatten out and often lose the ability to maintain a functional sleep–wake cycle. Gender differences also exist; older women have higher prevalence of difficulty falling asleep and waking up too early, and older men have a higher prevalence of daytime somnolence (Gislason, Reynisdottir, Kristbjarnarson, & Benediktsdottir, 2009). Bidirectional causality occurs between sleep and cognitive functioning; inadequate sleep contributes to cognitive impairment, and visa versa.

In the presence of a delirium, sleep patterns become more fragmented and unpredictable. Sleep deprivation is common with the hyperactive form of delirium, and excessive somnolence is characteristic of the hypoactive form. The tenuous relationship between sleep and cognition affects the integrity of the circadian system, which results in degrading of sleep architecture and disrupted circadian rhythms.

Sleep hygiene is very important in delirium. Maximizing sunlight, especially during early morning, helps regulate sleep–wake cycles. Getting out of bed for all meals helps promote orientation and provides cognitive stimulation. Darkening the room and drawing the shades at night helps promote restfulness. Applying a warm blanket at bedtime helps promote comfort and sleep (see **Table 13-7**).

When a "Sitter" is the Wrong Approach

One of the most common symptoms in delirium is psychosis, such as hallucinations or delusions (Trzepacz, 1996). When delirium takes the form of paranoia and suspiciousness, direct supervision may become challenging. The nurse must balance the needs of patient observation with provision of stimulus for delusions. For the patient with severe paranoia, the presence of an unfamiliar observer can cause worsening of psychosis. Family members or familiar friends of the patient should be enlisted if the patient requires a constant companion.

Close supervision may be appropriate to prevent injury in the patient with acute agitation, alleviate fear, or provide comfort. Many hospitals and care facilities have trained individuals to provide one-to-one supervision, commonly referred to as "sitters." For the patient with delirium, it is imperative that the use of a "sitter"

TABLE 13-7   When It's 3 A.M....
• Help the patient out of bed and assist with ambulation as needed to burn off excess energy
• Assist the patient to the bathroom
• Reduce as much stimulation as possible
• Turn off the television, turn off lights, provide a warm blanket, partially close door, and talk in a low monotone voice

support the patient's plan of care, rather than be used solely to observe. In a syndrome with a mortality rate that may be as high as 80%, stringent vigilance to the plan of care is essential. Rather than "sitting," (see **Box 13-2**) the one-to-one companion has an important role of assisting with hydration, monitoring for aspiration, providing cognitive stimulation during daytime hours and ensuring decreased stimulation at bedtime, providing frequent toileting, assisting with ambulation, and providing distraction and protection to avoid self-removal of tubes and devices.

BOX 13-2   Personal Reflection

If you were suffering from paranoia, would you want a stranger staring at you for 24 hours a day?

Safety Concerns

Individuals with delirium are at higher risk of injury. Reduce the risk of burns secondary to patients with delirium handling hot liquids by opening containers of hot liquids and allowing them to cool off before offering them to a delirious individual.

The nature of delirium is one of fluctuating levels of mentation. Individuals with the hypoactive form of delirium are at higher risk of aspiration because of decreased levels of consciousness. Maintain aspiration precautions and consider a mechanical soft diet until the delirium improves.

Delirious individuals are at high risk for falling. The human cost of a fall is immeasurable and life changing. Eighty-seven percent of all fractures among older adults are due to falls and half of all older people hospitalized for hip fractures cannot return home or live independently after their injury (Centers for Disease Control and Prevention [CDC], 2004). In fact, mortality rates range between 18% and 33% within the first year post-fracture (Magaziner et al., 2000). Place the bed in the lowest position and employ a bed alarm for restless patients. The use of physical restraints as a fall-prevention device is inappropriate, as they are associated with increased agitation and panic in confused individuals and can result in serious injury or death.

Falls among delirious patients are commonly related to toileting. It is important to provide scheduled toileting to reduce the risk of agitation and urinary retention. It is also important to provide direct supervision of delirious individuals while they are in the restroom or on a bedside commode. Privacy during toileting must be modified sufficiently to ensure a quick response to avoid a potential fall or injury.

Home Management After Discharge

It is not unusual for delirium to take weeks to entirely resolve. Most patients are discharged from the acute care setting before the delirium has entirely resolved. During this period, the patient's mental status will continue to wax and wane. In general, rehabilitation in a skilled nursing facility is beneficial during the recovery period.

For patients who are discharged directly to the community, it is important that the patient and their family know that the delirious individual needs 24-hour supervision until the delirium has completely resolved. Periods of inattention, disorganized thinking, and confusion may continue for several weeks. The patient recovering from delirium will need oversight of instrumental daily activities, including management of medications. They should refrain from driving until they are cleared by the primary care provider. Family members may need to help the patient make complex or abstract decisions, and may need to help provide substituted judgment until the delirium fully clears.

Prognosis

The nature of delirium is one of potentially long-term waxing and waning of cognition. Eventually, the periods of lucidity will become longer, and the periods of confusion will become less frequent and less severe. A consistent baseline will emerge.

Delirium accelerates the pace of underlying cognitive decline. It is not unusual for an individual with mild cognitive impairment to manage fairly well in a familiar environment, but have more pronounced impairment after an episode of delirium. An underlying dementia may "declare itself" with persistent cognitive deficits that do not remit. Outpatient cognitive evaluation should be performed a few months after the delirium has resolved to evaluate for an underlying dementia.

Although delirium is viewed as a temporary and reversible condition, many patients never return to their previous baseline. The longer the delirium persists, the poorer the outcomes, particularly when the delirium is superimposed on underlying dementia. Nursing assessment (see **Box 13-3**) and intervention are crucial (see **Case Study 13-1**).

Summary

Delirium is common problem among older adults, especially the frail and compromised elderly. Nursing care for the individual with delirium is aimed at discovering the underlying cause and treating it (see **Box 13-4**). Causes of delirium may be simple, such as a urinary tract infection, or complex and multifaceted. While most delirium is considered an acute geriatric syndrome, untreated delirium can have harmful effects on the person's health and quality of life.

BOX 13-3   Evidence-Based Practice Highlight

Go to http://consultgerirn.org/topics/delirium/want_to_know_more and review the resources available for assessing and treating delirium. A standard of practice guideline (Tullman, Fletcher, & Foreman, 2012), tools, and videos are available at this website.

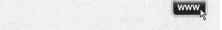

Case Study 13-1

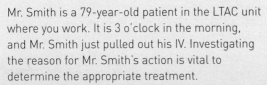

Mr. Smith is a 79-year-old patient in the LTAC unit where you work. It is 3 o'clock in the morning, and Mr. Smith just pulled out his IV. Investigating the reason for Mr. Smith's action is vital to determine the appropriate treatment.

Question:

Why did he pull out the IV?

- Because he is impulsive? Try diversion, an activity vest, or meaningful activity.

- Because he is restless? Ambulate around the nursing station to burn off energy.
- Because he had to go to the bathroom? Provide q2H toileting, check for urinary retention.
- Because he thought it was a worm or snake? He may benefit from a low-dose antipsychotic for psychosis.

BOX 13-4   Research Highlight

Aim: To determine if differences existed between doses of analgesia received by patients in pain who developed delirium and with those who did not develop delirium

Method: This study utilized a matched-group sample of 43 patients with and without delirium and examination of percentages of allowed analgesia. Patients with preexisting delirium were excluded. Patients were matched on age, gender, type of diagnosis, severity of illness, and number of delirium risk factors. Data were collected via retrospective chart review. Outcome criteria included the percentage of allowed analgesia received. Analysis of variance was used to compare groups.

Findings: The mean percentage of allowed analgesia received differed significantly between groups. Researchers found an association

between low dose of analgesia and development of delirium. The patients who developed delirium received a smaller amount of the total possible analgesic than those who did not develop delirium.

Application to Practice: This study supported earlier findings that undermanaged pain may be an additional precipitating factor in the development of delirium. Nurses should be aware of the need for adequate pain management in older adults. If the patient has risk factors for development of delirium, undermanaged pain may be the additional factor that precipitates delirium.

Source: Robinson, S., & Vollmer, C. (2012). Undermedication for pain and precipitation of delirium. *MEDSURG Nursing, 19*(2), 70–83.

Critical Thinking Exercises

1. If an older adult in your care presents with sudden onset of confusion, how does this influence your assessment? What risk factors and warning signs for delirium will you look for?

2. Identify a patient that you are caring for, or have cared for in the past, who could be at risk for delirium. List the risk factors for

this patient or resident and think about what interventions could be implemented to prevent delirium.

3. Go to http://www.consultgerirn.com and find the clinical guideline on delirium. Read through it, noting especially the statistics on delirium in older adults and the current standard of care.

Personal Reflection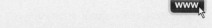

1. Have you ever cared for a patient that had delirium? If so, did you recognize it at the time? Was it a hyperactive, hypoactive, or mixed form? How was it treated?

2. What behaviors associated with delirium do you see as most problematic? Which are the

most difficult for you personally to handle in patients or residents?

3. How can you personally apply this information on delirium to your own clinical practice? Of what will you be more aware after studying the content of this chapter?

References

Alagiakrishnan, K. & Blanchette, P., (2012). Delirium. *Medscape Reference*. Retrieved from http://www.emedicine.medscape.com

Alagiakrishnan, K. & Wiens, C. A. (2004). An approach to drug induced delirium in the elderly. *Postgraduate Medical Journal, 80*, 388–393.

American Geriatrics Society Beers Criteria Update Expert Panel (2012). AGS updated Beers criteria for potentially inappropriate medication use in older adults. *Journal of the American Geriatric Society, 60*(4), 616–631. doi:10.1111/j.1532-5415.2012.03923.x

American Psychiatric Association (1999). Practice guideline for the treatment of patients with delirium. *American Journal of Psychiatry, 156*(5 Supp): 1–20.

American Psychiatric Association (2000). *Diagnostic and statistical manual of mental disorders* (4th ed., text rev.). Washington, DC: Author.

Beers, M. H. (1997). Explicit criteria for determining potentially inappropriate medication use by the elderly. An update. *Archives of Internal Medicine, 157*, 1531–1536.

Beers, M. H., Ouslander J. G., Rollingher I., Reuben, D. B., Brooks, J., & Beck, J. C. (1991). Explicit criteria for determining inappropriate medication use in nursing home residents. *Archives of Internal Medicine, 151*, 1825–1832.

Bergeron, N., Dubois, M. J., Dumont, M., Dial, S., & Skrobik, Y. (2001). Intensive care delirium screening checklist: Evaluation of a new screening tool. *Intensive Care Medicine, 27*(5), 859–64.

Bitsch, M., Foss, N., Kristensen, B., & Kehlet, H. (2004). Pathogenesis of and management strategies for postoperative delirium after hip fracture: A review. *Acta Orthopaedica Scandinavica, 75*(4), 378–389.

Boettger, S., & Breitbart, W. (2011). Phenomenology of the subtypes of delirium: Phenomenological differences between hyperactive and hypoactive delirium. *Palliative and Supportive Care, 9*(2), 129–135.

Brown, T. M. & Boyle, M. F. (2002). Delirium. *British Medical Journal, 325*, 644–647.

Campbell, N., Boustani, M., Limbil, T., Ott, C., Fox, C., Maidment, I.,....Gulati, R. (2009). The cognitive impact of anticholinergics: A clinical review. *Journal of Clinical Interventions in Aging, 4*, 225–233.

Camus, V., Burtin, B., Simeone, I., Schwed, P., Gonthier, R., & Dubos, G. (2000). Factor analysis supports the evidence of existing hyperactive and hypoactive subtypes of delirium. *International Journal of Geriatric Psychiatry, 15*, 313–316.

Carpenito-Moyet, L. J. (2008). *Nursing diagnosis: Application to clinical practice* (12th ed.). Philadelphia, PA: Lippincott Williams & Wilkins.

Centers for Disease Control and Prevention [CDC]. (2004). *A toolkit to prevent senior falls.* Atlanta, GA: National Center for Injury Prevention and Control.

Cole, M. G., Ciampi, A., Belzile, E., & Zhong, L. (2009). Persistent delirium in older hospital patients: A systematic review of frequency and prognosis. *Age and Ageing, 38*(1), 19–26.

DeCrane, S. K., Culp, K. R. & Wakefield, B. (2011). Twelve-month fall outcomes among delirium subtypes. *Journal for Healthcare Quality.* Advance online publication. doi: 10.1111/j.1945-1474.2011.00162.x

De Jonghe, J. F., Kalisvaart, K. J., Dijkstra, M., van Dis, H., Vreeswijk, R., Kat, M. G., … van Gool, W. A. (2007). Early symptoms in the prodromal phase of delirium: A prospective cohort study in elderly patients undergoing hip surgery. *American Journal of Geriatric Psychiatry, 15*(2), 112–121.

Duppils, G. S., & Wikblad, K. (2004). Cognitive function and health-related quality of life in connection with hip surgery: A six-month follow-up. *Orthopedic Nursing, 23*(3), 195–203.

Dyer, C.B., Ashton, C.M., & Teasdale, T.A. (1995). Postoperative delirium. A review of 80 primary data-collection studies. *Archive of Internal Medicine, 155*(5), 461–465.

Edlund, A., Lundstrom, M., Karlsson, S., Brannstrom, B., Bucht, G., & Gustafson, Y. (2006). Delirium in older patients admitted to general internal medicine. *Journal of Geriatric Psychiatry and Neurology, 19*(2), 83–90.

Ely, E. W., Shintani, A., Truman, B., Speroff, T., Gordon, S. M., Harrell F. E. Jr., … Dittus, R.S. (2004). Delirium as a predictor of mortality in mechanically ventilated patients in the intensive care unit. *JAMA: The Journal of the American Medical Association, 291*(14), 1753–1762.

Ely, E. W., Stephens, R. K., Jackson, J. C., Thomason, J. W., Truman, B., Gordon, S., … Bernard, G.R. (2004). Current opinions regarding the importance, diagnosis, and management of delirium in the intensive care unit: A survey of 912 healthcare professionals. *Critical Care Medicine, 32*, 106–112.

Fick, D. M., Agostini, J. V., & Inouye, S. K. (2002). Delirium superimposed on dementia: A systematic review. *Journal of the American Geriatric Society, 50*(10), 1723–1732.

Fick, D. M., Cooper, J. W., Wade, W. E., Waller, J. L., Maclean, J. R., & Beers, M. H. (2003). Updating the Beers criteria for potentially inappropriate medication use in older adults: Results of a US consensus panel of experts. *Archives of Internal Medicine, 163*, 2716–2724.

Flacker, J. M., & Lipsitz, L. A. (1999). Neural mechanisms of delirium: Current hypotheses and evolving concepts. *The Journals of Gerontology: Series A, 54*(6), B239–B246.

Fong, T. (2007, March 16). Man with Alzheimer's found in San Diego. *Rocky Mountain News.* Scripps Newspaper Group.

Foreman, M. D., Wakefield, B., Culp, K., & Milisen, K. (2001). Delirium in elderly persons: An overview of the state of the science. *Journal of Gerontological Nursing, 27*(4), 12–20.

George, M. A. (2007, April). Delirium in the elderly hospitalized patient. *OASIS 4th Annual Memory Event.* Tualatin, OR.

Girard, T. D., Pandharipande, P. P., & Ely, E. W. (2008). Delirium in the intensive care unit. *Critical Care, 12*(Suppl 3), S3.

Gislason, T., Reynisdottir, H., Kristbjarnarson, H., Benediktsdottir, B. (2009). Sleep habits and sleep disturbances among the elderly: An epidemiological survey. *Journal of Internal Medicine, 234*(1), 31–39.

Gordon, M. (1982). *Nursing diagnosis: Process and application.* New York, NY: McGraw-Hill.

Inouye, S. K. (1994). The dilemma of delirium: Clinical and research controversies regarding diagnoses and evaluation of delirium in hospitalized elderly medical patients. *American Journal of Medicine, 97*, 278–288.

Inouye, S. K. (2006). Delirium in older persons. *New England Journal of Medicine, 354*, 1157–1165.

Inouye, S. K., van Dyck, C. H., Alessi, C. A., Balkin, S., Siegal, A. P., & Horwitz, R. I. (1990). Clarifying confusion: The confusion assessment method. *Annals of Internal Medicine, 113*(12), 941–948.

Inouye, S. K., Viscoli, C. M., Horowitz, R. I., Hurst, L. D., & Tinetti, M. E. (1993). A predictive model for delirium in hospitalized elderly medical patients based on admission characteristics. *Annals of Internal Medicine, 119*, 474–481.

Kiely, D. K., Marcantonio, E. R., Inouye, S. K., Shaffer, M. L., Shaffer, M. L., Bergmann, M. A. ... Jones, R. N. (2009). Persistent delirium predicts greater mortality. *Journal of the American Geriatric Society, 57*, 55–61.

Kurlowicz, L. H. (2002). Delirium and depression. In V.T. Cogger & N.E. Strumpf (Eds.), *Advanced practice nursing with older adults: Clinical guidelines* (pp 141–162). New York, NY: McGraw-Hill.

Lakatos, B. E., Capasso, V., Mitchell, M. T., Kilroy, S. M., Lussier-Cushing, M., Sumner, L. ... Stern, T. A. (2009). Falls in the general hospital: association with delirium, advanced age, and specific surgical procedures. *Psychosomatics, 50*(3), 218–226.

Leonard, R., Tinetti, M. E., Allore, H. G., & Drickamer, M. A. (2006). Potentially modifiable resident characteristics that are associated with physical or verbal aggression among nursing home residents with dementia. *Archives of Internal Medicine, 166*(12), 1295–1300.

Magaziner, J., Hawkes W., Hebel J. R., Zimmerman, S. I., Fox, K. M., Dolan, M., & Kenzora, J. (2000). Recovery from hip fracture in eight areas of function. *The Journals of Gerontology. Series A, Biological Sciences and Medical Sciences. 55A*, M498–M507.

McCusker, J., Cole, M., Dendukuri, N., Han, L. & Belzile, É. (2003). The course of delirium in older medical inpatients. *Journal of General Internal Medicine, 18*, 696–704.

McNicoll, L., Pisani, M. A., Zhang, Y., Ely, E. W., Siegel, M. D., & Inouye, S. K. (2003). Delirium in the intensive care unit: Occurrence and clinical course in older patients. *Journal of the American Geriatric Society, 51*(5), 591–598.

Meagher, D. J., Hanlon, D. O., Mahony, E. O., Casey, P. R., & Trzepacz, P. T. (2000) Relationship between symptoms and motoric subtype of delirium. *The Journal of Neuropsychiatry & Clinical Neurosciences, 12*, 51–56.

Mach, J. R. Jr, Dysken, M. W., Kuskowski, M., Richelson, E., Holden, L., & Jilk, K. M. (1995). Serum anticholinergic activity in hospitalized older persons with delirium: A preliminary study. *Journal of the American Geriatrics Society, 43*, 491–495.

Micek, S. T., Anand, N. J., Laible, B. R., Shannon, W. D., & Kollef, M. H. (2005). Delirium as detected by the CAM-ICU predicts restraint use among mechanically ventilated medical patients. *Critical Care Medicine, 33*(6), 1260–1265.

Miller, L. (2011, April 1). A bus to nowhere. *Radiolab*. Podcast retrieved from http://www.radiolab.org/2011/apr/01/bus-nowhere/

Moore, A. R., & O'Keeffe, S. T. (1999). Drug-induced cognitive impairment in the elderly. *Drugs and Aging, 15*(1), 15–28.

Nash, M. C., & Rose, S. S. (2012). Using scales and measurement to improve quality in your geriatric practice. *Proceedings from the American Association for Geriatric Psychiatry 2012 Annual Meeting.* Retrieved from http://journals.lww.com/ajgponline/Fulltext/2012/03001/Session_Abstracts.1.aspx

Newton, P. A., Kuebrich, M. B., & Rose, S. S. (2012, January). Acute care of the elderly inpatient service. *Portland Area Geriatric Seminar Series: Excellence in Care, Research, and Education.* Portland, OR.

O'Keeffe, S. T., & Lavan, J. N. (1999). Clinical significance of delirium subtypes in older people. *Age and Ageing, 28*, 115–119.

Ouimet, S., Riker, R., Bergeron, N., Cossette, M., Kavanagh, B., & Skrobik, Y. (2007). Subsyndromal delirium in the ICU: Evidence for a disease spectrum. *Intensive Care Medicine, 33*(6), 1007–1013.

Peterson, J. F., Truman, B. L., Shintani, A., Thomason, J. W. W., Jackson, J.C., & Ely, E.W. (2003). The prevalence of hypoactive, hyperactive, and mixed-type delirium in medical ICU patients. *Journal of the American Geriatrics Society, 51*, S174.

Pompei, P., Foremen, M., Rudberg, M. A., Inouye, S. K., Braund, V., & Cassel, C. K. (1994). Delirium in hospitalized older persons: Outcomes and predictors. *Journal of the American Geriatrics Society, 42*(8), 809–815.

Robinson, S. & Vollmer, C. (2012). Undermedication for pain and precipitation of delirium. *MEDSURG Nursing, 19*(2), 70–83.

Rose, S. S. (2010). What's in your bag of tricks? Managing behavioral challenges in delirium and dementia. *Proceedings of the 11th Annual Oregon Geriatrics Society Conference.* Oregon Health & Sciences University: Portland, OR.

Rothschild, J. M., & Leape, L. L. (2000). *The nature and extent of medical injury in older patients: Executive summary.* Washington, DC: Public Policy Institute, AARP.

Schulte, J. J. Jr. (2003). Delirium: Confusional states. *Hospital Physician: Psychiatry Board Review Manual, 7*(4). Wayne, PA: Turner White Communications.

Siddiqui, N., House, A. O., & Holmes, J. D. (2006). Occurrence and outcome of delirium in medical in-patients: A systemic literature review. *Age and Aging, 35,* 350–364.

Sockalingam, S., Parekh, N., Bogoch, I. I., Sun, J., Mahtani, R., Beach, C., … Bhalerao, S. (2005). Delirium in the postoperative cardiac patient: A review. *Journal of Cardiac Surgery, 20,* 560–567.

Truman, B., & Ely, E. W. (2003). Monitoring delirium in critically ill patients. *Critical Care Nurse, 23,* 25–36.

Tullmann, D. F., Fletcher, K., & Foreman, M. D. (2012). Delirium: Nursing standard of practice protocol: Delirium: Prevention, early recognition, and treatment. Retrieved from http://consultgerirn.org/topics/delirium/want_to_know_more

Trzepacz, P. T. (1996). Delirium. *Psychiatric Clinics of North America, 19*(3), 429–448.

Trzepacz, P. T. (1994). The neuropathogenesis of delirium. A need to focus our research. *Psychosomatics, 35,* 374–391.

Trzepacz, P. T., Mittal, D., Torres, R., Kanary, K., Norton, J., & Jimerson, N. (2001). Validation of the Delirium Rating Scale-revised-98: Comparison to the delirium rating scale and cognitive test for delirium. *Journal of Neuropsychiatry and Clincal Neurosciences, 13,* 229–242.

Tune, L. E. (2001). Anticholinergic effects of medication in elderly patients. *Journal of Clinical Psychiatry, 62*(suppl 21), 11–14.

Uguz, F., Kayrak, M., Cicek, E., Kayhan, F., Ari, H., & Altunbas, G. (2010). Delirium following acute myocardial infarction: Incidence, clinical profiles, and predictors. *Perspectives in Psychiatric Care, 46*(2), 135–142.

Waardenburg, I.E. (2008). Delirium caused by urinary retention in elderly people: A case report and literature review on the 'Cystocerebral Syndrome.' *Journal of the American Geriatrics Society, 56,* 2371–2371.

Waszynski, C. M. (2007). How to try this: Detecting delirium. *AJN: American Journal of Nursing, 107*(12), 50–59.

Weber, J. R. (2010). *Nurses handbook of health assessment* (7th ed.). Philadelphia, PA: Lippincott Williams & Wilkins.

Wiesenfeld, L. (2008). Delirium: The ADVISE approach and tips from the frontline. *Geriatrics, 63*(5), 28–31.

Wise, M. G. (1986). Delirium. In R. E. Hales & S. C. Yudofsky (Eds.), *American Psychiatric Press Textbook of Neuropsychiatry* (pp. 89–103). Washington, DC: American Psychiatric Press.

For a full suite of assignments and additional learning activities, see the access code at the front of your book.

LEARNING OBJECTIVES

At the end of this chapter, the reader will be able to:

> Understand the behavioral changes associated with normal aging processes as related to mood.
> Recognize symptoms of anxiety and depression in older persons.
> Develop a plan of care for managing anxiety disorder in an older person.
> Distinguish among anxiety, sadness, and depression.
> Develop a plan of care for managing depression in an older person.
> Identify signs of suicidal risk in an older person.
> Explain an emergency plan for older persons who exhibit signs of suicidal ideation.

KEY TERMS

Anxiety
Anhedonia
Anxiety
Anxiolytic
General anxiety disorder (GAD)
Obsessive-compulsive disorder (OCD)
Panic disorders
Phobic disorders
Posttraumatic stress disorder (PTSD)
Substance-induced anxiety disorder

Depression
Antidepressant
Atypical antidepressants
Cognitive behavioral therapy (CBT)
Depression
Dysthymia
Late-onset depression
Major depression
Minor depression
Sadness
Self-neglect
Selective serotonin reuptake inhibitors (SSRIs)
Selective serotonin-norepinephrine reuptake inhibitors (SNRIs)
Suicidal ideation
Suicide

TABLE 14-4   Nursing Care for the Patient Experiencing Anxiety
Decrease environmental stimuli
Stay with the patient
Make no demands and do not ask the patient to make major decisions
Support current coping mechanisms (crying, talking, etc.)
Do not confront or argue with the patient
Speak slowly in a soft, calm voice
Avoid reciprocal anxiety (emotions can be contagious, and sensing anxiety in the nurse can worsen the patient's anxiety)
Reassure the patient you will help develop a solution to managing the problem
Reorient the patient to reality (unless this causes more anxiety)
Respect the patient's personal space

to rephrase the way they think about the cause of their anxiety and/or manage the anxious symptoms.

> *Routine.* Encourage anxious older patients to establish a daily routine so the individual can develop a sense of security in their ability to accomplish tasks and their safety in performing daily tasks. Engaging in routine activities will also assist the older person in developing familiarity in performance, which promotes independence. This is especially important in older patients with cognitive impairment, including Alzheimer's disease and other dementias, because they are less anxious when in a stable daily routine.

> *Cognitive-behavioral therapy.* The nurse may assist in **cognitive-behavioral therapy** to diminish anxiety in older patients—the cognitive part helps persons change their thinking patterns that support their fears, and the behavioral part helps change the way they react to anxiety-provoking situations. For example, if an individual has a fear of falling, exercise can improve balance and strength, while assistive devices may offer safety and security when walking. Physical and occupational therapists can help devise a plan to offer ways to ambulate and maneuver safely. If a person has a chronic medical condition or has had a traumatic medical event, the nurse may educate individuals about their condition and ways to decrease their problems, as well as provide strategies improve health. If an individual has chronic anxiety symptoms without an identifiable cause, the person may learn strategies to avert the anxious symptoms when they occur, including pursed breathing techniques and diversion maneuvers.

> *Medication.* Medical management of anxiety disorders may be necessary if the anxious episodes are exaggerated, prolonged, and incapacitating or if they worsen an individual's ability to function or other medical conditions. The goals of medication management are aimed at controlling the symptoms of anxiety to diminish their impact on an individual's life. The main classes

of medications used to treat anxiety disorders are antidepressants and anti-anxiety drugs, or *anxiolytics.*

> *Stress reduction.* Strategies to decrease stress as well as reduce the impact of illness or stress will assist in reducing anxiety. Stress reduction may be accomplished by distraction or diverting one's attention to a pleasant or non-anxiety-provoking topic. A monotonous sound may take someone's mind off what causes the individual anxiety—examples of monotonous sounds would be the whirl of a ceiling fan, the tick-tock of a clock, the sounds of the waves of the ocean, or rain—and a sound machine can help imitate some of these sounds. Stress management techniques include cognitive restructuring, imagery, meditation, prayer, relaxation exercises, and deep breathing exercises. Other methods include exercise, yoga, and Tai Chi.

> *Getting adequate and efficient sleep.* Inadequate sleep, whether it is trouble getting to sleep, waking throughout the night, or early morning awakenings, can lead to impaired attention, slowed response time, impaired memory, impaired concentration, and decreased performance. The nurse can encourage an older individual with anxiety to develop a more efficient sleep pattern and establish a sleep routine: go to bed the same time each day and awaken at the same time, decrease daytime napping, and cease drinking fluids 2–3 hours prior to bedtime and urinate immediately before bedtime to prevent nighttime urination (nocturia).

> *Staying active.* Activity of any kind, whether physical or intellectual, can offer distraction and ease anxiety symptoms. The nurse can encourage the older patient to perform repetitive exercises or activities as well as to stay socially active. Relaxing activities and hobbies should be encouraged; common activities in older individuals include gardening, reading, fishing, art, and music.

> *Avoiding triggers.* The nurse should encourage an older person to avoid things that cause or aggravate the symptoms of anxiety. Also, individuals with anxiety issues should avoid substances that may increase anxious symptoms, such as caffeine, nicotine, over-the-counter cold medications, and alcohol.

> *Support group therapy.* An older person and/or the family may benefit from support groups, which can offer not only psychological support but also be available for the person to discuss his/her problems and concerns in a nonjudgmental atmosphere. Other advantages of support groups are they allow individuals to vent their feelings and learn alternative methods to manage their issues from individuals who are experiencing similar problems.

Medication Management for Anxiety

Medication management of anxiety disorders in older individuals is often difficult because of the high incidence of side effects and contraindications of the multiple medications that elders are usually taking. Benzodiazepines have been the most commonly prescribed anxiolytic agent for managing anxious symptoms in the older population, but it should be used very cautiously and only when absolutely necessary. Benzodiazepines do have the potential for abuse and dependence. Possible side effects of benzodiazepines in an elderly individual include motor incoordination, cognitive impairment, dizziness, amnesia, and falls. When symptoms are severe and a benzodiazepine is necessary, the ones preferred are those with a short half-life, such as lorazepam or oxazepam. In certain individuals, longer-acting benzodiazepines may be required to manage chronic anxiety disorders.

Antidepressants are frequently used in older patients to assist in managing the symptoms of anxiety. They are recommended since some are efficacious in treatment of panic disorders, obsessive-compulsive disorders, general anxiety disorders, and posttraumatic stress disorder. Certain antidepressants must be used cautiously in elders since they can cause adverse cardiac effects or interact with other medications, especially the monoamine oxidase (MAO) inhibitors. The safest class of antidepressant agents, which is the most efficacious for use in older individuals with the least interactions with other medications and fewest side effects, is the *selective serotonin reuptake inhibitors (SSRIs)*. They are indicated for managing anxiety as well as depression (Auerhahn et al., 2007; Touhy & Jett, 2010). Commonly used antidepressants are discussed later in the section on managing depression (see **Case Study 14-1**).

All of these medications should be used with extreme caution in older individuals because they have anticholinergic properties, which can lead to cognitive decline, motor incoordination, dizziness, orthostatic hypotension, falls, urinary retention, and constipation. Effective psychotherapy may also assist in managing anxiety in older individuals. The combination of cognitive behavioral therapy and medications is often needed to optimize treatment (**Table 14-5**).

Behavioral Interventions for Managing Anxiety

Behavioral interventions to reduce stress and anxiety should be implemented to optimize treatment success in the older patient. Environmental structuring will assist in decreasing stress as well as diminishing triggers of anxiety. Techniques generally fall within three categories: relaxation, cognitive structuring, and exposure-response prevention (**Box 14-2** and **Box 14-3**).

TABLE 14-5 Anxiolytics	
Medication	**Suggested Geriatric Dosing (Preferred use is 'as needed')**
Alprazolam (Xanax)	0.25–0.5 mg every 6 to 8 hours
Clonazepam (Klonipin)	0.125–2 mg every 12 hours (has a very long half-life: stays in the older person's system longer than other agents)
Clorazepapte (Tranxene)	3.75–15 mg every 8 hours
Lorazepam (Ativan)	0.5–2 mg every 6 to 8 hours
Nonnarcotic alternative: Buspirone (Buspar)	5–15 mg up to three times a day

Potential Side Effects: ataxia, memory impairment, hypotension, falls, tremors, hallucinations.

BOX 14-2 Calming Maneuvers for Anxiety

Deep Breathing Exercises: Have the patient sit in a comfortable chair, with hands on the abdomen. Ask the patient to inhale slowly and deeply, feeling the abdomen rise. Hold the breath for a few seconds. Ask the patient to exhale slowly, allowing the abdomen to deflate. Repeat several times. Always speak in a soft, calm manner to assist the patient through the process.

Progressive Muscle Relaxation: The patient should lie down in a comfortable position. Ask the patient to tighten the muscles in his or her hand for a few seconds and then completely release the tension to relax the muscle. Focusing on a specific muscle by tightening and releasing tension provides greater relaxation response to the area. Progressively concentrate on the muscles of the arms, shoulders, face, chest, back, abdomen, legs, and feet. Again, use a soft, calm voice to assist the patient through the process.

BOX 14-3 Behavioral Strategies to Manage Anxiety

Relaxation Techniques	• Quiet environment, relaxed position • Have the individual focus on a monotonous sound or image to divert their attention and forget the anxious symptoms —Common items used are clocks, fans, and sound machines offering ocean waves or rain • Music Therapy: Listen to music the individual enjoys to distract their thoughts • Art Therapy: Participate in an activity which is nondemanding to distract the individual's thoughts • Exercise Therapy: Engage in repetitive exercises that do not exacerbate the anxious symptoms to offer distraction

Cognitive Restructuring	Identify dysfunctional attitudes and beliefs that lead to anxiety symptoms
	• Explore the validity of the fear or causative agent leading to anxiety by verbalizing statements about the anxiety
	• Replace dysfunctional attitudes and beliefs about the problem with more positive statements that are based on reality or ways to manage the problem
	• Allow time to 'worry'
	   —set aside a 'worry-time,' —a designated time the individual is allowed to think about their fear. Do not allow the individual to worry about the problem outside of the designated 'worry time.'
	   —Write down thoughts (brainstorm)
	   —Order priorities for attention
	   —Develop problem-solving strategies
	   —Regular practice is important (be proactive)

| Exposure-Response Prevention | • The person gradually encounters the object or situation that is feared, perhaps initially through pictures or tapes, then later face-to-face
• Often the therapist will accompany the person to a feared situation to provide support and guidance |

Sources: Ebersole, Hess, Touhy, Jett, & Schmidt-Luggen, 2008; Merck Manual of Geriatrics Online, 2012; Touhy & Jett, 2010

Relaxation techniques make an older person focus on sounds, smells, or thoughts other than the ones that make the individual nervous or anxious. These include distraction therapy, music therapy, visual imagery, aromatherapy, or imagination of relaxation through guided instructions.

Cognitive restructuring helps the person identify the trigger/stimuli that causes or maintains anxiety within the individual, making the person aware of the trigger so they may slowly gain control over the effect of the stimuli to develop a range of coping strategies and tools.

Exposure-response prevention may be used with individuals with both panic disorders and obsessive-compulsive disorder. The individual is exposed to thoughts of the trigger that causes his/her anxiety, is given strategies to cope with the problem, and eventually becomes desensitized to the trigger.

Depression

Elders often present with multiple challenges related to worsening health and a perceived lack of well-being, which can lead to depression. A significant number of older individuals experience *depression*, which can impact individual health and overall quality of life as well as decrease an individual's lifespan. Many older adults experience chronic medical conditions along with chronic pain and fatigue, all of which can lead to depression. Common causes of depression include:

> Exposure to multiple medications and their associated side effects, as well as drug–drug interactions, can cause elders to feel physically and mentally "down"
> Having outlived spouses, loved ones, and friends
> Having to move from private homes to assisted living or long-term care because of decreasing ability to live independently

However, isolating oneself, becoming more sedentary, and experiencing pervasive feelings of sadness are not normal consequences of aging. When these symptoms are present, seem severe, or last longer than expected, a diagnosis of depression must be considered.

Depression in older adult populations is often underdiagnosed and underreported, and can be confused with cognitive changes associated with dementia. Individuals over the age of 60 are often given a diagnosis of cognitive impairment or dementia when they become forgetful or present with symptoms of *self-neglect,* which include changes in eating habits, limited attention to personal hygiene, sleep disturbances that include excessive or diminished sleep, or overall changes in behavior (Byrd, 2011).

Prevalence of Depression in the Aging Population

Approximately 10% of men and 18% of women over the age of 65 in the United States report current symptoms associated with clinically significant depression. These findings have been relatively unchanged since 1998. Between men and women, men in the over-85 age group are at highest risk for depression (18%), and White males in this category are at the highest risk for suicide (National Institute of Mental Health [NIMH], 2012). Among women over the age of 65, those between the ages of 75 and 79 are noted to be at the highest risk (20%) for depression (Older Americans, 2010). In long-term care facilities the prevalence of depression has been reported as high as 29% (Seitz, Purandare, & Conn, 2010). From 1988 to 2008, use of prescription antidepressants by older adult males in the United States increased from roughly 2% to 10%; in the same time frame, older adult women increased their use of these medications from 4% to 17% (Pratt, Brody, & Gu, 2011).

Types of Depression and Presentation

Major Depression, Minor Depression, and Dysthymia

The American Psychiatric Association's (APA's) *Diagnostic and Statistical Manual of Mental Disorders* (4th edition, text revision) (2000), also known as the *DSM-IV-TR,* defines *major depression* as a depressive episode where an individual experiences pervasive feelings of anxiety and sadness that coincide with *anhedonia,* or loss of pleasure and interest in daily activities. Concurrently, at least five or more of the following symptoms must be present for a minimum of two consecutive weeks: increased fatigue with loss of energy, irritability and/or restlessness, oversleeping or trouble sleeping, poor concentration or difficulty with mental processing and decision making, inappropriate guilt or perception of worthlessness, changes in appetite that lead to weight gain or weight loss not related to dieting, and thoughts of suicide or death and/or attempts at suicide. Symptoms consistent with depression that occur for the first time later in life are referred to as *late-onset depression,* whereas older adults who report a history of depression at an earlier stage in life are often diagnosed with 'recurrent' depression. An older adult who presents with severe symptoms of sadness or other symptoms consistent with major depression will often report a history of one or more major depressive events at some point in their lifetime.

Major depression can change or distort the way older adults view themselves, their lives, and those around them. In addition, older adults with major depression often display functional activity impairments such as changes in regular activities of daily living, decreased socialization, and poor compliance with medication therapy and healthcare recommendations (Substance Abuse and Mental Health Services Administration, 2011).

Symptoms that are indicative of depression include the following:

> No interest or pleasure in enjoyable activities
> No interest in sexual activities
> Feeling sad or numb
> Crying easily or for no reason
> Feeling slowed down
> Feeling worthless or guilty
> Change in appetite; unintended change in weight
> Trouble recalling things, concentrating, or making decisions
> Problems sleeping, or wanting to sleep all of the time
> Feeling tired all of the time
> Thoughts about death or suicide (APA, 2000)

Minor depression is a subset of major depression and is defined as an episode of depressive thoughts that is less severe than major depression, but has a similar 2-week time frame for presentation. Individuals show evidence of only one to four of the eight cardinal symptoms of major depressive disorders. Minor depression may be a precursor to a major depressive illness (Soriano, 2007; APA, 2000).

Dysthymia is a chronic form of depression that is often diagnosed in older adults with prolonged illness or those who experience long-term challenges in their daily living. Older adults who present with dysthymia experience mild to moderate depressive symptoms that are present throughout most days over a 2-year period. In order to receive a diagnosis of dysthymia, individuals must also report two of the following symptoms: poor concentration or difficulty making decisions, poor appetite or overeating, fatigue, low energy, excessive sleep, or insomnia (APA, 2000).

Manifestations of Depression

Depression is manifested in both affective and somatic responses in varying patterns based on gender. Men often blame others for their current depressed mood, display increased irritability, and anger, and intentionally create conflicts. Males may act suspicious and guarded, display restlessness and agitation, display an extreme desire to be in control, and perceive that admitting self-doubt and despair are inherent weaknesses. In contrast, depressed women often blame themselves for their depressed state, feeling anxious, scared, apathetic, slowed down, and worthless. They often have trouble setting boundaries and avoid all conflicts, but do not have trouble talking with others about their self-doubt and despair (Helpguide.org, 2012).

Because the onset of depression in older adults can often coincide with onset of an illness, it is frequently misattributed to a somatic cause and not properly diagnosed (Fiske et al., 2009). Somatic symptoms such as persistent muscle aches, chronic headaches, palpitations, or insidious changes in stomach, bowel, or bladder function should be considered as possible symptoms of depressive disorders unless clearly attributable to a medical condition (Grohol, 2012).

Different Presentations of Depression

Symptoms of depression can also manifest in varying patterns of thought and behavior.

> *Catatonic depression:* Individual is very withdrawn; thinking, speech, and general activity may slow down, as well as the cessation of all voluntary activities; may not take care of him/herself, household, or pets; and may also mimic others' speech (echolalia) or movements (echopraxia).
> *Melancholic depression:* Individual does not receive pleasure from usual activities; may appear sluggish, sad, and withdrawn; may speak little, stop eating, and lose weight; often shows no emotions, or may feel excessively or inappropriately guilty.
> *Psychotic depression:* Individual has false beliefs (delusions) about having committed unpardonable sins or crimes, having incurable or shameful disorders, or being watched or persecuted; may have hallucinations, usually of voices accusing them of various misdeeds or condemning them to death; and some individuals may imagine that they see coffins or deceased relatives.

The scoring guide for the PHQ-9 is below (The MacArthur Initiative on Depression and Primary Care, 2009):

Score	Number of Days Reporting Symptoms in Past 2 Weeks
0	None
1	Several Days
2	More than 7 days
3	Almost every day

Total points scored for the screen determine the extent of depressive symptoms, can help guide therapy, and can determine possible suicide risk. A score between 5 and 9 indicates minimal depressive symptoms; supportive education and continued observation for worsening symptoms are warranted. Scores between 10 and 14 may indicate minor depression, dysthymia, or mild major depression; psychotherapy and antidepressant therapy may be indicated, but depending on situational exposures reported by the individual, supportive watchful waiting may be appropriate as well. Individuals who score between 15 and 19 report symptoms consistent with moderately severe major depression and will need psychotherapy or antidepressant therapy. Those individuals who score at or above 20 often need psychotherapy and antidepressant therapy to treat their depression (The MacArthur Initiative on Depression and Primary Care, 2009). At the completion of screening, it is important to assess the total time period that symptoms have been present. Those who report symptoms over a 2-year period are often diagnosed with chronic depression or dysthymia, which may require ongoing cognitive behavioral therapy and/or problem-solving therapy to maximize their treatment outcomes.

> *Atypical depression:* Individual may appear anxious and fearful (especially in the evening); may have an increased appetite, resulting in weight gain, and although initially unable to sleep, transitions to sleeping for increasingly longer periods of time; depressed mood may be lessened in response to positive events but individual is excessively sensitive to perceived criticism or rejection; may become agitated or very restless while exhibiting behaviors such as frequent wringing of the hands, rocking back and forth, or talking continuously.

Relationship of Depression to Chronic Disease

Chronic diseases remain pervasive in older adult populations and the incidence of morbidity and mortality from chronic disease increases with each decade of life. Currently, 80% of individuals over the age of 65 have one or more chronic conditions such as heart disease, vascular disease, hypertension, diabetes, cancer, arthritis, or lung disease (Centers for Disease Control and Prevention [CDC], 2011). Depressed individuals who present with heart disease, cancer, chronic obstructive pulmonary disease (COPD), or stroke have the highest incidence of mortality associated with their disease (Murphy, Jiaquan, & Kochanek, 2012). Concurrent depression in the presence of these four chronic diseases is strongly related to increased burden of illness and worsening overall outcomes.

Diagnosing Depression

Nurses providing care for older adults are currently being called to strongly consider screening for depression and assisting in the initiation of treatment as part of comprehensive holistic care for their patients. Primary screening of all at-risk older adults is the first step in diagnosing depression. A diagnosis of major depression in older adults is made with documentation of positive findings on a reliable depression screening tool (Low & Hubley, 2007). These findings revolve around eight cardinal symptoms: expression of guilt, loss of sexual interest, changes in nutritional intake, alterations in sleep patterns, decreased energy, poor concentration, agitation or apathy, and suicideality (Soriano, 2007). Symptoms must have been consistently present over the previous two-week period prior to the screening (Grohol, 2012).

The use of appropriate screening tools such as the 15-item Geriatric Depression Scale (Sheikh & Yesavage, 1986; Camus, Kraehenbuhl, Preisig, Bula, & Waeber, 2004) or the Patient Health Questionnaire nine-item screening tool (PHQ-9) (Spitzer, Kroenke, & Williams, 1999) demonstrate adequate sensitivity and specificity for older adults and provide avenues for intervention or referral depending on severity scores and suicidal risks.

Interpreting the Patient Health Questionnaire 9-Item Test

The PHQ-9 questions are designed to reflect the onset, in the previous 2 weeks at time of screening, of specific depression-related symptoms reported by individuals. Scoring is completed using a simple point system of 0 to 3, where 0 correlates with having no prior symptoms and 3 indicates having experienced the symptom almost every day (see **Figure 14-2**). The total score for the PHQ-9 is 27.

PATIENT HEALTH QUESTIONNAIRE-9 (PHQ-9)				
Over the last 2 weeks, how often have you been bothered by any of the following problems? *(Use "✓" to indicate your answer)*	**Not at all**	**Several days**	**More than half the days**	**Nearly every day**
1. Little interest or pleasure in doing things	0	1	2	3
2. Feeling down, depressed, or hopeless	0	1	2	3
3. Trouble falling or staying asleep, or sleeping too much	0	1	2	3
4. Feeling tired or having little energy	0	1	2	3
5. Poor appetite or overeating	0	1	2	3
6. Feeling bad about yourself — or that you are a failure or have let yourself or your family down	0	1	2	3
7. Trouble concentrating on things, such as reading the newspaper or watching television	0	1	2	3
8. Moving or speaking so slowly that other people could have noticed. Or the opposite — being so fidgety or restless that you have been moving around a lot more than usual	0	1	2	3
9. Thoughts that you would be better off dead or of hurting yourself in some way	0	1	2	3

FOR OFFICE CODING _____ + _____ + _____ + _____

=Total Score: _____

If you checked off any problems, how difficult have these problems made it for you to do your work, take care of things at home, or get along with other people?

Not difficult at all	**Somewhat difficult**	**Very difficult**	**Extremely difficult**
☐	☐	☐	☐

Figure 14-2 Patient Health Questionnaire-9 (Phq-9).

Source: Developed by Drs. Robert L. Spitzer, Janet B.W. Williams, Kurt Kroenke and colleagues, with an educational grant from Pfizer Inc. No permission required to reproduce, translate, display or distribute.

Screening in a Busy Practice

Initial use of a shortened two-item PHQ screening tool (PHQ-2), made up of the first two questions in the PHQ-9 (Spitzer et al., 1999; Arroll et al., 2010), to screen older adults at risk for depression may be completed with vital signs in both inpatient and outpatient care settings. Because time spent with patients in outpatient care is often limited, another productive method of obtaining this data would be to have a prepared self-screening tool (such as the PHQ-2) that could be completed by at-risk seniors while the nurse attends to other patient needs.

Older adults who score 2 or higher on one or both PHQ-2 questions often require some form of treatment for their depressed symptoms (The MacArthur Initiative on Depression and Primary Care, 2009). A positive two-item screening warrants further testing using expanded screening tools, and can be completed and reviewed by a nurse practitioner or other clinician for treatment planning. Data collected in the screening tool can also be used to ensure that appropriate referral for specialized interventional care is completed.

Differential Diagnoses for Depression

A thorough medical and cognitive assessment is necessary to determine whether the symptoms of depression are due to underlying neurologic diagnoses such as Alzheimer's disease or dementia. Depressive disorders must also be distinguished from other disorders such as anxiety disorders and late-life schizophrenia. Depression rating scales, cognitive screening instruments, and structural and functional neuroimaging studies may be implemented as determined by the individual patient.

Physical disorders, such as anemia, hypothyroidism, Parkinson's disease, and other neurologic disorders must also be ruled out since they may present with symptoms similar to depression (Merck Manual—Home Health Handbook, 2008a).

There are no definitive laboratory tests or neurologic imaging tests to diagnose depressive disorders; however, laboratory and radiographic testing should be performed to rule out other occult disorders that can be associated with depressive symptoms. Completion of a full laboratory screening includes a complete blood count (CBC), thyroid-stimulating hormone (TSH), complete metabolic panel (CMP), vitamin B_{12}, serum folate, and urinalysis. Magnetic resonance imaging of the brain to detect changes consistent with a mass or vascular lesion that may be causing depressive symptoms is also helpful in the diagnosis of depression (Lyness, 2012).

Depression and Dementia

Current estimates of mild cognitive impairment (MCI) presenting in older adults between the ages of 70 and 89 range from 13% to 18% (Petersen et al., 2008). Of those individuals with MCI, 10% to 15% will be diagnosed with progressive Alzheimer's-type dementia each year (Gauthier et al, 2006). Symptoms consistent with depression have been shown to precede dementia in both men and women (Goveas, Espeland, Woods, Wassertheil-Smoller, & Kotchen, 2011). Furthermore, as the number of recurrent depressive episodes increases throughout older adulthood, the prevalence of permanent cognitive changes suggestive of dementia also appears to increase. These neurological changes are thought to be similarly related to metabolic-induced hippocampal brain injury that can occur with traumatic brain injury and cerebrovascular insults. Early onset of treatment for depression may have important implications in decreasing onset and progression of dementia in older adult populations in the future (Dotson, Beydoun, & Zonderman, 2010).

Managing Depression

Effective treatment of depression involves using an interdisciplinary team approach, which includes the use of adaptive disease management to maximize quality of life; cognitive behavioral therapy; and pharmacologic therapy, as indicated, with antidepressants such as SSRIs, selective serotonin-norepinephrine reuptake inhibitors (SNRIs), and atypical antidepressants.

Counseling and Therapy

Cognitive behavioral therapy (CBT) is best performed by advanced practice mental health clinicians who specialize in geriatric care. Specialized counselors who are trained in senior care are able to assist older adults and their caregivers in reframing internal and external constructs in order to stabilize concepts of self in the presence of depression. Cognitive behavioral therapy, in combination with problem-solving therapy, is also effective in helping depressed older adults to identify problems in their daily living that contribute to depression, and formulate strategies for lifestyle and social modifications in the presence of chronic illness to improve overall quality of life (Arean et al., 2010).

Medication Management for Depression

Older adults, who have collected a lifetime of experiences in which to interpret new knowledge and ideas, often resist the use of an *antidepressant* medication. With a primary goal of initiating an antidepressant trial of therapy, nurses can affect care by assisting older adults in their understanding of all aspects of recommended medication therapy (see **Case Study 14-1**). In many cases, effective pharmacotherapy is necessary to manage major depression or depression that lasts for a prolonged period of time in older adults.

Selective Serotonin Reuptake Inhibitor Therapy. There are multiple classes of
   antidepressant medications; however, the selective serotonin reuptake
   inhibitors (SSRIs) are considered first-line therapy for managing depression
   in elders due to their limited side effect profile and overall performance in
   effectively treating depression. SSRIs inhibit cortical presynaptic serotonin
   5HT reuptake in the brain (**Box 14-4**). This pharmacologic response increases
   the amount of circulating serotonin in the neurosynapses, improves receptor
   binding to positively affect neurotransmission of serotonin (a potent mood
   stimulating neurotransmitter), and ultimately decreases symptoms of
   depression (Lundbeck Institute CNSforum, 2012).

Case Study 14–1

Ms. A is a 67-year-old female who has experienced a fall, which led to a fractured hip. After surgery to repair her fractured hip, she had a normal recovery period and was discharged to a rehabilitation center for improvement of balance and gait. However, her progression was extremely slow and she began crying hysterically during her physical therapy sessions. She stated she was extremely fearful of falling again. This fear of falling was justified, but would lead to incapacitation and further decline in her overall health if she became chair-bound or bed-bound. After the rehabilitation team discussed the problem of extreme anxiety with her healthcare provider, Ms. A was placed on a low dose of escitalopram (Lexapro) [an antidepressant that is also indicated for anxiety]. Ms. A also participated in cognitive behavioral therapy to assist in her understanding the cause of her anxiety attacks and helping her develop strategies to manage her fear of falling again. After 2 weeks, Ms. A was still fearful but she did not become hysterical during her therapy sessions. She was able to participate in her walking and gait exercises and slowly become less anxious when trying to walk. Ms. A was able to walk with the use of a walker and was discharged home again.

BOX 14-4   Antidepressants: Selective Serotonin Reuptake Inhibitors (SSRIs)

Medication	Suggested Geriatric Dosing
Citalopram (Celexa)	10–40 mg once a day
Escitalopram (Lexapro)	5–20 mg once a day
Fluoxetine (Prozac)	10–20 mg once a day
Paroxetine (Paxil)	10–40 mg once a day
Paroxetine controlled release (Paxil CR)	12.5–25 mg once a day
Sertraline (Zoloft)	25–100 mg once a day

Potential side effects: Weight gain, nausea, vomiting, dry mouth, dizziness, headache, nervousness, somnolence, decreased libido, tremors, akathesia, and sexual dysfunction

Sources: Auerhahn, Capezuti, Flaherty, & Resnick, 2007; Ebersole, Hess, Touhy, Jett, & Schmidt-Luggen, 2008; Touhy & Jett, 2010.

Selective Serotonin-Norepinephrine Reuptake Inhibitor Therapy. **Selective serotonin-norepinephrine reuptake inhibitors (SNRIs)** are other commonly used antidepressants (**Box 14-5**). SNRIs affect both serotonin and norepinephrine in the brain, through neuroregulation that helps brain cells send and receive messages important for improving mood. Medications in this group of antidepressants are sometimes called dual reuptake inhibitors and may also assist with managing the symptoms of fibromyalgia and chronic fatigue syndrome, thought to be related to low levels of serotonin and norepinephrine (Lee & Chen, 2010).

BOX 14-5   Antidepressants: Selective Serotonin-Norepinepherine Reuptake Inhibitors (SNRIs)

Medication	Suggested Geriatric Dosing
Duloxetine (Cymbalta)	10–40 mg once a day
Venlafaxine XR (Effexor XR)	20–60 mg once a day
Desvenlafaxine (Pristiq)	50 mg once a day

BOX 14-6   Atypical Antidepressants

Medication	Suggested Geriatric Dosing
Bupropion (Wellbutrin)	100 mg three times a day
Bupropion sustained release (Wellbutrin SR)	150 mg twice a day
Bupropion extended release (Wellbutrin XL)	300 mg once a day

Atypical Antidepressants. Another class of antidepressants commonly used in elders, often referred to as *atypical antidepressants,* includes dopamine-norepinephrine reuptake inhibitors (DNRIs), which work by primarily blocking the reuptake of dopamine and norepinephrine with no direct action on the serotonin system (**Box 14-6**). DNRIs may be utilized in the treatment of major depressive disorders (Byatt & Lundquist, 2012).

Nursing Interventions

As part of developing an optimal plan of care, nurses are responsible for completing assessments for evidence of depression in all older adults in their care; making sure that other somatic conditions have been ruled out; and developing strategies to optimize function, independence, and promote psychological health.

A comprehensive treatment plan may include the following (Kurlowicz & Havath, 2008):

> Providing a nonjudgmental atmosphere
> Instituting safety precautions for suicide risk for any patient who presents with severe symptoms or expresses suicidal ideation
> Monitoring and promoting nutrition, elimination, sleep/rest patterns, and physical comfort (especially pain control)
> Maintaining and/or enhancing physical function
   • Structuring regular exercise/activity
   • Considering referral to physical, occupational, and/or recreational therapies when necessary

- Encouraging the older patient to develop a daily routine/activity schedule
> Encouraging utilization of social support systems
  - Identifying/mobilizing a support person(s) such as family, confidants, friends, hospital resources, support groups, or patient visitors
  - Identifying if there is a need for spiritual support and contacting appropriate clergy, while being respectful of the patient's values and being cautious not to impart the one's personal and/or religious values upon a patient
> Maximizing independence and autonomy/personal control/self-efficacy by including the patient as an active participant in making daily schedules and short-term goals
> Identifying and reinforcing the patient's strengths and capabilities
> Providing structure to allow some familiarity in routine
> Encouraging daily participation in relaxation therapies or pleasant activities (art therapy, music therapy, etc.)
> Monitoring and documenting responses to medication and other therapies
  - Re-administering the depression-screening tool used initially to determine efficacy of medication(s)
> Assisting the patient with problem-solving strategies
> Providing emotional support
  - Being empathic
  - Engaging in active and supportive listening
  - Encouraging expression of feelings and working towards fostering hope
  - Supporting adaptive coping
  - Encouraging pleasant reminiscence
> Providing information about any physical illnesses and treatment(s)
> Providing information about depression, reinforcing that depression is common, treatable, and not the person's fault
> Educating the patient and family about the importance of adherence to the prescribed treatment regimen for depression (especially medication) to prevent recurrence
> Teaching about specific antidepressant side effects
> Ensuring mental-health community support, including psychiatric, nursing-home-care intervention

Education is paramount to the success of all treatment programs for depression (Saver, Van-Nguyen, Keppel, & Doescher, 2007). Depressed patients in all phases of treatment need to understand the biological and psychological indicators for depression associated with chronic illness and aging. A comprehensive education program provided by the nurse should encompass the beliefs that older adults are self-aware, dynamic, and use patterns of thought based on long-lived experiences to analyze, decide, and act on treatment recommendations. It is essential for nurses to understand and incorporate each patient's enduring patterns of living to enhance treatment outcomes, improve life satisfaction, and promote adaptation to changes associated with illness and aging. Using this knowledge will greatly assist nurses in helping patients assimilate depression care into their unique frameworks for optimal quality of life.

Notable Quotes

"For true happiness, you've got to have companionship—other people... in your life. It doesn't have to be a husband or a wife. It can be a friend or like us, as sister..."

—Sadie Delany. Delany & Delany, 1993, p. 83

Suicide

Older adults who are experiencing major depression are at risk for suicide. *Suicide* is defined as taking one's own life. An older person may be at risk for harm to self, which can lead to immediate or hastened death. Thoughts of death and ways to hasten death or even commit suicide are among the most serious symptoms of depression. Many depressed individuals want to die or feel extreme worthlessness and feel they should die. Fifteen percent of untreated depressed older adults end their own life by suicide. Men over the age of 70 have the highest rate of completed suicides (Merck Manual—Home Health Handbook, 2008b).

A suicide threat is an emergency situation and requires immediate action. It is imperative that the nurse recognizes suicidal ideation and seeks prompt intervention. When an older person presents with severe symptoms of depression, expresses thoughts of being better off dead, or threatens to kill him/herself, the individual may require hospitalization. This will provide supervision of the person until treatment reduces depression and the risk of suicide. The risk of an older person committing suicide is especially high in the following situations:

> When depression is not treated or is inadequately treated
> After initially beginning treatment (when an individual is becoming more active mentally and physically but their mood is still extremely sad)
> When people continue to feel excessively sad even while returning to normal routine and activities
> When the person has a significant anniversary such as the death of a spouse or during a holiday season
> When an individual alternates between depression and mania (bipolar disorder)
> When the person feels very anxious
> When an individual is drinking alcohol or taking recreational or illicit drugs

Assessing Suicidal Risks

When assessing an older person's risk for suicide, (**Box 14-7**) the nurse must determine if the patient has developed a plan. It is essential to directly ask the person if they have thought about what it would be like to be dead or if they have thoughts of killing themselves, and, if so, have they thought about how they would accomplish this (see Case Study 14-2). If the person has developed a plan, this is an emergent situation and the nurse should assist in getting the person immediate help.

Suicidal behavior may include three main types of self-destructive acts: completed suicide, attempted suicide, and suicide gestures. Thoughts and plans related to suicide are called *suicidal ideation*. Suicidal behavior includes the following:

> Completed suicide: Intentional acts of self-harm that result in death
  • Overmedicating self
  • Omitting medications

> **BOX 14-7   Risk Factors for Suicide**

- Over age 65 years of age
- Male
- Painful or disabling illness
- Living alone
- Perceived or real perception of inability to afford living expenses, medications, or other healthcare costs; debt or poverty
- Bereavement or loss
- Humiliation or disgrace
- Depression, especially when accompanied by psychosis or anxiety
- Persistent sadness even when other symptoms of depression are lessening
- A history of drug or alcohol abuse
- A history of prior suicide attempts
- A history of suicide in family members
- Traumatic childhood experiences, including physical or sexual abuse
- Preoccupation with and talk about suicide
- Well-defined plans for suicide

Source: Merck Manual—Home Health Handbook, 2008b

- Lifestyle choices that lead to worsening of health, which could lead to death
- Overt suicidal maneuvers such as shooting self with a gun or cutting self with a sharp object

> Attempted suicide: Acts of self-harm that are intended to result in death but do not. Frequently, many older persons who attempt suicide may have some ambivalence about wishing to die and the behaviors may be a cry for help.

> Suicide gesture: Acts of self-harm that are unlikely to result in death. For example, people may scratch their wrists only superficially or take an overdose of vitamins.

For successful or completed suicides, guns are most frequently used by both men (74%) and women (31%). The next most common methods include hanging for men and drug overdose for women.

The nurse should report any suicidal-type behaviors to the patient's primary healthcare provider, who may hospitalize the individual. Sometimes an older adult will not agree to hospitalization; in most states, a physician is allowed to hospitalize certain individuals against their wishes if they are at believed to be at high risk of harming themselves or others (Merck Manual—Home Health Handbook, 2008b).

Suicide Prevention

Any older person who presents with threatening suicide or attempts at suicide should be taken very seriously, and these behaviors regarded as a plea for help. If a threat or attempt is ignored, there is risk that a life may be lost. Once an older person is

Case Study 14-2

Mr. B is a 72-year-old male whose wife died 6 months ago. He presents to his healthcare provider's clinic for routine examination having lost 15 pounds since his last visit 1 year ago (he denies trying to lose weight). He states he lives by himself since his children live out-of-town. He states he doesn't like to cook because "it is so hard to make a meal for just one person." He looks at his feet and does not make eye contact. Mr. B states it has become really hard to keep going since he lost "the love of his life." The nurse is extremely concerned, as Mr. B is exhibiting signs of thoughts of suicide. The next step was to ask Mr. B if he had thought about dying; he states "I would be better off if I were not around." The nurse asks if Mr. B had thought about hurting himself or killing himself; he states that he has. The nurse next asks Mr. B if he has thought about how he would accomplish this. Mr. B states that he owns a gun and has been contemplating about shooting himself. The nurse initiates an emergency plan to have Mr. B admitted to the hospital for emergency treatment since he has a concrete plan to commit suicide and knows that elderly males who attempt suicide are often successful in accomplishing their goal of death. Mr. B is placed on paroxetine (Paxil) [an antidepressant] and is treated by a psychiatrist with individual as well as group therapy sessions. After 3 weeks of in-hospital management in a Geriatric-Psychiatric unit, he is discharged to live with his daughter and close supervision. Mr. B is still sad but his suicidal ideation has diminished and he is slowly improving. The nurse in this case saved Mr. B's life.

determined to have a high potential for suicide, help should be sought immediately and care should be taken to engage the individual by speaking in a calm, supportive manner while waiting for emergency interventional care (see **Case Study 14-2**).

An attempt should be made to develop a rapport with the individual by discovering common interests and repeatedly using their name in conversation. Allow the suicidal person to discuss their feelings and worries and, if appropriate, offer constructive suggestions for solving the problem that brought on the crisis. Remind the individual of loved ones who care about him or her and reinforce his or her value and importance to others. Finally, the nurse must ensure that the at-risk individual receives face-to-face interventional help as quickly as possible (Merck Manual—Home Health Handbook, 2008b). **Box 14-8** provides additional resources for nurses assisting persons with depression and anxiety.

Summary

Depression and anxiety are common among older adults, particularly those with limited social support or resources. Geriatric nurses play a role in examining all aspects of an older patient, including his or her mental and emotional health, to make appropriate referrals for treatment (**Box 14-9**). Early recognition and intervention for anxiety and depression can improve quality of life and help prevent unnecessary complications.

BOX 14-8 Recommended Resources

ConsultGeriRN: Provides free resources, including assessment instruments and specialty nursing Web links (http://www.consultgerirn.org)

Try This: Best practices in nursing care to the older adult. Offers assessment tools on a variety of topics relevant to the care of older adults. The *How to Try This* series is comprised of articles and videos presenting cases studies. (http://www.hartfordign.org)

Help Guide—Depression in Older Adults and the Elderly: Offers ways to recognize the signs and find treatment that works (http://www.helpguide.org/mental/depression_elderly.htm)

Anxiety Disorders Association of America (ADAA): Has as its mission to promote the prevention, treatment, and cure of anxiety, depression, and stress-related disorders through education, practice, and research. Excellent website for resources about understanding anxiety disorders and treatment strategies. (http://www.adaa.org)

My Mental Health Medication Workbook by Fran Miller RN, MSN, BC: Offers patients an excellent interactive resource for understanding their mental illness and medication treatment. Provides information for a wide variety of mental illnesses. Published by PESI, LLC, Eau Claire, WI

Nursing Standard of Practice Protocol: Depression: A resource for evidence-based and authoritative information about nursing care of older adults. ConsultGeriRN.org is the geriatric clinical nursing website of the Hartford Institute for Geriatric Nursing, New York University College of Nursing. ConsultGeriRN.org is an evidence-based online resource for nurses in clinical and educational settings. ConsultGeriRN.org is funded in part by a grant from The Atlantic Philanthropies (USA) Inc. and The John A. Hartford Foundation. http://consultgerirn.org/topics/depression/want_to_know_more

Personal Health Questionnaire-9: Screening tool for depression & how to interpret the results. http://www.phqscreeners.com/instructions/instructions.pdf

Geriatric Depression Scale: Screening tool for depression. http://www.nursingcenter.com/library/journalarticle.asp?article_id=744981

BOX 14-9 Research Highlight

Aim: To examine the relationship between activity level, fear of falling, and anxiety and depression.

Methods: Ninety-nine community-dwelling older adults over age 55 were given several surveys. These included a survey of activities and fear of falling, the Geriatric Depression Scale, and an anxiety scale.

Findings: The results showed a significant relationship between fear of falling and depression, anxiety, and activities. Depression and anxiety were related to activity restrictions.

Application to practice: Nurses should consider screening older adults for fear of falling, anxiety, and depression because these factors were associated with a restriction in activity.

Source: Painter, J. A., Allison, L., Dhingra, P., Daughtery, J., Cogdill, K., & Trujillo, L. (2012). Fear of falling and its relationship with anxiety, depression, and activity engagement among community-dwelling older adults. *American Journal of Occupational Therapy, 66*(2), 169–176.

Critical Thinking Exercises

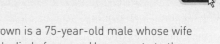

1. Mrs. Simmons, a 72-year-old widow living alone in her home, was recently admitted to the hospital after falling and fracturing her hip in her driveway. She underwent surgery to repair her hip fracture and was admitted to a nursing home for rehabilitation and gait training. She complains of not being able to sleep. She is not doing well in her rehabilitation—she states "I am afraid I am going to fall again." Should this be considered a problem? What additional information is needed to determine if changes should be made in her plan of care? What evidence can the nurse provide to Mrs. Simmons to support the need for further evaluation and treatment?

2. Mr. Brown is a 75-year-old male whose wife recently died of cancer. He presents to the emergency room with his daughter, who is concerned about his loss of 10 pounds since his wife's death. He does not make eye contact and appears to be in dirty clothes, the buttons on his shirt are not buttoned correctly, and presents with poor hygiene. He states that his kids would be better off if he were no longer around. Is this an emergent situation? What is the most important information to attain from this patient? What other information is necessary to determine an appropriate plan of care? How can the nurse provide the support this patient requires?

Personal Reflections

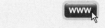

1. You are involved in a motor vehicle accident. You awaken in the ICU with both of your arms restrained. Discuss your emotions. What would you want the nursing staff to say or do?

2. Place the radio on a station, then set the dial where the station is not clear—there is a lot of background static and it is difficult to hear the announcer. Attempt to make a call or carry on a conversation with someone. Would you feel nervous? Would you be able to maintain the conversation? How does this experience affect your mood?

3. You present at an outpatient clinic where you are an established patient, to be seen for a routine follow up visit. You are being assessed by the nurse before being seen by your nurse practitioner. The nurse asks you how you are doing after the recent death of your spouse. You begin to cry. How would you want the nurse to respond? Would you feel comfortable being screened for depression at this time? Would you want to be educated about your risks for depression during this visit?

4. You are an older adult, living alone, and are aware that you are depressed. You have had recent thoughts of suicide but haven't made a plan to carry out the act yet. You are despondent and lacking energy to engage in any activities of daily living. A home health nurse comes to your home for a visit. What interactions, assessments, and plan of care would be necessary for the nurse to engage in to keep you from carrying out a suicide plan?

References

American Psychiatric Association [APA]. (2000). *Diagnostic and statistical manual of mental disorders* (4th ed., text rev.). Washington, DC: Author.

Arean, P. A., Rane, P., Mackin, R. S., Kanellopoulos, D., McCulloch, C., & Alexopoulos, G. S. (2010). Problem-solving therapy and supportive therapy in older adults with major depression and executive dysfunction. *American Journal of Psychiatry, 167*(11), 1391–1398.

Arroll, B., Goodyear-Smith, F., Crengle, S., Gunn, J., Kerse, M., Fishman, T., … Hatcher, S. (2010). Validation of PHQ-2 and PHQ-9 to screen for major depression in the primary care population. *Annals of Family Medicine, 8*, 348–353. doi:10.1370/afm.1139

Auerhahn, C., Capezuti, E., Flaherty, E., & Resnick, B. (2007). *The Geriatric nursing review syllabus.* New York, NY: American Geriatric Society.

Byatt, N., & Lundquist, R. (2012). Use of atypical antidepressants in elderly patients. *Abhazia: Institute for Social and Economic Research.* Retrieved from http://www.abkhazia.com/research-blogs/health/74-Therapeutic-Specialties/980-use-of-atypical-antidepressants-in-elderly-patients

Byrd, L. (2011). Caregiver Survival 101: Managing the Problematic Behaviors in Individuals with Dementia. PESI Publishing.

Camus, V., Kraehenbuhl, H., Preisig, M., Bula, C. J., & Waeber, G. (2004). Geriatric depression and vascular diseases: What are the links? *Journal of Affective Disorders, 81*, 1–16.

Cassidy, K., & Rector, N. (2008). The silent geriatric giant: Anxiety disorders in late life. *Geriatrics and Aging, 11*(3), 50–156.

Centers for Disease Control [CDC], Chronic Disease Prevention and Health Promotion. (2011). Healthy aging: Helping people to live long and productive lives and enjoy a good quality of life. Retrieved from http://www.cdc.gov/chronicdisease/resources/publications/aag/aging.htm

Dotson, V. M., Beydoun, M. A., & Zonderman, A. B. (2010). Recurrent depressive symptoms and the incidence of dementia and mild cognitive impairment. *Neurology, 75*, 27–34.

Delany, S. L., & Delany, A. E. (1993). Having our say: The Delany sisters' first 100 years. New York, NY: Dell.

Ebersole, P., Hess, P., Touhy, T., Jett, K., & Schmidt-Luggen, A. (2008). *Toward healthy aging: Human needs & nursing response* (7th ed.). St. Louis, MO: Mosby.

Fiske, A., Loebach Wetherell, J., & Gatz, M. (2009). Depression in older adults. *Annual Review of Clinical Psychology, 5*, 363–389. doi: 10.1146/annurev.clinpsy.032408.1536321\.

Gauthier, S., Reisberg, B., Zaudig, M., Petersen, R. C., Ritchie, K., Broich, K., … Winblad, B. (2006). Mild Cognitive Impairment. *Lancet, 367*(9518), 262–270.

Goveas, J. S., Espeland, M. A., Woods, N. F., Wassertheil-Smoller, S., & Kotchen, J. M. (2011). Depressive symptoms and incidence of mild cognitive impairment and probable dementia in elderly women: The women's health initiative memory study. *Journal of the American Geriatrics Society, 59*(1), 57–66.

Grohol, J. M. (2012). Symptoms and treatments of mental disorders. *PsychCentral.* Retrieved from http://psychcentral.com/disorders/

Helpguide.org (2012). Depression in women: Causes, symptoms, and treatment. Retrieved from http://www.helpguide.org/mental/depression/women.htm

Kurlowicz, L., & Harvath, T. (2008). Nursing standard of practice protocol: Depression in older adults. *ConsultGeriRN.org: Hartford Institute for Geriatric Nursing.* Retrieved from http://consultgerirn.org/topics/depression/want_to_know_more

Lee, Y., & Chen, P. (2010). A review of SSRIs and SNRIs in neuropathic pain. *Expert Opinion in Pharmacotherapy.17*, 2813–2825.

Low, G. D., & Hubley, A. M. (2007). Screening for depression after cardiac events using the Beck Depression Inventory II and Geriatric Depression scale. *Social Indicators Research. 82*(3), 527–543.

Lundbeck Institute CNSforum. (2012). *The mechanism of action of specific 5-HT re-uptake inhibitors.* Retrieved from http://www.cnsforum.com/imagebank/item/Drug_SSRI_2/default.aspx

Lyness, J. M. (2012). Clinical manifestations and diagnosis of depression. *UpToDate.* Retrieved on from http://www.uptodate.com/contents/clinical-manifestations-and-diagnosis-of-depression

Merck Manual of Geriatrics Online. (2012). *Overview of anxiety disorders.* Retrieved from http://www.merckmanuals.com/professional/psychiatric_disorders/anxiety_disorders/overview_of_anxiety_disorders.html

Merck Manual—Home Health Handbook. (2008a). Depression. Retrieved from http://www.merckmanuals.com/home/mental_health_disorders/mood_disorders/depression.html

Merck Manual—Home Health Handbook (2008b). Suicidal behavior. Retrieved from http://www.merckmanuals.com/home/mental_health_disorders/suicidal_behavior/suicidal_behavior.html

Murphy, S. L., Jiaquan, X., & Kochanek, K. D. (2012). Deaths: Preliminary data for 2010. *National Vital Statistics Reports, 60*(4), 1–68.

National Institutes of Mental Health [NIMH]. (2012). Suicide in the U.S.: Statistics and Prevention. Retrieved from http://www.nimh.nih.gov/health/publications/suicide-in-the-us-statistics-and-prevention/index.shtml

Older Americans. (2010). Key indicators of well-being. *Federal Interagency Forum on Aging-Related Statistics.* Retrieved from http://www.agingstats.gov/agingstatsdotnet/Main_site/default.aspx

Painter, J. A., Allison, L., Dhingra, P., Daughtery, J., Cogdill, K., & Trujillo, L. (2012). Fear of falling and its relationship with anxiety, depression, and activity engagement among community-dwelling older adults. *American Journal of Occupational Therapy, 66*(2), 169–176.

Pratt, L. A., Brody, D. J., & Gu, Q. (2011). CDC NCHS Data Brief – Antidepressant use in persons aged 12 and over- United States, 2005–2008. *Data from the NHANES, 2005–2008. #76.*

Petersen, R.C., Roberts, R.O., Knopman, D. S., Geda, Y. E., Cha, R. H., Pankratz, V. S. ... Rocca, W. A. (2008). Prevalence of mild cognitive impairment is higher in men: The Mayo Clinic Study of Aging Neurology, 75(10), 889–897. doi: 10.1212/WNL.0b013e3181f11d85

Salerno, M. (2005). Psychosocial disorders. In V. Millonig (Ed.), *Adult nurse practitioner certification review guide* (4th ed., pp. 548–581). Potomac, MD: Health Leadership Associates.

Saver, B. G., Van-Nguyen, V., Keppel, G., & Doescher, M. P. (2007). A qualitative study of depression in primary care: Missed opportunities for diagnosis and education. *Journal of the American Board of Family Medicine, 20*(1), 28–35.

Seitz, D., Purandare, N., & Conn, D. (2010). Prevalence of psychiatric disorders among older adults in long-term care homes: A systematic review. *International Psychogeriatrics, 22*(7), 1025–1039.

Shah, R. (2012). Major types of anxiety neuroses. Retrieved from http://www.anxietyneurosis.com/app/types.asp

Sheikh, J. I. & Yesavage, J. A. (1986). Geriatric Depression Scale (GDS). Recent evidence and development of a shorter version. In T. L. Brink (Ed.), *Clinical gerontology: A guide to assessment and intervention* (pp. 165–173). New York, NY: The Haworth Press.

Spitzer, R., Kroenke, K., & Williams, J. (1999). Validation and utility of a self-report version of PRIME-MD: The PHQ Primary Care Study. *Journal of the American Medical Association, 282,* 1737–1744.

Soriano, R. P. (2007). Depression, dementia, and delirium. In R. P. Soriano, H. M. Fernandez, C. K. Cassell, & R. M. Leipzig (Eds.). *Fundamentals of geriatric medicine: A case based approach.* New York, NY: Springer.

Substance Abuse and Mental Health Services Administration. (2011). *The treatment of depression in older adults: Depression and older adults: Key issues.* HHS Pub. No. SMA-11-4631, Rockville, MD: Center for Mental Health Services, Substance Abuse and Mental Health Services Administration, U.S. Department of Health and Human Services

The MacArthur Initiative on Depression and Primary Care. (2009). Retrieved from http://www.depression-primarycare.org/clinicians/toolkits/

Touhy, T., & Jett, K. (2010). Mental health and wellness in late life. In *Ebersole and Hess' gerontological nursing & healthy aging* (3rd ed., pp. 406–434). St. Louis, MO: Mosby.

Vink, D., Aartsen, M. J., & Schoevers, R. A. (2008). Risk factors for anxiety and depression in the elderly: A review. *Journal of Affective Disorders, 106,* 29–44.

For a full suite of assignments and additional learning activities, see the access code at the front of your book.

LEARNING OBJECTIVES www

At the end of this chapter, the reader will be able to:

> Describe the prevalence of urinary incontinence among older adults in community, acute care, and long-term care settings.
> Identify the negative social, psychological, physical, and economic implications of urinary incontinence.
> Understand that urinary incontinence is not a normal part of aging.
> Collect the appropriate data related to patients' urine control and plan evidence-based nursing care accordingly.
> Initiate evidence-based behavioral interventions to treat urinary incontinence and promote continence for those at risk for urinary incontinence.

KEY TERMS www

Bladder diary

Bladder training

Established (chronic) incontinence

Functional urinary incontinence

Mixed urinary incontinence

Nocturia

Overflow urinary incontinence

Pelvic floor muscle exercises

Pelvic muscle rehabilitation

Prompted voiding

Stress urinary incontinence

Transient (acute) urinary incontinence

Urge suppression techniques

Urge urinary incontinence

Chapter 15

Urinary Incontinence

B. Renee Dugger
Audrey Cochran

Urinary incontinence (UI) is a common problem of the elderly and has tremendous impact on both the morbidity and quality of life of older adults (Godfrey, 2008; Ko, Lin, Salmon, & Bron, 2005; Teunissen, Bosch, Weel, & Lagro-Janssen, 2006). It is often associated with aging, being female, and particularly as a sequela to bearing children. Other contributory factors of UI include urinary retention, urinary tract infection (UTI), fecal impaction, diseases such as diabetes and Parkinson's disease, as well as certain classes of medications such as anticholinergics and narcotics (Lewis, 1995; Newman, Gaines, & Snare, 2005; Wooldridge, 2000). Although UI may be a common problem, it is not a normal part of aging and requires evaluation.

Urinary incontinence, defined as the involuntary leakage of urine to a degree that it is troubling to the person, is a common health problem that affects more than 17 million Americans (AHRQ, 1996; Dowling-Castronovo & Bradway, 2008; Godfrey, 2008). This condition may exist in a variety of forms including stress urinary incontinence, urge urinary incontinence, mixed urinary incontinence, overflow urinary incontinence, and functional urinary incontinence (Dowling-Castronovo & Bradway, 2008; Dowling-Castronovo, 2008; Godfrey, 2008). However, approximately 80% of adults with UI can experience significant improvement or resolution of their symptoms with evaluation and treatment (AHRQ, 1996). The barrier to realization of UI improvement often is a failure of healthcare providers to: (1) identify those with continence problems, (2) conduct a comprehensive assessment, and (3) initiate targeted interventions to address causes and contributing factors. Professional nursing has the knowledge, skills, opportunity, and responsibility to provide aspects of continence care such as screening patients, performing basic evaluation, and initiating treatment or referring patients to a specialist, if indicated (Dowling-Castronovo & Bradway, 2008; Jirovec, Wyman, & Wells, 1998).

Prevalence

Urinary incontinence affects men and women of all ages, at all levels of health, in all settings. Prevalence estimates vary widely, primarily due to differences in the definition of incontinence, the population studied, sampling approaches, and data collection methods (Godfrey, 2008). An estimated 10% of the total population will have UI (Royal College of Physicians, 1995). The percentage of hospitalized elders expected to have UI is 10–43% (Fantl et al., 1996; Lincoln & Roberts, 1989), while up to 70% of residents in long-term care (LTC) settings experience this condition (Lekan-Rutledge, 2004; McCliment, 2002; Newman et al., 2005; Palmer, 2008; Sparks, Boyer, Gambrel, & Lovett, 2004). Between 30% and 40% of community-dwelling middle-aged women experience UI, increasing to 30–50% of older women living in the community (Hunskaar et al., 2002). Prevalence rates in community-dwelling men have a similar pattern, although the rates are lower, ranging from 1–5% in middle-aged men, and increasing to 9–28% in older men (Hunskaar et al., 2002).

Forty-five to 70% of residents in LTC experience UI (Lekan-Rutledge, 2004; McCliment, 2002; Newman et al., 2005; Palmer, 2008; Sparks et al., 2004) and it appears to be increasing (DuBeau, Simon & Morris, 2006). A National Institutes of Health (NIH) consensus and state-of-the-science paper places the prevalence of UI in nursing homes at 60–78% for women and 45–72% for men (Landefeld et al., 2008).

Although UI is not a normal consequence of aging, certain physiological changes that accompany aging increase the risk for development of voiding problems, and certain conditions that predispose to continence problems are more likely to occur in older persons. The reader can find information about normal aging changes in the urinary system and their significance in the older adult in Chapter 29.

Implications of Urinary Incontience
Physical, Psychological, and Social Implications

The vast majority of incontinent persons in the community do not seek help for their incontinence because they consider it a normal part of aging (Urinary Continence Guideline Panel, 1992). This raises questions about how people with this problem perceive UI and what determines the significance attributed to the issue. Many non-institutionalized individuals do not consider incontinence a major problem (Goldstein, Hawthorne, Engeberg, McDowell, & Burgio, 1992; Jeter & Wagner, 1990). However, it is clear that as the degree of incontinence increases, the negative impact on lifestyle and social isolation also increases. It is likely that the total picture of the impact of UI is unknown, because community-dwelling people with UI simply stay home.

Depression and anxiety are potential causes and consequences of incontinence (Dugan et al., 2000; Hajjar, 2004; Heidrich & Wells, 2004; Wells, 1984). Relationships, activities of daily living (ADLs), socialization, and self-concept are affected by UI (Godfrey & Hogg, 2007; Macauly, Stern, Holmes, & Stanton, 1987; Wyman, Harkins, Choi, Taylor, & Fantl, 1987). Urinary incontinence increases the risk of hospitalization and substantially increases the risk of admission to nursing homes in persons over 65 years of age (Newman et al., 2005; Thom, Haan, & Van Den Eeden, 1997). Urge incontinence occurring weekly or more frequently is associated with an increased risk of falls and non-spine, nontraumatic fractures in community-dwelling women age 65 years or older (Brown et al., 2000). Incontinence is one of the major risk factors for the development of skin breakdown (Doughty et al., 2012).

Studies have repeatedly shown a negative impact on quality of life when elderly should be Sitoh persons experience UI (DuBeau, 2005; DuBeau et al., 2006; Ko et al., 2005; Teunissen et al., 2006). Sitou and colleagues (2005) found from their research with elderly persons that the following conditions had the most harmful effect on health-related quality of life: "degree of frailty…., history of strokes, diagnosis of Parkinson's disease, previous falls or fractures and the presence of urinary incontinence" (p. 132). The International Continence Society recommended that any study involving UI should include assessing and measuring quality of life (Robinson & Shea, 2002).

Elderly persons who experience UI often suffer from physical and psychological distress. Some of the negative physical outcomes include dermatitis and possible skin ulceration, disruption of sleep patterns, urinary tract infections (UTIs) and falls, which can lead to fractures (Doughty et al., 2012; Lekan-Rutledge, 2004; Lewis, 1995; Newman et al., 2005; Wooldridge, 2000). Common psychological issues as a result of UI include feelings of loss of control, dependency, shame and guilt, social isolation, avoidance of activities, anxiety, impaired self esteem, and depression (Bradway, 2003; DuBeau et al., 2006; Ko et al., 2005; MacDonald & Butler, 2007; Teunissen et al., 2006) (see **Box 15-1**).

BOX 15-1   Research Highlight

Aim: An aspect of this pre-post quasi-experimental prospective design study was examination of urinary incontinence (UI) impact on nursing home residents' health-related quality of life.

Method: A multidisciplinary team conducted a study in four Midwestern nursing homes with 33 nursing home residents. The team examined the residents' health-related quality of life utilizing the Incontinence Stress Questionnaire for Patients (ISQ-P) instrument before and after interventions. The interventions included staff education and bladder scanner placement in each nursing home.

Findings: Figure 15-1 depicts relationships found between the following ISQ-P instrument variables (*try to hide UI from others, am worried about urine leakage, urine smell causes me to avoid others, having bedsores because of it*, and *keep myself clean*) with two additional ISQ-P variables (*am a burden to others* and *blue or depressed*). Calculation of Pearson correlation coefficient showed a strong positive correlation, suggesting a linear relationship between the first five variables culminating in feelings of being a burden and depression. These residents had an increased ISQ-P stress score leading to an assumption of decreased health-related quality of life (Coudret et al., 2009). During the interview process, residents made the statements shown in **Table 15-1** about their UI experience.

Application to practice: The relationships identified among the ISQ-P instrument variables show the residents with UI experience feelings of being a burden and depression. The resident comments captured in Table 15-1 also point to considerable stress and psychological pain. These findings give additional credence to the importance of caregiver sensitivity to these feelings and proper UI assessment and management to preserve or improve resident health-related quality of life.

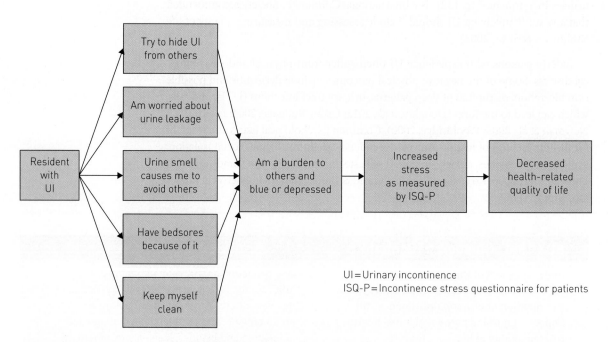

UI = Urinary incontinence
ISQ-P = Incontinence stress questionnaire for patients

Figure 15-1 Model of relationships of ISQ-P variables and resident health-related quality of life based on ISQ-P instrument.

Source: Coudret, N., Ehlman, K., Dugger, R., Eggleston, B., Wilson, A., Harrison, E. & Mathis, S. (October 30, 2009). *Assessing the benefits of bladder ultrasound scanners in nursing homes: Project funded by the Indiana State Department of Health - Final Report.* Unpublished manuscript, College of Nursing and Health Professions, University of Southern Indiana, Evansville, IN.

TABLE 15-1   Comments from Nursing Home Residents During Interviews

Select Comments from Nursing Home Residents During Interview Process about Their Experience of Urinary Incontinence

- *I get used to it and it doesn't bother me most of the time.*
- *It's inconvenient.*
- *I can't help it.*
- *This condition is the reason I am in the nursing home.*

- *I just accept it.*
- *I don't talk about it much.*
- *I don't want to see it or anybody else to see it.*
- *I felt everything was taken away. It's sad.*
- *I feel like a pest if I have to keep calling.*
- *Not too many people like talking about that.*
- *I have irritation all the time but nobody does nothing.*

Comments from Nursing Home Residents about the Variable *I Cry When I Think or Talk about the Incontinence*

- *I want to, but I can't.*
- *I feel that is something a person can't help.*
- *I do it softly.*
- *Inside when I'm alone.*
- *I am past that.*

Source: Coudret, N., Ehlman, K., Dugger, R., Eggleston, B., Wilson, A., Harrison, E. & Mathis, S. (October 30, 2009). *Assessing the benefits of bladder ultrasound scanners in nursing homes: Project funded by the Indiana State Department of Health—Final Report.* Unpublished manuscript, College of Nursing and Health Professions, University of Southern Indiana, Evansville, IN.

Economic Implications

Urinary incontinence carries a significant economic impact. The costs associated with UI management often are not covered by insurance and become an out-of-pocket expense (Wilson, Brown, Shin, Luc, & Subak, 2001). These expenses can interfere with the ability of persons on a fixed income to purchase medications and supplies to manage other health problems. In the United States, the direct costs associated with UI run as high $16 billion per year (Landefeld et al., 2008).

In addition to the adverse outcomes of UI for the nursing home resident, there are negative and costly effects for the nursing home facility as well. Estimated costs of UI care run as high as $5.2 billion annually for nursing homes in the United States (Frenchman, 2001; Landefeld et al., 2008). The cost of UI containment includes pads (both disposable and reusable), diapers, briefs, gloves, laundry products, and catheters, not to mention the time required by staff to provide care. Obviously, these materials and labor costs can add substantially to nursing home expenses. Frenchman (2001) estimated UI labor and materials costs as $17.21 per nursing home resident per day when examining two facilities in New Jersey. This resulted in over $6,200 of expense tied to UI per year per resident. Estimates are that 3–8% of nursing home costs and as much as 1 hour per day go toward each resident's incontinence care (Hu, Wagner, Bentkover, Leblanc, Zhou, & Hunt, 2004). The financial impact is even greater if residents experience falls, fractures, and pressure ulcers (Newman et al., 2005; Wooldridge, 2000). Wooldridge (2000) estimates institutions spend approximately $680 for each episode of UTI.

Assessment

An understanding of the types of incontinence and the factors associated with incontinence is necessary to guide evaluation and the development of appropriate targeted interventions. Urinary incontinence is categorized as *transient (acute)* or *established (chronic)* based on onset and etiology.

Assessment of Transient Urinary Incontinence

Transient or acute incontinence is caused by the onset of an acute problem that, once successfully, treated should result in the resolution of incontinence. Multiple causative and contributory factors have been associated with the development or exacerbation of voiding problems, in particular UI (Dowling-Castronova, 2007). **Table 15-2** lists common transient causes and potentially reversible factors of UI with a brief explanation of the basis for their impact on continence. If transient UI is not appropriately assessed and managed in a timely manner, it can become established or chronic UI, which is much more difficult to treat.

Assessment of Established Urinary Incontinence

Established or chronic incontinence encompasses four basic UI disorders. These bladder disorders include stress, urge, overflow, and functional incontinence.

Stress urinary incontinence refers to the involuntary loss of urine during activities that increase intra-abdominal pressure (e.g., lifting, coughing, sneezing, and laughing). Stress incontinence is distinguished from urge or overflow incontinence by the absence of bladder contraction or over-distention, respectively. The most common causes of stress incontinence are hypermobility of the bladder neck and urethral sphincter defects. Weakness of the pelvic floor muscles leads to loss of support for the bladder neck and disrupts the normal pressure gradient between the bladder and urethra, resulting in leakage of urine (AHRQ, 1996; Dowling-Castronovo & Bradway, 2012; MayoClinic.com, 2008).

Urge urinary incontinence is associated with a strong, abrupt desire to void and the inability to inhibit leakage in time to reach a toilet. Uninhibited bladder contractions usually, but not always, are a precipitating factor. Central nervous system disorders, such as stroke or multiple sclerosis, and local irritations such as infection or ingestion of bladder irritants (e.g., caffeine) are potential causes. Reflex incontinence, a variation of urge incontinence, results from uninhibited

TABLE 15-2   Transient Causes of Urinary Incontinence

The mnemonic DIAPPERS has been established to list common causes of transient incontinence.

Common Causes	Rationale
Delirium/dementia	Altered cognitive functioning interferes with the ability to recognize the need for toileting or respond in a timely manner.
Infection	The urinary frequency and urgency associated with symptomatic UTI may lead to urinary incontinence.
Atrophic vaginitis/urethritis	Decreased estrogen in women results in thin, dry, friable vaginal and urethra mucosa.
Psychological	Depression may interfere with an individual's motivation and desire to perform activities of daily living or attend to continence. Anxiety or fear that leakage will occur may contribute to frequency difficulties controlling urge
Pharmacological agents	Inadequate management of acute or chronic pain can interfere with the ability to attend to toileting needs. Narcotics, a component of many pain management regimens, can lead to constipation and fecal impaction that obstructs the bladder neck, leading to urine retention, overflow incontinence, and urgency. Narcotics can also decrease bladder muscle contraction resulting in urine retention, incomplete bladder emptying, increased risk for UTI, and overflow incontinence.
	Many medications have adverse or unintended side effects that may directly impact bladder function, bladder relaxation, urinary sphincter relaxation or obstruction, change in cognitive status (less awareness of an effective response to need to void), or urine production. Polypharmacy increases the risk for adverse drug effects and drug interactions.
Endocrine disease	Metabolic conditions (hyperglycemia, hypercalcemia, low albumin states, diabetes insipidus) associated with polyuria increase fluid load on the bladder and increase the risk for urge and stress incontinence.
Restricted mobility	Limited ability to move about interferes with the ability to reach a toilet in time to prevent leakage.
Stool impaction	Overdistention of the rectum or anal canal can obstruct the bladder neck, leading to urine retention, overflow incontinence, and urgency.

bladder contractions with no sensation of needing to void or urgency. This condition occurs most often in spinal lesions transecting the cord above T10–11. (AHRQ, 1996; Dowling-Castronovo & Bradway, 2012; MayoClinic .com, 2008). *Overflow urinary incontinence* refers to over-distention of the bladder due to abnormal emptying. The leakage may be continuous, or resemble the symptoms of stress or urge incontinence. Overflow incontinence results from a weak or areflexic bladder, neurologic conditions such as diabetes, spinal cord injury below T10–11, or obstruction of the bladder outlet or urethra (AHRQ, 1996; Dowling-Castronovo & Bradway, 2012; MayoClinic .com, 2008). *Functional urinary incontinence* refers to problems from factors external to the lower urinary tract such as cognitive impairments, physical disabilities, and environmental barriers (AHRQ, 1996; Dowling-Castronovo & Bradway, 2012; MayoClinic.com, 2008).

Although separate disorders clinically, patients may exhibit symptoms of more than one type of incontinence. The term *mixed urinary incontinence* refers to the existence of the symptoms of urge and stress incontinence at the same time (AHRQ, 1996; Dowling-Castronovo & Bradway, 2012; MayoClinic.com, 2008).

Diagnosis of the type(s) of UI experienced is essential in the development of appropriate interventions. These inventions should be designed to address the varying levels of cognitive and physical functioning of the patient. The elements of a basic evaluation of UI are outlined in **Table 15-3** and discussed in greater detail below with respect to the older patient.

TABLE 15-3   Components of a Basic Evaluation for Urinary Incontinence
History
Focused medical, neurologic, and genitourinary history
Assessment of risk factors
Review of medications
Detailed exploration of the symptoms of incontinence
Physical examination
General examination
Abdominal examination
Rectal examination
Pelvic examination in women
Genital examination in men
Postvoided residual volume
Urinalysis

Source: Fantl, J. A., Newman, D. K., Colling J., et al. Managing Acute and Chronic Incontinence in Adults. Clinical Practice Guideline, No. 2, 1996 Update. Rockville, MD: U.S. Department of Health and Human Services, Public Health Service, Agency of Health Care Policy and Research. AHCPRPub-No. 96-0686.

Data Gathering

History and Other Pertinent Data

The first step in the evaluation is a discussion of voiding patterns and problems. Initiating this line of questions by focusing on usual number of voids during the day and night, as well as other symptoms such as burning, hesitancy, pain, or low pelvic pressure, provides a less-threatening opening to this topic. It may be necessary to reword questions about the presence of incontinence to determine the occurrence of wetting accidents, their frequency, and volume of urine lost. Asking about the use of padding or protective garments may also provide important clues to the presence of incontinence or the fear of an accident. Gather information about the onset and duration of voiding problems and activities that precipitate or are associated with their occurrence. Of particular relevance is determining the status of bowel functioning and usual bowel habits since constipation and fecal impaction can precipitate UI.

A recall of daily food and fluid intake also provides important information in the evaluation of urological functioning and development of a treatment plan. It is typical for patients with urgency and urge incontinence to report a fluid intake that consists primarily of bladder irritants (e.g., diet drinks, carbonated and/or caffeinated beverages) and minimal to no water. Dietary modifications alone can reduce urge incontinence (Dowling-Castronovo & Bradway, 2012).

The initial interview should help identify potentially reversible causative factors and contributing risk factors for UI. The history should provide clues to the type(s) of incontinence involved. It may be necessary for the patient to complete a detailed bladder diary (discussed in the next section, see **Figure 15-2**) over a period of three days in order to obtain a complete picture of factors related to the UI.

Awareness of the specific symptoms experienced and the degree of discomfort associated with each can be useful in determining the priority for intervening. Identifying those aspects of daily life that UI or the fear of UI disrupts can provide the outcomes to evaluate. For example, if UI interferes with exercise, then participation in an exercise regimen three times a week might be the goal set with the patient; the nurse and patient would then develop a specific plan to achieve the exercise goal.

Urinary Incontinence Interview Instruments

Interviews and conversations with persons experiencing incontinence reveal the difficulty persons experience when thinking about and discussing this very personal, private matter. The use of a tool that provides words and choices for responses frequently facilitates the exchange of information. Short form versions of the Urogenital Distress Inventory/Incontinence Impact Questionnaire (UDI/IIQ) provide objective measurement of the life impact and symptom distress,

Your Daily Bladder Diary

This diary will help you and your health care team. Bladder diaries show the causes of bladder control trouble. The "sample" line (below) will show you how to use the diary.

ACCIDENTS

Time	Drinks		Urine	Accidental Leaks	Did you feel a strong urge to go?	What were you doing at the time?
	How much?	What kind?	How much? Circle one	How many times? How much? Use measuring cups (ml's or oz's)	(check one)	*Sneezing, exercising, having sex, lifting, etc.*
Sample	2 cups	Coffee	sm (med) lg	2 oz or 2 ml	Yes No	Running
6-7 a.m.					Yes No	
7-8 a.m.					Yes No	
8-9 a.m.					Yes No	
9-10 a.m.					Yes No	
10-11 a.m.					Yes No	
11-12 noon					Yes No	
12-1 p.m.					Yes No	
1-2 p.m.					Yes No	
2-3 p.m.					Yes No	
3-4 p.m.					Yes No	
4-5 p.m.					Yes No	
5-6 p.m.					Yes No	
6-7 p.m.					Yes No	
7-8 p.m.					Yes No	
8-9 p.m.					Yes No	
9-10 p.m.					Yes No	
10-11 p.m.					Yes No	
11-12 mid					Yes No	
12-1 a.m.					Yes No	
1-2 a.m.					Yes No	
2-3 a.m.					Yes No	
3-4 a.m.					Yes No	
4-5 a.m.					Yes No	
5-6 a.m.					Yes No	

Your name:
Date:

Figure 15-2 A sample voiding diary.

respectively, of UI and related conditions for women. With minor wording modifications of some items, the tool is appropriate for men and from hospitalization through reintegration into the community. A copy of this tool, along with modifications used with men and a hospitalized patient, is in **Table 15-4**. If the patient has communication or cognitive deficits, obtain information from family members, when possible. At times, previous medical records or observation of current behaviors may be the only data source available. An instrument specific to the nursing home resident setting that measures stress associated with UI is the Incontinence Questionnaire for Patients (ISQ-P) (Yu, 1987; Yu, Kaltreider, Hu, & Craighead, 1989).

TABLE 15-4   Urogenital Distress Inventory Short Form (UDI-6) and Incontinence Impact Questionnaire Short Form (IIQ-6)

Do you experience and, if so, how much are you bothered by:

1. Frequent urination
2. Urine leakage related to feeling of urgency
3. Urine leakage related to activity, coughing, or sneezing
4. Small amounts of urine leakage (drops)
5. Difficulty emptying your bladder
6. Pain or discomfort in lower abdominal or genital area

Has urine leakage affected your:

1. Ability to do household chores (cooking, housekeeping, laundry) (daily activities)
2. Physical recreation such as walking, swimming, or other exercise (therapy sessions)
3. Entertainment activities (movies, concerts, etc.)
4. Ability to travel more than 30 minutes from your room or unit
5. Participating in social activities outside your home
6. Emotional health (nervousness, depression, anger)
7. Feeling frustrated

Key to scoring

0 = Not at all
1 = Slightly
2 = Moderately
3 = Greatly

(Information in parentheses are modifications to reflect inpatient activities.)

Source: Uebersax, J. S., Wyaman, J.F., Schumaker, S. A., Fantl, J. A. Continence Program for Woman Research Group (1995). Short forms to assess life quality and symptom distress for urinary incontinence in women: The incontinence impact questionnaire and the urogenital distress inventory. *Neurourology and Urodynamics, 14,* 131, 139.

BOX 15-2   Evidence-Based Practice Highlight

The UDI-6 and IIQ-7 assessment instruments referred to in Table 15-4 are available at: http://consultgerirn.org/uploads/File/trythis/try_this_11_2.pdf, and a version of the 24-hour Bladder Diary in Figure 15-2 is available at: http://consultgerirn.org/uploads/File/trythis/try_this_11_1.pdf.

These resources are part of the *Try This: Best Practices in Nursing Care to Older Adults* series made available through the Hartford Institute for Geriatric Nursing at the http://www.ConsultgeriRN.org website. The website is an excellent source of evidence-based practice information and resources specific to multiple geriatric clinical nursing issues.

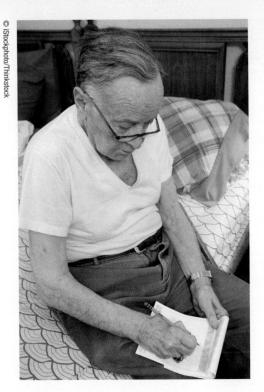

Figure 15-3 Keeping a bladder diary helps both the client and the nurse with assessment and management of UI.

Bladder Diary

The *bladder diary* is a critical component of a basic evaluation, regardless of the setting (Dowling-Castronovo, 2007; MayoClinic.com, 2008). By outlining the timing, amount, and type of fluid intake with the timing, amount, and continence status for each void, key UI data is collected, including severity, irritating or associated symptoms, precipitating events, and voiding problem patterns (Dowling-Castronovo, 2007; Wyman, 1994a). The patient should record bladder diary findings over 3–7 days; however, 72 hours typically provides sufficient data and is a more reasonable timeframe for data collection (Doughty, 2000). See **Figure 15-3** for a sample bladder diary. Patients or caregivers can also collect the bladder diary data. Many times patients or informal caregivers completing these records identify patterns to the occurrence of incontinence and can begin to make positive changes. The bladder diary is a reliable method for assessing the frequency of voluntary voiding and involuntary incidents of urine loss and can be a particularly important data source to differentiate factors contributing to nocturia (Wyman et al., 1988).

Nocturia, the awakening from sleep to urinate, is a frustrating and common problem for many older persons. Nocturia may result from alterations in normal circadian rhythm of urine output, physiological changes in the lower urinary tract that interfere with storage, or be an indication of sleep apnea (Donahue & Lowenthal, 1997; Umlauf, Burgio, Shettar, & Pillion, 1997). Nocturia can occur during sleep apnea when the heart, deprived of oxygen from soft airways obstruction, secretes beta natriuretic hormone, which causes diuresis as the body attempts to reduce the effort the heart is making to maintain normal blood pressure, oxygen, and carbon dioxide levels. Sleep apnea commonly occurs in individuals with cardiovascular disease, and is often the root cause of nocturia in this population. Comorbidities of diabetes and hypertension greatly increase the risk of sleep apnea (Umlauf & Chasens, 2003). The serious nature of sleep apnea necessitates a careful evaluation of the etiology of nocturia (Pressman, Figueroa, Kendrick-Mohamed, Greenspan, & Peterson, 1996). Additional information about nocturia treatment options appear later in this chapter.

Cognitive Status

A client's insight into voiding status, recall of pertinent health information, and ability to participate in an interview are the first clues to cognitive status. Objective cognitive data can be obtained with the Mini Mental State Examination (MMSE) (Folstein, Folstein, & McHugh, 1975), Mini-Cog (Borson, Scanlan, Brush,

BOX 15-3   Evidence-Based Practice Highlight

Proper cognitive status assessment of the patient experiencing urinary incontinence is critical. Two evidence-based instruments to utilize for this assessment include the Confusion Assessment Method (CAM) and Mini-Cog assessments. A copy of the CAM instrument, along with information about and proper use of the instrument, is at http://consultgerirn.org/uploads/File/trythis/try_this_13.pdf. A copy of the Mini-Cog and information about this instrument is located at http://consultgerirn.org/uploads/File/trythis/try_this_3.pdf. The availability of these instruments and accompanying assessment information, along with additional resources to support evidence-based practice, is part of the *Try This: Best Practices in Nursing Care of Older Adults* series of resources at the http://www.ConsultgeriRN.org website.

Vitallano, & Dokmak, 2000) and/or the Confusion Assessment Method (CAM) (Inouye et al., 1990). See **Box 15-3** for additional information about the Mini-Cog and CAM assessments. The cognitive impairment severity level alerts the healthcare professional to the client's increased risk for persistent incontinence. It also guides selection of options for interventions.

Physical Assessment

It is tempting to base the determination of incontinence type on the clinical signs and symptoms from the history; however, clinical symptoms alone are not sufficient to determine the pathophysiology of voiding problems (Rich & Pannill, 1999). Aspects of a general physical examination, with implications for voiding dysfunction, include focused physical examination of the genitourinary system, abdominal and rectal areas, and neurologic system.

General Physical Assessment

An overall physical examination is appropriate to detect conditions that contribute to incontinence, such as peripheral edema, or neurologic abnormalities that suggest stroke, Parkinson's disease, or other neurologic disorders. Gross motor skills (e.g., locomotion, transfer skills, sitting, and balance), dexterity (e.g., managing buttons, zippers, and toilet paper), and the ability to communicate the need for assistance or reliably respond to verbal or written words must be assessed. Evaluate functional deficits and capabilities to determine barriers and/or assets in continence promotion. Calculating the average time it takes the patient to access a toilet while suppressing the urge to void will assist in identification of therapeutic interventions to facilitate continence, specific intervention goals, and the degree of continence possible.

Hydration Assessment

Initial and ongoing evaluation of hydration is essential to diagnose dehydration and minimize its complications. Dehydration complications range from urine becoming concentrated and triggering UI due to bladder contractions from irritation of the bladder wall to more systemic problems including confusion and lethargy (Dowling-Castronovo & Bradway, 2012). Physical parameters of hydration status include condition of oral mucous membranes, sublingual saliva pool, weight changes, confusion, and muscle weakness. Monitoring the balance between fluid intake and urine output, urine color, and urine specific gravity (SG) for the second void of the day are useful indicators of fluid status (Mentes & Iowa Veterans Affairs Nursing Research Consortium [Iowa Veterans Affairs], 1998). Urine SG of greater than 1.020 and dark yellow or brownish-green urine indicate the need for increased fluid intake (Armstrong, 2000). Blood tests such as BUN/creatinine ratio, serum osmolality, and serum sodium are predictors of actual dehydration (Mentes & Iowa Veterans Affairs, 1998). Calculate body mass index (BMI) to identify persons at risk for hydration problems. Older adults with BMI of 21 or lower and 27 or higher are at risk for hydration issues (Mentes & Iowa Veterans Affairs, 1998). In addition, the BMI will provide an indication of the extent of obesity, which also contributes to voiding problems.

Genitourinary Examination

In women, the pelvic examination should include assessment of the perineal skin integrity, specifically looking for lesions, irritation, or inflammation. Evidence of atrophic vaginal changes including pale, thin, dry, friable mucosa with complaints of vaginal itching, dryness, burning, and dyspareunia are notable. Vaginal pH levels 5 or above in women without evidence of a vaginal infection are also indicative of poorly estrogenized tissues (Shull et al., 1999). A urethral carbuncle, a cherry-red lesion at the urinary meatus, is another indicator of estrogen deficiency. Atrophic urethritis and vaginitis contribute to urge and stress UI; topical estrogen therapy is usually the treatment of choice for these conditions. The presence of perineum sensation indicates intact sacral nerve roots for the external urethral and anal sphincters (Shull et al., 1999). Check for pelvic organ prolapse. If the organ prolapse is beyond the introitus or symptomatic, refer the woman for further evaluation and treatment. Multiple types and sizes of pessaries are available for correction of prolapse. In men, examination of the external genitalia should include inspection of the skin, location of the urethral meatus, and retractability of the foreskin, if present.

An evaluation of pelvic floor muscle strength is an important component of the examination. This is a particularly important evaluation for patients with diabetes due to possible neuropathy, which can interfere with normal sensory input resulting in bladder over-distention and urinary retention (Shull et al., 1999). However, consider the appropriateness of performing an invasive, uncomfortable, and embarrassing vaginal digital examination, particularly in frail older women and cognitively impaired elders (Lekan-Ruteledge, 2004). This evaluation also provides key information on the patient's ability to isolate and identify the correct muscles. In men and women with vaginal stenosis, pelvic floor muscle strength can be evaluated rectally. If the individual is capable of using pelvic muscles to inhibit urge or suppress urine flow, a vaginal or rectal digital examination may not be needed to evaluate pelvic muscle control.

Rectal Examination

Assess both resting and active anal sphincter tone. The ability to contract the anal sphincter indicates a functional pelvic floor with intact innervation (Shull et al., 1999). In men, palpate the prostate proximal to the internal anal sphincter through the anterior rectal wall, noting size, consistency, and tenderness. Remember that prostate size does not correlate well with bladder neck obstruction. During the digital rectal examination, evaluate pelvic floor muscle strength and assess the rectal vault for large-caliber, hardened stool, suggesting constipation or impaction. If found, treat the impaction prior to initiating a bladder program.

Abdominal Examination

Palpate the abdomen for tenderness, fullness, or masses that may be indicative of fecal impaction. Auscultate bowel sounds to evaluate bowel motility. Palpate the suprapubic area to detect bladder tenderness or distention (Shull et al., 1999).

Bladder Volume Evaluation

Evaluate for difficulties starting the urine stream, intermittent urine flow, strength of the urine stream, and the presence of post-void dribbling. Measure the patient's post-void residual (PVR) urine volume by in-and-out catheterization or with a bladder ultrasound scanner within a few minutes of voiding. A portable bladder ultrasound scanner is a useful indicator of the patient's ability to empty the bladder and is the preferable method since it is noninvasive (Lewis, 1995; McCliment, 2002). A PVR bladder volume of less than 150 milliliters in an elderly patient is considered normal. Consistent PVRs over 150 milliliters indicates incomplete bladder emptying and the need for further evaluation (Borrie et al., 2001).

Urine Examination

Urinalysis by dipstick or laboratory testing is a component of the initial evaluation of UI. Check urine for white blood cells, nitrites, glucose, and blood (Shull et al., 1999). A UTI should be treated prior to initiation of other treatment for UI, as treatment of a UTI may result in an improvement or resolution of urine leakage, frequency, and/or urgency.

Environmental Assessment

Evaluate the environment as a potential factor in the development and treatment of UI. Structural characteristics; the number, location, and accessibility of toileting facilities; the availability of physical assistance; and adaptive equipment and supplies for toileting are major considerations (Godfrey, 2008). Evaluate environmental characteristics of the hospital and potential discharge destinations and integrate the results into the treatment plan to achieve the optimal level of continence.

Interventions and Care Strategies

Categories of UI Treatment Strategies

Guidelines by national and international panels based on extensive literature reviews outline assessment and treatment of various types of UI in specific populations (Abrams, Khoury, & Wein, 1999; AHRQ, 1996; Dowling-Castronovo & Bradway, 2008, 2012; Fantl et al., 1996). The three primary categories of treatment for UI are behavioral management, pharmacological intervention (see **Box 15-4**), and surgical intervention (Godfrey, 2008). (see **Table 15-5**).

Behavioral management refers to interventions that modify the patient's behavior or environment. Strategies included in a behavioral approach are voiding scheduling regimens, dietary management, urge suppression techniques, and *pelvic floor muscle exercises* (PFME) with and without the addition of biofeedback, vaginal cones, and electrical stimulation. Pharmacological intervention involves medications that alter detrusor muscle activity or bladder outlet resistance. Surgical interventions primarily address increasing bladder outlet resistance resulting from intrinsic sphincter deficiency, as well as removal of bladder outlet obstruction, relieving overflow incontinence (Fantl et al., 1996).

Patient-Centered Urinary Incontinence Treatment Goals

Clarify all UI treatment goals and desired outcomes for evaluation with the patient first. It is important to keep in mind that an understanding of the patient's expectations for treatment outcomes will provide direction for intervention. Patient goals

---

BOX 15-4   Clinical Practice Example

"No Pads, No Pills, No Hurry, and No Leaks" is the title of a 3-hour class taught by Audrey Cochran, MSN, GCNS-BC, CCCN, at a community college for several years. At one class, attended by 20 people, she announced that she would like to phone them in 4 months to see what results they got from utilizing her suggestions. One of their assignments was to keep a diary of what they ate and drank and how that affected their bladder. In addition to learning how to do pelvic floor muscle exercises, the self-analysis helped all of them improve their bladder control.

Some findings from the group included that no one was bothered by coffee but one person had to rush to the bathroom more often after drinking tea. Another had a "twitchy bladder" when she ate tomatoes in any form, whether in salad or pizza or spaghetti sauce. Another had problems with honeydew melon. In Cochran's clinical practice, some patients report that if they eat watermelon they "had just better plan on staying home the rest of the day." After keeping track of what she ate and drank, another patient discovered when she had her usual cereal with milk and coffee and orange juice for breakfast she had trouble controlling her bladder, but not when she substituted apple juice for the orange juice. A post-prostatectomy patient discovered when he drank a diet soft drink (containing aspartame) he leaked more than when he drank a regular soft drink. Increased problems with urinary incontinence when using sugar substitutes was also reported by several other patients. These examples show the importance of patients keeping a diary of what goes in and when it comes out before and while making changes.

TABLE 15-5 Evidence-Based Practice Guidelines to Prevent and Manage All Types of Urinary Incontinence

Guidelines to prevent and manage all types of urinary incontinence (UI):

1. Identify and treat causes of transient UI.

2. Identify and continue successful prehospital management strategies for established UI.

3. Develop an individualized plan of care using data obtained from the history and physical examination and in collaboration with other team members.

4. Avoid medications that may contribute to UI.

5. Avoid indwelling urinary catheters whenever possible to avoid risk for urinary tract infection (UTI).

6. Monitor fluid intake and maintain an appropriate hydration schedule.

7. Limit dietary bladder irritants.

8. Consider adding weight loss as a long-term goal in discharge planning for those with a high body mass index (BMI).

9. Modify the environment to facilitate continence.

10. Provide patients with usual undergarments in expectation of continence, if possible.

11. Prevent skin breakdown by providing immediate cleansing after an incontinent episode and utilizing barrier ointments.

12. Pilot test absorbent products to best meet patient, staff, and institutional preferences, bearing in mind that diapers have been associated with UTIs.

Source: Dowling-Castronovo, A & Bradway, C. (2008). Urinary incontinence in older adults admitted to acute care. In: Capezuti, E., Zwicker, D., Mezey, M. & Fulmer, T. (eds.). Evidence-based geriatric nursing protocols for best practice, 3rd ed. New York, NY: Springer Publishing Company, 309–36.

are multidimensional and do not necessarily require total continence for patient satisfaction and improved health-related quality of life (Dowling-Castronovo & Bradway, 2007; Sale & Wyman, 1994).

Behavioral Management

Behavioral approaches should be the first line of treatment for UI. Eliminating reversible factors is a first step in treatment in order to optimize urological functioning. Clinical practice guidelines identify dietary modifications (hydration and avoidance of bladder irritants), scheduled voiding, *prompted voiding (PV), bladder training, pelvic muscle rehabilitation*, and *urge suppression techniques* as useful approaches in a comprehensive treatment regimen for UI (Abrams et al., 1999; Dowling-Castronovo & Bradway, 2008, 2012; Fantl et al., 1996; Godfrey, 2008).

Behavioral strategies differ in their mechanisms of action, the required level of patient participation, and the technology involved. Interventions should be selected for patients based on the patient's UI type, mental and physical abilities, any other limitations, and environmental resources available (Burgio & Burgio, 1986). The versatility of behavioral therapy enables the care providers to adapt and individualize the treatment plan according to the patient's level of functioning. If successful, behavioral approaches eliminate the added expense and potential risk of an adverse drug reaction from pharmacological intervention and the complications associated with surgery.

Hydration Management

Managing hydration focuses on maintaining fluid balance. Ensuring an adequate, timely, appropriate fluid intake is essential to a successful continence program (**Box 15-5**). Older adults concerned about UI may intentionally reduce their fluid intake, which can lead to concentrated urine and irritability of the bladder wall resulting in increased UI (Dowling-Castronovo & Bradway, 2007).

An individualized fluid goal must first be determined. To calculate fluid intake according to this standard, take 100 ml/kg for the first 10 kg of weight, 50 ml/kg for the next 10 kg, and 15 ml for the remaining kgs (Mentes & Iowa Veterans Affairs, 2000, 2004). Because this includes fluid from all sources, take 70% of the total to determine the goal for fluid volume intake alone (Mentes & Iowa Veterans Affairs, 2000, 2004).

Providing fluids throughout the day will help ensure meeting the fluid goal, yet minimize frequency and urgency resulting from rapid bladder filling from large fluid volume ingestion over a short period. The suggested percentage of fluid delivery is 75–80% of fluid at meals and 20–25% during nonmeal times, such as with medications and planned nourishment (Mentes & Iowa Veterans Affairs, 2000, 2004). For patients in a residential setting, this schedule offers the additional advantage of supervision, if necessary, for patients with swallowing problems. Fluid rounds midmorning and midafternoon, in conjunction with offers of assistance with toileting, have been effective in reducing incontinence and decreasing dehydration in bedfast elderly nursing home residents. Fluids should be limited in the evening hours prior to bedtime, especially if nocturia is present (Mentes & Iowa Veterans Affairs, 2000, 2004).

A final consideration in fluid intake concerns the type of fluids consumed. The fluids should be limited to those without a diuretic or irritant effect. Many common foods and beverages may be irritating to the bladder, causing or contributing to UI. Carbonated and caffeinated beverages, citrus juices, acidic foods, alcoholic

BOX 15-5   Evidence-Based Practice Highlight

Hydration Management Evidence-Based Practice Resources: The Nursing Standard of Practice Protocol for Oral Hydration Management is available at http://consultgerirn .org/topics/hydration_management/want_to_ know_more#Wrap on the Hartford Institute for Geriatric Nursing's website, http://www .ConsultGeriRN.org. In addition, a Dehydration Risk Appraisal Checklist is available at http:// rgp.toronto.on.ca/torontobestpractice/ Dehydrationriskappraisalchecklist.pdf.

beverages, and aspartame are among the products commonly considered bladder irritants or having a diuretic effect (Dowling-Castronovo & Bradway, 2012). A review of the bladder diary (see Figure 15-2) is especially useful in detecting possible agents that precipitate urgency or incontinence. Reducing the intake of caffeinated beverages to no more than two servings a day is recommended for individuals experiencing urgency or urge incontinence (Arya, Myers, & Jackson, 2000). Postum and sun teas are potential alternatives for coffee and tea, respectively. However, water is the better choice of a liquid since it is not an irritant or diuretic and does not interfere with diabetic control.

For patients with swallowing problems, providing the appropriate consistency can prevent choking or aspiration. Nectars and thick liquids such as buttermilk and V8 juice are usually acceptable alternatives. Any liquid may be thickened with commercial products or by mixing it with natural thickeners such as baby food, mashed bananas, or wheat germ (M. Kain, personal communication, September 6, 2001).

Bowel Function Management

Maintaining bowel regularity prevents bladder emptying problems that may result from constipation and fecal impaction. Irregular bowel habits, immobility, dehydration, decreased fiber intake, medication side effects, and emotional factors contribute to the development of constipation. Maintaining hydration is critical in promoting bowel function, which, in turn, aids bladder function. Many hospitalized patients identify the lack of privacy and change in daily routine as major factors contributing to their constipation. Consider adding fiber with adequate fluids, if stools are hard. A mild stimulant such as prunes or prune juice 6 to 8 hours prior to planned defecation can assist removal of stool that is difficult to pass. A mixture of applesauce, prune juice, and bran has been effective in decreasing constipation and for laxative use in nursing home patients (Smith & Newman, 1989) and has application in the treatment and prevention of constipation in at-risk patients (see **Box 15-6**). Its thick texture may facilitate administration to patients with swallowing problems. The use of regular grocery store items to prepare the mixture should decrease the overall cost of the bowel program when compared to prescription or over-the-counter products.

Prompted Voiding

Prompted voiding (PV) is an intervention for patients unable to recognize and act on the sensation of the need to void and exert neuromuscular control over voiding initiation. Prompted voiding has been successful in decreasing the frequency of

---

BOX 15-6 Evidence-Based Practice Highlight on Preventing Constipation

Best Practice Guideline: Prevention of Constipation in the Older Adult Population is available at http://rnao.ca/bpg/guidelines/prevention-constipation-older-adult-population

UI in clinical trials with physically and cognitively impaired nursing home residents (Colling, Ouslander, Hadley, Eisch, & Campbell, 1992; Fantl et al., 1996; McCormick, Cella, Scheve, & Engel, 1990; Schnelle, 1990). The use of PV is also effective in home settings. Persons with urge, stress, and mixed UI have responded positively to this intervention (Ouslander et al., 1995; Schnelle, 1990). Prompted voiding also has strong support for reducing UI in individuals with cognitive and physical deficits (Abrams et al., 1999; Fantl et al., 1996; Heavner, 1998).

Prompted voiding is a scheduling regimen that initially focuses on the caregiver's behavior in order to change the incontinent person's voiding behavior. This methodology involves the consistent use of three caregiver behaviors: monitoring, prompting, and praising. The caregiver adheres to a schedule of regular monitoring, asking if the incontinent individual needs to use the toilet, and checking to see if he or she is dry or wet. Prompting involves reminding the person to use the toilet and wait until the caregiver returns to void. Praise is the positive response or feedback given by the caregiver for appropriate toileting or dryness. The best predictor of an individual's likelihood to benefit is her or his success during a therapeutic trial, usually lasting 3 days (Lyons & Specht, 1999; Ouslander et al., 1995). A PV trial involves assessing the patient's ability to recognize the need to void and to respond to the need appropriately, either by asking to toilet or by agreeing to toilet when the bladder is full. See **Table 15-6**, **Box 15-7**, and **Table 15-7** and for the steps of the PV technique and associated caregiver behaviors.

Bladder Training

Bladder training is an important component for continence and focuses on the ability to delay urination and suppress urgency. Bladder training is an educational program of scheduled voiding to provide patients with the skills to improve the ability to control urgency, decrease frequency of incontinent episodes, and prolong the interval between voiding (Dowling-Castronovo & Bradway, 2007; Wyman, 1994b)

The steps in a bladder-training program include setting a voiding schedule, teaching strategies for controlling urgency, monitoring voiding, and positive reinforcement. The initial voiding schedule is determined from baseline voiding data and

TABLE 15-6 Bran Mixture Recipe for Treating or Preventing Constipation
1 cup applesauce
1 cup unprocessed coarse wheat bran
1/2 cup unsweetened prune juice
Mix together. Give 2 tablespoons a day with a glass of water or juice. May increase to 3 tablespoons twice a day gradually (weekly) until good bowel function is achieved. May be given in hot cereal or added to mashed bananas. Refrigerate the recipe.

TABLE 15-7   Steps in the Prompted Voiding Protocol

1. Greet the patient by name. Remember to always knock for resident privacy. Close the door and/or privacy curtain.

2. Ask the patient if she or he is wet or dry. Ask a second time if the patient doesn't respond.

3. Check clothes, bedding, or body to determine if he or she is wet or dry. Tell the patient if he or she is correct.

4. If the patient asks for help in toileting:

   a. Praise the resident.

   b. Assist him or her to the toilet.

5. If the patient does not ask for help toileting, you ask the patient if he or she wants to toilet.

   a. Ask a second time if he or she doesn't say yes the first time.

   b. Ask a third time if his or her response is other than yes or no.

6. Assist to toilet only if he or she says yes to your offer.

   a. Praise for appropriate toileting.

   b. Record outcome.

7. Ask if he or she wants something to drink and provide appropriate liquids.

8. Tell the resident when he or she can expect you to be back.

Source: Schnelle, J. F. (1991). Managing Urinary Incontinence in the Elderly. New York: Springer.

prescribed according to the guidelines presented in **Table 15-8**. A 5- to 10-minute window on either side of the scheduled voiding time is allowed for flexibility. The training regimen is followed during waking hours, and the time between voiding is gradually increased by 15–30 minutes until the goal interval between voiding is reached (Dowling-Castronovo & Bradway, 2007). Although a 3–4 hour voiding interval is considered a maximal goal, most patients report they best tolerate an interval of 2–2.5 hours (Wyman & Fantl, 1991). Strategies to suppress urge include relaxation and distraction techniques such as slow deep breathing, concentrating on a task such as talking to someone, and pelvic muscle contractions.

Bladder training has been evaluated and implemented primarily with independent, community-dwelling elderly women. Persons with physical and cognitive impairment have been considered unlikely candidates for bladder training

TABLE 15-8 Steps in Bladder Training

1. Complete a 72-hour bladder diary.

2. Review the bladder diary. Calculate the number of voids and bladder accidents in a 24-hour period. Determine fluid intake.

3. Examine data for patterns. Does urinary incontinence occur only during certain times of day? Are accidents associated with certain events (activities, intake of specific type of fluids, medications)? What is the average time between voids and what is the longest interval? Are behaviors different for weekdays or weekends, or workdays vs. nonworkdays, or time when you are at home or out of the home?

4. Establish an initial voiding interval and consider the optimal interval to be achieved. The typical interval for adults is every 4 hours during the day; however, data suggest for older persons every 2 hours may be optimum (Wyman, Choi, Harkins, Wilson, & Fantl, 1988). The objective is to start the voiding routine at the interval that is comfortable to separate urgency from voiding; then, as you develop urge suppression skills, to increase the time between voiding until the goal is reached.

5. Urinate when you wake, after meals, before bedtime, and at the prescribed intervals.

6. If you get the urge to void and it is too soon to void, use the relaxation technique to make the urge go away. Remember, this involves taking very slow deep breaths until the urge goes away. Relax and concentrate when doing this. Contract the pelvic floor muscles quickly 3–5 times. Relax. Contract again.

7. Void at the prescribed time even if you don't feel the need.

8. If after a week it is very easy to wait the assigned time interval, lengthen the time by 15–30 minutes.

9. Begin by only practicing this technique at home, when you are relaxed and the bathroom is nearby.

10. Fluid intake should be kept at 6 8-ounce glasses per day. If you awaken frequently during the night to void, drink the majority of your 8 ounces before 6 P.M.

Hints to remember:
- Do not go to the bathroom before you have the urge to void.
- Never rush or run to the bathroom—walk slowly.
- Use the relaxation technique in situations that cause you to have the urge to void before the assigned time interval. For example, if you get the urge to void whenever you start to unlock your front door, stop, relax, and take three slow deep breaths to let the urge pass. Then unlock the door and walk slowly to the bathroom.
- When you walk slowly to the bathroom, do some pelvic muscle exercises to prevent an accident.

techniques. However, the potential benefit to voiding supports an effort to try this approach. An exercise program to improve walking in cognitively impaired nursing home residents reduced daytime incontinence (Jivorec, 1991). Providing patients the skills to delay voiding until mobility improves or until assistance for toileting can be obtained is a missing element that may decrease incontinence regardless of the level of recovery of mobility.

Pelvic Muscle Rehabilitation

Pelvic muscle rehabilitation involves the use of pelvic floor muscle exercise (see **Box 15-8**) to increase the strength, tone, and control of pelvic floor muscles to facilitate urine flow control to suppress urgency. The pelvic floor muscles support the

---

BOX 15-8 **The Easy Way to Teach Pelvic Floor Muscle Exercises**

Most insurance companies now require documentation in the patient's records that she has tried pelvic floor muscle exercises (PFME) for 4 weeks before granting authorization for biofeedback training for urinary incontinence. Teaching PFME is very simple to do using the following method from Barbara Woolner, RN, CCCN. Teach it using the following script, which can be done by phone, letter, or in person with potential patients, senior citizen or women's groups, family, and friends.

"The bladder wall contains a muscle called the detrusor, and you can make it relax using a spinal reflex, just like when the doctor taps your knee and your foot goes up. By making it relax you can double the size of your bladder, which gives you time to get it to a toilet without it leaking en route.

You have to do it very quickly, about as fast as you can tap your finger on the table (ask them to do that). Since the muscles down there go in circles like the ones around your eyes it is sort of like winking your eye. Now let me see you do that, first your right eye, now your left eye, now your anus." That catches them by surprise and they either look shocked or giggle, but they do it. Explain, "be careful not to use your abdominal muscles, just the ones which go from your pubic bone to your tail bone."

If you are a position to do so, continue to work with them, teaching them how to make sure they are not also using their abdominal muscles, which would put pressure on their bladder. They can either hold their hand over their lower abdomen to feel or hum—that tone should not waver if they are correctly doing it.

In addition to doing 5 "winks" whenever their bladder says "run or else," they need to do this 10 times during the day. After a week of practicing they can begin holding the squeeze for a full second then rest for 2, and double the time each week for a maximum of a 5-second squeeze for older persons, or 10 seconds for younger persons. With seniors on the verge of dementia, attempting this can serve as a distraction, which is another way of slowing down their race to the toilet, which can be a cause of hip fractures if they trip or slip in a puddle of urine.

Men often have a problem with bladder control after prostate surgery. But when working with them a biofeedback machine is not needed because they have one built in. Tell them that after they have finished urinating, while still standing in front of the toilet or urinal, make their penis flop up and down 5 times. Then explain the timing and frequency of a brief pause between each flop, and gradually extending the muscle contraction and rest periods.

pelvic organs. Pelvic muscle rehabilitation refers to an exercise regimen to improve the integrity and function of the pelvic floor. The proposed mechanism of action for pelvic muscle training is that strong and fast pelvic muscle contractions close the urethra and increase urethral pressure to prevent leakage. Pelvic muscle contractions may inhibit bladder contractions, helping to suppress urgency (Dowling-Castronovo & Bradway, 2007).

To teach the individual to identify and isolate the correct muscles, instruct him or her to "draw in" and "lift up" the rectal/anal sphincter muscles. Instruct patients to lift up the perivaginal muscles and avoid contracting the abdominal, gluteal, and thigh muscles. To help the patient avoid a bearing down motion, have him or her practice pushing down to feel what not to do. Start with contracting for 2 seconds, and then gradually increase the length of the contraction to a maximum 10-second hold. A repetition includes relaxing or resting the pelvic floor muscles between contractions for the same amount of time the muscle is contracted. A typical training regimen involves 10 repetitions 2 to 3 times a day.

Once the patient learns the correct technique, instruct them to use pelvic muscle contraction to prevent urine flow. If leakage occurs with activities that increase intra-abdominal pressure, then a muscle contraction should precede the activity. If urgency is the primary problem, the pelvic floor muscles can be used to suppress the urge.

Biofeedback

Biofeedback is an adjunct to pelvic muscle rehabilitation and bladder contraction inhibition that has strong scientific support for effectiveness with stress and urge urinary incontinence (Abrams et al., 1999; Fantl et al., 1996; Hay-Smith, Herbison, & Morkved, 2002). The use of biofeedback-assisted bladder training for urge and stress incontinence has particular advantages since it is very low risk and has no documented side effects; however, because it relies on learning new behaviors, it may have limited application for cognitively impaired patients (Burgio et al., 1998).

Biofeedback, through either surface electrodes or vaginal or rectal probes, provides visual and/or auditory cues to facilitate incontinent patients' ability to isolate and identify pelvic floor muscles. It also helps decrease patients' tendency to use abdominal or gluteal muscles. In the absence of biofeedback equipment, digital checks can be used to teach and monitor ongoing performance.

The Health Care Financing Administration (HCFA) analyzed scientific data related to the use of biofeedback for treatment of stress, urge, and post-prostatectomy incontinence in a review of the Medicare coverage policy. A decision memorandum summarizing its findings and the recommendations of numerous professional organizations amended HCFA's policy to allow coverage for biofeedback with patients who had failed documented trials of PFME or who are unable to perform PFME (Tunis, Norris, & Simon, 2000). A failed trial is defined as no significant

BOX 15-9   Biofeedback in the Clinical Setting

Cochran stated she has encountered several patients who had been treated with Pelvic Floor Electrical Stimulation (PFES), but still were unable to initiate a pelvic floor muscle contraction on their own, when observed while using a standard biofeedback machine. Nor is biofeedback sufficient by itself to restore bladder and/or bowel control. One patient in her early seventies required 2 hours to identify contributing factors to her incontinence, including congenital scoliosis involving the lower spine through which the nerves to the bladder exit the spinal cord; a body mass index of 33, which put extra weight on the pelvic floor; insufficient fluid intake, allowing concentrated urine to irritate her bladder lining; and diabetes, which in theory can impair the nerves controlling the bladder but which Cochran has not encountered in 17 years of working with

patients using biofeedback. When the patient walked into the training room she asked, "May I use the bathroom first?" and Cochran said no. After the training session the patient commented (as many others have done), "You know, I don't need to go to the bathroom!"

A number of years ago Cochran had a patient who successfully was reeducated in the use of her pelvic floor muscles, but several years later returned to the program after an auto accident injured her lower back and left her with a worse case of incontinence than when originally seen. After one evaluation session Cochran referred her to a physical therapist to alleviate her back injury, then Cochran gave her several biofeedback training sessions to reeducate the injured neuromuscular connections.

improvement after completing a 4-week period of structured, ordered PFME to increase pelvic floor strength (Norris, 2001).

Pelvic Floor Electrical Stimulus

Pelvic floor electrical stimulation (PFES) is another adjunct to PFME (see **Box 15-9**). Pelvic floor electrical stimulation refers to the application of electric current to sacral and pudendal afferent fibers via a non-implantable vaginal or anal probe (Fantl et al., 1996). Variable rates of current are used to improve urethral closure by activating pelvic floor muscles, thus exercising and strengthening the pelvic floor (Tunis, Whyte, & Bridger, 2000). Pelvic floor electrical stimulation also can facilitate an individual's ability to identify and isolate pelvic floor musculature. The HCFA review panel concluded that PFES is effective for patients with stress and/or urge incontinence, and considers its use as necessary and reasonable if PFMEs have been unsuccessful (Tunis, Whyte, & Bridger, 2000). In addition, the ability of PFES to passively exercise the pelvic floor is a potentially valuable treatment for individuals unable to perform the exercises.

Pharmacological Management

Medications are available to help treat stress and urge incontinence. Because many older persons have multiple chronic health problems, medications to treat incontinence should primarily serve as an adjunct to behavioral interventions

BOX 15-10   Better Than "Power Pudding"

In the more than 17 years Audrey Cochran has been using biofeedback and counseling in activities of daily living as manager of a continence rehabilitation program for an OB/GYN office, she has noticed a trend of women getting heavier and their bladder control problems greater with all that weight pressing down on their pelvic floor. And they are constipated! (In contrast, her elderly patients in their eighties or early nineties tend to be thinner, and some only need three sessions before they are back in control.)

On the first visit she shows patients the Bristol Stool Form Scale (which can be found on Internet) and asks them to point to what they see when they look in the toilet, which most have never done. If they point to anything other than the smooth banana shape, she urges them to take one 250 mg magnesium tablet (not milk of magnesia)

with their evening meal. The only contraindication to magnesium would be the presence of kidney failure. The benefits of magnesium include help with sleep and relaxation of smooth muscles, which enables them to contract more forcefully. After doing that for a week, if they are still constipated they take two tablets. If necessary they can add one at breakfast, and finally two at breakfast.

Cochran only had one patient who needed that much. She was a retired nurse who had injured her back while lifting a patient, and was in so much pain that in addition to narcotics several times a day, she was getting epidural injections every few weeks. She ended up taking four magnesium tablets daily and was having daily bowel movements. This is all the more amazing because since the age of 10, she only had one bowel movement a week!

(see **Box 15-10**). Pharmacological management of urge UI added to the effectiveness of behavioral strategies in frail older persons (Benvenuti et al., 2002). However, consideration of the potential for adverse drug reactions and added cost must be discussed with the patient when a pharmacological intervention is considered. Medications prescribed for stress UI target the internal urinary sphincter or the urethral/vaginal tissues. The alpha agonist pseudoephedrine acts at the bladder neck, increasing urethral tone, which may decrease leakage and is often prescribed for mild cases of stress UI. However, pseudoephedrine potential side effects include insomnia, restlessness, nervousness, headache, and increased blood pressure and heart rate, which limit its usefulness in the older population. Duloxetine, a serotonin and norepinephrine reuptake inhibitor, increases external urethral sphincter tone and is used to treat stress UI. Estrogen is prescribed to treat urogenital atrophy, which increases stimulation of urogenital estrogen receptors and may increase urethral resistance. Evidence of its usefulness in stress UI is inconclusive (Fantl et al., 1996); however, estrogen's effectiveness in treating atrophic tissues can help alleviate irritative symptoms of urgency, which may decrease urge UI. The primary agents for uninhibited bladder contractions are anticholinergics or antispasmodics that decrease contraction of the detrusor muscle. **Table 15-9** presents an overview of the medications used for treatment of UI.

TABLE 15-9   Medications Commonly Used to Treat Urinary Incontinence

Medication	Dosage	Comments
Hyoscamine	0.375 mg twice daily orally	Has prominent anticholinergic side effects; available in alternate forms
Oxybutynin	2.5–5.0 mg three times daily orally (short-acting) 5–30 mg daily orally (long-acting) 3.9 mg over a 96-hr period (transdermal)	Long-acting and transdermal preparations have fewer side effects than short-acting preparations. Transdermal patch can cause local skin irritation in some patients
Propantheline	15–30 mg 4 times daily orally	Noted anticholinergic side effects
Tolterodine	1–2 mg twice daily orally (short-acting) 4 mg daily orally (long-acting)	Similar efficacy with long-acting and short-acting preparations.
Estrogen (for women)		
Vaginal estrogen preparations	Approximately 0.5 g cream applied topically nightly for 2 wk, then twice per week Estradiol ring, replaced every 90 days Estradiol, 1 tablet daily for 2 wk, then 1 tablet twice a week	Local vaginal preparations are probably more effective than oral estrogen; definitive data on effectiveness lacking
Alpha-Adrenergic Antagonists (for men)		
Alfuzosin	2.5 mg thrice daily orally	Useful in men with benign prostatic enlargement
Doxazosin	1–16 mg daily orally	Postural hypotension can be a serious side-effect
Prazosin	1–10 mg twice daily orally	Check blood pressure regularly
Tamsulosin	0.4–0.8 mg daily orally	Take 30 minutes after the same meal each day
Terazosin	1–10 mg orally each day at bedtime	Doses must be increased gradually to facilitate tolerance
Other medications		
Imipramine	10–25 mg thrice daily orally	May be useful for mixed urge-stress incontinence; can cause postural hypotension and bundle-branch block
Desmopressin	20–40 pg of intranasal spray daily at bedtime 0.1–0.4 mg orally 2 hr before bedtime	Intranasal spray used for primary nocturnal enuresis in children; hyponatremia occurs commonly in older adults; monitor serum sodium levels closely

Source: Adapted from Ouslander, J. G. (2004). Management of the overactive bladder. NEJM, 350, 786–799. Copyright (2004) Massachusetts Medical Society. All rights reserved.

Overflow incontinence in men that is the result of bladder neck obstruction from benign prostatic hypertrophy (BPH) may resolve with treatment of the prostate. Alpha antagonists (doxazosin, tamsulosin, and terazosin) relax the urinary sphincters, improving urine flow and decreasing urine retention and overflow incontinence. However, dizziness and orthostatic hypotension are potential side effects that must be addressed. Other options for BPH treatment are the 5-a reductase inhibitors finesteride and dutasteride. This class of medications blocks the conversion of testosterone to dihydrotestosterone, the form needed for prostate growth. The 5-a reductase inhibitors take about 3 to 6 months to take effect. An important consideration in the prescription and administration of these drugs is their tetraogenic effects.

It is important to review the patient's entire medication list to determine if any of their medications are actually contributing to the problem of UI. Such medications may include hypnotics, anti-anxiety drugs, and anticholinergics (including antimuscarinics and antinicotinics) (Godfrey, 2008).

Devices and Products

One of the first decisions made in the management of UI is the choice of protective undergarments. A variety of absorbent products is now available to contain urine. It is important that patients use products designed for urine; menstrual pads are a popular choice, but are not specifically designed to absorb and contain urine. The absorbent inner core of continence garments wicks the urine away from the skin and spreads it throughout the pad, increasing the volume of urine absorbed (Newman, 2002). The volume of urine that needs to be contained and the need for help toileting are important considerations in product selection. The use of briefs developed specifically for men and for women have several advantages to the traditional adult diaper. These garments are easier to manipulate to prepare for toileting and for repositioning clothing afterward. They also are more like usual underclothes, facilitating the expectation of a return to continence and promoting comfort. The introduction of products to accommodate moderate to heavy levels of incontinence has broadened the possibilities for successful containment. Many patients and family have been relieved (especially from an economic perspective) to learn of the availability of nondisposable garments that can be washed and reused.

Toileting equipment and collection devices are available for men and women to promote self-toileting, including female urinals, wheelchair urinals, and male reusable urinal/pant garments (Mueller, 2004). The National Association for Continence (2004) *Resource Guide* is an excellent resource for UI products and their manufacturers. This information can be accessed at http://www.nafc.org/.

Skin Care

Meticulous skin care is essential in the care of persons with incontinence. Moisture barriers and no-rinse incontinence cleansers are recommended over soap and water alone in preventing skin breakdown (Byers, Ryan, Regan, Shields, & Carta, 1995;

Dowling-Castronovo & Bradway, 2007). It is important to gently dry the skin after cleaning and to apply moisturizers. Petroleum-based products may be incompatible with some adult briefs, causing skin irritation (Newman, 2002).

Incontinence-associated dermatitis (IAD) describes skin irritation and impairment from exposure to urine and feces (Doughty et al., 2012). This condition is unique from pressure ulcer formation since it is caused by exposure to moisture and is not ischemic in nature. However, the presence of IAD increases the risk of pressure ulcer development (Doughty et al., 2012). Additional research is needed to better differentiate between types and grades of skin lesions (Doughty et al., 2012).

Environmental Intervention

Occupational therapy evaluations of the home may be helpful in modifying the environment to facilitate rapid access to the toilet. Although this may be only one component of UI treatment, it may facilitate urination, thus decreasing UI.

Indwelling Urinary Catheters

Indwelling urinary catheters, once the primary means for managing UI, are no longer accepted as the first step in an incontinence treatment regimen. However, there are situations that may require catheter use. The Centers for Medicare and Medicaid Services (CMS), an agency under the U.S. Department of Health and Human Services, developed regulations for guidance of long-term indwelling catheter use (see **Table 15-10**). With long-term use, care must be taken to monitor for common complications of polymicrobial bacteruria (universal by 30 days), fever (1 event per 100 patient days), nephrolithiasis, bladder stones, epididymitis, and chronic renal inflammation and pyelonephritis (Benvenuti et al., 2002). Maintaining hydration, urine flow, and cleanliness of the system are important components of care. Minimizing urethral trauma by using small-caliber catheters, a 5-cc retention balloon, and securing the catheter with a thigh strap will promote comfort and may help decrease complications. Emptying the catheter every 4–6 hours to avoid migration of bacteria up the lumen, cleaning the insertion site gently with soap and water daily, and avoiding irrigations may help decrease symptomatic UTI. Whenever the patient's status changes, such as healing of pressure ulcers or caregiver availability, then a trial without the indwelling catheter should be attempted.

Intermittent urinary catheterization is another supportive measure to manage urinary retention (Fantl et al., 1996). In and out catheterization allows regular bladder emptying, which reduces pressure within the bladder and improves circulation to the bladder wall, making the mucosa more resistant to infection (Newman, 2002). Sterile technique (ISC) is used in institutions, and clean technique (ICC) is used for catheterizations at home. No studies have been conducted comparing the use of intermittent urinary catheterization and long-term indwelling urinary catheterization in the frail elderly (Benvenuti et al., 2002). Dexterity and mobility

TABLE 15-10   Centers for Medicare and Medicaid Services Rules for Guidance of Indwelling Catheter Utilization
Urinary retention that cannot be treated or corrected medically or surgically, for which alternative therapy is not feasible, and which is characterized by:
•   Documented post void residual (PVR) volumes in a range over 200 milliliters (ml);
•   Inability to manage the retention/incontinence with intermittent catheterization;
•   Persistent overflow incontinence, symptomatic infections, and/or renal dysfunction.
•   Contamination of Stage III or IV pressure ulcers with urine, which has impeded healing, despite appropriate personal care for the incontinence; and
•   Terminal illness or severe impairment, which makes positioning or clothing changes uncomfortable, or which is associated with intractable pain.

Source: CMS Manual System, Publication 100-07, June 28, 2005, page 17, http://www.cms.gov/Regulations-and-Guidance/Guidance/Transmittals/downloads//r8som.pdf

problems may interfere with self-catheterizations. Comfort with intermittent catheterizations is a factor in ISC and ICC performed by caregivers.

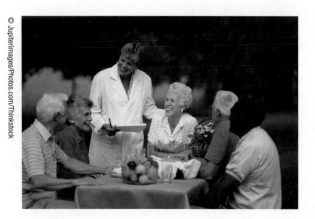

© Jupiterimages/Photos.com/Thinkstock

Figure 15-4 Nurses are in an ideal position to help educate older adults about current treatment for UI.

Summary

Urinary incontinence is a serious, potentially disabling condition with negative social, physical, psychological, and economic impacts. Incontinence is a common condition in the older population, but is not a part of the normal aging process. The majority of older adults who have UI can be successfully treated and experience improved health-related quality of life. The introduction of early, targeted behavioral interventions should improve urological functioning and limit the impact of uncontrolled incontinence. Therefore, older adults and their caregivers need education about evidence-based interventions to combat this all too prevalent health problem. Nurses are in a key position to assess, plan, intervene and evaluate to assure older adult patients prevent UI and maintain optimal urinary function (see **Figure 15-4**).

Critical Thinking Exercises

1. Mrs. O'Dell is having a problem with constipation since turning 70 years of age. She asks for advice about this. What would you suggest? What needs to be assessed before providing advice about this?

2. Choose one of the clinical practice guidelines provided in this chapter and review it. What can you take away from that guideline and apply to your clinical practice?

3. If you had to give a talk on urinary incontinence to a ladies' group from a church, what would you cover as the most important points on this topic? How could you make it interesting and engaging for the audience?

Personal Reflections

1. Have you ever cared for a person with urinary incontinence? If so, what was the setting and how did you feel about providing this care? What from this chapter might make you look at that situation differently?

2. Imagine that you have become an older adult and are beginning to experience problems with UI. What is the first action you would take after an incontinent episode? What, if anything, could you do earlier in your adult life to prevent UI?

3. Urinary incontinence is often thought of as more of a woman's problem than a man's. What would you recommend to a male who is experiencing UI as a result of spinal injury? Prostate problems? Dementia?

References

AHCPR Urinary Incontinence in Adults Guideline Update Panel. (1996). Managing acute and chronic urinary incontinence. *American Family Physician, 54*, 1661–72.

Abrams, P., Khoury, S., & Wein, A. (Eds). (1999). *Incontinence*. Plymouth, UK: Health Publication.

Armstrong, L. E. (2000). *Performing in extreme environments*. Champaign, IL: Human Kinetics.

Arya, L. A., Myers, D. L., & Jackson, N. D. (2000). Dietary caffeine intake and the risk of detrusor instability: A case-control study. *Obstetrics and Gynecology, 96*(1), 85–89.

Benvenuti, F., Cottenden, A., DuBeau, C., Kirshner-Hermanns, R., Miller, K., Palmer, M., & Resnick, N. (2002). Urinary incontinence and bladder dysfunction in older persons. In P. Abrams, L. Cardozo, S. Khoury, & A. Wein (Eds.), *Incontinence* (pp. 627–695). Plymouth, UK: Health Publication.

Borrie, M. J., Campbell, K., Arcese, Z. A., Bray, J., Labate, T., & Hesch, P. (2001). Urinary retention in patients in a geriatric rehabilitation unit: prevalence, risk factors, and validity of bladder scan evaluation. *Rehabilitation Nursing, 26*(5), 187–191.

Borson, S., Scanlan, J., Brush, M., Vitallano, P., & Dokmak, A. (2000). The Mini-Cog: A cognitive "vital signs" measure for dementia screening in multi-lingual elderly. *International Journal of Geriatric Psychiatry, 15*(11), 1021–1027.

Brown, J. S., Vittinghoff, E., Wyman, J. F., Stone, K. L., Nevitt, M. C., Ensrud, K. E., & Grady, D. (2000). Urinary incontinence: Does it increase risk for falls and fractures? *Journal of the American Geriatrics Society, 48*, 721–725.

Burgio, K. L., & Burgio, L. D. (1986). Behavioral therapies for urinary incontinence in the elderly. *Clinics in Geriatric Medicine, 2*(4), 809–827.

Burgio, J. L., Locher, J. L., Goode, P. S., Hardin, J. M., McDowell, B. J., Dombrowski, J. M., et al. (1998). Behavioral vs drug treatment for urge urinary incontinence in older women: A randomized controlled trial. *Journal of the American Medical Association,* 280, 1995–2000.

Byers, P. H., Ryan, P. A., Regan, M. D., Shields, A., & Carta, S. G. (1995). Effects of skin care cleansing regimens on skin integrity. *Journal of Wound, Ostomy, and Continence Nursing, 22*(4), 187–192.

Centers for Medicare and Medicaid Services. (2006, December 15). *CMS Manual System - Pub. 100-07 State Operations Provider Certification.* Retrieved from http://www.cms.gov/Regulations-and-Guidance/Guidance/Transmittals/downloads//r8som.pdf

Colling, J. C., Ouslander, J. G., Hadley, B. J., Eisch, T., & Campbell, E. (1992). The effects of patterned urge-response toileting on urinary incontinence among nursing home residents. *Journal of the American Gerontological Society, 40,* 135–141.

Coudret, N., Ehlman, K., Dugger, R., Eggleston, B., Wilson, A., Harrison, E. & Mathis, S. (2009). *Assessing the benefits of bladder ultrasound scanners in nursing homes: Project funded by the Indiana State Department of Health - Final Report.* Unpublished manuscript, College of Nursing and Health Professions, University of Southern Indiana, Evansville, IN.

Donahue, J. L., & Lowenthal, D. T. (1997). Nocturnal polyuria in the elderly person. *The American Journal of Medical Sciences, 314,* 232–237.

Doughty, D. (2000). *Urinary and fecal incontinence: Nursing management.* St. Louis, MO: Mosby.

Doughty, D., Junkin, J., Kurz, P., Selekof, J, Gray, M., Fader, M.,…Logan, S. (2012). Incontinence-associated dermatitis: Consensus statements, evidence-based guidelines for prevention and treatment, and current challenges. *Journal of Wound, Ostomy, Continence Nursing, 39*(3), 303–315.

Dowling-Castronova, A., & Bradway, C. (2003). Urinary incontinence. In M. Mezey, I. Abraham, D.A. Zwicker, (Eds.), *Geriatric nursing protocols for best practice* (2nd ed., pp. 83–98). New York, NY: Springer.

Dowling-Castronova, A., & Bradway, C. (2007). *Assessment and management of older adults with urinary incontinence.* [white paper] Presented at The National Gerontological Nursing Association and American Association of Colleges of Nursing Conference in St. Louis, MO in October 2008.

Dowling-Castronovo, A., & Bradway, C. (2008). Urinary incontinence in older adults admitted to acute care. In Capezuti, E., Zwicker, D., Mezey, M. & Fulmer, T. (eds.). *Evidence-based geriatric nursing protocols for best practice* (3rd ed., pp. 309–336). New York, NY: Springer.

Dowling-Castronovo, A., & Bradway, C. (2012). Urinary incontinence in older adults admitted to acute care. In Bolz, M., Capezuti, E., Fulmer, T, & Zwicker. (Eds.). *Evidence-based geriatric nursing protocols for best practice* (4th ed., pp. 363–387). New York, NY: Springer.

DuBeau, C. E. (2005). Improving urinary incontinence in nursing home residents: Are we FIT to be tied? *Journal of the American Geriatrics Society, 53*(7), 1254–1256.

DuBeau, C. E., Simon, S. E. & Morris, J. N. (2006). The effect of urinary incontinence on quality of life in older nursing home residents. *Journal of the American Geriatrics Society, 54*(9), 1325–1333.

Dugan, E., Cohen, S. J., Bland, S. R., Priesser, J. S., Davis, C. C., Suggs, P. K., McGann, P. (2000). The association of depressive symptoms and urinary incontinence among older adults. *Journal of the American Geriatrics Association, 48*(4), 413–416.

Fantl, J. A., Newman, D. K., Colling, J., DeLancey, J. O., Keeys, C., Loughery, R… Whitmore, K. (1996). *Urinary incontinence in adults: Acute and chronic management. Clinical practice guideline. No. 2.* AHCPR Pub No. 96-0682, Rockville, MD: U.S. Department of Health Care Policy and Research.

Folstein, M. F., Folstein, S. E., & McHugh, P. R. (1975). "Mini-mental state." A practical method for grading the cognitive state of patients for the clinician. *Journal of Psychiatric Research, 12,* 189–198.

Frenchman, I. B. (2001). Cost of urinary incontinence in two skilled nursing facilities: A prospective study. *Clinical Geriatrics, 9*(1), 49–52.

Godfrey, H. (2008). Older people, continence, and catheters: Dilemmas and resolutions. *British Journal of Nursing, 1*(3), S4–S11.

Godfrey, H. & Hogg, A. (2007). Links between social isolation and incontinence. *British Journal of Nursing, 1*(3), S1–S8.

Goldstein, M., Hawthorne, M. E., Engeberg, S., McDowell, B. J., & Burgio, K. (1992). Urinary incontinence—Why people do not seek help. *Journal of Gerontological Nursing, 18*(4), 15–20.

Hajjar, P. R. (2004). Psychosocial impact of urinary incontinence in the elderly population. *Clinical Geriatric Medicine, 20*(3), 55–564.

Hay-Smith, J., Herbison, P., & Morkved, S. (2002). Physical therapies for prevention of urinary and faecal incontinence in adults (review). *The Cochrane Database of Systematic Reviews.* Issue 2. Art. No.: CD003191. doi: 10.1002/14651858.CD003191

Heavner, K. (1998). Urinary incontinence in extended care facilities: A literature review and proposal for continuous quality improvement. *Ostomy/Wound Management, 44*(12), 46–53.

Heidrich, S., & Wells, T. J. (2004). Effects of urinary incontinence: Psychosocial well being and distress in older community dwelling women. *Journal of Gerontological Nursing 39*(5), 47–54.

Hu, T.W., Wagner, T.H., Bentkover, J.D., Leblanc, K., Zhou, S.Z., & Hunt, T. (2004). Costs of urinary incontinence and overactive bladder in the United States: A comparative study. Urology, 63(3), 461–465.

Hunskaar, S., Burgio, K., Diokno, A. C., Herzog, A. R., Hjalmas, K., & Lapitan, M. C. (2002). Epidemiology and natural history of urinary incontinence (UI). In P. Abrams, L. Cardozo, S. Khoury, & A. Wein (Eds.), *Incontinence* (pp. 167–201). Plymouth, UK: Health Publication.

Inouye, S.K., van Dyck, C.H., Alessi, C.A., Balkin, S., Siegal, A.P. & Horwitz, R.I. (1990). Clarifying confusion: the confusion assessment method. A new method for detection of delirium. *Annals of Internal Medicine.* 113(12), 941–948.

Jeter, K. F., & Wagner, B. A. (1990). Incontinence in the American home. *Journal of the American Geriatrics Society, 38*, 379–383.

Jirovec, M. M., Wyman, J. F., & Wells, T. I. (1998). Addressing urinary incontinence with educational continence care competencies. *Image: Journal of Nursing Scholarship, 30*(4), 375–378.

Jirovec, M. M. (1991). The impact of daily exercise on the mobility, balance, and urine control of cognitively impaired nursing home residents. *International Journal of Nursing Studies,* 28(2), 145–151.

Ko, Y., Lin, S., Salmon, J. W. & Bron, M. (2005). The impact of urinary incontinence on quality of life of the elderly. *The American Journal of Mananged Care, 11*(4), S103–S111.

Landefeld, C. S., Bowers, B. J., Feld, A. D., Hartmann, K. E., Hoffman, E., Ingber, M. U.,…Trock, B. J. (2008). National Institutes of Health state-of-the-science conference statement: Prevention of fecal and urinary incontinence in adults. *Annals of Internal Medicine, 148*(6), 449–458.

Lekan-Rutledge, D. (2004). Urinary incontinence strategies for frail elderly women. *Urologic Nursing, 24*(4), 281–301.

Lewis, N. (1995). Implementing a bladder ultrasound program. *Rehabilitation Nursing, 20*(4), 215–217.

Lincoln, R., & Roberts, R. (1989). Continence issues in acute care. Nursing *Clinics of North America, 24*(3), 741–754.

Lyons, S. S., & Specht, J. K. P. (1999). *Prompted voiding for persons with urinary incontinence.* Iowa City: University of Iowa, Gerontological Nursing Intervention Research Center.

Macauly, A. J., Stern, R. S., Holmes, D. M., & Stanton, S. L. (1987). Micturition and the mind: Psychological factors in the treatment of urinary symptoms. *British Medical Journal, 294*, 540–543.

MayoClinic.com. (2008). *Kegel exercises: A how-to guide for women.* Retrieved from http://www.mayoclinic.com/health/kegel-exercises/WO00119

McCliment, J. (2002). Non-invasive method overcomes incontinence. *Contemporary Long Term Care, 25*, Supplement.

McCormick, K. A., Cella, M., Scheve, A., & Engel, B. T. (1990). Cost effectiveness of treating incontinence in severely mobility-impaired long-term care residents. *Quality Review Bulletin, 16*, 439–443.

Mentes, J. C., & The Iowa Veterans Affairs Nursing Research Consortium. (1998). *Hydration management.* Iowa City: University of Iowa, Gerontological Nursing Intervention Research Center.

Mentes, J. C., & The Iowa Veterans Affairs Nursing Research Consortium. (2000). Hydration management protocol. *Journal of Gerontological Nursing, 26*(10), 6–15.

Mentes, J. C., & The Iowa Veterans Affairs Nursing Research Consortium. (2004). *Evidence-based practice guideline: Hydration management.* Iowa City: The University of Iowa Gerontological Nursing Interventions Research Center Research Translation and Dissemination Core.

Mueller, N. (2004). What the future holds for incontinence care. *Urologic Nurse, 24*(3), 181–186.

National Association for Continence. (2004). NAFC. Retrieved from http://www.nafc.org/library/search-our-articles/view-article/&id/695/

Newman, D. K. (2002). *Managing and treating urinary incontinence.* Baltimore, MD: Health Professions Press.

Newman, D., Gaines, T., & Snare, E. (2005). Innovation in bladder assessment: Use of technology in extended care. *Journal of Gerontological Nursing, 51*(12), 33–41.

Norris, A. (2001). HCFA correspondence, January 1, 2001.

Ouslander, J. G., Schnelle, J. F., Uman, G., Fingold, S., Nigam, J. G., Tuico, E., Jensen, B. B. (1995). Does oxybutynin add to the effectiveness of prompted voiding for urinary incontinence among nursing home residents? *Journal of the American Geriatrics Society, 43*(6), 610–617.

Palmer, M. H. (2008). Urinary incontinence quality improvement in nursing homes: Where have we been? Where are we going? *Urologic Nursing, 28*(6), 439–444.

Pressman, M. R., Figueroa, W. G., Kendrick-Mohamed, J., Greenspan, L. W., & Peterson, D. D. (1996). Nocturia: A seldom recognized symptom of sleep apnea and other occult sleep disorders. *Archives of Internal Medicine, 156,* 545–555.

Rich, S. A., & Panill, F. C. (1999). Urinary incontinence. In E. R. Black, D. R. Bordley, T. G. Tape, & R. J. Panzer (Eds.), *Diagnostic strategies for common medical problems* (2nd ed., pp. 527–539). Philadelphia, PA: American College of Physicians.

Robinson, J. P., & Shea, J. A. (2002). Development and testing of a measure of health-related quality of life for men with urinary incontinence. *Journal of the American Geriatrics Society, 50*(5), 935–945.

Royal College of Physicians. (1995). *Incontinence: Causes, management and provision of services.* London, UK: Author.

Sale, P. G., & Wyman, J. (1994). Achievement of goals associated with bladder training by older incontinent women. *Applied Nursing Research, 7*(2), 93–96.

Schnelle, J. F. (1990). Treatment of urinary incontinence in nursing home patients by prompted voiding. *Journal of the American Geriatrics Society, 38,* 356–360.

Shull, B. L., Halaska, M., Hurst, G., Laycock, J., Palmtag, H., Reilly, N., et al. (1999). Physical examination. In P. Abrams, S. Khoury, & A. Wein (Eds.), *Incontinence.* Plymouth, UK: Health Publication.

Smith, D., & Newman, D. (1989). Beating the cycle of constipation, laxative abuse, and fecal incontinence. *Today's Nursing Home,* 12–13.

Sparks, A., Boyer, D., Gambrel, A., & Lovett, M. (2004). The clinical benefits of the bladder scanner: A research synthesis. *Journal of Nursing Care Quality, 19*(3), 188–192.

Teunissen, D., Bosch, W., Weel, C., & Lagro-Janssen, T. (2006). "It can always happen": The impact of urinary incontinence on elderly men and women. *Scandinavian Journal of Primary Health Care, 24,* 166–173.

Thom, D. H., Haan, M. N, & Van Den Eeden, S. K. (1997). Medically recognized urinary incontinence and the risks of hospitalization, nursing home admission and mortality. *Age and Ageing, 26,* 367–374.

Tunis, S. R., Norris, A., & Simon, K. (2000). *Medicare coverage policy decisions. Biofeedback for treatment of urinary incontinence. (#CAG - 00020).* Washington, DC: Health Care Financing Administration.

Tunis, S. R., Whyte, J. J., & Bridger, P. (2000). *Medicare coverage policy decisions. Pelvic floor electrical stimulation for treatment of urinary incontinence. (#CAG-00021).* Washington, DC: Health Care Financing Administration.

Uebersax, J. S., Wyman, J. F., Schumaker, S. A., Fantl, J. A., & Continence Program for Woman Research Group. (1995). Short forms to assess life quality and symptom distress for urinary incontinence in women: The incontinence impact questionnaire and the urogenital distress inventory. *Neurourology and Urodynamics, 14,* 131, 139.

Umlauf, M. G., Burgio, K. L., Shetter, S., & Pillion, D. (1997). Nocturia and nocturnal urine production in obstructive sleep apnea. *Applied Nursing Research, 10*(4), 198–201.

Umlauf, M., & Chasens, E. (2003). Sleep disordered breathing and nocturnal polyuria: Nocturia and enuresis. *Sleep, 7*(5), 373–376.

Urinary Continence Guideline Panel. (1992). *Urinary incontinence in adults.* (AHCPR Pub. No. 92-0038). Rockville, MD: U.S. Department of Health and Human Services.

Wells, T. (1984). Social and psychological implications of incontinence. In J. C. Brocklehurst (Ed.), *Urology in the elderly* (pp. 107–126). New York, NY: Churchill Livingston.

Wilson, L., Brown, J. S., Shin, G. P., Luc, K., & Subak, L. L. (2001). Annual direct cost of incontinence. *Obstetrics & Gynecology, 98*, 398–406.

Wooldridge, L. (2000, June). Ultrasound technology and bladder dysfunction. *American Journal of Nursing*, 3–14.

Wyman, J. F. & Fantl, J. A. (1991). Bladder training in ambulatory care management of urinary incontinence. Urologic nursing : official journal of the American Urological Association Allied, 11(3), 11–17.

Wyman, J. F. (1994a). Level 3: Comprehensive assessment and management of urinary incontinence by continence nurse specialists. *Nurse Practitioner Forum, 5*(3), 177–185.

Wyman, J. F. (1994b). The psychiatric and emotional impact of female pelvic floor dysfunction. *Current Opinion in Obstetrics and Gynecology, 6*, 336–339.

Wyman, J. F., Choi, S. C., Harkins, S. W., Wilson, M. S., & Fantl, J. A. (1988). The urinary diary in evaluation of incontinent women: A test-retest analysis. *Obstetrics and Gynecology, 71*(6), 812–817.

Wyman, J., Harkins, S. W., Choi, S. C., Taylor, J. R., & Fantl, A. (1987). Psychosocial impact of urinary incontinence in women. *Obstetrics and Gynecology, 70*(1), 378–381.

Yu, L. C. (1987). Incontinence stress index: Measuring psychological impact. *Journal of Gerontological Nursing, 13*(7), 18–25.

Yu, L., Kaltreider, D., Hu, T. I., & Craighead, W. (1989). The ISQ-P tool: Measuring stress associated with incontinence. *Journal of Gerontological Nursing, 15*(2), 9–15.

For a full suite of assignments and additional learning activities, see the access code at the front of your book.

LEARNING OBJECTIVES

At the end of this chapter, the reader will be able to:

> Discuss the importance of sleep to successful aging.
> Describe the potential impact of sleep disturbance on quality of life in older adults.
> Explain common theories of sleep regulation.
> Identify the general effects of neurotransmitters associated with sleep and wakefulness.
> Describe basic sleep architecture, including stages of sleep.
> Discuss changes in sleep associated with the normal aging process.
> Obtain a basic sleep history, including identification of risk factors for sleep disturbance.
> Use basic and selected specific sleep screening instruments to assess sleep in older adults.
> Describe selected diagnostic tests used by sleep professionals to diagnose sleep disorders.
> Discuss common sleep disorders in older adults, including those associated with geropsychiatric disorders.
> Identify geriatric implications of pharmacologic interventions for sleep disorders.
> Discuss nonpharmacological interventions used in the management of sleep disorders in older adults, including cognitive, behavioral, and complementary alternative therapies.

KEY TERMS

Apnea

Actigraphy (ACTG)

Circadian rhythm

Circadian rhythm disorders

Cognitive behavioral therapy (CBT)

Complementary alternative therapy

Daytime sleepiness

Homeostatic sleep drive

Hypersomnias

Hypopnea

Insomnia

Neurotransmitters

Non-rapid eye movement (NREM) sleep

Obstructive sleep apnea (OSA)

Parasomnias

Periodic limb movements (PLMs)

Polysomnography (PSG)

Rapid eye movement (REM) sleep

REM sleep behavior disorder (RSBD)

Restless legs syndrome (RLS)

Sleep architecture

Sleep cycle

Sleep efficiency

Sleep fragmentation

Sleep quality

Sleep-related breathing disorders

Supraciasmatic nucleus

Total sleep time

Chapter 16

Sleep Disorders

Carol Enderlin
Melodee Harris
Karen M. Rose
Lisa Hutchison

Introduction

Healthy sleep plays an important role in successful aging. Decreased morbidity (Foley, Ancoli-Israel, Britz, & Walsh, 2004) and mortality (Dew et al., 2003) are associated with adequate sleep. In a cross-sectional study of nearly 2,800 people 100 years of age, 65% reported good or very good sleep quality and had a weighted average of 7.5 hours of sleep (Gu, Sautter, Pipkin, & Zeng, 2010). Although age-related changes predispose older adults to sleep disorders, according to the 2003 Sleep in America Poll (National Sleep Foundation, 2010), healthy older adults were less likely to report sleep disturbances compared with older adults with multiple comorbid conditions (Foley et al., 2004). The health benefits of adequate sleep and potential detriments of sleep disturbance should always be carefully considered in the nursing care of older adults.

While adequate sleep may promote health, approximately 50% of older adults have reported difficulty sleeping (Foley et al., 1999). Sleep disturbance may be related to poor sleep hygiene, including an irregular sleep schedule, environmental noise or light, and the use of stimulants (Ancoli-Israel, 2009). Nocturia, whether as a cause of awakening or in response to awakening for other reasons, is commonly associated with perceived poor sleep quality in older adults. Although nocturia may result in part from aging, it may also represent an overlooked pathologic disorder (Bliwise et al., 2009). Older adults with multiple chronic diseases such as depression, pain, cognitive or neurological disorders, and heart or lung disease may have difficulty falling or staying asleep or experience abnormal respiratory events during sleep (Foley et al., 2004). Lastly, older adults taking numerous medications (polypharmacy) may have disturbed sleep as a side effect of drug therapy (Neikrug & Ancoli-Israel, 2010). Increasing use of over-the-counter sleep

Notable Quotes

We are such stuff

As dreams are made on, and our little life

Is rounded with a sleep.

—Shakespeare. From The Tempest (4.1.168-170)

medications such as diphenhydramine (Basu et al., 2003) may also impact nighttime sleep indirectly through increased daytime sleepiness. Even the presence of mild insomnia symptoms is associated with poorer self-reported health status and quality of life than that enjoyed by good sleepers (Leger et al., 2001).

Sleep and Quality of Life

Sleep is a quality-of-life issue (Silva et al., 2009; Vitiello, 2006). Sleep impacts the physical, psychosocial, spiritual, economic, social, and spiritual well-being of older adults. Thus, impaired sleep can have serious consequences in multiple quality-of-life domains, which may jeopardize function and independence in this population (see **Box 16-1**).

BOX 16-1   Key Point

Sleep disturbance in older adults may lead to the loss of independence (Stone et al., 2008).

Older adults with sleep disturbances tend to have more difficulty meeting family, work, and self-care responsibilities. Poor sleep quality may contribute to decreased energy and motivation for the performance of everyday activities (Ancoli-Israel, 2009). Inadequate cognitive function to perform complex mental and decision-making tasks (Nebes et al., 2009; Haimov, Hanuka, & Horowitz, 2008), as well as the development of delirium (Misra & Malow, 2008) are associated with sleep disturbance and may result in institutionalization. There are also safety implications of sleep disturbance for older adults, such as drowsy driving, medication administration errors, or falls (Stone et al., 2008). Consequently, sleep has major implications for the nursing care of older adults (Vance et al., 2011).

Sleep Regulation

Sleep is thought to be regulated by multiple interacting processes, including a *homeostatic sleep drive* and *circadian rhythm* pacing. According to the Two-Process Model of Sleep (Borbely, 1982) sleep and wakefulness are theorized to exist in a homeostatic balance and are synchronized into circadian patterns of approximately 24-hour cycles. Sleep drive (propensity) is the proposed response to periods of extended wakefulness (Borbely, 1982), in concert with circadian response to environmental light stimulation of the retina and sleep pacemaker or *suprachiasmatic nucleus* (Chou et al., 2003; Scheer & Shea, 2009). The sleep pacemaker provides innervation of the ventrolateral preoptic and lateral hypothalamic areas, in which sleep and wake-promoting cells are respectively located (McGinty & Szymusiak, 2003). The Flip-Flop Switch Model of Homeostatic and Circadian Regulation of Sleep and Wake (see **Box 16-2**) proposes that these sleep and wake-promoting

---

BOX 16-2   Key Point

Proposed Models of Sleep Regulation:

The Two-Process Model of Sleep (Borbely, 1982) and The Flip-Flop Model of Homeostatic and Circadian Regulation of Sleep and Wake (Jun et al., 2006).

"systems" function similarly to a continuous feedback loop (Jun, Sherman, Devor, & Saper, 2006).

Neurotransmitters are released as a result of interaction between the specialized nerve cells of these systems, which either inhibit or stimulate wakefulness (arousal) (Fuller, Gooley, & Saper, 2006). Serotonin, norepinephrine, histamine, orexin, acetylcholine, dopamine, and glutamate are some of the main neurotransmitters, and pharmacologic therapies often target their actions or accessibility (McGinty & Szymusiak, 2011). Sleep and wake are also influenced by the hormones melatonin and cortisol. Melatonin promotes the initiation and maintenance of sleep. Levels of melatonin are highest before the sleep onset and are produced in response to sunlight exposure. In contrast, cortisol promotes wakefulness or arousal. Cortisol levels are inhibited during sleep and rise during wakefulness (Scheer & Shea, 2009). Disturbance of sleep homeostasis and circadian rhythms, such as through excessive daytime napping, frequent nighttime awakening, or decreased sunlight exposure, may result in sleep impairment. Neurological damage or deterioration may also alter sleep through reduced function or inability to produce adequate amounts of neurotransmitters, such as through strokes or degenerative disorders like Alzheimer's or Parkinson's disease. The general effects of neurotransmitters associated with sleep and wakefulness are summarized in **Table 16-1**.

Sleep Architecture

Sleep architecture refers to the "relative amounts of the different sleep stages composing sleep and timing of sleep cycles" (Berry, 2012, p. 649). Stage W refers to the shift from full alertness to drowsiness. *Non-rapid eye movement (NREM) sleep*, stages N1, N2 and N3, represent the transition from light to increasingly deep sleep. *Rapid eye movement (REM) sleep*, stage R, is commonly referred to as "dreaming" sleep. NREM sleep comprises approximately 75% of total sleep time (N1 = 5–10%, N2 = 50–60%, N3 = 15–20%), and REM makes up the remaining 25% in adults. NREM sleep stages N1, N2 and N3, plus sleep stage R, make up one *sleep cycle*, and one night of sleep is composed of 3 to 5 90–120 minute sleep cycles (see **Box 16-3**). The total minutes spent asleep during both NREM and REM is referred to as the *total sleep time* (Iber, Ancoli-Israel, Chesson, Quan, & The American Academy of Sleep Medicine [AASM], 2007).

During NREM sleep responsiveness to environmental stimuli decreases, but muscle tone is retained. REM sleep is characterized by dreaming with variable

Notable Quotes

"Sleep is a quality of life issue."

—Vitiello, 2006

TABLE 16-1   General Effects of Neurotransmitters Associated with Sleep and Wakefulness (Lee-Chiong, 2008)

Neurotransmitters	General Effects
Acetylcholine	Associated with EEG desynchronization during wake and REM sleep
Adenosine	Increased levels associated with sleep deprivation; action blocked by methylxanthines such as caffeine
Dopamine	Lesions of dopamine neurons are associated with decreased arousal; D2 and D3 receptor agonists are associated with sedation
Gamma-aminobutyric acid (GABA)	Promotes sleep (acts as a CNS depressant); primary inhibitory CNS neurotransmitter
Glutamate (glutamic acid)	Promotes wakefulness; primary excitatory CNS neurotransmitter
Glycine	Produces REM sleep-related paralysis
Histamine	Promotes wakefulness; N-1 receptor blockers (anti-histamines) increase sleepiness
Hypocretin (orexitin)	Promotes wakefulness; hypocretin system dysfunction is associated with narcolepsy and cataplexy
Melatonin (MT)	Promotes sleep onset; peaks before sleep; produced daily in response to sunlight stimulation of the suprachiasmatic nucleus; production decreases with aging
Norepinephrine (NE)	Promotes wakefulness
Serotonin or 5-hydroxytryptamine (5-HT)	Promotes wakefulness; highest during wake and lowest during sleep; serotonin inhibitors decrease REM sleep

BOX 16-3   Key Point

One night of sleep is composed of 3 to 5 90–120-minute sleep cycles (Iber et al., 2007).

responsiveness to environmental stimuli, voluntary muscle paralysis, and variable autonomic activity. During REM sleep, vital signs and cerebral blood flow are increased; however, temperature regulation is diminished (Carskadon & Dement, 2000).

Sleep and the Aging Process

The normal aging process is associated with some change in the sleep patterns and architecture of healthy older adults (Vitiello, 2006). In general, the bedtime and wake time of older adults are earlier than those of younger adults (Vitiello, 2006), and napping may increase (Driscoll et al., 2008; Foley, Ancoli-Israel, Britz, & Walsh, 2004). Sleep stages are characterized by decreased restorative NREM sleep (Carskadon & Dement, 2005) and REM or dreaming sleep (Bliwise, 2005). *Sleep efficiency* falls approximately 3% per decade, reflecting less time spent asleep while in bed attempting to sleep (Ohayon, Carskadon, Guilleminault, & Vitiello, 2004). This may be partly in response to changes in endogenous circadian temperature oscillation in older compared to younger adults, including a 60% lower mean amplitude and 2-hour-earlier minimum value (Czeisler & Dumont, 1992). Overall, sleep changes are similar in men and women after the age of 60 (Ohayon et al., 2004), and are associated less with actual aging than with existing disorders (Vitiello, Moe, & Prinz, 2002). Other normal developmental challenges that may impact the sleep of older adults include adaptation to retirement (Redeker, 2011) and grief (AASM, 2005). Overall, the normal aging process is not associated with a decreased need for sleep, but it is associated with decreased ability to sleep (Bliwise, 1993). This decreased ability to sleep is often related to the sleep, medical, or psychiatric disorders commonly found in this population (Crowley, 2011).

Assessment of Sleep

History

Assessment of sleep is important to the overall nursing care of the older adult. The SPICES (Sleep disorders, Problems with eating or feeding, Incontinence, Confusion, Evidence of falls, Skin breakdown) assessment tool (Fulmer, 2007) can be used to identify older adults with sleep disturbances. The onset, duration, and severity of the symptoms, along with previous treatments, should be determined. Risks for sleep disturbances should also be identified, including a personal or family history of sleep disturbance, obesity, smoking, hypertension, depression, and other factors. A subjective account about sleep quality should be elicited, and older adults should be asked to describe their usual sleep patterns and nighttime routines. Patient-maintained sleep diaries are helpful sleep assessment tools. Daytime work, exercise, and recreational activities should be included, as well as the older adults' perception of daytime sleepiness. A caregiver or partner is an important resource for the older adult who snores or who is a poor historian (see **Box 16-4**), such as older adults with a diagnosis of dementia (Ward, 2011).

Additionally, a thorough medication review is needed. Over-the-counter medications as well as herbal medications, supplements, alcohol, caffeine, nicotine, and substance abuse should be included. Special attention should be given to sedating medications such as antidepressants or anxiolytics. A schedule of medication administration such as diuretics is also important (Ward, 2011).

BOX 16-4 Key Point

A caregiver or partner is an important resource for the older adult who snores or who is a poor historian.

General Survey

An appearance of either hyperalertness or of a flattened affect in the older adult should be noted as a possible sign of anxiety or depression, respectively, both of which may be associated with *insomnia*. Excessive *daytime sleepiness* in the older adult may be suggested by yawning, rubbing of the face, dark circles under the eyes, lack of attentiveness, or dozing off during the assessment (Vaughn & D'Cruz, 2011).

Physical Assessment

During the physical assessment, the height and weight should be obtained and the body mass index calculated. The neck circumference should also be measured. *Obstructive sleep apnea (OSA)* is associated with a BMI greater than 30 kg/m^2 and/or a neck circumference exceeding 40 cm (Kushida & Efron, 1997). Simple visual inspection revealing a small or recessed mandible, dental malocclusion, a large tongue, or enlarged tonsils may suggest overcrowding of the oropharynx, which may contribute to OSA (Friedman et al., 1999; Mallampati et al., 1985). Mouth-breathing or asymmetry of the nose may suggest nasal obstruction, which may also contribute to OSA (Cao, Guilleminault, & Kushida, 2011).

Basic Sleep Assessment Instruments

There are several basic sleep assessment instruments that registered nurses may use as general screening tools to identify areas of concern. The presence and severity of daytime sleepiness can be assessed using the Epworth Sleepiness Scale (ESS). The ESS, composed of eight items using a Likert-type scale, takes 5 to 10 minutes to complete. While not diagnostic, high ESS scores suggest the possible presence of obstructive sleep apnea or narcolepsy (Johns, 1991, 1992, 1993, 1994).

Subjective *sleep quality* (the perception of sleep as restorative) can be assessed using the Pittsburgh Sleep Quality Index (PSQI). The PSQI, composed of 10 items that assess sleep disturbance and medication use, as well as daytime dysfunction, can be administered in approximately 10 minutes. A total or global sleep quality score can be computed, indicating adequate to poor sleep quality (Buysse, Reynolds III, Monk, Berman, & Kupfer, 1989).

Both of these instruments, along with background information, references, and online videos, can be accessed for free through the Hartford Institute for Geriatric Nursing General Assessment Series (Hartford Institute for Geriatric Nursing,

2012). If findings indicate severe daytime sleepiness or poor sleep quality, follow-up evaluation should be arranged with the primary healthcare provider for possible referral to a sleep specialist.

Specialized Sleep Assessment Instruments

A number of sleep assessment instruments may be used to screen for specific sleep disorders. The STOP BANG screening questionnaire surveys reported snoring, tiredness, and observed apnea (STOP) in addition to high blood pressure, body mass index, age, neck circumference, and gender (BANG). The presence of several of these risk factors suggests possible obstructive sleep apnea. The STOP BANG takes less than 10 minutes to administer, and is often included in preoperative assessments to identify patients at risk for postoperative obstructive sleep apnea (Chung et al., 2008; Chung & Elsaid, 2009).

The Cambridge-Hopkins Restless Legs Syndrome Questionnaire (CH-RLS-Q13) is used to screen for the presence of symptoms that suggest probable restless legs syndrome. The CH-RLS-Q13 consists of 13 items that survey the presence of a recurrent uncomfortable urge to move legs, the position in which this urge is experienced, influence of activity on symptoms, severity of distress with symptoms, frequency of symptoms, and age of symptom onset. This instrument takes 10 to 20 minutes to administer (Allen, Burchell, MacDonald, Hening, & Earley, 2009).

The Insomnia Severity Index (ISI) assesses the presence and severity of insomnia symptoms including difficulty falling or staying asleep, waking up too early, satisfaction with sleep, extent of sleep interference with function, how noticeable sleep impairment is to others, and amount of distress over sleep problems. The ISI can be completed in 5 minutes, and symptoms in the moderate to severe range suggest possible clinical insomnia (Bastian, Vallieres, & Morin, 2001).

It should be noted that the instruments described are intended for screening rather than diagnosis, and that positive findings should be evaluated by the primary care provider and possibly referred to a sleep medicine specialist for additional diagnostic testing.

Diagnostic Sleep Tests

Polysomnography (PSG), also referred to as an "overnight sleep test," records electroencephalographic changes during sleep and allows identification of sleep patterns and events (Dement, 2011). Multiple physiologic variables are also simultaneously recorded during sleep, including muscle activity, nasal airflow, chest and abdomninal effort, oxyhemoglobin saturation, and limb (leg) movement. Stages of sleep and sleep-related events can be detected with PSG, such as frequencies and durations of arousals, awakenings, apneas, and hypopneas (Collop, 2006). *Apnea* refers to absence of airflow at the nose or mouth for 10 seconds or longer, and is classifiable by type. Obstructive sleep apnea is associated with persistent pulmonary effort, whereas central apnea is characterized by an absence of

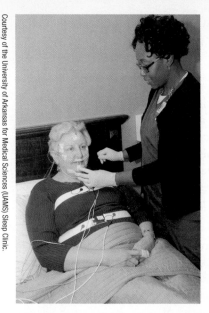

Figure 16-1 Dr. Carol Enderlin is prepared for overnight polysomnography by Valerie Wofford, registered PSG technologist (RPSGT).

respiratory effort. *Hypopnea* is broadly defined as partial reduction in airflow for 10 seconds or longer (Berry, 2012). Patient preparation for PSG is depicted in **Figure 16-1**, the PSG recording in **Figure 16-2**, and patient counseling in **Figure 16-3**.

Actigraphy (ACTG) detects motion as a proxy of wakefulness and the absence of motion as sleep (Tyron, 1991). An actigraph resembles a watch and is most commonly worn on the wrist during routine activity and sleep. Home monitoring of sleep for up to 60 days can be obtained with ACTG, depending upon the model used. More cost-effective and convenient than PSG, ACTG is a valid and reliable measure of sleep in normal healthy adults (Morgenthaler et al., 2007). The measurement of total sleep time is more accurate than of other sleep variables, and as sleep disturbance increases accuracy decreases (Ancoli-Israel et al., 2003). *Circadian rhythm disorders* and circadian rhythms and sleep–wake patterns of adults with insomnia can be assessed using ACTG. It may be used to measure total sleep time in adults with obstructive sleep apnea, and as an alternative in populations such as elderly adults who may not tolerate PSG (Morgenthaler et al., 2007). Care should be taken to avoid use of wrist ACTG in older adults with an arteriovenus shunt or with impaired lymphatic drainage. The frequency and pattern of periodic limb movements of sleep can be measured using ankle ACTG (Kazenwadel et al., 1995; Kemlink, Pretl, Sonka, & Nevsimalova, 2008); however, a history or risk of impaired peripheral perfusion or blood clots are contraindications to its use. Wrist ACTG is shown in **Figure 16-4**.

Common Sources of Geriatric Sleep Disturbance
Common Sleep Disorders

In order to effectively screen for potential sleep disorders in older adults, geriatric nurses must have a basic knowledge of the most common sleep disorders found in this population. Broadly, sleep disorders may be subdivided into insomnia, sleep-related breathing disorders, hypersomnias, circadian rhythm disorders, parasomnias, and sleep-related movement disorders.

Insomnia

Insomnia is defined as "repeated difficulty with sleep initiation, duration, consolidation, or quality despite adequate time & opportunity for sleep," and it is associated with some form of daytime impairment (AASM, 2005, p.1). Insomnia is more common in women than in men, and its prevalence increases with age (Ohayon, 2002). It has been estimated that 50% of older adults have insomnia, often comorbid with other sleep, medical, or psychiatric disorders. Symptoms of insomnia may be present in other sleep disorders including sleep-related breathing disorder, restless legs syndrome, and periodic limb movements (Morin, Mimeault, & Gagne, 1999).

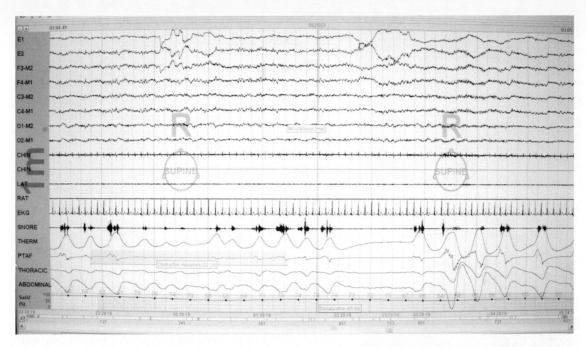

Figure 16-2 Polysomnography (PSG), or overnight sleep testing, records electroencephalographic changes during sleep (Dement, 2011). Muscle activity, nasal airflow, chest and abdominal effort, oxyhemoglobin saturation, and leg movements can also be recorded, and respiratory events (arousals, awakenings, apneas, hypopneas) detected (Collop, 2006).

Source: Courtesy of the University of Arkansas for Medical Sciences (UAMS) Sleep Clinic.

Insomnia symptoms may also accompany psychiatric disorders such as depression (Benca, Ancoli-Israel, & Moldofsky, 2004) or chronic pain disorders (Taylor et al., 2007), and can lead to dependence on sedative-hypnotics or on alcohol as a form of self-medication (Bliwise, 1993). Although older adults may experience insomnia that is acute (transient in nature), it is often chronic (lasting over 3 months) and persistent in up to 85% of cases (Morin, LeBlanc, Daley, Gregoire, & Merette, 2006).

Sleep-Related Breathing Disorders

Sleep-related breathing disorders are some of the most common sleep disorders found in the elderly population, and are characterized by "disordered respiration during sleep," (AASM, 2005, p. 33). They include central sleep apnea syndromes (Cheyne Stokes Breathing Pattern, medical conditions, drug or substance use), obstructive sleep apnea (obstruction of the airway with continued respiratory effort but inadequate ventilation), and hypoventilation/hypoxemia episodes (idiopathic or due to medical conditions). Central sleep apnea has been suggested to be familial in origin and to reflect a high ventilatory response to carbon dioxide. Central sleep apnea is diagnosed with PSG, based on documentation of

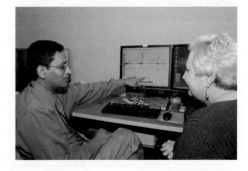

Figure 16-3 Dr. Raghu Reddy discusses the findings of the overnight PSG, pointing out episodes of apnea on the sleep recording.

Courtesy of the University of Arkansas for Medical Sciences (UAMS) Sleep Clinic.

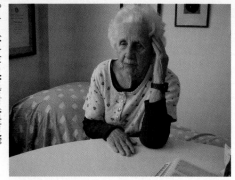

Courtesy of Ambulatory Monitoring (Ardsley, NY.

Figure 16-4 An actigraph resembles a watch and is most commonly worn on the wrist during routine activity and sleep. The actigraph detects motion as a proxy of wakefulness, and the absence of motion as sleep (Tyron, 1991).

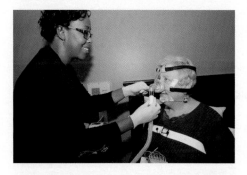

Figure 16-5 Multiple types of continuous positive airway pressure (CPAP) devices are available to maintain airway patency during sleep and are selected for patient comfort and maximum effectiveness.

Courtesy of the University of Arkansas for Medical Sciences (UAMS) Sleep Clinic.

recurrent episodes of cessation of ventilation and ventilatory effort (AASM, 2005).

Cheyne Stokes breathing pattern is associated with medical conditions such as congestive heart failure, stroke, or renal failure. This breathing pattern consists of a waxing and waning pattern of recurrent apneas (breathing cessation) and hypopneas (partial airflow reduction), which usually occur during NREM sleep when assessed with PSG (AASM, 2005).

Obstructive sleep apnea (OSA) refers to "repetitive episodes of complete or partial upper airway obstruction during sleep," (AASM, 2005, p. 51). The prevalence of OSA increases with aging; is more common in men; and is associated with obesity, hypertension, and daytime sleepiness (AASM, 2005). A Swedish study of sleep apnea in community-dwelling elders reported that CSA was associated with cardiovascular disease and impaired systolic function in adults older than 75 years, whereas OSA was not (Johansson, Alehagen, Svanborg, Dahlstrom, & Brostrom, 2012). Diagnosis of OSA is based on patient/partner report and PSG (AASM, 2005), although daytime sleepiness scales and sleep apnea scales may be used as preliminary screening tools. Treatment of OSA depends upon its severity, but most commonly includes continuous positive airway pressure (CPAP) (Neikrug & Ancoli-Israel, 2010). Although adherence to CPAP may present issues, older adults have demonstrated the ability to use it with multiple positive cardiovascular and cognitive benefits (Ancoli-Israel, 2007; Weaver & Chasens, 2007). Use of a CPAP device is shown in **Figure 16-5**.

Hypoventilation/hypoxemia syndromes are nonobstructive and are characterized by decreased alveolar hypoventilation with arterial oxygen desaturation during sleep. Hypoventilation/hypoxemia syndromes may occur in the presence of normal pulmonary mechanical properties and may be precipitated by central nervous system depressants. These syndromes often follow a slowly progressive course that can lead to pulmonary hypertension and cardiac failure. Hypoventilation/hypoxemia syndromes are diagnosed with PSG, based on recurrent episodes of cessation of ventilation and ventilatory effort with mild arterial oxygen desaturation (AASM, 2005).

Sleep-related breathing disorders are associated with frequent arousals from sleep, resulting in fragmented sleep and daytime sleepiness, which may be the presenting complaint (AASM, 2005). Patient education related to OSA is illustrated in **Figure 16-6**.

Hypersomnias

Hypersomnias of central origin refer to sleep disorders with the main complaint of daytime sleepiness unrelated to other causes of sleep disturbance such as circadian rhythm or sleep-related breathing disorders. Hypersomnias include the sleep disorder narcolepsy, with or without cataplexy (sudden bilateral loss of muscle tone elicited by strong, usually positive emotions such as laughter). Narcolepsy is defined as "rapid transition from wakefulness to REM sleep" (AASM, 2005, p. 81), and its etiology includes both genetic and nongenetic factors. The pathology of narcolepsy is associated with loss of hypothalamic neurons, which contain hypocretin (an excitatory neuropeptide). The onset of narcolepsy is usually in late adolescence or early adulthood, and is characterized by sleepiness and later by hypnagogic hallucinations (vivid perceptual experiences at sleep onset), sleep paralysis (a transient inability to move or speak during the sleep–wake transition), and disturbed nocturnal sleep. Diagnosis is based on patient-reported symptoms (AASM, 2005), and supported by a cerebrospinal fluid hypocretin-1 level of less than 110 pg/mL. Other confirming sleep findings include a short sleep latency (under 8 minutes taken to fall asleep) on the Multiple Sleep Latency Test (Carskadon et al., 1986; Carskadon & Dement, 1982), and/or a sleep-onset REM period (SOREMP) of 10 minutes or less after the onset of sleep, as measured by PSG. Narcolepsy can diminish quality of life by impairing school, work, and social functioning, and depression often develops (AASM, 2005). Treatment of narcolepsy includes pharmacologic agents; behavioral therapy, including sleep hygiene; and social support such as through groups (Guilleminault & Cao, 2011). Older adults who carry the human leukocyte antigen DQB1*0602 allele (associated with 95% of hypocretin-deficient narcolepsy) but who have no diagnosis of narcolepsy also have reported poorer perceptions of feeling rested than older adults without the allele with the same poor sleep efficiency. These findings suggest that there may be a "normal" phenotypic variation of REM sleep in DQB1*0602 allele carriers among older adults with insomnia (Zeitzer et al., 2011).

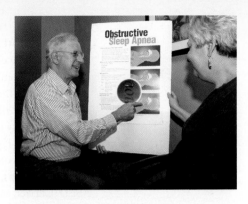

Figure 16-6 Dr. Greg Krulin discusses how the airway is closed in obstructive sleep apnea, and how CPAP works to relieve the obstruction.

Courtesy of the University of Arkansas for Medical Sciences (UAMS) Sleep Clinic.

Other types of hypersomnias may be idiopathic (of unknown etiology), due to medical conditions (Parkinson's disease, head trauma, brain tumors, endocrine disorders, toxic encephalopathies, genetic syndromes), or due to drugs or substances (stimulants, sedative-hypnotics). Hypersomnia may also be nonorganic (depression, conversion, or seasonal affective disorders). These medical and psychiatric disorders, as well as chronic sleep deprivation or chronic fatigue syndrome, should be considered in older adults with complaints of daytime sleepiness or reports of over 9 hours of sleep per day (AASM, 2005). Prolonged sleep duration (9 hours or more per day) in adults 68 years or older has been associated with daytime sleepiness, in contrast to short sleep duration (6 hours or less), which was associated with night sleep disturbance and poor sleep quality. However, this was only partly explained by associations with obesity and snoring, although obstructive sleep apnea must always be considered in the presence of daytime sleepiness (Mesas et al., 2011). Older adults with hypersomnia should be referred to their primary care provider for further evaluation and determination of the need for consultation with a specialist (AASM, 2005).

Circadian Rhythm Disorders

A circadian rhythm disorder (CRD) is defined as "a recurrent or chronic pattern of sleep disturbance (that) may result from alterations of the circadian timing system or a misalignment between the timing of the individual's circadian rhythm of sleep propensity and the 24-hour social and physical environments" (AASM, 2005, p.117). A CRD may be of the advanced or delayed phase type (ASPD or DSPD) based on the relative early or late onset patterns of sleep and wake time (Berry, 2012). While a morningness type of sleep pattern is associated with increased aging and poorer objective sleep quality (less total sleep time and increased wake time during last 2 hours of sleep), the morningness type alone, rather than age, is associated with ASPD (Carrier, Monk, Buysse, & Kupfer, 1997). Advanced phase-related complaints were twice that of delayed phase-related complaints in adults 40–64 years of age (Ando, Kripke, & Ancoli-Israel, 2002). Diagnosis is made based on sleep logs and actigraphy, and treatment may include evening light therapy (Sack et al., 2007).

Delayed sleep phase syndrome (DSPD) is relatively rare among adults 40–64 years of age (Ando et al., 2002), although less is known of its frequency among older adults. DSPD is also diagnosed with sleep logs and actigraphy, and may be managed with prescribed sleep scheduling. Insomnia should be considered as a possible underlying problem, as persons with ASPD have symptoms of delayed sleep onset (Sack et al., 2007).

Parasomnias

Parasomnias are described as "undesirable physical events or experiences that occur during entry into sleep, within sleep, or during arousals from sleep" (AASM, 2005, p. 137). Parasomnias reflect activation of the central nervous system and may be characterized by abnormal movements, behaviors, emotions, perceptions, dreams, and autonomic nervous system activity. They may also be demonstrated through aggressive behavior, locomotion, sleep-related eating disorder, or sexual behaviors. Parasomnias disrupt sleep and may result in injuries, negative health, and social effects for the person with the disorder and their bed partner (AASM, 2005).

Multiple subtypes are included under parasomnias. Sleepwalking and sleep terrors are two common parasomnias related to arousal from NREM sleep that occur most frequently in childhood but may also occur in older adults. Confusional arousals (mental and behavioral confusion upon awakening from sleep) are also related to arousal from NREM sleep, and similarly occur more frequently in children than in adults. Sleep-related abnormal sexual behaviors are a form of confusional arousal, which can result in inappropriate sexual activity or assault with subsequent amnesia of the behavior (AASM, 2005).

There are numerous parasomnias associated with REM sleep such as nightmare disorder, sleep-related dissociative disorder, and REM sleep behavior disorder. Nightmare disorder occurs most commonly in childhood but may also be related to acute stress or trauma. Recurrent nightmares are associated with psychopathology. Sleep-related dissociative disorder (screaming, walking, running, engaging in self-mutilating or violent behavior, reenactment of prior physical or sexual abuse) may reflect a history of trauma and psychiatric disorders. *REM sleep behavior disorder (RSBD)* is associated with the enactment of violent dreams, is most common in men older than 50 years with underlying neurological disorders (parkinsonism, dementia with Lewy bodies, narcolepsy, stroke), and is progressive in nature. Notably, 33% of persons newly diagnosed with Parkinson's disease have RSBD, as do 90% of persons with multiple system atrophy. Medications, including venlafaxine, selective serotonin reuptake inhibitors, mirtazapine, and other antidepressants may precipitate RSBD. This disorder is of particular concern in older adults due to the potential for self-injury or injury of the bed partner (AASM, 2005).

Restless Legs Syndrome

Restless legs syndrome (RLS) is defined as "a sensorimotor disorder characterized by a complaint of a strong, nearly irresistible, urge to move the legs" (AASM, 2005, p. 178). Parasthesias (abnormal skin sensation without a noticeable cause) may also be reported. These worsen when sitting or lying down, and are almost immediately relived by movement (AASM, 2005). Onset may be early (under 45 years of age) with slowly progressing symptoms, or late in life (40–65 years of age) with rapidly progressing symptoms. The prevalence of RLS is higher in women and varies by race/ethnicity, with 5–10% of Northern Europeans reporting symptoms. The etiology of RLS includes familial inheritance, brain iron dysregulation, and dopamine abnormalities. Conditions or disorders associated with iron deficiency (renal failure, iron deficiency anemia) precipitate symptoms, as do antihistamines, dopamine receptor antagonists, and many antidepressants (AASM, 2005).

Periodic limb movements (PLMs), which are repetitive, involuntary jerks or twitches of the legs, are present in 80–90% of persons with RLS. Combined, RLS symptoms impair the ability to fall or return to sleep after awakening, and PLMs repeatedly provoke arousals and awakenings from sleep, resulting in sleep disturbance and daytime sleepiness (AASM, 2005).

The diagnosis of RLS is based on patient report and established criteria (Allen et al., 2003), and PLMs are measured using PSG (AASM, 2005). Both RLS and PLMs tend to increase with aging (Ancoli-Israel et al., 1991).

Geropsychiatric Disorders and Sleep

Sleep disturbance is a common problem in older adults with mental health conditions. Sleep disturbance in older adults is considered a geriatric syndrome (see **Box 16-5**), and often occurs with depression, anxiety, dementia, and other neurological disorders such as Parkinson's disease, mental health conditions, and substance abuse (Vaz Fragoso & Gill, 2007). Older persons are living longer with underlying physical and mental health conditions (Crystal, Sambamoorthi, Walkup, & Akincigil, 2003). Therefore, it is critical that nurses are prepared to join the geropsychiatric workforce as leaders in the care of older persons with sleep disturbances and mental health conditions.

One in five older persons (26.3%) have a mental disorder, 16% have a primary mental health condition, and 3% also have dementia (Jeste et al., 1999).

BOX 16-5   Key Point

Sleep impairment in older adults is considered a geriatric syndrome, and it often occurs with depression, anxiety, dementia and other neurological disorders such as Parkinson's disease, mental health conditions, and substance abuse (Vaz Fragoso & Gill, 2007).

Because mental health disorders do not disappear with old age, conditions such as depression, bipolar disorder, and schizophrenia often worsen with chronic conditions or when superimposed on dementia.

Depression affects 11% of the general older adult population (Substance Abuse and Mental Health Services Administration [SAMHSA], 2007). Sleep disturbance places the older adult at high risk for depression (Schutte-Rodin, Broch, Buysse, Dorsey, & Sateia, 2008), and deficiencies in neurotransmitters such as serotonin are associated with both sleep disturbance and depression (Benca, 2005). Depressed older persons take longer to experience REM sleep, and early morning wakefulness with inability to fall back to sleep due to sadness and worry is also characteristic of depression. In addition, depression is associated with insomnia; dreaming; and a loss of deep, restorative sleep (Benca, 2005). Poor sleep efficiency (73%; normal > 85%) has been reported in depressed older persons (Bliwise, 2005).

Anxiety symptom prevalence is 20% in the population of older persons (SAMHSA, 2007). Anxiety often accompanies depression, along with nighttime panic attacks and the inability to fall asleep and stay asleep (Brenes et al., 2009; Stein & Mellman, 2005). A study (n = 110) of older persons with generalized anxiety disorder with or without depression showed a greater severity of sleep disturbance when compared with older persons without a psychiatric diagnosis (Brenes et al., 2009).

While only 1% of older adults suffer from bipolar disorder or schizophrenia (SAMHSA, 2007), older adults are living longer with these debilitating conditions associated with sleep disturbance. In the manic phase of bipolar disorder, there is a perceived decreased need for sleep and there may be a perception of feeling rested after only 3 hours of sleep (American Psychiatric Association, 2000). Schizophrenia may result in reversal of the sleep–wake cycle or long episodes of complete sleeplessness, decreased total sleep time, long sleep-onset latency, and fragmented sleep (Benson & Zarcone, 2005).

Sleep is heavily influenced by the central nervous system. Neurodegenerative changes in dementia cause fragmented sleep. Persons with dementia are at high risk for more severely disturbed sleep due to damaged neuronal pathways that interfere with the communication between the homeostatic and circadian rhythm processes that regulate sleep (Bliwise, 2005). There is decreased slow-wave sleep and less REM, making stages of sleep difficult to distinguish with PSG. Due to these changes, persons with dementia often present with a typical sleep pattern of nighttime wandering and daytime sleepiness (Petit, Montplaisir, & Boeve, 2005). Disturbed sleep is a common reason for institutionalization in persons with dementia. Consequently, *sleep fragmentation* is more severe in persons with dementia in the nursing home.

Subcortical damage to sleep-promoting neurons takes place in the cholinergic basal forebrain nuclei, serotonergic raphe nuclei, dopaminergic nigrostriatial and pallidostriatal pathways, and noradrenergic locus coeruleus (Neubauer, 2003; Vitiello & Borson, 2001). Neurodegenerative changes in the CNS alter circadian rhythm. Neurodeneration takes place in the efferent pathways from the retina, hypothalamic nuclei, limbic forebrain, raphe nuclei, and reticular formation. These neuronal pathways communicate with the CNS in response to melatonin and other hormones that regulate sleep in the sympathetic superior cervical ganglion and pineal gland (Vitiello & Borson, 2001). As neurons in the homeostatic mechanisms deteriorate, lesions are formed in the neuronal pathways causing the sleep–wake cycle response to weaken in the CNS (Cole & Richards, 2005).

Parkinson's disease is a neurodegenerative disorder that has a prevalence of 5% in persons 80 to 84 years of age. Parkinson's disease is caused by insufficient amounts of dopamine produced in the substantia nigra in the brain. REM Sleep Behavior Disorder is common in Parkinson's disease. In RBD, there is a loss of muscle atonia and an increase in motor activity such as kicking and biting. The person awakens suddenly and acts out their dream. REM Sleep Behavior Disorder is associated with degeneration in the synucleinopathies that occur in Parkinson's disease and dementia with Lewy bodies (Petit et al., 2005; Postuma et al., 2009). Research shows that RBD may predict Parkinson's disease (Postuma et al., 2009). Safety is the main nursing priority and nonpharmacological treatments are recommended because pharmacological therapy can worsen associated sleep apnea and dementia (Petit et al., 2005).

Sleep Management

Pharmacologic management of sleep disorders in older adults is sometimes needed for relief of symptoms not amenable to nonpharmacologic methods. However, older adults may be more sensitive to the potential side effects of sleep medications, especially those related to the central nervous system, which may predispose to cognitive impairment and falls (see **Box 16-6**).

As with other medications administered to this age group, the general rule is to start with a low dose and slowly increase it until the desired results are obtained. It should be noted that some medications have a risk profile that contraindicates their use in the elderly. Specialized references with geriatric doses and implications should always be consulted regarding the use of sleep medications in older adults. Medications often used to manage sleep disorders are summarized in **Table 16-2**,

Notable Quotes

"The normal aging process is not associated with a decreased need for sleep, but with a decreased ability to sleep."

—Bliwise, 1993

BOX 16-6 **Key Point**

Older adults may be more sensitive to the potential side effects of sleep medications, especially those related to the central nervous system, which may predispose to cognitive impairment and falls.

TABLE 16-2 Geriatric Implications of Sleep Medications

Sleep Disorder	Drug Classification	Medications	Mechanism of Action	Geriatric Implications
Sleep-Promotion Enhancers (Walsh & Roth, 2011)				
Insomnia	Sedative-Hypnotics	Non-benzodiazepines:	Theorized to enhance GABA	Avoid chronic use in elderly; increased risk of adverse events such as delirium, falls, fractures (AGS, 2012)
		Eszopicione (Lunesta)		Avoid use in elders with a history of falls or fractures (AGS, 2012); similar adverse reactions as in younger adults; 41% increase exposure for adults > 65 years (Semia, Beizer, & Hibgee, 2012); one-half of standard adult dose recommended in elderly http://www.drugs.com/pro/lunesta.html
		Zaleplon (Sonata)		Avoid use in elders with a history of falls or fractures (AGS, 2012); elderly responsive to one-half standard dose for younger adults (Semia et al., 2012); not recommended due to increased risk of falls, confusion, & daytime sleepiness (AGS, FHA, 2012)
		Zolpidem (Ambien)		Drug of choice in elders (only when a hypnotic is indicated (Semia et al., 2012); not recommended due to increased risk of falls, confusion & daytime sleepiness (AGS, FHA, 2012); avoid use in elders with dementia and cognitive impairment, or a history of falls or fractures (AGS, 2012)
		Zolpidem extended release		Use with caution in elderly; adverse events similar to younger adults with one-half standard dose (Semia et al., 2012)
		Benzodiazepines Long-acting:	Theorized to enhance GABA	Avoid use in elderly (AGS, 2012)
		Flurazepam (Dalmane) Quazepam (Doral)		Avoid use in elderly; extremely long half-life; prolonged sedation; increased falls and fractures (AGS, FHA, 2012; Semia et al., 2012)

Category	Drug	Mechanism	Notes
	Benzodiazepines Short-acting:	Theorized to enhance GABA	Avoid use in elderly (AGS, 2012); increased sensitivity in elderly; smaller doses potentially as effective and safer (if indicated) (Semia et al., 2012)
	Temazepam (Restoril)		Recommended (only) if benzodiazepine hypnotic is indicated; limit use to 10–14 days (Semia et al., 2012)
	Triazolam (Halcion)		Not drug of first choice due to high incidence of CNS adverse effects (Semia et al., 2012)

Other Sleep Promotion Enhancers (Krystal, 2011)

Category	Drug	Mechanism	Notes
Anti-anxiety	Buspirone (BuSpar)	Unknown; high affinity for 5HT receptors; moderate affinity for DA receptors	Recommended if anxiolytic is indicated (mild to moderate anxiety); less sedating than other anxiolytics (Semia et al., 2012)
Hormone	Melatonin *dietary supplement, OTC	MT1 & MT2 receptor agonist	No significant difference in safety for older as in younger adults (Semia et al., 2012)
	Ramelteon (Rozerem)		Total exposure of older adults to Ramelteon is 86–97% higher compared to younger adults; does not exacerbate mild to moderate obstructive sleep apnea http://www.drugs.com/pro/rozerem.html

Wake Promotion Blockers (Krystal, 2011)

Category	Drug	Mechanism	Notes
Sedating anti-depressants	Tricyclics:	5HT & NE receptor blockers; antagonize 5HT & NE receptors	Avoid use in elderly (AGS, 2012); strong sedative and anticholinergic properties in elderly (Semia et al., 2012)
	Amitriptyline (Elavil)		Avoid use in elderly (AGS, 2012); not drug of choice in elderly (Semia et al., 2012)
	Doxepin (Sinequan)		Avoid use in elderly (AGS, 2012); not drug of choice in elderly in doses >6 mg (Semia et al., 2012)

(Continues)

TABLE 16-2 Geriatric Implications of Sleep Medications (*Continued*)

Sleep Disorder	Drug Classification	Medications	Mechanism of Action	Geriatric Implications
		Trimipramine (Surmontil)		Avoid use in elderly (AGS, 2012); not drug of choice in elderly; one-half adult initial dose up to one-third adult max for elderly; CNS side effects, especially confusion (Semia et al., 2012)
		Other: Trazodone (Desyrel) Mirtazapine (Remeron)	5HT reuptake inhibitor; H1 & alpha adrenergic receptor blockers	Very sedating; few anticholinergic effects; limited data published regarding use in elderly (Semia et al., 2012)
	Anti-histamines	Diphenhydramine (Benedryl) *OTC	H1 receptor antagonist	Avoid use in elderly (AGS, 2012); strong sedative and anticholinergic properties; may cause confusion; not drug of choice in elderly; not recommended (AGS, FHA, 2012)
		Doxylamine succinate (Unisom) *OTC	Muscarinic cholinergic antagonist	Avoid use in elderly (AGS, 2012); increased risk of dizziness, sedation, and hypotension in elderly; anticholinergic effects—use cautiously with glaucoma, emphysema, prostatic hypertrophy http://www.drugs.com/monograph/doxylamine-succinate.html
	Antipsychotics	Olanzapine (Zyprexa) Quetiapine (Seroquel)	Antagonize DA, H1, 5HT, muscarinic, cholinergic, & adrenergic receptors	Avoid use in elderly (AGS, 2012); not recommended for elderly except for actual diagnosis of psychosis; increased risk of stroke, death, tremors, & falls (AGS, FHA, 2012)

Wake-Promotion Enhancers (Guilleminault & Cao, 2011)

Sleep Disorder	Drug Classification	Medications	Mechanism of Action	Geriatric Implications
Narcolepsy	Stimulants	Amphetamines:	↑MAO release (dopamine, norepinephrine, & 5-HT)	

	Methamphetamine	Similar to amphetamine, less peripheral side effects	Avoid use in elderly due to CNS stimulant effects (AGS, 2012); may cause cardiovascular effects including palpitations, tachycardia, and hypertension http://www.drugs.com/sfx/methamphetamine-side-effects.html
	Methylphenidate (Ritalin)	Blocks MAO uptake at lower dose than amphetamine	Avoid use in elderly due to CNS stimulant effects (AGS, 2012)
	Selegiline (Eldepryl)	MAO-B inhibitor; converts to amphetamine	Use of orally disintegrating tablet (Zelapar) associated with increased adverse effects (hypertension, hypotension, dizziness, somnolence); lowest dose possible recommended if used in elderly (Semia et al., 2012)
	Modafinil (Provigil) Armodafinil (Nuvigil)	Unknown mode of action	Reduced excretion of modafinil and its metabolites in elderly; safety and effectiveness not established over 65 years of age (Semia et al., 2012)
Anti-cataplectics	Venlafaxine (Effexor)	5HT & NE reuptake inhibitor	Low anticholinergic and sedative properties; recommended in elderly when a stimulant is indicated; adjust dose for renal function (Semia et al., 2012)
	Atomoxetine (Strattera)	NE reuptake blocker	Potentially fatal cardiovascular side effects with underlying cardiac disorders; no data regarding geriatric use (Semia et al., 2012)
	Fluoxetine (Prozac)	5HT reuptake inhibitor	Potential stimulating and anorexic effects; long half-life in elderly; associated with hyponatremia in elderly; high severity risk of side effects in elderly (Semia et al., 2012)
	Protriptyline (Vivactil)	MAO uptake inhibitor	Strong anticholinergic properties; one-third standard maximum adult dose in elderly (Semia et al., 2012)

(Continues)

TABLE 16-2   Geriatric Implications of Sleep Medications (*Continued*)

Sleep Disorder	Drug Classification	Medications	Mechanism of Action	Geriatric Implications
		Imipramine (Tofranil) Desipramine (Norpramin)	5HT & NE reuptake inhibitor; down regulation of beta-adrenergic and 5HT receptors	Potential orthostatic hypotension and arrhythmias; avoid in elderly (AGS, FHA, 2012)
				Mild side effect profile; a preferred agent (if needed) in elderly; one-half standard maximum adult dose in elderly (Semia et al., 2012)
		Clomipramine (Anafranil)	Affects 5HT & NE uptake	Anticholinergic and hypotensive side effects (Semia et al., 2012); higher plasma concentrations in elderly; avoid use in elderly (AGS, FHA, 2012)
Dopamine Promoters or Enhancers (Montplaisir, Allen, Arthur, & Ferini-Strambi, 2011)				
Restless Legs Syndrome (RLS)	Dopamine agonists	Pramipexole (Miripex) Ropinirole (Requip)	Bind to DA receptors(D3) in place of DA; directly stimulate DA receptors	Half-life 1.5 times longer in elderly; renal clearance decreased in elderly; postural hypotension and confusion (Semia et al., 2012) Dosage not adjusted for elderly; postural hypotension and daytime somnolence (Semia et al., 2012)
	Dopamine precursors:	Levodopa/carbidopa	↑ available DA	Greater sensitivity to CNS side effects in elderly (confusion, somnolence, insomnia, nightmares) (Semia et al., 2012)
	Benzo-diazepines	Clonazepam (Klonopin) Temazepam (Restoril)	Depress nerve transmission in the motor cortex (decrease PLMs and PLMs-associated	Potential decreased hepatic clearance and renal excretion in elderly; CNS (confusion, somnolence, insomnia, nightmares)

		arousals in RLS; given for insomnia symptoms secondary to dopaminergic agents)	and pulmonary (respiratory congestion and depression) toxicities Recommended (only) when indicated; use should be limited to 10–14 days (Semia et al., 2012)
Opiates	Oxycodone Codeine	Possible ↑opiate receptor binding and opioid levels to counter-balance endogenous opioid system dysfunction	Increased sensitivity to CNS and constipating effects; higher serum levels at same dose in older as in younger adults (Semia et al., 2012) Increased sensitivity to CNS depression and confusion, and constipating effects (Semia et al., 2012)
Anti-convulsants	Gabapentin (Neurontin)	↑brain DA levels directly (decrease peripheral neuropathy-related pain in RLS)	Decreased renal clearance with increasing age; CNS side effects of somnolence and fatigue in >10% (not specific to elderly) (Semia et al., 2012)

Key: 5HT = serotonin
CNS = central nervous system
DA = dopamine
GABA = gamma-hydroxybutyrate
H = histamine
MAO = monoamine oxydase
MT1, MT2 = melatonin 1 and 2 receptors
NE = Norepinephrine
PLMs = Periodic Limb Movements of Sleep
RLS = Restless Legs Syndrome

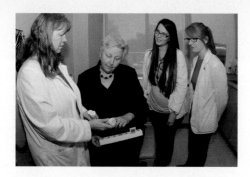

Figure 16-7 Dr. Lisa Hutchison, PharmD and pharmacy students provide sleep medication counseling.

Courtesy of Thomas and Lyon Longevity Clinic, Donald W. Reynolds Institute on Aging, UAMS.

with current geriatric implications. Patient sleep medication counseling is critical to successful management of sleep disturbance or disorders (see **Figure 16-7**).

Complementary Alternative Medicine

For all adults, national surveys indicate that as many as 38% use a complementary and/or alternative medicine (CAM) modality to improve some aspect of their health and well-being (Barnes, Bloom, & Nahin, 2008). CAM practices are used by older adults for reasons that may have implications related to improvement in sleep: to relive pain, to improve quality of life, and to maintain health and fitness (Williamson, Fletcher, & Dawson, 2003).

CAM practices are organized into several classifications according to the National Center of Complementary and Alternative Medicine (NCCAM), a component of the National Institutes of Health (NCCAM, 2012). According to NCCAM, CAM practices and products are classified in to these categories: whole medical systems (e.g., acupuncture); mind–body modalities (e.g., cognitive behavior therapy); biological-based products (e.g., herbs and natural substances); manipulative and body-based modalities (e.g., massage, Tai Chi); and energy modalities (e.g., cranial electrical stimulation). While not every CAM practice and product has been shown to be efficacious in improving sleep in older adults, there are promising results in some areas and these will be discussed.

Acupuncture

Acupuncture is practiced by providers who insert small needles into different points on the body, with or without the use of electrostimulation (NCCAM, 2007). While acupuncture has shown promise in decreasing sleep disturbances in older adult females who are experiencing distressing symptoms related to menopause, including hot flashes that interrupt sleep; in insomnia in persons who have experienced a stroke; and in persons with fibromyalgia, there is insufficient evidence to support its widespread use to improve sleep in older adults (Borud, Grimsgaard, & White, 2010; Gooneratne, 2008). Further research in this area is ongoing and may provide more solid evidence for its use in older adults.

Mind-Body Modalities

Cognitive behavioral therapy (CBT) refers to a number of therapeutic approaches that focus on the influence of thinking on feelings and actions. Although approaches may differ, they are all based on the premise that clients can learn to think differently, act on that learning, and change behaviors. Cognitive behavioral therapy is collaborative, time-limited in nature, and provides clients with the rationale and methods necessary to develop self-management skills (National Association of Cognitive Behavioral Therapists, 2007). Multicomponent CBT approaches are often used for sleep disturbance (Bootzin, 2005), and effective standard modalities include cognitive therapy, stimulus control therapy and relaxation therapy. Sleep hygiene may also be included, although it is not considered effective as a single modality (Morgenthaler et al., 2006). Cognitive (restructuring) therapy is aimed at helping clients to recognize maladaptive thoughts (cognitions) and beliefs about their sleep and to reframe or "restructure" them more positively (Perlis & Gehrman, 2011). Stimulus control therapy focuses on helping clients to re-associate the bed and bedroom with falling asleep, rather than bedtime being a stimulus for wakefulness (Bootzin & Perlis, 2011). The aim of relaxation therapy is to reduce somatic and/or cognitive arousal (Berry, 2012). Sleep hygiene education (Hauri, 1991) addresses knowledge deficits related to sleep processes and behaviors that may promote or inhibit sleep (Posner & Gehrman, 2011). One established form of CBT is CBT-Insomnia (CBT-I), which is administered by a behavioral sleep medicine specialist and includes stimulus control therapy plus sleep restriction therapy (limiting the time in bed to the average time spent asleep, with progressive increases). A shortened version, called Brief Behavioral Treatment of Insomnia (BBTI), may be administered in primary care settings (Espie et al., 2007; Germain & Buyssee, 2011).

Cognitive behavioral therapy interventions for sleep disturbance offer some advantages for older adults who are at risk for polypharmacy and potential side effects of pharmacologic interventions that may impair cognitive function or contribute to the risk of falls (Montgomery & Dennis, 2009b)(see **Box 16-7**). Moreover, CBT is recommended as equivalent to pharmacologic interventions, with more sustained effectiveness over time, for the treatment of insomnia (Riemann & Perlis, 2009; Smith et al., 2002). Concern expressed by the client about adverse consequences, causes, and emotions related to sleep disturbance has been suggested to predict interest in CBT-I (Cahn et al., 2005), and should be noted when initiating discussion of treatment options. The majority of nonpharmacologic interventions require specialized training in behavioral sleep medicine for safe and effective delivery, especially in older adults with medical or psychiatric comorbidities such as psychosis or bipolar disorder. However, some standardized formats of CBT have been recommended as appropriate for nurses to deliver under the supervision of a sleep specialist (Espie et al., 2007). Relaxation techniques and sleep hygiene education may be delivered by nurses familiar with the techniques and information. Nurses may also apply sleep hygiene to the care of hospitalized older adults by implementing relaxing bedtime routines (LaReau, Benson, Watcharotone & Manguba, 2008), and minimizing adverse environmental noise and light (Missildine, 2008). Common methods of cognitive behavioral therapy and their purposes are summarized in **Table 16-3**.

A number of studies have described the effective use of various forms of CBT for adults and older adults with insomnia (Brenes et al., 2012; Buysse et al., 2012;

BOX 16-7   Key Point

Cognitive behavioral therapy is recommended as equivalent to pharmacologic interventions, with more sustained effectiveness over time, for the treatment of insomnia (Riemann & Perlis, 2009; Smith et al., 2002).

TABLE 16-3   Cognitive Behavioral Therapies for Sleep Promotion

Therapy	Purpose
Cognitive (Restructuring)	Promotes identification of maladaptive cognitions or beliefs that stimulate worry (catastrophic thinking about the consequences of poor sleep) with their subsequent analysis and more positive restructuring (Buysse & Perlis, 1996; Perlis & Gehrman, 2011; Schutte-Rodin et al., 2008).
Stimulus Control	Re-associates the bed and bedroom with falling asleep rather than with anxiety over not being able to fall asleep (Bootzin, Epstein, & Ward, 1991; Bootzin & Perlis, 2011).
Relaxation	Decreases cognitive arousal and somatic tension (Berry, 2012; Lichstein, Taylor, McCrae, & Thomas, 2011). Includes multiple approaches including guided imagery, progressive muscle relaxation, and biofeedback.
Paradoxical Intention	Decreases or eliminates performance anxiety through intentional avoidance of falling asleep (Espie, 2011).
Sleep Restriction	Sharply limits the time in bed to the total sleep time, then progressively increases time in bed through earlier bedtimes until it is equivalent to total sleep time (Spielman, Saskin, & Thorpy, 1987); contraindicated in persons requiring maximal vigilance for activities like driving, in conditions exacerbated by sleepiness (epilepsy, parasomnias, sleep-disordered breathing) (Epstein & Bootzin, 2002; Spielman, Yang, & Glovinsky, 2011), and in conditions potentially exacerbated by lack of sleep (bipolar disorder) (Espie et al., 2007; Germain & Buysse, 2011).
Sleep Compression	An alternative to sleep restriction in older adults with serious medical comorbidities; sleep is increasingly restricted in small increments over approximately 5 weeks through delayed bedtime or earlier wake time, until the time spent in bed is equivalent to the time asleep (Lichstein, Thomas, & McCurry, 2011).
Multi-component	Combines stimulus control, relaxation, and sleep restriction therapies with or without cognitive therapy (Berry, 2012), such as Cognitive Behavioral Therapy for Insomnia (CBT-I) and Brief Behavioral Treatment of Insomnia (BBTI), which are designed to provide intensive therapy over 6–8 weeks by a behavioral sleep medicine specialist, or less-intensive therapy over a shorter time period in a group format delivered by a specially trained nurse in a primary care setting; containindicated if sleep restriction is contraindicated (Espie et al., 2007; Germain & Buysse, 2011).
Sleep Hygiene Education	Increases knowledge of homeostatic and circadian processes, and sleep-promoting behaviors (sleep schedule, stimulants, environment, etc.) that influence sleep (Chesson, Jr. et al., 2000; Hauri, 1991; Posner & Gehrman, 2011); most effective if individually tailored (Perlis, Jungquist, Smith, & Posner, 2005); used in combination with other cognitive behavioral therapies for sleep initiation or maintenance problems.

Edinger et al., 2001; Lichstein et al., 2001; McCrae, McGovern, Lukefahr, & Stripling, 2011). These approaches have also demonstrated some success in the treatment of older adults with insomnia and such comorbid disorders as chronic obstructive pulmonary disease (Kapella et al., 2011), coronary artery disease, osteoarthritis (Rybarczyk et al., 2005; Rybarczyk, Mack, Harris, & Stepanski, 2009; Vitiello, Rybarczyk, VonKorff, & Stepanski, 2009), and hot flushes and night sweats following breast cancer treatment (Mann et al., 2012).

Biological-Based Products

The two most widely studied biological-based products for sleep are melatonin and valerian (see **Box 16-8**). Melatonin is an endogenous neurohormone that is believed to play a role in the sleep–wake cycle. Lower levels of melatonin are found in older adults as compared to young adults (Sharma, Palacios-Bois, Schwartz, & Iskandar, 1989). A large meta-analysis on the efficacy of melatonin therapy concluded that melatonin did not have a significant benefit for insomnia in older adults, despite small improvements in sleep latency (Buscemi et al., 2004). Data on the efficacy of melatonin for sleep are mixed (Arendt, 2006). Valerian, an extract of the plant species *Valeriana officinalis*, has been studied to determine its effect on sleep–wake patterns. While statistically significant results have been found in some clinical trials using Valerian in older adults, additional study is warranted in this area as the authors of a meta-analysis of the use of the Valerian compound concluded that it was safe but ineffective (Taibi, Landis, Petry, & Vitiello, 2007).

BOX 16-8   Acupuncture, Valerian, Melatonin, Tai Chi, and Cranial Electrical Stimulation

Acupuncture, Valerian, melatonin, Tai Chi, and Cranial electrical stimulation need further research to support their use in older adults. A 3-minute slow-stroke back massage was associated with a 36-minute increase in minutes of nighttime sleep in persons with dementia residing in the nursing home (Harris, 2010).

Manipulative Modalities

Back massage has been efficacious in a variety of older adult populations, including those in intensive care units (Richards, 1998), those with dementia in long-term care facilities (Harris, 2010), and in hospitalized patients following coronary artery bypass surgery (Nerbass, Feltrim, Souza, Ykeda, & Lorenzi-Filho, 2010). In a review of the evidence of massage for improvement of sleep in older adults, physiological and psychological indicators suggest the effectiveness of slow-stroke back massage and hand massage in promoting relaxation in older people across all settings (Harris & Richards, 2010). In a randomized controlled trial investigating

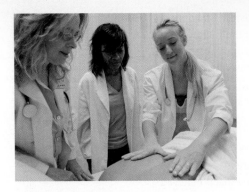

Figure 16-8 Dr. Melodee Harris instructs nursing students in the method of slow-stroke back massage.

Courtesy of Carr College of Nursing, Harding University.

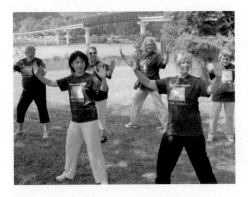

Figure 16-9 Dr. Pao-feng Tsai (front left), Alice An-Loh Sun Endowed Professor in Geriatric Nursing, provides instruction in Tai Chi.

Courtesy of UAMS College of Nursing.

the sleep effects of a 3-minute slow-stroke back massage in persons with dementia residing in the nursing home, Harris (2010) found an increase of 36 minutes in the group receiving massage compared to controls. Slow-stroke back massage can be easily used by nurses and other patient care providers to promote sleep (see **Figure 16-8**).

Body-Based Modalities

Tai Chi is referred to as "moving meditation" as persons who use this modality move their bodies slowly, gently, and with awareness, while breathing deeply (National Sleep Foundation, 2010). Tai Chi is a modality that is easily adaptable to a wide range of physical limitations, making it suitable for older adults. Tai Chi has been shown to be effective in improving self-reported sleep quality in older adults with sleep complaints (Irwin, Olmstead, & Motivala, 2008) and in older adults with heart failure (Yeh et al., 2008). A systematic review of the effects of Tai Chi, including those clinical trials that enrolled older adults, concluded that the strongest evidence for Tai Chi is in the prevention of falls and in improvement in psychological health, not in sleep parameters, per se (Lee, Ernst, & Choi, 2010). Tai chi can be adapted for use by older adults (see **Figure 16-9**).

Cranial Electrical Stimulation

Cranial electrical stimulation (CES) refers to the delivery of small, imperceptible amounts of microcurrent via clips to the ears. While the precise mechanisms of action of CES are unknown, it is hypothesized that CES may inhibit the reuptake of norepinephrine, serotonin, and dopamine (Shealy, Cady, Culver-Veehoff, Cox, & Liss, 1998). Studies of CES are mixed, with no conclusive evidence to suggest the widespread use of this modality to improve sleep in older adults. Rose, Taylor, and Bourguignon (2009) reported improvement of daily sleep disturbances trending toward statistical significance and clinical improvement in sleep onset latency in elders receiving CES, although overall findings were inconclusive. A CES device is shown in **Figure 16-10**.

Energy Fields

Light therapy is a form of CAM that involves the manipulation of energy or "biofields" (NCCAM, 2011a). It is based on the circadian rhythm-related response to long-wavelength (green) light and short wavelength (blue) light levels (Gooley et al., 2010; NCCAM, 2011a). Light therapy has been used for some time in the management of seasonal affective disorder (Terman, 2007), but there is limited high-quality evidence to support the use of light therapy for sleep disturbance in healthy older adults (Montgomery & Dennis, 2009a, 2009b). Early-morning awakening insomnia, subjective and objective sleep measures, and daytime functioning were improved for up to 1 month after two evenings of bright light therapy in a small sample of adults and older adults (Lack, Wright, Kemp, & Gibbon, 2005).

A number of small, randomized controlled trials have also explored light therapy in the management of sleep in older persons with dementia. Overall, their findings suggest no significant sleep improvements for this population (Forbes et al., 2009), although 1 hour of morning or evening bright light exposure did facilitate entrainment to the 24-hour day (Dowling, Mastick, Hubbard, Luxenberg, & Burr, 2005). A study using brief bright or dim morning light exposure in persons with dementia and their caregivers found improved sleep in the caregivers only, whether receiving bright or dim light therapy (Friedman et al., 2012).

Older adults may be intolerant of bright light therapy and they should have opthalmological eye exams prior to its use. It should be used with caution in older adults with mania, retinal photosensitivity, or migraine headaches (Bloom et al., 2009).

Consequently, light therapy for sleep disturbance or circadian sleep disorders in either healthy older adults or in those with dementia has not yet been clearly established as effective. Possible adverse consequences of light therapy also require further investigation.

While other CAM modalities have been investigated to document their efficacy for improving sleep in older adults, because research is limited in these areas, no formal recommendations for use of these other modalities in older adults is warranted at this time.

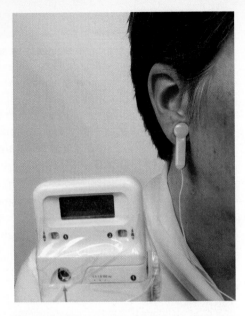

Figure 16-10 Dr. Karen Rose demonstrates the use of a Cranial Electrical Stimulator device.

Courtesy of the University of Virginia, School of Nursing, and Alpha-Stim (Mineral Wells, TX).

Summary

Geriatric nurses should be aware of the positive implications of sleep for health promotion in older adults, as well as the potential negative implications of sleep disturbance for quality of life in this population. Disturbed sleep appears to have a bidirectional relationship with many common disease processes in older adults such as depression, anxiety, heart disease, hypertension, and diabetes, as well as with many of the medications used to treat these disorders. Consequently, the care of older adults with sleep disturbance and multiple chronic diseases/disorders requires a holistic approach, in close collaboration with other healthcare providers. Sleep should be routinely included in nursing assessments of older adults, and should be monitored periodically to detect changes that may indicate emerging alterations in health status or in response to therapy. **Boxes 16-9, 16-10**, and **16-11** provide additional resources on sleep in older adults.

BOX 16-9 Research Highlight

Aim: This study investigated subjective sleep quality in women aged 50 years and older as predicted by breast cancer or noncancer status, age, number of comorbidities, and symptoms of depressed mood. Objective sleep characteristics, insomnia symptom severity, and daytime sleepiness were also compared in this population of women with and without breast cancer.

Methods: Sixty-seven community-dwelling older women aged 50 to 90 years (mean 65 years) met study criteria and comprised the final sample. Demographic data was collected using an investigator-developed form, and clinical data was collected for the breast cancer group using electronic medical record review. Subjective sleep quality was assessed using the Pittsburgh Quality of Sleep Index (PSQI) (Buysse, Reynolds, Monk, Berman, & Kupfer, 1989), and depressed mood was assessed using the Profile of Mood States (POMS) (McNair & Heuchert, 2005). Objective sleep was assessed using 72 hours of home wrist actigraphy combined with a patient-maintained Pittsburgh Sleep Diary (Monk et al., 1994). Insomnia and daytime sleepiness symptoms were assessed using the Insomnia Severity Index (ISI) (Morin, 1993), and the Epworth Sleepiness Scale (ESS) (Johns, 1991, 1992), respectively. All subjective data was collected by two phone or face-to-face interviews, approximately 1 month apart, and the results were averaged.

Findings: Only depressed mood significantly predicted poor subjective sleep quality (p < 0.00005). Breast cancer and comparison groups demonstrated similar objective sleep characteristics. Both groups demonstrated frequent nighttime awakenings (mean 9.2 versus 7.3). The breast cancer group had longer sleep onset latency than the comparison group (mean 34.8 versus 15.6 minutes). The breast cancer group reported insomnia severity scores in the subthreshold insomnia range, while the comparison group reported no clinical significant insomnia symptoms (mean 8.9 versus 6.4). Both groups reported similar daytime sleepiness scores within the normal range (7 versus 6).

Application to Practice: Exacerbated sleep disturbance in older women with breast cancer may be prevented by early identification and intermittent monitoring of sleep disturbance.

Source: Adapted from Enderlin, C.A., Coleman, E. A., Cole, C., Richards, K. C., Kennedy, R. L., Goodwin, J. A., ... Mack, K., 2011, Subjective sleep quality, objective sleep characteristics, insomnia symptom severity, and daytime sleepiness in women aged 50 and older with nonmetastatic breast cancer. *Oncology Nursing Forum, 38,* E314–E325.

BOX 16-10 Recommended Resources

Resource	Website
American Academy of Dental Sleep Medicine	http://www.dentalsleepmed.org http://www.aadsm.org/PatientResources.aspx http://www.aadsm.org/PubResearch.aspx
American Academy of Sleep Medicine	http://www.aasmnet.org/ http://www.aasmnet.org/practiceparameters.aspx http://www.sleepeducation.com/

Resource	Website
American Sleep Apnea Association	http://www.sleepapnea.org/
American Sleep Association	http://www.sleepassociation.org/
Association for Behavioral and Cognitive Therapies	http://www.abct.org/Home/ http://www.abct.org/docs/Members/FactSheets/Aging%200907.pdf http://www.abct.org/docs/Members/FactSheets/INSOMNIA%200707.pdf
Geriatrics at Your Fingertips Sleep Disorders	http://www.geriatricsatyourfingertips.org/
Hartford Institute for Geriatric Nursing	http://consultgerirn.org/topics/sleep/
Narcolepsy Network, Inc.	http://www.narcolepsynetwork.org/
National Sleep Foundation Sleep in America Poll 2003, Sleep in Aging	http://www.sleepfoundation.org/primary-links/how-sleep-works http://www.sleepfoundation.org/article/sleep-america-polls/2003-sleep-and-aging
Oncology Nursing Society	www.ons.org/Research/PEP/Sleep
Restless Legs Syndrome Foundation	http://www.rls.org/
Society of Behavioral Sleep Medicine	http://www.behavioralsleep.org/ http://www.behavioralsleep.org/WhatIsBSM.aspx

BOX 16-11   Evidence-Based Practice

Aim: The aim of this meta-analysis was to evaluate the effectiveness of current studies using dietary weight loss interventions to treat obstructive sleep apnea (OSA) in obese patients.

Methods: PubMed, EMBASE, CINAHL, Web of Science, and The Cochrane Central Register of Controlled Trials were searched through September 2011 using study design, patient characteristics, pre- and post-dietary weight loss measures of OSA, and body mass index (BMI). Two independent analysts extracted the data.

A random-effects model was used to weight the averages using 95% confidence intervals.

Findings: A total of nine articles were selected, representative of 577 patients. A BMI reduction of 4.8 kg/m^2 (95% confidence interval [CI] 3.8–5.9) was found for the dietary weight loss interventions. Pre- and postintervention random effects pooled apnea-hypopnea indices were 52.5 (range 10.0–91.0) and 28.3 events/hour respectively (range 5.4–64.5; $p < 0.001$). The dietary weight loss intervention resulted in a weight mean difference of an AHI decrease of −14.3 events/hour (95% CI -23.5 to -5.1; p = 0.002), in comparison with the control intervention.

Practice Implications: Although dietary weight loss interventions reduce the severity of OSA, they do not result in total resolution of respiratory events. However, dietary weight loss interventions may be implemented as adjunct interventions in the management of OSA.

Note. Adapted from Anandam, A., Akinnus, M., Kufel, T., Porhomayon, J., & El-Solh, E. A. (2012). Effects of dietary weight loss on obstructive sleep apnea: A meta-analysis. *Sleep and Breathing,* Advance online publication.

Critical Thinking Exercises

1. Your patient is a 69-year-old widow who is having her routine blood pressure checked. In the conversation she mentions that she is exhausted and has been having trouble sleeping. You notice that she is very slow in her speech and movement, and that her facial expression appears flat. How would you approach investigating her sleep disturbance further?

2. A 78-year-old gentleman has a follow-up visit for his congestive heart failure. While you are getting his vital signs you notice he appears sleepy. When questioned, he states that he has been very sleepy during the day, often dozes off when he gets still, and takes several naps a day. He reports no difficulty falling asleep, but does recall that he often awakens during the night for no specific reason in addition to getting up to urinate several times. His wife adds that he snores loudly and sometimes stops breathing for a time. What screening assessments should you consider in assessing his daytime sleepiness and snoring?

3. A 62-year-old woman is being seen for difficulty falling asleep. She reports that although she feels tired and ready for sleep at night, her legs bother her and often keep her awake for hours. She describes "crawling" sensations in her legs that become most noticeable in the evening, and often require her to get up and walk around to obtain relief. Although walking relieves her discomfort, she states that the sensations in her legs return when she tries to lie down and sleep. What additional information do you need to ask regarding these problematic symptoms?

Personal Reflection

1. Maintain a sleep diary for your own sleep, by going to Sleep Diary NIH Office of Science Education, available at http://science .education.nih.gov/supplements/nih3/sleep/ guide/nih_sleep_masters.pdf

2. Scan through the materials provided at this site, and test your knowledge of sleep by taking the quiz: What Do You Know (or Think You Know) about Sleep?

References

Allen, R. P., Burchell, B. J., MacDonald, B., Hening, W. A., & Earley, C. J. (2009). Validation of the self-completed Cambridge-Hopkins questionnaire (CH-RLSq) for ascertainment of restless legs syndrome (RLS) in a population survey. *Sleep Medicine, 10*(10), 1097–1100. doi: 10.1016/j.sleep.2008.10.007

American Academy of Sleep Medicine [AASM]. (2005). *The international classification of sleep disorders: Diagnostic and coding manual* (2nd ed.). Westchester, IL: Author.

American Geriatrics Society [AGS], Foundation for Health in Aging [FHA]. (2012). Ten medications older adults should avoid or use with caution. *The Foundation for Health in Aging.* Retrieved from http://www.healthinaging.org/files/documents/tipsheets/meds_to_avoid.pdf

American Geriatrics Society [AGS] 2012 Beers Criteria Update Expert Panel (2012). American Geriatrics Society updated Beers criteria for potentially inappropriate medication use in older adults. *Journal of the American Geriatrics Society, 60*(4), 616–631. doi: 10.1111/j.1532-5415.2012.03923.x

American Psychiatric Association. (2000). *Diagnostic and statistical manual of mental disorders* (4th ed.). Washington, DC: Author.

Anandam, A., Akinnusi, M., Kufel, T., Porhomayon, J., & El-Solh, A. A. (2012). Effects of dietary weight loss on obstructive sleep apnea: A meta-analysis. *Sleep and Breathing,* Advance online publication. doi: 10.1007/s11325-012-0677-3

Ancoli-Israel, S. (2007). Sleep apnea in older adults: Is it real and should age be the determining factor in the treatment decision matrix? *Sleep Medicine Reviews, 11*(2), 83–85. doi: 10.1016/j.smrv.2006.11.002

Ancoli-Israel, S. (2009). Sleep and its disorders in aging populations. *Sleep Medicine, 10,* S7–S11. doi:10.1016/j.sleep.2009.07.004

Ancoli-Israel, S., Cole, R., Alessi, C., Chambers, M., Moorcroft, W., & Pollak, C. P. (2003). The role of actigraphy in the study of sleep and circadian rhythms. *Sleep, 26*(3), 342–392. Retrieved from http://www.aasmnet.org/Resources/PracticeReviews/cpr_Actigraphy.pdf

Ancoli-Israel, S., Kripke, D. F., Klauber, M. R., Mason, W. J., Fell, R., & Kaplan, O. (1991). Periodic limb movements in sleep in community-dwelling elderly. *Sleep, 14*(6), 496–500.

Ando, K., Kripke, D. F., & Ancoli-Israel, S. (2002). Delayed and advanced sleep phase symptoms. *Israel Journal of Psychiatry and Related Sciences, 39*(1), 11–18. Retrieved from http://ukpmc.ac.uk/abstract/MED/12013705

Arendt, J. (2006). Does melatonin improve sleep? Efficacy of melatonin. *BMJ: British Medical Journal (International Edition), 332*(7540), 550.1. doi: 10.1136/bmj.332.7540.550

Barnes, P. M., Bloom, B., & Nahin, R. L. (2008). Complementary and alternative medicine use among adults and children: United States, 2007. *National Health Statistics Reports,*(12), 1–23.

Bastian, C. H., Vallieres, A., & Morin, C. M. (2001). Validation of the Insomnia Severity Index as an outcome measure for insomnia research. *Sleep Medicine,*(2), 4–297. doi:10.1016/S1389-9457(00)00065-4,

Basu, R., Dodge, H., Stoehr, G.P. & Ganguli, M. (2003). Sedative-hypnotic use of diphenhydramine in a rural, older adult, community-based cohort: effects on cognition. American Journal of Geriatric Psychiatry, *11*(2), 205–213. Retrieved from http://journals.lww.com/ajgponline/Abstract/2003/03000/Sedative_Hypnotic_Use_of_Diphenhydramine_in_a.11.aspx

Benca, R. (2005). Mood disorders. In M.H. Kryger, T. Roth, & W. C. Dement (Eds.), *Principles and practice of sleep medicine* (pp. 1311–1326). Philadelphia, PA: Elsevier Saunders.

Benca, R. M., Ancoli-Israel, S., & Moldofsky, H. (2004). Special considerations in insomnia diagnosis and management: Depressed, elderly, and chronic pain populations. *Journal of Clinical Psychiatry, 65*(Suppl8), 26–35.

Benson, K. L., & Zarcone, V. P. (2005). Schizophrenia. In M.H. Kryger, T. Roth, & W. C. Dement (Eds.), *Principles and Practice in Sleep Medicine* (pp. 1327–1336). Philadelphia, PA: Elsevier Saunders.

Berry, R. B. (2012). *Fundamentals of Sleep Medicine.* Philadelphia, PA: Elsevier Saunders.

Bliwise, D. L. (1993). Sleep in normal aging and dementia. *Sleep: Journal of Sleep Research & Sleep Medicine, 16*(1), 40–81.

Bliwise, D. L. (2005). Normal aging. In M. H. Kryger, T. Roth, & W. C. Dement (Eds.), *Principles and practice of sleep medicine* (pp. 24–38). Philadelphia, PA: Elsevier Saunders.

Bliwise, D. L., Foley, D. J., Vitiello, M. V., Farzaneh, P. A., Ancoli-Israel, S., & Walsh, J. K. (2009). Nocturia and disturbed sleep in the elderly. *Sleep Medicine, 10* (5), 540–548. doi: 10.1016/j.sleep.2008.04.002

Bloom, H.G. Ahmed, I., Alessi, C.A., Ancoli-Israel, S., Buysse, D.J., Kryer, M.H., ...Zee, P.C. (2009). Evidence-based recommendations for the assessment and management of sleep disorders in older persons. *Journal of American Geriatric Society, 57*(5), 761–769. doi:10.1111/j.1532-5415.2009.02220.x

Bootzin, R. R. (2005). Preface. In M. L. Perlis, C. Jungquist, M. T. Smith, & D. Posner (Eds.), *Cognitive behavioral treatment of insomnia: A session-by-session guide.* New York, NY: Springer.

Bootzin, R. R., Epstein, D., & Ward, J. M. (1991). Stimulus control instructions. In P. Hauri (Ed.), *Case studies in insomnia* (pp. 19–28). New York, NY: Plen Press.

Bootzin, R. R., & Perlis, M. L. (2011). Stimulus control therapy. In L. Perlis, M. Aloia, & B. Kuhn (Eds.), *Behavioral treatments for sleep disorders: A comprehensive primer of behavioral sleep medicine interventions* (pp. 21–30). Boston, MA: Elsevier.

Borbely, A. A. (1982). A two process model of sleep regulation. *Human Neurobiology, 1*(3), 195–204.

Borud, E., Grimsgaard, S., & White, A. (2010). Menopausal problems and acupuncture. *Autonomic Neuroscience: Basic & Clinical, 157*(1–2), 57–62. doi: 10.1016/j.autneu.2010.04.004

Brenes, G. A., Miller, M. E., Stanley, M. A., Williamson, J. D., Knudson, M., & McCall, W. V. (2009). Insomnia in older adults with generalized anxiety disorder. *The American Journal of Geriatric Psychiatry, 17*(6), 465–472.

Brenes, G.A., Miller, M.E., Williamson, J.D., McCall, W.V., Knudson, M. & Stanley, M.A. (2012). A randomized controlled trial of telephone-delivered cognitive-behavioral therapy for late-life anxiety disorders. *American Journal of Geriatric Psychiatry, 20*(8), 707–716. doi: 10.1097/JGP.0b013e31822ccd3e

Buscemi, N., Vandermeer, B., Pandya, R., Hooton, N., Tjosvold, L., Hartling, L., ... Klassen, T. (2004). Melatonin for treatment of sleep disorders. *Agency for Healthcare Research and Quality Evidence Report/Technology Assessments, 108*, 1–7.

Buysse, D.J., Germain, A., Moul, D.E., Franzen, P.L., Brar, L.K., Fletcher, M.E....Monk, T.H. (2012). Efficacy of brief behavioral treatment for chronic insomnia in older adults. *Archives of Internal Medicine, 171*(10), 887–895. doi:10.1001/archinternmed.2010.535

Buysse, D. J., & Perlis, M. E. (1996). The evaluation and treatment of insomnia. *Journal of Practical Psychiatry and Behavioral Health, 2*(2), 80–93.

Buysse, D. J., Reynolds III, C. F., Monk, T. H., Berman, S. R., & Kupfer, D. J. (1989). The Pittsburgh sleep quality index: A new instrument for psychiatric practice and research. *Psychiatry Research, 28*(2), 193–213. doi: 10.1016/0165-1781(89)90047-4

Cahn, S.C., Lanenbucher, J.W., Friedman, M.A., Reavey, P., Falco, T. & Pallay, R.M. (2005). Predictors of interest in psychological treatment or insomnia among older primary care patients with disturbed sleep. *Behavioral Sleep Medicine, 3*(2), 87–98. doi:10.1207/s15402010bsm0302_3

Cao, M. T., Guilleminault, C., & Kushida, C. A. (2011). Clinical features and evaluation of obstructive sleep apnea and upper airway resistance syndrome. In M. Kryger, T. Roth, & W. Dement (Eds.), *Principles and practice of sleep medicine* (5th ed., pp. 1206–1218). Philadelphia, PA: W.B. Saunders.

Carrier, J., Monk, T. H., Buysse, D. J., & Kupfer, D. J. (1997). Sleep and morningness-eveningness in the 'middle' years of life (20–59 y). *Journal of Sleep Research, 6*(4), 230–237. doi: 10.1111/j.1365-2869.1997.00230.x

Carskadon, M., & Dement, W. (2000). Normal human sleep: An overview. In M. Kryger, T. Roth, & W. Dement (Eds.), *Principles and practice of sleep medicine* (3rd ed., pp. 15–25). Philadelphia, PA: Elsevier Saunders.

Carskadon, M. A., & Dement, W. C. (1982). The Multiple Sleep Latency Test: What does it measure? *Sleep: Journal of Sleep Research & Sleep Medicine, 5*(Suppl 2), 67–72.

Carskadon, M. A., Dement, W. C., Mitler, M. M., Roth, T., Westbrook, P. R., & Keenan, S. (1986). Guidelines for the Multiple Sleep Latency Test (MSLT): A standard measure of sleepiness. *Sleep, 9*(4), 518–524.

Chesson, A., Jr., Hartse, K., Anderson, W. M., Davila, D., Johnson, S., Littner, M., ... Rafecas, J. (2000). Practice parameters for the evaluation of chronic insomnia. An American Academy of Sleep Medicine report. Standards of practice committee of the American Academy of Sleep Medicine. *Sleep, 23*(2), 237–241.

Chou, T. C., Scammell, T. E., Gooley, J. J., Gaus, S. E., Saper, C. B., & Lu, J. (2003). Critical role of dorsomedial hypothalamic nucleus in a wide range of behavioral circadian rhythms. *The Journal of Neuroscience, 23*(33), 10691–10702. Retrieved from http://www.jneurosci.org/content/23/33/10691.full.pdf+html

Chung, F., & Elsaid, H. (2009). Screening for obstructive sleep apnea before surgery: Why is it important? *Current Opinion in Anesthesiology, 22*(3), 405–411. doi: 10.1097/ACO.0b013e32832a96e2

Chung, F., Yegneswaran, B., Liao, P., Chung, S. A., Vairavanathan, S., Islam, S., … Shapiro, C. M. (2008). STOP questionnaire: A tool to screen patients for obstructive sleep apnea. *Anesthesiology, 108*(5), 812–821. doi: 10.1097/ALN.0b013e31816d83e4

Cole, C. S., & Richards, K. C. (2005). Sleep and cognition in people with Alzheimer's disease. *Issues in Mental Health Nursing, 26*(7), 687–698. doi: 10.1080/01612840591008258

Collop, N. A. (2006). Polysomnography. In T. Lee-Chiong (Ed.), *Sleep: A comprehensive handbook* (pp. 973–976). Hoboken, NJ: Wiley-Liss.

Crowley, K. (2011). Sleep and sleep disorders in older adults. *Neuropsychology Review, 21*(1), 41–53. doi: 10.1007/s11065-010-9154-6

Crystal, S., Sambamoorthi, U., Walkup, J. T., & Akincigil, A. (2003). Diagnosis and treatment of depression in the elderly Medicare population: Predictors, disparities, and trends. *Journal of the American Geriatrics Society, 51*(12), 1718. doi: 10.1046/j.1532-5415.2003.51555.x

Czeisler, C. A., & Dumont, M. (1992). Association of sleep–wake habits in older people with changes in output of circadian pacemaker. *Lancet, 340*(8825), 933. doi: 10.1016/0140-6736(92)92817-Y

Dement, W. C. (2011). History of sleep physiology and medicine. In M. Kryger, T. Roth, & W. Dement (Eds.), *Principles and practice of sleep medicine* (5th ed., pp. 3–15). Philadelphia, PA: W.B. Saunders.

Dew, M. A., Hoch, C. C., Buysse, D. J., Monk, T. H., Begley, A. E., Houck, P. R., … Reynolds III, C.F. (2003). Healthy older adults' sleep predicts all-cause mortality at 4 to 19 years of follow-up. *Psychosomatic Medicine, 65*(1), 63–73. doi: 10.1097/01.PSY.0000039756.23250.7C

Dowling, G.A., Mastick, J., Hubbard, E.M., Luxenberg, J.S. & Burr, R.L. (2005). Effect of timed bright light treatment for rest-activity disruption in institutionalized patients with Alzheimer's disease. *International Journal of Geriatric Psychiatry, 20*(8), 738–743. doi:10.1002/gps.1352

Driscoll, H. C., Serody, L., Patrick, S., Maurer, J., Bensasi, S., Houck, P. R.… Reynolds III, C.F. (2008). Sleeping well, aging well: A descriptive and cross-sectional study of sleep in "successful agers" 75 and older. *American Journal of Geriatric Psychiatry, 16*(1), 74–82. doi: 10.1097/JGP.0b013e3181557b69

Edinger, J. D., Wohlgemuth, W. K., Radtke, R. A., Marsh, G. R., & Quillian, R. E. (2001). Cognitive behavioral therapy for treatment of chronic primary insomnia: A randomized controlled trial. *Journal of the American Medical Association, 285*(14), 1856–1864.

Enderlin, C.A., Coleman, E. A., Cole, C., Richards, K. C., Kennedy, R. L., Goodwin, J. A., … Mack, K. (2011). Subjective sleep quality, objective sleep characteristics, insomnia symptom severity, and daytime sleepiness in women aged 50 and older with nonmetastatic breast cancer. *Oncology Nursing Forum, 38*(4), E314–E325. doi: 10.1188/11.ONF.E314-E325

Epstein, D. R., & Bootzin, R. R. (2002). Insomnia. *The Nursing Clinics of North America, 37*(4), 611–631. doi: 10.1016/S0029-6465(02)00028-2

Espie, C. A. (2011). Paradoxical intention therapy. In *Behavioral Treatments for Sleep Disorders* (pp. 61–70). San Diego, CA: Academic Press.

Espie, C. A., MacMahon, K. M., Kelly, H. L., Broomfield, N. M., Douglas, N. J., Engleman, H. M., … Wilson, P. (2007). Randomized clinical effectiveness trial of nurse-administered small-group cognitive behavior therapy for persistent insomnia in general practice. *Sleep, 30*(5), 574–584.

Foley, D., Ancoli-Israel, S., Britz, P., & Walsh, J. (2004). Sleep disturbances and chronic disease in older adults: Results of the 2003 National Sleep Foundation Sleep in America Survey. *Journal of Psychosomatic Research, 56*(5), 497–502. doi: 10.1016/j.jpsychores.2004.02.010

Foley, D.J., Monjan, A., Simonsick, E.M., Wallace, R.B., & Blazer, D.G. (1999). Incidence and remission of insomnia among elderly adults: an epidemiologic study of 6,800 persons over three years. *Sleep: Journal of Sleep Research & Sleep Medicine, 22*(Suppl 2), S366–S372.

Forbes, D., Culum, I., Lischka, A.R., Morgan, D.G., Peacock, S., Forbes, J.,...Forbes, S. (2009). Light therapy for managing cognitive, sleep, functional, behavioral, or psychiatric disturbances in dementia. *Cochrane Database of Systematic Reviews*, Issue 4. doi: 10.1002/14651858.CD003946.pub3

Friedman, L., Spira, A.P., Hernandez, B., Mather, C., Sheikh, J., Ancoli-Israel, S.,... Zeitzer, J. M. (2012). Brief morning light treatment for sleep/wake disturbances in older memory-impaired individuals and their caregivers. *Sleep Medicine*, 13, 546–549. doi:10.1016/j.sleep.2011.11.013

Friedman, M., Tanyeri, H., La Rosa, M., Landsberg, R., Vaidyanathan, K., Pieri, S., & Caldarelli, D. (1999). Clinical predictors of obstructive sleep apnea. *The Laryngoscope, 109*(12), 1901–1907. doi:10.1097/00005537-199912000-00002

Fuller, P. M., Gooley, J. J., & Saper, C. B. (2006). Neurobiology of the Sleep-Wake Cycle: Sleep architecture, circadian regulation, and regulatory feedback. *Journal of Biological Rhythms, 21*(6), 482–493. doi: 10.1177/0748730406294627

Fulmer, T. (2007). How to try this. Fulmer SPICES: A framework of six 'marker conditions' can help focus assessment of hospitalized older patients. *American Journal of Nursing, 107*(10), 40–49. doi: 10.1097/01.NAJ.0000292197.76076.e1

Germain, A., & Buysse, D. J. (2011). Brief behavioral treatment of insomnia. In L. Perlis, M. Aloia, & B. Kuhn (Eds.), *Behavioral treatments for sleep disorders* (pp. 143–150). San Diego, CA: Academic Press.

Gooley, J. J., Rajaratnam, S. M., Brainard, G. C., Kronauer, R. E., Czeisler, C. A., & Lockley, S.W. (2010). Spectral responses of the human circadian system depend on the irradiance and duration of exposure to light. *Science Translational Medicine, 2*(31), 1–9. doi:10.1126/scitranslmed.3000741

Gooneratne, N. S. (2008). Complementary and alternative medicine for sleep disturbances in older adults. *Clinics In Geriatric Medicine, 24*(1), 121. doi: 10.1016/j.cger.2007.08.002

Gu, D., Sautter, J., Pipkin, R., & Zeng, Y. (2010). Sociodemographic and health correlates of sleep quality and duration among very old Chinese. *Sleep, 33*(5), 601–610.

Guilleminault, C., & Cao, M. T. (2011). Narcolepsy: Diagnosis and management. In M. Kryger, T. Roth, & W. Dement (Eds.), *Principles and practice of sleep medicine* (5th ed., pp. 957–968). Philadelphia, PA: W.B. Saunders.

Haimov, I., Hanuka, E., & Horowitz, Y. (2008). Chronic insomnia and cognitive functioning among older adults. *Behavioral Sleep Medicine, 6*(1), 32–54. doi: 10.1080/15402000701796080

Harris, M. (2010). The effects of slow-stroke back massage on minutes of nighttime sleep in persons with dementia in the nursing home: A pilot study. *Geriatric Nursing, 31*(1), 70.

Harris, M., & Richards, K. C. (2010). The physiological and psychological effects of slow-stroke back massage and hand massage on relaxation in older people. *Journal of Clinical Nursing, 19*(7/8), 917–926. doi: 10.1111/j.1365-2702.2009.03165.x

Hartford Institute for Geriatric Nursing. (2012). *Assessment tools: Try this and how to try this resources.* Retrieved from http://consultgerirn.org/resources

Hauri, P. (1991). *Case studies in insomnia.* New York, NY: Plenum.

Iber, C., Ancoli-Israel, S., Chesson, A., Quan, S. F., & The American Academy of Sleep Medicine. (2007). *The AASM manual for the scoring of sleep and associated events: Rules, terminology and technical specifications.* Westchester, NY: American Academy of Sleep Medicine.

Irwin, M. R., Olmstead, R., & Motivala, S. J. (2008). Improving sleep quality in older adults with moderate sleep complaints: A randomized controlled trial of Tai Chi Chih. *Sleep, 31*(7), 1001–1008.

Jeste, D. V., Alexopoulos, G. S., Bartels, S. J., Cummings, J. L., Gallo, J. J., Gottlieb, G. L. ... Lebowitz, B. D. (1999). Consensus statement on the upcoming crisis in geriatric mental health: Research agenda for the next 2 decades. *Archives of General Psychiatry, 56*(9), 848–853.

Johansson, P., Alehagen, U., Svanborg, E., Dahlstrom, U., & Brostrom, A. (2012). Clinical characteristics and mortality risk in relation to obstructive and central sleep apnoea in community-dwelling elderly individuals: a 7-year follow-up. *Age and Ageing,* Advance online publication. doi: 10.1093/ageing/afs019

Johns, M. W. (1991). A new method for measuring daytime sleepiness: The Epworth Sleepiness Scale. *Sleep, 14*(6), 540–545.

Johns, M. W. (1993). Daytime sleepiness, snoring, and obstructive sleep apnea. The Epworth Sleepiness Scale. *Chest, 103*(1), 30–36.

Johns, M. W. (1992). Reliability and factor analysis of the Epworth Sleepiness Scale. *Sleep: Journal of Sleep Research & Sleep Medicine, 15*(4), 376–381.

Johns, M. W. (1994). Sleepiness in different situations measured by the Epworth Sleepiness Scale. *Sleep: Journal of Sleep Research & Sleep Medicine, 17*(8), 703–710.

Jun, L., Sherman, D., Devor, M., & Saper, C. B. (2006). A putative flip-flop switch for control of REM sleep. *Nature, 441*(7093), 589–594. doi: 10.1038/nature04767

Kapella, M. C., Herdegen, J. J., Perlis, M. L., Shaver, J. L., Larson, J. L., Law, J. A., & Carley, D. W. (2011). Cognitive behavioral therapy for insomnia comorbid with COPD is feasible with preliminary evidence of positive sleep and fatigue effects. *International Journal of Chronic Obstructive Pulmonary Disease, 6*, 625–635. doi:10.2147/COPD.S24858

Kazenwadel, J., Pollmcher, T., Trenkwalder, C., Oertel, W. H., Kohnen, R., Kunzel, M., & Kruger, H. P. (1995). New actigraphic assessment method for periodic leg movements (PLM). *Sleep, 18*(8), 689–697.

Kemlink, D., Pretl, M., Sonka, K., & Nevsimalova, S. (2008). A comparison of polysomnographic and actigraphic evaluation of periodic limb movements in sleep. *Neurological Research, 30*(3), 234–238. doi: 10.1179/016164107X229911

Krystal, A. D. (2011). Pharmacologic treatment: Other medications. In M. Kryger, T. Roth, & W. Dement (Eds.), *Principles and practice of sleep medicine* (5th ed., pp. 916–930). Philadelphia, PA: W.B. Saunders.

Kushida, C. A., & Efron, B. (1997). A predictive morphometric model for the Obstructive Sleep Apnea Syndrome. *Annals of Internal Medicine, 127*(8), 581–587.

LaReau, R., Benson, L. & Kuanwong, W. (2008). Examining the feasibility of implementing specific nursing interventions to promote sleep in hospitalized elderly patients. *Geriatric Nursing, 29*(3), 197–206. doi:10.1016/j.gerinurse.2007.10.020

Lack, L., Wright, H., Kemp, K. & Gibbon, S. (2005). The treatment of early-morning awakening insomnia with 2 evenings of bright light. *Sleep, 28*(5), 616–623.

Lee, M. S., Ernst, E., & Choi, T. Y. (2010). Tai Chi for breast cancer patients: A systematic review. *Breast cancer research and treatment, 120*(2), 309–316. doi: 10.1007/s10549-010-0741-2

Lee-Chiong, T. (2008). *Sleep medicine: Essentials and review*. Oxford, UK: Oxford University Press.

Leger, D., Scheuermaier, K., Philip, P., Paillard, M., & Guilleminault, C. (2001). SF-36: Evaluation of quality of life in severe and mild insomniacs compared with good sleepers. *Psychosomatic Medicine, 63*(1), 49–55.

Lichstein, K. L., Riedel, B. W., Wilson, N. M. Lester, K. W., & Aguillard, R. N. (2001). Relaxation and sleep compression for late-life insomnia: A placebo-controlled trial. *Journal of Consulting and Clinical Psychology, 69*(2), 227–229. doi: 10.1037/0022-006X.69.2.227

Lichstein, K. L., Taylor, D. J., McCrae, C. S., & Thomas, S. J. (2011). Relaxation for insomnia. In L. Perlis, M. Aloia, & B. Kuhn (Eds.), *Behavioral treatments for sleep disorders: A comprehensive primer of behavioral sleep medicine interventions* (pp. 45–54). Boston, MA: Elsevier.

Lichstein, K. L., Thomas, S. J., & McCurry, S. M. (2011). Sleep compression. In L. Perlis, M. Aloia, & B. Kuhn (Eds.), *Behavioral treatments for sleep disorders: A comprehensive primer of behavioral sleep medicine interventions* (pp. 55–60). Boston, MA: Elsevier.

Mallampati, S. R., Gatt, S. P., Gugino, L. D., Desai, S. P., Waraksa, B., Freiberger, D., & Liu, P. L. (1985). A clinical sign to predict difficult tracheal intubation: a prospective study. *Canadian Anaesthetists' Society Journal, 32*(4), 429–434. doi:10.1007/BF03011357

Mann, E., Smith, M. J., Hellier, J., Balabanovic, J. A., Amed, H., Grunfeld, E. A., & Hunter, M. S. (2012). Cognitive behavioural treatment for women who have menopausal symptoms after breast cancer treatment (MENOS 1): A randomised controlled trial. *Lancet Oncology, 13*(3), 309–318. doi:10.1016/S1470-2045(11)70364-3

McCrae, C. S., McGovern, R., Lukefahr, R., & Stripling, A. M. (2011). Research Evaluating Brief Behavioral Sleep Treatments for Rural Elderly (RESTORE): A preliminary examination of effectiveness. *American Journal of Geriatric Psychiatry, 15*(11), 979–982. doi:10.1097/JGP.0b013e31813547e6

McGinty, D., & Szymusiak, R. (2003). Hypothalamic regulation of sleep and arousal. *Frontiers in Bioscience, 1*(8s), 1074–1083. doi:10.1196/annals.1417.027

McGinty, D., & Szymusiak, R. (2011). Neural control of sleep in mammals. In M. Kryger, T. Roth, & W. Dement (Eds.), *Principles and practice of sleep medicine* (5th ed., pp. 76–91). Philadelphia, PA: W.B. Saunders.

McNair, D. M. & Heuchert, J. W. P. (2005). Profile of Mood States (POMS), Technical Update. North Tonawanda, NY: Multi-Health Systems.

Mesas, A. E., Lopez-Garcia, E., Leon-Munoz, L. M., Graciani, A., Guallar-Castillon, P., & Rodriguez-Artalejo, F. (2011). The association between habitual sleep duration and sleep quality in older adults according to health status. *Age & Ageing, 40*(3), 318–323. doi: 10.1093/ageing/afr004

Misra, S. & Malow, B.A. (2008). Evaluation of sleep disturbances in older adults. *Clinical Geriatric Medicine, 24*(1), 15–26. doi:10.1016/j.cger.2007.08.011

Missildine, K. (2008). Sleep and the sleep environment of older adults in acute care settings. *Journal of Gerontological Nursing, 34*(6), 15–21.

Monk, T. H., Reynolds, C. F., Kupfer, D. J., Buysse, D. J. Coble, P. A., Hayes, A. J., Machen, M. A., Petrie, S. R. and Ritenout, A. M. (1994). The Pittsburgh Sleep Diary. *Journal of Sleep Research*, 3, 111±120.

Montgomery, P. & Dennis, J.A. (2009a). Bright light therapy for sleep problems in adults aged 60+. *Cochrane Database of Systematic Reviews*, Issue 1. doi:10.1002/14651858.CDC003403

Montgomery, P. & Dennis, J.A. (2009b). Cognitive behavioral interventions for sleep problems in adults aged 60+. *Cochrane Database of Systematic Reviews*, Issue 1. doi:10.1002/14651858.CD003161

Montplaisir, J., Allen, R. P., Arthur, W., & Ferini-Strambi, L. (2011). Restless legs syndrome and periodic limb movements during sleep. In M. Kryger, T. Roth, & W. Dement (Eds.), *Principles and practice of sleep medicine* (5th ed., pp. 1026–1037). Philadelphia, PA: W.B. Saunders.

Morgenthaler, T., Alessi, C., Friedman, L., Owens, J., Kapur, V., Boehlecke, B. … American Academy of Sleep Medicine. (2007). Practice parameters for the use of actigraphy in the assessment of sleep and sleep disorders: An update for 2007. *Sleep, 30*(4), 519–529.

Morgenthaler, T., Kramer, M., Alessi, C., Friedman, L., Boehlecke, B., Brown, T. … Academy of Sleep Medicine. (2006). Practice parameters for the psychological and behavioral treatment of insomnia: An update. An American Academy of Sleep Medicine report. *Sleep, 29*(11), 1415–1419.

Morin, C. M., LeBlanc, M., Daley, M., Gregoire, J. P., & Merette, C. (2006). Epidemiology of insomnia: prevalence, self-help treatments, consultations, and determinants of help-seeking behaviors. *Sleep Medicine, 7*(2), 123–130. doi: 10.1016/j.sleep.2005.08.008

Morin, C. M., Mimeault, V., & Gagne, A. (1999). Nonpharmacological treatment of late-life insomnia. *Journal of Psychosomatic Research, 46*(2), 103–116. doi:10.1016/S0022-3999(98)00077-4

Morin, C. M. (1993). Insomnia: Psychological Assessment and Management. New York, NY: Guilford Press.

National Association of Cognitive Behavioral Therapy. National Online Headquarters. (2007). *Cognitive Behavioral Therapy* (2007). Retrieved from http://www.nacbt.org/whatiscbt.htm

National Center for Complementary and Alternative Medicine [NCCAM]. (2007). *Acupuncture*. Retrieved from http://nccam.nih.gov/health/acupuncture/introduction.htm

National Center for Complementary and Alternative Medicine [NCCAM]. (2011a). *Light therapy: The intensity and duration of exposure to light can affect the circadian rhythm*. Retrieved from http://nccam.nih.gov/research/results/spotlight/051710.htm

National Center for Complementary and Alternative Medicine [NCCAM]. (2011b). *Tai Chi*. Retrieved from http://nccam.nih.gov/health/taichi/introduction.htm

National Center for Complementary and Alternative Medicine [NCCAM]. (2012). *What is CAM?* Retrieved from http://nccam.nih.gov/health/whatiscam

National Sleep Foundation. (2010). *2003 Sleep in America Poll*. Washington, DC: Author.

Nebes, R. D., Buysse, D. J., Halligan, E. M., Houck, P. R., & Monk, T. H. (2009). Self-reported sleep quality predicts poor cognitive performance in healthy older adults. *Journal of Gerontology Psychological Sciences, 64B*(2), 180–187. doi:10.1093/geronb/gbn037

Neikrug, A. B., & Ancoli-Israel, S. (2010). Sleep disorders in the older adult: A mini-review. *Gerontology, 56*(2), 181–189. doi: 10.1159/000236900

Nerbass, F. B., Feltrim, M. I. Z., Souza, S. A. D., Ykeda, D. S., & Lorenzi-Filho, G. (2010). Effects of massage therapy on sleep quality after coronary artery bypass graft surgery. *Clinics (Sao Paulo, Brazil), 65*(11), 1105–1110. doi:10.1590/S1807-59322010001100008

Neubauer, D. (2003). *Understanding sleeplessness: Perspectives on insomnia.* Baltimore, MD: John Hopkins University Press.

Ohayon, M. M. (2002). Epidemiology of insomnia: What we know and what we still need to learn. *Sleep Medicine Reviews, 6*(2), 97–111. doi:10.1053/smrv02002.0186

Ohayon, M. M., Carskadon, M. A., Guilleminault, C., & Vitiello, M. V. (2004). Meta-Analysis of quantitative sleep parameters from childhood to old age in healthy individuals: Developing normative sleep values across the human lifespan. *Sleep, 27*(7), 1255–1273.

Perlis, M. L., Jungquist, C., Smith, M. T., & Posner, D. (2005). *Cognitive behavioral treatment for insomnia: A session-by-session guide.* New York: Springer.

Perlis, M. L., & Gehrman, P. R. (2011). Cognitive restructuring: Cognitive therapy for catastrophic sleep beliefs. In L. Perlis & B. Kuhn (Eds.), *Behavioral treatments for sleep disorders: A comprehensive primer on behavioral sleep medicine interventions* (pp. 119–126). Boston, MA: Elsevier.

Petit, D., Montplaisir, J., & Boeve, B. F. (2005). Alzheimer's disease and other dementia. In M. Kryger, T. Roth, & W. Dement (Eds.), *Principles and practice of sleep medicine* (pp. 853–862). Philadelphia, PA: Elsevier Saunders.

Posner, D., & Gehrman, P. R. (2011). Sleep hygiene. In L. Perlis, M. Aloia, & B. Kuhn (Eds.), *Behavioral treatments for sleep disorders: A comprehensive primer of behavioral sleep medicine interventions* (pp. 31–44). Boston, MA: Elsevier.

Postuma, R. B., Gagnon, J. F., Vendette, M., Fantini, M. L., Massicotte-Marquez, J., & Montplaisir, J. (2009). Quantifying the risk of neurodegenerative disease in idiopathic REM sleep behavior disorder. *Neurology, 72*(15), 1296–1300. doi: 10.1212/01.wnl.0000340980.19702.6e

Redeker, N. S. (2011). Developmental aspects of sleep. In N.S. Redeker & G. P. McEnany (Eds.), *Sleep disorders and sleep promotion in nursing practice* (pp. 19–32). New York, NY: Springer.

Richards, K. C. (1998). Effect of a back massage and relaxation intervention on sleep in critically ill patients. *American Journal of Critical Care: An Official Publication, American Association of Critical-Care Nurses, 7*(4), 288–299.

Riemann, D., & Perlis, M. L. (2009). The treatments of chronic insomnia: A review of benzodiazepine receptor agonists and psychological and behavioral therapies. *Sleep Medicine Reviews, 13*(3), 205–214. doi: 10.1016/j.smrv.2008.06.001

Rose, K. M., Taylor, A. G., & Bourguignon, C. (2009). Effects of cranial electrical stimulation on sleep disturbances, depressive symptoms, and caregiving appraisal in spousal caregivers of persons with Alzheimer's disease. *Applied Nursing Research: ANR, 22*(2), 119–125. doi: 10.1016/j.apnr.2007.06.001

Rybarczyk, B., Stapanski, E., Fogg, L., Lopez, M., Barry, P. & Davis, A. (2005). A placebo-controlled test of cognitive-behavioral therapy for comorbid insomnia in older adults. *Journal of Consulting and Clinical Psychology, 73*(6), 1164–1174. doi:10.1037/0022-006X.73.6.1164

Rybarczyk, B., Mack, L., Harris, J.H. & Stepanski, E. (2011). Testing two types of self-help CBT-I for insomnia in older adults with arthritis or coronary artery disease. *Rehabilitation Psychology, 56*(4), 257–266. doi: 10.1037/a0025577

Sack, R. L., Auckley, D., Auger, R. R., Carskadon, M. A., Wright, K. P., Jr., Vitiello, M. V., & Zhdanova, I. V. (2007). Circadian rhythm sleep disorders: Part II, advanced sleep phase disorder, delayed sleep phase disorder, free-running disorder, and irregular sleep-wake rhythm: An American academy of sleep medicine review. *Sleep, 30*(11), 1484–1501.

Scheer, F. A., & Shea, S. A. (2009). Fundamentals of the circadian system. In C. J. Amlaner & P. M. Fuller (Eds.), *Basics of Sleep Guide* (2nd ed., pp. 199–221). Westchester, NY: Sleep Research Society.

Schutte-Rodin, S., Broch, L., Buysse, D., Dorsey, C., & Sateia, M. (2008). Clinical guideline for the evaluation and management of chronic insomnia in adults. *Journal of Clinical Sleep Medicine, 4*(5), 487–504.

Semia, T. P., Beizer, J. L., & Hibgee, M. D. (2012). *Geriatric dosage handbook* (17th ed.). Hudson, NY: Lexicomp.

Sharma, M., Palacios-Bois, J., Schwartz, G., & Iskandar, H. (1989). Circadian rhythms of melatonin and cortisol in aging. *Biological Psychiatry, 25*(3), 305–319. doi:10.1016/0006-3223(89)90178-9

Shealy, C. M., Cady, R. K., Culver-Veehoff, D., Cox, R., & Liss, S. (1998). Cerebrospinal fluid and plasma neurochemicals: Response to cranial electrical stimulation. *Journal of Neurological and Orthopaedic Medicine and Surgery, 18*(2), 94–97.

Silva, G. E., An, M. W., Goodwin, J. L., Shahar, E., Redline, S., Resnick, H. … Quan, S. F. (2009). Longitudinal evaluation of sleep-disordered breathing and sleep symptoms with change in quality of life: The Sleep Heart Health Study (SHHS). *Sleep, 32*(8), 1049–1057.

Smith, M. T., Perlis, M. L., Park, A., Smith, M. S., Pennington, J., Giles, D. E., & Buysse, D. J. (2002). Comparative meta-analysis of pharmacotherapy and behavior therapy for persistent insomnia. *The American Journal of Psychiatry, 159*(1), 5–10.

Spielman, A. J., Yang, C.-M., & Glovinsky, P. B. (2011). Sleep restriction therapy. In L. Perlis, M. Aloia, & B. Kuhn (Eds.), *Behavioral treatments for sleep disorders: A comprehensive primer of behavioral sleep medicine interventions*. Boston, MA: Elsevier.

Spielman, A. J., Saskin, P., & Thorpy, M. J. (1987). Treatment of chronic insomnia by restriction of time in bed. *Sleep, 10*(1), 45–56.

Stein, M. B., & Mellman, T. A. (2005). Anxiety disorders. In M. Kryger, T. Roth, & W. Dement (Eds.), *Principles and practice of sleep medicine* (pp. 418–434). Philadelphia, PA: Elsevier Saunders.

Stone, K. L., Ancoli-Israel, S., Blackwell, T., Ensrud, K. E., Cauley, J. A., Redline, S. S. … Cummings, S. R. (2008). Poor sleep is associated with increased risk of falls in older women. *Archives of Internal Medicine, 168*, 1768–1775.

Substance Abuse and Mental Health Services Administration [SAMHSA]. (2007). *An action plan for behavioral health workforce development*. Retrieved from http://www.samhsa.gov/Workforce/Annapolis/WorkforceActionPlan.pdf

Taibi, D. M., Landis, C. A., Petry, H., & Vitiello, M. V. (2007). A systematic review of valerian as a sleep aid: Safe but not effective. *Sleep Medicine Reviews, 11*(3), 209–230. doi: 10.1016/j.smrv.2007.03.002

Taylor, D. J., Mallory, L. J., Lichstein, K. L., Durrence, H. H., Riedel, B. W., & Bush, A. J. (2007). Comorbidity of chronic insomnia with medical problems. *Sleep, 30*(2), 213–218.

Terman, M. (2007). Evolving applications of light therapy. *Sleep Medicine Reviews, 11*(6), 497–507. doi:10.1016/j.smrv.2007.06.003

Tyron, W. W. (1991). *Activity measurement in psychology and medicine*. New York, NY: Plenum Press.

Vance, D. E., Heaton, K., Eaves, Y. & Fazeli, P. L. (2011). Sleep and cognition on everyday functioning in older adults: Implications for nursing practice and research. *Journal of Neuroscience Nursing, 43*(5), 261–271. doi:10.1097/JNN.0b013e318227efb2

Vaughn, B. V., & D'Cruz, O. F. (2011). Cardinal manifestations of sleep disorders. In M. Kryger, T. Roth, & W. Dement (Eds.), *Principles and practice of sleep medicine* (5th ed., pp. 647–657). Philadelphia, PA: W.B. Saunders.

Vaz Fragoso, C. A., & Gill, T. M. (2007). Sleep complaints in community-living older persons: A multifactorial geriatric syndrome. *Journal of the American Geriatrics Society, 55*(11), 1853–1866. doi: 10.1111/j.1532-5415.2007.01399.x

Vitiello, M. V. (2006). Sleep in normal aging. *Sleep Medicine Clinics, 1*(2), 171–176.

Vitiello, M. V., & Borson, S. (2001). Sleep disturbances in patients with Alzheimer's disease: Epidemiology, pathophysiology and treatment. *CNS Drugs, 15*(10), 777–796.

Vitiello, M. V., Moe, K. E., & Prinz, P. N. (2002). Sleep complaints cosegregate with illness in older adults. Clinical research informed by and informing epidemiological studies of sleep. *Journal of Psychosomatic Research, 53*(1), 555–559.

Vitiello, M. B., Rybarczyk, B. Von Korff, M. & Stepanski, E. J. (2009). Cognitive behavioral therapy for insomnia improves sleep and decreases pain in older adults with co-morbid insomnia and osteoarthritis. *Journal of Clinical Sleep Medicine, 5*(4), 355–362. doi:10.1016/S0022-3399(02)00435-X

Walsh, J. K., & Roth, T. (2011). Pharmacologic treatment of insomnia: Benzodiazepine receptor agonists. In M. Kryger, T. Roth, & W. Dement (Eds.), *Principles and practice of sleep medicine* (5th ed., pp. 905–915). Philadelphia, PA: W.B. Saunders.

Ward, T. M. (2011). Conducting a sleep assessment. In N.S. Redeker & G. P. McEnany (Eds.), *Sleep disorders and sleep promotion in nursing practice* (pp. 53–70). New York, NY: Springer.

Weaver, T. E., & Chasens, E. R. (2007). Continuous positive airway pressure treatment for sleep apnea in older adults. *Sleep Medicine Reviews, 11*(2), 99–111. doi: 10.1016/j.smrv.2006.08.001

Williamson, A. T., Fletcher, P. C., & Dawson, K. A. (2003). Complementary and alternative medicine. Use in an older population. *Journal of Gerontological Nursing, 29*(5), 20–28.

Yeh, G. Y., Mietus, J. E., Peng, C. K., Phillips, R. S., Davis, R. B., Wayne, P. M. ... Thomas, R. J. (2008). Enhancement of sleep stability with Tai Chi exercise in chronic heart failure: Preliminary findings using an ECG-based spectrogram method. *Sleep Medicine, 9*(5), 527–536. doi: 10.1016/j.sleep.2007.06.003

Zeitzer, J. M., Fisicaro, R. A., Grove, M. E., Mignot, E., Yesavage, J. A., & Friedman, L. (2011). Faster REM sleep EEG and worse restedness in older insomniacs with HLA DQB1*0602. *Psychiatry Research, 187*(3), 397–400. doi: 10.1016/j.psychres.2011.01.00

For a full suite of assignments and additional learning activities, see the access code at the front of your book.

LEARNING OBJECTIVES www

At the end of this chapter, the reader will be able to:

> Assess for dysphagia at the bedside.
> Develop a plan to meet the nutritional and hydration needs of a patient with dysphagia.
> Differentiate between anorexia of aging and malnutrition.
> Describe the steps necessary to adequately assess an older adult for malnutrition.
> Develop a plan to meet the nutritional needs of a homebound older adult suffering from weight loss and malnutrition.

KEY TERMS www

Albumin
Anorexia of aging
Anthropometric measures
Bioelectrical impedance analysis
Body mass index
Cachexia
Diet history review
Deglutition
Dysphagia
Dysphagia diet
Esophageal dysphagia

Leptin
Malnutrition
Mid-upper arm circumference
Nasogastric tube
Oropharyngeal dysphagia
Percutaneous endoscopic gastrostomy
Prealbumin
Sarcopenia
Triceps skin fold
Weight loss

Chapter 17

Dysphagia and Malnutrition

Neva L. Crogan

Food is basic to life. For the older adult, food means family, togetherness, and quality of life. In response to a decrease in energy needs and expenditures, older age leads to a physiological change referred to as *anorexia of aging* (Morley, 2007). This physiological anorexia results from alterations in taste and smell, earlier satiation, and other changes related to normal aging (Morley, 2011b). The professional nurse needs to be able to successfully identify, evaluate, and treat problems affecting food intake. In this chapter, we will present the diagnoses and treatments of dysphagia and malnutrition. To start, we will pay special attention to the problem of dysphagia, a key causative and contributory factor of malnutrition for many older adults.

Dysphagia
Prevalence

We swallow approximately 600 times per day (Herskowitz, 2012). Swallowing is an automatic response to food or liquid in the mouth. *Dysphagia*, or problems with swallowing, is "an underrecognized, poorly diagnosed, and poorly managed health problem" that negatively impacts the quality and potentially quantity of life (Ekberg, Hamby, Woisard, Wuttge-Hanning, & Ortega, 2004, p. 143). Although dysphagia may occur at any age, it is more prevalent in the elderly (Morris, 2004; Roy, Stemple, Merrill, & Thomas, 2007; White, O'Rourke, Ong, Cordato, & Chan, 2008). Prevalence data suggest that 13–35% of elderly persons living in the community report dysphagia symptoms (Kawashima, Motohashi, & Fujishima, 2004; Lindgren & Janzon, 1991; Roy et al., 2007). Between 25% and 30% of hospitalized patients, and approximately 40–60% of persons in nursing homes, experience dysphagia (Brin & Younger, 1988; Layne, Losinski, Zenner, & Ament, 1989; Stevenson, 2002). Most importantly, the prevalence of dysphagia increases with age; thus, it is a major health problem in older adults.

Implications of Dysphagia

The physiological sequelae of dysphagia have traditionally received the greatest attention. Untreated dysphagia places a person at greater risk for nutritional deficiencies and respiratory problems. Dehydration and malnutrition from inadequate intake predispose persons to the development of many medical problems. Dehydration thickens secretions, increasing the risk for respiratory problems, and aspiration may lead to pneumonia and death. The ability and motivation to be active and involved in daily activities may also be adversely impacted. The development of these complications is dependent on the nature and severity of the dysphagia and the overall health status of the individual.

The social and psychological consequences of dysphagia must also be considered in the treatment and evaluation of care. The effects of dysphagia on quality of life were evaluated in 360 adults with subjective dysphagia complaints living in nursing homes or clinics in four European countries (Ekberg et al., 2004). The findings confirm the serious physiological impact of dysphagia. Fifty-five percent reported their eating habits were affected by their swallowing problems; over 50% ate less, 44% experienced weight loss, and over 30% were still hungry or thirsty after a meal. From a psychosocial perspective, 45% no longer found eating to be enjoyable, and more than half indicated dysphagia made life less enjoyable. Loss of self-esteem and an increasing sense of isolation also were reported. Over one-third (36%) avoided eating with others, and 41% experienced anxiety or panic during meals. Of the individuals interviewed, 40% had a confirmed diagnosis, only 32% had received treatment, and just 39% believed dysphagia could be treated (Ekberg et al., 2004). An individual's ability to be nourished physically, emotionally, and socially is threatened by dysphagia. The findings from this study are supported by other literature (Morris, 2004; Roy et al., 2007).

Warning Signs/Risk Factors for Dysphagia

Deglutition is the act of swallowing in which a food or liquid bolus is transported from the mouth through the pharynx and esophagus into the stomach. Swallowing is a complex neuromuscular process that occurs in stages. Dysphagia is usually identified as being either oropharyngeal or esophageal, designating the phase in which dysfunction occurs. In the oropharyngeal phase, food is prepared for swallowing by mastication and mixing with saliva, and then is moved posteriorly, triggering the pharyngeal swallow reflex, which moves the bolus down the pharynx (Logemann, 1998; Morris, 2004). During the pharyngeal swallow, the larynx closes and the epiglottis redirects the bolus around the airway, protecting the respiratory tract (Logemann, 1998; Morris, 2004). The esophageal phase begins when the bolus enters the esophagus at the cricopharyngeal juncture or upper esophageal sphincter (UES). Peristaltic waves propel the bolus through the esophagus to the lower esophageal sphincter, which opens into the stomach (Logemann, 1998). Because swallowing is a complex, coordinated event, causes of dysphagia are multiple and diverse. Each type of dysphagia is characterized by specific symptoms and associated with specific disorders.

Oropharyngeal dysphagia is usually related to neuromuscular impairments affecting the tongue, pharynx, and upper esophageal sphincter (Kennedy-Malone, Fletcher, & Plank, 2004). Stroke is the leading cause of oropharyngeal dysfunction (Agency for Health Care Policy and Research, 1999). Persons experiencing oropharyngeal dysphagia often complain of difficulty initiating a swallow. A cough early in the swallow and nasal regurgitation are symptoms associated with oropharyngeal dysphagia (Kennedy-Malone et al., 2004). The oropharyngeal phase of dysphagia is voluntary and utilizes the motor and sensory pathways to move food posteriorly to the oropharaynx, which then triggers the reflexive/involuntary phase in which the larynx and epiglottis are elevated and lowered, respectively, to prevent aspiration into the trachea (White et al., 2008). Dysphonia and dysarthria indicate motor dysfunction in the structures involved in the oral and pharyngeal phases and may be accompanied by dysphagia (Glenn-Molali, 2002). Inadequate saliva production can also interfere with the formation and movement of the food bolus. Candidiasis, or thrush, a fungal infection identified by white plaques on the mucous membranes of the oral cavity, can cause pain and discomfort when swallowing.

Esophageal dysphagia results from motility problems, neuromuscular problems, or obstruction that interferes with the movement of the food bolus through the esophagus into the stomach (Logemann, 1998; White et al., 2008). Common symptoms of esophageal dysphagia include complaints of food sticking after a swallow and coughing late in the swallow (Kennedy-Malone et al., 2004). Muscular dystrophy, myasthenia gravis, scleroderma, achalasia, and esophageal spasms may cause motility problems. Inflammation of the esophagus, secondary to gastroesophageal reflux disease (GERD) or a retained pill, is another etiology for esophageal dysphagia. Medications associated with pill-induced irritation or injury include tetracycline, potassium chloride, quinidine, iron, nonsteroidal anti-inflammatory drugs, alendronate sodium, and vitamin C (Amella, 1996). Common medical conditions associated with dysphagia are outlined in **Table 17-1**.

Assessment

Clinical evaluation of swallowing skills in patients with conditions that predispose to dysphagia or who voice complaints that suggest a swallowing disorder should be a priority for nursing. Evaluation as it relates to dysphagia can refer to screening or diagnostic testing. Screening involves determining if the patient has signs or symptoms of dysphagia for the purpose of referring for diagnostic evaluation to identify physiological components of swallowing (Smith & Connolly, 2003). Nursing plays a pivotal role in the early detection of swallowing problems and intervening to prevent complications from dysphagia. The findings from a screening evaluation allow prompt referral for diagnostic workup and implementation of interventions to promote safe eating/feeding practices.

Castell (1996) suggests that 80% of dysphagia can be diagnosed through a history. A careful history of the dysphagia should be obtained during the nursing assessment. Open-ended questions that the nurse can ask of the patient or the caregiver

TABLE 17-1 Common Medical Conditions Associated with Dysphagia

Classification of Dysphagia	Neuromuscular Causes	Mechanical Causes
Oropharyngeal dysphagia	Cerebrovascular accident Parkinson's disease Multiple sclerosis Amyotrophic lateral sclerosis (ALS) Traumatic brain injury (TBI)	Tumors Inflammatory masses
Esophageal dysphagia	Zenker's diverticulum Achalasia Scleroderma	Tumors Strictures Tracheosophageal fistula Foreign bodies Medication irritation Gastroesophageal reflux disease (GERD)

might include: How often do you cough after eating or drinking? How often do you feel that food is caught in your throat or chest? Show me where it sticks. How long does it take for you to eat a meal? Is this a change for you? (Morris, 2004). The patient or caregiver should be asked about the presence of predisposing conditions or warning signs and symptoms. Additional questions might include: What type of food causes the symptoms? Is the swallowing problem intermittent or progressive? Is heartburn present? Specific signs and symptoms of both oropharyngeal and esophageal dysphagia are listed in **Table 17-2** (Paik, 2012).

The physical examination involves a cognitive, neuromuscular, and respiratory assessment (**Box 17-1**). Important cognitive factors include interest in eating, ability to focus on and complete a meal, and the ability to remember and follow directions for safe eating. Neurological assessment involves testing sensory and motor components of the cranial nerves, in particular cranial nerves V, VII, IX, X, XI, and XII. Breath sounds, the strength of the person's cough, and his or her ability to clear the throat are clues to the integrity of the respiratory structures and the presence of protective mechanisms. Although commonly considered to be protective, the gag reflex is not an indication of the patient's ability to swallow (Logemann, 1998). However, detection of laryngeal elevation during a swallow maneuver grossly suggests airway closure (Amella, 1996). Medications should be reviewed for those that can decrease saliva production (antihistamines, anticholinergics, antihypertensives, cold medications), decrease cognition (sedatives, hypnotics), and/or decrease the strength of the muscles involved in swallowing (antispasticity drugs) (See **Box 17-2**).

TABLE 17-2   Signs and Symptoms of Dysphagia by Classification

Oropharyngeal:
- Coughing or choking with swallowing
- Difficulty initiating swallowing
- Food sticking in the throat
- Sialorrhea
- Unexplained weight loss
- Change in dietary habits
- Recurrent pneumonia
- Change in voice or speech (wet voice)
- Nasal regurgitation

Esophageal:
- Sensation of food sticking in the chest or throat
- Oral or pharyngeal regurgitation
- Change in dietary habits
- Recurrent pneumonia

BOX 17-1

Monitor abdominal distention by measuring the abdominal circumference from iliac crest to iliac crest. An increase in measurement of 8–10 cm beyond baseline is considered distention.

BOX 17-2

Older adults take more medications than any other age group. Medications can cause loss of appetite, reduced taste and smell, painful swallowing, nausea and vomiting, and can affect the absorption and use of nutrients.

Source: http://nutritionandaging.fiu.edu/aging_network/malfact2.asp

A standard procedure for bedside evaluation has not been formulated (Smith & Connolly, 2003); however, screening protocols have been developed and evaluated. Screening generally involves a checklist for warning signs and symptoms (Logemann, 1998). See Table 17-2 for signs and symptoms of dysphagia.

The effectiveness of trained nurses to screen for dysphagia after stroke was evaluated in the Collaborative Dysphagia Audit (CODA) Study. Nurses on a stroke unit received training in a simple water-screening test and screened acute stroke patients. The findings demonstrated a decrease in the number of patients who kept nothing by mouth (NPO), a decrease in the number of patients with inappropriate feeding orders, and improved referrals (Davies, 2002; Stroke Research Unit, 2001). The Gatehead Dysphagia Management Model (GDMM), developed from the results of the CODA, provides a decision tree to guide assessment and management of dysphagia (see **Case Study 17-1**).

Case Study 17-1

Mr. C., an 81-year-old widower, is admitted for stroke rehabilitation. He underwent a cystoscopy and transurethral resection of the prostate (TURP) for benign prostatic hypertrophy (BPH) one week ago. After the procedure he experienced a hypotensive episode and mental status changes. A workup revealed a large left middle-cerebral artery stroke. His stroke deficits include expressive aphasia, left neglect, dysphagia, and left hemiplegia. Concurrent health problems include coronary artery disease, hypertension, and hyperlipidemia under good control prior to surgery. Prior to transfer, Mr. C. had a low HCT and hemoccult-positive stool and received a blood transfusion. He was also suspected to have pneumonia and was started on an antibiotic.

On examination, Mr. C. is noted to be thin, pale, and lethargic. He has a weak cough, facial weakness, and a mild case of thrush. An indwelling urinary catheter is draining amber urine. Nonpitting edema is noted in his right hand; his arms have multiple bruises and dry, flaky skin. The transfer report indicates he requires minimal assistance with bed mobility and moderate assistance with transfers including toilet transfers; his sitting balance is fair; and he can self-propel his wheelchair 150 ft. with standby assistance. His son and daughter live out of town and have had to return home. They were not able to accompany him at transfer and will not be able to visit until the weekend (4 days from now).

Orders on admission include a pureed texture diet with moderate thick liquids; Isosource 1.5 cans at 0800 and 1600 and 1 can at 1200 and 2000 with 325 cc free water flush every shift via PEG tube. One scoop of Benefiber is added to tube feeding three times a day. His medication orders include Tenormin, 25 mg once a day; Lipitor, 20 mg at bedtime; Prevacid, 30 mg once a day; ASA, 81 mg once a day; Plavix, 75 mg once a day; amiodarone, 200 mg once a day; and clindamycin, 600 mg 3 times a day.

Questions:

1. Mr. C. presents multiple challenges. Which of the common health problems discussed in this chapter are relevant to his nursing care?

2. What are the priorities for Mr. C.'s care plan during his first week of rehabilitation?

3. What are key interventions to promote recovery and prevent complications?

After 3 days, the physician orders to discontinue his indwelling catheter. He experiences frequency, urgency, and incontinence. He has developed symptoms of an allergy—he is suffering from runny nose and dry cough. His tube feeding is being decreased as his dietary intake increases. When his family arrives, they ask about putting him on that medicine advertised on TV for overactive bladder and bring his over-the-counter (OTC) allergy medicine (Sudafed) for his cold. They also bring him his favorite soda.

Questions:

4. How would you respond to the family?

5. What actions would you take to address the problems and concerns raised?

6. How would your goals for care evolve over the next weeks of his stay?

7. What interventions would you institute to prevent the development of common health problems during his hospitalization and upon return to the community?

BOX 17-3

Nearly one-half of the nation's low-income elders have lost all or most of their teeth, leading to problems with chewing and swallowing.

Source: http://nutritionandaging.fiu .edu/aging_network/malfact2.asp

A careful assessment (see **Box 17-3**) of the individual eating a meal also is an essential component of an evaluation, even if the initial screening does not suggest a swallowing problem (Davies, 2002). Observations of a prolonged time required to complete a meal, "picking" at food, and active attempts to avoid eating (pushing the food away, turning away from offered food, refusing to open the mouth) may indicate a swallowing problem. Environmental factors that influence intake and eating behaviors, such as distractibility, fatigue, or even compatibility with dining companions or assistants, will not be apparent in a bedside evaluation. Amella (1999) emphasizes the importance of contextual issues in an evaluation, pointing out that fatigue, pain, and anxiety may mask an older person's true abilities.

Assessment for aspiration is also important. Aspiration occurs when material passes into the larynx below the true vocal cords; silent aspiration refers to situations in which aspiration does not produce the typical cough or change in voice quality (Smith & Connolly, 2003). Pulse oximetry has been found to be an effective, efficient tool to detect aspiration while eating. In a review of trends in the evaluation and treatment of dysphagia after stroke, Smith and Connolly report that a 2% drop in oxygen saturation levels from baseline detects 86% of penetration/aspiration. When followed by a 10 ml water swallow test at the bedside, the ability to detect aspiration increases to 95%.

Persons at risk should be assessed upon admission to a facility or community caseload; if deterioration occurs after admission, the individual should be reassessed at that time. Persons with degenerative conditions should be reassessed on a regular basis and when the condition progresses. (Monitoring lung sounds, respiration rate and quality, and other vital signs remains an important component of ongoing assessment and evaluation of care.) If screening suggests dysphagia, a referral for diagnostic evaluation should be ordered. A speech-language therapist (SLT) will conduct a more focused examination, and occupational therapists (OTs) also may be requested to complete an extensive examination. Further testing to confirm the diagnosis and determine the presence of and conditions surrounding aspiration are conducted by radiology or gastroenterology subspecialists.

Interventions/Strategies for Care

Actual treatment of the dysphagia depends on the specific diagnosis and the level of dysfunction. Restoration of swallowing has been attempted using a variety of strategies ranging from electrical stimulation to thermal stimulation, muscle exercises, and even black pepper oil—all with varying success at restoring muscular function and normal swallowing. Forthcoming should be the results of trials of Shaker exercises (which provide another way to open the upper esophageal sphincter through postural maneuvering) vs. standard treatment and muscle exercises vs. sensory postural therapy. Those studies may shed new light on the problem of restoration of normal swallowing function (White et al., 2008). Nursing interventions to manage dysphagia in order to minimize the risk of aspiration and promote nutrition and hydration involve compensatory eating techniques, diet modification, and oral care, and may require adaptive equipment.

Compensatory Eating Techniques

Specific interventions are developed for persons with dysphagia based on the swallowing problems identified. The results of a diagnostic workup or referral to an SLT or OT should provide specific recommendations for eating techniques. However, appropriate positioning is critical for safe eating and swallowing for all individuals. An upright position with the arms and feet supported, the head midline in a neutral position, and the chin slightly tucked is recommended to minimize the possibility of aspiration. The upright position should be maintained for at least 30 to 60 minutes after eating (the longer interval is necessary for esophageal dysphagia) (Avery-Smith, 1992). The location of food placement in the mouth as well as the size, consistency, and temperature of food items are important sensory cues to promote safe swallowing. If the individual has a sensory loss or oral muscular weakness, placing food on the unaffected or least affected side may help improve control over the bolus and its movement to the back of the mouth. If movement of the food to the back of the mouth is the problem, then placement of the bolus at the back of the tongue may be necessary to trigger the swallow (Martin-Harris & Cherney, 1996). The bolus size also influences swallow. A small bolus will not enter the pharynx as quickly as a large bolus, decreasing the risk of aspiration. However, a large bolus improves movement through the oral cavity in persons with delayed oral transit and also prolongs laryngeal elevation and closure (Martin-Harris & Cherney, 1996). For persons with decreased oral sensation or the impaired oral movement of food, cold items may improve posterior tongue movements and laryngeal swallow; for other persons, a warm bolus facilitates swallowing (Glenn-Molali, 2002). Careful questioning and observation of the conditions that result in optimal intake without evidence of swallowing problems and those associated with apparent problems will help guide eating techniques and feeding strategies. Having said this, a study looking at dysphagia between Parkinson's and dementia patients found that honey-thick foods were more effective than nectar-thick foods in preventing aspiration; the chin-down swallowing posture was least effective (Logemann et al., 2008).

Characteristics of the environment, including assistive personnel and dining partners, are factors that can facilitate or interfere with a safe, efficient swallow and adequate intake. For the first meal or eating/feeding session (and subsequent meals in some cases), a quiet room is preferable to decrease distractions and allow greater concentration on eating. The healthcare provider should sit down to assist with eating, positioning herself or himself and the food tray directly across from the patient in order to maintain the proper posture for the patient and ensure that she or he can see and reach food items and utensils (Avery-Smith, 1992). An unhurried, calm demeanor is important. Conversation should be limited to after a swallow is completed and before the next bite is taken. However, interaction that requires a response from the person eating is necessary to provide information about changes in voice quality as well as to promote a more pleasant social experience.

Diet Modifications

Modifying the texture of the food and fluids consumed is a common response to suspected swallowing problems. Alterations in diet consistency should be tailored to the type of swallowing disorder. An example of levels for food consistency is provided in **Table 17-3**. Foods can be prepared in blenders or food processors to the approved consistency or purchased in the infant–child food section. Attention to seasoning may improve flavor and therefore adherence to and intake of a modified diet (see **Box 17-4**).

Thickened fluids frequently present a challenge to adequate hydration. Complaints about the texture, taste, and ability to quench thirst are common. The Dysphagia Diet Task Force has standardized food and fluid textures for the *dysphagia diet* (see **Table 17-4**). Certain fluids have a thicker consistency naturally, whereas others will require thickening to the appropriate consistency with commercial or natural thickeners. Instant potato flakes, instant baby rice cereal, and mashed bananas are natural thickeners, but may not meet special diet requirements and may change the taste of the thickened items. Commercial thickening agents differ with respect to the directions for preparation and the effect of time on consistency. The type and temperature of the fluid to be thickened also affects mixing directions, so it is important to be familiar with the product used by the facility or individual at home.

TABLE 17-3   Dysphagia Diet According to Viscosity

Level I: pudding, crushed potato, and ground meat
Level II: curd-type yogurt, orange juice (3% thickener mixed), cream soup, and thin soup with starch
Level III: tomato juice; fluid-like yogurt; and thick, fluid rice
Level IV: water and orange juice

Source: Adapted from Paik, N. (2012, March 26). *Dysphagia.* [Web online article]. Retrieved from http://emedicine.medscape.com/article/324096-overview.

BOX 17-4

Therapeutic diets should be avoided if at all possible.

Sources: Tariz, S. H., Karcic, E., Thomas, D. R., et al. (2001). The use of a no-concentrated-sweets diet in the management of type 2 diabetes in nursing homes. *Journal of the American Dietetic Association, 101,* 1463–1466.

Coulston, A. M., Mandelbaum, D., & Reaven, G. M. (1990). Dietary management of nursing home residents with non-insulin-dependent diabetes mellitus. *American Journal of Clinical Nutrition, 51,* 67–71.

TABLE 17-4   The National Dysphagia Diet (NDD)

The National Dysphagia Diet (NDD) provides guidelines for progressive diets to be used nationally in the treatment of dysphagia. The following are some examples:

- Dysphagia Pureed (NDD 1): "Pudding-like" consistencies; pureed, no chunks or small pieces; avoid scrambled eggs, cereals with lumps.
- Dysphagia Mechanically Altered (NDD 2): Moist, soft foods; easily formed into a bolus; ground meats; soft, tender vegetables; soft fruit; slightly moistened dry cereal with little texture. No bread or foods such as peas and corn. Avoid skins and seeds.
- Mechanical Soft: Same as the mechanically altered but allows bread, cakes, and rice.
- Dysphagia Advanced (NDD 3): Regular textured foods except those that are very hard, sticky, or crunchy. Avoid hard fruit and vegetables, corn, skins, nuts, and seeds.

Liquid consistencies:
- Spoon thick
- Honey-like
- Nectar-like
- Thin: All beverages such as water, ice, milk, milkshakes, juices, coffee, tea, and sodas

Source: Adapted from *Journal of the American Dietetic Association, 103*(3), McCallum S.L. (2003). American Dietetic Association.

Encouraging fluid intake with thickened liquids often requires creativity and persistence. Some facilities allow dysphagia patients to drink plain water between meals when requiring thickened liquids with meals. There are contradictory beliefs about the likelihood that allowing plain water will lead to aspiration pneumonia (Garon, Engle, & Ormison, 1997; Panther, 2005). Oral care appears to be a crucial link in the aspiration to pneumonia process (Langmore et al., 1998; White et al., 2008). Frequent oral care to ensure the oral cavity is clear of food particles and to prevent the growth of bacteria is a critical component of liberalized fluid programs and an essential strategy to minimize the risk for pneumonia.

Oral Hygiene

Examination of the relative risk of multiple factors (medical/health status, functional status, dysphagia/gastroesophageal reflux, feeding/mode of nutritional intake, and oral/dental status) in the development of pneumonia in older persons suggests that colonization and host resistance are key contributors (Langmore et al., 1998). Oropharyngeal colonization from inadequate oral care, decayed teeth, or periodontal disease is the initial process that can lead to the development of pneumonia. Aspiration of these organisms in liquids, food, or saliva, combined with decreased immunity, increases the risk for development of pneumonia.

Regular cleaning of the teeth or dentures, gums, and tongue and maintaining moisture in the mouth are essential components of an oral hygiene protocol.

(See Johnson and Chalmers [2002] for tools and strategies to address various problems in providing oral care.) A soft toothbrush, gauze-covered swabs, or foam toothettes may be used to scrub the surfaces of the oral cavity after meals. Electric toothbrushes may also be useful tools and, depending on the person's physical and cognitive abilities, may enable the older person with limited hand grasp and movement to more adequately and independently clean the mouth's surfaces. Individuals who receive non-oral feedings also need to have regular oral care to remove debris. The teeth and mouth should be cleaned upon awakening, after meals (or snacks for persons with dysphagia), and before bed. Dentures should be taken out and scrubbed at least daily with a brush; chemical denture cleaner tablets may be used in addition to brushing with soap or toothpaste (Johnson & Chalmers, 2002). Soaking dentures in a solution of white wine vinegar and cold water (a 50:50 solution) will help remove built-up calculus. Denture cups must also be cleaned or replaced regularly. A weekly cleaning and soaking of the denture cup in a diluted hypochlorite solution for an hour followed by thorough washing with soap and water will help sterilize the container (Johnson & Chalmers, 2002) if frequent replacement is not feasible.

Maintaining moist mucous membranes is essential to the health and integrity of the oral cavity. Dry membranes contribute to an increased rate of plaque accumulation (Almstahl & Wikstrom, 1999), and dental and denture plaque serves as a major reservoir for pathogenic organisms in the elderly (Aiden et al., 2004). Many of the medications prescribed for chronic conditions result in a dry mouth. Limited fluid intake and infrequent oral care, especially for persons who are ordered nothing by mouth, contribute to dryness. Meticulous oral care as outlined previously is crucial; however, additional measures may be needed. Saliva substitutes, toothpaste and mouth rinses without alcohol or excessive additives such as in the Biotene range, water or mouthwash in spray bottles to spritz inside the mouth, water-soluble lubricants applied to the tongue and cheeks, and Vaseline or lanolin applied frequently to the lips are among the strategies recommended for combating dry mouth in the physically dependent or cognitively impaired older adult (Johnson & Chalmers, 2002).

Adaptive Equipment

The modification of utensils or use of adaptive equipment is frequently necessary to promote independence in eating and to facilitate safe swallowing. However, careful evaluation of eating is needed for each person to ensure safe and effective tools are used. Using a straw to drink moves a fluid bolus quickly through the mouth and can exacerbate problems with swallowing. Drinking from a cup requires the head to be tilted to empty the glass; this maneuver (hyperextension) can increase the risk of aspiration. Specially designed cups with a cutout for the nose can be purchased or made to prevent the need to tilt the head back. Similarly, shallow bowls on spoons may be helpful in preventing hypertension when eating with a spoon (Glenn-Molali, 2002). An ongoing assessment of abilities and problems at mealtime will help ensure that necessary changes to the plan of care are made in a timely manner. Rehabilitation nurses and texts and continuing education programs focusing on swallowing evaluation and feeding techniques are resources for new tools and techniques. Physical, occupational, and speech-language therapists can recommend specific techniques and equipment for safe intake and can help modify available tools. Their expertise and assistance should be sought.

Enteral Feeding

The initiation of tube feedings is a complicated decision made by the patient, healthcare provider, and family or healthcare surrogate. Often prescribed to maintain adequate nutrition and hydration levels and prevent aspiration, persons receiving enteral feedings are still at risk for aspiration (Logemann, 1998; White et al., 2008) and inadequate nutritional intake. The most appropriate mode and method of administering enteral feeding (e.g., continuous or intermittent, intestinal or gastric) remains controversial (Paik, 2012) (see **Box 17-5**).

Nasogastric tube. **Nasogastric tube** (NGT) feeding is a commonly used method of enteral feeding for patients with a short-term life expectancy. Insertion of a nasogastric tube is a quick, easy, relatively noninvasive procedure; however, many patients find the tube uncomfortable and pull the tube out. Prolonged use of nasogastric tubes can lead to complications such as lesions to the nasal mucosa, chronic sinusitis, gastroesophageal reflux, and aspiration pneumonia (Paik, 2012).

Percutaneous endoscopic gastrostomy. **Percutaneous endoscopic gastrostomy** (PEG) requires the invasive insertion of a feeding tube through the anterior abdominal wall, which can be complicated by bleeding, peritonitis or perforation of other abdominal organs, chest infections, insertion site infection, and ease of tube removal (Paik, 2012). PEG has several advantages over surgical gastrostomy, including reduced procedure time, cost, and recovery time and it requires no general anesthesia. Contraindications for PEG are aspiration pneumonia due to gastroesophageal reflux, significant ascites, and morbid obesity (Paik, 2012). Whether or not to insert a PEG can be an ethical and quality-of-life issue. Nearly 50% of patients die within 6 months following PEG insertion, often from insertion complications such as peritonitis or severe wound infections (Wirth et al., 2012).

BOX 17-5

Weight loss can be predictive of mortality and is considered clinically significant when there is a →2% decrease in baseline body weight in 1 month, a →5% weight loss in 3 months, or a →10% weight loss in 6 months.

Sources: Morley, J. E. (2011a). Assessment of malnutrition in older persons; A focus on the Mini Nutritional Assessment. *Journal of Nutrition, Health, and Aging, 15*(2), 87–90.

Kaiser, M. J., Bauer, J. M., Ramsch, C., & MNA-International Group. (2009). Validation of the Mini Nutritional Assessment short-form (MNA-SF); A practical tool for identification of nutritional status. *Journal of Nutrition, Health, and Aging, 13*(9), 782–788.

Attention to positioning during and after a feeding and meticulous oral hygiene are very important in preventing or minimizing the risk for aspiration in persons receiving enteral nutrition. In a literature review on GI motility, feeding tube site, and aspiration, Metheny, Schallom, and Edwards (2004) reported that the

> aspiration risk exists to some extent in all tube-fed patients, depending on GI dysmotility patterns and individual patient characteristics. However, regardless of the feeding site, it is ultimately regurgitated gastric contents that are aspirated into the lungs. For this reason, the assessment of greatest interest for tube-fed patients is the evaluation of gastric emptying. (p. 131)

Although the need for additional research is indicated, Edwards and Metheny (2000) suggest McClave et al.'s (1999) recommendation that a residual volume (RV) greater than or equal to 200 cc for nasogastric tubes and greater than or equal to 100 cc for gastrostomy tubes should raise concern about intolerance. Although these volumes were associated with dysmotility, McClave and colleagues emphasize the importance of giving consideration to other symptoms of intolerance before holding feedings. Interruptions and incomplete feedings interfere with the nutritional adequacy of non-oral diets. Nausea/vomiting, absent bowel sounds, abdominal distention, and stool pattern are clues to intolerance that should be evaluated and factored into the decision.

The administration of medications to patients with dysphagia remains a challenge for nurses. If a patient is eating but needs changes in food consistency to promote swallowing, the problem then arises—should medications be crushed? The answer is simple and has been identified as being the best practice in delivering medications to patients with dysphagia: Only medications that have been specifically designed to be crushed or opened (in the case of capsules) may be administered in that way. To crush or open capsules not designed for that purpose alters the pharmacodynamics and pharmacokinetics of the drug and must not be done. If the patient cannot take the medications, the nurse's responsibility is to contact the prescribing practitioner and seek a different medication. To not do so is negligence on the part of the nurse and potentially life threatening for the patient (Griffith, 2008).

Managing Gastroesophageal Reflux Disease

The relationship between gastroesophageal reflux disease (GERD) and enteral nutrition remains unclear; however, interventions to prevent the development of reflux or esophageal irritation and treat GERD are supported by data implicating reflux in the development of aspiration. An individual's diet pattern, in particular food or fluids associated with heartburn or discomfort, should be evaluated. Coffee, spicy foods, fatty foods, citrus fruits, alcohol, and smoking may weaken the lower esophageal sphincter and contribute to the development of the symptoms of reflux (Kennedy-Malone et al., 2004). Diet modification can be a simple, effective strategy. Sitting up for at least an hour after eating and/or raising the head of the bed 4 to 6 inches with blocks may help control the onset of symptoms, too. An oral proton pump inhibitor taken 60 minutes before a meal may be indicated (Kennedy-Malone et al., 2004). Be sure an adequate amount of fluid is consumed before and after oral medications are administered to avoid esophageal irritation.

Malnutrition
Prevalence

As described earlier, anorexia of aging is a physiological process that occurs with older age. This physiological anorexia increases the risk of developing malnutrition and weight loss when an older adult develops a physical or psychological illness (Hajjar, Kamel, & Denson, 2004). *Malnutrition* is defined as "the state of being poorly nourished" (Hickson, 2006, p. 4) and can be caused by a lack of nutrients (undernutrition) or an excess of nutrients (overnutrition). For the older adult, the cause is usually a lack of nutrients, or undernutrition. The prevalence of malnutrition in community-dwelling older adults is 15%, increasing to 5–44% if the older adult is homebound (Hajjar et al., 2004). The prevalence among those living in nursing homes is 30–85% (Omran & Morely, 2000; Hajjar et al., 2004), and 20–65% if hospitalized (Hajjar et al., 2004).

Two major markers of malnutrition in older adults are sarcopenia and cachexia (Cruz-Jentoft et al., 2010). *Sarcopenia* is defined as "a syndrome of progressive and generalized loss of skeletal muscle mass and strength, which increases the risk of adverse outcomes, such as physical disability, poor quality of life, and even death" (Loreck, Chimakurthi, & Steinle, 2012, p. 20). Diagnosis is confirmed with findings of decreased muscle mass and either decreased muscle strength or decreased physical performance. *Cachexia* is defined as complex metabolic processes associated with an underlying terminal illness (e.g., cancer, end-stage renal disease) and is characterized by loss of muscle mass with or without loss of fat mass (Thomas, 2007). Cachexia is usually characterized by severe wasting, and is frequently associated with inflammation, insulin resistance, and breakdown of muscle protein. Most older adults with cachexia also have sarcopenia, but those with sarcopenia frequently do not have cachexia (Loreck, Chimakurthi, & Steinle, 2012).

Implications

A lack of food or nutrients can affect nearly every organ system (Hajjar et al., 2004). Malnutrition can lead to delayed wound healing, the development of pressure ulcers, increased susceptibility to infections, functional decline, cognitive decline and depression, delayed recovery from acute illness (Hajjar et al., 2004), difficulty in swallowing, and dehydration (Shatenstein, 2002). Poor nutritional status also can result in decreased lean body mass; lessened muscular strength and aerobic capacity, which can lead to chronic fatigue; and alterations in gait and balance, increasing the risk for falls and fractures. For many older adults, this sequence of events leads to a deterioration in their overall quality of life, causing dependence on others (Shatenstein, 2002) (see **Box 17-6**).

BOX 17-6

Body mass index (BMI) is a useful measurement for assessing nutritional status and can be calculated using the following formula: BMI = Weight (kg)/height (m)^2

Source: Hajjar, R. R., Kamel, H. K., & Denson, K. (2004). Malnutrition in aging. *The Internet Journal of Geriatrics and Gerontology, 1*(1), 1–16.

Factors Influencing Nutritional Risk

Many factors contribute to malnutrition and weight loss in elders. These factors can be classified into three major groups: social, psychological, and biological (see **Table 17-5**).

Social Causes

The most significant social cause of malnutrition and weight loss in older adults is poverty. Affording expensive medications is a common problem for older adults with limited incomes. If insurance does not cover all or most of this expense,

TABLE 17-5 Factors Influencing Nutritional Risk in Older Adults

Social
- Isolation
- Loneliness
- Poverty
- Dependency

Psychological
- Depression
- Anxiety
- Dementia
- Bereavement

Biological
- Dentition
- Loss of taste or smell
- Gastrointestinal disorders
- Muscle weakness
- Dry mouth
- Olfaction
- Renal disease
- Physical disability
- Infections
- Chronic obstructive pulmonary disease (COPD)
- Drug interactions

Source: Loreck, E., Chimakurthi, R., & Steinle, N. I. (2012). Nutritional assessment of the geriatric patient: A comprehensive approach toward evaluating and managing nutrition, *Clinical Geriatrics, 20*(4), 20–26.

older adults are faced with going without medications or reducing their food budgets to afford the prescribed medication. Social isolation, loneliness, and grieving due to the death of family or friends have long been known as an important risk factors for malnutrition and weight loss (McIntosh, Shifflet, & Picou, 1989). In a study by De Castro et al. (1990), socialization with others resulted in increased food intake at meals. Other social risk factors or causes of malnutrition and weight loss in older adults are their inability to shop, cook, or feed themselves (Hajjar et al., 2004).

Psychological Causes

Depression is one of the most common treatable causes of weight loss in older adults. Elders suffering from depression can have many symptoms that can lead to weight loss, including weakness (61%), stomach pains (37%), nausea (27%), anorexia (22%), and diarrhea (20%) (Kivela, Nissinen, & Tuomiiehto, 1986). Successful treatment of depression has been shown to reverse weight loss in nursing home residents (Morley & Kraenzle, 1995).

Dementia is commonly associated with weight loss. Older adults with dementia often forget or refuse to eat, and feeding can become a time-consuming process. Elders with late-stage dementia may wander excessively, express paranoid ideation, and may be prescribed psychotropic medications that cause anorexia. Some demented older adults develop apraxia of swallowing and must be reminded to swallow after each mouthful of food (Morley & Morley, 1995).

Biological Causes

Numerous medical conditions can cause malnutrition and weight loss by one or more of the following mechanisms: hypermetabolism, anorexia, swallowing difficulty, or malabsorption (Hajjar et al., 2004). Diseases such as stroke, tremors, or arthritis can affect an older adult's ability to eat or prepare food, thereby leading to decreased food intake; swallowing disorders (dysphagia) are associated with increased risk of aspiration and food aversion, which may be conscious or subconscious (Hajjar et al., 2004). Infections are another cause of weight loss in older adults, especially those who live in nursing homes. Infections may result in confusion, anorexia, and negative nitrogen balance (Hajjar et al., 2004). Another physical cause is chronic obstructive pulmonary disease (COPD). Older adults with COPD experience a decrease in arterial oxygen tension when eating due to the thermic energy of eating and the brief interruption of respiration with swallowing. They frequently are unable to eat their meals because of dyspnea (Schols, Mostert, Cobbin, Soeters & Wouters, 1991). Further, their condition is aggravated by hyperventilation and use of accessory muscles, leading to increased metabolism. Hyperthyroidism and Parkinson's disease also cause hypermetabolism, which can lead to weight loss (Hajjar et al., 2004). Finally, there are several medications associated with poor appetite and weight loss (see **Table 17-6**).

TABLE 17-6   Medications Associated with Weight Loss
• Digoxin
• Theophylline
• Metformin
• Antibiotics
• Nonsteroidal anti-inflammatory drugs (NSAIDS)
• Psychotropic drugs: Prozac (fluoxetine), Lithium, Phenothiazines

Source: Hickson, M. (2006). Malnutrition and ageing. *Postgraduate Medical Journal, 82,* 2–8.

Assessment

Nutritional risk screening should be integrated into the comprehensive geriatric assessment (Bauer, Kaiser, & Sieber, 2010). Many screening methods are available, including specific clinical screening tools, anthropometric and body composition measurements, laboratory tests, a review of clinical data, and examination of an individual's diet history. Each method has its pros and cons, so a combination of assessments may be necessary to provide a more accurate picture of a patient's nutritional status (Loreck, Chimakurthi, & Steinle, 2012).

Clinical Screening Tools

Mini Nutritional Assessment (MNA): The MNA is a simple and reliable tool for assessing nutrition status in older adults. Originally developed by Vellas and Guigoz in 1989 (Guigoz, Vellas, & Garry, 1996), it has become the tool of choice for many healthcare providers. The original MNA is an 18-item questionnaire that takes 10–15 minutes to administer. A shortened version (MNA-SF) includes six items and takes less than 5 minutes to administer. The questions examine food intake, weight loss, mobility, psychological stress/acute disease incidence, neuropsychological problems, and BMI or calf circumference (Loreck, Chimakurthi, & Steinle, 2012). Calf circumference was provided as an option because BMI can be difficult to assess in older adults. On the MNA-SF, a score between 8 and 11 indicates an increased risk of malnutrition, and a score < 7 reflects malnutrition (Loreck, Chimakurthi, & Steinle, 2012).

Instant Nutritional Assessment (INA): The INA is a simple and practical nutrition screening tool. It was developed by Seitzer and colleagues (1979) and combines three easily obtainable elements: lymphocyte count, albumin, and weight change (referred to as "LAW") (Hajjar et al., 2004). Each item, if used alone, has limited predictive value, but when combined has a high degree of accuracy (Hajjar et al., 2004).

Nutritional Screening Initiative and the DETERMINE Checklist: The DETERMINE checklist was developed by the Nutritional Screening Initiative (NSI), an interdisciplinary multi-organizational effort aimed at introducing nutritional screening into the healthcare system (Detsky, et al., 1984). The checklist is self-administered and includes 10 questions about risk factors for malnutrition. Total scores of 6 or higher (highest score is 21) indicate a need for further assessment. The checklist is a screening tool, not a reliable diagnostic tool, but has had some success in promoting public awareness of malnutrition.

Malnutrition Risk Scale (SCALES): The malnutrition risk scale was developed by Morley (1989) as an outpatient screening tool. The acronym SCALES represents the six elements in the tool (Sadness, Cholesterol, Albumin, Loss of weight, Eating problems, and Shopping) that cover common known-risk factors for malnutrition, including depression, which has emerged as a major risk factor for malnutrition and mortality (Blazer & Williams, 1980). A score of three or higher suggests high risk for malnutrition.

Malnutrition Screening Tool (MST): A quick, valid and reliable two-item tool developed by Ferguson et al. (1999), this free tool can be used by any health professional and does not require any anthropometrical or biochemical measurements. The tool simply asks about unplanned weight loss and poor appetite. If the patient reports weight loss or poor appetite, he or she may be at risk for malnutrition.

Food Expectations—Long Term Care (FoodEx-LTC): FoodEx-LTC is a 28-item, 4-domain instrument developed to measure nursing home-resident food satisfaction (Crogan, Evans, & Velasquez, 2004; Crogan & Evans, 2006). The instrument can be self-administered or administered by an evaluator who reads each item and marks the resident's response. During development and pilot testing of the FoodEx-LTC, internal consistency reliability (Cronbach's alpha) estimates ranged from 0.65, "Exercising Choice" to 0.82, "Providing Food Service." All alpha coefficients were above the 0.50 criterion for a new scale and 3 of 4 scales met the more stringent criterion of 0.70. Two-week test–retest coefficients ranged from 0.79 for "Enjoying Food and Food Service" to 0.88 or "Providing Food Service" and "Exercising Choice."

Other Tools

Anthropometric and Body Composition Measures

Anthropometric measures are important indicators of an elder's nutritional status. The following is a list of anthropometric measures with a simple explanation of each measure.

Serial Body Weight. Serial body weight is a useful way to identify a change in overall nutritional status. However, body weight can be unreliable if the patient also suffers from congestive heart failure, hepatic disorders, or renal disease (Loreck et al., 2012).

Body Mass Index. *Body mass index* (BMI) is used to determine body fat levels, with a BMI < 18.5 kg/m^2 indicating underweight and in increased risk of mortality (Loreck et al., 2012). A BMI of 18.5 to 24.9 kg/m indicates normal weight, 25 to 29.9 kg/m^2 overweight, and >30 kg/m^2 obesity (Loreck et al., 2012). In older adults, BMI may be problematic, in that an inaccurate height may be obtained and BMI does not accurately predict body composition. In this population, inaccurate heights may be due to vertebral collapse, change in posture, or loss of muscle tone. In these cases, height can be estimated by measuring knee height or arm span (Hickson & Frost, 2003).

Triceps Skin Fold. *Triceps skin fold* (TSF) is reflective of fat stores. It is measured using a skinfold caliper by measuring the mid-point between the acromion process and the alecranon process of the upper arm. The clinician palpates the site to distinguish fat from muscle, grasps a fold of skin approximately 1 cm above the mid-point, and performs three readings. The average of these readings is used. Nutritional depletion is defined as a skinfold measure of < 11.3 mm in women and < 4.3 mm in men (Burr & Phillips, 1984).

Mid-Upper Arm Circumference. *Mid-upper arm circumfrence* (MUAC) is a predictor of mortality in older adults living in long-term care facilities (Allard et al., 2004). To determine MUAC, the mid-point of the upper arm is measured with a tape measure placed snugly against the skin. Once the TSF and MUAC are measured, a mid-arm muscle circumference (MAMC), an indicator of lean mass, can be calculated using the following equation $MAMC = AC - (TSF \times 0.314)$ (Burr & Phillips, 1984). Older adults are considered nutritionally depleted when their measure falls below the tenth percentile, which are <17.2 cm in women and <19.6 cm in men.

Bioelectrical Impedance Analysis. *Bioelectrical impedance analysis* (BIA) is an expensive, quick, and noninvasive tool used in clinical practice to estimate fat mass versus lean mass. BIA-enabled devices send a low current through the body to determine the electrical impedance of body tissues, which provides an estimate of total body water (TBW). Total body water measures are then plugged into an equation that can determine body composition (Loreck et al., 2012). The ideal percentage body fat for older adults is 27.6–34.4% for women and 20.3–26.7% for men. Accuracy of BIA can be affected by patient obesity, body position, hydration status, recent consumption of food, ambient air and skin temperature, recent physical activity, and conductance of the examining table (Loreck et al., 2012).

Laboratory Assessments

Laboratory assessment is another component of a comprehensive nutritional assessment (see **Table 17-7**). Even though serum proteins such as *albumin* and *prealbumin* are widely used to assess nutritional status, their levels are impacted by non-nutritional factors. Proteins are influenced by cellular processes, including inflammation and renal disease, so their use are limited in definitively establishing nutritional status in older adults (Morley, 2011a). Total lymphocyte count (TLC) also has been used as a marker of nutritional status, but there is limited evidence that low TLC levels reflect malnutrition in older adults (Kuzuya et al., 2005). In cross-sectional studies, low total cholesterol (<150 mg/dL) is often seen among individuals with poor nutritional status (Loreck et al., 2012). Two additional studies evaluated the use of *leptin* as a clinical predictor of nutritional status in older adults

TABLE 17-7 Laboratory Studies Associated with Poor Nutrition
Serum albumin ←3.5 g/dL
Serum prealbumin ←11 mg/dL
Cholesterol ←150 mg/dL
Leptin ←4.0 ug/L in men, ←6.48 ug/L in women

Source: Loreck, E., Chimakurthi, R., & Steinle, N. I. (2012). Nutritional assessment of the geriatric patient: A comprehensive approach toward evaluating and managing nutrition, *Clinical Geriatrics, 20*(4), 20–26.

(Amirkalali et al., 2010; Bouillanne et al., 2007). Leptin levels decrease as malnutrition becomes more pronounced in older adults.

Clinical Data Review

Clinical data specific to nutritional assessment in older adults includes a review of current medications, evaluation of oral and swallowing problems, review of gastrointestinal problems, and a review of psychiatric and neurologic disorders (Bauer et al., 2010).

Diet History Review

The final component of the nutritional assessment is an evaluation of the older adult's diet history. Numerous strategies could be used to complete a *diet history review*. For example, the older adult could be asked to keep a food diary, the healthcare provider could conduct a 24-hour recall, or a questionnaire could be administered to determine the frequency with which foods from various food groups are consumed (Thompson & Subar, 2012).

Evidence-Based Strategies to Improve Nutrition

Previous accepted strategies to improve nutrition in older adults included educating them on diet and providing various supplements, including vitamins, minerals, and meal replacements. However, more recent research findings do not support all of these past strategies. For example, in a population-based study of 38,772 older women from the Iowa Women's Health Study (Mursu, Robien, Harnack, Park, & Jacobs, 2011), vitamin and mineral supplementation was associated with increased mortality risk (see **Boxes 17-7** and **17-8**). This association was strongest with supplemental iron. In contrast to these findings, calcium was associated with decreased risk. In short, dietary supplementation should not be routinely recommended, but rather used only to treat symptomatic nutrient deficiency disease.

The consumption of food is always preferable to meal replacements. If this is not possible or realistic, between-meal snacks (Morley, 2010) or liquid caloric supplements can increase energy intake (Wilson, Purushothaman, & Morley, 2002). Maintenance of good oral hygiene, sensible treatment of dysphagia and depression, and decreasing or limiting the number of prescribed and over-the-counter medications also play an important role in enhancing food intake (Morley, 2010).

BOX 17-7

Antioxidant use could be harmful to older women.

Source: Crogan, N. L. (2012). Various vitamin and mineral supplements are observed to increase mortality risk in older women, with the exception of calcium, which decreases risk [Peer commentary on the paper Dietary supplements and mortality rate in older women: The Iowa Women's Health Study, by Mursu et al., (2011). *Archives of Internal Medicine, 171*(18), 1625–1633] *Evidence-Based Nursing,* Mar 22. Advance online publication.

BOX 17-8

Try This: Best Practices in Nursing Care to Older Adults from the Hartford Institute for Geriatric Nursing, Division of Nursing, New York University. Addresses topics such as preventing aspiration, avoiding restraint use in patients with dementia, and oral assessment. Material may be downloaded and/or distributed in electronic format (http://www.hartfordign.org).

University of Iowa Gerontological Nursing Interventions Research Center. Research-based protocols on a variety of common health problems including prompted voiding, restraint use, prevention of falls, oral care, and depression (http://www.nursing.uiowa.edu/excellence/ nursing_interventions/ index.htm).

An illustrative tool that could be used to demonstrate what constitutes healthy eating and portion size is the USDA's My-Plate method, which divides a plate into quarters, with one-fourth appropriated to grains, one-fourth to protein, and the remaining half to fruits and vegetables (see **Figure 17-1**). Older adults should be advised that their nutrient intake might be inadequate if they are not eating close to this food composition.

Nutrients found to be essential to older adults are protein and vitamin D. Deficiencies in these nutrients are associated with higher risk of falls in this population (Zoltick et al., 2011). Zoltick and colleagues examined food intake in 807 men and women, aged 67 to 93 years, from the Framingham Study. Higher protein intake was associated with decreased odds of falling. In those with a >5% weight loss from baseline, higher protein intake significantly decreased fall incidents. The researchers concluded that protein intake might be a modifiable factor for fall prevention in older adults.

A systematic review and meta-analysis of older adults investigated the effectiveness of vitamin D in the prevention of falls and found that vitamin D therapy (200–1000 IU) resulted in 14% fewer falls (Kalyani et al., 2010).

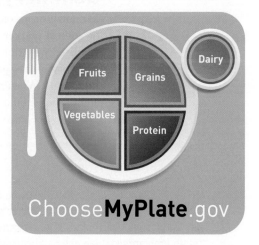

Figure 17-1 USDA's My-Plate Method.
Source: U.S. Department of Agriculture. ChooseMyPlate.gov website. Washington, DC.

Older adults who reside in nursing homes are especially at risk for malnutrition. Improving the dining experience by offering food choice, select menus, and buffet dining, as well as ice cream parlors, have been successful in increasing food intake and decreasing weight loss (Heaton et al., 2011; Nijs, de Graaf, van Staveren, & de Groot, 2009; Simmons, Zhuo, & Keller, 2010).

Finally, it may be necessary to refer the older adult to other healthcare providers after completing a nutritional assessment. A speech-language pathologist can be invaluable in assessing and treating dysphagia and swallowing problems. A registered dietitian can be of value in the assessment and treatment of reversible nutritional issues, such as by determining the adequacy of intake, developing a custom meal plan, making recommendations for increasing oral intake, or developing a plan to initiate nutrition support. A social worker can assist elders and families to obtain access to home-delivered meals, congregate feeding programs, food stamps, and other assistance programs. A referral to a dentist for oral health issues or to a geriatric psychiatrist for mental health issues may also be warranted. An occupational or physical therapist consultation may be of value for older adults with physical limitations. A pharmacist can provide assistance with nutrition-related medication management issues (Loreck et al., 2012). Nutritional assessment and the selection of specific interventions are not just the responsibility of the nurse, but rather, the responsibility of the interdisciplinary team.

Summary

Malnutrition in older adults is a multifaceted and complex issue. No single tool or clinical marker accurately predicts nutritional status. However, integrating a validated nutrition screening tool with anthropometric and laboratory data, the geriatric nurse or provider can get a more accurate picture of the older adult's nutrition status. When reversible causes of malnutrition are identified, evidence-based approaches should be undertaken, which may require referral to other disciplines.

Critical Thinking Exercises

1. Mrs. Jones, an 80-year-old widow living alone in the community, was recently diagnosed with congestive heart failure. Concurrent health problems include osteoarthritis and osteoporosis. During the initial home health visit, the nurse notices that Mrs. Jones is very thin. Upon questioning, Mrs. Jones reports she rarely gets out to buy food. She says that she is not a big eater and has neighbors that bring her food. Should this be considered a problem? What additional information is needed for decision making? What evidence can the nurse provide to Mrs. Jones to support a need for further evaluation and treatment of this problem?

2. A 60-year-old African American woman has been admitted to the rehabilitation hospital for treatment following a stroke. Her past medical history includes congestive heart failure, type 2 diabetes mellitus, and hypertension. While obtaining her history, you note that she has difficulty speaking. You suspect she may also suffer from dysphagia. What would be your next step? What referrals may be needed? What nursing interventions may help improve her ability to swallow?

Personal Reflections

1. Have someone feed you an entire meal. What was your interaction like (who talked, what were the topics of conversation)? How did it feel to be fed? Did your pattern for eating or the amount of food and fluid consumed differ from normal?

2. Have you ever cared for a person with dysphagia? Malnutrition? After reading this chapter, reflect on that experience and think about some strategies that may have helped to improve care for that person.

References

Agency for Health Care Policy and Research. (1999). *Diagnosis and treatment of swallowing disorders (dysphagia) in acute care stroke patients: Evidence report/technology assessment, 8. AHCPR 99-EO23*. Rockville, MD: Author.

Aiden, E., Feldman, P. A., Madeb, R., Steinberg, J., Merlin, S., Sabo, E.,…Srugo, I. (2004). Candida albicans colonization of dental plaque in elderly dysphagia patients. *IMAGE, 6*, 342–345.

Allard, J. P., Aghdassi, E., McArthur, M., McGeer, A., Simor, A., Abdolell, M.,…Liu, B. (2004). Nutrition risk factors for the survival in elderly living in Canadian long-term care facilities. *Journal of the American Geriatric Society, 52*(1), 59–65.

Almståhl, A., & Wikström, Mm. (1999). Oral microflora in subjects with reduced salivary secretion. *J Dent Res 78*, 1410–1416.

Amella, E. J. (1996). Choking—Aspiration in the elderly. In C. W. Bradway (Ed.), *Nursing care of geriatric emergencies* (pp. 154–169). New York, NY: Springer.

Amella, E. J. (1999). Dysphagia—The differential diagnosis in long-term care. *Primary Care Practice, 3*(2), 135–149.

American Dietetic Association. (2003). National Dysphagia Diet. *Journal of the American Dietetic Association, 103*(3) 748–765.

Amirkalali, B., Sharifi, F., Fakhrzadeh, H., Mirarefein, M., Ghaderpanahi, M., Badamchizadeh, Z., & Larijani, B. (2010). Low serum leptin serves as a biomarker of malnutrition in elderly patients. *Nutrition Research, 30*(5), 314–319.

Avery-Smith, W. (1992). Management of neurologic disorders: The first feeding session. In M. E. Groher (Ed.), *Dysphagia: Diagnosis and management* (2nd ed., pp. 219–236). Boston, MA: Butterworth-Heinemann.

Bauer, J. M., Kaiser, M. J., & Sieber, C. C. (2010). Evaluation of nutritional status in older persons: Nutritional screening and assessment. *Current Opinion on Clinical Nutrition Metabolic Care, 13*(1), 8–13.

Blazer, O., & Williams, C. D. (1980). Epidemiology of dysphagia and depression in an elderly population. *American Journal of Psychiatry, 137*, 439.

Bouillanne, O., Golmard, J. L., Coussieu, C., Noel, M., Durand, D., Piette, F., & Nivet-Antione, V. (2007). Leptin a new biological marker for evaluating malnutrition in elderly patients. *European Journal of Clinical Nutrition, 61*(5), 647–654.

Brin, M. F., & Younger, D. (1988). Neurologic disorders and aspiration. *Otolaryngeal Clinics of North America, 21*, 691–699.

Burr, M. L., & Phillips, K. M. (1984). Anthropometric norms in the elderly. *British Journal of Nutrition, 51*(2), 165–169.

Castell, D. O. (1996). The efficient dysphagia work-up. *Emergency Medicine, 58*(2), 73–77.

Coulston, A. M., Mandelbaum, D., & Reaven, G. M. (1990). Dietary management of nursing home residents with non-insulin-dependent diabetes mellitus. *American Journal of Clinical Nutrition, 51*, 67–71.

Crogan, N. L. (2012). Various vitamin and mineral supplements are observed to increase mortality risk in older women, with the exception of calcium, which decreases risk [Peer commentary on the paper Dietary supplements and mortality rate in older women: The Iowa Women's Health Study, by Mursu, J., Roblen, K., Harnack, L.J., Park, K., & Jacobs, D. R. Jr. (2011). *Archives of Internal Medicine, 171*(18), 1625–1633] *Evidence-Based Nursing*, Mar 22 [Epub ahead of print].

Crogan, N., Evans, B., & Velasquez, D. (2004). Measuring nursing home resident satisfaction with food and food service: Initial testing of the FoodEx-LTC. *Journals of Gerontology: Medical Sciences, 59A*(4), 370–377.

Crogan, N., & Evans, B. (2006). The shortened food expectations – Long-Term Care questionnaire: Assessing nursing home residents' satisfaction with food and food service. *Journal of Gerontological Nursing, 32*(11), 50–59.

Cruz-Jentoft, A. J., Baeyens, J. P., Bauer, J. M., Boirie, Y., Caderholm, T., Landi, F.,…European Working Group on Scarcopenia in Older People. (2010). Sarcopenia: European consensus on definition and diagnosis: Report of the European Working Group on Sarcopenia. *Age and Ageing, 39*(4), 412–423.

Davies, S. (2002). An interdisciplinary approach to the management of dysphagia. *Professional Nurse, 18*(1), 22–25.

De Castro, J. M., Brewer, E. M., Elmore, D. K., & Orazco, S. (1990). Social facilitation of the spontaneous meal size of humans occurs regardless of time, place, alcohol or snacks. *Appetite, 15*, 89–101.

Detsky, A. S., Baker, J. P., Mandelson, R. A., Wolman, S. L., Wesson, D. E., & Jeejeebhoy, K. N. (1984). Evaluating the accuracy of nutritional assessment techniques applied to hospitalized patients: Methodology and comparisons. *Journal of Parenteral and Enteral Nutrition, 8*, 153–159.

Edwards, S. J., & Metheny, N. A. (2000). Measurement of gastric residual volume: State of the science. *MEDSURG Nursing, 9*(3), 125–128.

Ekberg, O., Hamby, S., Woisard, V., Wuttge-Hanning, A., & Ortega, P. (2004). Social and psychological burden of dysphagia: Its impact on diagnosis and treatment. *Dysphagia, 17*, 139–146.

Ferguson, M., Capra, S., Bauer, J., & Banks, M. (1999). Development of a valid and reliable malnutrition screening tool for adult acute hospital patients. *Nutrition, 15*(6), 458–464.

Garon, B. R., Engle, M., & Ormison, C. (1997). A randomized control study to determine the effects of unlimited oral intake of water. *Journal of Neurological Rehabilitation, 11*, 139–148.

Glenn-Molali, N. H. (2002). Nourishment and swallowing. In S. P. Hoeman (Ed.), *Rehabilitation nursing* (3rd ed., pp. 322–346). St. Louis, MO: Mosby.

Guigoz, Y., Vellas, B. & Garry, P. J. (1996). Assessing the elderly: The mini nutritional assessment as part of the geriatric evaluation. *Nutrition Review, 54*(1 Pt 2):S59–65.

Hajjar, R. R., Kamel, H. K., & Denson, K. (2004). Malnutrition in aging. *The Internet Journal of Geriatrics and Gerontology, 1*(1), 1–16.

Heaton, G., Crogan, N., Short, R., & Dupler, A. (2011). Resident food choice: Evolution of the facility menu using Rate the Food. *Dietary Manager, 20*, 30–34.

Herskowitz, J. (2012). *Do you have a swallowing problem?* [Web online article]. Retrieved from: http://EzineArticles.com/?expert=Joel_Herskowitz

Hickson, M. (2006). Malnutrition and ageing. *Postgraduate Medical Journal, 82*, 2–8.

Hickson, M., & Frost, G. (2003). A comparison of three methods for estimating height in the acutely ill elderly population. *Journal of Human Nutrition & Dietetics, 16*(1), 13–20.

Johnson, V., & Chalmers, J. (2002). *Oral Hygiene Care for Functionally Dependent and Cognitively Impaired Older Adults. Research Dissemination Core.* Iowa City, IA: University of Iowa.

Kalyani, R. R., Stein, B., Valiyil, R., Manno, R., Maynard, J. W., & Crews, D. C. (2010). Vitamin D treatment for the prevention of falls in older adults: Systematic review and meta-analysis. *Journal of the American Geriatric Society, 58*(7), 1299–1310.

Kaiser, M. J., Bauer, J. M., Ramsch, C., & MNA-International Group. (2009). Validation of the Mini Nutritional Assessment short-form (MNA-SF): A practical tool for identification of nutritional status. *Journal of Nutrition, Health & Aging, 13*(9), 782–788.

Kawashima, K., Motohashi, Y., & Fujishima, I. (2004). Prevalence of dysphagia among community-dwelling elderly individuals as estimated using a questionnaire for dysphagia screening. *Dysphagia, 19*, 266–271.

Kennedy-Malone, L., Fletcher, K. R., & Plank, L. M. (2004). *Management guidelines for nurse practitioners working with older adults* (2nd ed.). Philadelphia, PA: F. A. Davis.

Kivela, S. L., Nissinen, A., & Tuomiiehto, J. (1986). Prevalence of depressive and other symptoms in elderly Finnish men. *Acta Psychiatrica Scandinavica, 73*, 93–100.

Kuzuya, M., Kanda, S., Koike, T., Suzuki, Y., & Iguchi, A. (2005). Lack of correlation between total lymphocyte count and nutritional status in the elderly. *Clinical Nutrition, 24*(3), 427–432.

Langmore, S. E., Terpenning, M. S., Schork, A., Chen, Y., Murray, J. T., Lopatin, D., ...Loesche, W. J. (1998). Predictors of aspiration pneumonia: How important is dysphagia? *Dysphagia, 13*, 69–81.

Layne, K. A., Losinki, D. S., Zenner, P. M., & Ament, J. A. (1989). Using the Flemish index of dysphagia to establish prevalence. *Dysphagia, 4*, 39–42.

Lindgren, S., & Janzon, L. (1991). Evaluating dysphagia. *American Family Physician, 61*(12), 147–152.

Logemann, J. A. (1998). *Evaluation and treatment of swallowing disorders* (2nd ed.). Austin, TX: Pro-ed.

Logemann, J. A., Gesler, G., Robbins, J., Lindblad, A. S., Brandt, D., Hind, J A.,...Gardener, P. J. (2008). A randomized study of three interventions for aspiration of thin liquids in patients with dementia or Parkinson's disease. *Journal of Speech, Language, and Hearing Research, 5*(1), 173–183.

Loreck, E., Chimakurthi, R., & Steinle, N.I. (2012). Nutritional assessment of the geriatric patient: A comprehensive approach toward evaluating and managing nutrition. *Clinical Geriatrics, 20*(4), 20–26.

Martin-Harris, B., & Cherney, L. R. (1996). Treating swallowing disorders following stroke. In L. R. Cherney & A. S. Halper (Eds.), *Topics in stroke rehabilitation* (3rd ed., pp. 27–40). Frederick, MD: Aspen.

McIntosh, W. A., Shifflet, P. A., & Picou, J. S. (1989). "Social" support stressful events, strain, dietary intake, and the elderly. *Medical Care, 27*, 140–153.

McClave, S. A., Sexton, L. A., Spain, D. A., Adams, J. L., Owens, N. A., Sullins, M. B., Blandford, B. F. & Snider, H. L. (1999). Enteral tube feeding in the intensive care unit: factors impeding adequate delivery. *Critical Care Medicine, 27*(7), 1252–1256.

Metheny, N. A., Schallom, M. E., & Edwards, S. J. (2004). Effect of gastrointestinal motility and feeding tube site on aspiration risk in critically ill patients: A review. *Heart and Lung, 33*(3), 131–145.

Morley, J. E. (1989). Death by starvation: A modern American problem? *Journal of the American Geriatric Society, 37*, 184.

Morley, J. E. (2007). Weight loss in the nursing home. *Journal of the American Medical Directors Association, 8*, 201–204.

Morley, J. E. (2010). Anorexia, weight loss, and frailty. *Journal of the American Medical Directors Association, 11*, 225–228.

Morley, J. E. (2011a). Assessment of malnutrition in older persons: A focus on the Mini Nutritional Assessment. *Journal of Nutrition, Health, and Aging, 15*(2), 87–90.

Morley, J. E. (2011b). Undernutrition: A major problem in nursing homes. *Journal of the American Medical Directors Association, 12*, 243–246.

Morley, J.E., & Kraenzle, D. (1995). Weight loss. *Journal of the American Geriatrics Society, 43*, 82–83.

Morley, J. E., & Morley, P. M. K. (1995). Psychological and social factors in pathogenesis of weight loss. *Annual Reviews of Gerontology and Geriatrics, 15*, 83–109.

Morris, H. (2004). Dysphagia in the elderly: A management challenge for nurses. *British Journal of Nursing, 15*(10), 558–562.

Mursu, J., Robien, K., Harnack, L. J., Park, K., & Jacobs, D. R. (2011). Dietary supplements and mortality rate in older women. *Archives of Internal Medicine, 171*(18), 1625–1633.

Nijs, K., de Graaf, C., van Staveren, W.A., & de Groot, I.C. (2009). Malnutrition and mealtime ambiance in nursing homes. *Journal of the American Medical Directors Association, 10*, 226–229.

Omran, M. L., & Morely, J. E. (2000). Assessment of protein energy malnutrition in older persons, part 1: History, examination, body composition, and screening tools. *Nutrition, 16*, 50–63.

Paik, N. (2012, March 26). *Dysphagia* [Web online article]. Retrieved from http://emedicine.medscape .com/article/324096-overview

Panther, K. (2005). The Frazier free water protocol. *Perspectives on Swallowing and Swallowing Disorders (Dysphagia), 14*(1), 4–9.

Roy, N., Stemple, J., Merrill, R. M., & Thomas, L. (2007). Dysphagia in the elderly: Preliminary evidence of prevalence, risk factors and socioemotional effects. *Annals of Otology, Rhinology and Laryngology, 111*(11), 858–865.

Schols, A., Mostert, R., Cobbin, N., Soeters, P., & Wouters, E. (1991). Transcutaneous oxygen saturation and carbon dioxide tension during meals in patients with chronic obstructive pulmonary disease. *Chest, 100*, 1287–1292.

Seitzer, M. H., Bastidas, J. A., Cooper, D. M., Engler, P., Slocum, B., & Flatcher, H. S. (1979). Instant Nutritional Assessment. *Journal of Parenteral and Enteral Nutrition, 3*(3), 157–159.

Shatenstein, B. (2002). Malnutrition. *Encyclopedia of aging*. Retrieved from http://www.encyclopedia .com/doc/1G2-3402200250.html

Simmons, S. F., Zhuo, X., & Keller, E. (2010). Cost-effectiveness of nutrition interventions in nursing home residents: A pilot intervention. *Journal of Nutrition, Health & Aging, 14*, 367–372.

Smith, H. A., & Connolly, M. J. (2003). Evaluation and treatment of dysphagia following stroke. *Topics in Geriatric Rehabilitation, 19*(1), 43–59.

Spieker, M. R. (2000). Evaluating dysphagia. *American Family Physician, 61*(12), 3639–3648.

Stevenson, J. (2002) Meeting the challenge of dysphagia. *Nurse2Nurse, 3*, 2–3.

Stroke Research Unit, Queen Elizabeth Hospital, Gateshead. (2001). *Collaborative Dysphagia Audit (CODA) Study*. Retrieved from http://www.nursingtimes.net/nursing-practice-clinical-research/ an-interdisciplinary-approach-to-the-management-of-dysphagia/199842.article

Tariz, S. H., Karcic, E., Thomas, D .R., Thomson, K., Philpot, C., Chapel, D. L., & Morley, J. E. (2001). The use of a no-concentrated-sweets diet in the management of type 2 diabetes in nursing homes. *Journal of the American Dietetic Association, 101*, 1463–1466.

Thomas, D. R. (2007). Loss of skeletal muscle mass in aging: Examining the relationship of starvation, sarcopenia and cachexia. *Clinical Nutrition, 26*(4), 389–399.

Thompson, F. E., & Subar, A. F. (2012). *Dietary assessment methodology*. Retrieved from http://www.indiana .gov/isdh/files/4_TAB__3.pdf

Wirth, R., Voss, C., Smoliner, C., Sieber, C.C., Bauer, J.M., & Volkert, D. (2012). Complications and mortality after percutaneous endoscopic gastrostomy in geriatrics: A prospective multicenter observational trial. *Journal of the American Medical Directors Association, 13*, 228–233.

Wilson, M. M., Purushothaman, R., & Morley, J. E. (2002). Effect of liquid dietary supplements on energy intake in the elderly. *American Journal of Clinical Nutrition, 75*, 944–947.

White, G., O'Rourke, F., Ong, B. S., Cordato, D. J., & Chan, D. Y. K. (2008). Dysphagia: Causes, assessment, treatment and management. *Geriatrics, 63*(5), 15–20.

Zoltick, E. S., Sahni, S., McLean, R. R., Quach, L., Casey, V. A., & Hannan, M. T. (2011). Dietary protein intake and subsequent falls in older men and women: the Framingham study. *Journal of Nutrition, Health, and Aging, 15*(2), 147–152.

For a full suite of assignments and additional learning activities, see the access code at the front of your book.

LEARNING OBJECTIVES

www

At the end of this chapter, the reader will be able to:

> Describe the etiology of pressure ulcers.
> Discuss the implications and relevance of pressure ulcers.
> Classify pressure ulcers using the staging system.
> Identify key components of pressure ulcer prevention and management.
> List the components of assessment of skin and wounds.
> Identify interventions for pressure ulcer prevention and management.
> Describe critical factors in wound management.
> Develop a care plan for potential/impaired skin integrity.

KEY TERMS

www

Avoidable/unavoidable pressure ulcers
Braden Scale for Pressure Ulcer Risk
   Assessment
Causative factors
Facility acquired (FA) pressure ulcers
National Pressure Ulcer Advisory Panel
   (NPUAP)

Pressure ulcers
Pressure ulcer risk assessment
Pressure ulcer staging system
Pressure redistribution
Pressure ulcer management

Pressure Ulcers

Sandra Higelin

Introduction

Pressure ulcers are now recognized as a significant healthcare threat to patients with restricted mobility or chronic disease and to older patients. A pressure ulcer can cause serious complication, pain, decreased quality of life, increased morbidity and mortality, a significant increase in caregiver time, and an increase in the spending of healthcare dollars. Patients with pressure ulcers have a higher rate of morbidity and mortality. Research indicates that approximately 60,000 patients die each year from complications of pressure ulcers; the most common major complication is infection, which can result in sepsis (Salcido, 2012). It has recently been reported that over 445,000 pressure ulcers developed in Medicare patients from 2005 to 2007, at a cost in excess of $2.41 billion in healthcare costs (VanGilder, Amlung, Harrison, & Meyer, 2009). Pressure ulcer prevention and management is important to hospitals, skilled nursing facilities, community-based healthcare services, and other community settings. Over the past 20 years there has been a burgeoning of knowledge related to pressure ulcer prevention and management, as well as a significant increase in the types of wound care products and treatment modalities that can be used in the management of pressure ulcers.

Etiology

"A pressure ulcer is localized injury to the skin and/or underlying tissue usually over a bony prominence, as a result of pressure, or pressure in combination with shear. A number of contributing or confounding factors are also associated with pressure ulcers; the significance of these factors is yet to be elucidated" (National Pressure Ulcer Advisory Panel [NPUAP] & European Pressure Ulcer Advisory Panel [EPUAP], 2009, p. 7).

The most common sites for pressure ulcers to occur are the coccyx, sacrum, ischial tuberosity, trochanter, and the calcaneus. These sites have less soft tissue present between the bone and the skin. There are also device-related pressure ulcers that develop as a result of nasal cannulas, urinary catheters, casts, orthotics, and other types of medical equipment or tubing.

The major *causative factor* in pressure ulcer formation is pressure. Several factors are involved to determine what pathologic effect pressure has on soft tissue to create ischemia, which results in tissue anoxia and cell death. Depending on the physical health of the individual, pressure ulcers can develop within 1–24 hours of the insult and may take up to 7 days to present themselves. Factors that influence pressure ulcer development are (1) intensity of pressure, (2) duration of pressure, and (3) tissue tolerance, which is the ability of skin and its supporting structures to endure pressure (Bryant & Nix, 2012).

Shear and friction are also extrinsic causative factors that are involved in pressure ulcer development. Shear is caused by a force, working parallel to the skin, that is exerted when gravity is pushing down on the body and there is resistance between the patient and a surface such as a chair or bed. As a result of this resistance, the skin is held in place while the weight of the skeleton pulls the body downward; thus, injury to deeper tissues overlying bony prominences occurs. Friction is resistance to motion in a parallel direction and acts in concert with shear. If friction is the only factor present, the injury to the skin is confined to the epidermis and upper dermal layers of the skin (Bryant & Nix, 2012).

Moisture, usually caused by incontinence, is another extrinsic factor for pressure ulcer development. Moisture alters the resiliency of the epidermis to external forces by weakening the lipid layer of the stratum corneum and collagen. In the presence of urinary or fecal incontinence, the skin's pH is alkalinized and the normal skin flora are altered (Bryant & Nix, 2012).

Intrinsic factors that influence the development of pressure ulcers include advanced age, nutritional deficiency, smoking, medications, and other comorbidities such as chronic obstructive lung disease, cardiac disease, musculoskeletal disorders, renal disease, diabetes, and cognitive impairment. The normal skin changes associated with aging, combined with the effects of illness, contribute to the higher risk of ulcer development in the older population. Skin becomes thinner, has less collagen and moisture, and can lose the ability to protect itself against invading organisms. Blood flow to the dermis is reduced, resulting in fewer nutrients reaching the skin and less waste removal. It is also more susceptible to friction and shear injuries (Bryant & Nix, 2012).

Implications/Prelevance of Pressure Ulcers

Hospitalizations involving patients with pressure ulcers increased at least 80% between 1993 and 2006, according to the Healthcare Cost and Utilization Project (Levit, Stranges, Ryan & Elixhauser, 2008). When pressure ulcer care is involved, hospitalizations are longer and more expensive: Inpatient hospital admissions with a pressure ulcer diagnosis totaled $11.0 billion in 2006. When a pressure ulcer is diagnosed, the average hospital stay extends from 5 days to 14 days, with additional costs between $16,700 and $20,400, depending on the medical condition of the patient. In adult patients, 56.5% were age 65 or older. Hospital patients with a diagnosis of pressure ulcer are discharged to long-term care facilities at a rate of approximately 54%. In older adults with pressure ulcers, comorbidities such as fluid and electrolyte disorders, nutritional disorders, diabetes, multiple system failure, and dementia are also part of the patient's medical condition (Wound, Ostomy and Continence Nurses Society [WOCN], 2010).

Pressure ulcer prevalence is defined as the number of patients with at least one pressure ulcer who exist in a given patient population at a given point in time. Research indicates pressure ulcer prevalence in acute care settings ranges from 14% to 17% in the United States. In long-term care, the prevalence of pressure ulcers has been reported as high as 27%, with approximately 8% of these being nosocomial. In home care, prevalence of pressure ulcers is 3–10% (Bryant & Nix, 2012).

Prevalence surveys are conducted to provide a method for healthcare institutions to benchmark their facilities against national prevalence rates. *Facility-acquired (FA) pressure ulcers* are also surveyed in this process. A prevalence survey that was conducted in 2008 reported the prevalence rates for all acute care facilities was 13.5% and that FA pressure ulcer rates were 6%; in 2009, the rates decreased to 12.3% and 5%, respectively. Overall prevalence rates in long-term acute care facilities were 22%. In adult intensive care units, the FA pressure ulcer rates were the highest ranging from 9.2–12.1% in 2008 and from 8.8–10.3% in 2009. In long-term care facilities the rates were 11.7 and 4.9% in 2008 and 11.8 and 5.2% in 2009. Patients in intensive care developed Stage III, Stage IV, unable to stage, or deep tissue injuries at a rate of 3.3%. In 2009, device-related pressure ulcers developed at a rate of 10%. The ear (20%) and the sacro/coccyx area (17%) were the most common location for the development of device-related pressure ulcers (VanGilder et al., 2009).

Incidence is defined as the number of patients who were initially ulcer free and developed a pressure ulcer within a particular time period in a defined population. According to the research, the incidence of pressure ulcers in acute care ranges from 7–9%; in long-term care, 3–31%; and in home care, 0–17% (Bryant & Nix, 2012).

A 2006 prevalence survey reports an overall acute care facilities FA pressure ulcer incidence rate of 6.7%. This rate decreased in 2009 to 5%. The overall FA pressure ulcer rate for long-term acute care was 8% in 2006; this rate decreased to 3.8% in 2009. The FA pressure ulcer rate for long-term care was reported as 6.7% in 2006 and 5.2% in 2009 (VanGilder et al., 2009). Data from these types of surveys suggest that the overall pressure ulcer prevalence and incidence rates are improving. Research is continuing in pressure ulcer etiology, risk assessment, prevention, and treatment strategies.

A pressure ulcer impacts quality and duration of life. Pressure ulcers can be painful, odorous, and disfiguring; social isolation can frequently result. Hospital mortality for patients with pressure ulcers as a secondary diagnosis is approximately

11%, and greater than 4% if pressure ulcer is the primary diagnosis. Research further indicates approximately 60,000 patients die each year from pressure ulcer-related complications. These deaths occurred more frequently in patients over 75 years of age. Septicemia was reported in 39.7% of the reported deaths from pressure ulcer complications (Bryant & Nix, 2012).

Pressure ulcer development is considered an indicator for quality of care. The Centers for Medicare and Medicaid Services (CMS) added Stage III and Stage IV pressure ulcers to the list of reportable Never Events in 2008. Never Events are defined as errors in medical care that are clearly identifiable, preventable, and have serious consequences for patients (Miller, 2009); the costs associated with these Never Events are nonreimbursable by Medicare and Medicaid. In 2004, CMS addressed the prevention of pressure ulcers in long-term care residents by defining *avoidable* and *unavoidable pressure ulcers*. When pressure ulcers develop during admission and are identified as avoidable, civil monetary penalties can be assessed in the long-term care setting (Black et al., 2011). According to CMS, *avoidable* means that a resident developed a pressure ulcer when the facility did not evaluate the resident's clinical condition and pressure ulcer risk factors; did not define and implement interventions consistent with the resident's needs, goals, and recognized standards of practice; or did not monitor and evaluate the impact of the intervention or did not revise the interventions as appropriate to the findings of the evaluation. *Unavoidable* means that a resident developed a pressure ulcer even though the facility had appropriately and comprehensively assessed the residents clinical condition and risk factors, implemented appropriated interventions, monitored and evaluated the effectiveness of these interventions, and revised them as indicated by the care plan (CMS, 2004).

Pressure Ulcer Prevention

The overall goal for the prevention of pressure ulcers is to identify persons at risk and initiate early prevention strategies to maintain intact skin, prevent complications, optimize potential for wound healing, and involve the patient and the caregiver in the plan of care. It is also an important goal to implement cost-effective strategies in the plan of care.

Assessment

A complete medical history should be included in the ***pressure ulcer risk assessment***. Risk factors for pressure ulcer development include advanced age; immobility; malnutrition; incontinence; diminished level of consciousness; impaired sensation; history of pressure ulcers; multiple comorbidities such as diabetes, chronic obstructive pulmonary disease, renal disease, and arterial/vascular disease; medication history; and previous treatment with steroids, radiation, or chemotherapy.

Risk assessment instruments are utilized to ascertain pressure ulcer risk and should be completed on all patients. The ***Braden Scale for Pressure Ulcer Risk Assessment*** is the most widely used instrument that determines risk of pressure ulcer development.

The scale assesses sensory perception, skin moisture, activity, mobility, nutrition, and friction/shear. Each area is scored on a scale of 1–3 or 4, with a possible total score of 23 points—the lower the Braden score, the higher the risk of pressure ulcer development (Braden & Bergstrom, 1987). A Braden score of 16 or less indicates a high risk of pressure ulcer development in the general population, while a score of 18 or less is indicative of high risk in older adults or persons with darkly pigmented skin. Subset scores of 2 or less in any one category also places one in a high-risk category even if the patient has an overall score greater than 16 (see **Box 18-1**).

BOX 18-1   Braden Scale for Pressure Ulcer Risk Assessment

Sensory Perception

Ability to respond meaningfully to pressure-related discomfort

1. Completely Limited: Unresponsive (does not moan, flinch, or gasp) to painful stimuli, due to diminished level of consciousness or sedation.

OR

Limited ability to feel pain over most of body surface.

2. Very Limited: Responds only to painful stimuli.

Cannot communicate discomfort except by moaning or restlessness.

OR

Has a sensory impairment, which limits the ability to feel pain or discomfort over half of body.

3. Slightly Limited: Responds to verbal commands but cannot always communicate discomfort or need to be turned.

OR

Has some sensory impairment, which limits ability to feel pain or discomfort in one or two extremities.

4. No Impairment: Responds to verbal commands. Has no sensory deficit that would limit ability to feel or voice pain or discomfort.

Moisture

Degree to which skin is exposed to moisture

1. Constantly Moist: Perspiration, urine, etc. keep skin moist almost constantly. Dampness is detected every time patient is moved or turned.

2. Moist: Skin is often but not always moist.

3. Linen must be changed at least once a shift.

4. Occasionally Moist: Skin is occasionally moist, requiring an extra linen change approximately once a day.

5. Rarely Moist: Skin is usually dry; linen requires changing only at routine intervals.

Activity

Degree of physical activity

1. Bedfast: Confined to bed.

2. Chairfast: Ability to walk is severely limited or nonexistent. Cannot bear own weight and/or must be assisted into chair or wheelchair.

3. Walks Occasionally: Walks occasionally during day but for very short distances, with or without assistance. Spends majority of each shift in bed or chair.

4. Walks Frequently: Walks outside the room at least twice a day and inside room at least once every 2 hours during waking hours.

Pressure Ulcers

Ability to change and control body position

1. Completely Immobile: Does not make even slight changes in body or extremity position without assistance.

2. Very Limited: Makes occasional slight changes in body or extremity position but unable to make frequent or significant changes independently.

3. Slightly Limited: Makes frequent though slight changes in body or extremity position independently.

4. No Limitations: Makes major and frequent changes in position without assistance.

Nutrition

Usual food intake pattern

1. Very Poor: Never eats a complete meal. Rarely eats more than one-third of any food offered. Eats two servings or less of protein (meat or dairy products) per day. Takes fluids poorly. Does not take a liquid dietary supplement.

OR

Is NPO and/or maintained on clear liquids or IV for more than 5 days.

2. Probably Inadequate: Rarely eats a complete meal and generally eats only about half of any food offered. Protein intake includes only three servings of meat or dairy products per day. Occasionally will take a dietary supplement.

OR

Receives less than optimum amount of liquid diet or tube feeding.

3. Adequate: Eats over half of most meals. Eats a total of four servings of protein (meat, dairy products) each day. Occasionally will refuse a meal, but will usually take a supplement if offered.

OR

Is on a tube feeding or TPN regimen, which probably meets most of nutritional needs.

4. Excellent: Eats most of every meal. Never refuses a meal. Usually eats a total of four or more servings of meat and diary products. Occasionally eats between meals. Does not require supplementation.

Friction and Shear

1. Problem: Requires moderate to maximum assistance in moving. Complete lifting without sliding against sheets is impossible. Frequently slides down in bed or chair, requiring frequent repositioning with maximum assistance. Spasticity, contractures, or agitation leads to almost constant friction

2. Potential Problem: Moves feebly or requires minimum assistance. During a move, skin probably slides to some extent against sheets, chair, restraints, or other devices. Maintains relatively good position in chair or bed most of the time but occasionally slides down.

3. No Apparent Problem: Moves in bed and in chair independently and has sufficient muscle strength to lift up completely during move. Maintains good position in bed or chair at all times.

TOTAL SCORE:

Source: Copyright Barbara Braden and Nancy Bergstrom, 1988. Reprinted with permission.

Baseline Braden scores should be determined upon admission to the healthcare facility, and the assessment should be repeated at regular intervals or when the patient's condition changes. Hospitals, long-term care facilities, and community healthcare facilities should implement nursing care policies to determine the frequency of assessment.

The standard of care is to perform accurate and routine skin inspections and assessments. A total-body skin inspection should be completed on admission to the healthcare facility to determine if there are any skin impairments, including reddened areas, rashes, abnormal lesions, abrasions, bruises, skin tears, traumatic injuries, and pressure ulcers. The temperature of the skin should also be assessed. Any area of skin that deviates from what is normal needs to be compared to the adjacent skin, and the findings should be documented. Skin assessment includes the skin inspection, the interpretation of the findings from the inspection, and the synthesis of the inspection information combined with information from the comprehensive assessment of the patient, such as comorbidities, medication history, nutrition, perfusion, and pressure ulcer history.

Evidence-based practice includes nutritional status as part of the total assessment. Assessment of nutritional status is critical to identify the risk of malnutrition, as malnutrition is associated with poor wound healing and overall morbidity and mortality (Demling, 2009). A nutritional assessment should be performed upon entry to a new healthcare setting and whenever there is a change in the individual's condition. A comprehensive nutritional assessment includes:

1. Current weight and usual weight (an actual weight, not a stated weight)
2. History of unintended weight loss or gain
3. Body mass index (BMI)
4. Determining possible protein energy malnutrition
5. Food intake
6. Dental health
7. Oral and gastrointestinal history, including chewing and swallowing difficulties and the ability to feed one's self
8. Medical/surgical history or interventions that influence nutrient intake or absorption of nutrients
9. Drug/nutrient interaction
10. Psychosocial factors affecting food intake
11. Cultural and lifestyle influences on food selection

Laboratory parameters for nutritional status should be evaluated. Serum albumin levels are frequently used to assess nutritional status, but they are a poor indicator of protein status as multiple factors decrease albumin levels even when protein intake is adequate. Factors that affect albumin levels include infection, acute stress, surgery, cortisone excess, dehydration, and kidney disease. Normal albumin levels are approximately 3.5–5, which reflects what protein levels were approximately 14–21 days prior to the exam. Prealbumin is a more current reflection of protein stores, indicating status for the past 2–3 days, though it may be artificially low in the presence of severe inflammation or infection. Normal prealbumin levels range from 18 to 28.

Interventions for the Prevention of Pressure Ulcers

Evidence-based practice indicates the interventions that should be present in a pressure ulcer prevention program include *pressure redistribution* and offloading, maintaining skin health, nutrition and hydration, and patient/family education. Because prevention and treatment interventions overlap, both prevention and treatment strategies are addressed for tissue redistribution in this section.

Tissue Load Management

Tissue load is the distribution of friction, pressure, and shear on the tissue. Pressure redistribution is the ability of a support surface to distribute load over the contact areas of the human body to reduce the overall pressure and avoid areas of focal pressure. Offloading is provided by turning and repositioning the patient. Both pressure redistribution and offloading are necessary activities for the at-risk patient and the patient with existing pressure ulcers while in bed, in a chair, on a gurney, or in the operating room. Support surfaces should be utilized on beds and chairs to redistribute pressure, but they should be used only as adjuncts and do not replace the need for manual turning and repositioning. The type of support surface to be used is determined by the patient's condition, the healthcare setting, the cost, and the availability of product. Properly sized equipment should be used for morbidly obese patients; these are classified by the weight limits of the equipment. The terms and definitions developed by the National Pressure Ulcer Advisory Support Surface Standard Initiative in 2007 should be used when choosing support surfaces (Bryant & Nix, 2012) (see **Table 18-1**).

TABLE 18-1	**Specialty Support Surface Selection Guide**						
Therapeutic Support Surface	**Prevention At Risk**	**Trunk Stage I**	**Trunk Stage II**	**Multiple Trunk Stage II**	**Trunk Stage III**	**Trunk Stage IV**	**Multiple Trunk Stage III/IV**
Mattress overlay (alternating pressure, self-adjusting mattress	X	X	X	X			
Low Air Loss			X	X	X	X	
Gel Overlay			X	X	X	X	
Low Air Loss Bed (total bed system)			X	X	X	X	X
Air Fluidized						X	X

Many factors affect product choice such as complex comorbidities, patient size, product cost, and user environment. The criteria for use of a support surface are usually defined in the facility's policies and procedures. Table 18-1 illustrates a therapeutic support surface selection guide. When a support surface is indicated by the patient's clinical condition, the physician order is obtained and the facility vendor or product supplier is notified (Oklahoma Foundation for Medical Quality, 2009).

Repositioning reduces the duration and intensity of pressure over a bony prominence (see **Box 18-2**). The standard has been turning and repositioning at least every 2 hours; however, evidence for the optimal frequency of repositioning is lacking. The current research suggests that repositioning every 4 hours when combined with any pressure redistribution mattress is just as effective for prevention of pressure ulcers (Lyder & Ayello, 2008). The patient's activity/mobility level and overall clinical condition should be considered to determine the frequency of repositioning. The frequency of repositioning must be individualized per the patient's needs and outlined in the patient's plan of care, and the plan of care should be evaluated frequently per the facility's policy and procedures and revised according to changes in the patient's clinical condition. Frequent small position changes can be achieved by using pillows and wedges. To avoid skin surfaces rubbing together, such as at the knees, a pad placed between the legs can be effective (WOCN, 2010).

While in bed, the head of the bed should be maintained at 30 degrees or below. Use a 30-degree, side-lying position and alternate positions (right, back, left); these techniques will prevent sliding, shearing, and pressure-related injuries. Other methods to minimize friction and shear include the use of dry lubricants, transparent films, foams, or hydrocolloids to bony prominences. Avoid pulling or dragging the patient by using lift sheets and lift equipment for repositioning or transfer activities. Friction and shear are enhanced in the presence of moisture, so the skin should be cleaned and dried as soon as possible after each incontinent episode (WOCN, 2010).

For chair-bound patients it is important to redistribute the weight frequently. Pay special attention to the individual's anatomy, postural alignment, and support of the feet. While the patient is sitting in a chair it is recommended that the patient be repositioned at least every hour with small shifts in position every 15–30 minutes. A pressure redistribution cushion should be placed in the chair. When pressure ulcers are present on the sacrococcyx area, sitting should be limited to 3 times a day in periods of 60 minutes or less (WOCN, 2010).

BOX 18-2   Evidence-Based Practice Highlight

A Cochrane systematic review and metaanalysis (McInnes, Jammali-Blasi, Bell-Syer, Dumville, & Cullum, 2011) concluded that there is good evidence that "higher specification foam mattresses, sheepskins, and that some overlays in the operative setting are effective in preventing pressure ulcers, there is insufficient evidence to draw conclusions on the value of seat cushions, limb protectors, and various constant low pressure devices" (p. 1).

Heels are the second most common location of pressure ulcer development and should be completely offloaded using pillows, cushions, or other heel suspension pressure-reducing devices. The recommended placement of the pillow is longitudinally underneath the calf with the heel suspended in the air. Heel protectors are effective for reducing friction to the heels, but they provide no pressure redistribution. If heel protectors are used, a frequent heel inspection should be performed to evaluate for skin breakdown. Consulting a physical therapist in clinical situations where the above modalities have failed is recommended (WOCN, 2010).

Maintaining Skin Health

Maintaining skin health through good skin care is another important intervention for prevention of pressure ulcers. Managing incontinence and cleansing the skin gently at each incontinent episode using a pH-balanced perineal skin cleanser will be more effective for the prevention and treatment of incontinence-associated dermatitis (IAD) than soap and water. Avoid vigorous cleansing as it leads to erosion of the epidermis. Incontinence skin barriers such as creams, ointments, and paste are effective in protecting and maintaining intact skin. The use of briefs to manage incontinence increases the risk of IAD, and a patient with IAD is at higher risk for pressure ulcer development. The use of external containment systems for urine (e.g., condom catheters) and external and internal containment systems for feces should be considered to reduce moisture's effect on the skin. **Box 18-3** provides a summary of strategies to prevent pressure ulcers.

BOX 18-3 Preventing Pressure Ulcers

1. Assess all clients for risk of pressure ulcer development.

2. Identify all factors of risk to determine specific interventions.

3. Inspect the skin at least daily and document results.

4. Use mild cleansing agents for bathing, avoiding hot water, harsh soaps, and friction.

5. Moisturize after bathing and minimize environmental factors that lead to dry skin.

6. Avoid massaging bony prominences.

7. Assess for incontinence. Use skin barriers after cleansing, absorbent underpads or briefs, and monitor frequently for episodes of incontinence.

8. Use dry lubricants, such as cornstarch, on transfer surfaces (linens) to prevent friction.

9. Assess for compromised nutrition, particularly protein and caloric intake. Consider nutritional supplements and support for clients at risk.

10. Maintain or improve client's mobility and activity levels.

11. Reposition bed-bound clients at least every 2 hours and chair-bound clients every hour. Patients should be instructed or assisted to shift their positions more frequently (i.e., every 15 minutes for chair-bound patients and at least every hour for bed-bound).

12. Place at-risk clients on pressure-reducing devices. (Donut devices should not be used—they simply displace the pressure and friction

to the periphery of the area that is meant to be protected.)

13. Use lifting devices to transfer clients.

14. Pillows or foam wedges should be used to keep bony prominences from direct contact with each other (e.g., knees, ankles).

15. Avoid positioning the client on the trochanter when lying on his or her side. (Use a 30-degree lateral inclined position.)

16. Elevate the head of the bed at 30 degrees or less. (Shearing injuries can occur at elevations higher than 30 degrees.)

17. Evaluate and document the effectiveness of interventions, and modify the plan of care according to client response.

18. Provide education to clients, family, and caregivers for the prevention of pressure ulcers.

Nutrition and Hydration

Nutritional deficiencies should be addressed. A dietary consult should be ordered for all patients at moderate to high risk for pressure ulcer development or if there is a change in the patient's condition. Assessment of the adequacy of nutritional intake is essential. Weight should be monitored; a weight loss of >5% in 30 days or >10% in 180 days is considered significant (NPUAP & EPUAP, 2009). When the patient has a pressure ulcer and is underweight or losing weight, calories need to be enhanced and protein supplementation needs to be provided.

Adequate hydration is essential to maintaining skin health. Dehydration causes skin to become fragile and prone to breakdown; decreases the circulating blood volume; and reduces peripheral blood flow, impairing the delivery of nutrients and oxygen to wounds. Risk factors for dehydration should be assessed in all patients. The risk factors for dehydration include fluid loss, fluid restriction, altered cognition, poor oral intake of food or fluids, functional impairments, dysphagia, medications, incontinence, and acute illness. When a patient is at risk for or has a pressure ulcer, a comprehensive nutritional assessment should be conducted by a registered dietician (RD). The average adult requires 30–40 mL/kg of body weight in daily fluid intake. When a patient has a pressure ulcer, additional fluids are required to compensate for losses including wound exudates, fever, vomiting, or diarrhea. The RD will evaluate the patient's fluid needs based on the patient's clinical condition and make recommendations (Kondracki & Collins, 2009).

Patient and Family Education

Patient and family education in pressure ulcer prevention is very important to help reduce the incidence of pressure ulcers in any care setting. Through education, the patient and the family are empowered to participate in the prevention of pressure ulcers.

Documentation of the assessments, interventions, and outcomes is an integral part of the prevention program and should be completed according to the institution's nursing policies for documentation.

Pressure Ulcer Management

Pressure ulcer management includes nursing assessment, accurate staging (classification) of the pressure ulcer, and documentation of the onset and assessed stage. Appropriate interventions and frequent evaluations of the healing progress are implemented with changes made to the plan of care as indicated by changes in the wound.

Classification of Pressure Ulcers

The International Association for Enterostomal Therapy, now known as the WOCN Society, modified the Shea *pressure ulcer staging system*, originally developed in 1975. The *National Pressure Ulcer Advisory Panel* (NPUAP) updated the staging system to provide clarity and accuracy by including more descriptors and defining suspected deep tissue injury and unstageable pressure ulcers (NPUAP, 2007). **Figures 18-1** through **Figure 18-6** provide examples of each stage of pressure ulcer. International guidelines released in 2009 added the term *category* and specified that the suspected deep tissue injury and unstageable pressure ulcer are categories used in the United States (see **Box 18-4**) (NPUAP & EPUAP, 2009).

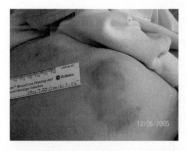

Figure 18-1 Stage I Pressure Ulcer.

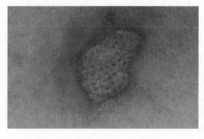

Figure 18-2 Stage II Pressure Ulcer.

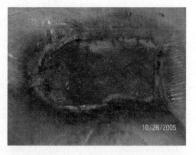

Figure 18-3 Stage III Pressure Ulcer.

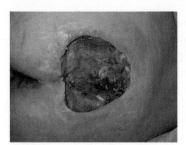

Figure 18-4 Stage IV Pressure Ulcer.

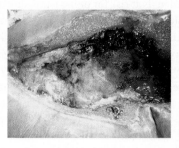

Figure 18-5 Unstagable Pressure Ulcer.

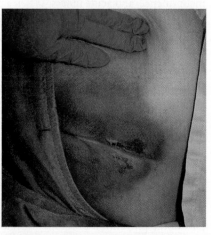

Figure 18-6 Deep Tissue Injury.

BOX 18-4   International NPUAP-EPUAP Pressure Ulcer Classification System

Category/Stage I: Non-blanchable redness of intact skin

Intact skin with non-blanchable erythema of a localized area usually over a bony prominence. Discoloration of the skin, warmth, edema, hardness or pain may also be present. Darkly pigmented skin may not have visible blanching.

Further description: The area may be painful, firm, soft, warmer or cooler as compared to adjacent tissue. Category/Stage I may be difficult to detect in individuals with dark skin tones. May indicate "at risk" persons.

Category/Stage II: Partial thickness skin loss or blister

Partial thickness loss of dermis presenting as a shallow open ulcer with a red pink wound bed, without slough. May also present as an intact or open/ruptured serum-filled or serosanguinous filled blister.

Further description: Presents as a shiny or dry shallow ulcer without slough or bruising. This category/stage should not be used to describe skin tears, tape burns, incontinence associated dermatitis, maceration or excoriation.

Category/Stage III: Full thickness skin loss (fat visible)

Full thickness tissue loss. Subcutaneous fat may be visible but bone, tendon or muscles are **not** exposed. Some slough may be present. **May** include undermining and tunneling.

Further description: The depth of a Category/Stage III pressure ulcer varies by anatomical location. The bridge of the nose, ear, occiput and malleolus do not have (adipose) subcutaneous tissue and Category/Stage III ulcers can be shallow. In contrast, areas of significant adiposity can develop extremely deep Category/Stage III pressure ulcers. Bone/tendon is not visible or directly palpable.

Category/Stage IV: Full thickness tissue loss (muscle/bone visible)

Full thickness tissue loss with exposed bone, tendon or muscle. Slough or eschar may be present. Often include undermining and tunneling.

Further description: The depth of a Category/Stage IV pressure ulcer varies by anatomical location. The bridge of the nose, ear, occiput and malleolus do not have (adipose) subcutaneous tissue and these ulcers can be shallow. Category/Stage IV ulcers can extend into muscle and/or supporting structures e.g., fascia, tendon or joint capsule) making osteomyelitis or osteitis likely to occur. Exposed bone/muscle is visible or directly palpable.

Additional Categories for the USA

Unstageable/Unclassified: Full thickness skin or tissue loss—depth unknown

Full thickness tissue loss in which actual depth of the ulcer is completely obscured by slough (yellow, tan, gray, green or brown) and/or eschar (tan, brown or black) in the wound bed.

Further description: Until enough slough and/or eschar are removed to expose the base of the wound, the true depth cannot be determined; but it will be either a Category/Stage III or IV. Stable (dry, adherent, intact without erythema or fluctuance) eschar on the heels serves as "the body's natural (biological) cover" and should not be removed.

Suspected Deep Tissue Injury-depth unknown

Purple or maroon localized area of discolored intact skin or blood-filled blister due to damage of underlying soft tissue from pressure and/or shear.

Further description: The area may be preceded by tissue that is painful, firm, mushy, boggy, warmer, or cooler as compared to adjacent tissue. Deep tissue injury may be difficult to detect in individuals with dark skin tones. Evolution may include a thin blister over a dark wound bed. The wound may further evolve and become covered by thin eschar. Evolution may be rapid exposing additional layers of tissue even with treatment.

Assessment and Monitoring

Nursing assessment and documentation of pressure ulcers should include onset, location, staging (classification), measurement, exudate description, wound bed characteristics, pain, condition of surrounding tissue, and any undermining or tunneling factors. The healing process is described by the Pressure Ulcer Scale for Healing (PUSH) tool, which provides a consistent method of recording the effectiveness of treatment. The scale has three subscales with a possible total score of 17; the score will trend downward when treatment is effective, and a score of 0 indicates the pressure ulcer has completely healed. Wound assessments should be performed on admission and at least weekly to monitor the healing or deterioration of the pressure ulcer (see **Table 18-2**).

If eschar is present, it must be debrided before staging can occur. The ulcer shoud be documentd as an eschar-covered pressure ulcer. Structures beneath the epidermis and dermis, including muscle, are more susceptible to the effects of ishemia. Pressure ulcers are usually much worse than they appear on the surface; therefore, staging should be to the maximum anatomical depth after necrotic tissue debridement is performed. This is also the case for a deep tissue injury (DTI). These types of wounds should be documented as a suspected DTI, and doucmentation should indicate that the wound will likely develop into a stage III or stage IV pressure ulcer.

The length, width, and depth of pressure ulcers should be measured and documented with distinctions made between the healed and nonhealed areas of the ulcer.

TABLE 18-2 PUSH (Pressure Ulcer Scale for Healing)

Length	0	1	2	3	4	5	Sub-
×	$0\ cm^2$	$<0.3\ cm^2$	$0.3–0.6\ cm^2$	$0.7–1.0\ cm^2$	$1.1–2.0\ cm^2$	$2.1–3.0\ cm^2$	score
Width		6	7	8	9	10	
		$3.1–4.0\ cm^2$	$4.1–8.0\ cm^2$	$8.1–12.0\ cm^2$	$12.1–24.0\ cm^2$	$>24.0\ cm^2$	
Exudate	0	1	2	3			Sub-
Amount	None	Light	Moderate	Heavy			score
Tissue	0	1	2	3	4		Sub-
Type	Closed	Epithelial tissue	Granulation tissue	Slough	Necrotic tissue		score

Length × Width: Measure the greatest length (head to toe) and the greatest width (side to side) using a centimeter ruler. Multiply these two measurements (length 3 width) to obtain an estimate of surface area in square centimeters (cm^2). Caveat: Do not guess! Always use a centimeter ruler, and always use the same method each time the ulcer is measured.

Source: Copyright NPUAP, 2003. Reprinted with permission.

Photographs are often used to document the occurrence and healing of pressure ulcers. The quantity and characteristics of any exudates and the types of wound bed tissue—necrotic, slough, or granulation—are also documented. The sorrounding skin should be assessed for any maceration, induration, crepitus, or injury, including abrasions. Pressure ulcers with undermining or tunnels often lead to further skin breakdown.

Pain related to a pressure ulcer should be assessed. It is also important to identify and document pain relief measures and provide analgesia prior to dressing changes or other interventions.

Reevaluation of the pressure ulcer, the plan of care, and the individual should be done at least every 2 weeks, if there is a significant change in the wound, or if progress towards closure is not observed.

Treatment Modalities

A central component of pressure ulcer care is wound dressing. The dressing used should be based on the tissue in the wound bed, the condition of the skin around the pressure ulcer, and the desired outcomes (see **Table 18-3**). A clean, moist wound bed is ideal to promote healing. When selecting a dressing, the following guidelines should be considered:

1. Assess pressure ulcers at every dressing change and confirm the appropriateness of the current treatment plan.
2. Follow the manufacturer recommendations, especially regarding the frequency of dressing changes.

Exudate Amount: Estimate the amount of exudate (drainage) present after removal of the dressing and before applying any topical agent to the ulcer. Estimate the exudate (drainage) as none, light, moderate, or heavy.

Tissue Type: This refers to the types of tissue that are present in the wound (ulcer) bed. Score as a 4 if there is any necrotic tissue present. Score as a 3 if there is any amount of slough present and necrotic tissue is absent. Score as a 2 if the wound is clean and contains granulation tissue. A superficial wound that is reepithelializing is scored as a 1. When the wound is closed, score as a 0.

4—Necrotic tissue (eschar): Black, brown, or tan tissue that adheres firmly to the wound bed or ulcer edges and may be either firmer or softer than surrounding skin.

3—Slough: Yellow or white tissue that adheres to the ulcer bed in strings or thick clumps, or is mucinous.

2—Granulation tissue: Pink or beefy red tissue with a shiny, moist, granular appearance.

1—Epithelial tissue: For superficial ulcers, new pink or shiny tissue (skin) that grows in from the edges or as islands on the ulcer surface.

0—Closed/resurfaced: The wound is completely covered with epithelium (new skin).

TABLE 18-3	Wound Care Product Guide		
Types/Examples	Indications	Advantages	Change Frequency
Polymeric Film (Transparent film)	• Superficial, partial thickness wounds • Wounds with necrosis and slough • Wounds with little or no exudate	• Can visualize the wound • Control gas exchange • Promotes autolytic debridement • Impermeable to contaminates	24–72 hours
Impregnated Non-Adherent Dressings	• Abrasions • Burns • Graft Donor Sites • Skin Tears	• Covers, soothes and protects underlying tissues where exudate is light	Every 8–12 hours
Polyurethane Foam	• Partial and full thickness wounds with minimal to moderate exudate. May be used as a secondary dressing for wound packing and fillers	• Non-adherent, repels contaminants • Hydrophilic-absorbs a moderate amount of exudate	1–5 days depending on drainage amount
Hydrogels (Water based sheets or amorphous gel)	• Dry wounds • Burns or radiation necrosis or injuries	• Pain reduction • Rehydrates dry wounds • Promotes autolytic debridement • Fills the dead space	1–5 days depending on drainage amount
Types/Examples	Indications	Advantages	Change Frequency
Hydrocolloid	• Superficial, partial thickness wounds • Shallow, full thickness wounds • Wounds with slough or eschar	• Promotes autolytic debridement • Self-adherent • Protects wounds from contaminants	1–7 days depending on drainage amount
Calcium Alginates (ropes and sheets)	• Partial and full thickness wounds • Wounds with slough and necrosis • Wounds with undermining and tunneling	• Fills dead spaces, tunnels and undermining • Absorbs large amount of drainage • Promotes autolytic debridement • Forms a gel interacting with the drainage	1–4 days depending on the drainage amount

3. The care plan should be used to guide the frequency of dressing changes.
4. A dressing that maintains a moist wound bed should be chosen.
5. The dressing should remain in contact with the wound bed and the periwound protected to prevent maceration. There are several moisture retentive dressings available to maintain a moist wound bed.
6. Dressings should be used to help decrease the bioburden in the wound bed and prevent infection. These include a variety of antimicrobial ointments and silver dressings.
   > Silver-impregnated dressings are used for pressure ulcers that are infected or heavily colonized with bacteria. Most of the wound care products utilized today are impregnated with silver.
7. Secondary dressings are to secure a dressing in place and are selected based upon patient comfort.
   > Gauze dressings are mainly used as secondary dressings. As primary dressings they are labor-intensive and can cause pain when removed if they dry out. Desiccation of viable tissue can occur when gauze dressings dry out and adhere to the wound bed.

There are several biophysical agents used in the management of pressure ulcers. These include electrical stimulation, phototherapy, ultrasound, hydrotherapy, laser, negative pressure wound therapy, and hyperbaric oxygen therapy (see **Box 18-5**).

Debridement of devitalized tissue in the wound bed is essential for healing to progress. If necrotic tissue is present, it must be debrided before staging can occur.

BOX 18-5   Guidelines for Pressure Ulcer Treatments

1. Cleanse the wound with a noncytotoxic cleanser (saline) during each dressing change.

2. If necrotic tissue or slough is present, consider the use of high-pressure irrigation.

3. Debride necrotic tissue.

4. Do not debride dry, black eschar on heels.

5. Perform wound care using topical dressings determined by wound and availability.

6. Choose dressings that provide a moist wound environment, keep the skin surrounding the ulcer dry, control exudates, and eliminate dead space.

7. Reassess the wound with each dressing change to determine whether treatment plan modifications are needed.

8. Identify and manage wound infections.

9. Clients with stage III and IV ulcers that do not respond to conservative therapy may require surgical intervention.

Source: Adapted from National Guideline Clearinghouse Guideline for Prevention and Management of Pressure Ulcers (http://www .guideline.gov).

TABLE 18-4 Methods of Pressure Ulcer Debridement	
Extrinsic	**Factors**
Sharp	Devitalized tissue is removed with a scalpel, scissors, or other sharp instrument. The most rapid form of debridement, and can be used for removing areas of thick eschar.
Enzymatic	Topical debriding agents are applied to devitalized tissue areas.
Autolytic	Appropriate for noninfected ulcers only. Synthetic dressings that aid self-digestion of devitalized tissue.
Mechanical	Wet-to-dry dressings, hydrotherapy, and irrigation.

The main types of debridement include autolytic, mechanical, enzymatic, and sharp/surgical debridement (refer to **Table 18-4** for a description of these types of debridement). The debridement method utilized should be determined by the condition of the wound. The wound should be assessed for the presence or absence of infection, amount of necrotic tissue, vascularity of the wound, pain tolerance, setting, and availability and access to various debridement methods. A thorough vascular assessment should be performed prior to debridement of lower extremity ulcers. Dry, hard, stable eschar in ischemic limbs should not be debrided. When using an enzymatic debriding ointment on dry eschar, the eschar should be scored or crosshatched prior to applying the ointment. Maintenance debridement on a chronic wound should be performed until the wound bed is covered with granulation tissue. Sharp debridement is performed by clinicians who have been trained in sharp debridement, which would be a wound consultant, a physician, or a physical therapist. When undermining, tunneling, and extensive necrotic tissue are present in the wound, it may be necessary for a physician to perform surgical debridement (WOCN, 2010).

Critical Factors

There are many critical factors that must be considered in the management of pressure ulcers, including nutrition, pain, infection, and goals of treatment. These factors must be evaluated and care plans must be implemented to address these factors based on the individual needs of the patient. Nutrition is fundamental for cellular integrity, tissue repair, and tissue regeneration. Wound healing is an anabolic process that requires specific nutrients for the biochemical processes in wound healing. The prevalence of malnutrition in hospitals throughout the United States is between 20% and 50%, and further deterioration in nutritional status often occurs during hospitalization. In addition, malnutrition is associated with increased morbidity of 25% and mortality of 5% in patients with acute or chronic diseases. Undernutrition is often called protein malnutrition, which occurs when intake is inadequate, from poor absorption or metabolism that occurs with chronic illnesses, or from acute and traumatic injuries. With malnutrition, the patient experiences severe weight loss, muscle wasting, and loss of adipose tissue. Nutrition screening is essential to identify if the patient is at risk for malnutrition. This screening should be performed by a registered dietician and should be performed on admission and every week (or as often as indicated by the patient's clinical condition). Plasma protein levels are frequently used to determine the patient's protein status. Serum albumin (3.5–5.0 normal level) is the most frequently used blood test to evaluate nutritional status. It has a long half-life of 17–21 days and is not sensitive to rapid changes in nutritional status. Serum prealbumin (18–28 normal range) has a short half-life of 2 days and reflects the decreased intake of protein or calories more rapidly. Serum prealbumin is expected to reflect not only what has been ingested but also what the body has been able to absorb, digest, and metabolize. Serum albumin and prealbumin results may be low even when protein intake is adequate if the patient is suffering from severe inflammation, infection, acute stress, dehydration, and surgery-related cortisone excess. Protein needs are increased after injury and prolonged illness, and a protein deficiency prolongs wound healing time. As much as 100 grams of protein per day can be lost through wound exudate. More calories are also needed to improve healing potential. Nutrients involved in wound healing include protein; arginine; zinc; and vitamins A, B, and C. If dietary intake is inadequate, nutritional support should be used to provide approximately 35 calories/kg per day and 1.5 grams of protein/kg per day. The registered dietician will recommend the calories and protein based on the patient's nutritional status, weight, and other variables (Bryant & Nix, 2012) (see **Box 18-6**).

BOX 18-6 Laboratory Studies Associated with Poor Nutrition

Serum albumin	3.5 g/dl
Serum transferrin	200
Prealbumin	11 mg/dl
Cholesterol	160
Lymphocytopenia	1,500 (100 indicates severe malnutrition)

Source: Adapted from Best Practices for Care of Older Adults (Clark & Baldwin, 2004).

Wound pain has a negative effect on physiologic processes including oxygenation and infection control, as well as on the quality of life. Undertreatment of patients with chronic wound pain is far too common. If undertreated, wound pain can lead to poor wound healing and increased risk of infection; therefore, assessment of all individuals for pain related to a pressure ulcers and their treatment is essential to promote healing. A validated pain scale should be used when assessing pain. The assessment of pain should also include assessment of body language and nonverbal cues. Care delivery should be coordinated with pain medication administration and minimal interruptions while providing patient care. Pressure ulcer pain can be reduced by using nonadherent dressings and maintaining a moist wound bed. Encourage repositioning as a means to reduce pain.

Infection does not usually occur in Stage I or II ulcers, as ischemic tissue is more susceptible to the development of infection. The level of bacteria inhibiting wound healing is not always manifested by the clinical signs of infection. Critically colonized or infected pressure ulcers may exhibit signs of infection such delayed healing, poor or friable granulation tissue, changes in odor or increased exudate, and wound tissue discoloration. Induration may also be present. Culturing of the wound for infection is not recommended if acute signs of infection are not present, since bacteria are present on all wounds and a positive culture would likely result even in the absence of infection. A diagnosis of spreading acute infection should be considered if there is erythema extending from the ulcer edge, induration, new or increasing pain, warmth, or purulent drainage. Crepitus, fluctuance, an increase in size, and discoloration in the surrounding skin may also be signs of acute infection in the wound. There may be systemic signs of infection such as a fever, malaise, lymph node enlargement, confusion, and anorexia. To determine the bacterial bioburden of the pressure ulcer, a tissue biopsy or quantitative swab technique might be performed. Management of infection includes prevention of contamination of the pressure ulcer. Cleansing and debridement of necrotic tissue removes loose debris and planktonic, free-floating bacteria. Debridement can also remove biofilms. Antimicrobials are used to decrease the bacterial bioburden on the wound bed and may slow the rate of biofilm development. Antiseptics can be used for a limited time to control the bacterial bioburden, clean the ulcer, and reduce surrounding inflammation. Topical antimicrobial silver, cadexomer iodine, hypertonic saline, methylene blue/genitial violet-impregnated foams, or medical-grade honey dressings can be used for pressure ulcers infected with multiple organisms. Make sure to assess the patient for allergies to honey, bee products, and bee stings before using honey dressings. Systemic antibiotics are used for patients with clinical evidence of a system infection such as cellulitis, fasciitis, osteomyelitis, and positive blood cultures. Osteomyelitis should be suspected and evaluated if bone is exposed, or the ulcer has failed to heal (WOCN, 2010).

Special Populations

The principles of effective wound management must utilize a holistic approach that is individualized to the patient's clinical and psychosocial situation. Effective wound care identifies and intervenes to minimize or abate the underlying etiology, including coexisting contributing factors. Cost effectiveness of the treatment plan must also be taken into account when recommending wound care products and devices. There are special patient populations that can be very complex when developing their wound management care plan. These include obese patients and terminally ill patients. The goals of treatment for these patient populations must be clearly defined.

The obese patient has special skin care needs that need to be evaluated and planned. There are many common problems in the obese patient that interfere with skin integrity. These include pressure ulcers, intertrigo, and IAD. Difficulty with off-loading pressure is a significant problem in the obese patient. Friction, shear, and pressure existing in locations unique to the obese patient compound the problem. As a result, atypical pressure ulcers result from tubes, catheters, and ill-fitting chairs and beds (see **Box 18-7**). Pressure within skin folds can also result in pressure ulcers. It is vital that frequent, careful assessments are performed of these atypical areas of potential skin breakdown. Make sure proper interventions are implemented to reduce the risk of skin breakdown as well as to properly manage wounds that are already present. The use of bariatric beds with pressure redistribution mattresses and other appropriate bariatric equipment will reduce the risk of pressure ulcers, promote patient independence, decrease staff workload, help control costs, and improve clinical outcomes (Bryant & Nix, 2012).

BOX 18-7   Key Point

Tubes and catheters burrow into skin folds. Reposition tubes and catheters every 2 hours. Place tubes so that patient does not rest on them. Use tubes and catheter holders.

Another special-needs patient is the patient in palliative care or hospice. Palliative care and hospice are associated with the end of a patient's life. The wound management goals for this patient population are relief from distressing symptoms, easing pain, and enhancing the quality of life. Preventing wound deterioration or healing the wound are not realistic goals; instead, the goal in this patient is palliation or maintenance. The focus of wound management in the terminally ill is management of symptoms such as odor, exudate, pain, infection, bleeding, and skin integrity. The wound management care plan should be developed and implemented to encourage comfort and prompt symptom management with consistency between the care provided and consideration of the patient's and the family's goals (NPUAP & EPUAP, 2009).

Summary

Pressure ulcers are a global health concern commonly encountered in both hospital and community settings. Research in pressure ulcer development and management has historically been lacking, though there has been improvement in this area. Continued research will result in a better understanding of the etiology and management of these wounds. Pressure ulcers are considered an avoidable, costly complication caused by unrelieved pressure and inappropriate care.

A comprehensive, multidisciplinary plan that includes risk assessment; comprehensive assessment; regular and routine skin assessment; frequent evaluations; collaboration; safe handoffs; continuity of care across all healthcare settings; and patient, family, and staff education is required to appropriately prevent and manage pressure ulcers. (see **Case Study 18-1**) A team approach with clear communication (see **Box 18-8**), incorporating all of the above components, is essential to accomplishing good clinical outcomes for pressure ulcer prevention and management.

Case Study 18-1

Peter Douglas is a 77-year-old nursing home resident with congestive heart failure and insulin-dependent diabetes mellitus. He is alert and oriented times three and needs maximum assistance with all mobility needs. He was recently admitted to the nursing home after a 6-week hospitalization for pneumonia and congestive heart failure. When he was admitted to the nursing home, the nurse admitting Mr. Douglas documented that he had a pressure ulcer on his sacrum. She described this pressure ulcer as measuring 3 cm by 5 cm by 0 cm. The wound bed presented with 100% yellow necrotic tissue, a moderate amount of drainage, and a foul odor. He was underweight and his albumin level was 2. He was admitted to the nursing home for physical therapy to provide a program to improve strength, balance, and mobility after his long hospital stay. A nutritional consult and a wound consult were ordered by the physician.

Questions

1. What factors put Mr. Douglas at greater risk of developing pressure ulcers?

2. What factors would delay wound healing for this patient?

3. What stage would you classify this wound?

4. What are the signs and symptoms of an active infection in a wound?

5. What products would you use on this type of wound?

BOX 18-8   Research Highlight

Aim: The researchers wanted to determine if the type of organizational culture, team climate, and quality management of pressure ulcer prevention were associated with the prevalence of pressure ulcers.

Methods: A cross-sectional observational study with data from 1,274 patients and 460 health professionals in 37 general hospital wards and 67 nursing home wards in the Netherlands was used. The researchers measured nosocomial pressure ulcers and preventive quality management, looking at the prevalence of pressure ulcers at the ward level.

Findings: No significant correlations were found between organizational culture, team climate, or preventive quality management (at the ward level) and nosocomial pressure ulcer prevalence. However, there was a positive association between institutional quality management and ward quality management with regard to nosocomial pressure ulcer development.

Application to practice: These results from the Netherlands did not support the widely suggested importance of team factors in improving health care that is generally espoused in the United States. However, different research designs and methods in various geographic locations and healthy systems might provide different results in better exploring the relationships between these factors and pressure ulcer outcomes.

Source: Bosch, J., Halfens, J. G., van der Weijden, T., Wensing, M., Akkermans, R, & Grol, R. (2011). Organizational culture, team climate, and quality management in an important patient safety issue: nosocomial pressure ulcers. *Worldviews on Evidence-Based Nursing*, (1), 4–14.

Critical Thinking Exercises

1. Of the types of wounds discussed in this chapter, which have you seen the most of in your experience?

2. What information discussed in this chapter can you apply to your daily practice in order to promote skin integrity and prevent pressure ulcers?

3. What type of risk assessment tool is used at your facility? Is it helpful? Effective?

Personal Reflections

1. Have you ever cared for an older adult with a pressure ulcer? If so, what stage wound did the patient/resident have? What steps might have prevented it? How was it being treated?

2. Visit http://www.consultgerirn.com and review the clinical practice guideline on pressure ulcers. How can you apply this to your practice?

3. Look at the photographs provided in this chapter. How do you think these wounds occurred? What measures can you think of that might have prevented initial breakdown and/or subsequent deterioration of wounds?

4. According to current best practice guidelines, how would you stage a closed, black wound on a person's heel?

References

Black, J. M., Edsberg, L. E., Baharestani, M. M., Langemo, D., Goldberg, M., McNichol, L., …National Pressure Ulcer Advisory Panel. (2011). Pressure ulcers: Avoidable or unavoidable? Results of the national pressure ulcer advisory panel consensus conference. *Ostomy Wound Management, 57*(2), 24–37.

Bosch, J., Halfens, J. G., van der Weijden, T., Wensing, M., Akkermans, R, & Grol, R. (2011). Organizational culture, team climate, and quality management in an important patient safety issue: Nosocomial pressure ulcers. *Worldviews on Evidence-Based Nursing,* (1), 4–14.

Braden, B., & Bergstrom, N. (1987). A conceptual schema for the study of the etiology of pressure sores. *Rehabilitation Nursing, 12,* 8–12, 16.

Bryant, R. & Nix, D. (2012). *Acute and chronic wounds: Current management concepts.* St. Louis, MO: Mosby.

Centers for Medicare & Medicaid Services [CMS]. (2004). *CMS manual system.* Pub. 100-07 State Operations.

Clark, A. P. & Baldwin, K. (2004). Best practices for care of older adults. *Clinical Nurse Specialist, 18*(6), 288–299.

Demling, R. H. (2009). Nutrition, anabolism, and the wound healing process: An overview. *Eplasty, 9,* e9.

Kondracki, N. L. & Collins, N. (2009). The importance of adequate hydration. *Ostomy Wound Management, 55*(12), 16–20.

Levit, K., Stranges, E., Ryan, K., & Elixhauser, A. (2008). *HCUP Facts and Figures, 2006: Statistics on Hospital-based Care in the United States*. Rockville, MD: Agency for Healthcare Research and Quality. Retrieved from http://www.hcup-us.ahrq.gov/reports/factsandfigures/facts_figures_2006.jsp

Lyder, C. H., & Ayello, E. A. (2008). Pressure ulcers: A patient safety issue. In *Patient Safety and Quality: An Evidence-based Handbook for Nurses*. Agency for Healthcare Research and Quality, Publication No. 08-0043: Vol. 2. Washington, DC: U.S. Government Printing Office.

McInnes, E., Jammali-Blasi, A., Bell-Syer, S.E.M., Dumville, J.C., & Cullum, N. (2011). *Support surfaces for pressure ulcer prevention* (Review). Retrieved from http://www.eswell.eu/files/Supportsurfacesforpressureulcerprevention_0.pdf

Miller, A. (2009). Hospital reporting and "Never Events". Retrieved from http://www.medicarepatientmanagement.com/issues/04-03/mpmMJ09-NeverEvents.pdf

National Pressure Ulcer Advisory Panel (NPUAP) and European Pressure Ulcer Advisory Panel (EPUAP). (2009). *Pressure ulcer prevention & treatment*. Quick Reference Guide. Retrieved from http://www.npuap.org/Final_Quick_Prevention_for_web_2010.pdf

National Pressure Ulcer Advisory Panel (NPUAP). (2007). NPUAP Pressure Ulcer Stages/Categories. Retrieved from http://www.npuap.org/resources/educational-and-clinical-resources/npuap-pressure-ulcer-stagescategories/

Oklahoma Foundation for Medical Quality. (2009). *Pressure ulcer prevention and treatment*. Retrieved from http://www.ofmq.com/Websites/ofmq/Images/SOS%20PU%20Toolkit/Cover.pdf

Salcido, R. (2012). *Pressure ulcers and wound care*. Retrieved from http://emedicine.medscape.com/article/319284-overview

VanGilder, C., Amlung, S., Harrison, P., & Meyer, S. (2009). Results of the 2008–2009 international pressure ulcer prevalence survey and a 3-year, acute care unit specific analysis. *Ostomy Wound Management, 55*(11), 39–45.

Wound, Ostomy and Continence Nurses Society [WOCN]. (2010). *Clinical practice guidelines for prevention and management of pressure ulcers*. Mount Laurel, NJ: Author. Retrieved from http://guideline.gov/content.aspx?id=23868

For a full suite of assignments and additional learning activities, see the access code at the front of your book.

Unit VI
Leadership and Responsibility

(COMPETENCIES 1, 11, 12, 13)

LEARNING OBJECTIVES

At the end of this chapter, the reader will be able to:

> Identify characteristics of effective nurse managers and leaders.
> Compare and contrast the roles of nurse manager and leader.
> Compare various leadership styles and strategies.
> Describe effective communication strategies.
> Describe the process of delegation, including how it is used in the management of unlicensed assistive personnel.
> Compare various leadership roles available to nurses who care for older adults.
> Analyze the characteristics of the major generations of nurses.
> Recognize the value of professional associations to the nurse manager and leader.
> Evaluate one's own strengths and weaknesses as a future nurse manager or leader.

KEY TERMS

21st century leadership
Behavior theory
Communication
Complexity leadership
Conflict resolution
Culture of safety
Delegation
Employee retention
High-performance work team

Kotter's Change Model
Leaders
Nurse manager
Nurse Manager Leadership Partnership (NMLP) Learning Domain Framework
Servant leadership
Transactional leadership
Transformational or charismatic leadership

Chapter 19

(Competencies 1, 11, 13)

The Gerontological Nurse as Manager and Leader

Brenda Tyczkowski
Kristen L. Mauk
Dawna S. Fish
Marilyn Ter Maat

The nursing profession has changed significantly in the past decade, with advances in technology, knowledge, and healthcare demands. Nursing is a highly skilled profession, with growing opportunities in all healthcare settings. Exciting breakthroughs in medicine occur daily, and with those breakthroughs come greater responsibilities, challenges, and competence requirements for nurses. Nurses are in constant contact with patients, caregivers, family members, and medical staff, and they play a key role in the dynamics of meeting the complex healthcare needs of older adults. In this chapter, the roles and skills of the nurse as manager and leader in settings where care is provided to older adults will be explored.

The Nurse Manager

Over the last decade, the role of the *nurse manager* has evolved from a focus on clinical expertise to one that focuses on the administrative management of a unit (McCallin & Frankson, 2010). Responsibilities now include management and leadership of unit staff, stewardship of organizational resources, and meeting clinical concerns. The span of control has increased significantly, increasing the importance of having nurse managers who are well-prepared to meet the challenges inherent in the role. Today, the role of the nurse manager is complex, ambiguous, and demanding (McCallin & Frankson, 2010).

The nurse manager is sometimes selected for the position based on his or her skill as a clinician. Nurse managers need a wider variety of skills to meet the challenges of healthcare delivery today. Trial-and-error is not a safe or efficient manner of becoming familiar with the role. While it is ideal to participate in a formal development program to gain self-understanding, when this is not available, working with an experienced manager in a coaching relationship is helpful.

The *Nurse Manager Leadership Partnership (NMLP) Learning Domain Framework* (American Organization of Nurse Executives [AONE], 2006) (see **Figure 19-1**) describes essential functions of nurse managers and outlines opportunities that may be useful to achieve mastery of these functions. The framework includes three domains: (1) the leader within: creating the leader in yourself; (2) the art of leadership: leading the people; and (3) the science of leadership: managing the business.

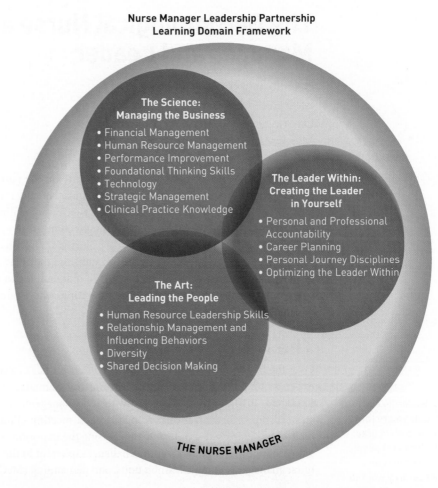

Figure 19-1 Nurse manager Leadership Partnership (NMLP) Learning Domain Framework.

The Leader Within: Creating the Leader in Yourself

In domain one, the new leader develops a personal understanding, gaining self-confidence and learning to trust and empower others. Specific tasks included in this domain are: (1) personal and professional accountability; (2) career planning; (3) personal journey disciplines; and (4) optimizing the leader within (AONE, 2006).

A good place to start with gaining this understanding of self is to do a self-assessment. For example, the Center for Creative Leadership (CCL, n.d.) has a variety of tools to provide a baseline self-assessment. These assessments provide focus on areas that may need additional attention as the manager becomes comfortable in the new role.

New managers should set goals for themselves that will lead to growth in the role. Relationships with employees are established and networks of peers are built. Managers develop an awareness of self, see how their actions impact the unit, and learn to find the style that is comfortable for them and works well for the unit.

The Art of Leadership: Leading the People

In the second domain, the focus is on building effective teams. Specific areas include: (1) human resource leadership skills; (2) relationship management and influencing behaviors; (3) diversity; and (4) shared decision making (AONE, 2006).

Nurse managers use effective communication, conflict resolution skills, and motivation techniques to move the team beyond day-to-day conflicts (see **Case Study 19-1**). Building a *high-performance work team* is critical to providing high-quality patient care. Teams are usually comprised of high, middle, and low performers (Rushing, 2008). High-performing individuals have brilliance and drive, with the ability to propose solutions to problems. Middle performers are supportive of the team, but often lack the knowledge, expertise, or self-confidence to put solutions forward. Low performers place blame on others, fear change, and spread discontentment. Effective nurse managers will recognize the strengths, talents, and skills of each individual on the team and strive to assist them to become even better performers.

High performers should be encouraged to bring concerns and solutions forward. The manager can foster this by conducting rounds and interacting with the high performers, soliciting their input and offering praise for proposed solutions. To encourage middle performers to become high performers, the manager needs to be visible to them, empowering them by offering support and encouragement. Low performers can be encouraged to become better performers by arranging private meetings where direct and decisive plans for improvement should be described. The plans should be attached to a specific timeline for improvement, with clear consequences for continued low improvement. Follow-up meetings should be scheduled to monitor progress (Rushing, 2008).

Notable Quotes

"Surround yourself with the best people you can find, delegate authority, and don't interfere as long as the policy you've decided upon is being carried out."

—Ronald Reagan

Case Study 19–1: Change and Conflict Resolution

Ms. Casey, RN, BSN, is the unit manager of a geriatric medical floor in a large acute-care hospital. The hospital is introducing a new electronic medical records (EMR) system that requires the staff to attend training to be approved to use it. All of her 44 staff members are required to attend a 4-hour training class within 1 month to prepare for the switch to the EMR. Most of the nursing staff who have been working on this unit for years are resistant to the idea of a new charting system and wish to continue using the traditional paper and pencil means of charting. Ms. Casey hears many complaints about this change in policy and sees that it threatens morale.

Questions:

1. What are some practical ways that Ms. Casey can facilitate change to the new computerized charting system?

2. Can you think of any incentives that might help the staff be more open to this change in policy?

3. How might the resistance of the nursing staff to this change affect morale? Patient care?

4. Devise a plan for how Ms. Casey would be able to send each of her 44 nurses to attend computer class and continue to adequately staff her unit.

5. What problems can you foresee that might arise? Are there any resources that Ms. Casey could use to aid in this transition?

Specific strategies that are useful to foster improved teamwork among all unit staff include establishing a common goal for the team (Vogelsmeier & Scott-Cawiezell, 2011), conducting briefings for staff, and using team huddles to ensure that the lines of communication are open. In order to have effective communication, staff members need to trust the manager. When the manager seeks out staff members' opinions, the staff feel valued and empowered and trust is established (Vogelsmeier & Scott-Cawiezell, 2011).

Conflict resolution is often an uncomfortable task for new managers, though it is a task that is essential to the functioning of the unit. When dealing with conflict, the manager should focus on mutual goals among the team and encourage collaborative decision making to move the team beyond the conflict.

Relationship management, described in the second domain, includes fostering a *culture of safety* within the unit. The composition of teams providing care for older adults may include staff with a wide variety of educational preparation and skill development, ranging from registered nurses (RNs), to certified nursing assistants (CNAs), to unlicensed assistive personnel (UAP), such as medication aides. The RN is responsible for safely delegating care to appropriate members of the team.

In 2005, the National Council of State Boards of Nursing (NCSBN) and the American Nurses Association (ANA) issued a joint statement on *delegation*, (2005) defining delegation as "the process for a nurse to direct another person to perform nursing tasks and activities" (p. 1). Steps to the delegation process include (see **Figure 19-2**): (1) assessment of the client, the staff, and the context of the situation; (2) communication to provide direction and opportunity for interaction during the completion of the delegated task; (3) surveillance and monitoring to assure compliance with standards of practice, policies, and procedures; and (4) evaluation to consider the effectiveness of the delegation and whether the desired client outcome was attained (NCSBN & ANA, 2005) (see **Case Study 19-2**).

In order to safely delegate a task, the nurse needs to be familiar with the certification, educational preparation and skill level of the staff member to whom they are delegating a task. Asking questions of the staff member about the task, seeking clarification of their knowledge about the task, or requesting a return demonstration of the task prior to delegating are all good ways of determining if a task can be safely delegated to a specific team member (NCSBN, 2005a). **Box 19-1** outlines the "Five Rights of Delegation."

Though the nurse practice acts vary from state to state, RNs should be aware that in most states licensed

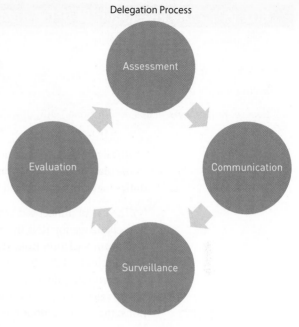

Figure 19-2 The delegation process.

Source: Adapted from https://www.ncsbn.org/Working_with_Others.pdf

Case Study 19-2: Nursing Management and Delegation

Ms. Brown, RN, is the night charge nurse for an inpatient geriatric rehabilitation unit with 30 beds in a small acute-care hospital. She is making her nightly assignments and finds that she has herself, one LPN, and two CNAs to care for 28 patients with relatively high acuity. Ms. Brown does not feel this staffing is adequate, because the evening charge nurse reported that one of the patients was receiving a blood transfusion and might need to be transferred to intensive care, and another patient was complaining of atypical shortness of breath, so tests were being run to determine the cause. The LPN is experienced, but one of the CNAs is still in orientation to the night shift and has little experience.

Questions:

1. What is Ms. Brown's best course of action?

2. If she feels she needs more help to provide quality care to her patients, whom should she contact?

3. What should she do if told no more help is available?

4. What is the most assertive response in this situation?

5. How should Ms. Brown divide assignments between herself and the LPN? Between the CNAs?

6. Is there a certain nursing model of care that might work better than another in this situation?

7. How should Ms. Brown apply the delegation process to this situation?

BOX 19-1   The Five Rights of Delegation

1. Right task
2. Right circumstance
3. Right person
4. Right direction/communication
5. Right supervision

Source: https://www.ncsbn.org/Working_with_Others.pdf

practical nurses (LPNs) do not independently develop the plan of care, make changes in the plan of care, or perform telephone triage (NCSBN, 2005a). Therefore, these duties may not be delegated to them.

The use of unlicensed assistive personnel (UAP) provides an additional delegation challenge for RNs in the long-term care setting. The NCSBN (2005a) found significant variation from state to state with regard to the educational preparation of and roles for UAP. In some states, UAP pass medications, while in others they do not; when states do allow UAP to pass medications, they do receive some training, but this also varies greatly from one state to another. If UAP will be passing medications, the RN is responsible for ensuring that the UAP is competent enough to do so, since it is a complex process that holds the potential for serious complications if not completed safely.

It is the manager's responsibility to provide sufficient resources for care, such as adequate staff members, and to set up systems and policies that foster appropriate delegation. Some nursing functions may not be delegated; these include assessment, planning, evaluation, and nursing judgment (NCSBN, 2005a). The principle of patient safety must be the behind every delegated act.

Another role of the nurse manager, included in the second domain of the NMLP (AONE, 2006), is to provide intentional acknowledgement of the work and contributions of staff to the unit. Staff members need to feel valued and respected by the manager. Specific strategies range from a simple thank you, to providing rewards to celebrate achievements, to nominating staff for awards.

The Science of Leadership: Managing the Business

The third domain in the NMLP focuses on developing effective business practices for the unit. Specific competencies include: (1) financial management; (2) human resource management; (3) performance improvement; (4) foundational thinking skills; (5) technology; (6) strategic management; and (7) clinical practice knowledge (AONE, 2006).

Staff members are being asked to do more, with fewer resources. The manager needs to understand how to provide high-quality care in an efficient manner in their unit. One of the most important aspects of this is having a clear understanding of how staffing decisions impact the financial stability and health of the organization as a whole. Managers need to become familiar with the graphs and reports used within the organization to monitor budgets. To facilitate this, it is helpful for the manager to find someone in the organization to serve as a budget-specific coach.

There are many tasks often specifically associated with the role of nurse manager; **Table 19-1** outlines some of these tasks. The role and responsibilities charged to the nurse manager are varied and complex, requiring many skills. The nurse manager balances the needs of the patients, unit staff, and the overall organization with the provision of safe, high-quality care. While many aspects of the manager's role are skill-focused, the effective manager will also exhibit the qualities of a leader.

TABLE 19-1 **Tasks Associated with the Role of Nurse Manager**
1. Staffing for patient care
2. Developing goals and objectives for the unit
3. Establishing standards of care
4. Developing budgets and using resources in a cost-effective manner
5. Implementing quality improvement activities to affect patient outcomes
6. Engaging in problem solving
7. Planning, organizing, managing, controlling, and directing unit activities
8. Hiring, orienting, evaluating, and educating staff
9. Mentoring and developing staff
10. Identifying systems problems and suggesting solutions
11. Acting as a resource for clinical issues
12. Ensuring compliance with policies, procedures, and accrediting or regulatory agencies
13. Recruiting and retaining staff
14. Participating in organizational committees and task forces
15. Acting as a corporate supporter

Source: Morelli (as cited in Richmond, Book, Hicks, Pimpinella and Jenner, 2009).

The Nurse Leader

"Management is doing things right; leadership is doing the right things" (Drucker, n.d.). This implies that there are subtle differences between the roles of managers and leaders. Kotter International's "Change Leadership" (n.d.) describes managers as those who "make systems of people and technology work well day after day, week after week, year after year" (p. 1) and *leaders* as those who create the systems that managers manage and changes them in fundamental ways to take advantage of opportunities and to avoid hazards (p. 1). Bennis (1989) provides comparisons between managers and leaders, which appear in **Box 19-2**.

BOX 19-2   Comparisons Between Managers and Leaders

Managers	Leaders
Administer	Innovate
Ask how and when	Ask what and why
Focus on systems	Focus on people
Do things right	Do the right things
Maintain	Develop
Rely on control	Inspire trust
Short-term perspective	Long-term perspective
Accept status quo	Challenge status quo
Have eye on the bottom line	Have eye on the horizon
Imitate	Originate
Classic "good soldiers"	Own person
A copy	The original

Source: Bennis, W. (1989). *On Becoming a Leader*. New York, NY: Addison-Wesley.

Leadership is the "ability to effectively move a group of people to successfully achieve the mission and vision of the organization" (American Health Care Association and National Center for Assisted Living [AHCA/NCAL], n.d., p. 1). Effective management requires leadership skills, and effective leadership requires management skills. However, leaders tend to be visionaries who focus on the larger picture, while managers focus on day-to-day operations. Managers are appointed, but leaders arise from within a group.

The AHCA/NCAL (2009) describe long-term-care leaders as the a central resource for staff, residents and families, integral to providing quality care. **Box 19-3** describes seven major roles and the competencies associated with leaders, which are explored in more depth here.

Leader

The first role described by AHCA/NCAL (2009) is that of leader. The effective leader is able to develop and articulate a clear vision of the future of the organization. To achieve this, the leader must be able to create a mental picture of the vision that can be easily communicated to others. For example, the Healthy People (n.d.) "About Healthy People" is committed to the vision of a "society in which all people live long, healthy lives." This simple, yet descriptive, statement allows a vision of the future to be easily seen. This vision is translated into strategies or processes, which are designed to turn the vision into action. When the vision is successfully conveyed, all

BOX 19-3   Leader Roles and Associated Competencies

Role	Associated Competencies
1. Leader	The leader models, advocates, communicates, and leads in creating systems, processes, and programs all within the focus of the facility/organizational mission and vision.
2. Performance Improvement Catalyst	Acts as a catalyst to systematically analyze and evaluate performance, design and implement strategies, and empower staff toward performance improvement.
3. Interpersonal Relations Facilitator	Models healthy communications, interacts sensitively, and promotes cooperative behaviors.
4. Human Resources Developer	Develops strategies to recruit and retain, coaches, assures quality education/training, and ensures meaningful work to maximize job satisfaction of the facility's human resources.
5. Resource and Finance Manager	Budgets, manages resources, and monitors revenues and expenses in order to optimize available resources and finances.
6. Standards and Compliance Expert Resource	Is a regulatory (expert) resource, institutes proactive strategies to meet and exceed standards, and assures meeting ongoing compliance standards and high standards of care.
7. Customer Service Advocate	Is continually customer-focused, builds and maintains trust relationships, initiates/seeks satisfaction feedback, and implements/evaluates improvement in customer services.

Source: Adapted from AHCA/NCAL (2009).

members of the organization know how their role fits the vision of the organization (Baker & Orton, 2010).

Merely passing on the vision is not enough. Heuston and Wolf (2011) describe inspiring a shared vision as the "ability to get staff nurses engaged in aligning the vision of their unit to that of the [facility]" (p. 248). To achieve this, they indicate that the nurse leader should encourage others to join in spreading the vision, discuss with staff any potential barriers to this, and solicit their ideas for improvement. Leaders should present changes with enthusiasm and spend time explaining to staff why changes need to occur. Communication about proposed changes should occur early in the process, so staff has time to absorb the changes.

Utilizing a change management model can help plan for a successful transition through the change process. *Kotter's Change Model*, described in Campbell (2008), helps leaders generate positive feelings among employees toward the change. It also allows leaders to instill feelings of action in employees' hearts, by helping them to envision the problem and identify solutions to the problem (Campbell, 2008). Kotter's Change Model is seen in **Box 19-4**.

BOX 19-4 Kotter's Change Management Model

Phase 1—Creating a climate for change
- Increase urgency
- Build guiding teams
- Get the vision right

Phase 2—Engaging and enabling the whole organization
- Communicate for buy-in
- Enable action
- Create short-term wins

Phase 3—Implementing and sustaining the change
- Don't let up
- Make it stick

Source: Campbell, R. J. (2008). Change management in healthcare. *The Health Care Manager, 27,* 23–39.

Performance Improvement Catalyst

The second role is that of "performance improvement catalyst" (AHCA/NCAL, 2009). Improvements in quality of care have been noted when staff have been empowered, feel engaged in decision making, and are satisfied in their work (Brody, Barnes, Ruble, & Sakowski, 2012). One way that leaders can facilitate these outcomes is through a shared governance structure. This type of structure gives staff nurses control over practice-related decision making. It also holds them accountable for quality patient outcomes. Shared governance often includes the development and support of staff-led councils. Brody et al. (2012) found that council members had a greater sense of ownership in the organization and pride in their work. Staff also reported an increase in the meaningfulness of their work and a heightened sense of the impact they had on the organization. Empowerment through staff nurse-led councils also positively impacted job satisfaction, trust in management, labor relations, turnover, and commitment to the organization.

Like managers, leaders need to foster a culture of resident safety, where a commitment to safety permeates the organization. Open discussion of errors, without fear of reprisal, should occur. Process improvements are ongoing and system issues can be discussed without fear of attack or criticism. In addition, there is an expectation that there will be compliance with established procedures. Common safety-related concerns in the population of frail elders include medication errors, falls, pressure ulcers, and urinary tract infections (Arnetz et al., 2011).

Interpersonal Relations Facilitator

Leaders need to be an interpersonal relations facilitator, according to AHCA/NCAL (2009). Effective leaders "tune in" to the needs of individual employees, recognizing the contributions they make to providing quality care. This is accomplished using a guiding and nurturing approach to communication with employees. The use of keen listening skills, soliciting feedback from employees, and eliminating communication barriers facilitate creating an environment where staff voices are heard (Harvarth et al., 2008). Effective nurse leaders are visible to staff, creating opportunities for one-to-one interaction and holding regular meetings to discuss care issues.

Nursing leaders spend considerable time crafting effective messages, using quality care as a cornerstone to convey the need for action (Keys, 2011). They distance themselves from their own emotions, viewing situations objectively and from various perspectives. Leaders must be persistent in keeping a message alive (see **Box 19-5**). Messages must be delivered with presence and confidence, in order to be effective.

Nurse leaders must set professional *communication* standards and then role model these standards in their interactions with others. Examples of these standards include responding quickly to staff questions and following up on concerns. Nonverbal messages are also sent to staff when nurse leaders answer call lights, pick up trash, and present a calm demeanor when dealing with others (Heuston & Wolf, 2011).

BOX 19-5   Evidence Based Practice Highlight

Resident Advocacy

Miles (2010) argued that elderly nursing home residents are likely to have a higher risk for hospitalization due to non-action of physicians because of cognitive bias. The author explained that physicians may not be sufficiently educated about the benefits of using evidence-based medicine with frail older adults in long-term care settings, and that this lack of knowledge is resulting in poorer outcomes and increased hospitalizations for this population. Common pitfalls were identified as to why physicians often do not practice evidence-based medicine in nursing homes. A bias toward undertreatment of nursing home residents has resulted from physicians' uncertainty over the appropriateness of evidence-based medical treatment in this setting. Such treatment may be viewed by medical doctors as life-extending when in fact it is preventive of medical complications. Gerontological nurses should be aware of this potential pitfall in the long-term care setting and actively advocate for the practice of evidence-based medicine in the nursing home to prevent medical complications and reduce hospitalizations. Nurse leaders should look for opportunities to serve as resident advocates and encourage their staff to do the same.

Source: Miles, R. W. (2010). Cognitive bias and planning error: Nullification of evidence-based medicine in the nursing home. *Journal of the American Medical Directors Society, 11*(3), 194–203.

Human Resources Developer

The next role of the leader described by AHCA/NCAL (2009) is that of human resource developer. *Employee retention* has become even more crucial in the long-term care environment, as turnover among direct care workers in the long-term care environment has been reported to range from 40% to 100% (Robert Wood

Johnson Foundation [RWJF], 2011), and the cost to replace a registered nurse can range from two to three times the annual salary (Brody et al., 2012). Because of this high turnover, fewer employees are challenged to provide high-quality care, using fewer resources. At the same time, resident care needs have become more complex and demanding.

Shifting demographics and workforce demands lead to the prediction that additional nurses will be needed. Brody and colleagues (2012) note the potential to empower, engage, and satisfy nurses through the formation of staff-led evidence-based practice (EBP) councils. By giving nurses a voice in the implementation of EBP findings, there is potential to improve quality outcomes and reduce turnover.

Employee retention is enhanced when leaders create satisfying work environments. To achieve this, the leader needs to help employees to feel valued, acknowledged, challenged, and engaged in unit decision making (Utley, Anderson, & Atwell, 2011).

These findings were echoed by those of Tourangeau, Cranley, Spence Laschinger, and Pachis (2010), who found that staff turnover was tied to psychological and global empowerment, as well as perceived organizational support. These are all areas over which the leader has the ability to exert influence. When an employee identifies with and feels accepted as a member of a work group, this leads to increased job satisfaction and retention. Sponsoring celebrations and social events are one way to accomplish this. Opportunities for ongoing education can also foster workgroup cohesion. Leaders can foster feelings of personal accomplishment among the staff by recognizing and rewarding employee accomplishments, which is just one method of addressing staff turnover.

Emotional exhaustion is detrimental to job satisfaction. Finding ways to make sure that staff takes their coffee and meal breaks can prevent emotional exhaustion and boost feelings of satisfaction (Tourangeau et al., 2010). The work environment should also assist employees to find a better quality of work–life balance (Curtis & O'Connell, 2011).

Resource and Financial Manager

An important leader role is that of resource and financial manager (AHCA/NCAL, 2009). In these difficult economic times, the focus in health care has been learning towards doing more with less. The nurse leader's role is crucial to maintaining a balance between high-quality care and cost-effective care. This is achieved by setting the right goals for the organization and motivating others to achieve the goals (Goetz, Janney, & Ramsey, 2011). As funding cuts continue to occur, it takes thoughtful planning, adequate resources, support, innovation, and strong partnerships among nursing, finance, administration, and medical leaders to bring about achievement of financial goals while maintaining safe and high quality care (Valentine, Kirby, & Wolf, 2011).

In most healthcare facilities, salary and benefits for nurses and unlicensed assistive personnel make up the largest portion of the budget, which puts nursing at the center of most budget decisions. Nursing is ultimately responsible for identifying, developing, and implementing plans to meet annual productivity forecasts. These plans are achieved through accountability for outcomes at all levels in the nursing department. Expectations must be clearly communicated to nursing staff, and nurses must know that their role is essential to the provision of high-quality care and to the achievement of financial viability of the entire organization. In order for staff to "buy in" to the financial goals, the nurse leader must be able to clearly articulate not only what needs to be achieved, but why it is important (Goetz et al., 2011).

Progress toward goals must be frequently reviewed with staff, so their contributions may be acknowledged. If goals are not being met, plans are revisited by the nurse leader and alterations to the work plan may be made.

Standards and Compliance Expert Resource

Leaders are responsible for acting as a standards and compliance expert resources (AHCA/NCAL, 2009). While this responsibility is present in many healthcare settings, it is of particular importance in the long-term care and assisted living settings. Health care is highly regulated in these industries and facilities providing this care undergo frequent regulatory oversight reviews, which can be in the form of survey visits or other monitoring efforts by the state and federal governments. A variety of federal and state regulations are in place to ensure that minimum standards of safe care are provided.

For example, nursing homes must be in compliance with over 180 federal regulations at all times (Centers for Medicare and Medicaid Services [CMS], n.d.). State survey agencies regularly inspect facilities to ensure compliance. Health inspections consist of a review of the care of residents and processes used to give care, how the staff and residents interact, and the overall nursing home environment. The second component of inspections is the fire safety inspection, which ensures compliance with the Life Safety Code (LSC) standards and the National Fire Protection Agency (NFPA) standards (CMS, n.d.). If the facility does not meet the standards of the health or Life Safety Code inspections, a deficiency citation is issued. This may result in fines or denial of payment for new admissions whose payer source is Medicare or Medicaid until the deficiency has been remedied.

Leaders need to create a culture of compliance, comprised of three components (Abell, 2011). The first is the development and implementation of policies and procedures that reinforce compliance with the regulations. Secondly, it is important to maintain an awareness of quality-of-care issues, through a rigorous quality compliance program—Abell (2011) points out that "you never want to be in a situation where the government is discovering things before you are" (p. 36). The final component of a culture of compliance is an effective training program, designed to reinforce compliance in areas of potential concern.

Customer Service Advocate

Leaders serve as customer service advocates, according to AHCA/NCAL (2009). The key to customer service is maintaining a proactive, rather than a reactive, position. Anticipating patients' needs instead of waiting for them to arise sets this proactive tone. When you go beyond the expected, providing exceptional care, customer loyalty is built (Basom, 2012). Making regular contact with patients and their family is crucial to building trusting relationships. This allows them the opportunity to express concerns, if there are any. Lack of communication is one of the biggest customer dissatisfiers in health care (Abbott-Shultz, 2010). Making regular rounds to engage with patients and their families is an important task for the leader.

Staff members also need to be on board with a proactive stance toward customer service. Empowering staff to make decisions related to customer service goes a long way in making this happen. A feeling of "family" needs to be established among the patients, families, and staff. By allowing staff to make customer service decisions at the bedside, instead of through the bureaucratic structure of the facility, a quick resolution to concerns can be achieved, which is important to patients and their families.

Keys to customer satisfaction include doing things right the first time, welcoming and encouraging complaints, and apologizing for the issue and for any inconvenience (Abbott-Shultz, 2010). A satisfied patient or family member will be a wonderful advocate for the facility, drawing more potential patients to the organization. On the other hand, a dissatisfied patient can drag an organization down, particularly when that person is spreading their concerns out in the community.

Leadership Qualities and Theories

Qualities of Effective Leaders

While no one can possess every quality of an effective leader, he or she should be able to demonstrate most of them. Effective leaders maintain an awareness of these qualities and strive to grow and gain knowledge in any areas where they may identify weaknesses. Sims (2009) provides a list of these qualities, found in **Table 19-2**.

There are numerous leadership theories that are useful for nurse leaders. Sometimes an organization may embrace a specific theory and expect that all staff use this theory as a basis for relationships and decision making. At other times, a leader may be free to select whatever theory is comfortable for them. This chapter takes a look at some of the more widely used leadership theories.

TABLE 19-2 Qualities of Effective Leaders
Knowledgeable in their area of expertise and willing to share that knowledge
Willing to collaborate with others
Having self-awareness and a conviction of beliefs
Goal oriented
Lifelong learners
Take responsibility for their actions and for those of their staff
Trustworthy
Create a healthy work environment where staff are free to contribute to the work
Possess vision and is willing to share it with others
Foster an environment in which staff feels free to contribute
Have a good relationship with the staff
Create a sense of relationship with staff
Create a sense of community
Have good oral communication skills
Have a positive attitude
Has the ability to make hard choices
Takes advantage of teachable moments
Flexible
Assists others to develop their practice
Acts as a mentor
Recognizes the strength of others
Recognizes their own strengths

Source: Sims, J. M. (2009). Styles and qualities of effective leaders. *Dimensions of Critical Care Nursing, 28,* 272–274.

Transactional Leadership

Transactional leadership has been described as "you scratch my back, I'll scratch yours" (National Research Council [NRC], 2003, p. 110). Leaders and followers exchange economic, political, or physical items of value, which ties them loosely together. Sims (2009) indicates that an individual employee's strengths are identified and a system of rewards and punishments is established by the leader. The ties between the leader and their employee are loose at best and relationships are superficial. Transactional leaders may exhibit behaviors associated with management-by-exception, where action is taken only after problems occur or mistakes are made. They intervene only when issues are obvious, seeking to maintain the status quo

(Gardner, 2010). When transactional leadership is used, control is maintained at the top of the hierarchy (Weberg, 2010).

Behavior Theory

Behavior theory is comprised of four types of leadership styles (Sims, 2009). Unique behaviors are associated with each style.

The first style is autocratic; it is sometimes known as authoritarian style. These leaders make most of the decisions, with little decision-making authority being extended to the followers. The authoritarian leader is generally viewed as aloof or impersonal (Lewin, Lippitt, & White, 1939). Under this style of leadership, efficiency is foremost. These leaders need to be highly confident and competent in their skills.

The second style is bureaucratic leadership. Bureaucratic leaders expect that rules will be followed at all times. They value structure and uniformity. Bureaucratic leaders focus attention on irregularities and mistakes.

Participative, or democratic leaders, allow others to have input into decision making and problem solving. The leader is perceived as objective and focused on facts (Lewin et al., 1939). In this style, the decision-making process is time-consuming and the leader must be willing to give up control over decisions.

Free rein, or laissez-faire, style of leadership centers on the concept that employees are able to set their own goals or tasks, with minimal interference from the leader. These leaders offer little direction or support to employees, appearing indifferent to their needs. Laissez-faire leaders avoid making decisions and often refuse to take sides in disputes (Gardner, 2010).

The final model drawn from behavioral theories is situational leadership. The premise is that there is no one single leadership style that is appropriate for every situation, so a leader needs to draw from several styles, depending on the situation at hand. Situational leaders identify the needs of the job, determine successful ways of dealing with people to meet these needs, and then select a leadership style that will match the needs of the organization with the abilities of the staff. Situational leaders use directing, coaching, supporting, and delegating behaviors to be flexible in the style they select to meet the needs of the organization (Lynch, McCormack, & McCance, 2011).

21st Century Leadership

As we transition from an industrial age to a "socio-technical age," leaders need to rethink their approach to *21st Century leadership*, adopting new strategies to meet the changing scene in health care (Porter-O'Grady & Malloch, 2009). There is an emerging need for visionary leaders who can facilitate innovation and change within the organization. Porter-O'Grady and Malloch indicate that these leaders must display characteristics of innovative leaders, summarized in **Table 19-3**.

TABLE 19-3　Characteristics of 21st Century Leaders

Understands complexity, diversity, context, theory, and format
Personal knowledge of dynamics and processes of innovation
The desire to collaborate with many stakeholders
The ability to see connections, flow, and movement between processes
The ability to place innovation within the financial and strategic processes of the organization
Possession of the knowledge necessary to maintain the integrity of the innovation and system
The ability to serve as a mentor and coach to advance new leadership capacity

Source: Porter-O'Grady, T. & Malloch, K. (2009). Leaders of innovation: transforming postindustrial healthcare. *Journal of Nursing Administration, 39,* 245–248.

Transformational or Charismatic Leadership

The landmark work by the Institute of Medicine (IOM) (NRC, 2003) indicates that transformational leaders "seek to engage individuals in the recognition and pursuit of a commonly held goal—in this case, patient safety" (p. 111). Transformational leaders seek to attain a collective goal for the organization, rather than a series of potentially disjointed goals, as found in translational leadership. Transformational leaders stimulate innovative thinking and transform followers' beliefs. They understand the need for change in the organization and clearly communicate the vision to achieve the change. In doing so, they motivate and empower the followers to commit to the vision (Curtis & O'Connell, 2011). Emphasis is placed on inspirational messages, moral values, individual attention, and intellectual stimulation (Avolio, Walumbwa, & Weber, 2009).

Transformational or charismatic leadership has been particularly useful in the long-term care environment. According to Utley, Anderson, and Atwell (2011), improved resident outcomes, such as a reduction in falls and pressure ulcers, has been shown in institutions with transformative leaders. Employees felt valued and empowered in their work; the work environment was perceived as more positive, resulting in greater job satisfaction. In particular, certified nursing assistants (CNAs) were more likely to stay employed at the facility. Residents also reported increased satisfaction with the quality of life. In facilities where leaders used transformational leadership, effective communication techniques, teamwork, leadership, and quality of care were stressed. Weberg (2010) found that transformational leadership created a healthy work environment. Improved employee satisfaction and reduced staff turnover rates were noted in the acute care setting. **Table 19-4** displays characteristics of transformational leaders.

Servant Leadership

Robert K. Greenleaf, the founder of the servant leadership movement, describes *servant leadership* as "the servant-leader is servant first... It begins with the natural feeling that one wants to serve, to serve first. Then conscious choice

TABLE 19-4 Characteristics of Transformational Leaders

Inspire a Shared Vision
- Clearly articulate the vision
- Discuss barriers to change and solicit ideas for improvement
- Explain why changes are needed
- Communicate regularly about proposed plans, so changes are not as surprising to staff

Model the Way
- Model enthusiasm and optimism to employees
- Provide frequent feedback and recognition
- Praise good communication and teamwork
- Promote employee independence and empowerment
- Encourage employees to do their best

Challenge the Process
- Challenge the norm when indicated
- Encourage staff development by encouraging creativity, problem solving, and learning
- Acknowledge the importance of employees' knowledge and skills

Enable Others to Act
- Be visible and approachable
- Demonstrate competency and integrity
- Coach and mentor, give staff the tools for the job, but do not do the work for them

Encourage the Heart
- Get to know employees and create feelings of being cared about as a person
- Create opportunities to succeed
- Show concern for employees' needs

Source: Adapted from Utley, R., Anderson, R. & Atwell, J. (2011). Implementing transformational leadership in long-term care. *Geriatric Nursing, 32,* 212–219.
Heuston, M. M. & Wolf, G. A. (2011). Transformational leadership skills of successful nurse managers. *Journal of Nursing Administration, 41,* 248–251. doi:10.1097/NNA.0b013e31821c4620.
Brady Schwartz, D., Spencer, T., Wilson, B. & Wood, K. (2011). Transformational leadership: implications for nursing leaders in facilities seeking Magnet® designation. *AORN Journal, 93,* 737–748. doi:10.1016/j.aorn.2010.09.032.

brings one to aspire to lead. That person is sharply different from one who is leader first, perhaps because of the need to assuage an unusual power drive or to acquire material possessions" (Greenleaf Center for Servant Leadership, n.d., para. 2).

Servant leadership differs from other leadership models, in that the focus is on the leader meeting the needs of the followers before the needs of the leader or the organization are met. In the healthcare setting, the needs of the patients and staff are of utmost importance.

Spears (as cited in Avolio et al., 2009) lists the characteristics of a servant leader as the following:

1. listening,
2. empathy,
3. healing,
4. awareness,
5. persuasion,
6. conceptualization,
7. foresight,
8. stewardship,
9. commitment, and
10. building community (p. 436).

Complexity Leadership

Avolio and colleagues (2009) describe how research has led to the development of complexity theory, which attempts to account for the dynamic state of leadership in a knowledge-driven society. Leadership is viewed as "an interactive system of dynamic, unpredictable agents that interact with each other in complex feedback networks, which can then produce adaptive outcomes such as knowledge dissemination, learning, innovation and further adaptation to change" (Uhl-Bien, Marion, & McKelvey, 2007, p. 299). Complexity leadership roles within a bureaucratic structure include adaptive roles, such as facilitating brainstorming sessions to overcome challenges; administrative roles, such as formal planning; and enabling roles, such as minimizing bureaucratic restraints to enhance follower potential (Avolio et al., 2009). The very nature of *complexity leadership* is that it embraces adaptation and innovation.

Summary

Regardless of the leadership model used, the relationship between the nurse leader and his or her followers is important. Followers do not simply follow, but rather leaders and followers are interdependent (Kean & Haycock-Stuart, 2011). Nurse leaders should carefully consider the style that suits their own needs, the needs of the nurses and the needs of the organization.

Effective Communication

Issues such as working in interdisciplinary teams, leading a multigenerational workforce, and dealing with shrinking budgets necessitate strong communication skills and effective conflict resolution strategies (see **Box 19-6**). Disruptive communication may occur between nurses, between nurses and physicians, or between nurses and other stakeholders, raising the potential of negatively impacting patient safety.

The hierarchal authority structure and sexism in the healthcare environment further complicate the issues (Robinson, Gorman, Slimmer, & Yudkowsky, 2010). In

---

BOX 19-6 Research Highlight

Aim: To examine the research surrounding geriatrics and evaluation management units (GEMUs) and their effectiveness.

Methods: The authors used systematic reviews, meta-analyses (from multiple databases), and personal discussion with research article authors to examine the literature and rate the quality of studies on 10 criteria. Meta-analysis was used to evaluate the effectiveness of GEMUs in current research.

Findings: GEMUs were found to have a significantly positive effect on decreasing the rate of hospitalization after 1 year and reducing functional decline at discharge. A need for more and better quality studies in this area was noted.

Application to practice: Having dedicated units that focus on the management of hospitalized older adults, with proper assessment and evaluation provided by an educated team, was shown to improve patient outcomes. Frail elderly may especially benefit from an interdisciplinary team approach to care. However, more research is needed to establish specific outcomes for various types of older patients.

Source: Van Craen, K., Braes, T., Wellens, N., Denhaerynck, K., Flamaing, J., Moons, P, Boonen, S.... Milisen, K. (2010). The Effectiveness of Inpatient Geriatric Evaluation and Management Units: A Systematic Review and Meta-Analysis. *Journal of the American Geriatric Society, 58*, 83–92.

---

some settings, nurses do not feel supported by the bureaucratic structure of the organization, perceiving that decisions are made at higher levels in the organization and then imposed upon them. They do not feel they have a voice in the organization. In addition, in some environments, there is a perception that female nurses are not on the same level as male members of the interdisciplinary team. This can be a barrier to effective and collegial communication.

Robinson et al. (2010) asked focus groups comprised of nurses and physicians to reflect on effective communication strategies. They found that the need for straightforward and unambiguous communication is paramount. In order to be effective, there needs to be an opportunity to verify what was heard and ask clarifying questions. Visibility and open communication among the leader, subordinates, and colleagues provide this opportunity.

Collaborative problem solving emerged as the next theme. By bringing people together to discuss concerns, a sense of team camaraderie emerged, instead of an us-versus-them mindset. This has implications for patient safety. Team members were open to hearing different perspectives and weighing various options. The opinions of others were highly valued and sought after as respect grew among the team members.

Robinson et al. (2010) also found that maintaining a calm and supportive demeanor, even in stressful situations, was integral to effective communication. This included displaying a collegial tone and normal volume of voice. Positive reinforcement, expressed as appreciation, was also part of this strategy.

Establishing a sense of trust and building mutual respect also emerged as a theme. A comfortable rapport among members of the team ensures that even uncomfortable issues can be raised with the knowledge that they will be dealt with in a professional manner.

Developing an authentic understanding of and appreciation for the unique role of each member of the team was the final theme described by Robinson and colleagues (2010). Each profession experiences unique challenges and brings unique contributions to the team process. When everyone works in isolated silos, instead of in teams, they lose the richness that comes with welcoming others to the table for discussion. By developing an understanding of these varied contributions, each profession will establish a sense of respect for the other.

Gil (2010) describes aspects of communication styles that lead to effective communication by leaders. These include: "listen[ing] to the concerns of stakeholders, maintain[ing] professional integrity, adher[ing] to ethical standards, balanc[ing] stakeholders interests, and be[ing] aware of the emotional barriers (preconceived opinions and beliefs, prejudices, biases, egos and politics)" (p. 451). Gil also describes four additional key attributes of effective communication. The first is assertiveness, which is the ability to forcefully state your own position, despite opposition from influential others. Leaders need to exhibit strategic influence, which is the ability to build coalitions with influential others, gaining their support and mutually overcoming obstacles. Spending time and energy getting to know influential others is referred to as relationship development. Political awareness is the final area of effective communication, wherein the leader understands who the influential people are and how to work effectively with them.

The role of the nurse leader in the process of establishing effective communication is to facilitate the establishment of a collegial relationship among the team members, whether the team is comprised of all nurses or is more interdisciplinary. When the nurse leader sets clear expectations for the atmosphere of professionalism, respect, and collegiality, this fosters effective communication and patient safety. The nurse leader should serve as a role model for effective communication and promote opportunities for ongoing education about effective communication strategies. Patient safety and quality care can flourish in an environment where the leader actively pursues establishing effective communication among the team.

Nursing Leadership Roles in Caring for Older Adults

Nurses who work with older adults show a strong motivation to provide high-quality care (Dwyer, 2011). Geriatric nursing is considered a specialty area, as the care needs of older adults are complex. Because care for older adults is provided in a variety of settings, the range of leadership roles available to nurses is extensive. Though not an exhaustive list, the most common leadership roles are discussed.

Executive Roles

Nurses hold great potential to excel in executive roles in many settings where care is provided to older adults. Their broad background allows them to meet the five areas of expected leadership competency in health care, determined by the Healthcare Leadership Alliance (HLA) and described in VanDriel, Bellack, and O'Neil (2012). These include communication and relationship management, leadership, professionalism, knowledge of the healthcare environment, and business knowledge and skills.

Nurses may be owners of nursing homes, assisted living facilities, adult daycare centers, and more. Nurses often hold dual licensure as Nursing Home Administrators (NHA). They may be hospital administrators or serve as administrators of public health departments. In these positions, they have the ability to exert positive influence over the quality of care provided to older adults in a variety of settings.

Director of Nurses

The role of Director of Nurses (DON) has been called pivotal to the ensuring that the long-term care industry is ready for the impending increase in the aging population (Siegel, Mueller, Anderson, & Dellefield, 2010). The DON must shape high-quality and cost-effective care, in the face of such challenges as culture change, regulatory issues, shrinking revenues, and staff turnover. Turnover rates for this position have been reported to range from 38–147% (Siegel et al., 2010). This is attributed to the depth and breadth of role requirements for DONs. Though opportunities for ongoing leadership and management training are available, many DONs instead rely on their nursing education as a foundation for their practice, without taking advantage of these additional educational opportunities. The time is right for nurses with leadership and management skills to take on this challenging and important role and make a difference in the lives of older adults.

Charge Nurse

Wojciechowski, Ritze-Cullen, and Tyrrell (2011) define a charge nurse as someone who "provides leadership to staff by being an effective resource, role model, mentor, and change agent…they positively influence the quality and delivery of patient care in [nursing units]" (p. E11). Charge nurses represent leadership at the unit level of the organization and are typically responsible for day-to-day concerns and ensuring that the unit operates efficiently and effectively. Critical skills for charge nurses include communication, supervision, delegation, conflict management, and team building (Wojciechowski et al., 2011).

Though an essential part of a successful nursing unit, charge nurses are often expected to fulfill their duties with very little attention to training in leadership skills. This offers an excellent opportunity for a nurse leader to coach and mentor charge nurses. Ongoing professional development should be encouraged—competency-based education and assessments, training programs, and certification exams are readily available through various professional organizations.

Staff Nurse

Staff nurses are responsible for supervising care for older adults that has been delegated to paraprofessionals, such as certified nursing assistants (CNAs). Often, they are unprepared to delegate or supervise (Harvarth et al., 2008). Strong clinical skills are needed to meet the complex care needs of older adults and to adequately supervise the care provided. Staff nurses should have a clear understanding of the responsibility associated with delegating care.

Gerontological Nurse Practitioner

Gerontological Nurse Practitioners (GNPs) are "advanced practice nurses with specialized education in the diagnosis, treatment, and management of acute and chronic conditions often found among older adults and generally associated with aging" (Gerontological Advanced Practice Nurses Association [GAPNA], 2003, p. 2). Gerontological nurse practitioners are found in a variety of practice settings, including ambulatory care clinics, hospitals, private homes, and long-term care. In the nursing home setting, regulatory visits to examine residents may alternate between the physician and the GNP (CMS, 2011).

Clinical Nurse Leader

The clinical nurse leader (CNL) is relatively new to the healthcare scene, first developed in the early 2000s in response to the Institute of Medicine's quality and safety reports (Reid & Dennison, 2011). The CNL role focuses on enhancing safety across diverse settings. The CNL role has been most prevalent in the hospital setting, where it provides direct clinical leadership, most often on a unit-based level. Clinical nurse leaders ensure that care delivery is safe and evidence-based, and that it achieves optimal quality outcomes (Reid & Dennison, 2011). Though not yet widely seen in settings such as long-term care, according to Reid and Dennison, as the number of CNL graduates rises and the role matures, they are expected to expand to the home health, rehab, long-term care, community, and ambulatory care settings, where care is provided for many older adults.

Registered Nurse Assessment Coordinator

The Minimum Data Set (MDS) is a standardized, primary screening and assessment tool, used in Medicare and/or Medicaid-certified long-term care facilities (CMS, 2012). The MDS assessment includes measures of physical, psychological, and psychosocial aspects of resident needs. According to the State Operations Manual (SOM) (CMS, 2011), a registered nurse must conduct or coordinate each MDS assessment in nursing homes. The MDS forms the foundation of assessment and care planning. In many facilities, the MDS coordinator serves as the leader of the interdisciplinary care planning team. The RN assessment coordinator is vital to the facility, since the payment rate for residents whose nursing home stay is being paid for by Medicaid is generated based on responses on the MDS. The length of eligibility for Medicare coverage is also documented using the MDS. This is a highly specialized and important role within the nursing home setting, offering RNs an opportunity to utilize leadership skills within the interdisciplinary team.

Multigenerational Workforce Issues

As the population of older adults in need of healthcare services continues to climb, the need for an adequate supply of nurses prepared to meet their specialized needs will increase as well. Maintaining a stable staff is important and retention of staff is essential. The workforce is made up of nurses from several generations, each with unique views, attributes, and concerns.

The first group is often referred to as the veterans and includes people born before 1945 (Stanley, 2010). The number of nurses in this group is declining as they retire, but the influence of their presence is still felt in the structure and policies that remain in the workplace. Those that remain in the workforce bring a lifetime of experience. Many are in formal and informal leadership positions. These nurses generally are loyal, often working for one organization for their entire career. Values held by this group include maintaining the professional image of nursing, respect for authority, dedication, and sacrifice (Stanley, 2010).

Baby boomers are those people born between 1946 and 1964 (Stanley, 2010). Many are approaching retirement age. Nurses of this generation are usually optimistic and value personal growth and interpersonal communication, often questioning the status quo (Stanley, 2010). Baby boomers bring a strong work ethic to the workplace.

Generation X nurses were born between 1965 and 1980 and experienced a rapidly changing society, including two-career families, divorced parents, and an explosion of technology (Stanley, 2010). Generation X nurses value independence, informality, technological literacy, and having fun, with less emphasis placed on work (Stanley, 2010).

Generation Y, or millennials, were born between 1981 and 1999 (Stanley, 2010). They bring a mastery of all things technical to the workplace. These nurses are adept at multitasking and wish to collaborate in decision making. Group membership is highly valued, as is achievement; members of this generation present themselves in a confident manner (Stanley, 2010).

Leaders need to recognize and leverage the different values and strengths of each generation. According to Stanley (2010), in the former chain of command, older nurses were the supervisors and the younger nurses were the apprentices. This has been replaced by teams of all generations. Younger nurses are more likely to make demands, speak their mind, and voice opinions.

Leaders must use caution to avoid stereotyping of individuals. Lack of recognition of employees as individuals may lead to further misunderstandings and tension. Generational differences may lead to misunderstandings and conflicts surrounding communication styles, values, problem-solving methods, and work ethics. If left unresolved, the organization may see absenteeism, interpersonal conflict, communication breakdown, and turnover (Stanley, 2010).

To deal with these differences, several strategies should be used (Stanley, 2010). Core nursing values that transcend the generations, such as quality care, respect, and ethical decision-making, should be emphasized. The mission and values of the organization should also be reinforced. Each employee should be held to the same standards as described in the goals, policies, and procedures in the organization. Opportunities should be made available for nurses to have a voice in the organization.

Leaders need to be open, flexible, and approachable. Hahn (2011) suggests that leaders conduct a self-assessment of their own managerial style and generational cohort; this can help with achieving a greater understanding of their own values, in relation to those of the nurses in their unit. Efforts must be made to deal with conflict and differences through dialogue and solutions that retain respect for all employees.

In summary, nurses from all generations should be given the opportunity to make contributions to the organization that recognize and celebrate their unique perspectives, insights, and views. Engaging nurses from all generations will improve retention and facilitate quality care.

Professional Associations

Knowledge about professional associations will assist in providing quality care to patients and offers the latest information in gerontology for staff and the community. There are many organizations for the gerontological nurse manager or leader. A few of the more common associations pertaining to this field are presented in this section.

All of the associations provide useful education and have websites that are easily accessed. Information provided by the associations ranges from certification exams, continuing education, standards of care, best practices, and political updates (important legislation impacting long-term care) to research and publications. The gerontological nurse manager or leader can use information from these individual websites to provide the latest information to staff, improve care for residents, and empower caregivers in a variety of settings.

Coalition of Geriatric Nursing Organizations

The Coalition of Geriatric Nursing Organizations (http://hartfordign.org/advocacy/cgno/) was formed in 2001 to establish a common voice to benefit care of older adults (Hartford Institute for Geriatric Nursing, n.d.). A summary of the member organizations, many of whom are presented in this section, can be found online at http://hartfordign.org/advocacy/cgno/. Collectively, this organization represents 28,700 geriatric nurses seeking to improve the healthcare of older adults across care settings.

National Gerontological Nursing Association

The National Gerontological Nursing Association (NGNA, http://ngna.org) was founded in 1984 and is dedicated to the clinical care of older adults across diverse care settings (NGNA, n.d.). Members include clinicians, educators, and researchers with vastly different educational preparation, clinical roles, and interest in practice issues. A striking feature is the substantial number of certified gerontological clinical nurse specialists who select NGNA for membership. Members of the NGNA work in the following roles: staff nurse, clinical nurse specialist, manager, administrator, clinical educator, academic educator, nurse practitioner, and researcher. Membership benefits include:

> A subscription to *Geriatric Nursing* magazine
> Reduced rates to attend the annual NGNA convention and other educational offerings
> Bi-monthly newsletter: *SIGN* (*Supporting Innovations in Gerontological Nursing*)
> NGNA local chapter networking opportunities
> Research and education to promote professional development of gerontological nurses
> NGNA fellows program
> Discounted certification exams through a cooperative arrangement between NGNA and the American Nurses Credentialing Center (ANCC) for gerontological nurse, clinical specialist in gerontological nursing (CNS), and gerontological nurse practitioners (GNP)

National Association of Directors of Nursing Administration in Long Term Care

The National Association of Directors of Nursing Administration in Long Term Care (NADONA/LTC, http://www.nadona.org) has been an advocate and educational organization for directors of nursing (DONs), assistant directors of nursing (ADONs), and RNs in long term care. Membership is in both the United States and Canada. Membership benefits (NADONA, n.d., pp. 1–2) include:

> Mentor system that allows directors to speak with a veteran DON in administration
> Education, including conferences both regional and national, and other professional materials
> A quarterly journal, which provides continuing education units (CEUs) and has both clinical and newsworthy items
> Scholarships for all educational stages
> Director of nursing certification program

American Association for Long Term Care Nursing

The American Association for Long Term Care Nursing (AALTCN, http://aaltcn .org) promotes the importance of and advances excellence in practice for the entire nursing department of long-term care facilities (AALTCN, n.d.). By addressing issues that affect the entire nursing team and promoting measures to foster unity in meeting shared goals, AALTCN removes fragmenting silos to promote working relationships that support a caring culture. AALTCN advocates for long-term care nursing staff with consumers, agencies, the business community, and other groups, and it provides a strong voice in casting a positive image for long-term care nursing and ensuring that others understand the complexities and importance of this specialty. Some of the membership (for the entire nursing department) benefits include:

> Comprehensive association website
> Monthly e-newsletters, current news, and education articles
> Discounts on certification programs and Health Education Network Position statements and Core competencies
> Training modules on major clinical issues
> Opportunities for networking and sharing of resources
> Special education grants to the College Network
> Representation on national committees and with national initiatives
> Website job market to find and post job opportunities

American Association of Nurse Assessment Coordinators

The American Association of Nurse Assessment Coordinators (AANAC, http://www.aanac.org) is a not-for-profit professional association that provides access to accurate and timely information on clinical assessment, regulatory requirements, reimbursement, computer automation, research, and the law (AANAC, n.d.). Membership benefits include:

> Access to their website with must-know updates
> Networking opportunities with formal mentoring programs for Minimum Data Set/Prospective Payment System (MDS/PPS) neophytes
> Online question and answer service through the AANAC website
> Online discussion group
> Online seminars
> Easy access to recognized experts
> Management and in-service aids—forms and protocols
> Online archive of most frequently asked questions
> Reasonably priced conferences and continuing education
> Career recognition and development
> Newsletter and bulletins
> Membership certificate

American Health Care Association

The American Health Care Association (AHCA, http://ahcancal.org) is a not-for-profit group of state health organizations representing a variety of long-term care providers that care for more than one and a half million elderly and disabled individuals across the country (AHCA, 2012). AHCA "represents the long-term care community to the nation at large—to government, business leaders, and the general public. It also serves as a force for change within the long term care field, providing information, education, and administrative tools that enhance quality at every level" (AHCA, 2012, para. 2).

Membership benefits (through state affiliates only) include:

> Up-to-date news and publications including *Provider* magazine
> Research and data on areas such as surveys, facility trend reports, and completed studies
> Legislative information including issue briefs and testimonies
> Conferences and educational offerings
> Quality improvement programs including "Advancing Excellence in Nursing Homes" and "Radiating Excellence," which focus on the assessment of specific leadership roles and competencies essential to nurse leaders
> Access to members-only sections of the website

Leading Age

Leading Age (http://www.leadingage.org/) is an association of not-for-profit organizations dedicated to making America a better place to grow old (Leading Age, n.d.). They advance policies, promote practices, and conduct research that supports, enables, and empowers people to live fully as they age. The work of Leading Age is focused on advocacy, leadership development, and applied research and promotion of effective services, home health, hospice, community services, senior housing, assisted living residences, continuing care communities, nursing homes, as well as technology solution for seniors, children, and others with special needs.

Membership benefits vary based on the type—provider, business, or associate. Some of the benefits are:

> Publications such as *Leading Age*, weekly newsletters, and other publications helpful to the consumer and the professional
> Serves as a hub for articles, analyses and information about legislative and political action related to services for aging
> The facts on aging services
> Consumer information
> Discounts on national and international conferences
> Access to members-only sections on the website
> Provides a link to services and programs such as Center for Aging Services Technology, International Association of Homes, and Services for the Aging that advocate for older adults and the disabled

National Association of Health Care Assistants

The National Association of Health Care Assistants (NAHCA, http://www.nahcacares.org/) began as the National Association of Geriatric Nursing Assistants. This organization was started by former certified nursing assistants Lori Porter and

Lisa Cantrell, both of whom later became senior managers and realized that nursing assistants are both the backbone and the heart and soul of the nursing home profession (NAHCA, n.d.). The name was changed in 2006 to meet the growing needs of all healthcare assistants including those in nongeriatric facilities. NAHCA member benefits include:

> Association shirt
> Educational opportunities
> "Key to Quality" national annual CNA awards
> National annual convention and expo
> Scholarship program for higher education

American Medical Directors Association

The American Medical Directors Association (AMDA, http://www.amda.com) is the professional association of medical directors, attending physicians, and others practicing in the long-term care continuum (AMDA, n.d.). Many nurse leaders also belong to this organization to help deal with difficult clinical, administrative, and ethical issues in long-term care. Membership benefits include:

> Educational programs
> Print and online resources, including *Caring for the Ages, Journal of the American Medical Directors Association*, and AMDA Reports
> Exclusive member rates and members-only access
> State chapters
> AMDA Foundation Research Network Answers the Long-term Care Questions

American College of Health Care Administrators

The American College of Health Care Administrators (ACHCA, http://www.achca.org) is a non-profit membership organization that provides superior educational programming, certification in a variety of positions, and career development for its members (ACHCA, n.d.). Membership benefits include:

> Peer2Peer network
> Education opportunities such as the annual convention and the ACHCA Winter Marketplace
> Self-study programs
> Various publications such as the *ACHCA Continuum* and *ACHCA E-News*

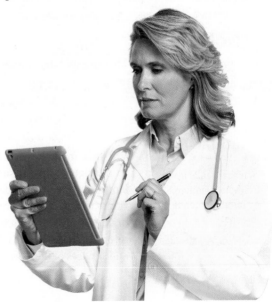

© kurhan/ShutterStock, Inc.

Figure 19-3 Nurse managers and leaders have the ability to positively influence the care of older adults.

> Professional development catalog
> Computer-based testing for certification

Summary

In conclusion, both nurse managers and nurse leaders are needed in gerontological nursing. While managers focus on direction of the details of a unit, leaders are visionaries who see the larger picture. Both must develop good communication skills and healthy interpersonal relationships. Specific strategies discussed in this chapter can be used to assist staff in feeling engaged in the operations of the unit or organization, to foster recruitment and retention, and ultimately to result in safe care and better health outcomes for patients and residents. Developing sound management strategies requires the desire to change and maintain a constant state of self-reflection (see **Case Study 19-3**).

Case Study 19-3: Standards of Care and Disciplinary Policies

Mr. Gonzalez, RN, is the charge nurse on the evening shift of the skilled care unit at a long-term care facility. The day shift nurses have complained to Mr. Gonzalez that the evening shift CNAs have not been showering the residents as scheduled. They tell him that family members of the residents have complained about poor hygiene of their loved ones.

Questions:

1. What is the first step Mr. Gonzalez should take in resolving this situation?

2. To which staff members should he speak?

3. What immediate steps must be put in place to remedy this situation?

4. If no action is taken by Mr. Gonzalez and the complaints are true, what could happen?

5. Who has responsibility in this situation for the quality of patient care?

Notable Quotes

"A leader leads by example, whether he [or she] intends to or not."

—John Quincy Adams

Nurse managers and leaders of today are faced with unique challenges related to multigenerational staffing patterns. Professional organizations can be excellent resources to provide support and information to those in management positions. Gerontological nurses should choose the most appropriate professional organization(s) in which to be active. As nursing leaders in the specialty of gerontology (see **Case Study 19-4**), they can also contribute to advancing the mission and services of their organization through scholarly activities and political activism.

Case Study 19–4: Leadership, Vision, and Staffing

Mrs. Petty, RN, BSN, is the director of nursing (DON) for the assisted living portion of a for-profit healthcare facility. One of her jobs is to hire an assistant director of nursing (ADON), a new position created to help the DON with the growing number of residents in the facility.

Questions:

1. What qualifications should Mrs. Petty look for in an assistant director of nursing?

2. Describe the ideal candidate for this position. What types of experience, background, and education would be expected in this position?

3. Where does the ADON position fall in the organizational structure of this facility?

4. Where does the DON position fall in the organizational chart?

Critical Thinking Exercises

1. Examine the organizational chart of a facility where you work or have your clinical experiences. Analyze the hierarchical levels in comparison to the discussion of leadership roles in this chapter.

2. Follow a nurse manager for a day. Make a list of duties that you observe and what skills seem important.

3. Map out your own personal strategic plan for your career goals. Set goals for 1 year, 5 years, and 10 years.

4. Make a list of your own strengths and weaknesses as a manager or leader. Determine which of your weaknesses you wish to improve upon and how you will accomplish this.

5. Think of a nurse whom you admire as a good role model of a leader or manager. Write down the qualities you have observed in this person. Compare them to the list in Table 19-2.

Personal Reflections

1. Where do you presently see yourself in the hierarchy of management in nursing? Where do you want to be in 5 years? Ten years? What is your ultimate goal related to advancement in your nursing career? Do you have a plan to accomplish this?

2. Is management an avenue you have considered? What are your personal strengths and weaknesses with regard to the qualities of leaders and managers discussed in this chapter?

3. Do you see yourself more as a leader or as a manager? What leadership styles fit your personality the best? How do you feel about delegating tasks to other nurses and UAP? What skills do you feel you need to develop in order to be comfortable in a charge nurse position?

4. To which nursing organizations do you belong? Have you ever considered applying for a leadership position? Why or why not?

5. Which of the organizations discussed at the end of this chapter would be most appropriate for you to become involved in to help you reach your goals?

References

Abbott-Shultz, B. (2010). Engaging families: Enhancing the relationship among residents, their families, and your community. *Long Term Living Magazine, October,* 36–39.

Abell, T. (2011). Creating a compliance/QA culture: Training to achieve corporate compliance and quality assurance. *Long Term Living Magazine, May,* 36–37.

American Association for Long Term Care Nursing [AALTCN]. (n.d.). Retrieved from AALTCN "About Us," http://www.aaltcn.org/longterm-care-nursing-education.htm

American Association of Nurse Assessment Coordinators [AANAC]. (n.d.). Retrieved from http://www.aanac.org

American College of Health Care Administrators [ACHCA]. (n.d.). Retrieved from ACHCA "About Us," http://www.achca.org/index.php/about-achca

American Health Care Association [AHCA]. (2012). Retrieved from "About AHCA," http://www.ahcancal.org/about_ahca/Pages/default.aspx

American Health Care Association and National Center for Assisted Living [AHCA/NCAL]. (n.d.). *NCAL's guiding principles for leadership.* Retrieved from http://www.ahcancal.org/ncal/about/Documents/GPLeadership.pdf

American Health Care Association and National Center for Assisted Living [AHCA/NCAL]. (2009). Leadership excellence. Retrieved from http://www.ahcancal.org/quality_improvement/leadership_excellence/Documents/Section2-RolesAndCompetencies.pdf

American Medical Directors Association [AMDA]. (n.d.). Retrieved from "About AMDA," http://www.amda.com/about/mission.cfm

American Organization of Nurse Executives [AONE]. (2006). Nurse manager leadership partnership learning domain framework (NMLP). Retrieved from http://www.aone.org/resources/leadership%20tools/NMLPframework.shtml

Arnetz, J. E., Zhdanova, L. S., Elsouhag, D., Lichtenberg, P., Luborsky, M. R., & Arnetz, B. B. (2011). Organizational climate determinants of resident safety culture in nursing homes. *The Gerontologist, 51,* 739–749. doi:10.1093/geront/gnr053.

Avolio, B. J., Walumbwa, F. O. & Weber, T. J. (2009). Leadership: Current theories, research and future directions. *Annual Review of Psychology, 60,* 421–449.

Baker, E.L. & Orton, S.N. (2010). Practicing management and leadership: Vision, strategy, operations and tactics. *Journal of Public Health Management Practice, 16,* 470–471.

Basom, J. (2012). Proactive customer service: strong customer service sends positive message to residents, families and the community at large. *Long Term Living Magazine, February,* 28–29.

Bennis, W. (1989). *On Becoming a Leader.* New York, NY: Addison-Wesley.

Brady Schwartz, D., Spencer, T., Wilson, B. & Wood, K. (2011). Transformational leadership: Implications for nursing leaders in facilities seeking Magnet® designation. *AORN Journal, 93,* 737–748. doi:10.1016/j.aorn.2010.09.032.

Brody, A. A., Barnes, K., Ruble, C., & Sakowski, J. (2012). Evidence-based practice councils: Potential path to staff nurse empowerment and leadership growth. *Journal of Nursing Administration, 42,* 28–33.

Campbell, R. J. (2008). Change management in healthcare. *The Health Care Manager, 27,* 23–39.

Center for Creative Leadership [CCL]. (n.d.). Retrieved from "About CCL," http://www.ccl.org/leadership/about/index.aspx

Centers for Medicare and Medicaid Services [CMS]. (n.d.). *Nursing home compare.* Retrieved from http://www.medicare.gov/NursingHomeCompare/search.aspx

Centers for Medicare and Medicaid Services [CMS] (2011). State operations manual. Retrieved from http://www.cms.gov/Regulations-and-Guidance/Guidance/Manuals/downloads/som107ap_pp_guidelines_ltcf.pdf

Centers for Medicare and Medicaid Services [CMS]. (2012). *Minimum Data Set (MDS).* Retrieved from https://www.cms.gov/Research-Statistics-Data-and-Systems/Files-for-Order/IdentifiableDataFiles/LongTermCareMinimumDataSetMDS.html

Curtis, E. & O'Connell, R. (2011). Essential leadership skills for motivating and developing staff. *Nursing Management, 18*, 32–35.

Drucker, P. (n.d.). *Peter F. Drucker quotes*. Retrieved from http://thinkexist.com/quotes/peter_f._drucker/

Dwyer, D. (2011). Experiences of registered nurses as managers and leaders in residential aged care facilities: A systematic review. *International Journal of Evidence-Based Healthcare, 9*, 388–402.

Gardner, B. (2010). Improve RN retention through transformational leadership styles. *Nursing Management, August*, 8–12.

Gerontological Advanced Practice Nurses Association [GAPNA]. (2003). Position statement: Clinical practice of gerontological nurse practitioners. Retrieved from http://enp-network.s3.amazonaws.com/Gulf_Coast_GNP/pdf/Clinical%20Practice%20of%20GNP_2003.pdf

Gil, N. A. (2010). Language as a resource in project management: A case study and a conceptual framework. *IEEE Transactions on Engineering Management, 57*, 450–462.

Goetz, K., Janney, M. & Ramsey, K. (2011). When nursing takes ownership of financial outcomes: Achieving exceptional financial performance through leadership, strategy, and execution. *Nursing Economic$, 29*, 173–182.

Greenleaf Center for Servant Leadership. (n.d.). *What is servant leadership?* Retrieved from http://www.greenleaf.org/whatissl/

Hahn, J.A. (2011). Managing multiple generations: Scenarios from the workplace. *Nursing Forum, 46*, 119–127.

Hartford Institute for Geriatric Nursing. (n.d.). *Coalition of geriatric nursing organization*. Retrieved from http://hartfordign.org/advocacy/cgno/

Harvarth, T. A., Swafford, K., Smith, K., Miller, L. L., Volpin, M., Sexson, K.,…Young, H. A. (2008). Enhancing nursing leadership in long-term care: A review of the literature. *Research in Gerontological Nursing, 1*, 187–196.

Healthy People (n.d.). Retrieved from "About Healthy People," http://www.healthypeople.gov/2020/about/default.aspx

Heuston, M. M. & Wolf, G. A. (2011). Transformational leadership skills of successful nurse managers. *Journal of Nursing Administration, 41*, 248–251. doi:10.1097/NNA.0b013e31821c4620.

Kean, S., & Haycock-Stuart. E. (2011). Understanding the relationship between followers and leaders. *Nursing Management, 18*, 31–35.

Keys, Y. (2011). Perspectives on executive relationships. *Journal of Nursing Administration, 41*, 347–349. doi:10.1097/NNA.0b013e31822a717d.

Kotter International (n.d.). Retrieved from "Change leadership," http://www.kotterinternational.com/our-principles/change-leadership

Leading Age. (n.d.). Retrieved from "About Leading Age," http://www.leadingage.org/About_LeadingAge.aspx

Lewin, K., Lippitt, R. & White, R. K. (1939). Patterns of aggressive behavior in experimentally created "social climates". *Journal of Social Psychology, 10*, 271–298.

Lynch, B. M., McCormack, B., & McCance, T. (2011). Development of a model of situational leadership in residential care for older people. *Journal of Nursing Management, 19*, 1058–1069. doi:10.1111/j.1365-2834.2011.01275.x

McCallin, A. M., & Frankson, C. (2010). The role of the charge nurse manager: A descriptive exploratory study. *Journal of Nursing Management, 18*, 319–325. doi:10.1111/j.13652834.2010.01067.x.

Miles, R. W. (2010). Cognitive bias and planning error: Nullification of evidence-based medicine in the nursing home. *Journal of the American Medical Directors Society, 11*, 194–203.

National Association of Directors of Nursing Administration in Long Term Care [NADONA/LTC]. (n.d.). Retrieved from "Benefits of Membership," http://www.nadona.org/pdfs/Benefits_Membership.pdf

National Association of Health Care Assistants [NAHCA]. (n.d.). Retrieved from http://www.nahcacares.org/.

National Council of State Boards of Nursing. [NCSBN]. (2005a). *Practical nurse scope of practice white paper*. Retrieved from https://www.ncsbn.org/Final_11_05_Practical_Nurse_Scope_Practice_White_Paper.pdf

National Council of State Boards of Nursing [NCSBN]. (2005b). *Working with others: A position paper*. Retrieved from https://www.ncsbn.org/Working_with_Others.pdf

National Council of State Boards of Nursing [NCSBN] and the American Nurses Association [ANA]. (2005). *Joint statement on delegation*. Retrieved from https://www.ncsbn.org/Delegation_joint_statement_NCSBN-ANA.pdf

National Gerontological Nursing Association [NGNA]. (n.d.). Retrieved from "About the NGNA," http://ngna.org/

National Research Council [NRC]. (2003). Transformational leadership and evidence-based management. In *Keeping Patients Safe: Transforming the Work Environment of Nurses* (pp. 108–161). Washington, DC: The National Academies Press. Retrieved from http://books.nap.edu/openbook.php?record_id=10851&page=108

Porter-O'Grady, T., & Malloch, K. (2009). Leaders of innovation: Transforming postindustrial healthcare. *Journal of Nursing Administration, 39*, 245–248.

Reid, K. B., & Dennison, P. (2011). The clinical nurse leader (CNL): Point-of-care safety clinician. *Online Journal of Issues in Nursing, 16*. doi:10.3912/OJIN.Vol16No03Man04.

Richmond, P. A., Book, K., Hicks, M., Pimpinella, A., & Jenner, C. A. (2009). C.O.M.E. be a nurse manager. *Nursing Management, February*, 52–54.

Robert Wood Johnson Foundation [RWJF]. (2011). *Better jobs, better care: Building a strong long-term care workforce*. Retrieved from http://www.rwjf.org/en/research-publications/find-rwjf-research/2011/04/better-jobs-better-care-.html

Robinson, F. P., Gorman, G., Slimmer, L. W., & Yudkowsky, R. (2010). Perceptions of effective and ineffective nurse-physician communication in hospitals. *Nursing Forum, 45*, 206–216.

Rushing, J. (2008). Transforming staff through leadership excellence. *Nursing Management, 39*, 8–10.

Siegel, E. O., Mueller, C., Anderson, K. L., & Dellefield, M. E. (2010). The pivotal role of the Director of Nursing in Nursing Homes. *Nursing Administration Quarterly, 34*, 110–121.

Sims, J. M. (2009). Styles and qualities of effective leaders. *Dimensions of Critical Care Nursing, 28*, 272–274.

Stanley, D. (2010). Multigenerational workforce issues and their implications for leadership in nursing. *Journal of Nursing Management, 18*, 846–852. Doi:10.1111/j.1365-2834.01158.x.

Tourangeau, A., Cranley, L., Spence Laschinger, H. K., & Pachis, J. (2010). Relationships among leadership practices, work environments, staff communication and outcomes in long-term care, *Journal of Nursing Management, 18*, 1060–1072.

Uhl-Bien, M., Marion, R., & McKelvey, B. (2007). Complexity leadership theory: Shifting leadership from the industrial age to the knowledge age. *The Leadership Quarterly, 18*, 298–318.

Utley, R., Anderson, R. & Atwell, J. (2011). Implementing transformational leadership in long-term care. *Geriatric Nursing, 32*, 212–219.

U.S. Department of Health and Human Services. (n.d.). *Healthy people 2020*. Retrieved from http://www.healthypeople.gov/2020/

Valentine, N. M., Kirby, K. K. & Wolf, K. M. (2011). The CNO/CFO partnership: Navigating the changing landscape. *Nursing Economic$, 29*, 201–210.

Van Craen, K., Braes, T., Wellens, N., Denhaerynck, K., Flamaing, J., Moons, P., …Milisen, K. (2010). The effectiveness of inpatient geriatric evaluation and management units: A systematic review and meta-analysis. *Journal of the American Geriatric Society, 58*, 83–92.

VanDriel, M. K., Bellack, J. P., & O'Neil, E. (2012). Nurses in the C-Suite: Leadership beyond chief nurse. *Nursing Administration Quarterly, 36*, 5–11. doi:10.1097/NAQ.0b013e318238b9e4.

Vogelsmeier, A. & Scott-Cawiezell, J. (2011). Achieving quality improvement in the nursing home: Influence of nursing leadership on communication and teamwork. *Journal of Nursing Care Quarterly, 26*, 236–242.

Weberg, D. (2010). Transformational leadership and staff retention: An evidence review with implications for healthcare systems. *Nursing Administration Quarterly, 34*, 246–258.

Wojciechowski, E., Ritze-Cullen, N. & Tyrrell, S. (2011). Understanding the learning needs of the charge nurse. *Journal for Nurses in Staff Development, 27*, E10–E17.

For a full suite of assignments and additional learning activities, see the access code at the front of your book.

LEARNING OBJECTIVES

At the end of this chapter, the reader will be able to:

> Define key ethical constructs as they relate to the care of geriatric patients.
> Relate concepts of ethics to their implications in the care of geriatric patients.
> Recognize the influence of personal values, attitudes, and expectations about aging on care of older adults and their families/extended families.
> Analyze the impact of fiscal, sociocultural, and medico-legal factors on decision making in the care of geriatric patients.
> Identify strategies for facilitating appropriate levels of autonomy and supporting the right to self-determination decisions in the care of geriatric patients.

KEY TERMS

Advance directives
Advocacy
Autonomy
Beneficence
Codes of ethics
Competence
Confidentiality
Conflict
Conflict of interest
Dilemma
Ethics of care
Failure to rescue
Fidelity
Fiduciary responsibility

Informed consent
Justice
Moral dilemma
Moral distress
Moral principles
Moral sensitivity
Moral uncertainty
Nonmaleficence
Patient rights
Quality of life
Reciprocity
Sanctity of life
Values
Veracity

Chapter 20

(Competencies 1, 11, 12)

Ethical/Legal Principles and Issues

Janice Edelstein

As the population ages and technology advances in health care, the need for nurses to be skilled in geriatric ethics care will grow. The *ethics of care* in the geriatric population is complex and provides many decision-making challenges. As with other nursing specialties, geriatric care includes concerns for compassion, equity, fairness, dignity, and confidentiality. Continual development of skills in ethical decision-making processes is a requirement in meeting competence levels in geriatric care. Nursing practice requires mindfulness of a person's autonomy within the realm of the person's abilities and mental capacity, which may change as one ages. It is impossible to care for this population without being faced with difficult choices surrounding the varied issues relating to the ability to live and care for oneself independently. Independence in the community requires some level of self-sufficiency in the management of activities of daily living, medication usage, health literacy, transportation, and maintaining and running a home (self-care, pet care, meals, housekeeping, shopping, banking, etc.). Self-sufficiency, issues of finance, and personal choices directly impact adherence to and understanding of a plan of care for health maintenance.

These basic issues of autonomy are further challenged by the biological effects of aging and chronic disease on cognitive functioning and decision making. The ability to make decisions related to advance directives, informed consent, and refusal of treatment are dependent on clarity of mind. Difficult choices call for judgments and serious consideration of what is right or best for patients, their families, and their communities. These personal choices are further compounded by social pressures associated with technological developments, options for end-of-life care, genetic research, transplantation options, mechanical devices, and resource allocation as one ages. The advances in healthcare science and technology have raised legal and ethical concerns and dilemmas that the elderly and their families shoud discuss today. The additional need for legal documents, such as a power of attorney for health care and finances, required by healthcare agencies also requires thoughtful consideration.

BOX 20-1	**Ethical/Moral Principles**
Advocacy	Justice
Autonomy	Quality of life
Beneficence/nonmaleficence	Reciprocity
Confidentiality	Sanctity of life
Fidelity	Veracity
Fiduciary responsibility	

Ethical concepts are principles that facilitate decision making and guide our professional behavior. (See **Box 20-1**). They evolve from our beliefs and *values,* and therefore have their foundations in religion, culture, and family expectations. Ethical decision making is driven by moral reasoning—our determination of what is right and wrong. Ethical concepts and personal values define our character and are expressed in our conduct and actions. Professional codes or standards within the profession of nursing help to define ethical actions. Changes in our social networks, including global awareness, cultural diversity, and advances in science, medicine, and technology, have created increasingly complex conflicts and dilemmas. Therefore, nurses must have a clear understanding of their own values and a strategy for decision making as a care provider. As pointed out by Chinn and Kramer (2008), ethical decision trees provide a tool for thinking through options and action plans. Values clarification and values analysis is also noted by Chinn and Kramer (2008) as important components in moral/ethical decisions. A nurse's personal and spiritual beliefs are unique to them and may be quite different from the patient's, the organization's values and expectations, or society's social norms. Ethics is also referred to as the "moral code for nursing and is based on obligation to service and respect for human life" (McEwen & Willis, 2002, p. 14). It is the foundation of practice in nursing, since nurses are perceived (and perceive themselves) as caregivers. On June 14, 2010, the American Nurses Association (ANA, 2010b) revised the position statement of the nurse's role in ethics and human rights, outlining the ethical obligation of nursing in practice settings; this created a clear statement for nursing practice.

Conflict and Dilemma

An ethical *conflict* occurs when a choice must be made between two equal possibilities. The three types of moral conflict described by Redman and Fry (1998) are moral distress, moral uncertainty, and moral dilemma. *Moral distress* (MD) occurs when someone wants to do the right thing but is limited by the constraints of the organization or society. Moral distress in nurses who provided end-of-life care to geriatric patients was studied by Piers et al. (2012), who noted a link between MD

BOX 20-2   Web Exploration

Agency for Healthcare Research and Quality: http://www.ahrq.gov. An excellent site for tracking and learning about quality of care initiatives that support autonomy, safety, and appropriate access to care. Also includes information on elderly health care and end-of-life care.

American Hospital Association: http://www.aha.org. A site emphasizing better health care for persons and communities; contains multiple links related to health policy, research, and advocacy.

American Nurses Association: http://www.nursingworld.org. Contains multiple sections on ethics in nursing. Position papers can be found here.

Berman Institute of Bioethics at Johns Hopkins University: http://www.bioethicsinstitute.org. A wealth of information on bioethics, including discussions on genetic research. Also includes research news and seminar information.

Hospital Compare: http://www.hospitalcompare.hhs.gov. Allows comparison of hospitals in your area of choice on a range of outcome measures.

National Hospital and Palliative Care Organization: http://www.caringinfo.org/i4a/pages/index.cfm?pageid=3289. Provides downloadable copies of advance directives by state.

National Quality Measures Clearinghouse: http://www.qualitymeasures.ahrq.gov. Learn about the quality measures that reflect data on failure to rescue and many other topics. Evidence-based practice and instruments are identified.

Medicare: http://www.medicare.gov/NHCompare. Specific information on coverage.

The Patient Care Partnership: Understanding Expectations, Rights and Responsibilities: http://www.aha.org. An excellent resource for involving patients in their care. Available in multiple languages.

National Healthcare Disparities Report (2011): http://www.ahrq.gov/qual/nhdr11/nhdr11.pdf

---

and burnout and termination of employment. *Moral uncertainty* defines the confusion surrounding situations in which a person is uncertain what the moral problem is or which moral principles or values apply to it. A *moral dilemma* arises when two or more moral principles apply that support mutually inconsistent actions. A true dilemma occurs when it appears there are no acceptable choices. To qualify as a *dilemma*, there must be active engagement in the situation that forces an evaluation of and need for choices. *Moral sensitivity* in graduate and undergraduate nursing students was studied by Comrie (2012), focusing on the stress and burnout associated with the "ethic of caring" (p. 116).

Dilemmas are inherent in the health care of the geriatric population because of the biology of aging and chronic health care issues creating ethical problems for those providing care. **Case Study 20-1** provides an example of a dilemma. Differences in values and opinions can lead to conflicts between caregivers and healthcare providers and are more common in diverse communities where cultural values may be quite different (Ellis & Hartley, 2012). There are seldom perfect solutions to ethical dilemmas. Those forced to make decisions are often required to justify their choices and actions. Some conflicts are resolved through dialogue, others are

Case Study 20-1

Mr. Bowen is 64 years old. He has been very healthy by report and very active working as a farmer. He had a right-sided cerebral vascular accident (CVA) 14 days ago and currently has a moderate leg weakness with a more significant arm weakness, slurred speech, and mild dysphagia (swallowing difficulty). He is predicted to be ambulatory with a cane, though prognosis of arm function returning is more guarded. It is likely he will improve speech function and swallowing ability but will require some specialization of diet to prevent aspiration.

Mr. Bowen has chosen to stop eating, stating that he does not want to live as an invalid. His family is very distressed and wants the nursing staff to force him to eat. The staff cannot imagine why he has made this choice, given that his prognosis is so good compared to others they have seen in the rehabilitation setting with much more severe deficits. He has been evaluated for depression and an antidepressant has been ordered, which he refuses to take, along with all other medications for his newly diagnosed cardiovascular disease. Mr. Bowen is oriented to time, place, and person. He has never had his competence questioned prior to taking this stand on self-determination.

Some of the staff supports his decision and others do not. Discussion with the family reveals that Mr. Bowen has frequently made deriding remarks about persons with disability, including remarks like "If I ever end up that way, just take me out behind the barn and shoot me." The psychologist comments that Mr. Bowen is clinically depressed and that part of this depression is related to the location of his stroke, which prevents him from going back to working on the farm. He also points out that, in his strong opinion, should the depression be resolved, Mr. Bowen would most likely change his opinion.

Questions:

1. What is the healthcare dilemma?

2. What principles of healthcare ethics can be identified in this case study?

3. Does Mr. Bowen have the right to refuse to eat and take medications when he is clearly not in an end-of-life situation?

4. How does the team resolve the situation when the depression is so prevalent and he refuses treatment for it?

5. As the nurse, how will you approach and direct the care for Mr. Bowen?

6. What elements (provisions) from the code of ethics come to mind as you prepare to care for Mr. Bowen?

7. Can you apply theory related to the concept of grief to the care of Mr. Bowen?

legislated, and others are defined by agreements regarding basic rights. Healthcare organizations utilize ethics committees to resolve such dilemmas, where opposing values can be discussed openly by a variety of people. Nurses with geriatric expertise may be asked to serve on a hospital ethics committee as a healthcare representative.

Moral Principles

Moral principles are incorporated into professional *codes of ethics*, organizational value statements, and position statements published by professional groups such as the American Nurses Association (ANA). Lachman (2009) reports the importance of a code of ethics for any profession and states that a code of ethics represents a "social contract with society" (p. 55). *The Guide to the Code of Ethics for Nurses: Interpretation and Application*, published by the ANA (2010a), outlines the ethical standards for the nursing profession. This code forms the cornerstone of all nursing practice. The ANA has issued many position statements speaking to ethics and human rights and is active in addressing issues of genetic research, confidentiality, privacy, managed care, health services for undocumented persons, and the healthcare system's impact on the profession of nursing, using moral principles as a guide while the healthcare system undergoes change. A nurse's understanding of moral principles facilitates decision making based on the code of ethics in daily practice and professional relationships.

Advocacy

ANA's (2010c), *Scope and Standards of Practice Nursing*, describes *advocacy* as "a fundamental aspect of nursing practice" (p. 20). Advocacy in nursing practice may be related to ethical considerations as well as legal considerations (Guido, 2010). Nurses act as client advocates, protecting the health and safety of their clients by communicating needs, promoting safe environments, and helping with assertion of legal rights (Craven & Hirnle, 2008). Our increasingly complex healthcare system often calls for advocacy efforts to help patients and families negotiate and receive appropriate services. By influencing society through political action, nurses also advocate for patients by supporting them in their efforts to retain as much autonomy as their abilities allow. At times, nurses advocate for the expressed desires of the patient within the context of team and family discussions in which the patient is not present, ensuring true representation of the patient's desires when known. Other situations require advocacy efforts to prevent elder abuse, neglect, and exploitation of vulnerable individuals.

Advocacy also refers to maintaining the status of safe care. The nurse is committed to the well-being of the patient and thus must take appropriate action in the event that incompetent, illegal, unethical, or impaired practice puts a patient at risk. Nurses are first obligated to address the issue with the person involved and, if necessary, with higher authorities so that patients are not placed in jeopardy (ANA, 2010a). Most healthcare organizations have processes in place for reporting and managing such behaviors. Utilization of official channels reduces the risk of reprisal against the reporting nurse (ANA, 2010a).

Autonomy

Autonomy is the concept that each person has a right to make independent choices and decisions. It is reflected in guidelines and laws regarding patient rights and self-determination. Inherent in the concept of autonomy is respect for others and their decisions and that each person should be treated with dignity as a unique individual with inherent worth (see **Figure 20-1**). Evidence of respect for autonomy is found in care that considers the patient's lifestyle, value system, and religious beliefs. Such respect does not mean that the nurse condones those beliefs or choices, but rather that

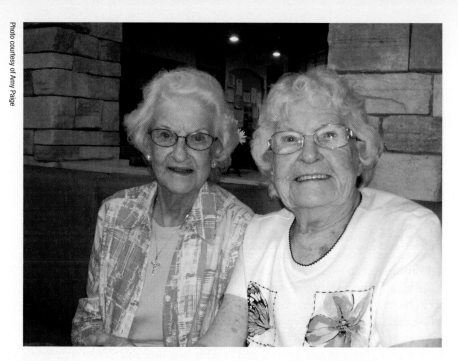

Figure 20-1 Supporting the autonomy of competent older adults is an important component of the ethical code for nurses.

the nurse respects the patient as a person with autonomy and rights (ANA, 2010a). Autonomy may be limited by cognitive deficits that impair clarity of thought and the ability of the patient to make decisions. A growing concern today related to self-determination is self-neglect in older adults, creating a dilemma to care (Mauk, 2011).

Autonomous choices are based on values and experiences. In order for patients and their families to make sound choices, they must have appropriate resources and information available. Thus, autonomy is supported by informed consent and patient and family education. *Informed consent* means making sure that consent has been granted, not assumed, following an educational process that facilitates the weighing of benefits, risks, and available options (Aveyard, 2005). Informed consent is not compliance, but ensuring that voluntariness is honored. (See **Box 20-3**).

When caring for elderly individuals, Guido (2010) points out that it is important to ensure that patients both understand the care they receive and appreciate the consequences of their decisions. All too often nurses discover that patients do not really understand why they are doing something that was prescribed by a healthcare provider. We often err by assuming they understood and provided consent because they were participating (Aveyard, 2005).

Autonomy also means that nurses and other health professionals can educate, provide support, and provide resources, but they cannot force compliance with recommended treatment. Thus, it is important to recognize that informed consent

BOX 20-3   Informed Consent

Elements to include in discussion:

- The specific condition requiring treatment

- The purpose and distinct nature of the procedure or treatment

- Potential complications or risks associated with the procedure or treatment

- Reasonable alternatives with a discussion of their relative risks and benefits

- Discussion of the option of taking no action

- The probability of success of the recommended treatment or procedure

Source: Adapted from Quallich, S. A. (2004). The practice of informed consent. *Urologic Nursing,* 24(6), 513–515.

also means that consent can be denied, can be withdrawn after it has been given, and that such requests should be respectfully honored. Refusal of treatment is a patient right. Care should be taken that healthcare providers do not abuse their power in the relationship by persuading patients to comply with recommended treatment. Any influencing factors such as "pain, depression, psychiatric illness, or effects of medications, can affect this decision-making capacity" (Guido, 2010, p. 525). Furthermore, "decisions should not be made under duress or under great stress" (Guido, 2010, p. 525). Patients and their families have been badgered into agreeing to an intervention that they did not want to pursue (Aveyard, 2005). It is important to recognize the impact of previous experiences on choices made by patients and to actively address barriers through support and education.

Ethical conflicts around autonomy can occur with issues of chronic or life-threatening illness, when patients and family members fail to conform to expected behavior patterns, or when they disagree with the recommendations of professionals. Patients are labeled noncompliant and families are labeled dysfunctional. Paternalism has been prevalent in the medical field, and healthcare providers, including nurses, are at risk for paternalistic behavior when patients are perceived as difficult to work with. Paternalism is easily supported by the distribution of power in relationships with patients and families in many healthcare settings, but it fails to support autonomy and limits the development of trusting partnerships. The best outcomes are achieved when autonomy is supported through a shared responsibility for decision making that allows the patient and family to be vested in the plan.

Health care for the elderly has been steadily shifting from acute-care hospitals to the community and community-based residential facilities. Nurses and other healthcare providers would be wise to invest in the development of strong relationships and partnerships with relational and nonrelational caregivers. Case management roles allow for coordination of care from acute to community settings (Nies & McEwen, 2011). This ethic of negotiation and accommodation means providing information in a timely manner in a way that addresses concerns for health literacy.

It also means allocating time to prepare and educate the client and caregiver on both the technical and emotional aspects of their changing roles with regards to advanced aging and disease.

As models of healthcare reform change and resource allotment shifts or diminishes, autonomy can be lost by the directives or requirements of those who control the flow of resources. The elderly are often overwhelmed by the multiple choices they must make regarding health insurance, prescription coverage, healthcare access, and disability support. Decisions regarding living arrangements, transportation, and support services also stress resources and potentially limit autonomy.

Elderly patients may need support from healthcare professionals to be assertive regarding their needs and expectations. Healthcare professionals across the continuum of care should actively include elders in decision making and care planning as long as they are able to participate. Some elders may have the resources to work around the system and its regulations, but many will not. Resources can be quickly diminished in a very expensive healthcare industry. Healthcare professionals are in a unique position of being able to direct elders to community resources and to educate and support them should they appeal the system. Feedback to regulatory bodies regarding patient needs by patients and healthcare professionals alike provides opportunities for changing regulations. At this time, Congress is considering changes to the 2006 version of the Older Americans Act of 1965. Among the proposed 11 targeted changes is the inclusion of evidence-based disease prevention and health promotion services and expanded eligibility for long-term care ombudsman services and abuse reporting (Administration on Aging, 2012).

Nurses may face ethical dilemmas when they advocate for autonomy in the face of being forced to comply with regulatory guidelines (Hoeman, Duchene, & Vierling, 2007). Nurses can facilitate autonomy in elder patients by:

> Encouraging completion of advance directives, living wills, powers of attorney, or other documents that can ensure that personal preferences are met should cognitive capacity decline
> Providing patient-centered care
> Providing appropriate education and training
> Ensuring that consents are truly informed
> Actively supporting and educating patients about their rights
> Staying informed of regulatory guidelines and appeal processes and knowing how to help patients access resources to navigate insurance and healthcare systems
> Staying politically informed and active in providing feedback to those developing laws and allotting patient access and resources
> Creatively devising care strategies that support autonomy while complying with regulations
> Referring patients to ombudsmen, community care managers, or other resources to help them navigate issues of insurance, living arrangements, transportation, and healthcare access

Beneficence/Nonmaleficence

These concepts of do good (*beneficence*) and do no harm (*nonmaleficence*) are integral to health care. Nurses intend to do good for their patients, and nurses are also concerned about situations that can result in harm to patients, such as understaffing. Consider the situation of a busy medical unit where a nurse does a cursory assessment on rounds due to heavy workload demands. One patient is a very social and talkative elderly woman who has had a recent crisis with heart failure and is having her medications adjusted. She has become significantly deconditioned and has spent much of the last couple of weeks in her recliner prior to admission. Near the end of the shift the patient complains of severe chest pain and anxiety. An emergent work-up determines that she has a deep vein thrombosis with pulmonary embolism. Is this an example of maleficence (doing harm)? Obviously, purposeful behavior such as administering a lethal dose of medication is an example of maleficence, but also consider failure to rescue on the ethical scale. How does this impact quality and safety in care?

Quality and patient safety are major concerns when providing care to older adults. The National Quality Measures Clearinghouse (NQMC) is a component of the Agency for Health Care Research and Quality, which is part of the U.S. Department of Health and Human Services. NQMC is a public resource for evidence-based measures and measure sets. One set of measures collected is related to the failure to rescue data, which refers to the effectiveness of healthcare facilities in rescuing a patient from a complication vs. preventing a complication. *Failure to rescue* data are collected by measuring the number of deaths occurring out of those discharges with potential complications of care listed in the failure to rescue definitions (pneumonia, deep vein thrombosis/pulmonary embolism, sepsis, acute renal failure, shock/cardiac arrest, or gastrointestinal hemorrhage/acute ulcer). Failure to rescue has many causes, from situations as simple as educational background, inexperience, and lack of knowledge to more complex issues such as attitudes toward work, staffing patterns, and resource allocation (see **Case Study 20-2**). It can be an issue of

---

Case Study 20-2

Mr. Jacobs, a young-acting 72-year-old who is rather obese, was admitted for trauma following a motorcycle accident in which he broke his femur. He is 24 hours post-op and has requested pain meds at 0400. The medications were given, and the nurse glanced in the room 2 hours later and noted he appeared to be sleeping. At 0700, the nurse on the next shift enters the room and turns on the light to see the patient is cyanotic and difficult to arouse. Aggressive stimulation and oxygen revived him. Discussion with the patient noted a history of sleep apnea that appeared to be worsened by the effects of the pain medication.

Questions:

1. Was this a near miss or failure to rescue?

2. Did the night shift nurse adhere to principles of beneficence and nonmaleficence?

3. What should the nurse have done differently? Consider a decision tree for your answers.

omission as much as an issue of commission. The ethics relating to nonmaleficence are certainly of concern for nursing, given the possible relationship between non-maleficence and failing to rescue.

Confidentiality

The ANA Code of Ethics (2010a) emphasizes respect for human dignity that is demonstrated in daily work. This includes respect for privacy and maintaining confidentiality. So much value is placed on the concept of *confidentiality* that it is considered a right—the right to privacy. The right to privacy has been inferred from the U.S. Constitution, but has been legislated more directly since 1996 by the Health Insurance Portability and Accountability Act (HIPAA), which includes a section concerning protected health information.

Driving forces for these laws relate to the spread of socially stigmatized diseases such as HIV/AIDS and concerns over the large volumes of information transmitted electronically, including sensitive material, detailed descriptions of interactions with healthcare workers, and genetic data that can result in potential invasions of privacy or be utilized for discrimination in the workplace or denial of insurance coverage (Ellis & Hartley, 2012). HIPAA requires that providers educate their patients regarding their rights under HIPAA and that they release only information the patient specifically designates as sharable with others. HIPAA regulations protect privacy so strongly that even admitting the patient is in your care is a violation unless the patient has expressly agreed that such information can be shared. This has changed many practices related to confidentiality in healthcare settings.

HIPAA has legislated the concept of confidentiality inherent in practice by requiring that only persons with a need to know access the patient's record or receive information about the patient. Nurses are entrusted with personal information in the course of providing care that should be shared only as necessary to facilitate that patient's care. In addition to the personal responsibility for protecting privacy, legal ramifications for failure to comply with this law are steep; the nurse should be well informed of organizational guidelines for compliance with this regulation. Health-care providers can be held liable for harm that results from sharing information without permission. Nurses should be able to easily access appropriate administrative personnel in the event that a request for patient information is questionable. As pointed out by Mitty and Post (2008), "although it is important to respect patient preferences and cultural traditions, a patient's waiver of the disclosure obligation must be explicitly confirmed, not presumed" (p. 528).

Fidelity

Fidelity refers to keeping promises or being true to another—being faithful to established agreements, commitments, and responsibilities (Ellis & Hartley, 2012). Fidelity is particularly important in the care of geriatric patients because of the amount of trust they put into the healthcare system. Fidelity is also important in relationships with team members and the organization with which the nurse works.

The team and the organization need to be able to trust the nurse to keep promises and honor relationships with them. Trust is earned, and fidelity is demonstrated in daily work and the relationships therein.

Fiduciary Responsibility

Financial responsibility as one ages becomes an important concern for both the elderly and their family. Power of attorney for finances provides an opportunity to identify persons who can address finances on behalf of the individual. Nurses need to be alert to the potential for abuse and fraud with vulnerable older adults.

As healthcare reform impacts available resources, it is important that all nurses have an understanding of the costs and benefits of care that is given. Healthcare professionals have an ethical obligation to good stewardship of both the patient's and the organization's funds—*fiduciary responsibility*. This refers to using both fiscal reserves and caregiving resources wisely, potentially requiring a cost–benefit analysis to facilitate decision making. It becomes more difficult to deal with persons who are noncompliant or who have conditions that could have been prevented through healthier lifestyles as resources and manpower decline (Hoeman & Duchene, 2002). For many, rehabilitation and other special healthcare programs are not a right, they are a privilege that is rationed and controlled by those who control funding.

Justice

Fiduciary responsibility and fidelity are some of the moral principles that help to determine what is just. *Justice* refers to the fairness of an act or situation. Health care is replete with issues of justice. Residents of nursing homes, in particular, have varying degrees of physical and cognitive needs in which a variety of ethical concerns develop (Bolmsjo, Sandman, & Anderson, 2006). Questions may arise as to whether or not it is justified for one patient to receive rehabilitation following a stroke and another to be sent to a nursing home without acute rehabilitation. Is it justified for a person who has attempted suicide and severely damaged his liver to receive a transplant before another who has been patiently waiting for the same liver? Who decides what is just and right? Does age make a difference in care? Why should one person receive more resources than another? Is the government responsible for providing resources to those unable to provide for themselves? Another concern pointed out by Guido (2010) is the issue of partial care by nursing staff in long-term care. The concern for providing equal care for all residents should be addressed so time is allocated to all, not just to a few.

Many geriatric patients depend on Medicare and Medicaid for insurance, so nurses in the field of geriatrics should conscientiously follow the government's efforts to determine just distribution of its dollars. The Medicare Prospective Payment System has been mandated by the Balanced Budget Act of 1997 and requires strict accounting for where its dollars go in post-acute care. This has led to a redistribution of services and limiting of access to home health, outpatient, and rehabilitation services for the geriatric population.

This situation quickly reinforces the issue of access, of whether we all deserve the same sort of care and who should decide what that care should be. Care of geriatric patients is burdened with age-related biases regarding resource allocation and rationales for resource allotment. Resources are limited. Elderly persons are usually on fixed incomes with restricted benefits and strict criteria for access to services, especially supportive assistance in the home. This increases the burden on caregivers, creating a difficult, isolated, and often unsupported role (Hoeman & Duchene, 2002). Success in this role is further hampered by the complexities of the system and limitations on time spent with patients and caregivers.

Quality and Sanctity of Life

The issues of justice and access to care remind us that many decisions regarding self-determination and autonomy are related to *quality of life*, or one's personal perception of the conditions of life, and *sanctity of life*, referring to the value of life and the right to live. Quality of life is a perception based on personal values and beliefs. Views on quality of life are widely variable and likely to change when circumstances differ. They are influenced by emotional, physical, economic, and social needs. Quality of life is enhanced by prevention and management of chronic disease through preventive care, support for healthy lifestyle choices, education, and home evaluations to reduce risk of injury. However, even the best nurse cannot prevent injury or reduce risk of complications in those who continue to make unhealthy choices or fail to heed health or safety recommendations (Hoeman & Duchene, 2002). Some quality-of-life decisions are made in direct relation to the burden being placed on others. Sometimes it is not the big things such as limitations in mobility that cause the greatest burden on quality of life, but rather the indignity and emotional burden associated with problems such as incontinence and dependency.

Sanctity of life supports the belief that all life is of value and that this value is not based on how functional or effective a person's life is, but simply because we all have a right to life. The meeting of personal perspectives on quality and sanctity of life can thus be expressed in an individual's advance directives. Conflicts in health care are rife with issues related to values surrounding sanctity of life and end-of-life care issues. The ANA (2010a) has addressed this directly in the *Code of Ethics for Nurses*, stating that nurses may not act with the intent to end life but may support and act on well-thought-out decisions regarding resuscitation status, withholding and withdrawing of life-sustaining care including nutrition and hydration, and aggressively managing pain and other symptoms at the end of life even if such care hastens death.

Reciprocity

Reciprocity is a feature of integrity concerned with the ability to be true to one's self while respecting and supporting the values and views of another; it is also commonly known as the "golden rule." Living according to this principle is particularly important when values and views are different. Nurses need to be impartial once a plan of care is agreed on, actively facilitating achievement of intended goals and outcomes. Passive resistance does not support reciprocity or trust. If a nurse or other healthcare provider cannot demonstrate reciprocity, another should take his or her place in the care of the patient.

Veracity

Veracity means truthfulness and refers to telling the truth, or, at the very least, not misleading or deceiving patients or their families. Veracity forms the basis of informed consent—without truthfulness and an explanation of options, the patient cannot possibly make the best choice. Failure to be truthful impairs trust and reliability (Ellis & Hartley, 2012). But issues of truthfulness create conflict as well. Do you tell the truth when you know it will cause harm or distress? How do you maintain hope while sharing a poor prognosis? It is possible to support hopefulness and decrease stress with truthfulness through careful choice of words. It is as simple as the difference between stating, "You will not likely walk again considering the severity of this stroke" and compassionately saying, "It will take considerable work and fortunate healing of your brain in order for you to walk again, but we will work with you and see what happens." Careful consideration must be made in verbal and nonverbal communication while not compromising the truth.

Patient Rights

Patient rights direct actions on ethical issues in the care of geriatric populations. The concept of rights forms the basis of many of our laws and is indeed the basis for the foundation of the U.S. Constitution. Rights are considered basic to human life, and each person is entitled to them on a legal, moral, or ethical basis (Ellis & Hartley, 2012). Over the last several decades considerable effort has been put into defining patients' rights. These rights are defined by organizational values, accreditation standards, professional codes, and legislative guidelines. The American Hospital Association has published a document addressing patient rights and hospital responsibility, entitled The *Patient Care Partnership: Understanding Expectations, Rights and Responsibilities*, in an effort to define these rights and to hold hospitals and patients accountable to them. This document is available in plain language and has been translated into multiple languages at http://www.aha.org/advocacy-issues/communicatingpts/pt-care-partnership.shtml.

Rights also evolve as values within a cultural or social group change. The right to decide what can and cannot be done to a person evolved as a legal definition due to a malpractice lawsuit in 1957 (Quallich, 2004). The right to effective pain management has evolved due to changes in perception and studies assessing the impact of poor pain management on outcomes. This is supported by The Joint Commission, which identifies pain assessment and effective pain management as a right and is part of the survey and accreditation process. As pointed out by Horgas and Yoon (2008), older adults have a high prevalence of pain due to the increase in chronic conditions. Thus, the concern for pain in older adult care is important.

Advance Directives and Living Wills

The most fundamental patient right is the right to decide. The Patient Self-Determination Act of 1990 was enacted to reduce the risk that life would be shortened or prolonged against the wishes of the individual. Following the belief that each person has a fundamental right to decide (autonomy), this law requires that patients are provided the opportunity to express their preferences regarding life-saving or life-sustaining care on entering any healthcare service, including hospitals, long-term care centers, and home care agencies. The law also requires that adequate information be supplied to the patient so that he or she can make informed decisions regarding self-determination.

Decisions regarding life-saving or life-sustaining care are recorded in legal documents known as advance directives. *Advance directives* describe actions to be taken in a situation where the patient is no longer able to provide informed consent. Living wills are alternative documents that direct preferences for end-of-life care issues, providing an "if . . . then . . ." plan. They often include what type of care to provide and whether resuscitation measures should be taken. The "if" condition (e.g., If I am terminally ill and not expected to recover) must be confirmed by a physician (Ellis & Hartley, 2012). Laws vary from state to state regarding living wills, and some require two physicians to agree to the status of the patient before enacting directives. In states where living wills have been enacted into law, healthcare providers who do not agree with a patient's directives must remove themselves from the case (Ellis & Hartley, 2012). Remember that living wills are equally as likely to indicate that resuscitation efforts be limited as they are that all possible efforts be taken. Similar to advanced directives is the physician orders for life-sustaining treatment (POLST), which is intended for those who do not want to be resuscitated in an emergency (Guido, 2010). Not all states recognize a POLST at this time, but it is suggested that both advance directives and a POLST should be completed. This also allows an opportunity for one's wishes to be discussed in advance. However, not only should a patient's preferences be discussed, but they also must be recorded. In a study supported by the Agency for Healthcare Research and Quality (HS17621), Yung, Walling, & Min (2010) reported the lack of documentation in electronic health records even though patient preferences were identified in advance. This supports the need for up-to-date information in charting, especially when medical conditions change.

Durable Power of Attorney

A durable power of attorney for health care (DPAHC) is a legal document designating an alternative decision maker in the event the person is incapacitated. This document supersedes all other general legal designations for decision makers. In other words, a patient may designate a close friend with durable power of attorney, superseding the designation of immediate family members in decision making in a situation where the patient is incapacitated. The reasoning behind having a proxy appointment is that the person's wishes have been discussed with the proxy prior to incapacitation (Mitty & Ramsey, 2008). If there is no designated proxy, a living will provides direction to the decision maker. The use of a durable power of attorney can decrease conflicts between family members and allows the designated decision maker to perform in roles negotiated in advance with the patient (Ellis & Hartley, 2012).

The absence of a living will or "do not resuscitate" order requires that all possible efforts at resuscitation should be initiated. Care of the incapacitated person is greatly simplified by an advance directive or living will. However, the issues of paternalism and boundary violations can cause ethical conflicts in the pursuit of such directives if not handled empathetically. It is imperative that information be supplied in an ethically appropriate manner for each patient because the manner in which alternatives are discussed greatly influences choices made (Elliot & Hartley, 2012). Cultural values influence decisions made as well as the way in which decisions are made. Whereas one family may see the decision as solely up to the individual involved, others may feel it is a family decision because of duty, compassion, or the concern of those ultimately assuming the burden of care. The nurse supports the preferences of the patient in resolving self-determination issues (**Box 20-4**).

BOX 20-4   Recommended Reading

American Nurses Association [ANA]. (2008). Some nurses still need end-of-life education. Retrieved from http://ana.nursingworld .org/MainMenuCategories/EthicsStandards/ Resources/IssuesUpdate/UpdateArchive/ IssuesUpdateSpring2001/EndofLifeEducation.aspx

Anthony, J. S. (2007). Self-advocacy in health care: Decision-making among elderly African Americans. *Journal of Cultural Diversity 17*(2), 88–97.

Beauchamp,T. L. & Childress, J. F. (2009). *Principles of biomedical ethics.* (6th ed.). New York: NY: Oxford University Press.

Butts, J. B., & Rich, K. L. (2008). *Nursing ethics across the curriculum and into practice* (2nd ed.). Sudbury, MA: Jones and Bartlett.

Dauwerse, L., Van der Dam, S., & Abma, Y. (2012). Morality in the mundane: Specific needs for ethics support in elderly care. *Nursing Ethics 19*(1), 91–103.

Dunbar, B. (2011). Ethical perspectives of sustaining residential autonomy: A cultural transformation best practice. *Nursing Administration Quarterly 28*(2), 126.

Joint Commission. (2007). *"What did the doctor say?": Improving health literacy to protect patient safety.* Oakbrook Terrace, IL: Author.

Winterstein, T-B, (2012). Nurses' experiences of the encounter with elder neglect. *Journal of Nursing Scholarship, 44*(1), 55–62.

Competence

Competency refers to one's mental clarity and appropriateness for decision making based on a mental status exam (Vogel, 2010). *Competence* must be present for persons to exercise autonomy and their right to decide. Inherent in autonomy is the right to choose, the right to be informed, and the right to refuse treatment, including whether to participate in research. Loss of competence due to impaired memory or sensory function significantly impacts one's ability to make such informed decisions. There is a difference between being declared legally incompetent and situations where there is evidence of impaired competence that may be transient due to health problems or side effects of medications. Legal competence is determined by the courts, and if a person is deemed legally incompetent, a legal guardian is appointed.

Informed consent means that the person clearly understands the choices offered. Problems develop when one no longer has the capacity to make healthcare decisions. Nurses should involve patients in the planning of their own health care to the extent that they are able to participate. But what do we do when the patient is confused and refusing care that is necessary for both comfort and health? Do we perform that care against the person's will, documenting that clarity of thought was limited? We do. Under our ethical standards, we are equally obligated to provide the best care under the circumstances (ANA, 2010b). Each state has laws indicating who is designated as a decision maker in the event a person becomes confused, unconscious, or considered incompetent to make informed decisions. Organizational guidelines are established in line with these laws to guide staff in management of such situations. If a physician determines a person is no longer competent for such decision making, it should be noted in writing with an explanation of the probable cause and its likely duration.

BOX 20-5   Research Highlight

Aim: To examine moral distress (MD) in geriatric nursing care and identify factors related to moral distress.

Methods: In this study, 222 nurses from 20 nursing homes and 3 acute geriatric wards in Belgium were surveyed. A 18-item moral distress questionnaire, adapted from the moral distress scale was used. Multivariate linear regression analysis was used for analysis of data.

Findings: With a response rate of 57%, the frequency mean score of MD was 1.1 (range 0–4) and the intensity mean score was 2.3 (range 0–4). Situations identified as causing the most MD included unjustifiable life support, unnecessary tests and treatment, and working with incompetent colleagues. Working in an acute care setting, nurses with elevated MD were factors of lack of involvement in end-of-life decisions, lack of ethical debate, and burnout (emotional exhaustion and personal accomplishment).

Application to practice: The authors concluded that providing futile and inadequate care contributes to MD, which in turn impacts burnout and termination of employment.

Source: Piers, R. D., Van den Eynde, M., Steeman, E., Vlerisck, P., Benoit, D. D., & Van Den Noortgate, N. J., (2012). End-of-life care of the geriatric patient and nurses' moral distress. *American Medical Directors Association, 13,* 80e7–80e13.

Assisted Suicide

Another ethical issue of self-determination and autonomy is that of assisted suicide. In most states, intentionally aiding a person in death is considered a crime of manslaughter. The ANA published a position statement on assisted suicide in 1994 that still applies today, stating that it is a violation of the *Code of Ethics for Nurses*. Instead, it suggests that nurses focus on providing competent, comprehensive, and compassionate end-of-life care.

Oregon enacted the Death with Dignity Act in 1997 to allow terminally ill residents of Oregon to use voluntary self-administration of lethal medications to end their lives. These medications are expressly prescribed by physicians for this purpose. The law applies only to mentally competent adults who must:

> Provide written documentation of their intentions
> Be diagnosed as terminally ill
> Participate in a prescribed waiting period
> Take the prescribed medication themselves—medications must be taken orally

The Death with Dignity Act specifically disallows lethal injection, mercy killing, or active euthanasia and protects those who participate in the process from liability and criminal prosecution (Oregon Department of Human Services, 1997). There were many concerns that outsiders would flock to Oregon to take advantage of the law, but that has not happened (Oregon Department of Human Services, 2007). Guido (2010) reports that 341 people have died under the law, citing reasons for their choice as "loss of autonomy, decreasing ability to participate in activities that made life enjoyable, and loss of dignity" (p. 187).

Ethics in Practice

Ethical dilemmas and conflicts surround us in real life, and ethical principles alone are not likely to address many of the quandaries and dilemmas occurring in the care of geriatric patients. Living by these principles requires reflection and consideration of one's own beliefs and values along with how they interface with the professional code of ethics, organizational statements, and beliefs of patients in the community in which the nurse practices. The ethics of care is complex and ever-changing, requiring critical thinking skills. Nurses must prepare for such dilemmas by considering the influence of their own personal values, attitudes, and expectations about aging on the care of older adults and their families. Without such reflections, the patient may lose autonomy, the right to self-determination, and justice.

Nurses must know how to assess competency as related to specific features of care in the geriatric population. Developing skills in probing the expressed wishes of patients and advocating for those wishes to be followed facilitates respect and the honoring of self-determination. Nurses also need to recognize that clarity of thought is fluid, and lucid moments can return or appear. These moments should be recognized and viewed as opportunities for discussion. Nurses, as patient advocates, also bear responsibility for effective communication of a patient's preferences through documentation and reporting processes. They are also responsible for creatively thinking about and problem-solving situations that limit functional status and safety to support quality of life and independent living (**Box 20-6**).

BOX 20-6   Evidence-Based Practice Highlight

The authors provide an overview of the international literature on ethical considerations in the field of assistive technology (AT) related mainly to older adults (especially those with dementia) who live in the community. Assistive technology is generally considered to be useful in terms of promoting independence (as with assistive devices or monitoring), but ethical aspects are not commonly studied. A systematic literature review on the topic of AT and ethics yielded 46 papers that met the inclusion criteria. The authors found three major themes: (1) personal living environment, (2) the outside world, and (3) the design of AT devices. The evidence revealed that there was

not much ethical debate surrounding the use of AT with older adults living at home; instead, most discussions centered around the concepts of autonomy and the right of elderly persons to be have self-determination. The authors noted there was a lack of clarity in concepts and assumptions in the literature, and more research is needed to shed light on different ethical aspects of the use of AT.

Source: Zwijsen, S. A., Niemeijer, A. R., & Hertogh, C. M. P. (2011). Ethics of using assistive technology in the care for community-dwelling elderly people: An overview of the literature. *Aging & Mental Health, 15*(4), 419–427.

Medical Errors

Because of the increased awareness regarding the frequency and cost of medical mistakes, as reported in *Preventing Medication Errors: Quality Chasm Series* (2007), considerable effort has been put into reducing mistakes and improving patient safety. As noted in the Institute of Medicine (2007) report, *Informing the Future: Critical Issues in Health*, "the average hospital patient can expect to be subjected to at least one medication error per day" (p. 14). Consider the potential number of errors in long-term care where multiple treatments and medications are part of care! Nurses can become more proactive in preventing medical errors by recognizing and reporting the multiple areas in which system failures may occur. Designing prevention strategies, rather than responding to mistakes, must be a priority in care delivery (see **Case Study 20-3**).

Conflict of Interest

Conflict of interest situations arise from competing loyalties and opportunities. These may include conflicts of values between the nurse's value system and choices made by the patients, their families, other healthcare team members, the organization, or the insurance company. This is particularly evident in discussions related to resource allocation and end-of-life care. Other conflicts occur when incentive

Case Study 20-3

Jane is a junior-level baccalaureate nursing student who is doing her clinical rotation in a long-term care facility. She is assigned to care for a resident who occupies a double room, 111-2. The resident assigned to Jane is named Iva Wittacker, and Iva's roommate is Ida Wallace. Both residents are elderly women and have the same initials. While passing out medications, Jane asks the nursing assistant to identify Ms. Wittacker because the residents do not wear armbands, Ms. Wittacker's picture is missing from the medication book, and Jane has not cared for this resident in the past. The CNA points to a white-haired woman in room 111. Jane administers the medications to the resident, and then her roommate enters the room and asks where her pills are. Jane asks the woman's name and she states she is Iva Wittacker. Jane realizes that she has administered medications to the wrong resident.

Questions:

1. What should Jane do immediately in this situation?

2. What could and should have been done to prevent such an error from occurring?

3. Who is responsible for Jane's mistake? What about accountability of the facility, the CNA, and/or the clinical instructor?

4. What are the ethical and legal implications in this situation?

5. Discuss what might happen if this mistake occurred in the facility where you are practicing.

---

systems or other financial gains create conflict between professional integrity and self-interest. Nurses should facilitate resolution of conflicts by disclosing potential or actual conflicts of interest or withdraw from participation in care or processes that are causing the conflict (ANA, 2010b).

Summary

As trusted professionals, nurses must continue to respect the worth, dignity, and rights of the elderly as they provide care that meets their patients' comprehensive needs across the life span continuum. Nursing's fundamental commitment to the uniqueness of the person creates opportunities for participation in planning and directing care with patients, their families, and the community. Nursing's vigilance in advocating for dignified, just, and humane care establishes a standard that can be appreciated by all. It is not through rules and regulations that ethical care delivery is created—it is through the actions of every nurse in every day of practice.

Understanding the uniqueness of the geriatric population as it relates to age-related changes, psychosocial pressures, spiritual needs, and adapting to change provides the nurse with multiple ethical challenges as one prepares for the end of the life span. The *Scope and Standards of Practice* (ANA, 2010c) in nursing identifies the code of ethics as the framework of practice, "regardless of the practice setting, role, and provides guidance for the future" (p. 26). Providing respectful care that

Notable Quotes

"Pride in a job well done is the one kind of pride God allows you to have. I earned that pride. Nothing brings more satisfaction than doing quality work, than knowing that you've done the very best you can. Reach high!"

—Bessie Delany (Delany & Delany, 1993, p. 39)

puts the patient's safety and welfare first helps us to avoid situations that can result in failure to rescue, abuse of power, exploitation, and over-involvement (Ellis & Hartley, 2012). Developing a framework for ethical decision making provides a foundation for discussion when dilemmas present themselves, smoothing the way for integrity-saving compromise. The nurse's conscientious effort to follow professional ethical standards in daily practices supports the quality of care we all strive to provide and experience.

Critical Thinking Exercises

1. Are your patients truly informed about their care? Ask five patients why they are taking the medications they are prescribed, and evaluate their responses.

2. Mrs. Gomez is confused and at times combative. Her family regularly visits and is actively involved in her care. She has been agitated and wandering the unit for the last several days and has not had a bowel movement for 6 days. She is constantly complaining of stomach pain and refuses all oral or rectal medications to facilitate bowel emptying. Her bowel sounds are diminished, and a hard mass, suspected to be stool, can be felt in the descending colon. Will you restrain her and give her an enema to prevent further complications?

3. You see a good friend while you are shopping at the mall. She inquires, "Hey, is my aunt on your unit? Can you tell me how she is doing? I just haven't had the time to get over and see her." How do you respond?

4. You answer the phone and a woman, indicating she is the daughter of your patient, asks you about her status. How will you respond considering confidentiality and privacy issues?

5. You observe a fellow nurse undressing an elderly woman and restraining her hands. The woman has been crying and yelling out for much of the night and is obviously confused. She leaves the woman naked on the stripped bed and walks out of the room, closing the door behind her and commenting as she passes you, "There, let her wet herself all night, I am done with her." What should you do?

Personal Reflections

1. As you prepare to care for older adults, what values, conflicts, or ethical dilemmas do you anticipate you will face?

2. Assess your feelings about the right to die and assisted suicide. Do you agree with the ANA's stand on this issue? How would you respond in the event that an elderly patient asks "please help me die" when death is not near?

3. An elderly person is becoming unsafe living alone and has been identified as being at risk for serious injury. During admission to an alternative living setting, the person appears oriented and appropriate. Furthermore, the person expresses disagreement with the recommendations for this admission. How would you respond in this situation?

References

Administration on Aging. (2012). *AOA Reauthorization Targeted Areas*. Retrieved from www.aoa.gov/AoARoot/AoA_programs/OAA/Reauthorization/Target_change.aspx

American Nurses Association [ANA]. (1994). *Position statement on assisted suicide*. Washington, DC: Author.

American Nurses Association [ANA]. (2010a). *Guide to the code of ethics for nurses: Interpretation and application*. Washington, DC: Author.

American Nurses Association [ANA]. (2010b). *Position statement: The nurse's role in ethics and human rights: Protecting and promoting individual worth, dignity, and human rights in practice settings*. Retrieved from http://gm6.nursingworld.org/gm-node/33771.aspx

American Nurses Association [ANA]. (2010c). *Scope and standards of practice* (2nd ed.). Silver Spring, MD: Nursebooks.org.

Aveyard, H. (2005). Informed consent prior to nursing care procedures. *Nursing Ethics, 12*(1), 19–29.

Bolmsjo, I. A., Sandman, L., & Anderson, E. (2006). Everyday ethics in the care of elderly people. *Nursing Ethics, 13*(3), 249–263.

Chinn, P. L., & Kramer, M. K. (2008). *Integrated theory and knowledge development in nursing* (7th ed.). St. Louis, MO: Mosby/Elsevier.

Comrie, R. W. (2012). An analysis of undergraduate and graduate student nurses' moral sensitivity. *Nursing Ethics, 19*(1), 116–127.

Craven, R. F., & Hirnle, C. J. (2008). *Fundamentals of nursing: Human health and function*. Philadelphia, PA: Lippincott, Williams, & Wilkins.

Delany, S. L. & Delany, A. E. (1993). Having our say: The Delany sisters' first 100 years. New York, NY: Dell.

Ellis, J. R., & Hartley, C. L. (2012). *Nursing in today's world: Trends, issues and management* (10th ed.). Philadelphia, PA: Lippincott, Williams, & Wilkins.

Guido, G, W. (2010). *Legal and ethical issues in nursing* (5th ed.). Upper Saddle River, NJ: Pearson.

Hoeman, S. P., & Duchene, P. M. (2002). Ethical matters in rehabilitation. In S. P. Hoeman (Ed.), *Rehabilitation nursing process, application, and outcomes* (3rd ed., pp. 28–35), St. Louis, MO: Mosby.

Hoeman, S. P., Duchene, P. M., & Vierlin, J. D. (2007). Ethical and legal issues in rehabilitation nursing. In S. P. Hoeman (Ed.), *Rehabilitation nursing process, application, and outcomes* (4th ed., pp. 30–44). St. Louis, MO: Mosby Elsevier.

Horgas, A. L., & Yoon, S, L. (2008). Pain management. In E. Capezuti, D., Zwicker, M. Mezey, & T. Fulmer (Eds.), *Evidence-based geriatric nursing protocols for best practice* (3rd ed., pp. 199–222). New York, NY: Springer.

Institute of Medicine [IOM]. (2007). *Informing the future: Critical issues in health* (4th ed.). Washington, DC: National Academies Press.

Lachman, V. D. (2009). Practical use of the nursing code of ethics: Part I, *MEDSURG Nursing, 18*(1), 55–57.

Mauk, K. L. (2011). Ethical perspective on self-neglect among older adults. *Rehabilitation Nursing, 36*(2), 60–65.

McEwen, M., & Wills, E. M. (2002). *Theoretical basis for nursing*. Philadelphia, PA: Lippincott, Williams, & Wilkins.

Mitty, E. & Ramsey, G. (2008). Advance Directives. In E. Capezuti, D. Zwicker, M. Mezey, & T. Fulmer (Eds.), *Evidence-based geriatric nursing protocols for best practice* (3rd ed., pp. 539–564). New York, NY: Springer.

Mitty, E. L. & Post, L. F. (2008). Health care decision making. In E. Capezuti, D. Zwicker, M. Mezey, & T. Fulmer (Eds.), *Evidence-based geriatric nursing protocols for best practice* (3rd ed., pp. 521–538). New York, NY: Springer.

Nies, M. A., & McEwen M. (2011). *Community/public health nursing*. St. Louis, MO: Elsevier.

Oregon Department of Human Services. (1997). Death with Dignity Act. Retrieved from http://www.oregon.gov/DHS/ph/pas/

Oregon Department of Human Services. (2007). Oregon's Death with Dignity Act—2007. Retrieved from http://public.health.oregon.gov/ProviderPartnerResources/EvaluationResearch/Deathwith DignityAct/Documents/year10.pdf

Piers, R. D., Van den Eynde, M., Steeman, E., Vlerick, P., Benoit, D., & Van Den Noortgate, N. J. (2012). End-of-life care of the geriatric patient and nurses' moral distress. *Journal of American Medical Directors Association (JAMDA) 13*, 80.e7–e13.

Quallich, S. A. (2004). The practice of informed consent. *Urologic Nursing, 24*(6), 513–515.

Redman, B., & Fry, S. (1998). Ethical conflicts reported by certified registered rehabilitation nurses. *Rehabilitation Nursing, 23*(4), 179–184.

Vogel, T. M. (2010). Legal and financial issues related to health care for older people. In R. H. Robnett & W. C. Chop (Eds.), *Gerontology for the health care professional* (2nd ed.). Sudbury, MA: Jones & Bartlett.

Yung, V. Y., Walling, A. M., & Min, L. (2010). Elder's preferences for end-of-life are not captured by documentation in their medical records. *Journal of Palliative Medicine, 13*(7), 861–867.

Zwijsen, S. A., Niemeijer, A. R., & Hertogh, C. M. P. (2011). Ethics of using assistive technology in the care for community-dwelling elderly people: An overview of the literature. *Aging & Mental Health, 15*(4), 419–427.

For a full suite of assignments and additional learning activities, see the access code at the front of your book.

Unit VII

Gerontological Care Issues

(COMPETENCIES 3-6, 8-11, 13-16, 18)

LEARNING OBJECTIVES

At the end of this chapter, the reader will be able to:

> Cite cultural demographic trends in United States.
> Discuss the importance of assessing health literacy and usage of translation services.
> List components of a cultural questionnaire.
> Discuss various interventions to provide culturally aware care to elders from culturally diverse groups.
> Differentiate between religiosity and spirituality.
> Identify how nurse's attitudes and beliefs about spiritually impact nursing practice in relation to holistically caring for the older client.
> Identify strategies that could assist the nurse to be productive in conducting a spiritual assessment with the older client.
> Recognize resources available to the professional nurse working with an older client assessed and diagnosed with a "loss of spiritual integrity."

KEY TERMS

Acculturation	Holistic
African Americans	Immigrant
American Indian	Interpretation
Asian Americans	Limited English proficiency (LEP)
Assimilation	Minority
Continuity theory	Myth
Core values	Native Americans
Cultural awareness	Non-Hispanic White
Cultural congruence	Older adult
Culture	Religiosity
Ethical principles	Spiritual assessment
Ethnogeriatrics	Spiritual baseline assessment
European Americans	Spiritual resources
Health disparities	Spiritual well-being
Health–illness continuum	Spirituality
Hispanic Americans	Translation

Culture and Spirituality

MaryAnne Pietraniec Shannon

Linda J. Hassler

Educational programming for the professional nurse includes a varied course and clinical curriculum in the context of an ever-changing healthcare knowledge base (Eliopoulos, 2010). The goal of nursing education is to prepare the nurse to be a safe, competent, and effective member of the healthcare team. This is accomplished through the utilization of evidence-informed nursing behaviors, which are intended to assist the client in achieving his optimal level of physical and mental functioning.

To be successful, the nurse must have a strong clinical knowledge base for professional practice, as well as value the client's important role in the process toward achieving optimal health. The nurse must be aware that client health behaviors are based on a variety of client-centered factors unique to each individual; these factors can impact health, healthcare decision making, and/or healthcare delivery. The purpose of this chapter is to explore culture and spirituality, including what it means to provide sensitive care in these areas to older clients. This chapter prepares the nurse to envision culture and spirituality as two essential client-centered factors to be considered when assessing, planning, implementing, and evaluating nursing care with older clients.

Culture and Cultural Awareness

Hola, soy una estudiante de enfermeria. **(Spanish—Hello, I am a nursing student.)**

There is a growing body of literature that proposes that patients whose *culture* is taken into consideration have better outcomes than those whose culture is not. The Institute of Medicine (IOM, 2003) stated that nursing education needs to support the development of patient-centered care that identifies, respects, and addresses differences in patients' values, preferences, and expressed needs. The CDC (2011) indicated that healthcare organizations continue to need to eliminate health disparities; to accomplish this goal, nurses will need to be prepared to function in a global environment, in partnership with other healthcare disciplines. Calvillo and colleagues (2009) developed a series of cultural competency guidelines for nurses that apply to a variety of healthcare settings, to patients across the health–illness continuum, and to patients across the lifespan.

While it is unrealistic to expect a nursing student to be proficient in working with every category and subgroup of minority older persons, it is possible to develop levels of awareness, skills, and sensitivity that can be applied to interactions with ethnic minority older persons and their families (McBride, 2006). This chapter challenges nursing students and nurses to develop *cultural awareness*.

Cultural Diversity in the United States

For many years, America had been called "the melting pot," wherein people would melt (blend) together into one culture, assimilating into the mainstream culture of their new home. They would adopt the values, beliefs, behaviors, and attitudes of the majority culture. Recently, America has been called a "tossed salad:" Many cultures are still coming together, but they are keeping their unique identities. The new groups experience some majority-culture *assimilation* but keep the group affiliations, traditions, and values of their original culture. Due to this "tossed salad," there is a need in nursing to both accept and appreciate the differences among people. In this way, nurses can better understand and care for their patients, rather than making them choose between their cultural heritage and their care (Spector, 2009).

According to the U.S. Department of Homeland Security (2011), when statistics were first gathered in 1820, there were 8,385 people who immigrated to the United States, as compared to 2011, when there were 1,062,040 immigrants, an 89% increase in 191 years. **Table 21-1** shows the number of legal,

TABLE 21-1	Statistics on Immigrants				
Continent of Origin	**1820–1849**	**1850–1899**	**1900–1949**	**1950–1999**	**2000–2011**
Africa	152	2,203	30,395	596,598	955,409
Asia	210	357,015	750,741	7,152,188	4,319,624
Europe	1,891,894	15,592,768	16,035,248	5,383,656	1,535,750
North and Central America	92,094	1,129,118	3,498,453	12,351,111	5,101,287
Oceania	6	19,931	51,378	173,193	77,564
Other America	18	7440	25,411	82,939	23
South America	2,424	9,557	127,868	1,573,100	1,026,978
Not specified	109,864	102,396	35,046	347,251	223,961

Source: U.S. Department of Homeland Security. (2011). Available at http://www.dhs.gov/sites/default/files/publications/immigration-statistics/yearbook/2011/ois_yb_2011.pdf

permanent resident *immigrants* into the United States over the past 191 years. It is interesting to note how the pattern of immigration has changed. From 1820–1949, the continent of origin was mainly Europe, though there were fluctuations in the regional immigration patterns (Western Europe versus Eastern Europe, for example). Starting in 1950, there was an increase in the number of immigrants from Latin America (which includes Mexico, much of the Caribbean, and Central and South America). By reviewing these immigration statistics, nurses can be better prepared to care for the many different cultures in their own geographic area. **Table 21-2** shows the age distribution of the foreign born as a percentage of the total foreign-born population for the United States from 1870–2010.

TABLE 21-2 Age Distribution of the Foreign Born as a Percentage of the Total Foreign-Born Population, for the United States: 1870 to 2010

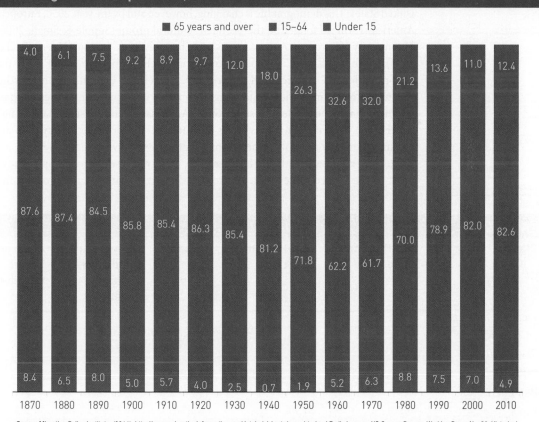

	65 years and over	15–64	Under 15

Year	65 years and over	15–64	Under 15
1870	4.0	87.6	8.4
1880	6.1	87.4	6.5
1890	7.5	84.5	8.0
1900	9.2	85.8	5.0
1910	8.9	85.4	5.7
1920	9.7	86.3	4.0
1930	12.0	85.4	2.5
1940	18.0	81.2	0.7
1950	26.3	71.8	1.9
1960	32.6	62.2	5.2
1970	32.0	61.7	6.3
1980	21.2	70.0	8.8
1990	13.6	78.9	7.5
2000	11.0	82.0	7.0
2010	12.4	82.6	4.9

Source: Migration Policy Institute. (2011). http://www.migrationinformation.org/datahub/charts/age.shtmland Emily Lennon, US Census Bureau, Working Paper No. 29, Historical Census Statistics on the Foreign-Born Population of the United States: 1850 to 1990, US Government Printing Office, Washington, DC. 1999. This report is available online.

Characteristics of the Five Major Ethnic Groups in the United States

The five major ethnic groups in the United States will be discussed here: *European Americans, African Americans, Hispanic Americans, Asian Americans, and Native Americans*. Some basic health and religious beliefs of each group will be explored, followed by the top five *health disparities* (see **Table 21-3**) for each group. Disparities, according to Keppel (2007), "were measured as the percentage difference between each of the other group rates and the rate for the best group" (p. 98), with "all indicators being expressed as adverse events" (p. 97). So, to simplify the discussion, one might consider the disparities discussed here as the most significant health-related differences found among ethnic groups, based on Keppel's research. Brief summaries of culturally sensitive nursing research to promote health in each ethnic group are also discussed in this section.

European Americans

Currently, European Americans constitute the majority of the population in the United States. This demographic is changing, however, and by the year 2050, European Americans will no longer be the prevalent cultural group (Supple & Small, 2006). The majority of European Americans describe themselves as Christian (Nelson-Becker, 2005). Within this sect, European Americans include the two major Christian denominations: Catholics and Protestants. Protestant denominations further fracture into, among others, Lutherans (Scandinavian Americans), Presbyterians (German Americans), Methodists (Scottish Americans), and Episcopalians (Anglo Americans). Of note is that these sects are not hard-and-fast rules; many Irish and Italian Americans are not Catholics, but Protestants; likewise many German and Anglo Americans are Catholic. Furthermore, many of these churches, upon movement to the United States, split off from their parent churches and evolved into

TABLE 21-3	Place of Death by Race and Ethnicity				
Place	Non-Hispanic White	Non-Hispanic Black	Hispanic	American Indian or Alaskan Native	Asian or Pacific Islander
Inpatient hospital	31.1%	38.2%	41.1%	40.5%	43.6%
Nursing home/ long-term care facility	28.4%	18.8%	15.8%	19.4%	17.2%
Residence	24.3%	21.3%	28.4%	26.5%	24.4%
Other	16.2%	21.7%	14.8%	13.5%	14.8%

NOTE: *Other* refers to outpatient or emergency department, including dead on arrival, inpatient hospice facilities, and all other places and unknown. Reference population: These data refer to the resident population.

Source: National Vital Statistics System. Mortality public use files, 2009, as printed in *Older Americans 2012*, page 154.

nondenominational Christian churches (Kelley, Small, & Tripp-Reimer, 2004). European Americans are less likely to turn to religion or *spirituality* as coping or problem-solving mechanisms. European Americans tend to rely on science to explain health and illness, rather than one's communion with God. European Americans also are more likely to turn to the government as the responsible caretaker for the infirm and/or elderly (Walker, Lester, & Joe, 2006).

European Americans generally do not have as close ties to their extended families as other cultural groups within the United States. European Americans tend to be individualistic when it comes to health care, often presenting a stoic attitude about illness, so as not to "be a burden" on others. This is represented by the value system of European Americans as "doers." Upon reaching retirement, European Americans can lose their sense of self-worth (Giger & Davidhizar, 2004). European Americans are more accepting of the paternalistic nature of the healthcare system, are generally more trusting of authority, and therefore tend to follow the advice of healthcare providers to engage in more physical and mental activity than other cultural groups within the United States (Njoku, Jason, & Torres-Harding, 2005).

The top five health disparities for European Americans (*non-Hispanic White*) are (1) smoking by pregnant women, (2) drug-induced deaths, (3) deaths from poisoning, (4) deaths from melanoma, and (5) deaths from chronic lower respiratory disease before age 45 (Keppel, 2007). Notice that only one of these, deaths from melanoma, is a specific concern for older adults. The U.S. healthcare system is primarily designed to meet the needs of European Americans.

Crespo and Arbesman's (2003) analysis of the differences in factors associated with obesity in different cultural and ethnic groups is an excellent way to emphasize the importance of cultural assessments when providing nursing care. The prevalence of obesity is higher among African American (35%) and Hispanic (33%) women than among European American women (22%). In African Americans and Hispanics, obesity is associated with poverty: It may not be safe to walk or run for exercise in poorer neighborhoods, and there may not be affordable gyms nearby. Poverty is associated with higher fat diets, as higher fat foods are less expensive. In African Americans and Hispanics with higher education and higher income levels, obesity levels are similar to European Americans. On the other hand, obesity in European Americans is associated with higher income and less education, or truly a disease of excess living. In all groups, increased time watching television is associated with obesity. Thus, when intervening with older adults who are obese, it is important to identify specific factors that are contributing to obesity, and make culturally sensitive recommendations to exercise more, reduce fat and calorie intake, and watch television less.

African Americans

As seen in Chapter 2, African Americans make up the second-largest *minority* population in the United States, only recently being overtaken by Hispanics. The majority of African Americans live in the South (54.8%); in the remaining regions of the country, the majority of African Americans live in large metropolitan areas such as New York City, Chicago, Detroit, Philadelphia, and Baltimore (Cherry & Giger, 2004). African Americans' religions vary as much as European Americans, but most African Americans are Protestant (Baptist, Pentecostal, and others). A fair number of African Americans are Muslim, or followers of Islam. It is therefore of vital importance not to generalize about any particular culture, but to inquire about religious beliefs and practices instead of making assumptions (Nelson-Becker, 2005).

The role of religion and spirituality plays an important part in the African American health and wellness belief system. Often, African Americans equate good luck, good fortune, and good health with "being right with God." Therefore, disease and illness can be thought of as being in disfavor with God, and incurring His wrath. Likewise, African Americans believe they have less control over their health and well-being than God, and illness and disease are part of "God's plan" (Walker et al., 2006). This is, however, an oversimplification of a much more complex locus of control discussion that is beyond the scope of this chapter.

Despite the systematic destruction of the family unit by 200 years of slavery in the United States, African Americans have much closer ties to their extended families as compared to other cultural groups within the United States. African Americans tend to rely on their close family ties or close neighbors when in need of support rather than turning inward, as with other cultural groups. Along with slavery, other historical injustices, such as segregation and economic disparity, have influenced African Americans' distrust of authority. African Americans are particularly distrustful of healthcare personnel because of discrimination in medical care and because most authority figures in health care are not African Americans. Wallace et al. (2007) found that the "Tuskegee Syphilis Study continues to influence the relationship of the African American patient and the biomedical community" (p. 722). A study of older, community-dwelling African Americans identified the following categories of coping strategies for chronic health conditions: dealing with it, engaging in life, exercising, seeking information, relying on God, changing dietary patterns, medicating, self-monitoring, and self-advocacy (Loeb, 2006).

Notice the dramatic difference in health disparities for African Americans when compared to those noted earlier for European Americans. The top five health disparities for African Americans are (1) and (2) new cases of gonorrhea, (3) congenital syphilis, (4) new cases of AIDS, and (5) deaths due to HIV infection. None of these are even in the top 10 for European Americans. Obviously, as a nation, we are much better at identifying and treating sexually transmitted diseases in European Americans than African Americans. For example, some nurses worked with a community housing project that had an outbreak of syphilis and gonorrhea among elderly residents who did not think they were at risk, and thus engaged in unprotected sex. Culturally sensitive educational efforts by African American staff and volunteers quickly controlled the outbreak, which has not reoccurred.

The impact of racism towards African Americans has long been considered one of the factors that contribute to decreased longevity and increased chronic illnesses (see **Table 21-4**). Moody-Ayers, Stewart, Covinsky, and Inouye (2005) studied the prevalence and correlates of perceived societal racism in African American adults age 50 or older with type 2 diabetes mellitus. The investigators found that 92% of the sample experienced social racism, which correlated with fair or poor health. The investigators caution healthcare providers that day-to-day societal racism may affect patients' trust in healthcare providers, adherence to medical advice, and self-management of chronic health problems.

Hispanic Americans

Hispanic Americans have recently become the second largest population demographic in the United States, and as a result of immigration and higher-than-average birth rates, the number of Hispanic Americans (people of Latin descent) is projected to comprise 29% of the U.S. population by the year 2050 (Passel & Cohn, 2008; Supple & Small, 2006). It is for these reasons, and others, that it is important for healthcare providers to understand the needs of this population and find ways to meet those needs.

Most Hispanic Americans place a high value on family, religion, and community. Hispanic cultures emphasize family interdependence over independence. For this population, self-care is not as important as receiving care in recovery

TABLE 21-4 Percentage of People Age 65 and Over Who Reported Having Selected Chronic Health Conditions, by Sex, 2007–2008

	Heart disease	Hypertension	Stroke	Asthma	Chronic bronchitis or Emphysema	Any cancer	Diabetes	Arthritis
				Percent				
Total	31.9	55.7	8.8	10.4	9.0	22.5	18.6	49.5
Men	38.2	53.1	8.7	8.9	8.6	23.9	19.5	42.2
Women	27.1	57.6	8.9	11.5	9.2	21.4	17.9	54.9
Non-Hispanic White	33.7	54.3	8.7	10.2	9.7	24.8	16.4	50.6
Non-Hispanic Black	27.2	71.1	10.8	11.3	5.9	13.3	29.7	52.2
Hispanic	23.8	53.1	7.7	10.9	6.2	12.4	27.3	42.1

NOTE: Data are based on a 2-year average from 2007–2008.

Source: Centers for Disease Control and Prevention, National Center for Health Statistics, National Health Interview Survey.

from illness. An individual who becomes ill will turn to the family first before seeking outside health care. The Hispanic culture, especially among the elderly, will seek the use of homeopathic remedies in conjunction with religious artifacts before engaging a healthcare professional. Additionally, direct disagreement with a healthcare provider is uncommon; the usual response to a decision that the patient or the family disagrees with is silence and noncompliance. Other Hispanic Americans may choose not to seek health care because they, like members of other cultures and religions, feel that their affliction is a punishment for sins. However, a growing number of Hispanic Americans do not seek health care because they do not have access to health care. This could be because they lack health insurance, have communication difficulties, or fear legal ramifications for residing in the country illegally (Gonzalez & Kuipers, 2004; Padilla & Villalobos, 2007).

Most Hispanic Americans are Catholic, but as with most cultures, the role that religion plays in health practices varies greatly from person to person. Those Hispanic Americans who have experienced *acculturation* to the United States generally accept the scientific theory of health and illness, although many subscribe to a more naturalistic approach. This approach in the Hispanic American culture strives to achieve a balance between "hot" and "cold" within the body. Illnesses are categorized as either hot or cold, and treated with the reciprocal type of substance, found in either medicine or food (Gonzalez & Kuipers, 2004).

The top five health disparities for Hispanic Americans are (1) congenital syphilis, (2) new cases of tuberculosis, (3) new cases of AIDS, (4) exposure to particulate matter, and (5) cirrhosis deaths (Keppel, 2007). Note that all except congenital syphilis affect older adults, and exposure to infectious disease, particulate matter, and liver disease all have increased consequences the longer one's body is exposed and/or not treated.

Diabetes and heart disease are two health problems that have an increased prevalence and mortality (see **Table 21-5**) in Hispanic Americans. Whittemore (2007) conducted a systematic review of the literature to identify culturally competent interventions for Hispanic adults with type 2 diabetes. In reviewing 11 studies, Whittemore found that providing educational sessions and written materials in both English and Spanish; employing bilingual Hispanic staff; including family members in an informal atmosphere in healthcare encounters; incorporating cultural traditions in interventions; developing culturally relevant program literature; and providing fact sheets about risks and potential poor outcomes of chronic conditions such as diabetes will increase the effectiveness of interventions.

Asian Americans

Often, immigrants from China, India, the Philippines, Vietnam, Korea, and the Middle East are grouped together as Asian Americans (see **Table 21-6**). However, to do so not only is a gross oversimplification, but also does an injustice to the ancient histories of these cultures, with recorded history going back 10,000 years

TABLE 21-5 Leading Causes of Death Among Men Age 65 and Over, by Race and Hispanic Origin, 2006

	All races, men	White	Black	Asian or Pacific Islander	American Indian	Hispanic
1	Diseases of heart	Diseases of heart	Diseases of heart	Diseases of heart	Diseases of heart	Diseases of heart
2	Malignant neoplasms	Malignant neoplasms	Malignant neoplasms	Malignant neoplasms	Malignant neoplasms	Malignant neoplasms
3	Chronic lower respiratory diseases	Chronic lower respiratory diseases	Cerebrovascular diseases	Cerebrovascular diseases	Diabetes mellitus	Cerebrovascular diseases
4	Cerebrovascular diseases	Cerebrovascular diseases	Diabetes mellitus	Chronic lower respiratory diseases	Chronic lower respiratory diseases	Diabetes mellitus
5	Diabetes mellitus	Diabetes mellitus	Chronic lower respiratory diseases	Influenza and pneumonia	Cerebrovascular diseases	Chronic lower respiratory diseases

Source: Centers for Disease Control and Prevention, National Center for Health Statistics, National Vital Statistics System.

TABLE 21-6 Leading Causes of Death Among Women Age 65 and Over, by Race and Hispanic Origin, 2006

	All races, women	White	Black	Asian or Pacific Islander	American Indian	Hispanic
1	Diseases of heart	Diseases of heart	Diseases of heart	Diseases of heart	Diseases of heart	Diseases of heart
2	Malignant neoplasms	Malignant neoplasms	Malignant neoplasms	Malignant neoplasms	Malignant neoplasms	Malignant neoplasms
3	Cerebrovascular diseases	Cerebrovascular diseases	Cerebrovascular diseases	Cerebrovascular diseases	Diabetes mellitus	Cerebrovascular diseases
4	Chronic lower respiratory diseases	Chronic lower respiratory diseases	Diabetes mellitus	Diabetes mellitus	Cerebrovascular diseases	Diabetes mellitus
5	Alzheimer's disease	Alzheimer's disease	Nephritis	Influenza and pneumonia	Chronic lower respiratory diseases	Alzheimer's disease

Source: Centers for Disease Control and Prevention, National Center for Health Statistics, National Vital Statistics System.

(Spector, 2009). The majority of Asian Americans in the United States are Chinese Americans, and this section will briefly cover health and religious practices of the Chinese culture.

Most Asian Americans' health beliefs and practices follow the same trajectory as other cultures within the United States—that is, the more acculturated to Western traditions, the more they move toward the scientific theory of health and illness. Hsiung and Ferrans (2007) identified four Chinese American groups in the acculturation continuum: the most traditional and least acculturated elderly immigrants; less acculturated elderly immigrants of working class; bi-acculturated professionals; and Chinese Americans born and raised in the United States. The most traditional and least acculturated elderly Asian Americans may still practice holistic (naturalistic) medicine and may incorporate this as an adjunct to allopathic (Western) medicine. Some of these herbal supplements may have undesired effects when combined with prescribed medications; therefore, it is vital that all complementary medicine and treatment be taken into consideration in directing care for individuals (Giger & Davidhizar, 2004).

Chinese cultural beliefs are influenced by forms of Buddhism, Confucianism, and Taoism, but the majority of the influence comes from Confucianism. Confucianism stresses accommodation and avoids confrontation, and heavily influences health beliefs and practices. Confucianism follows a naturalistic perspective, defining health and illness as a balance between the individual and the world around the individual. Individuals are a component of the universe, and it is believed that the individual should strive to be in harmony with the universe in which he or she lives. The basic concept of Chinese medicine is that all things, including the body, are composed of opposing forces called yin and yang. Health is said to depend on the balance of these forces. Chinese medicine focuses on maintaining the yin–yang balance to maintain health and prevent illness. If the balance between yin and yang is broken, it is essential to restore this balance to bring about health. To regain balance, the belief is that the balance between the internal body organs and the external elements of earth, fire, water, wood, and metal must be adjusted.

Treatment to regain balance may involve:

> Acupuncture
> Moxibustion (the burning of herbal leaves on or near the body)
> Cupping (the use of warmed glass jars to create suction on certain points of the body)
> Massage
> Herbal remedies
> Movement and concentration exercises (such as Tai Chi) (Xu & Chang, 2004)

Some elderly Chinese patients may forgo life-sustaining treatment because of the principle of *ren*. Ren is considered the golden rule of Chinese decision making, and is embodied in Confucius's axiom, "Do not do to others what you do not want done to yourself" (Hsiung & Ferrans, 2007, p. 135).

Keppel (2007) lists the top five health disparities for Asian Americans as (1) new cases of tuberculosis, (2) congenital syphilis, (3) no Papanicolaou (Pap) tests among females older than 18 years, (4) exposure to particulate matter, and (5) carbon monoxide exposure. All of these problems except congenital syphilis have an increased impact on adults as they age. Of note is that the lack of Pap tests, which does not rank in the top 10 for any other racial or ethnic group in the United States. This is an excellent example of the need for culturally sensitive approaches for health promotion measures in Asian Americans, most likely individualized for different subgroups of Asian Americans (see **Table 21-7**), as is illustrated by the following studies.

Two nursing studies of health promotion interventions to prevent breast and cervical cancer among Asian Americans confirm that nurses need to modify interventions for subgroups of Asian Americans, because the strongest correlations were within the specific subgroups of Chinese, Filipino, Korean, Japanese, or Vietnamese decent; however, there were no correlations with Asian Americans when lumped together in a single group (Kim, Ashing-Giwa, Singer, & Tejero, 2006; Lee-Lin & Menon, 2005). These studies show how important it is to not lump together people who may look alike to the European American, when the differences among diverse Asian cultures may be even greater than the differences between European American culture and all Asian cultures.

One example of a nursing study that focused specifically on the needs of a subgroup, Taiwanese Americans, is Suen and Morris's (2006) study of depression. The investigators found depression was underdiagnosed in Taiwanese American older adults, and recommended the establishment of support groups and health promotion activities at local Taiwan Centers because many elders go to these centers every day to talk to friends, sing, and participate in leisure activities. The investigators believe that the resulting discussion and sharing will promote mental health, and assist in both preventing and treating depression, which often accompanies chronic illness in this population.

Native Americans

There are about 500 different Native American tribes within the United States, and nearly half of these 2.4 million people reside in the western part of the country due to forced migration. The two predominant tribes are the Cherokee and the Navajo, each with more than a quarter million people (Spector, 2004). *American Indians* did not immigrate to the United States; therefore, the process of acculturation does not apply. In fact, many American Indians' culture is insulated from the rest of the country, either literally (by way of land reservation) or in other ways, such as linguistically. For example, the majority of Navajo people speak both English and Navajo, but many speak Navajo alone and require an interpreter when interacting with someone who does not speak Navajo (Hanley, 2004).

Like other cultures throughout the world, Native Americans follow a naturalistic approach to health and illness, believing that health is a balance of the mind, body, and spirit, and illness occurs when there is an imbalance or disharmony with nature (Spector, 2004). Native American religion is centered on legends of sacred spirits that take many forms, some human and some animal. Native American health beliefs and practices are blended with religion, thus carrying a magic facet as well as holistic and naturalistic approaches (Hanley, 2004).

The top five health disparities for Native Americans and Alaska Natives are (1) fetal alcohol syndrome, (2) smoking by pregnant women, (3) alcohol-related motor vehicle deaths, (4) cirrhosis deaths, and (5) new cases of gonorrhea (Keppel, 2007). All of

TABLE 21-7 Asian American Information at a Glance

	Asian Indians (third largest)	Chinese (largest sub-group)	Filipino (second largest)	Japanese	Korean (fastest growing sub-group)	Pakistani	Vietnamese
Abuse *statistics from APIIDV and NAPAWF	Spousal abuse private between husband and wife; in-law emotional abuse; 36–65% women report abuse	Coin rubbing may look like abuse; women more tolerant; "do not tell"—certain times "may be justified"; 18–22% women report abuse	Vulnerable group— WWII veterans, esp.; sexual exploitation; spousal abuse ignored; 20–31% women report abuse	Human trafficking for sex work, domestic servitude, hotel work, agricultural labor, sweatshop factories; 32.9% women report abuse;** Moxibustion: resultant bruising may look like abuse	Coin rubbing may look like abuse. 30–60% women report abuse	Domestic violence not explicitly prohibited, considered "a private family matter"	Family violence related to "thinking too much"; healing *coin rubbing* (superficial abrasions) may appear as abuse; 30–47% women report abuse
Advance directives	Aggressive intervention; unlikely to use AD; talking may make reality	Reluctance due to karma; lack of information; don't want to burden children	May avoid conversation as this may bring on death; approach gradually; may be resistive	More open as death is natural process; approach with courteous respect	Involve family members; discussing death may bring sadness and depression; unlikely to have written documents	May be reluctant to discuss as this may make it a reality; withholding food is forbidden in Islam	Death is natural phase, make concrete preparations but not AD due to lack of knowledge
Alcohol	15–20% abuse; whiskey popular; prohibited some areas	Lower rates	*Tuba* (philippin beer) and hard liquor; Islam forbids alcohol	2% population	Moderate risk of abuse	Rare according to Islamic laws	Abuse related to "thinking too much"
Decision makers	Men and family; mother-in-law has special status; Youngest son takes care of elders	Husband, son, or physician; Father head of family; filial piety—oldest son	Husband; may have surrogate decision maker	"Master of the home": husband or oldest adult son; family consulted before medical decisions made	Men have more status; more concern over men's illness	Older women may defer to their sons or daughters; family may want to shield the patient from negative diagnosis: ask patient if family can make decisions for patient; do not use word cancer; males make decisions	Oldest male

Dementia	Lower rates of Alzheimer's and vascular dementia: 1.8–3.6%	Vascular	Very small amount	Vascular higher in men; undiagnosed and untreated; 1.8–5.4%	Noted	Al-Harim (severely debilitated or demented elderly): fourth major health problem	Natural part of aging and the lifecycle
End of Life/ Dyng	Family-centered decision; do not tell elder poor prognosis; die at home. Move to floor—family wash body and wrap in red cloth. Belief in resurrection; may want to return to India to die	Bad luck to talk about death; Karma; surgery may be avoided as it disrupts life cycle; want patient alert till time of death. Bathe after death, three grains of rice on tongue for journey to next life, may not visit friends for 30–100 days. Buddhist: stay with body for 3 days and pray; won't show emotion; believe in euthanasia	Tell family first of poor prognosis as they may wish to spare elder suffering; "Last Rites"; resistant to stop life support. Family washes body before transport	Defer decisions to children/oldest son; concept of shiata go ni: it cannot be helped; family may not tell of poor prognosis; commit suicide with terminal illness	Prefer to die at home or return to Korea to die; death is a virtue; burial. Descendants visit ancestors' tombs on Korean Thanksgiving Day; inform family of poor prognosis first, they may/may not tell elder; may chant or burn incense; wash body of deceased	Focus spiritually on preparing soul for life after death; withholding food is forbidden in Islam; same-sex caregiver dealing with dead body. Extensive death rituals: ceremonies, washing body, positioning on left or right side towards Mecca [southeast in North America], recitation of the Holy Qur'an by fakirs [holy men]. Never give up hope; inform family of poor prognosis before elder; resistance to postmortem exam; burial within 24 hours linked to prayer timing	Sudden Unexpected Nocturnal Death Syndrome: nightmare or attack of evil spirits, press the life of terrified victim; hospital strangers at death may be viewed as negative for a "Bad Death"; withdrawal of life support may be viewed as causing or speeding up death; palliative care more acceptable. Cultural difference in truth telling about death: may cause elder to lose hope, lack of respect, upsetting, may bring death sooner

(continues)

TABLE 21-7 Asian American Information at a Glance (continued)

	Asian Indians (third largest)	Chinese (largest sub-group)	Filipino (second largest)	Japanese	Korean (fastest growing sub-group)	Pakistani	Vietnamese
Family system	Men play major role; decisions by family; men arrange marriages	Family and society over individual; different between rural and urban areas; may wash patient in hospital; may never leave patient alone	Respect and love for parents and elders; group harmony; loyalty; family reunification and elders with children; adherence to health practice related to desire to participate in family group; core value *kapwa*: shared identity, interacting as equals; extended family membership; females stay with patient in hospital.	Provide physical care to patient; individuals less important than family	Family collectivity; clearly divided family roles; blood relatives important; children of mixed ethnicity are undesirable to elders; believe family and friends over medical practitioner; education important; self-esteem tied to identification with family; males more status; family stay in hospital	Marriages between first cousins; family important to identity; extended families live in one home	Eldest male head of family; if adults work, elders take care of grandchildren and cook
Folk lore/ Folk healers Indigenous Health beliefs	*Ayurvedic medicine:* knowledge of life; holistic, balance, natural remedies; body, mind, senses, spiritual; soul; *Karma:* law of behavior and consequence; *Mangalsutra:* sacred thread around neck (women) or chest (men); consult astrologist; apply	Illness results from imbalance of yin/yang; vital energy; organs associated with illness: lung (worry), gallbladder/ liver (anger), heart (happy), kidney (fear), spleen (desire); acupuncture (may cause skin irritations);	*Timbang:* principles of balance, range of hot/cold beliefs; prevention and curing; elders use dual systems; rice porridge during illness; may refuse oxygen because it means serious illness; bowel movement means good health; for stomach ache: toast, uncooked rice, add water, drink liquid.	*Kampo:* strives to restore energy flow; herbs, acupuncture; acupressure; massage; *moxibustion:* burning a cone or cylinder of downy or woolly material; *shiatsu:* healing massage; green or Chinese teas remedy; ginger, sake, eggs help during a cold; don't want to	*Hanbang* or *hanyak:* balance between *um* (yin) and yang and balance of fire, earth, metal, water, wood; use of acupuncture, herbs, moxibustion, and cupping; may alternate between Eastern medicine and Western	Traditional folk medicine first, then Western medicine when disease is intolerable; *Unani:* therapy based on humeral theory of Hippocrates; three body states: health, disease, neutral state: six primary factors: air, food/beverage, movement/rest, sleep/wake, eat/	Opium or backache remedies used to cope with acculturation stress; speaking of vomiting or bowels not common and uncomfortable; don't touch head; holistic concept of health; illness as suffering has value as a catalyst for change and development; herbal medicines; coining (coin rubbing);

poultices; folk medicine; home remedies prior to physician; food for hot and cold illnesses; water and cumin for indigestion; black pepper and licorice to protect health; combine with Western medicine; yoga, meditation, prayer to achieve balance; may not wear gown worn by another; nod = no, shake = yes; woman with a red dot on forehead are married; spirituality, fashion

Cupping (vacuum on skin); Coining (hot coins on skin); moxibustion (burn mugwart burn near skin); herbology; meditation; blood work will cause weakness; dyspnea and vomiting treat with soup and liquids; ginseng for anemia, colic, depression, indigestion, impotence, rheumatisms; exorcism; good luck articles worn; aromatherapy; rice teas treat diarrheas; congee (rice porridge) to help recover from illness

Illness theories:
Mystical: retribution from ancestors for unfilled obligations; *Bangungot:* nightmares after heavy meal result in death; *Personalistic:* Social punishment or retribution by supernatural beings, such as *Mankukulam* (sorcerer); wears anting anting (a amulet or talisman) for protection; Naturalistic: nature events, stress, incompatible food, drugs, infection. Same sex care provider; aromatherapy; once illness effects functional capacity, then seek medical treatment; may not perform IADLs as part of living with family; rest after surgery is important

look for something bad, so no screenings

medicine; *shamans* remove evil spirits; illness is interruption of flow of life energy: lack of control of food, physical exertion, blood, elements; spiritual causes of illness; may not trust patent medications; traditional Korean medicine aimed at relieving symptoms and not treating underlying condition; natural ways of improving health; fatalistic; vomiting and bowel issues embarrassing and not discussed

evacuate; emotions; *hakim: unani* practitioner; certain hot/cold foods promote recovery from certain illnesses; do not believe in self-care during illness

cupping; *moxibustion* (therapeutic burning); accupuncture; Vietnamese three models of health: 1. *Am-Duong* – illness imbalance of yin and yang, clear by acupuncture; 2. *Than kinh suy nhuoc:* neuroses or illness of nerves; *Than kinhthac loan:* psychosis or turmoil of nerves; for "weak nerves," prescribe nerve tonic or tranquilizer; 3. Supernatural interventions: *Ten deities:* protection; humoral imbalance from Ayurvedic medicine: five basic elements (ether, wind, water, earth, fire) are upset; ritual ceremonies to deal with spirits and pay homage; practitioners of "black magic." Hmong *Shaman* (leader and healer) can communicate with spirits; spirit illness and soul loss a factor in illness; Laotians Chinese Taoist, healing Lao-tsu and his priests; spirit influence; accumulated merits

(continues)

TABLE 21-7 Asian American Information at a Glance (*continued*)

	Asian Indians (third largest)	Chinese (largest sub-group)	Filipino (second largest)	Japanese	Korean (fastest growing sub-group)	Pakistani	Vietnamese
Folk lore/ Folk healers Indigenous Health beliefs (*cont.*)							in life; 12 souls relate to 12 parts of body; *hwen*: illness created by malevolent ancestors in one part of body or soul; *Dia*: hereditary illness; *Tsiang*: ceremonies by grand master priests, other priests, or spirit mediums for supernatural illness; Eastern and herbal remedies
Health Disparities	Tuberculosi, malaria, and CAD rates higher; 1:8 have breast cancer; high risk for osteoporosis; insulin resistance; Lathyrism: paralysis from eating plant; diarrheas related to intestinal parasites; HIV; Chikungunya viral dengue hemmorrhaggic fever; bacterial meningitis; hepatitis A, B, C, & E	"Model minority", (all Asians are affluent and healthy) myth; Increased rates of cancers of the breast, colon and prostate; hepatitis B and associated liver cancer; tuberculosis; naso-pharyngeal cancer; lower smoking rates; thalassemia and glucose 6 dehydrogenase deficiency; CVD; COPD; malaria; poor air quality and pollution; Less likely to get mammograms	HTN, CHD, DM (3X), Lower rates of cancer and cancer survival of women; higher rates of gout in men; tuberculosis; HIV; hepatitis B; vitamin A and iron deficiency;	Longest life expectancy in world; risk of most diseases lower than for other elders; lower heart disease, CAD, and strokes; cancer; diabetes higher in America; Higher type II diabetes	Low risk for obesity; moderate risk for adjustment problems; High risk for Type II diabetes (4x risk); HTN; CVD; hepatitis B carriers; malaria; cirrhosis of liver; tuberculosis; oxygen means a life-threatening illness, so patients may not want to use; acupressure and massage; sensitive to cold feelings; air and water pollution concern in Korea	High risk for coronary heart disease and DM; oral sub-mucous fibrosis (from *paan/* chewing tobacco); women risk for dyslipidemia; tuberculosis; HTN; higher risk breast cancer; asking questions about sex may be insult to widow	High risk for osteoporosis and HTN; high total cholesterol; obesity; cigarette smoking; seizures; men have high risk of cancer of nasopharnx, liver, stomach; women have high risk for cancer of the cervix, stomach, thyroid; insulin resistance; hepatitis B; Agent Orange exposure; chewing *betel nut quid* (stimulant/narcotic) causes oral squamous cell cancer in women; low participation in screening programs

Historical Events	1908: Alienation of Land Act in India forced immigration; 1947: M. Gandhi lead non-violent protests for independence; 1980s: Family Reunification laws	1941: Japan invaded, many war crimes committed; post WWII immigration to United States; 1945: U.S. War Bride Act; Southeast Asia: Chinese refugees	1930s: *Pinoys*— overt racism, discrimination, oppressive farm management practices; WWII: war brides; 1965: Family Reunification Act, health professions, veterans; 1970s: refugees from Marcos regime; 1990: amendment to Naturalization Act, WWII veterans; negative attitudes may be passed on by generations	Hawaiian sugar industry; internment during WWII; Japanese wives of U.S. servicemen	1948: war, split to North and South; Hawaiian sugar industry; 1950: Korean War, war orphans sent to United States; 1965: Immigration Act; elders are "followers of children"	1947: Pakistan separated from India; 1971: Bangladesh separated from Pakistan	1975: Vietnam War, refugees left country; boat people. <u>Cambodia</u>: genocide— Pol Pot and Khmer Rouge; killing fields; 1987: Amerasian Homecoming Act; 1996 – Welfare Reform Act: funds withheld for elders
Languages	LEP: English Hindu Gujarati Punjabi Bengali Urdu Marathi Oriya Kannada Tamil Maylayalam	LEP: English Mandarin Yue (Cantonese) Wu (Shanghainese) Minbei (Fuzhou) Minnan (Hokkien— Taiwanese) Xiang Gan Hakka Many dialects	English Over 170 languages: Pilipino Tagalog "Tag-lish" (combo of Tagalong and English) Cebuano Ilocano Ilonggo Bicolano Waray Kampangan Pangasinanes Ask if medical interpreter needed	English Japanese dialects: Okinawan	Korean LEP: English	Urdu Punjabi Pashto Saraiki Sindhi Kashmiri Balochi English; Same sex professional interpreters (for modesty)	Vietnamese Hmong Mong English
Living arrangements	Financially dependent on children who they followed; grandparents raise grandchildren	Sickly live with son	Multigenerational households	Elderly cared for in their homes; close family network	Children provide physical care to elders	Elderly cared for at home and shown great respect; extended family members live together in a family home	Extended families; polygamous; elders as "followers of children"

(continues)

TABLE 21-7 Asian American Information at a Glance (*continued*)

	Asian Indians (third largest)	Chinese (largest sub-group)	Filipino (second largest)	Japanese	Korean (fastest growing sub-group)	Pakistani	Vietnamese
Long-Term Care (Overall: 1.5% of long term care population are Asian/Pacific Islanders)	Elderly cared for in home	Reluctance: filial piety	Children take care of elders in their home	Reluctance due to filial piety, unless dementia; care for in home of adult children; retirement homes increasing	Seen as last resort; financial support lacking; adult children guilt; women take care of elder in home; extended family criticize family decision	Elderly cared for in home; extended families live together in one home	Demented elderly cared for by sons in home; LTC only when sanctioned by entire extended family
Mental Health	Due to possession of the evil eye; high stigma; high suicide rate; may complain vague symptoms when depressed; lower (castes) believe they did bad things in former life	Depression; 3x suicide rate women (hanging); Buddhist believe shame family; medications; underdiagnosed and undertreated; psychosomatic and hypochondriac for emotional distress or attention; psychotherapy for seriously mental ill only; lower does of psychiatric medications	Situational depression; headache, loss of appetite, sleeplessness, fatigue, low energy; medication preferred over talk therapy; psychiatry perceived for affluent; mental problems result of witchcraft or demons; shameful; stigma	Stigma; avoid shame to family name (*hazukashii*); shame a powerful driver; shaming family is devastating; social stigma; no therapy; problems caused by own behavior; suicide a major problem; *kamikaze*: honorable suicide; physical problems instead of stress complaints	*Hwabyung*: fire illness results from failure to keep emotions from being expressed, especially in women; suicide rates are high; depression; stress of adaption; caregiver stress and guilt;	Stigma; may describe illness in physical terms; anxiety and depression high; *pir or fakir* (holymen) will visit shrines and tombs to prevent and cure physical and mental illness	Horrific life events during Vietnam War; refugee migration lead to depression, loss, and trauma (PTSD); elderly at higher risk due to above; *PruitChiit/ KiitChraen*: thinking too much; sadness, depression related to killing fields events; severe headaches and dizziness may lead to family violence; "weak nerves" cause anxiety, depression, mental deterioration; social stigma; may be due to lack of spiritual harmony—ancestors coming back to visit. Vision loss related to conversion hysteria from wartime experience

Nutrition	Ramadan (fasting from sunrise to set); fasting by women improves welfare of family; often vegetarians; no beef or pork; risk of malnutrition; eat rice, beans, chicken, nuts, vegetables, fish, coconut; eat with fingers; overweight gives stature.	Hot and cold foods: must have proper balance to maintain health; Risk for malnutrition and anemia; eat rice, vegetables, seafood, tofu, soy sauce; high-sodium meals; tea is the main drink; burned rice is bad luck; lactose intolerant; use of chopsticks	*Arbularyo* (herbalist) has special treatment skills with liquid infusion and dietary measures; use of salty condiments, pork fat, and coconut milk; being overweight is a sign of wealth; many lactose intolerant; roasted pig, sausage, chicken; dog meat a delicacy	Rice, vegetables, fruit, noodle, tofu, and seafood (raw and cooked); high sodium; low obesity rates.	Rice, vegetables, meat, and fruit as dessert; diet high in salt; preserved foods; lactose intolerant; "hot" and "cold" foods to restore balance; *kimchi*: pickled cabbage; hot liquids preferred	Poor nutrition; foods high in saturated fat; *halal*: lawful or sanctified meat; all forms of pork forbidden; withholding food is forbidden in Islam; wheat flatbread, lentils, vegetables; at mealtime, express gratitude and be serious; sweet foods not common; fish, red meat, certain fruits not with dairy; Ramadan fast sunrise to sunset; anemia in women	Rice, meats, vegetables, French bread, noodles; soft, warm foods for ill patients; iced drinks not accepted; lactose intolerance
Organ donation/ Transplants / Autopsy	Not common	Resistant (keeping body whole after death); rare	May be difficult due to religious beliefs (resurrection) and that body parts should be buried	Not favored, as there is an importance of dying intact; body should be clean and orifices be blocked with cotton or gauze; assisted suicide legalized in Japan (1995) for severe pain or impending death; cremation; practice Buddhist rituals after death: wetting lips with water, flowers, incense, and candle on table, a knife on the body to drive away evil spirits; head facing north or west, towards the realm of Buddha.	Not commonly accepted	Subject of great debate in Muslim faith; some feel it mutilates the body and shows disrespect to a gift from Allah	Less likely because donors would be reborn without their vital organs in the next life (reincarnation); Vietnamese may be more willing for barter of medical care or monetary awards

(continues)

TABLE 21-7 Asian American Information at a Glance (*continued*)

	Asian Indians (third largest)	Chinese (largest sub-group)	Filipino (second largest)	Japanese	Korean (fastest growing sub-group)	Pakistani	Vietnamese
Pain	Stoic; Hinduism believes that suffering is positive and leads to spirituality; fear drug abuse and addiction	Not readily expressed, offer pain medication frequently as it is impolite to accept something first time it is offered	Physical or emotional pain is challenge to ones spirituality; "will of God"; prefer IV or oral to IM	Belief ub tolerating pain and not expressing discomfort; may refuse pain medication; oral medications preferred	Men may not express; pain medication accepted	Not comfortable expressing pain; ask specific questions to determine pain; Islam prohibits narcotics; pain relievers may not be utilized on religious holidays	Tolerant of pain; smile or appear happy to cover pain; warm compresses are acceptable
Religion	Hinduism Islam Sikhism Buddhism Jainism Christianity Rites are preformed at death; Sikhs don't cut hair; black, white, blue are colors of death and funeral	Confucianism (achieve harmony); Buddhism (dignity); Taoism (the way: selflessness, cleanliness, emotional calm, conformity); Christianity; Islam; Ancestor worship; numbers are of great significance: 4,7 = unlucky; 8,6,2 = lucky; People's Republic of China's official religion is atheism	Catholic Protestant Aglipay Muslims (Mindanao and Sulu regions); Mysticism; church affiliation may encourage health promotion; importance of prayer, church affiliation, spiritual fellowship and faith; God as "divine physician"; religious jewelry to promote healing; *babaylan*: practitioner uses prayers and rituals, herbal plants, and massage manipulation for health and wellness; prayer and spiritual counseling part of treatment plan; "Soul Loss" due to shock, fear, or desire, requires prayer or exorcism	*Shintoism*: belief in *Kami* (spirit gods); *Buddhism*: code of ethics, harmony with themselves, universe, and society for good health; *Confucianism*: importance of family and social order; Christianity; may combine religious customs; many agnostic	Buddhist; Christian (Protestant, Catholic); churches/ temples play important role; Korean church ties; 50% do not claim a religious affiliation; fatalistic; luck or past doings create illness; *shamans* remove evil spirit or promote spiritual healing	Islam; Christianity; Hinduism; spiritual peace part of health; disease a direct punishment from God; wear *taawiz*: amulet with holy Qur'an verses; sickness is a test from God; avoid complaining about sickness; illness is for atonement of sins; may wear *taawiz* or *topi* (religious cap); *Ramadan*: self-purification by a fast from eating, drinking, smoking, or sex sunrise to sunset (not applicable to children, pregnant women, or *Al-Harim* (severely debilitated or demented elderly); at sunset,	Buddhist; Cambodians: Theravada Buddhism; in United States, Catholic; Delays in obtaining relief from illness may be a Buddhist stoic response to religious awakening; *tiendietes*: errant spirit ancestors not properly venerated by descendants with worship or offerings and cause mental illness; spirit mediums and sorcerers deal with spirits; Buddhist priests and monks give amulets and medicines for physical ailments or do exorcism for spiritual ailments; spirit world can influence health; placing rice, coins, or jewels in

Religion (cont.)

	fast is broken with prayers and *iftar* (meal), then visit with friends and family; *Namaz*: obligatory prayers five times per day; facing Mecca, after washing themselves; Fridays go to *masjid* (mosque or church) offer special prayers; *Wudu*: ceremonial washing before prayers	mouth of deceased to help travel after death; Last Rites for Catholics; Buddhists: death ritual last 3 days, include praying and burning incense

Respect

| Same sex caregivers; patient is passive; direct eye contact from women to men limited; remove shoes before entering home; physical contact limited; older person has high respect | *Li*: proper way, control of emotions, restraint, obedience to authority, conforming, and "face" are highly valued and important; authority and elders; filial piety: protect elders from poor prognosis; may hesitate to ask questions as not to appear disrespectful or inconvenient; proper title and name; older adults called auntie and uncle; direct eye | Address by Mr/Mrs/Miss; with permission *Lola* (grandma) or *Lolo* (grandpa); protect elders from external forces; respect for elders and authority; children should be taught to care for elders and take care of aging parents; firm handshake and greet elder first; ask to repeat instructions as a sign of respect (instead of asking if they understand); healthcare provider respected and may not be questioned or challenged; sit at eye level; keep personal | *Filial piety*: taking care of one's own parents; courtesy and thoughtfulness; great respect for elders and authority; introduce self to elder first; children provide physical care to elderly; may call by title | Proper title and bow; filial piety; same sex provider; respect for authority; no direct eye contact or physical contact; silence; modesty; use both hands when giving object; silence | Old age is respected; same sex care providers; do not use first names; direct eye contact not common; expansive personal space; silence; elders may respond to stories as opposed to direct questions; feel unsure about signing consents | May not make direct compliment as this may bring attention to evil spirits; proper titles; no eye contact; large area of personal space; elders highly respected |

(continues)

TABLE 21-7 Asian American Information at a Glance (*continued*)

	Asian Indians (third largest)	Chinese (largest sub-group)	Filipino (second largest)	Japanese	Korean (fastest growing sub-group)	Pakistani	Vietnamese
Respect (cont.)		contact avoided; no head touching; no winking	space; covering mouth = shyness or embarrassment; don't want to be burden so won't seek health care; saving face is important				
Utilization of Health Care	Surgery only on auspicious days	Language barriers, geography, economic barriers	Lack of health insurance; lack of mobility; LEP; adherence to own cultural health beliefs	Medical problems, not mental illness	Decreased due to LEP, unfamiliar systems and food in hospitals; utilize "Korean" hospitals in United States, which are unlicensed private homes	Lack of health insurance (50%)	Buddhists may avoid hospitals where "lost souls gather"; souls of dead people linger and may create havoc upon living as they have no place to rest

*NAPAWF - National Asian Pacific American Women's Forum http://napawf.org

*APIDV -Asian and Pacific Islander Institute on Domestic Violence http://www.apiidv.org/violence/ethnic-specific-information.php

**The Yomiuri Shimbun 2012 (Tokyo) One-third of married Japanese women are victims of domestic abuse http://www.standard.net/stories/2012/05/02/one-third-married-japanese-women-are-victims-domestic-abuse

The Rise of Asian Americans video: http://www.pewsocialtrends.org/2012/06/19/video-the-rise-of-asian-americans/

these disparities point to the lack of effective programs to reduce alcohol consumption among those Native American individuals who are at high risk of alcoholism. There continues to be a pressing need for culturally sensitive interventions to address major health problems in Native Americans. The authors are aware of a project in a tribe in Wisconsin to promote walking and a return to a traditional diet, which includes wild rice, venison, trout, and salmon, all harvested locally. The concept is to promote weight maintenance and glycemic control in order to reduce the incidence of diabetes, heart disease, and alcoholism. The prevention of high and low blood sugar in those who are at risk of alcoholism may be an effective prevention strategy. Poor glycemic control is also considered a risk factor for diabetes and heart disease. In a review of cardiovascular research in Native Americans, Eschiti (2005) found only one study, conducted by nurses; that the existing research of other disciplines relies on only a few tribes of the more than 500 tribes in the United States; and very little intervention research. Eschiti recommends that studies focus on the establishment of trust with providers as well as those working in governmental agencies by involving tribal members in all aspects of program design, implementation, and evaluation. Miller and Clements (2006) also call for active partnerships between healthcare providers and tribal communities to identify the extent of elder abuse and effective treatment measures that are sensitive and responsive to tribal cultures and conditions in order to assist Native Americans in their desire to care for and honor their elders.

English Language Proficiency

According to the Migration Policy Institute (Pandya, Batalova, & McHugh, 2011), the number of *Limited English Proficiency (LEP)* persons is steadily increasing (see **Table 21–8**) as the number of foreign born immigrants increases. In 1990, 6.1% of the total United States population had LEP, in 2000 the LEP share was 8.1% and in 2010 the number has grown to 8.7%. The highest states in the country with LEP individuals were California (27%) and Texas (13.3%).

In the Hispanic population, English is not spoken in 12% of Puerto Rican homes, 14% of Mexican American, 15% of other Hispanic, and 33% of Cuban homes. Anywhere from 28–54% of Hispanics are linguistically isolated (Mutchler and Brailler, 1999). The top ten languages spoken by LEP individuals in 2010 were Spanish (65%), Chinese (6.1%), Vietnamese (3.3%), Korean (2.5%), Tagalong (1.9%), Russian (1.7%), French Creole and Arabic (1.3% each), and Portuguese/Portuguese Creole or African languages (1.1% each).

TABLE 21-8 English Proficiency According to the U.S. Census Bureau, American Community Survey 2010	
Speak only English	79.4%
Speak language other than English	20.6%
Speak English "very well"	11.9%
Speak English less than "very well" (LEP)	8.7%

In order to meet the needs of immigrants with LEP, policies have been put into place for *translation* services for all patients at the bedside. Healthcare organizations have an obligation to provide LEP patients, and patients with disabilities, with a meaningful access to care through effective communication free of charge. It is important to note that is **not** appropriate to ask a family member, especially a child, to interpret your healthcare activities. Asking a non-trained interpreter can lead to risk management issues and litigation. The Department of Health and Human Services Office for Civil Rights considers inadequate *interpretation* as a form of discrimination.

There are four different types of translation services:

1. In-person interpreters: Each facility should have trained interpreters in languages that are common to their demographic area. Typically, trained interpreters complete 45 hours of training in order to be certified.
2. Sign language interpreters: For those who are deaf or hard of hearing utilizing the American Sign Language (ASL).
3. Over the phone interpretation (see **Figure 21-1**): For this type of service, the nurse would call a toll-free number, give the facility identification number, state which language is needed, and then be connected via phone to the interpreter.

MARTI (my accessible real time trusted interpreter) video remote interpretation: For deaf, hard of hearing, and over 150 languages. The television monitor provides an on-screen interpreter (see **Figure 21-2**) (for more information, visit http://www.languageaccessnetwork.com).

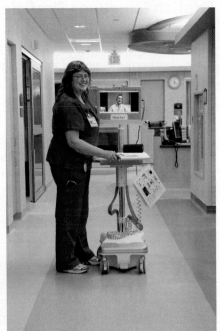

Courtesy of Bryan Health

Figure 21-2 Technological advances such as MARTI may assist when interpretation/translation is needed.

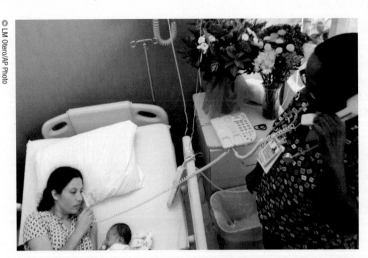

© LM Otero/AP Photo

Figure 21-1 Over-the-phone interpretation phone.

Culture and Nursing Care History

The Transcultural Nursing Society (TCNS) was organized in 1974 (see **Figure 21-3**) and has as its mission to enhance the "quality of culturally congruent, competent, and equitable care that results in improved health and wellbeing for people worldwide" (Transcultural Nursing Society, 2013, p. 1). The Society has developed standards for cultural competence in nursing practice as seen in **Box 21-1**. Knowledge of Cultures, Standard #3 states, "Nurses shall gain an understanding of the perspectives, traditions, values, practices, and family systems of culturally diverse individuals, families, communities and populations for whom they care, as well as a knowledge of the complex variables that affect the achievement of health and wellbeing" (Transcultural Nursing Society, 2011, p. 1).

Gerontological nurses need to be culturally aware, which is a dynamic, life-long, learning process. Understanding the process for assessing cultural patterns and factors that influence individual and group differences is critical in preventing overgeneralization and stereotyping. The following are essential in order to provide culturally competent, evidence-based care for *older adults*, otherwise known as *ethnogeriatrics*:

A. Awareness of one's personal biases through critical self-reflection
B. Understanding of
  1. Culturally diverse health-related values, beliefs, and behaviors
  2. Disease incidence, prevalence, or mortality rates
  3. Population-specific treatment outcomes
  4. Individuals, families, communities, and populations for whom they care
C. Skills in working with culturally diverse populations (Transcultural Nursing Society, 2011)

Assessment of Culture

The culturally aware nurse should assure that the assessment tool being utilized has been researched in the cultural population as a reliable and valid instrument. One tool to assess cultural needs was developed by Arthur Kleinman and colleagues (1978). They developed eight questions to recognize and validate patients' conceptions, explanations, and expectations of their own illness experiences, many of which are based on cultural beliefs. This patient illness narrative is also termed the "Explanatory Model of Illness."

Another questionnaire that can be utilized is from the SCAN Health Plan (2012) website and is aptly called the *D-I-V-E-R-S-E, A Mnemonic for Patient Encounters*. This mnemonic can assist the nursing student in developing a personalized care plan based on aspects of cultural diversity. After it is completed, it should be placed on the patient chart for future reference.

Notable Quotes

"If we are to achieve a richer culture, rich in contrasting values, we must recognize the whole gamut of human potentialities, and so weave a less arbitrary social fabric, one in which each diverse human gift will find a fitting place."

—Margaret Mead

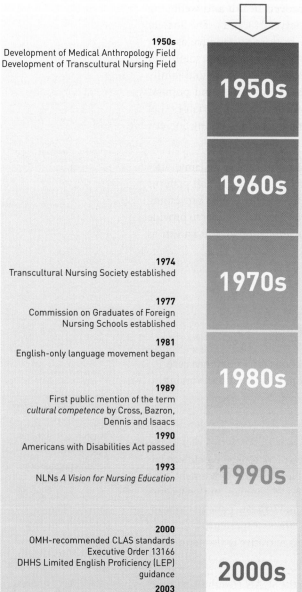

1897
Nurses Associated Alumnae of the
United States and Canada established
(renamed American Nurses Association
or ANA in 1911)

1950s
Development of Medical Anthropology Field
Development of Transcultural Nursing Field

1950s

1950
ANA *Code of Ethics* released

1951
Integration of African Americans into
American Nurses Association

1960s

1964
Title VI. Civil Rights Act

1974
Transcultural Nursing Society established

1977
Commission on Graduates of Foreign
Nursing Schools established

1970s

1971
National Black Nurses Association founded

1975
National Association of Hispanic Nurses
founded

1981
English-only language movement began

1989
First public mention of the term
cultural competence by Cross, Bazron,
Dennis and Isaacs

1990
Americans with Disabilities Act passed

1980s

1984
National Alaskan Native American Indian
Nurses Association formed

1986
Release of **original** ANA position statement
of cultural diversity in nursing practice

1991
Release of **new** ANA position statement
on cultural diversity in nursing practice

Asian American/Pacific Islander
Nurses Association established

1993
NLNs *A Vision for Nursing Education*

1990s

1998
Philippine Nurses Association founded

2000
OMH-recommended CLAS standards
Executive Order 13166
DHHS Limited English Proficiency (LEP)
guidance

2003
Office of Civil Rights
LEP policy guidance

2000s

2001
US Department of Justice (DOJ)
LEP policy guidance
Revised CLAS standards
American Arab Nurses Association founded

2002
Revised DOJ LEP policy guidance
Institute of Medicine report

Figure 21-3 Transcultural nursing.

Source: Office of Minority Health, U.S. Department of Health & Human Services.

BOX 21-1   Standards for Cultural Competence in Nursing

Standard 1. Social Justice

Standard 2. Critical Reflection

Standard 3. Knowledge of Cultures

Standard 4. Culturally Competent Practice

Standard 5. Cultural Competence in Healthcare Systems and Organizations

Standard 6. Patient Advocacy and Empowerment

Standard 7. Multicultural Workforce

Standard 8. Education and Training in Culturally Competent Care

Standard 9. Cross Cultural Communication

Standard 10. Cross Cultural Leadership

Standard 11. Policy Development

Standard 12. Evidence-Based Practice and Research

BOX 21-2   Questions to Validate Illness Experiences

1. What do you call the problem?

2. What do you think has caused the problem?

3. Why do you think it started when it did?

4. What do you think the sickness does? How does it work?

5. How severe is the sickness? Will it have a short or long course?

6. What kind of treatment do you think you (or your loved one) should receive? What are the most important results you hope to receive from this treatment?

7. What are the chief problems the sickness has caused?

8. What do you fear most about the sickness?

9. What do you want most from your work with me?

Care Interventions and Cultural Awareness

(Malama – Hawaiian "to care for")

A key strategy for achieving *cultural congruence* is to learn about different cultural and religious preferences, customs, and restrictions, and then use this knowledge in planning and providing care. In the journal *Minority Nurse*, ElGindy (2004) has written guides to meeting the special dietary needs of those of several faiths, including Jewish, Muslim, Hindu, and Buddhist. When an elder is in the hospital or extended care facility, encourage the family to bring in favorite foods from home, unless there are dietary restrictions that prevent this. Encourage the family to eat together. Hostler (1999) found that bringing in food promoted both recovery and family integrity in hospitalized children, and it is likely bringing in food for elders will also promote recovery. Again, remember that food preferences within a cultural group, even within families, vary greatly.

Economic diversity is also great among elders: Some are barely getting by, whereas others are among the wealthiest in society. Ensuring that all have adequate food, shelter, and health care has always been a societal problem. The effects of age also differ. Some 60 year olds who have lived with chronic illness may be frail and disabled, though the majority of persons at this age are active, productive, and independent. Likewise, 80 year olds are frail, yet a growing number are still active, productive, and independent. The key for nurses is to assess each individual's level of activity, health status, and heritage and plan care accordingly, rather than relying simply on age in planning care.

Another aspect of diversity is in religion and faith practices. Again, the elderly are a very diverse group. Some have practiced only one faith for their entire lives, whereas others may have made many changes in a lifelong spiritual quest. Faith communities provide a great deal of support for some elderly. These communities are active in promoting health for elders and in overcoming health disparities.

Health care for elders is also diverse. Those who are wealthy, well educated, and used to having power have access to the best care. Those who are poor, poorly educated, and used to living on the margins of society suffer from health disparities and often have poor access to care.

A 2002 issue of *Generations* contained an interview with E. Percil Stanford and Fernando Torres-Gil, two leaders in the field of aging who have long focused on diversity. This interview (Kaufman, 2002) contains several points crucial to consider when caring for diverse older adults. The first is that diversity has been mainstream for over a decade in the field of aging, and elders with diverse points of view have long been in leadership positions in the American Society on Aging, the Gerontological Society of America, and AARP. Some minority elders who were once overlooked now have a well-heard voice. The first lesson for nurses here is that to ensure culturally competent care, elders who are being cared for need to have a voice in their care and give regular input into how care is delivered, both for themselves and their loved ones. The second point is the need to use well elders as volunteers and as paid staff when providing care, as well as ensuring that they have educational and training opportunities and the support to remain active members of their communities and their healthcare organizations. Virtually all elders will eventually require some level of assistance or health care, so helping them stay healthy as long as possible and then helping them plan for their own care is key to the financial survival of our healthcare system. We need to help elders make sound healthcare decisions early on, before a crisis occurs, and to ensure that all family members are in agreement with the decision. A third point is the need to seek out individuals who are not being served, who are still marginalized, and who lack resources, and to target care to those who really need it. Not all elders need all resources; the focus needs to be on those who are in the greatest need.

Table 21-9 provides general guidelines to promote a better understanding of a cultural group, but remember that the members of a culture are not necessarily homogenous. Always ask the patient/family if you have any questions that pertain to providing culturally congruent care (see **Figure 21-4**).

感谢您的阅读 (Chinese – Thank you for reading.)

Notable Quotes

"If art is to nourish the roots of our culture, society must set the artist free to follow his vision wherever it takes him."

—John F. Kennedy

TABLE 21-9 Comparison of Cultural Groups

	American Indian	Hispanic and Latino	African American	Native Hawaiian/Pacific Islanders
Abuse incidence and type – if noted (White 77%)(NCEA % of all cases)	0.6% Neglect; financial	10.5%	21.2%	0.7% Spousal and child, ignored
Advance directives	Develop trust relationship before asking	Involve family; Trust physician; Complex	Less likely; God is ultimately in charge	Reluctant
Decision makers	Clan leaders, matriarchs, patriarchs, religious or medicine	Nuclear and extended family, fictive kin (non-relatives), friends, church members	Loved one; fictive kin: long-standing family relationships	*Ohana*: family
Dementia deaths (White 25.4%) (Health, US 2011)	11.4% Rare	15% Lower rates	19.7% Vascular dementia; higher rates	8.9% Guam Parkinsonism dementia (*lytico-bodig*); lower rates
Education (all older adults: 76.5% high school; 20.2% bachelor's or higher)	All ages: 77% high school 13% bachelor's 4.5% advanced degree; doing rather than talking	All ages: 60.9% high school 12.6% bachelor's or higher; Cubans: higher levels	Older adults: 44% high school; 7% bachelor's or higher	All ages: 85.3% high school 49.7% bachelor's or higher
End of Life/ Dying	Death natural part of life; home care; family may not visit – spiritually bad for living & dying; death rituals: dressing and positioning body, burning herbs and grasses, funerals and burials	Protect from cancer dx; more likely to use heroic measures; *El Dia de Los Muertos* (Day of Dead) celebrate and honor lives; *dicos* – sayings about God; hospice less likely; die at home	Death rates higher till crossover; reluctant to participate due to mistrust; certain diseases and prognosis withheld	Keep at home; hospice; home care; *Ohana*: family stay at side of sick; *uwe*: death chant, wailing to express grief; money and cards given at funerals

(continues)

TABLE 21-9 Comparison of Cultural Groups (*continued*)

	American Indian	Hispanic and Latino	African American	Native Hawaiian/Pacific Islanders
Family system	Extended; mixed tribal heritage; many single-parent homes	Live with children; *familismo*; fictive kin (*compadres*)	Dependant care from children, grandchildren, or fictive kin; many raising grandchildren	Importance of group: multi-generational; value society; revere elders; defer to judgment of adult children; men live alone
Folk lore/folk healers	558 tribes/nations; allopathic medicine, but "healer" used first; chanting to promote healing and remove evil; do not cut hair	Over-the counter; home remedies; *curanderos* (general practitioners); *yerbistas* (herbalists) *sobadores* (massage]; *empacho:* locked bowels	Herb and root doctors; *conjurer:* place a hex or ward off evil; spiritual healers; natural illness—physical cause; occult illness—supernatural forces/evil spirits; spiritual illness—willful violation of sacred beliefs or sin	*Kahuna lapaʻau:* priest heals with medicines; tattoos denote significant achievement in rank; illness is seen as curse; *noni:* plant to heal bowel problems and menstrual cramps; *lokani triangle:* physical body, environment, relationships with others, mental and emotional states; *poi:* taro root used for illness; talking about illness hastens death
Functional status	Assess if they have ever performed ADLs first; self-care limitations and health-related mobility problems	More disabilities; dear of admitting one's dependence; report greater activity limitations; needed more help with personal and routine activities, and more used of assistive devices for walking; women appeared to be higher than for men [HE1]	Higher rates of walking difficulties and higher rates of activity limitation	Higher levels of physical limitation

Health disparities	Diabetes; heart disease; gallbladder disease; poor survival rates with all types of cancer; low incidence of brain cancer; kidney disease; liver disease; tuberculosis; rheumatoid arthritis; hearing and vision problems	Border medications; complimentary and alternative medicine; heart disease; cancer; cerebrovascular disease; respiratory disease; increased hip fractures specifically in Mexican Americans	Diabetes; prostate cancer; HTN; blindness: specifically glaucoma; John Henryism: making it because of sheer determinism against overwhelming odds	Obesity; diabetes and lower extremity infections; HTN; tuberculosis death; rheumatic fever and heart disease; cancer; Women: high rates of HIV; Simoan men: cancer; rehab less likely; *Vog*: respiratory disease from volcano smoke
Historical Events	Indian Self Determination and education Act 1975; Indian Health Service	1910: Mexican revolution; 1940: Mexicans for labor (Cesar Chavez); 1996: welfare reform; Puerto Rico: overcrowding; Cuba: Fidel Castro, Bay of Pigs, Mariel Boatlift	Exploitation: South—legalized discrimination, North—covert discrimination; suspicious of healthcare providers (see Tuskegee Experiment)	
Languages	106 Indian dialects; Indian sign language; LEP	Spanish; LEP	English	English; Hawaiian; Pidgin
Life expectancy (Whites: 78.9 years)	72.6 years	81.3 years; Centenarians by 2050 = 19%	75 years; Shorter "Crossover Phenomenon" (Reversal in average life expectancy after age 80)	68.3 years; Lowest
Long-Term Care	No provision in Indian Health Service; 12 tribally run nursing homes, but are a long distances for most families; social adult daycare centers	Less likely; Cultural Aversion Hypothesis: myth of aversion to LTC and "they take care of own"	Less likely; remain at home with support of family, church ` paid home caregivers; higher over age 85	Half the rate of White elders; last resort

(continues)

TABLE 21-9 Comparison of Cultural Groups (*continued*)

	American Indian	Hispanic and Latino	African American	Native Hawaiian/Pacific Islanders
Mental Health	Increased rate of major depression—Indian Depression Scale is highest Apache tribe with 1.5x suicide rate; "bad spirits"	Depression (woman); GDS less valid	Depression usually not treated	Decreased suicide rate; many homeless; drug abuse
Nutrition	Food expression of taking care of people; high fat, high sugar, processed food, corn	*Tapas*: snacks; *sobremesa*: sitting after meal and talking; wine with meals; coffee important with meals: *café con leche* (coffee with milk), *café solo* (coffee without milk), or *café cortado* (coffee with some milk); *churros*: twisted donut sprinkled with sugar or dunked in hot chocolate; large lunch; *arroz*: rice with meals; *chimichangas*: large, deep-fried burritos; spices in food and drinks	"Soul food": during slavery, had to cook with leftovers; okra, collard greens, black-eyed peas and sweet potato; pigs feet, chicken livers, beef neck bones and chitterlings (cleaned pig intestines); fried fish and chicken; corn as cornbread and grits	Rice; *musubi*: Spam, rice, and seaweed wrap; bar-b-que; meats; macaroni salad; soda

Organ transplant need and donations (White: 45% need; 68.2% donors)	Do not desire; ESRD possibly: 1% need; 0.4% donors.	18% need; 13.4% donors: deceased donors; mistrust of the medical profession; religious acceptance concern; perceptions of inequity in the distribution of donated organs; women more likely than men	Largest group in need of transplants: 29%; 14% donors	0.5% need; 0.2% donors; deceased donors
Pain	Withstand the pain: survival	Stoic; folk beliefs and non-drug; do not understand scales	Higher pain intensity	Stoic; use massage, relaxation, and prayer
Religion	Indian spiritual beliefs and Christianity	*Espiritismo* (Puerto Rican): belief that good/evil spirits can affect well-being; *santeros* (Cuban faith healers)	Protestant, Catholic, Muslim; Part of life fabric; Church community plays important role	Catholic, LDS, Baptist, Pentacostal; Worship god and goddesses, nature, human spirit; Mana: spiritual essence of protection
Respect	Listening; calmness; slow down; nondirect eye contact; may be guarded; modesty and privacy; obtain permission	Early attention to build rapport; use titles and last name	Titles: Mr/Mrs	Revere elders: *filial piety*; indirect communication; negative not expressed; females: *Aunties*
Utilization of health care (White: 11.7% uninsured)	29.2% uninsured; Indian Health Service; LEP concern; cautious of nontribal health care	30.7% uninsured; LEP concern	20.8% uninsured	17.4% uninsured

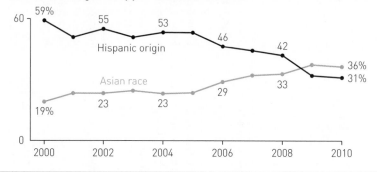

FIGURE 21-4   Social Trends

Meet the new immigrants: Asians overtake hispanics
Percent of immigrants, by year of arrival, 2000–2010

Source: http://www.pewsocialtrends.org/files/2012/06/2012-sdt-asian-americans-001a.png

Spirituality and Religiosity

When the nurse addresses the client in a *holistic* way, attention needs to be directed to assess the mind, the body and the spirit (Anderson, 2007). Viewing all three of these components individually and recognizing that they are in dynamic relation with one another is an important responsibility for all nurses, regardless of their nursing role in relation to client care. As with the body and mind, the spirit is recognized to be a universal, intrinsic, and integrated basic human component of the patient's being, transcending socioeconomic status, race, gender, culture, and age (Taylor, 2002). Even though attention to the spirit should occur in the care of all clients, this chapter will focus on the role of the nurse in addressing the needs of the older client.

Spirituality encompasses but is not limited to religiosity (Ebersole, Touchy, Hess & Jett, 2007). Our spirit incorporates our sense of identity and our understanding about our place and status in the world (Thompson, 2007). Demonstrations of the spirit are reflective of the individual's perception of quality and meaning of life, and can be explicit or implicit in nature. In the literature, spirituality has been associated with a variety of terms (beliefs, faith, morals, values, ethics, standards, symbols, rituals, culture, religion, balance, nature, connectedness, centeredness, homeostasis, mystic, resiliency, transcendence, hope, well-being, God, deity, etc.). Some clients report that their spirituality is fully in the context of dogmatic guidelines affiliated with a specific formal religious group. For these clients, the terms *religiosity* and spirituality may appear to be synonymous. However, the nurse must be cautious against stereotyping and accepting the common *myth* that the practices proposed by one religious sect are perceived and practiced the same way by each group member, since complex variations in adherence to religious practices can actually range from excessively strict compliance for some, to being lax or even

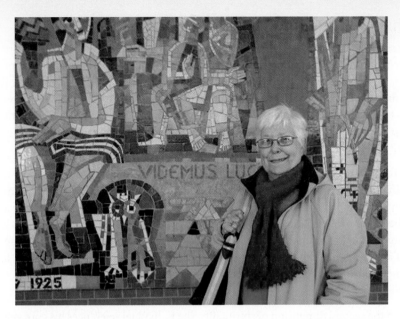

Figure 21-5 Nurses should be sensitive to spiritual and cultural differences among families.

nonexistent for others. For this reason, the nurse should be open and respond in a nonstereotypic manner when questioning religious preference notations in the patient's chart or seeing a religious symbol on the patient's bedside stand (Miller, 2009) (see **Figure 21-5**).

It is helpful in considering an older client's spirituality for the nurse to be aware of some practices and rituals outlined by formal religious groups in terms of expected behaviors that may have an impact on health and/or healthcare decisions for older clients or for their significant others (see Appendix A). Although such "resources at a glance" can serve as valuable starting points in education on factors that can influence health, the professional nurse must supplement such guides with anecdotal comments from the individual client's perspective if the goal for designing an individualized holistic nursing plan of care is to be met.

Finally, the nurse must be aware that even though spirituality and religiosity may be perceived as the same by some elderly clients, others may view these concepts as two distinct entities, and still others may report that neither plays any role in impacting their health or their healthcare decision making. This refutes a set of commonly held myths that all people need spirituality as a way to provide meaning for their lives, and that spirituality must be tied to a formal religion for beliefs to be moved into practice. Regardless of the view held by the older client, it is the responsibility of the nurse to take the direction provided by the client and respect that client's point of reference for his or her spirituality.

Three Dimensions of Spirituality

Since the purpose of this chapter is to explore the dynamic and complex nature of spirituality for consideration in planning holistic nursing care, it is important to consider all dimensions of the concept perceived by the older client. By putting this term in full context, the nurse will gain a better understanding of spirituality in view of (1) the client's relationship with himself (intrapersonal), (2) the client's relationship with others (interpersonal), and (3) the client's relationship with another higher entity greater than himself (transpersonal).

In the first spiritual dimension, the focus is on the individual and how that individual feels about and relates to himself as a human being. This first dimension of a person's spirituality consists of uniquely wrapped inner *core values* and beliefs that provide "meanings" that the individual holds to be true and just. It is through the individual's reflection on these "meanings" that he gains a sense of self and purpose (Thompson, 2007). The nurse is witness to the status of this first dimension in assessing how the client addresses his personal needs and how he cares for "self."

In the second dimension of spirituality, the individual references his core values and uses them as standards to guide his behaviors and relationships with other people. These contacts can be personal in nature (e.g., the client provides attention and respect to others during his conversations with them) or impersonal (e.g., observing how the client chooses to treat property that belongs to someone else). It is the individual alone who decides which standards he will apply in his dealings with other people.

Finally, in the third dimension of spirituality the view is broadened to focus on the relationship between the individual and a greater entity or power (God, Deity, Allah, Mother-Earth, Nature, etc.). Again, tied back to the inner core of the individual's values and beliefs, this third dimension relies strongly on the individual's faith and confidence in self within the context of a "bigger picture" that transcends life on earth as we know it, viewing life purpose in an even larger context (Koenig, 2006).

The Role of Spirituality for Some Older Clients

Even if one chooses to view spiritual development as universal and lifelong, the process remains unique for each individual (Miller, 2009). The interpretation of the "age factor" in the study of religion and spirituality has proven to be difficult for researchers, who cite the need for more longitudinal research studies on the topic (Atchley, 2009; Carson & Koenig, 2008; Dalby, 2006, Koenig, 2006). Although there have been many hypotheses proposed that address religion in later life (Moberg, 2001), there is no evidence to support the common myth that people become more spiritual and/or religious as they age (Dalby, 2006).

It has been suggested, however, that elders may use their existing spirituality differently in old age than they did in their youth (Krause, 2011). The sociological frame using a type of *continuity theory* is one way to help the nurse understand the relationship some elders have with their spirituality and/or religious practices over time (Moberg, 2001). When spirituality of the older client is viewed within a historic context, the nurse needs to consider the amount of time accrued with advancing age, and the role developmental life experiences have on the normal aging process. With this focus, the nurse recognizes that older clients are more likely to have had (a) more life experiences, especially in relation to different types and intensities of loss (Krause, 2011), (b) more time for introspective reflection in efforts to make meaning of those life experiences in relation to life purpose, and (c) that they most likely had an early life experience with religion and/or spiritually during a period of time in our society where the religious spirit of the individual was highly valued, accepted, and expected (Moberg, 2001).

Individuals who have had success utilizing their spirituality to cope with difficult times in the past are apt to attempt to access these *spiritual resources* when confronted with difficulties in their present (Eliopoulos, 2010). Beyond these historic factors, the nurse must understand that the older client's present health/illness status may also influence how the older client implicitly and/or explicitly engages with spirituality. Though older clients are likely to attach profound meanings to their illness states (Atchley, 2009), there is little evidence in the literature to support the myth that elders seek out religious/spiritual supports more often at times of reported loss of control over their health (Koenig, 2006). Even if spiritual resources are not utilized by elders more often during difficult times, Krause (2011) suggests that clients (and their family members) may approach spiritual resources differently as they see the elder move along the *health–illness continuum*—during times of wellness, illness, and at end-of-life.

Demonstrations of Spirituality

Even if the older client has an encouraging support system to assist him in strengthening his spirit, it is the older client alone who determines if, when, and how he may choose to demonstrate his spirituality. As noted earlier, sometimes outward displays of the spirit evolve from the client's affiliation with a specific religion and the practices and rituals associated with that religion (Moberg, 2001). However, it is not uncommon for the nurse to conduct a *spiritual assessment* with an elder who associates with one religious group only to find that the client selectively accepts and adopts only those religious practices that are congruent with his core values. This client may also report spiritual practices from a nonreligious perspective that he feels strengthens his spiritual self. Examples of these vary and can include such things as promoting the holistic self through behaviors aimed at promoting "energy balance" (e.g., yoga, use of crystals), "centeredness" (e.g., deep patterned breathing, meditation), and/or "connectedness to key elements of nature" (e.g., use of nature visualization, spiritual quigong).

Regardless of which (if any) practices the older client uses to express his spirituality, the nurse caring for the client must evaluate each carefully before supporting its use in the client's care plan. In this evaluation, the nurse must consider the client practice in terms of *ethical principles*, legality, and client safety (e.g., the nurse would not support the religious use of peyote by a mentally ill elder with a previous diagnosis of hallucinations, nor would the nurse support the desire of the older client to fast from all foods and fluids if he was already diagnosed with malnutrition and dehydration). However, if a client practice is found to have no scientific evidence indicating that it would harm or put the client at risk for harm, then the nurse must demonstrate spiritual competence in remaining open and nonjudgmental toward including that spiritual practice into the client's plan of care (Miller, 2009).

Spirituality and the Nursing Profession

Not only does the profession of nursing have a strong foundation for spiritual care giving (Taylor, 2002; Beckman, Harges, Sorge, & Salmon, 2007), but the essence of nursing practice also has a strong spiritual component not related to doctrine or dogma (Mauk & Schmidt, 2004). The practice of nursing centers on caring for and caring about the holistic well-being of others. In the infancy of our profession, nurse training was tightly linked to religion, as it was provided by members of a religious group who viewed nursing as a "call to service."

Over the years, the importance of the nurse facilitating a client's *spiritual well-being* has been addressed in the work of many nurse theorists (Nightingale, Henderson, Watson, Neuman, Orem, etc.), as well as many supportive theorists from other disciplines. It has also been suggested that spiritual nursing care is not merely an option, but a responsibility for all nurses (Beckman et al., 2007), with mandates for assessing the client's spirituality noted in both organizational and professional nursing guidelines (health agency/organizational standards, codes and guidelines, professional nursing codes for ethical practice, Joint Commission on Accreditation of Healthcare Standards, nursing care specialty competencies such as those noted in the American Holistic Nurses Association, the Oncology Nursing Society, etc.).

In efforts to maintain a holistic nursing practice and follow mandates to address the spiritual needs of clients, it is essential for the nurse to make time to first assess his or her own personal attitudes, values, and beliefs regarding spirituality. It is only in becoming self-aware of his or her own spirituality that the nurse is able to make a conscious effort to be accepting of other points of view and to work to refrain from the dangers of becoming spiritual-centric in nursing practice. In addition to determining how spirituality is incorporated into practice, it is essential to consider how spirituality can assist in building personal strength and resiliency for both the client and the nurse.

When considering the second dimension of the nurse's spirituality, it is important to recognize that the nurse uses a therapeutic self to enter the intimate world of others (clients). It is after this relationship with the client is established that the nurse provides evidence-informed professional care aimed at meeting client needs. Oftentimes, nursing procedures that are a part of professional nursing practice can themselves create pain and/or sickness for a client. This result can create a spiritual and/or ethical conflict for the nurse as caregiver (e.g., the nurse administers the chemotherapy infusion with the intent to help the client get well, only to see side effects that create initial harm as the client becomes physically ill from the treatment). Unless the nurse is able to personally and professionally resolve such conflicts, the nurse is at risk for a spiritual depletion of his or her own energy (Myers, 2009). For this reason, it is essential that the nurse constantly monitors his or her personal energy level in relation to professional nursing practice, addressing personal concerns for providing client care before they become problems (e.g., professional burnout).

Incorporating Spirituality into the Nursing Process

If the nurse is expected to take an active role in nursing care with older clients, it is essential that he or she assembles accurate, current information and documents all data to present a complete picture of the older client. Although some feel that client spirituality is a personal topic best left for discussions between clients and their chaplains, others report that nurses are in the best position for this conversation with clients at admission and throughout the course of nursing care (O'Brien, 2008).

When nurses employ successful observational and interview techniques with the older client (client-directed communication, developing trust, use of appropriate timing and concern for readiness to share, active listening, providing a comfortable and private setting for discussions, control over resources to maximize vocal and written information in consideration for the normal sensory changes with advancing age, use of valid and reliable assessment tools and documentation formats, etc.) in efforts to obtain client admission information on the status of the body, mind, and spirit, two important messages are relayed to the older client. The first message is that the human spirit is an important part of the client's health, and the second message is that the nurse is available and interested in helping the client work to improve his health status.

Hussey (2009) noted that although spiritual caregiving is individualized, some nursing roles are universal when it comes to caring for older clients (roles of assessor, friend, advocate, caregiver, case manager, and researcher). The nursing role in this process is supported by professional and agency mandates that recognize spirituality as an important component of client care that help to guide best practice for nursing.

Assessment and Nursing Diagnosis

When one considers the dynamic nature of the health–illness continuum (Neuman 1990), it is easy to see that in addition to obtaining the first *spiritual baseline assessment* upon admission, there is an essential need for the nurse to re-assess the spiritual status of the client at various points during the care experience. As with all other categories of client assessment, it is important that a systematic approach be utilized for conducting the spiritual assessment (Miller, 2009). The literature provides a variety of tools for the nurse to use when conducting a spiritual evaluation of the older client (forms based on care competencies, spiritual inventories, and spiritual assessments), noting that there is no one standardized "best" tool to date that can be used for conducting a spiritual assessment (Eliopoulos, 2010). Admission resources for the nurse should include a set of agency-determined tools for screening and history taking, as well as a form to address the next level, which calls for a more detailed and focused spiritual assessment. Information obtained from the spiritual assessment should be placed in the client's record so that a baseline data set for comparison purposes is available whenever a spiritual re-assessment is conducted.

As a part of the assessment process, it is essential for the nurse be alert to any changes in client behavior that may signal spiritual distress, spiritual risk, or the client's need for a more focused spiritual re-assessment (Mauk & Schmidt, 2004). Because of this, on-going evaluation is best accomplished by the nurse who has strong client observational and communication skills. A good knowledge base in these areas helps the nurse become aware of subtle client behaviors that can signal early client difficulties: identifying what the older client does and/or says, as well as what he does not do and/or does not say, over the course of daily nurse–client contacts.

To insure a consistent and speedy referral process, it is to everyone's benefit to have a written agency-supported referral procedure in place before any client spiritual screenings or spiritual assessments begin. If the older client can read and is provided an easy-to-understand, large-print form to complete with the nurse as a part of his spiritual assessment, both client and nurse are more apt to complete the form and begin spiritual dialogue. If a form is given to the client to complete independent of the nurse, it is important for the nurse to verify that it was indeed the older client who supplied the information contained in that form (as some family members complete such forms without the client's knowledge).

First-level spiritual screening questions (see **Box 21-3**) can be those where the client provides a yes/no response to a simple set of five close-ended questions asked by the nursing professional. Following client direction (based on responses to these first level questions), the nurse can choose to conduct a second level screening utilizing five open-ended questions aimed at clarifying or expanding this part of the spiritual intake process (see **Box 21-4**). The client's response to two sets of screening questions will inform the nurse if questions for a spiritual history need

BOX 21-3 Spiritual Screening Tools Level 1

FIVE **FIRST-LEVEL** SPIRITUAL SCREENING QUESTIONS FOR THE NURSE TO ASK THE OLDER CLIENT:

1. "Do you see yourself as a spiritual person at this time?"

2. "Do you have any spiritual/religious behaviors or practices that are important to you at this time?"

3. "Do you associate with a religious or spiritual community or group at this time?"

4. "Does your spirituality play any role in helping you to understand your health or illness condition(s) at this time?"

5. "Is there anything here that you see would get in the way of having your personal spiritual needs met?"

Source: Adapted from Mauk & Schmidt, 2004, p. 213.

BOX 21-4 Spiritual Screening Tools Level 2

FIVE **SECOND-LEVEL** SPIRITUAL SCREENING QUESTIONS FOR THE NURSE TO ASK THE OLDER CLIENT:

1. "One of our jobs to help you while you are here is to keep you comfortable. I am hoping that you can share information about what things are meaningful in your life so I can try to help you access those while you are here with us?"

2. "Life can be difficult at times, and we all cope with our difficulties in different ways. Please tell me what strategies you use to help you to understand and make sense about your current health situation."

3. "If faith is a part of your life, how does your faith fit for you right now?"

4. "Do you feel that your present health situation has created any disturbance in your core values or belief system?"

5. "How are your energy reserves holding up when you consider your health status at the present time?"

Source: Adapted from O'Brien, M. (2008). *Spirituality in Nursing: Standing on Holy Ground.* Sudbury, MA: Jones & Bartlett Learning. p. 111.

to be obtained and/or if a more detailed and focused spiritual assessment needs to be completed for the client's chart.

Data obtained from the spiritual assessment process can be placed in a large-print spiritual continuum form, which will support on-going communication between the nurse and the older client for re-assessments of spiritual status over time (see **Table 21-10**). This continuum form has a quantifiable score card determined by the older client with a range from zero to three. A perceived score of zero represents that the older client either does not identify with spirituality or perceive any spiritual need at that assessment point in time. If a spiritual need is expressed by the older client, the need is identified and reported to the nurse,

TABLE 21-10 Example of Data from Spiritual Assessment

	No Spiritual Need Identified	Identified Spiritual Need	Spiritual Continuum Client Preceived Need Level			
			(low)	(medium)	(high)	
Date	0	**Diagnosis**	1	2	3	**Signature**
		Loss of spiritual integrity				
Narrative:						

SAMPLE SPIRITUAL CONTINUUM ENTRY

	No Spiritual Issues Identified	Identified Spiritual Issue	Client Perceived Spiritual Continuum Level			
			(low)	(medium)	(high)	
Date	0	**Diagnosis**	1	2	3	**Signature**
04/23/12		Loss of spiritual integrity		X		Jane Doe, RN

Narrative:

S. "My doctor said he was very hopeful that the stem cell treatment would help put me in remission. I prayed hard for the last few months that this would buy me a little more time so I can hold on to see my son one more time. Today I found out that there has been no change in my bloodwork levels as I had hoped, and the doctor said there is little more he can do but keep me comfortable. He said that he is confused by my lack of progress. I don't blame him but do feel that God is no longer listening to my prayers... so I will be alone at the end. I have been a faithful and religious person all my life, but this lack of progress is really wearing down my faith."

O. Labwork on 04/23/12 post stem cell treatment shows continued deterioration of client's health state. Physician put client on pallitive list today after talking with him about his active cancer status. Rates physical pain level at 2 (scale 0–10) and spiritual integrity need at 2 (scale 0–3). Refused to see pastor at regularly scheduled visit this afternoon.

A. Client reports loss of spiritual integrity at level 2 during spiritual assessment today.

P. Re-assess client needs when wife arrives during afternooon shift later this evening. Contact hospital chaplain with current spiritual assessment results. Provide active listening with client during dressing change this evening and then reassess for planning using spiritual continuum form.

who works with the client in determining an appropriate nursing diagnosis for its communication to other members of the client's health team (see **Case study 21-1**).

After identification of the spiritual need via the documented nursing diagnosis, the client determines the level of need at that time, using a scale of one to three (one identifying a low spiritual need level, two identifying a medium spiritual need level,

Case Study 21-1

Seventy year old Mr. Hutt has attended the local Presbyterian church regularly since he was 14 years old. He has maintained his spiritual strength through his religious participation over the years, and has worked his way up to "church elder." When admitted he said that one of his proudest accomplishments is that he and his wife raised four sons who actively practice their Presbyterian faith.

When he was admitted post-stroke to the long-term-care (LTC) facility 6 months ago, he noted on his initial spiritual assessment form that "attending Sunday services was most important to him," ranking that as his #1 "personal strength factor." Together, he and his wife have regularly attended Sunday services at the LTC chapel, until a couple of months ago. It was at that time that Mr. Hutt told his wife that she should go to the services alone because he was just too tired, and would rather read his Bible alone in his room at that time.

This Sunday you are assigned to work on Mr. Hutt's LTC wing. You acknowledged Mr. Hutt's wife before she entered the chapel for Sunday service, and she told you Mr. Hutt wanted to stay in his room again today. She said that she has tried everything to get him to join her at Sunday again, but he refuses. When you go in to see Mr. Hutt later in the day, he tells you "I thought we had a merciful God, but He hasn't shown me much mercy in the last couple months. It has been 6 months since my stroke and I expected to be out of here by now. I guess I probably have to do more suffering yet for all the bad things I have done in my lifetime—that is, if he is even listening to my prayers anymore."

Questions:

1. What would be your nursing diagnosis for Mr. Hutt at this time?

2. What signs and symptoms provide the evidence to support your diagnosis?

3. What would be the goal you would identify with Mr. Hutt to improve his present state?

4. What spiritual care intervention options are available for the nurse to assist Mr. Hutt at this time?

5. What other words and/or behaviors would be important for the nurse to be alert to when working with Mr. Hutt?

6. What would be the nurse's response if Mr. Hutt refuses to participate in any activities intended to assist in his spiritual recovery?

7. What nonverbal behaviors by the nurse would communicate a nonjudgmental response to Mr. Hutt's vocal expressions of despair?

8. Should the nurse work to incorporate Mrs. Hutt in activities intended for improving Mr. Hutt's spiritual status? What might be some positive factors for involving her? What might be some negative factors if she were involved?

9. What other contributing factors (besides the slower than expected stroke progress) may be impacting Mr. Hutt's spirituality strength?

or three, which recognizes a high spiritual need level). By reviewing this large-print continuum form with the older client over the course of his stay, the nurse can seek clarification from the client directly as to his status over time, as well as identify any emerging needs that can be addressed early in the process. The goal for the older client who values spirituality is that his spirit will serve as an inner resource to provide hope and faith in times of need while giving an inner serenity and resilience to promote health (Wold, 2012).

It is important to consider putting nursing interventions in place to help support older clients who are "spiritually thriving" at assessment (spiritual continuum score of 0), as well as for those who report they are in spiritual need (spiritual continuum score of 1, 2, or 3). Determining the level of a spiritual need is based upon the client's perception, but would be reflected in the client who reports that he is unable to forgive himself or others for perceived failures. He may also report or demonstrate a low spiritual reserve or a low self-esteem and feelings of being immobilized, apathetic, hopeless, worthless, depressed, or a bother to others: all disturbances that can threaten his meanings of life (Atchley, 2009). Early case finding may result in an "at risk" nursing diagnosis for loosing spiritual integrity, with these older clients expressing guilt, fear, anxiety, or frustration directly related to their spiritual self.

Planning

Once the initial assessment and diagnosis segments of the nursing process are completed, the nurse works with the older client (and a significant other of the elder's choosing if indicated) to begin a plan intended to shift the client towards the "spiritually thriving" category on the spirituality continuum. In addition to providing a list of the older client's strengths and needs at that point, spiritual resource building can serve to empower the older client in decision making if he is able. If it is determined that the older client has limited capacity at this time, a significant other (family member, client advocate, etc.) may assist the nurse in the planning process if the client allows for such.

It is important in this phase of the nursing care plan that spiritual resource banks (activity ideas, support agencies and websites, spirituality tools, "people" contacts, etc.) be identified and individualized. The nurse needs to work with the client (or his representative) on his care planning by incorporating his desired practices as long as there is evidence to support that these would not put the client at a health risk. In addition to incorporating this written plan as a part of the client's formal record, providing start and re-evaluation dates next to each activity and linking each with the name of the responsible planning team member will foster good communication among all those who have a vested interest in the health of the older client.

Nursing Interventions

Nursing interventions are as unique as the individuals receiving and providing them (Carson & Koenig, 2008). In the planning process, the client may report his desire to use environmental supports (e.g., time out of the facility to sit outside in nature) to strengthen his inner spiritual core. With the guidance of the older client (or his planning representative), nurse interventions could include a variety of activities to assist the client to gain a better sense of himself in this first dimension of spirituality (use of music, sounds of nature, journaling, aroma therapy, painting, deep breathing exercises, hygiene care, visit from a barber or hair dresser, quiet time, pictures or symbols that have spiritual meaning for the older client, prayer, animal therapy, meditation, humor therapy, guided imagery exercises, deep breathing activities, exercise therapy, etc.).

To focus on the second dimension of spirituality (relationship with others), the nurse may wish to consider interventions that include scheduling visits with the older client's family and friends in ways that would strengthen energy levels. If there are few or no visitors for the older client, with client approval the nurse can make a referral to a volunteer or friendly visitor program. If the client is able, the nurse may suggest that the older client considers participation in group activities where clients are able to share their feelings with others in similar life situations (common, shared practices as a part of spiritual caregiving). In addition, the nurse may choose to provide a personal spiritual care strategy by scheduling a 10-minute visit with the older client where the nurse could utilize therapeutic communication skills (e.g. active listening, nonverbal tools of appropriate touch, and silence) to support a "connectedness" that can help to provide feelings of worth and value for the withdrawn or isolated elder (Ebersole et al., 2007).

Efforts to strengthen the third dimension of spirituality for the older client start with the nurse's demonstrated respect for the client, his values, his beliefs, and his privacy. Nursing interventions to support this dimension can be achieved by gaining contact (through nurse referrals) with the client's preferred spiritual advisor/coach if one is identified. This procedural example of spiritual care by the nurse refers out the patient contact, but keeps the nurse actively involved through support of such visits by scheduling daily routines. The nurse can help to maintain these contacts through indirect involvement with mailings, television, telephone, radio or emailing services.

The nurse can also suggest some supplemental options via referrals to a social worker, parish nurse, activity director, or pastoral care service group at the client's agency of choice. This culturalistic type of nursing intervention incorporates what the nurse knows of the client's spiritual history, taking client direction and finding adaptations for the environment or an activity to fit the client situation (e.g., arranging for a client's re-activation into prayer contacts/groups, arranging wheelchair tai chi sessions for a man who no longer can attend his stand up tai-chi program, etc.). This type of spiritual nursing care can provide a renewed spiritual energy for the older client, providing greater reflection of him in a larger life context (Koenig, 2006).

Evaluation

Evaluation is the nursing action that sets the stage for on-going reassessment (formative evaluation) through a review of both goal achievement and the client plan of care (Mauk & Schmidt, 2004). As with all interventions aimed at strengthening the mind, body, or spirit of the older client, it is important for the nurse to work closely with the client to monitor the impact of the intervention strategies employed. This process requires a focus on both the desired outcomes (summative evaluation) from the plan as well as the unexpected outcomes that occurred with the process. By incorporating the use of the spiritual continuum grid as a part of the on-going evaluation process, the client and nurse can share a visual display of spiritual progress or regression over time. Including the older client (or his representative) as a member of the planning team reinforces client empowerment in selected care decisions, which in itself can work to strengthen the older client's spiritual core (Moberg, 2001).

Summary

If the nurse is to practice in a holistic way with older clients, it is important to recognize that a complete client picture must be obtained through the careful utilization of nursing assessments. Although culture (see **Box 21-5**) and spirituality have different meanings for members in our society, it is reflective of the individual client's core values and beliefs, and therefore can play an important role in health and healthcare decision making for our healthcare clients. For this reason, the professional nurse must recognize the value of conducting cultural assessments, spiritual screening, spiritual health histories, and focused spiritual assessments for all clients in the nurse's care, identifying spiritual strengths and planning with the client to meet any spiritual needs that impact health **Boxes 21-6 to 21-8** provide additional resources for nurses seeking to incorporate cultural and spiritual awareness into their practice.

BOX 21-5   Cultural Research Highlight

Aim: The goal of the study was to provide insight into the cultural beliefs and ways of people, thus providing the knowledge needed to design and implement culturally congruent nursing care.

Method: Underpinned by Dr. Madeleine Leininger's Theory of Culture Care Diversity and Universality, as well as the ethnonursing method, 8 key elderly informants and 16 general informants participated in the study through detailed interviews.

Findings: This study uncovered many botanical practices and multiple themes including (1) defining health as getting up and going about your business and illness as the inability to go on; (2) staying well by caring about self and doing right; (3) recalling past times of need, healing with what nature provided, and making do; (4) caring

and healing in modern times still involved roots, herbs, and plants of a bygone era; (5) caring and healing from God as the answer to everything; (6) caring and healing from the hands of women—woman as healer; and (7) preserving the old ways of caring and healing: the treasure of the past.

Application to practice: Gerontological nurses can use the field of ethnonursing to enlighten and inform their practice. Each culture may have subcultures in various geographic areas that have their own unique needs and practices.

Source: Gunn, J. & Davis, S. (2011) Beliefs, meanings, and practices of healing with botanicals recalled by elder African American women in the Mississippi Delta. *Online Journal of Cultural Competence in Nursing and Healthcare, 1*(1), 37–49

BOX 21-6   Recommended Readings

Artifacts of Cultural Change Tool:

http://paculturechangecoalition.org/Resources/Articles/Cms%20-%20Culture%20Change%20Artifact%20Tool%20Explanation.Pdf

Stages of Change:

http://www.context.org/iclib/ic09/gilman1/

Culture of Medicine:
Taylor, J. S. (2003). Confronting "Culture" in Medicine's "Culture of No Culture. *Academic Medicine, 78*(6), 555–559. Retrieved from

http://journals.lww.com/academicmedicine/

Fulltext/2003/06000/Confronting__Culture__in_Medicine_s__Culture_of_No.3.aspx

Stuart, B., Cherry. C., & Stuart, J. (2011). *Pocket guide to culturally sensitive health care*. Philadelphia, PA: FA Davis.

Yeo, G. (2000). Ethnogeriatrics: Overview, Introduction. In V. S. Periyakoil (Ed.), *eCampus-Geriatrics* [online], Stanford, CA. Retrieved from

http://geriatrics.stanford.edu/culturemed/overview/introduction/

BOX 21-7   Aging Elders Specific Cultural Websites

- National Asian Pacific Center on Aging:
  http://www.napca.org/
- National Caucus and Center on Black Aged:
  http://www.ncba-aged.org/
- National Center for Native Hawaiian Elders:
  http://manoa.hawaii.edu/hakupuna/

- National Hispanic Council on Aging:
  http://www.nhcoa.org/
- National Indian Council on Aging and Alaska Native Elders:
  http://nicoa.org/

BOX 21-8   Websites

Care Transitions:

http://www.caretransitions.org/definitions.asp

Center for Minority Veterans:

http://www.va.gov/centerforminorityveterans

Center for Spirituality and Aging:

http://www.spiritualityandaging.org

Cultural Competence Project:

http://www.cultural-competence-project.org/en/index.html

Culturally Competent Nursing Care:
A Cornerstone for Caring:

https://ccnm.thinkculturalhealth.hhs.gov/

Developing Nurses Cultural Competencies,
Train-the-Trainer program:

www.cultural-competence-project.org

DiversityRX:

www.diversityrx.org

John Hartford Institute for Geriatric Nursing
Assessment of Spirituality in Older Adults: FICA
Spiritual History Tool:

http://consultgerirn.org/uploads/File/trythis/try_this_sp5.pdf

Standards for Accreditation Programs (n.d.).
Spiritual assessment:

http://www.jointcommission.org/AccreditationPrograms/HomeCare/Standards

Madeleine Leininger, Transcultural nursing
and leader in transcultural nursing education,

administration, and practice:

http://www.madeleine-leininger.com/en/index.shtml

Medical Anthropology:

http://www.medanthro.net

Network of Multicultural Aging:

http://www.asaging.org/noma/

Online Journal of Cultural Competence:

http://www.cultural-competence-project.org/ojccnh/2(1).shtml

Quality Improvement in our Nation's Nursing
Homes:

http://www.cms.gov/Medicare/Provider-Enrollment-and-Certification/CertificationandComplianc/Downloads/2012-Nursing-Home-Action-Plan.pdf

Registry for Interpreters of the Deaf:

http://www.rid.org/aboutRID/overview/index.cfm

Stanford School of Medicine, ecampus Geriatrics,
Health and Healthcare of Multi-Cultural Older Adults:

http://geriatrics.stanford.edu/ethnomed/

National Adult Protective Services Association:

www.ncea.aoa.gov/ncearoot/Main_Site/pdf/021406_60PLUS_REPORT.pdf

Transcultural Care Associates:

http://www.transculturalcare.net/

Transcultural Nursing Society:

http://www.tcns.org

Critical Thinking Exercises

1. Explore one of the common cultural groups served in your area. Discuss your findings with another student nurse in your clinical groups. How is this culture different than your own?

2. Interview YOUR family. What is your family background, nationality, and religion? How does your family's heritage affect health practices for health maintenance, health protection, and health restoration? What year did your family first come to America? Share with the class.

3. Utilizing the Transcultural Nursing Society's Standards of Practice for Culturally Competent Nursing Care – Standard 3, do one of the following:

   a. Generate and/or provide staff education modules on the general principles of culturally competent care.

   b. Generate and/or provide staff education modules focusing on increasing specific knowledge of the most common cultural groups served.

   c. As a group of student nurses on a clinical unit or in a clinical agency, establish journal clubs/staff in-service sessions to review current literature about the most common cultural groups served to ensure evidence based practice.

   d. As a group of student nurses on a clinical unit or in a clinical agency, generate monthly cultural awareness activities for you and your colleagues that promote cultural competence (i.e., culturally diverse speakers, media, ethnic food).

   e. As a student nurse working with colleagues and a science librarian (if available), gain information literacy skills in order to access electronic sources to gain current knowledge of cultures and cultural assessment tools (diversity websites, cross cultural health care case studies) as well as multimedia sources and professional webinars.

Personal Reflections

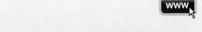

1. What role does spirituality play in your life?

2. It is important that nurses assess spirituality for themselves before they can be successful assessing this domain with their clients. Think about your answers to each of the following questions:

   • How would I describe my spirituality?

   • How would I describe the dynamic interaction of my physical, social, mental, and spiritual selves?

   • What formal and informal organizations have helped me to develop my spirituality over time?

   • What factors have contributed to my "spiritual" status today?

   • How much do I value my own spirituality?

   • How much do I value the spirtuality of others?

   • How comfortable am I speaking about the topic of spirituality with others? What resources can I use to assist in helping me discuss spirituality with others?

   • What role does my spiritual self play in my professional practice of nursing?

   • What behaviors do I utilize to strengthen my spiritual reserve?

- What tools do I utilize to measure my spiritual strength?

3. As the nurse, what would you do or say to the following older adult clients? On what factors do you base your response?

    1. Client asks to hold your hand and pray aloud with him before he goes down for surgery.

    2. Client's nutritionist from home provides a smelly bark tea for the client to drink each evening in the hospital. The tea was approved by the client's physician; however, storage is a problem because of its bad smell in the kitchen on the floor.

    3. Native American client asks if he can have his traditional healer "smudge" his patient room. Because smudging involves burning sage, cedar, and other herbs in the room, you are unsure if this can be done in the hospital setting.

    4. Catholic client asks to keep his rosary pinned to his hospital gown while on the floor.

    5. Client asks to switch bed positions in the two-patient room so that he can face east instead of staying in his assigned bed that faces west.

    6. The client is due for gallstone removal and asks if she can keep the gallstones that are retrieved from her surgery to make a set of "worry beads" to help in her meditation practice.

References

Anderson, M. (2007). *Caring for older adults holistically* (4th ed.). Philadelphia, PA: F.A. Davis.

Atchley, R. (2009). *Spirituality and aging*. Baltimore, MD: The John Hopkins Press.

Beckman, S., Harges, S., Sorge, C., & Salmon, B. (2007). Five strategies that heighten nurses' awareness of spirituality to impact client care. *Holistic Nursing Practice, 21*(3), 135–139.

Calvillo E., Clark, L., Ballantyne, J. E., Pacquiao, D., Purnell, L. D., & Villarruel, A. M. (2009). Cultural competency in baccalaureate nursing education. *Journal of Transcultural Nursing, 20*(2), 137–145.

Carson, V. & Koenig, H. (Eds.). (2008). *Spiritual dimensions of nursing practice*. Conshohocken, PA: Templeton Foundation Press.

Centers for Disease Control and Prevention. (2011). CDC Health Disparities and Inequalities Report, United States, 2011. Retrieved from http://www.cdc.gov/mmwr/pdf/other/su6001.pdf.

Cherry, B., & Giger, J. N. (2004). African-Americans. In J. N. Giger & R. E. Davidhizar (Eds.), *Transcultural nursing assessment and intervention* (4th ed., pp. 177–219). St. Louis, MO: Mosby.

Crespo, C. J., & Aresman, J. (2003). Obesity in the United States: A worrisome epidemic. *Physician and Sports Medicine, 31*(11), 23–28.

Dalby, P. (2006). Is there a process of spiritual change or development associated with aging: A critical review of the research. *Aging & Mental Health, 10*(1), 4–12.

Ebersole, P., Touchy, T., Hess, P., & Jett, K. (2007). *Toward healthy aging: Human needs and nursing response* (7th ed.). St. Louis, MO: Mosby.

ElGindy, G. (2004, Fall). We are what we eat: Cultural competence and dietary needs. *Minority Nurse*, 54–55.

Eliopoulos, C. (2010). Spirituality. In *C. Eliouploulos' Gerontological Nursing* (7th ed., pp. 150–158). Philadelphia, PA: Lippincott-Raven.

Eschiti, V. S. (2005). Cardiovascular disease research in Native Americans. *Journal of Cardiovascular Nursing, 20*(3), 155–161.

Giger, J. N. & Davidhizar, R. E. (2004). Transcultural Nursing Assessment and Intervention (4th ed.). St. Louis: MO.

Giger, J., Davidhizar, R. E., Purnell, L., Harden, J. T., Phillips, J., & Strickland, O. (2007). American Academy of Nursing expert panel report: Developing cultural competence to eliminate disparities in ethnic minorities and other vulnerable populations. *Journal of Transcultural Nursing, 17,* 95–102.

Gonzalez, T., & Kuipers, J. (2004). Hispanic-Americans. In J. N. Giger & R. E. Davidhizar (Eds.), *Transcultural nursing assessment and intervention* (4th ed., pp. 221–253). St. Louis, MO: Mosby.

Hanley, C. (2004). Navajos. In J. N. Giger & R. E. Davidhizar (Eds.), *Transcultural nursing assessment and intervention* (4th ed., pp. 255–277). St. Louis, MO: Mosby.

Healthy People 2020. (2012). About Healthy People 2020. Retrieved from http://healthypeople.gov/2020/

Hostler, S. L. (1999). Pediatric family-centered rehabilitation. *Journal of Head Trauma Rehabilitation, 14,* 384–351.

Hsiung, Y. & Ferrans, C. (2007). Recognizing Chinese Americans cultural needs in making end-of-life treatment decisions. *Journal of Hospice and Palliative Nursing,* 9(3),132–140.

Hussey, T. (2009). Nursing and spirituality. *Nursing Philosophy, 10,* 71–80.

Institute of Medicine [IOM]. (2003). *Health professions education: A bridge to quality.* Washington, DC: National Academies Press. Retrieved from http://www.iom.edu/Reports/2003/Health-Professions-Education-A-Bridge-to-Quality.aspx

Kelley, L. S., Small, C. C., & Tripp-Reimer, T. (2004). Appalachians. In J. N. Giger & R. E. Davidhizar (Eds.), *Transcultural nursing assessment and intervention* (4th ed., pp. 279–299). St. Louis, MO: Mosby.

Keppel, K. G. (2007). Ten largest racial and ethnic health disparities in the United States based on Healthy People 2010 objectives. *American Journal of Epidemiology, 166,* 97–103.

Kim, J., Ashing-Giwa, K. T., Singer, M. K., & Tejero, J. S. (2006). Breast cancer among Asian-Americans: Is acculturation related to health-related quality of life? *Oncology Nursing Forum, 33,* 1071.

Kleinman, A., Eisenberg, L., & Good, B. (1978). Culture, illness and care. *Annals of Internal Medicine, 88,* 251–258.

Koenig, H. (2006). Religion, spirituality and aging. *Aging and Mental Health, 10*(1), 1–3.

Krause, N. (2011). Age stereotypes. In K. W. Schaie & S. L. Willis (Eds.), *Handbook of the psychology of aging* (7th ed., pp. 249–262). San Diego, CA: Elsevier.

Kaufman, J. (2002). Looking at the past and the future of diversity and aging: An interview with E. Percil Stanford and Fernando Torres-Gil. *Generations, 26*(3), 74–78.

Lee-Lin, F., & Menon, U. (2005). Breast and cervical cancer screening practices and interventions among Chinese, Japanese, and Vietnamese Americans. *Oncology Nursing Forum, 32,* 995–1003.

Leininger, M. (1997). Overview and reflection of the theory of culture care and the ethnonursing research method. *Journal of Transcultural Nursing, 8,* 32–52.

Loeb, S. J. (2006). African-American older adults coping with chronic health conditions. *Journal of Transcultural Nursing, 17,* 139–147.

Mauk, K. & Schmidt, N. (2004). *Spiritual care in nursing practice.* Philadelphia, PA: Lippincott, Williams, & Wilkins.

McBride, M. (2006). *Ethnogeriatrics and cultural competence for nursing practice.* Retrieved from http://consultgerirn.org/topics/ethnogeriatrics_and_cultural_competence_for_nursing_practice/want_to_know_more

Miller, C. (2009). *Nursing for wellness in older adults* (5th ed.). Philadelphia, PA: Lippincott Williams & Wilkins.

Miller, R. I., & Clements, P. T. (2006). Fresh tears over old griefs: Expanding the forensic nursing research agenda with Native American elders. *Journal of Forensic Nursing, 2,* 147–153.

Moberg, D. (Ed.). (2001). *Aging and spirituality: Spiritual dimensions of aging theory, research, practice and policy.* New York, NY: Haworth Pastoral Press.

Moody-Ayers, S. Y., Stewart, A. L., Covinsky, K. E., & Inouye, S. K. (2005). Prevalence and correlates of perceived societal racism in older African-American adults with type 2 diabetes mellitus. *Journal of the American Geriatrics Society, 53,* 2202–2208.

Mutchler, J. E., & Brailler, S. (1999). English language proficiency among older adults in the United States. *The Gerontologist, 39*(3), 310–319.

Myers, J. (2009). Spiritual calling. *Nursing Standard, 23*(40), 22.

National Center for Health Statistics. (2012). *Health, United States 2011: With special feature on socio-economic status and health.* Hyattsville, MD: Centers for Disease control and Prevention. Retrieved from http://www.cdc.gov/nchs/data/hus/hus11.pdf#024

Nelson-Becker, H. (2005). Religion and coping in older adults: A social work perspective. *Journal of Gerontological Social Work, 45*(1/2), 51–67.

Neuman, B. (1990). Health as a continuum based on the Neuman Systems Model. *Nursing Science Quarterly, 3,* 129.

Njoku, M. G. C., Jason, L. A., & Torres-Harding, S. R. (2005). The relationships among coping styles and fatigue in an ethnically diverse sample. *Ethnicity and Health, 10*(4), 263–278.

O'Brien, M. (2008). *Spirituality in nursing: Standing on holy ground* (3rd ed.). Sudbury, MA: Jones & Bartlett.

Online Journal of Cultural Competence in Nursing. (2012). *Cultural competence project.* Retrieved from http://www.ojccnh.org/project/about.shtml

Padilla, Y. C., & Villalobos, G. (2007). Cultural responses to health among Hispanic American women and their families. *Family and Community Health, 30*(18), S24–S33.

Pandya, C., Batalova, J., & McHugh, M. (2011). *Limiting English proficient individuals in the United States: Number, share, growth, and linguistic diversity.* Washington, DC: Migration Policy Institute. Retrieved from www.migrationinformation.org/integration/LEPdatabrief.pdf

Passel, J. S., & Cohn, D. (2008). *U.S. population projections 2005–2050.* Pew Research Center. Retrieved from http://pewhispanic.org/files/reports/85.pdf

SCAN Health Plan. (2012). D-I-V-E-R-S-E—A mnemonic for patient encounters. Retrieved from http://www.scanhealthplan.com/provider-tools/benefits-resources/multi-cultural-resources/communication/diverse/?

Spector, R. (2009). *Cultural diversity in health and illness* (7th ed.). Upper Saddle River, NJ: Prentice Hall.

Suen, L.-J. W., & Morris, D. L. (2006). Depression and gender differences: Focus on Taiwanese-American older adults. *Journal of Gerontological Nursing, 34*(4), 28–36.

Supple, A. J., & Small, S. A. (2006). The influence of parental support, knowledge, and authoritative parenting on Hmong and European American adolescent development. *Journal of Family Issues, 27*(9), 1214–1232.

Taylor, E. (2002). *Spiritual care: Nursing theory, research and practice.* Upper Saddle River, NJ: Prentice Hall.

Thompson, S. (2007). Spirituality and old age. *Illness, Crisis, & Loss, 15*(2), 167–178.

Transcultural Nursing Society. (2011). Standards of Practice. Retrieved from http://www.tcns.org/TCNStandardsofPractice.html

Transcultural Nursing Society. (2013). Transcultural Nursing. Retrieved from http://www.tcns.org

United States Department of Homeland Security. (2011). *Yearbook of immigration statistics: 2011.* Retrieved from http://www.dhs.gov/files/statistics/publications/LPR11.shtm

Wallace M. W. J., Pekmezaris R. et al. (2007). "Physician Cultural Sensitivity in African American Advance Planning: A Pilot Study." *Journal of Palliative Care, 10*(3), 721–727.

Walker, R. L., Lester, D., & Joe, S. (2006). Lay theories of suicide: An examination of culturally relevant suicide beliefs and attributions among African Americans and European Americans. *Journal of Black Psychology, 32*(3), 320–334.

Whittemore, R. (2007). Culturally competent interventions for Hispanic adults with type 2 diabetes: A systematic review. *Journal of Transcultural Nursing, 18,* 157–166.

Wold, G. (2012). *Basic geriatric nursing* (5th ed.). St. Louis, MO: Mosby.

Xu, Y., & Chang, K. (2004). Chinese Americans. In J. N. Giger & R. E. Davidhizar (Eds.), *Transcultural nursing assessment and intervention* (4th ed., pp. 407–427). St. Louis, MO: Mosby.

Xu, J. Q, Kochanek, K. D., Murphy, S. L., & Tejada-Vera B. (2010). Deaths: Final data for 2007. National vital statistics reports; vol 58 no 19. Hyattsville, MD: National Center for Health Statistics. Yeo, G. (2000). Ethnogeriatrics: Overview, Introduction. In V. S. Periyakoil (Ed.), *eCampus-Geriatrics* [online], Stanford, CA. Retrieved from http://geriatrics.stanford.edu/culturemed/overview/introduction/

Appendix A

Baha'i

Abortion	Forbidden
Artificial insemination	No specific dictate
Autopsy	Acceptable if medical or legal need
Birth control	Individual can choose best family planning method
Blood and blood products	No restrictions
Diet	Alcohol and drugs forbidden
Euthanasia	Destruction of life not allowed
Healing beliefs	Harmony between religion and science
Healing practices	Pray
Medications	No vaccine restrictions; medications acceptable with prescriptions
Organ donations	No restrictions
Right-to-die issues	Forbidden
Surgical procedures	No restrictions
Visitors	Community members assist and support

Buddhist Churches of America

Abortion	Dependent on condition of patient
Artificial insemination	Acceptable
Autopsy	Individual choice
Birth control	Individual choice
Blood and blood products	Acceptable
Diet	Restricted food combinations
Euthanasia	Allowed
Healing beliefs	Do not believe in healing through faith
Healing practices	No restrictions
Medications	No vaccine or any medication restrictions
Organ donations	Considered act of mercy; all means can be taken if hope for recovery
Right-to-die issues	With hope, all means encouraged
Surgical procedures	Acceptable except for extremes
Visitors	Family and community assist and support

Roman Catholics

Abortion	Prohibited
Artificial insemination	Illicit, even between husband and wife

Autopsy	Permissible
Birth control	Natural rhythm method is only option acceptable
Blood and blood products	Permissible
Diet	No restrictions except during Lenten season before Easter (holy week fast and abstain from meat)
Euthanasia	Direct life-ending procedures prohibited
Healing beliefs	Many within religious belief system
Healing practices	Sacrament and anointing of the sick/dying, use of candles and religious articles, laying of hands
Medications	No vaccine restrictions; medications may be taken if benefit outweighs risks
Organ donations	Acceptable
Right-to-die issues	Obligation to take ordinary (but not extraordinary) means to prolong life
Surgical procedures	Acceptable except for abortion and sterilization
Visitors	Family, friends, priest, deacons, lay ministers assist and support
Christian Science	
Abortion	Incompatible with faith
Artificial insemination	Unusual
Autopsy	Unusual but family can decide to do so
Birth control	Individual choice
Blood and blood products	Ordinarily not used
Diet	Generally no restrictions except abstain from alcohol and tobacco and some abstain from tea and coffee
Euthanasia	Forbidden
Healing beliefs	Looks at physical and moral healing
Healing practices	Full-time healing ministers, active practice of spiritual healing
Medications	No vaccine restrictions that comply with laws; no medication restrictions
Organ donations	Individual choice
Right-to-die issues	Unlikely to seek medical help to prolong life
Surgical procedures	No medical ones practiced
Visitors	Family, friends, Christian Science community and healers, Christian Science nurses assist and support
Church of Jesus Christ of Latter Day Saints	
Abortion	Forbidden
Artificial insemination	Acceptable between husband and wife

(continues)

Appendix A   (*continued*)

Church of Jesus Christ of Latter Day Saints

Autopsy	Permitted with consent by next of kin
Birth control	Forbidden
Blood and blood products	No restrictions
Diet	Alcohol, tea (except herbal), coffee, and tobacco are forbidden; fasting (24 hours without food or drink) is required once a month
Euthanasia	Forbidden
Healing beliefs	Power of God can bring healing
Healing practices	Anointing with oils, sealing, prayer, and laying-on of hands
Medications	No restrictions for vaccines, prescribed medications, or folk medicine use
Organ donations	Permitted
Right-to-die issues	If death is inevitable, promote a peaceful and dignified death
Surgical procedures	Individual choice
Visitors	Family, friends, Church members (especially Elder & Sister), and the Relief Society assist and support

Hinduism

Abortion	No policy
Artificial insemination	No restrictions
Autopsy	Acceptable
Birth control	All types are acceptable
Blood and blood products	Acceptable
Diet	Eating of meat is forbidden
Euthanasia	Forbidden
Healing beliefs	Some believe in faith healing
Healing practices	Traditional faith healing system
Medications	Vaccines and all medication uses are acceptable
Organ donations	Acceptable
Right-to-die issues	No restrictions as death is viewed as one step toward nirvana
Surgical procedures	With an amputation, view is that this happened due to sins from an earlier life
Visitors	Family, friends, and priest assist and support

Islam

Abortion	Acceptable
Artificial insemination	Permitted between husband and wife

Autopsy	Permitted for medical and legal purposes
Birth control	Acceptable
Blood and blood products	No restrictions
Diet	Alcohol and pork prohibited
Euthanasia	Forbidden
Healing beliefs	Faith healing is generally not acceptable
Healing practices	Some use herbal remedies and faith healing
Medications	Vaccines and all prescribed and folk medicines are acceptable
Organ donations	Acceptable
Right-to-die issues	Attempts to shorten life is prohibited
Surgical procedures	Most permitted
Visitors	Family and friends assist and support
Jehovah's Witnesses	
Abortion	Forbidden
Artificial insemination	Forbidden
Autopsy	Acceptable if required by law
Birth control	Sterilization forbidden but all other methods are of the individual's choice
Blood and blood products	Forbidden
Diet	Abstain from tobacco; moderate use of alcohol accepted
Euthanasia	Forbidden
Healing beliefs	Faith healing is forbidden
Healing practices	Use of scriptures to comfort and lead to spiritual and mental healing
Medications	Vaccines and all other medications not derived from blood products are accepted
Organ donations	Forbidden
Right-to-die issues	Individual choice
Surgical procedures	Not opposed but administration of blood strictly prohibited
Visitors	Family and friends assist and support; congregation members and Elders pray for the sick person
Judaism	
Abortion	Therapeutic permitted by all groups; some groups accept abortion on demand
Artificial insemination	Permitted
Autopsy	Permitted under certain circumstances; all body parts must be buried together
Birth control	Permitted for all groups except Orthodox Jews

(*continues*)

Appendix A (*continued*)

Judaism

Blood and blood products	Acceptable
Diet	Variability among groups, when kosher rules followed, milk and meat products cannot be mixed or served on the same plates; predatory fowl and shellfish, as well as all pork products, are forbidden; many will request only kosher products
Euthanasia	Prohibited
Healing beliefs	Medical care is an expectation
Healing practices	Prayers for the sick
Medications	Vaccines and all medications are accepted
Organ donations	Complex issue; some groups do accept this based on situation
Right-to-die issues	Right to die with dignity; if death inevitable, no new procedures but continue with present ones
Surgical procedures	Most allowed
Visitors	Family, friends, rabbi, and many community members and services to assist and support

Mennonite

Abortion	Therapeutic is acceptable
Artificial insemination	Individual conscience for husband and wife
Autopsy	Acceptable
Birth control	Acceptable
Blood and blood products	Acceptable
Diet	No restrictions
Euthanasia	Not condoned
Healing beliefs	Part of God's work
Healing practices	Prayers and anointing with oils
Medications	Vaccines and all other medications allowed
Organ donations	No restrictions
Right-to-die issues	Forbidden as "life must continue at all costs"
Surgical procedures	No restrictions
Visitors	Family, friends, and community assist and support

Seventh-day Adventists

Abortion	Therapeutic is acceptable
Artificial insemination	Acceptable between husband and wife
Autopsy	Acceptable

Mennonite

Birth control	Individual choice
Blood and blood products	No restrictions
Diet	Vegetarian diet is encouraged
Euthanasia	Not practiced
Healing beliefs	Divine healing
Healing practices	Prayers and anointing with oils; opposes use of hypnotism
Medications	Vaccines and all medications are acceptable
Organ donations	Acceptable
Right-to-die issues	Follow the ethic of prolonging life
Surgical procedures	No restrictions
Visitors	Pastor and elders pray and anoint the sick person; because there is a SDA world-wide health system of both hospitals and clinics, some clients will seek care only from these facilities

Unitarian/Universalist Church

Abortion	Acceptable
Artificial insemination	Acceptable
Autopsy	Recommended
Birth control	Acceptable
Blood and blood products	No restrictions
Diet	No restrictions
Euthanasia	Favor nonaction; acceptable to withdraw treatment if death imminent
Healing beliefs	Sees faith healing as superstitious
Healing practices	Use of science to facilitate healing
Medications	No restrictions
Organ donations	Acceptable
Right-to-die issues	Favor the right to die with dignity
Surgical procedures	No restrictions
Visitors	Family, friends, and church members assist and support

Source: Adapted from Spector, R. (2009). Selected religion responses to health events. In Cultural diversity in health and illness (7th ed., pp. 120–125). Upper Saddle River, NJ: Prentice Hall.

For a full suite of assignments and additional learning activities, see the access code at the front of your book.

LEARNING OBJECTIVES

At the end of this chapter, the reader will be able to:

> Discuss the sexual development of older adults and changes in the sexual response due to aging and chronic illness.
> Identify strategies to overcome vaginal dryness and erectile dysfunction.
> Implement appropriate policies that promote intimacy in community and long-term care settings.
> List strategies to extinguish sexually inappropriate behavior.

KEY TERMS

Dyspareunia
Erectile dysfunction (ED)
Sexual intimacy

Sexuality
Triphasic model of human
    sexual response

Sexuality

Donald D. Kautz
LaShonda Barnett

Enhancing Sexual Intimacy

This chapter addresses sexual issues in providing holistic nursing care for older adults. A basic human need of people of all ages is intimacy with others. Loneliness, loss, and lack of meaningful social relationships have been addressed in other chapters in this text. This chapter is designed to assist the nurse in enhancing romantic intimacy and sexual function in older adults. Those over 50 are a very diverse group, and when it comes to romantic intimacy and sexual expression, they are probably more diverse than any other age group.

Despite decades of research showing that older adults want to discuss intimacy and sexual concerns (Alterovitz & Mendelsohn, 2009; Elias & Ryan, 2011), these needs continue to be ignored by healthcare professionals, for several reasons. Sex is not seen as a priority for either the patient or the provider, and sexual concerns have not traditionally been addressed in health care encounters. As nurses, we do not see any consequences to not addressing sexual concerns. The problem is that *sexuality* is seen as separate from healthcare concerns, rather than integral to quality of life. Anxiety and fear of embarrassment prevent both patients and nurses from bringing up sexual concerns. Further, we fear that we may not have the resources to assist patients to overcome sexual problems.

Most sexual concerns that result from aging or chronic health problems are within the realm of nursing practice (Heath, 2011; Kaplan, 2011; Wallace, 2012). Yet instead of helping, we may contribute to sexual dysfunction by ignoring the underlying health problems that lead to sexual problems. For example, urge or stress incontinence in women may lead to vaginal infections and *dyspareunia*, or painful intercourse; in addition, the woman or her partner may be turned off by the smell. Yet hospital nurses rarely ask about this type of incontinence when a patient is admitted. Acute respiratory infections, abdominal surgery, and mobility limitations following surgery may all lead to temporary urge or stress incontinence, but nurses do not routinely warn patients about this possibility, or treat or refer those with problems. For example, sending a patient home with an indwelling Foley catheter will certainly interfere with sexual intercourse. Teaching a woman to tape the catheter up on her abdomen and wear some type of t-shirt to prevent the catheter from rubbing during intercourse, or to wear a crotchless teddy or crotchless panties, will keep the catheter out of the way; men can fold the catheter back over an erect penis, and then put on a condom. Partners report not being able to feel the catheter during intercourse, and ejaculation will occur unimpeded around the catheter. Both of these techniques have been recommended for decades, and they are not thought to increase the chances of urinary tract infection (Cournan, 2012), but nurses regularly fail to teach clients who are discharged with catheters these effective and safe techniques.

We also miss many opportunities to assist our clients in overcoming problems. Most health promotion strategies have the potential to make a positive impact on sexual relationships and sexual function. Quitting smoking, limiting fat in the diet, losing weight, and exercising all may reverse the sexual changes that occur due to aging. If our patients realized that heightened intimacy and regained sexual function may result from these lifestyle changes, they may be more motivated to make the changes.

Sexuality and Quality of Life

In 2004, AARP conducted a survey with 1,682 respondents, whose average age was 61 years. The majority of participants were non-Hispanic whites. AARP (2005) found that sexuality was an essential part of the life of those 45 or older. Approximately two-thirds of the participants were married or living with a partner, and most had been with their partner for over 10 years. Approximately one-third reported sexual intercourse once a week or more often. Robinson and Molzahn (2007) found that satisfaction with personal relationships, health status, and sexual activity strongly contributed to quality of life in a sample of 426 older adults, regardless of gender, marital status, and education. These studies add to the evidence that intimacy and sexuality are important regardless of age.

Romantic Relationships in the Elderly

Elders differ greatly in their romantic relationships. Some older adults have been in the same romantic relationship for 50 years and have developed a profoundly deep relationship. (See **Box 22-1** in which Tim, an 81-year-old man, and Teresa, a 79-year-old woman, discuss how they feel about their 50-year relationship.)

Some people become involved in a romantic relationship for the first time after retiring. Alterovitz and Mendelsohn's (2009) study of Internet personal ads found that many over the age of 60 years, even those over 75 years, were seeking partners. Some older adults have been married many times; others not at all. Some have had

BOX 22-1   Tim and Teresa

Tim (81): "I think she feels about me just about the same way I feel about her. I'm sure I come first in her life and I'm sure she's first in my life. It's always been that way. She was the girl that I wanted. I got her and I still want her. Both of us try to please each other. One of the most important things in a marriage is a connection. That if you do [have a connection] show your relationship in love and with expressions of love. We say it every day, two or three times. I love you."

Teresa (79): "I couldn't live without him. I like to know where he is every minute. I like to touch him, I like him by me in bed. I like him. I just like him. Tim married for keeps and so did I. We're always together, and most of the time either holding hands or he has his arm around me or I have my hand on his knee. And there's not just one, it's not just Teresa, and it's not just Tim, it's Teresa and Tim."

Source: Kautz, D. D. (1995). *The maturing of sexual intimacy in chronically ill, older adult couples.* (Doctoral dissertation, University of Kentucky). Dissertation Abstracts International (UMI Order #PUZ9527436), p. 55.

literally hundreds of partners over their lifetime; others only a few, others one, and still others none. Some were nuns and priests or celibate for other reasons, who then gave up being celibate in order to be in a romantic relationship. Others became nuns or priests or otherwise became celibate after being married when younger. May–September relationships also occur, and an elder may have a partner who is 30 or even 40 years younger. Some elders have been gay or straight for their whole lives; others are bisexual and were in gay or lesbian relationships when younger, then later got married and had children. The opposite is true as well. The 2010 movie *Beginners* portrays a 75-year-old man who, after the death of his wife of over 40 years, reveals that he has always been gay, and becomes active in the local gay community and enters a relationship with a much younger man. Gender identity may be an issue that a man or woman struggles with all his or her life, and then acts on the desire to become the opposite gender when older. A poignant example is a man who had transsexual surgery at age 74 (Docter, 1985). When asked why he had not pursued the change earlier, he said that he was married to the love of his life for decades, and if she had known that he wanted to be a woman, it would have crushed her. Several years after her death, he had the surgery and lived out his last 3 years as a woman.

As a society, we continually try to come to terms with the diversity of romantic relationships. As nurses, remaining nonjudgmental will ensure that our care includes and is respectful of those who are most important to our patients, regardless of whether we believe their romantic relationships to be healthy or morally or politically correct. Indeed, excluding the love or loves of a patient's life when the person is ill or dying may potentiate complications or hasten death, while including the love may speed recovery. We need to ask, "Who should I call?" rather than asking about marital status. Unfortunately, those who are most important to our patients may stay away out of fear or unease when their partner is admitted to a healthcare facility. Nurses have a unique opportunity to be welcoming to those our patients love.

The loss of one's romantic partner is common for older adults, through both divorce and death. However, the sexual loss is overlooked by most of society. Research on grieving completely ignores how people who lose a lifelong romantic partner adjust to the loss of sex and what we as health professionals can do to assist them in coping with and overcoming their loss. Of course, not all experience grief; the last years of a long-term relationship may have been sexless and filled with anger and pain. Nevertheless, nurses need to assess for the loss of intimacy and sex, acknowledge the loss, and listen to our patients as they express grief and anger.

Sexual Development in Older Adults

Contrary to what some think, adults continue to develop sexually throughout their lives. Chronic illnesses have the potential to affect sexual function, and those who are older who continue to have sex have to adapt to many changes. Most adults who are now over 65 were raised not to talk about sex, and they may not talk with their partners about their sexual desires or preferences. They may see this silence as a way of protecting their partner, even though the silence results in loss of intimacy. The oldest among us have lived through several sexual revolutions. The first was in the roaring 20s, when women gained the right to vote and gained a great deal of sexual freedom. The second came shortly after World War II, when Kinsey published *Sexuality in the Human Male* in 1948 and *Sexuality in the Human Female* in 1952. The third was in the 1960s and early 1970s, with the advent of the birth control pill and legalization of abortion. A fourth revolution occurred with the discovery of HIV, which led to the promotion of safe sex and the use of condoms (see **Box 22-2**). Some might argue that another sexual revolution is occurring now due to the advent of better treatments for erectile dysfunction (ED) and vaginal dryness.

Triphasic Human Response and Changes with Aging

Kaplan (1990), building on early work by Masters and Johnson, identified a *triphasic model of human sexual response*. The three phases are desire, excitement, and orgasm. The desire phase includes the sensations that move one to seek sexual pleasure. Sexual desire is probably stimulated by endorphins; pleasure centers are stimulated by sex, whereas pain inhibits sexual desire. Love is a powerful stimulus to sexual desire. The excitement phase primarily occurs due to myotonia, or increased muscle tone and vasodilation of the genital blood vessels: In men the penis becomes erect; in women the vagina becomes lubricated, the clitoris and vagina become longer and wider, and the labia minora extend outward. Sexual excitement is controlled by the sympathetic nervous system, and fear will inhibit sexual excitement. The orgasm phase is a climactic release of the genital vasodilation and myotonia of the excitement phase. Orgasm is an automatic spinal reflex response. Typically sexual problems can be classified as either desire, excitement, or orgasm phase disorders, or combinations of the three.

BOX 22-2   Research on Older Adults with HIV

- People over 50 comprise over 30% of the people living with HIV, largely due to the success of anti-HIV drugs (HAART), which increase the quality of life and life expectancy of those with HIV.

- Heterosexual sex is the dominant mode of HIV transmission in older adults.

- African American and Hispanic women report higher levels of risk-taking behaviors.

- The poor make up a disproportionate number of those with HIV.

- Elders may not reveal risky behaviors that are socially unacceptable.

- Depression is undertreated in older adults with HIV infection.

- Comorbid conditions (heart disease, arthritis, hypertension, diabetes), normal aging, and age-related changes in drug absorption and distribution may increase adverse drug reactions, drug interactions, and mortality among those with HIV.

Nursing strategies:

- Identify those at risk and provide referrals, social support, and educational materials.

- Target HIV prevention efforts to older adults.

- Increase public education to reduce HIV stigma, homophobia, and ageism in health care.

- Promote more qualitative and quantitative research on elders and HIV.

Changes in sexual response have for decades been considered normal consequences of aging. Desire may or may not change with aging; levels of desire may remain the same throughout life (see **Box 22-3**). However, both men and women experience changes in excitement with age. Achieving an erection may require more direct stimulation and take longer, and the erection may be softer. Ejaculation may not be as forceful, and it may not occur with every sexual encounter. Vaginal lubrication is often decreased, and women find the need for more direct stimulation. Orgasms for women include uterine contractions, and changes in the uterus may change the way an orgasm feels.

Elders differ greatly in their response to these changes. Some couples adapt by increased genital fondling and caressing, taking more time, and paying more attention to each other's needs. In this way, sex may be better than when they were younger. Other couples may welcome an end to sex. Still others may transcend the need for sex and actually become closer (Kautz, 1995). If an elder abstains from sex for months to years when in a sexless relationship or due to loss of a sexual partner, desire will eventually decrease. This loss of sexual desire has been thought to be permanent; however, there are anecdotal reports that when a person who has not been involved in a sexual relationship for many years meets a new partner, desire will return. When those who have stopped having sex for many years start with a new partner, some regain erectile function and vaginal lubrication after several weeks of manual or oral genital stimulation. Still others may seek help from their healthcare provider, which has led to what some call the Viagra revolution, or "Viagra Mindset" (Barnett, Robleda-Gomex, & Pachana, 2012).

BOX 22-3 Harry and Alice Kautz

Harry (1920 – 2009) and Alice (1920 – 2008) were classmates in high school in the rural town of Custer, South Dakota, where they both graduated in 1938. Alice held various jobs, and during WWII moved to Denver, where she became a nurse. She married Morris Lang and had three children while living in rural Colorado, until Morris died of cancer in May, 1957. Harry worked his way through engineering school at the School of Mines in South Dakota and remained a bachelor while working in a variety of engineering jobs in Florida, New York, West Virginia, Michigan, and Colorado. When Alice's brother told Harry that his old classmate and friend, Alice, was a widow, they began to correspond. After a courtship of only a few months, in December 1957, Harry married Alice, taking on a ready-made family with three small children. Both were 37 years old.

When their son Don got married in 1983, Harry's advice was, "To be successful in marriage, it is important to show your love, every day, whether you are feeling that love or not."

After Harry retired in his early 60s and they moved to Sun City, Arizona. Harry began to drink every day. Alice said that his interest in sex waned. However, they still were very active socially together, especially through their church and social clubs.

When they were 75, Alice told her son Don that at 75, life was better than ever. They had moved into a new condo in the retirement community where they were both very active. She said "All of my clothes fit" and "Harry had quit drinking and has a renewed interest in sex." They continued to be active in their church, where Alice adopted the nickname "Bad Alice" because she was a constant flirt.

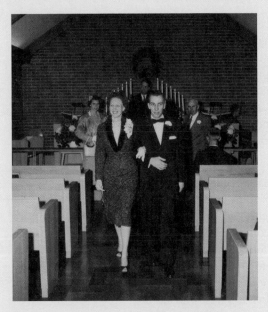

Alice and Harry's wedding in 1957 when they were both 37 years old

Both were devoted to their family, and they enjoyed camping and other outdoor activities.

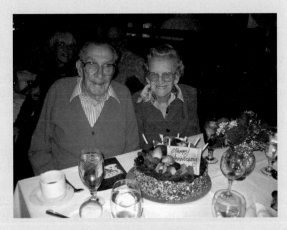

Harry and Alice in 2007 celebrating their 50th wedding anniversary when they were both 87 years old

Due to health problems in their mid-80s, Harry and Alice moved into an independent living community where they celebrated their 50th wedding anniversary in December 2007.

Shortly after their 50th wedding anniversary, Alice was diagnosed with metastatic breast cancer. In the last months, Alice was cared for by hospice. Because of his dementia, the hospice nurse asked Harry who Alice was. He responded, "That's my Alice." When asked who she was to him, he responded, "She is the world to me." Alice died at home, with Harry by her side. The hospice nurse, who was there for her death, said that Harry's goodbye to Alice after she died was very tender. Harry was moved to an Alzheimer's unit, where he died the next year.

Vaginal Dryness and Erectile Dysfunction (ED)

The decreased ability of a man to achieve and maintain an erection and the decreased ability for a woman to achieve vaginal lubrication have, for decades, been considered normal consequences of aging (Touhy & Jett, 2011). As with most changes associated with aging, changes in sexual function may begin as early as age 40, and they occur in almost every adult by age 80. Lindau and colleagues (2007) studied a diverse sample of 3,005 adults ages 57 to 85 and identified several sexual problems. Among women, 43% complained of low desire, 39% complained of vaginal dryness, and 34% had problems with orgasm. *Erectile dysfunction (ED)* was the most common problem among men (37%). Yet some have estimated that less than 50% of men and women seek treatment for sexuality-related issues, either because of embarrassment or because they are not bothered by the problems; in addition, many do not discuss the issue with their partners (Barnett et al., 2012).

Erectile dysfunction and vaginal dryness are also associated with diabetes, heart disease, hypertension, and arthritis (Barnett et al., 2012). Current recommendations for the therapeutic management of ED and vaginal dryness include stopping smoking; drinking only a moderate amount of alcohol; exercising more; and reducing obesity, especially belly fat. The physiologic rationale for this is that smoking, obesity, and a sedentary lifestyle increase atherosclerosis in genital blood vessels, and there is excellent evidence that stopping smoking, losing weight, and doing aerobic exercises reverse this process. Vaginal dryness in women is the physiologic correlate of ED in men, and thus it is possible that the same illnesses and lifestyle habits are correlated with vaginal dryness in women.

The introduction of sildenafil (Viagra) in 1998, followed by vardenafil (Levitra) and tadalafil (Cialis), have changed the norms for sexual dysfunction. The constant barrage of ads in print media and junk mail, on television, and through Internet providers imply that ED is common, almost expected, and the norm is to seek treatment. Twenty years ago, ED and vaginal dryness may have been a private matter for a couple; however, it is now literally impossible for couples to escape these ads. Ads put pressure on men and women who otherwise might not have considered treatment or not thought the problem was important to seek treatment. The ads are still being produced because an estimated 50% of all men over age 40 are experiencing some sexual dysfunction, yet less than 10% have sought treatment (Barnett et al., 2012). Traditionally, vaginal dryness has been treated with lubricants or the oral or cream form of estrogen. Although there are no medications for women that are direct corollaries of Viagra, Levitra, and Cialis, women are bombarded with ads to relieve vaginal dryness and increase sexual desire with hormonal medications and nutritional/natural supplements. There are also constant ads for nutritional supplements and natural remedies for erectile dysfunction.

Clinical literature has long recommended that maintaining a healthy lifestyle will lead to more satisfying sexual relationships. Many reputable websites, maintained by healthcare organizations and providers including the Mayo Clinic and Dr. Dean Ornish, and self-help groups such as the Diabetes and Heart Associations, advocate healthy behaviors as a first step in overcoming problems with erections and vaginal dryness. Books such as *Sex After 60: Tips for Enjoying a Healthy and Happy Sex Life Into Your 60s* (Viljoen, 2012) and *Sex in the Golden Years: The Best Sex Ever* (Bilett & Seiden, 2008) recommend aerobic exercise, a low-fat diet, and stopping smoking as ways to improve sexual performance for both men and women. Nurses can focus patient education on the adoption of healthy behaviors as one step in overcoming sexual dysfunction. Because both erectile dysfunction and vaginal dryness may be early signs of hypertension, heart disease, dementia, or diabetes (Jackson, Rosen, Kloner, & Kostis, 2006), all patients should be told to see their physician for problems with erectile dysfunction or vaginal dryness to ensure that there are no underlying problems and to explore all treatment options.

One approach to adopting healthy behaviors to prevent or alleviate sexual dysfunction is the popular South Beach Diet by Agatston (2003). One of the diet's claims to fame is the loss of belly fat first. Belly fat, especially a waist of over 40 inches in either men or women, has been associated with both erectile dysfunction and vaginal dryness. Loss of belly fat, when combined with exercise, is an effective treatment for erectile dysfunction in men and vaginal dryness in women (Barnett et al., 2012). Similarly, adopting a Mediterranean diet, which also decreases belly fat, has been shown to increase erectile ability (Giugliano, Giugliano, & Espositio, 2006).

Although studies have examined the effectiveness of Viagra in improving both erectile function and quality of life in men, little is known about couples' experiences with these medications. Men receive the prescription for Viagra, but it is possible that women may be the ones taking the medication. Researchers have studied the effectiveness of Viagra in women (Barnett et al., 2012) and found that it is effective if vaginal dryness is the only problem. However, most women with vaginal dryness also have a decrease in sexual desire, and for this Viagra is not helpful. It is also unclear whether couples use lubricants during intercourse to help the man achieve an erection through stimulation or to assist the woman to overcome vaginal dryness. Finally, the differences in views and experiences of men and women are unknown. Most studies of Viagra have only examined the men taking it, not their partners. Barnett and colleagues (2012) point out that "Viagra is the little blue pill with big repercussions" (p. 84). Some women may push their husbands to take Viagra, others may find it a "bother," and still others may experience several detrimental effects, including unwanted changes in their sexual relationship, tension, communication difficulties, fears of infidelity, and, in some cases, vaginal trauma. The authors point out that nurses and physicians need to ask women if their partners take Viagra, and if so, do they have any concerns or need treatment for vaginal dryness.

Promoting Sexual Function in Community-Dwelling Elders

Nurses can have a tremendous impact in assisting elders who reside in the community and wish to maintain sexual function in spite of a myriad of health problems and physical limitations due to aging. Those who wish to maintain an active sex life will need to learn to overcome and compensate for the changes. Articles have been written by nurses to assist clients to overcome sexual problems due to stroke (Kautz, Van Horn, & Moore, 2009), heart and lung disease (Steinke, Barnason, Mosack, & Wright, 2011), and the sexual problems of psychotropic medications taken to treat depression (Higgins, 2007). Whatever the underlying cause(s), the three major obstacles to *sexual intimacy* that elders need to overcome are fatigue, pain, and finding comfortable positions for giving and receiving of pleasure. These obstacles may occur for either men or women, and for either one partner or both. However, there are practical ways to help overcome these problems.

Overcoming Fatigue and Pain

Overcoming fatigue and pain is essential to feeling desire and having the stamina to give and receive pleasure. The specifics of fatigue and pain are addressed in detail elsewhere in this text. Common ways to overcome fatigue are to plan for sex when rested, which is often in the morning—Kautz (1995) and others have found that elders who continue to have sex tend to have sex in the morning. Another key factor is to plan one's activities to save some time and energy for pleasure.

Pain is a hallmark of aging. Arthritis and other chronic illnesses have a chronic pain component that lasts until one dies. Most pain management strategies leave some residual pain, which may interfere with sexual desire and sexual excitement. The irritability, fatigue, and depression that accompany chronic pain can also have an impact on a couple's sexual relationship. Recommendations include planning for sex at a time when the pain is at its lowest level, often mid-morning for those with rheumatoid arthritis, or when pain medications have their peak action. Incorporating massage, a hot bath for chronic arthritic pain, cold packs for acute inflammation, or using an electric massager or vibrator may relax sore muscles, relieve stiffened joints, and, when done with a partner, stimulate sexual excitement. Women may focus the water jets from a hot tub on their clitoris, and both men and women may use the vibrator for sexual stimulation. Anecdotal reports from those with arthritis suggest that the relaxing effects of these pain relief strategies and orgasm

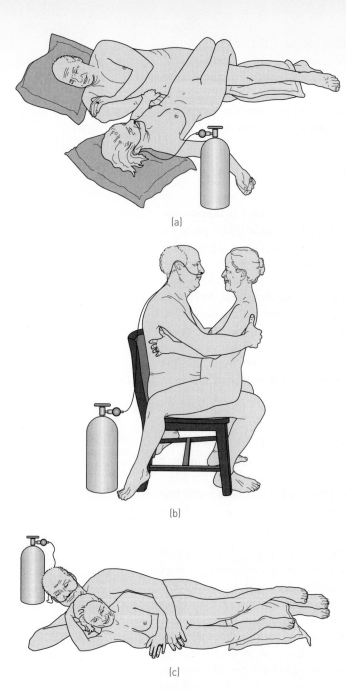

(a)

(b)

(c)

Figure 22-1 These positions may be used by men and women when either or both have limited endurance, COPD, hip or knee replacement, stroke. Those with GERD may find sitting in the chair will not exacerbate their symptoms.

actually relieve chronic pain for many hours. This effect is thought to be due to endorphin release during the relaxing treatment and sexual stimulation.

Adopting New Positions and Learning New Techniques for Lovemaking

Because of limitations from disease and disability, some elders need to adopt new positions for lovemaking. **Table 22-1** lists resources that provide suggestions for comfortable positions as well as additional information about sex and intimacy with specific chronic illnesses. The illustrations in **Figure 22-1** provide examples of positions for intercourse when adapting to chronic illness or disability. **Table 22-2** lists resources where couples can obtain educational materials and products through reputable sex education websites.

Promoting Romantic and Sexual Relationships in Long-Term Care Facilities

Another issue that is rarely addressed in the literature is intimacy and sex among elders residing in long-term care facilities. Barriers exist in virtually all facilities, including lack of privacy and door locks, lack of queen size beds, and the literal lack of opportunities for romance. Inability to leave a facility overnight without "losing the bed" prevents couples who have had long-term relationships from getting away for even one night. Although it is important for staff to protect patients from sexual abuse and ensure safety, policies and environmental design go overboard to prevent intimacy. Studies confirm that staff continue to be uncomfortable with residents' sexual behavior (Elias & Ryan, 2011; Heath, 2011). A timeless story of love in a nursing home, *The*

TABLE 22-1 Resources for Information and Comfortable Positions for Intercourse

- *COPD and Sex.* Available from http://www.webmd.com/lung/copd/features/copd-sex
- *Sex and Arthritis*. Available from: http://www.orthop.washington.edu
- *Sex and Cancer* (several articles by American Cancer Society). Available from: http://www.cancer.org
- *Sex After Stroke*. Available from: http://www.strokeassociation.org
- *Intimacy and Diabetes*. Available from: http://www.netdoctor.co.uk

TABLE 22-2 Web Links: Sex Education Websites

The following are a few professional websites that are highly recommended by the authors for older people to obtain sex education materials. Reassure older adults these are legitimate sex education websites and are not "porno sites."

- http://www.hivwisdom.org (HIV Wisdom for Older Women)
- http://www.womenshealth.org (Estronaut: A Forum for Women's Health)
- http://www.erectile-dysfunction-impotence.org
- http://marriage.about.com (Intimacy and sexuality information for couples)
- http://www.sexualhealth.com (Sexual Health Network)

Notebook by Nicholas Sparks (1999), shows us what is possible if nursing staff respect the rights and privacy of those who have entrusted us with the last years of their lives. Some staff may actually promote romance and sex in long-term care, but they do not reveal these efforts for fear of reprisal.

The American Medical Directors Association (AMDA), a professional organization for directors of long-term care facilities, has developed policies that are available on the AMDA website, Caring for the Ages, at http://www.amda.com/publications/caring/may2002/sex.cfm. Heath (2011) provides guidelines for sex in the nursing home, taking into account the issues of what to do if a resident is cognitively impaired, the health needs of the residents, and how to keep the staff informed so that the privacy of the couple can be maintained. The authors recommend the video *Freedom of Sexual Expression: Dementia and Resident Rights in Long Term Care Facilities*, developed by the Hebrew Home for the Aged, a facility that is nationally known for its policies promoting intimacy between residents. (Their current policies can be obtained at http://www.hebrewhome.org.) This film and many others on a wide range of topics on aging, including intimacy and sexuality, are available through Terra Nova Films, http://www.terranova.org.

Evidence-based practice guidelines that balance safety with the lifelong need for intimacy are needed. The need to be touched and held by someone who loves us, and the need to feel loved, not just cared for, does not diminish with age or with physical or cognitive impairment (Heath, 2011).

Extinguishing Sexually Inappropriate Behavior

Unfortunately, nursing staff may sometimes be confronted with an older adult, either a man or a woman, who displays sexually inappropriate behavior. Most of the incidents reported involve men, but women may display these behaviors as well. Sexually inappropriate behaviors include inappropriate language ("Won't you get in the bed with me?"), inappropriate requests for personal care ("Make sure and wash my penis really good"), inappropriate gestures (such as sticking the tongue out and wiggling it at staff), exposing one's self or masturbating in public places, and inappropriate touching (grabbing a breast or buttock when in close proximity). All of these behaviors constitute sexual harassment and are not to be tolerated. These behaviors may reflect a power issue, a loss of inhibition due to cognitive impairment, or a combination of factors. The behaviors make it difficult or impossible to care for the patient exhibiting them.

The goal is to extinguish the behavior while maintaining the dignity of the patient. Nursing staff need to confront the patient calmly and firmly, saying, "This behavior is inappropriate, interferes with me doing my job, and will not be tolerated." Laughing it off, reacting violently, or showing anger are all likely to encourage the behavior. Saying, "Oh, Mr. Smith, you wouldn't know what to do even if you could," although meant light-heartedly, is demeaning and may encourage the patient to try the behavior with someone else. Ask other staff if the behavior is a pattern and be sure to inform others so that they will not be caught off guard. One quadriplegic client told the authors he had rubbed the breasts of every nursing staff member on the unit with his upper arm when they were leaning over him to assist in dressing. He had gotten away with this behavior for weeks because the staff had not talked with each other about this behavior. We informed the staff, two nursing staff firmly and compassionately confronted him together, and the behavior ended. Confronting him led several staff to talk with him about his fears of dating and being seen as attractive, which was the underlying need behind this behavior.

Although extinguishing sexually inappropriate behavior is necessary to care for older adults, there is some "good news" about this behavior, as it is an indicator of recovery in a client who has been too ill to think or worry about his or her sexuality. It may be an expression of power or anger, both of which are expressions of independence. Interest in sexuality can aid in the rehabilitation process. After confronting a patient and ensuring that the client is not going to act out again, the nurse can initiate discussions about recovery and how to take an active role in that process.

Confronting cognitively impaired clients who act out may be effective in extinguishing the behavior. If this strategy does not work, other strategies may extinguish the behavior. If a client has a habit of inappropriately touching staff during a bath or bed-to-chair transfer, put a washrag in the client's hand during the bath, or place the patient's hand on the armrest to assist in the transfer. Approach a client from the weaker side, which will both protect the staff member and discourage the client from acting out. Another strategy is to encourage appropriate behaviors and ignore inappropriate behaviors (see **Box 22-4**). In rehabilitative settings, rewarding appropriate behaviors can be included as a part of a behavioral modification program. If possible, get a client's family involved in extinguishing the behavior. Do not assume that the behavior is a premorbid

> **BOX 22-4   Sexuality and Alzheimer's Disease: Can the Two Go Together?**
>
> In an article in Nursing Forum, Tabak and Shemesh-Kigli (2006) examine the ethical issue of sexual relations in nursing homes among those who are demented. The authors demonstrated that staff is often untrained and may be confused about patient/resident rights related to sexual relations within a nursing home. Two case studies are used to illustrate the dilemmas confronting nurses. Recommendations are given for nurses, the nursing profession, owners of nursing homes, and those making policy.
>
> ***Source:*** Tabak, N., & Shemesh-Kigli, R. (2006). Sexuality and Alzheimer's disease: Can the two go together? *Nursing Forum*, 41, 158–166.

or lifelong behavior, and try not to feed into perceptions of the client as a "dirty old man." Another strategy is to avoid using language the client may misinterpret as sexual. Nurses typically say, "I am your nurse today," or "I am going to take care of you," both of which may be misinterpreted as flirting. Instead say, "I am going to work with you" or "I am going to assist you," which sound much more businesslike. Lesser, Hughes, Jemelka, and Griffith (2005) outline pharmacologic therapies that may be necessary when sexually inappropriate behaviors continue despite the interventions outlined previously.

Dealing with Masturbation in Public Places in Hospitals or Long-Term Care

Masturbation is self-limiting and has no known harmful effects. It does not spread sexually transmitted diseases, and it can be performed with minimal cognitive and hand function. The comedian Phyllis Diller has been quoted as saying that another advantage is "You don't have to get dressed up." However, masturbation is only appropriate in private. Public masturbation is best extinguished using the strategies described previously for sexually inappropriate behaviors. The goal is to allow privacy, yet not draw undue attention. If "privacy" signs are necessary, keep them inconspicuous. Try to provide privacy even if clients' rooms are only semi-private, such as by giving the client some private time. Schover and Jenson (1988), who worked extensively with head injury survivors, noted that some clients benefited from an inflatable doll to have intercourse with. Clients using sex toys or explicit materials should do so in private and store them in their own private space, away from public view.

Patients Displaying Sexually Explicit Materials on the Unit or in the Home

Display of sexually explicit materials is a problem that is ignored in the nursing literature. Nursing staff may need to set some ground rules with patients in regard to posters, jokes, magazines, or cards on display on the patient's room wall or on dressers or over-bed tables. Staff need to recognize that although having these materials is the patient's choice, openly displaying them is a form of sexual harassment. A good rule is that materials with a PG-13 rating, such as the *Sports Illustrated* swimsuit issue, are acceptable, but those with naked bodies are not. Rules apply equally to men and women and apply regardless of the patient's sexual orientation. Rules also apply

BOX 22-5   Evidence-Based Practice Highlight

The authors conducted a systematic review of the literature on the topic of primary prevention of HIV/AIDS in those over 50, resulting in 21 articles. Three major challenges to education in this area were identified: 1) ageism in health professionals, 2) reluctance on the part of older adults to discuss sexuality, and 3) older adults' perception of risk of HIV/AIDS. Three educational models were identified: 1) educational programs delivered by health professionals, 2) peer education, and 3) one-to-one early intervention, including screening for HIV/AIDS. More research is needed to develop effective models for education on these topics.

Source: Milaszewski, D., Greto, E., Klochkov, T., & Fuller-Thompson, E. (2012). A systematic review of education for the prevention of HIV/AIDS among older adults. *Journal of Evidence-based Social Work*, 9(3), 213–230.

Notable Quotes

"In times of grief and sorrow I will hold you and rock you, and take your grief and make it my own. When you cry, I cry, and when you hurt, I hurt. And together we will try to hold back the floods of tears and despair and make it through the potholed streets of life."

—From a character in *The Notebook* by Nicholas Sparks

to staff areas; the inside of a staff member's locker may be his or her private space, but when the door is open in a public lounge and others have to view the pictures, that is a form of sexual harassment. Pictures are not the only problem; get-well cards that overtly encourage sexual relationships with patients and nursing staff are also inappropriate. If a patient has displayed these materials, calmly tell the patient why they are inappropriate and encourage the patient or family to remove them. Use respect when approaching a patient about offensive material. It is the patient's home too, especially in a long-term care setting. Try a compassionate approach first, focusing on your feelings. Keep the confrontation one-on-one if possible.

Occasionally, nursing staff who visit patients in their homes may encounter sexually explicit materials on display. Tell patients you cannot work with them in the rooms in which the materials are displayed. Negotiate with the patient for one room of the house where treatment can occur where there are no explicit materials.

Summary

This chapter has addressed a wide variety of areas related to sexuality and intimacy. The goal is to promote intimacy when appropriate by assisting older adults to overcome the effects of age and chronic illness (see **Box 22-5**).

Critical Thinking Exercises

1. You are caring for an older man with dementia who keeps wandering into the rooms of female residents in the long-term care facility. How would handle this issue?

2. What have you read about HIV and AIDS among the older adult population? Do you think this is a real problem? Why or why not?

3. An older client in assisted living asks you to buy him a pornographic magazine because he cannot drive to the store and get one for himself. As an employee of the place where the client lives, what is your responsibility in this situation?

Personal Reflections

1. If an older patient was having problems dealing with sexuality after a life-changing event, how could you assist him or her?

2. What is your comfort level with discussing sexual information with patients? How could you become more comfortable with this important aspect of nursing?

3. What resources are available in your area for older persons or those with disabilities who may need additional information and counseling about sexuality after an event such as a stroke or heart attack?

References

AARP. (2005). *Sexuality at midlife and beyond.* Retrieved from http://www.aarp.org

Agatston, A. (2003). *The South Beach diet.* Emmaus, PA: Rodale Press.

Alterovitz, S. R., & Mendelsohn, G. A. (2009). Partner preferences across the life span: Online dating by older adults. *Psychology and Aging, 24,* 513–517.

Barnett, Z. L., Robleda-Gomez, S., & Pachana, N. A. (2012). Viagra: The little blue pill with big repercussions. *Aging & Mental Health, 16,* 84–88.

Billett, J. L. & Seiden, O. J. (2008). Sex in the Golden Years: The Best Sex Ever. Parker, CO: Books To Believe In.

Cournan, M. (2012). Bladder management in female stroke survivors: Translating research into practice. *Rehabilitation Nursing, 37*(5), 220–230. doi: 10.1002/rnj.054.

Docter, R. F. (1985). Transsexual surgery at 74: A case report. *Archives of Sexual Behavior, 14,* 271–277.

Elias, J., & Ryan, A. (2011). A review and commentary on the factors that influence expressions of sexuality by older people in care homes. *Journal of Clinical Nursing, 20,* 1668–1676.

Giugliano, D., Giugliano, F., & Esposito, K. (2006). Sexual dysfunction and the Mediterranean diet. *Public Health Nutrition, 9,* 1118–1120.

Heath, H. (2011). Older people in care homes: Sexuality and intimate relationships. *Nursing Older People, 23*(6), 14–20.

Higgins, A. (2007). Impact of psychotropic medication on sexuality: Literature review. *British Journal of Nursing, 16,* 545–549.

Jackson, G., Rosen, R. C., Kloner, R. A., & Kostis, J. B. (2006). The second Princeton consensus on sexual dysfunction and cardiac risk: New guidelines for sexual medicine. *Journal of Sexual Medicine, 3,* 28–36.

Kaplan, H. S. (1990). Sex, intimacy, and the aging process. *Journal of the American Academy of Psychoanalysis, 18,* 185–205.

Kautz, D. D. (1995). *The maturing of sexual intimacy in chronically ill, older adult couples.* (Doctoral dissertation, University of Kentucky). Dissertation Abstracts International (UMI Order #PUZ9527436).

Kautz, D. D., Van Horn, E. R., & Moore, C. (2009). Sex after stroke: An integrative review and recommendations for clinical practice. *Critical Reviews in Physical and Rehabilitation Medicine, 21*(2), 99–115.

Lesser, J. M., Hughes, S. V., Jemelka, J. R., & Griffith, J. (2005). Sexually inappropriate behaviors: Assessment necessitates careful medical and psychological evaluation and sensitivity. *Geriatrics, 60,* 34–37.

Lindau, S. T., Schumm, L. P., Laumann, E. O., Levinson, W., O'Muircheataigh, C. A., & Waite, L. J. (2007). A study of sexuality and health among older adults in the United States. *New England Journal of Medicine, 357,* 762–774.

Milaszewski, D., Greto, E., Klochkov, T., & Fuller-Thompson, E. (2012). A systematic review of education for the prevention of HIV/AIDS among older adults. *Journal of Evidence-based Social Work, 9*(3), 213–230.

Robinson, J. G., & Molzahn, A. E. (2007). Sexuality and quality of life. *Journal of Gerontological Nursing, 33*(3), 19–27.

Schover, L. R., & Jensen, S. B. (1988). Sexuality and chronic illness: A comprehensive approach. New York, NY: Guilford.

Sparks, N. (1999). *The notebook*. New York, NY: Warner Books.

Steinke, E., Mosack, V., Barnason, S., & Wright, D. (2011). Progress in sexual counseling by cardiac nurses, 1994–2009. *Heart & Lung, 40*(3), e15–e24.

Tabak, N., & Shemesh-Kigli, R. (2006). Sexuality and Alzheimer's disease: Can the two go together? *Nursing Forum, 41*, 158–166.

Touhy, T. A., & Jett, K. K. (2011). *Ebersole & Hess' toward healthy aging: Human needs and nursing response* (8th ed.). St. Louis, MO: Mosby.

Viljoen, P. O. (2012). *Sex after 60: Tips for enjoying a healthy and happy sex life into your 60s.* Amazon Digital Services, Inc.

Wallace, M. (2012). *Want to know more. Issues regarding sexuality. Protocol: Sexuality in the older adult.* Hartford Institute for Geriatric Nursing. Retrieved from: http://consultgerirn.org/topics/sexuality_issues_in_aging/want_to_know_more

For a full suite of assignments and additional learning activities, see the access code at the front of your book.

LEARNING OBJECTIVES

At the end of this chapter, the reader will be able to:

> Distinguish between elder abuse and self-neglect.
> Describe several categories of the mistreatment of older adults.
> Recognize risk factors for elder abuse.
> Identify characteristics of perpetrators of mistreatment.
> Recognize signs that an older adult is being mistreated.
> Name two screening tools for elder abuse.
> Discuss strategies to prevent the mistreatment of older adults.
> Synthesize interventions in various cases of abuse.

KEY TERMS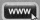

abandonment
Direct physical abuse
Elder abuse
Elder mistreatment
Emotional/psychological abuse
Financial abuse
Financial exploitation
Financial or material
    exploitation

Hwalek–Sengstock Elder Abuse
    Screening Test
physical abuse
Psychological or emotional abuse
Psychological or emotional neglect
Self-neglect
Sexual abuse
Neglect
Violation of personal rights

Chapter 23

(Competencies 3, 4, 6, 15)

Abuse and Mistreatment of Older Adults

Kristen L. Mauk
Kathleen Urban

Background

Elder abuse is "a single, or repeated act, or lack of appropriate action, occurring within any relationship where there is an expectation of trust which causes harm or distress to an older person" (World Health Organization [WHO], n.d., para.1). Elder abuse is connected with a wide variety of adverse health outcomes. There is evidence of risk of greater mortality (Baker et al., 2009; Lachs, Williams, O'Brien, Pillemer, & Charlson, 1998); higher dependence in performance of activities of daily living (Cohen, 2008); and increased dementia, delusions, and depression (Cooper et al., 2006; Cooper, Manela, Katona, & Livongston, 2008; Dyer, Pavlik, Murphy & Hyman, 2000; Pillemer & Suitor, 1992). Other findings suggest that older women who have experienced abuse are likely to report to their physicians with fatigue, headache, myalgias, depression, anxiety, and gastrointestinal disorders, as well as with gynecological issues and physical injuries.

Elder abuse or mistreatment is an often-underestimated problem. Statistics on abuse of older adults may not be reliable, due to underreporting or a lack of scientific evidence. There is no national reporting system, so statistics may be based on varying definitions of abuse. Combined with the fact that older adults may be hesitant to report abuse because of fear of reprisal, the American system of gathering data and reporting abuse is woefully inadequate. The statistics that are available are outdated.

Data from the 1990s estimated that 5–10% of older adults experienced abuse (Pritchard, 1995), with translates to 1–2 million people (Frost & Willette, 1994; Thobaben, 1996). In 2010, the National Center on Elder Abuse (2010) cited that one in 10 older adults experiences some form of abuse, but less than one in five report it. Fulmer cited that

"Elder abuse and neglect is a serious and prevalent problem that is estimated to affect 700,000 to 1.2 million older adults annually in this country" (2012, p. 1) There is a wide variation between sources as to the extent of elder mistreatment or abuse and much of our information is outdated.

For the purposes of this discussion, elder abuse will be defined simply as "the mistreatment of an older adult that threatens his or her health or safety" (Hildreth, 2011, p. 568). There are several types of elder abuse that will be discussed in this chapter. Prevention, identification, and intervention strategies will also be reviewed.

Types of Elder Abuse

Elder mistreatment may be classified into several different categories. These include neglect; *financial exploitation*; and emotional, physical, or sexual abuse (Daly, 2011). Some authors include violation of personal rights as another category of abuse. Neglect of older adults and financial exploitation seem to be the two most commonly reported types of mistreatment (Fulmer & Greenberg, 2012). Several types of abuse may be present at once, and abuse or neglect tends to be recurring (Quinn & Tomita, 1986). Abuse is often ongoing, may be eventually tolerated by the person being mistreated, and can have long-lasting negative consequences on health and emotional well-being (McGarry & Simpson, 2011).

Sengstock and Barrett (1992) distinguished six types of abuse or neglect; these distinctions are still applicable today because they distinguish between degrees of abuse or neglect and can be helpful in providing specificity to reporting and documentation. These include psychological or emotional neglect, psychological or emotional abuse, violation of personal rights, financial abuse, physical neglect, and direct abuse or neglect. These are discussed in the next section.

Psychological or Emotional Neglect

Psychological or emotional neglect may be present when a person receives good or adequate physical care, but is socially isolated. The older adult in such a situation may stay in his/her room, have decreased socialization with others outside of the home, and express little purpose for living. This may present as a type of "failure to thrive" in older adults.

Psychological or Emotional Abuse

Sometimes preceded by psychological or emotional neglect, *psychological or emotional abuse* shows a greater degree of severity of mistreatment. This type of abuse includes verbal or nonverbal insults, such as hurtful things said or done to damage the person's self-esteem. Humiliation, intimidation, and harassment fall into this category (Fulmer & Greenberg, 2012). Common assaults in this category of abuse include telling the older person that he is a burden and threatening to send him to a nursing home.

Violation of Personal Rights

Ignoring the rights of an older person who is capable of decision making can be considered a *violation of personal rights*. Healthcare facilities may be guilty of this type of mistreatment. For example, addressing questions to a younger adult about the older adult in his presence or making wrong assumptions that an older adult is not mentally competent are common violations. In long-term-care settings, not allowing persons to marry or assuming lack of competence if a person answers too slowly are other examples. Within families, if a relative goes into Grandma's purse or on her cellphone to retrieve information without permission, this is also a violation of personal rights.

Financial Abuse

Financial abuse is one of the most common types of mistreatment and may be easier to quantify than other forms of abuse. Also referred to as material abuse, *financial abuse* can include stealing money or property, making the person feel obligated to the abuser in some way in order to obtain goods or possessions, or borrowing money and not repaying it.

Another avenue leading to financial abuse of older adults on a larger scale is mail fraud. This may occur through attractive fliers and brochures that promise prizes or the chance to win large amounts of money over time. Such "contests" frequently target susceptible older people with limited means. They may win small items that lead them to think they are more likely to win big prizes, so they send money to remain in the contest. Older adults who fall prey to this misleading advertising may spend thousands of dollars for little return, much like more traditional gambling.

A study by MetLife (2012b) estimated that over one million older adults are victims of financial abuse. The same study estimated that $2.6 billion was lost annually in the United States to this type of abuse. The most common characteristics of victims included: White, frail, ages 70–89 years, cognitively impaired, isolated, and trusting. About 55% of financial abuse cases were due to exploitation from family members (MetLife, 2012b). In a later examination of the data, women were twice as likely as men to experience financial abuse. These women tended to be between the ages of 80 and 89, live alone, and require some type of assistance for health problems. Sixty percent of perpetrators were men between the ages of 30 and 59 (MetLife, 2012a). Financial abuse appeared to be worse during the holidays as a result of friends and family members taking advantage of older adults. Financial exploitation can have negative effects on an older adult, including credit problems, depression, and loss of independence (MetLife, 2012b).

Physical Neglect

Physical neglect is not providing what the older adult needs, such as glasses, dentures, medications, food, or adaptive equipment. Though stopping short of direct physical abuse, signs of this type of neglect could be insect or vermin bites, overgrown toenails, overuse of restraints, pressure ulcers, malnutrition, and poor hygiene.

It should be noted that some older adults engage in self-neglect, so care should be taken to complete a thorough assessment of the living situation. Self-neglect among older adults is a difficult problem to manage, particularly when a competent elder chooses to live in this way.

Self-Neglect

Self-neglect is defined as the inability to provide basic needs for oneself (Dyer, Goodwin, Pickens-Pace, Burnett, & Kelly, 2007) and is associated with poor nutrition and functional decline (Reyes-Ortiz, 2006). Persons who do not maintain a socially acceptable level of self-care would be considered to be engaging in self-neglect (Gibbons, Lauder, & Ludwick, 2006). Signs of self-neglect may include inadequate physical hygiene, poor diet, missing medical appointments, medication mismanagement, and lack of follow-up with prescribed medical care (Mauk, 2011).

Although gerontological nurses strive to uphold the autonomy and independence of older adults, "dilemmas result when people's poor health behaviors put them or others at risk for negative consequences" (Mauk, 2011, p. 64). Careful assessment is needed if self-neglect is suspected, as reporting such a case to adult protective services could eventually result in an older adult being forcibly removed from his or her place of residence. An "interdisciplinary team of professionals should be consulted and decisions should be made that are in the ultimate best interest of the older adult" (Mauk, 2011, p. 64) when self-neglect is serious enough to produce negative health outcomes.

Direct Abuse

This is the most obvious type of mistreatment seen in older adults. *Direct physical abuse* involves the use of physical force to purposefully inflict pain or harm to another. Direct abuse includes assault and aggressive violence such as hitting, kicking, biting, punching, pushing, shoving, burning, restraining, overmedicating, and slapping. Sexual assault and rape are also included in this category. Female victims are more likely to experience significant injury, especially if the abuser is a male.

Case Studies

Within this section of the chapter are several case studies to test your knowledge related to assessment of elder mistreatment. Look at each situation and see if you can correctly distinguish the type of elder abuse as described in this section.

Case Study 23-1

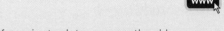

You are working in the emergency room. A 65-year-old woman comes in with bruises to her inner thighs and small burns on her the bottom of her feet. Her major complaint is abdominal pain. She is 5'7" and weighs 100 pounds. She has no teeth. She is accompanied by her son, a 40-year-old man who appears unkempt, belligerent, and does not want you to examine his mother without him in the room. What is your best course of action? What is your initial impression of this situation? What interventions should be taken?

Case Study 23-2

You are working in your backyard and hear yelling from the house next door. You hear a woman screaming and glass breaking. All you know about your neighbors is that their mother, 80 years old, has Alzheimer's disease and they have recently brought her to live with them. A few minutes later you see the old woman running outside in her underwear with a middle-aged woman chasing after her. What is your best course of action? What is your initial impression of this situation? What interventions should be taken?

Case Study 23-3

You are living in a small suburban neighborhood. You notice that the younger couple from down the street frequently visit the older man who lives across the street from you. They seem to be taking care of him, mowing his lawn and driving him to the doctors. When you take cookies over to this gentleman, he tells you that the neighbors down the street charge him a lot of money to look after him, but he has nobody else to do it. Upon questioning him further, he confesses that they have threatened to stop helping him if he doesn't give them $1,000 each week for their troubles. He is perplexed but does not know what else to do. He says he now feels scared of them. What is your best course of action? What is your initial impression of this situation? What interventions should be taken?

Case Study 23-4

You come from a large family of 7 children and 30 grandchildren. Your elderly parents do not have much money, but one of their children, your brother, seems to always be borrowing money from them. You learn, rather by accident through another sibling, that your mom and dad cosigned a loan for your brother and he defaulted. Now your mom and dad are in financial trouble but do not want the rest of the family to know. What is your best course of action? What is your initial impression of this situation? What interventions should be taken?

Case Study 23-5

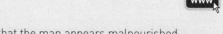

A woman is admitted to the emergency room where you are working. She has large bruises across her left shoulder, abdomen, and chest to her right hip. Her face has some cuts and bruises. She states that she was in a car accident. The accident report states she was wearing her seatbelt. What is your best course of action? What is your initial impression of this situation? What interventions should be taken?

Case Study 23-6

You are working at an underserved clinic where an 81-year-old man comes in for treatment of a cough that has lingered for weeks. The man seems quiet and withdrawn. He is accompanied by his wife, who is 15 years younger than he is, and who displays loud, aggressive behavior, speaking rudely to the staff. During your assessment, you find that the man appears malnourished, underweight, and dehydrated. He is reluctant to answer any questions about his living situation at home with his wife and he cowers when she is in the room. What is your best course of action? What is your initial impression of this situation? What interventions should be taken?

Characteristics of Victims

The majority of early elder abuse studies in the 1980s characterized the "typical" victim as being an older female, vulnerable, and having functional impairment and dementia (DeCalmer & Glendenning, 1993; Hocking, 1988; Pritchard, 1996; Tomlin, 1989). Although it is important to avoid stereotyping, these early data gave a relatively accurate picture that is often still true today. There are several factors emerging in the literature that have been consistently associated with a higher risk of being a victim of mistreatment or abuse. **Table 23-1** lists risk factors associated with being a victim of elder abuse or neglect. Persons who have memory problems or physical disabilities and those who are socially isolated are at increased risk. More specifically, "lower levels of global cognitive function, MMSE, episodic memory, and perceptual speed are associated with an increased risk of elder abuse" (Dong, Simon, Rajan, & Evans, 2011, p. 209).

Older persons who are substance abusers, who experience depression or loneliness, and have a lack of social support are also at risk (Hildreth, 2011). In addition, if an older adult who is dependent on others for care is verbally or physically abusive to the caregiver, then the risk for being a victim of mistreatment is higher. There is generally more evidence to suggest that females tend to be more likely victims of abuse than males proportionately, although spousal abuse from either gender is

TABLE 23-1   General Risk Factors for Elder Abuse or Mistreatment (Victim)
Lives alone or with another person (shared living arrangement)
Elderly (with financial abuse, between 80 and 89 years of age)
Poor or of limited means
Physical disability
Significant functional or cognitive limitations (such as memory loss or dementia)
Impaired psychosocial health
Female
Socially isolated, depressed, or lacking social support
Substance abuse issues
Dependent on others for care or assistance
Verbally or physically combative

Source: Daly, 2010; Fulmer & Greenberg, 2012; Hildreth, 2011; MetLife, 2012a.

likely underreported but represents a growing trend (Fulmer & Greenberg, 2012; Sengstock & Barrett, 1992; Hildreth, 2011; MetLife, 2012a).

The elderly most at risk are those who live in a shared living situation, whether in a home or in a residential situation. Zhang et al. (2011), in the *Journal of Elder Abuse and Neglect*, stated that some studies indicate that an older person's mental, physical, and cognitive impairments are related to neglect both in the community and in institutions. According to Rosen and associates (2008), resident-to-resident aggression is "negative and aggressive physical, sexual, or verbal interactions between long-term care residents that in a community setting would likely be construed as unwelcome and have high potential to cause physical or psychological distress to the recipient" (p. 1398).

Characteristics of Perpetrators of Elder Abuse

One of the most popular older theories used to explain elder abuse is the caregiver stress model, which stated that elders who become abused have created extreme levels of stress on their caregiver, resulting in an intolerable burden, which leads to mistreatment. Wilson (1992) summarized caregiver stress theory by stating that the hypothesis is that "elders' physical, emotional, and financial dependency needs create an unfair and inescapable relationship with the caregiver" (p. 69), which leads to abuse. Other research, however, suggested that "the dependency of the victim may simply be a catalyst for abuse in a caretaker who cannot cope effectively" (Barnett, Miller-Perrin, & Perrin, 1997, p. 26).

TABLE 23-2   General Characteristics of Perpetrators of Elder Mistreatment or Abuse

Substance abuse, especially alcoholism
Increased stress
Lack of social support
Depression, anxiety, or other mental health issues
Lack of knowledge or training about caring for an older adult
Overwhelmed caregiver
Poor coping skills
History of family violence
Maladaptive personality traits
Other social, psychological or emotional problems

Source: Centers for Disease Control and Prevention, 2010; Fulmer & Greenberg, 2012.

Some common characteristics of those who mistreat older adults have emerged through several studies in the 1990s and more recently (see **Table 23-2**). Maladaptive personality characteristics, anxiety, a history of family violence, inability of the caregiver to meet the demands of the elder, and lack of knowledge have all been associated with abusers (Buckwalter, Campbell, Gerdner, & Garand, 1996; Fulmer & Greenberg, 2012; Saveman, Hallberg, & Norberg, 1996; Wierucka & Goodridge, 1996). The perpetrator is often someone who knows the victim and upon whom the victim may be dependent. Nurses must be alert to the fact that "children, family members, friends, and formal caregivers are prospective perpetrators of elder abuse" (Stark, 2011, p. 431).

Prevention of Abuse or Mistreatment

The best prevention is education, so education about elder abuse should be a priority. Laws regarding elder abuse are not standard from state to state, and the magnitude of elder abuse is not fully realized due to few population-based studies. All gerontological nurses, social workers, healthcare workers, law enforcement workers, and the general public should be educated about the signs and symptoms, screening, identifying, reporting, and support services for the elderly abused and the abuser (see **Table 23-3**).

Communities should look at developing outreach programs that involve elders, respite care, and education. Families and friends need to understand and realize how important it is to give support to the caregiver and help them with rest on a regular basis.

TABLE 23-3 Nursing Interventions in the Prevention of Elder Abuse
Establish a trusting relationship with the elder.
Know about community resources and be able to appropriately refer people for help.
Strengthen social supports and networking of older adults.
Encourage regular respite for the caregiver.
Identify and refer to appropriate caregiver support groups.
Identify caregivers who are at high risk to be abusers and target interventions to prevent stress from caregiver burden.
Interview the patient and family or caregiver to find out normal patterns for stress management.
Identify possible scenarios and facilitate strategies to cope with those.
Observe family interactions, dynamics, and body language.
Encourage single older adults to remain involved and connected to society.
Be aware of risk factors and contributing factors.
Perform thorough physical assessments and carefully document findings, including appearance, nutritional state, skin condition, mental attitude and awareness, and need for aids to enhance sensory perception.
If abuse is suspected, interview caregivers and other possible informants separately to confirm or refute suspicions.
Know the reporting laws for your own state.
Encourage the older person to let a trusted person know where valuable papers are stored.

Community education is necessary for everyone to realize how important and valuable it is to plan financially for one's own care in his/her "golden years." Older adults can be taught to decrease their risk of being victimized (see **Table 23-4**). Remaining involved and engaged in the community, participating in outside interests, and maintaining connections with family and friends can help provide older adults with a buffer against the potential for abuse.

Gerontological nurses have a great opportunity to educate representatives, senators, and other policymakers on the issues of elderly abuse, encouraging them to make legislative changes that can impact effective services for the elderly and their caregivers (Stark, 2011).

TABLE 23-4   Suggestions for Older Adults to Reduce the Potential for Abuse
Stay active—keep involved in social activities.
Have access to a telephone and use of it in private.
Store important contact information in two separate places (for example: in a cellphone and a phone directory).
Maintain contact with family and friends.
Know your financial situation and when to expect deposits and automatic withdrawals.
Have a secure, private place where your important files are kept.
Have a family members or friends visit regularly and unannounced.
Have an emergency safety plan if you are concerned about potential abuse.
Let a trusted person know where you are going if you are traveling or visiting out of town.

Assessment and Screening

The following criteria indicate those older adults most likely to benefit from further assessment:

> Physical, functional, or cognitive impairment
> Mental illness, alcoholism, or drug abuse problems
> Socially isolated, have a poor social network, or low social support
> Dependent on others
> Past history of abusive relationships
> Financial problems or other family problems
> Reside in inadequate housing or other unsafe conditions
> Depression
> Delusions
> Previous traumatic exposure
> Poor health
> Caregiver is stressed/frustrated with the difficulties of caring for an older person
> Caregiver has mental illness, alcoholism, or drug abuse problems
> Caregiver has inadequate financial resources
> Caregiver has health problems (Acierno et al., 2010; American Medical Association, 1992; Cohen, 2008; Cooper et al., 2006; National Research Council, 2003; Shugarman et al., 2003; Vida, Monks, & Des Rosiers, 2002)

Elder abuse can occur across all settings and can be recognized by nurses and other healthcare workers, as well as others not in the healthcare field (see **Table 23-5**). It affects elders without respect to their residence, socioeconomic status, or geographic

TABLE 23-5   Indications of Possible Mistreatment or Abuse
Poor hygiene
Unexplained bruises of different stages of healing
Broken bones
Malnutrition
Dehydration
Depressed mood
Withdrawn, fearful, cowering
History of treatment in a variety of facilities and by different physicians
Person is left alone in the home frequently
Person is brought for treatment by someone other than the caregiver
Elder expresses feelings of hopelessness, helplessness
Elder expresses ambivalent feelings toward family

location. As the baby boomer population continues to increase, the potential for elder abuse is certain to rise.

There are many screening tools or suggested questions for assessment related to elder abuse. Most tools share common questions directed to the older adult regarding feelings of safety, having basic needs met, feeling threatened, and the like. A careful physical exam with observation of behavior, emotion, and cognition is also common to most instruments used for screening. Most elder abuse screening tools appeared in publication in the mid-1990s and early 2000s. The National Center for Elder Abuse/Administration on Aging (n.d.) provides an annotated list of nearly 75 tools developed between the dates of 1995 and 2005, available at http://www.ncea .aoa.gov/main_site/library/cane/CANE_Series/CANE_EA_Assessment2.aspx. A few examples of screening tools will be discussed in this section.

One example of an early screening tool is the the *Hwalek–Sengstock Elder Abuse Screening Test* (Davies, 1993). It has 3 categories for a total of 15 of questions: violation of personal right or direct abuse, characteristics of vulnerability, and potentially abusive situation. Davies (1993) developed the Elder Abuse Assessment Protocol. This one-page form includes prompts for general assessment physical assessment (lists spaces to write about bruises, abrasions, lesions, alopecia, burns) with empty body figures to note locations of injuries. Davies's tool also requires a cognitive emotional assessment, an observation for sexual abuse, and discussion of the relationship with the carer. A complimentary tool called the Carer Abuse Assessment Protocol (Davies, 1993) also prompts the nurse to assess the carer; observe the caregiver's attitude; look for evidence of dependence on drugs or alcohol, family violence, or mental illness; and assess behavior with the patient while visiting. The caregiver's knowledge and living situation is also assessed. These tools provide an excellent place to begin when addressing the potential for abuse or mistreatment of an older adult.

Fulmer (2012) developed the Elder Assessment Instrument (EAI) to help nurses identify elder abuse and neglect. The EAI is a 41-item Likert scale that has been used in research since the 1980s and is appropriate for use in all clinical settings. The tool has good reliability and validity. The instrument takes about 12–15 minutes to use (Fulmer, 2012). The EAI can be easily accessed at no cost through the Hartford Foundation's *Try This Series* at http://consultgerirn.org/uploads/File/trythis/try_this_15.pdf.

Regardless of what tool is chosen to screen for elder abuse or mistreatment, it is important that facilities adopt some type of consistent measure to assess for this common problem. Some organizations have a few specific questions about abuse built into their admitting documentation. Those facilities providing care to older adults are responsible for assuring that this issue is not overlooked. Gerontological nurses can help to facilitate the use of appropriate screening tools but sharing information with their peers and administrators.

Recognizing the Signs and Symptoms of Elder Abuse or Mistreatment

To recognize the signs and symptoms of elder abuse or mistreatment, is may be helpful to think of the categories mentioned earlier and reviewed in general here. The reader will recall that *physical abuse* is the use of physical force that may result in bodily injury, physical pain, or impairment. Signs and symptoms may include bruising, welts, fractures, and/or open wounds. Bruises of various colors (in various stages of healing) are a key sign of abuse. There may be internal injuries present. The description of the injury should fit what is observed by the health professional; if it does not match, then suspicion of abuse should arise. Laboratory results may indicate medication overuse or underuse. The elder adult may exhibit a sudden change in behavior or the caregiver may refuse to allow visitors to see the older adult alone. (National Center on Elder Abuse [NCEA], 2010) (see **Table 23-6**).

Sexual abuse is the nonconsensual sexual contact of any kind with an older adult. This can include unwanted touching, rape, sodomy, forced nudity, and sexual photography. Signs and symptoms include sudden withdrawn behavior, bruising around breasts and genitals, unexplained sexually transmitted diseases, unexplained vaginal or anal bleeding, or torn or bloody undergarments. The nurse should observe the patient walking and sitting to assess for any signs of pain or discomfort that might indicate sexual abuse.

Neglect is the refusal or failure to fulfill any part of a person's obligations or duties to an older adult. It can be manifested in many ways, such as through failure to provide for the basic necessities of care. Some of the common signs are dehydration and malnourishment. Also included are untreated pressure

---

TABLE 23-6 **The Three Rs In Detecting and Reporting Elderly Abuse**

RECOGNIZE

- Risk Factors: Older age, dementia, depression, isolation, caregiver strain
- Types of Abuse: Physical, sexual, emotional, financial exploitation, neglect, and abandonment
- Signs and symptoms: Signs of physical harm (e.g., bruising), agitation, withdrawn behavior, under/overuse of medications, malnutrition, dehydration, unkempt appearance, poor living conditions, sudden changes in financial matters, unmet needs despite financial ability to provide.
- Never ignore an older adult's report of abuse.

RESPOND

- Perform a thorough assessment.
- If abuse is suspected, follow facility protocol.
- Meet with care team or social worker for further guidance.
- Check state laws regarding mandatory reporting and how to handle if adult is competent and able to report abuse, but doesn't wish to.

REPORT

- The care team or social worker will meet with patient/abuse reporter regarding intent to report.
- The type of abuse will determine which departments will be involved and notified of the case (e.g., adult protective service, law enforcement).
- After intent to report has been made, follow up according to facility policy.
- Provide accurate and detailed documentation.
- Provide assistance for nonmedical personnel in reporting abuse by referring them to abuse hotlines, which can be found on National Center on Elder Abuse website.
- Refer to local adult protective agencies and/or ombudsman programs.

---

ulcer sores and untreated/unattended health problems. Unsafe and unclean living conditions are also a form of neglect.

Emotional/psychological abuse is the infliction of anguish, pain, or distress through verbal or nonverbal acts. This would include humiliating or isolating the older adult, as well as berating. It can also include threats or treating an older adult like a child. Passive-aggressive behavior on the part of the caregivers can also be emotionally abusive when they deliberately change the expected routine to upset the elderly. Older adults may exhibit symptoms such as being emotionally upset and agitated, along with withdrawing from social interactions. They may even exhibit unusual behaviors, such as rocking in place or biting.

Desertion of an older person by an individual who has assumed responsibility for providing care for the older adult, or by a person with physical custody is considered **abandonment**. The deserter can be a family member, caregiver, or employee of a facility. This is considered "dumping" and can occur at a hospital, nursing home, or mall.

Financial or material exploitation is the illegal or improper use of the older adult's funds, property, or assets. A sudden change in banking practice or bank accounts is often the first sign. Beware of an abrupt change in the will or other financial documents. Financial exploitation could be stealing an older adult's money or cashing an older adult's checks without permission. Lack of appropriate clothing, food, or housing when the older adult has the resources available to be financially stable is a key sign of financial exploitation. Sometimes caregivers or families force or deceive an older adult into signing documents.

The Role of the Gerontological Nurse in Reporting Elder Abuse

Reporting elder abuse is an obligation of healthcare providers. Elder adults, by the nature of the increased health problems, visit hospitals and doctors' offices frequently. This means that healthcare providers, and especially nurses, have a greater opportunity than others to recognize when elder abuse may be occurring (see **Boxes 23–1** and **23–2**).

Specific laws for reporting elder abuse vary from state to state. The Older Americans Act of 1965 in the United States (U.S. Administration on Aging, 2010), and the Theft Act 1968 and Mental Capacity Act 2005 in the United Kingdom (Griffith & Tengnah, 2008), are some of the laws in place to protect the elderly.

Abuse hotlines are listed on the NCEA website at http://www.ncea.aoa.gov for state resources. In life-threatening situations, utilize the 911 emergency alert system. When in a professional setting, the facility's protocol for reporting elder abuse to the proper authorities should be followed. It is worthwhile to note that accurate and detailed documentation of events and assessments is critical in such cases. Table 23-6 provides strategies for nurses when dealing with possible elder abuse.

For cases that occur in institutions, often the agency that licenses the residential facility is the state Department of Health. It is the gerontological nurse's responsibility to know the appropriate course of action in the state in which he or she practices. Proper follow through, with adequate security protection for the abuse victim and the abuse reporter and with appropriate interventions, must be in place.

BOX 23-1   Web Resources

Elder Abuse Prevention Clinical Practice Guideline:

http://www.guideline.gov/content.aspx?id=34018&search=elder+abuse

Hartford Institute for Geriatric Nursing:

http://www.consultgerirn.com/topics/elder_mistreatment_and_abuse/want_to_know_more

JAMA Patient Teaching Page:

http://jama.ama-assn.org/content/306/5/568.full.pdf+html

MetLife Study of Elder Financial Abuse:

https://www.metlife.com/mmi/research/elder-financial-abuse.html#key%20findings

National Center on Elder Abuse:

http://www.ncea.aoa.gov/Main_Site/pdf/publication/FinalStatistics050331.pdf

The National Center on Elder Abuse/Administration on Aging:

http://www.ncea.aoa.gov/main_site/library/cane/CANE_Series/CANE_EA_Assessment2.aspx

---

BOX 23-2   Clinical Practice Guidelines: Elder Abuse Prevention

This clinical practice guideline (CPG) for elder abuse prevention provides a synthesis and evaluation of existing evidence on elder abuse, with a focus on nursing interventions for prevention. The CPG was developed through the University of Iowa College of Nursing, John A. Hartford Foundation Center for Geriatric Excellence, in Iowa City, Iowa. The levels of evidence are provided and the methods discussed. The literature was searched using key terms via databases and hand searches through December 31, 2008 for the most current evidence available at the time. A systematic review of current evidence was performed using expert external reviewers who were selected by a panel. In addition, two outside expert reviewers examined the CPG prior to publication. The practice guideline was updated in 2010 and is available at http://www.guideline.gov/content.aspx?id=34018&search=elder+abuse#Section405

Sometimes healthcare providers do not report abuse because of fear of repercussion, especially if the investigation turns out to be negative. To combat this fear, geriatric nurses need to become very knowledgeable and comfortable with the laws in their state and adult protective services regulations. A person will likely not get into trouble for reporting suspicions of abuse. In fact, there will be greater blame for failure to report if the scenario turns out to be real. Forty-four states have a provision for penalties for failure to report elder abuse. Iowa is the only state that has mandatory education for reporters.

The gerontological nurse should also work in collaboration with other members of the healthcare team, notably physicians, social workers, chaplains, and psychiatrists to help determine whether elder abuse is present. Interviews with the victim and the possible offender should be done separately. Benefits of the care team include support during difficult decisions; reduction of duplicity, burnout, and workload; improved safety for the victims; and earlier intervention (Brandt, Dyer, Heisler, Otto, & Thomas, 2007). The team should meet with victim and the reporter, notifying him/her of the intent to report.

The nurse's core responsibility is to report suspected elder abuse, not to confirm the abuse. The nurse does not need to analyze the intention of the abuser. The nurse's role is to protect the rights of older adults, treating them with dignity and respect, while providing appropriate care.

Summary

All gerontological nurses should be educated in the prevention, detection, and treatment of elder abuse. Content on this topic should be included in all basic nursing programs. Better mechanisms are needed for reporting abuse and neglect of older adults. Nurses should be aware of the reporting laws for the state in which they reside and practice.

Elder abuse occurs across many socioeconomics groups and settings. Older adults, particularly those with dementia, are often marginalized and stripped of their dignity in today's society. This is our duty, our obligation, and our privilege as gerontological nurses to protect the treasure of our older generation and value all that they have to offer us. The responsibility rests with all of us. The gerontological nurse can lead the way.

Critical Thinking Exercises

1. Have you ever worked with a patient, resident, or older adult living in the community who was a victim of mistreatment or abuse? If so, what type of mistreatment was it?

2. Using the case studies presented in this chapter, identify the various types of elder abuse.

3. Read the Fact Sheet from the National Center on Elder Abuse at http://www.ncea.aoa.gov/Main_Site/pdf/publication/FinalStatistics050331.pdf. What statistics are particularly striking to you as a nurse?

4. What type of abuse do you think is most prevalent in the areas where you live and work? Why?

5. Of the risk factors for elder abuse identified in this chapter, which are the ones that you have seen the most in older adults in the clinical setting? In the community? In long-term care?

6. Find the phone number and website for Adult Protective Services for your state. Browse the website.

7. Analyze the patient educational page from the *Journal of the American Medical Association* (JAMA) found at http://jama.ama-assn.org/content/306/5/568.full.pdf+html. Is this a tool that you could use in your practice? How would you improve upon it?

Personal Reflections

1. What is one strategy that you could use from this chapter to prevent elder abuse or mistreatment in the patient or resident population where you work?

2. How do you feel when you hear about abuse of older adults in the media?

3. If you recognized financial abuse of an older parent or grandparent occurring in your family, what action would you take?

4. What are the laws regarding reporting suspected abuse in the state in which you live?

References

Acierno, R., Hernandez, M. A., Amstadter, A. B., Resnick, H. S., Steve, K., Muzzy, W., & Kilpatrick, D. G. (2010). Prevalence and correlates of emotional, physical, sexual and financial abuse and potential neglect in the United States: The National Elder Mistreatment Study. *American Journal of Public Health, 100*, 292–297.

American Medical Association [AMA]. (1992). *Diagnostic and treatment guidelines on elder abuse and neglect.* Chicago, IL: Author.

Baker, M. W., LaCroix, A.Z., Wu, C., Cochrane, B. B., Wallace, R., & Woods, N. F. (2009). Mortality risk associated with physical and verbal abuse in women aged 50 to 79. *Journal of the American Geriatrics Society, 57*, 1799–1809.

Barnett, O. W., Miller-Perrin, C. L., & Perrin, R. D. (1997). *Family violence across the lifespan.* Thousand Oaks, CA: Sage.

Brandt, B., Dyer, C. B. Heisler, C. J., Otto, J. M., & Thomas, R. W. (2007) *Elder abuse detection and intervention: A collaborative approach,* New York, NY: Springer.

Buckwalter, S. C., Campbell, J., Gerdner, L.A., & Garand, L. (1996). Elder mistreatment among rural family caregivers of persons with Alzheimer's disease and related disorders. *Journal of Family Nursing, 2*(3), 249–265.

Centers for Disease Control and Prevention [CDC]. (2010). *Understanding elder mistreatment.* Retrieved from http://www.cdc.gov/violenceprevention/pdf/EM-FactSheet-a.pdf

Cohen, M. (2008). Research assessment of elder neglect and its risk factors in a hospital setting. *Internal Medicine Journal, 38*, 704–707.

Cooper, C., Katona, C., Finne-Soveri, H., Topinkova, E., Carpenter, G. I., & Livingston, G. (2006). Indicators of elder abuse: A crossnational comparison of psychiatric morbidity and other determinants in the Ad-HOC study. *American Journal of Geriatric Psychiatry, 14*, 489–497.

Cooper, C., Mandela, M., Katona, C., & Livingston, G. (2008). Screening for elder abuse in dementia in the LASER-AD study: Prevalence, correlates and validation of instruments. *International Journal of Geriatric Psychiatry, 23*, 283–288.

Daly, J. M. (2010). *Elder abuse prevention.* Retrieved from http://www.guideline.gov/content.aspx?id=34018&search=elder+abuse#Section405

Daly, J. M. (2011). Evidence-based practice guideline: Elder abuse prevention. *Journal of Gerontological Nursing, 37*(11), 11–17.

Decalmer, P., & Glendenning, F. (Eds). (1993). *The mistreatment of elderly people.* London, UK: Sage.

Dong, X., Simon, M., Rajan, K., & Evans, D. A. (2011). Association of cognitive function and risk for elder abuse in a community-dwelling population. *Dementia & Geriatric Cognitive Disorders, 32*(3), 209–215.

Frost, M. H. & Willette, K. (1994). Risk for abuse/neglect: Documentation of assessment data and diagnoses. *Journal of Gerontological Nursing, 29*(8), 37–45.

Fulmer, T. & Greenberg, S. (2012). *Elder mistreatment and abuse.* Retrieved from http://www .consultgerirn.com/topics/elder_mistreatment_and_abuse/want_to_know_more

Fulmer, T. (2012). *Elder mistreatment assessment.* Retrieved from http://consultgerirn.org/uploads/File/trythis/try_this_15.pdf

Gibbons, S. Lauder, W., & Ludwick, R. (2006). Self-neglect: A proposed new NANDA diagnosis. *International Journal of Nursing Terminologies and Classifications, 17*(1), 10–18.

Davies, M. (1993). Recognizing abuse: An assessment tool for nurses. In P. Decalmer & F. Glendenning (Eds.) *The mistreatment of elderly people,* (p. 116). London: Sage.

Dyer, C. B., Goodwin, J. S., Pickens-Pace, S. Burnett, J., & Kelly, P. A. (2007). Self-neglect among the elderly: A model based on more than 500 patients seen by a geriatric medicine team. *American Journal of Public Health, 97*(9), 1971–1676.

Dyer, C. B., Pavlik, V. N., Murphy, K. P., & Hyman, D. J. (2000). The high prevalence of depression and dementia in elder abuse or neglect. *Journal of the American Geriatrics Society*, 48(2), 205-208.

Griffith, R., & Tengnah, C. (2008). *Mental capacity act 2005:* lasting powers of attorney. *British Journal of Community Nursing*, 12, 577–81.

Hildreth, C. J. (2011). Elder abuse. *Journal of the American Medical Association, 306*(5), 568.

Hocking, E. D. (1988). Miscare: A form of abuse in the elderly. *Update, 15,* 2411–2419.

Lachs, M. S., Williams, C. S., O'Brien, S., Pillemer, K. A., & Charleson, M. E. (1998). The mortality of elder mistreatment. *Journal of the American Medical Society, 280,* 428–432.

McGarry, J., & Simpson, C. (2011). Domestic abuse and older women: Exploring the opportunities for service development and care delivery. *Journal of Adult Protection, 13*(6), 294–301.

MetLife. (2012a). *The MetLife Study of Elder Financial Abuse.* Retrieved from https://www.metlife.com/mmi/research/elder-financial-abuse.html#key%20findings

MetLife. (2012b). *Broken trust: Elders, family, & finances.* Retrieved from http://www.metlife.com/mmi/research/broken-trust-elder-abuse.html#findings

Mauk, K. L. (2011). Ethical perspectives on self-neglect among older adults. *Rehabilitation Nursing, 36*(2), 60–65.

National Center on Elder Abuse. (n.d.). Identifying Elder Abuse: Tools, techniques, and guidelines for screening and assessment. Retrieved from http://www.ncea.aoa.gov/main_site/library/cane/CANE_Series/CANE_EA_Assessment2.aspx

National Center on Elder Abuse. (2010). *Why should I care about elder abuse?* Retrieved from http://www .ncea.aoa.gov/ncearoot/Main_Site/pdf/publication/NCEA_WhatIsAbuse-2010.pdf

National Research Council. (2003). *Elder mistreatment: Abuse, neglect and exploitation in an aging America.* Retrieved from http://www.nap.edu/openbook.php?isbn=0309084342

Pillemer, K. A., & Suitor, J. J. (1992). Violence and violent feelings: What causes them among family caregivers? *Journal of Gerontology: Social Sciences, 47*(4), 165–172.

Pritchard, J. (1995). *The abuse of older people: A training manual for detection and prevention.* London, UK: Jessica Kingsley.

Pritchard, J. (1996). Darkness visible…elder abuse. *Nursing Times, 92*(42), 26–31.

Quinn, M. J., & Tomita, S. K. (1986). Elder abuse and neglect. New York, NY: Springer.

Reyes-Ortiz, C. A. (2006). Self-neglect as a geriatric syndrome. *Journal of the American Geriatrics Society, 54*(12), 1945–1975.

Rosen, T., Pillemer, K., & Lachs, M. (2008). Resident-to-resident aggression in long-term care facilities: An understudied problem. *Aggression and Violent Behavior, 13*(2), 77–87.

Saveman, B., Hallberg, I. R., & Norberg, A. (1996). Narratives by district nurses about elder abuse within families. *Clinical Nursing Research*, 5, 220–236.

Sengstock, M. C. & Barrett, S. A. (1992). Abuse and neglect of the elderly in family settings. In J. Campbell & J. Humphreys (Eds.), *Nursing care of the survivors of family violence* (pp. 173–208). St. Louis, MO: Mosby.

Shugarman, L. R., Fries, B. E., Wolf, R. S. & Morris, J. N. (2003). Identifying older people at risk of abuse during routine screening practices, *Journal of the American Geriatric Society, 51,* 24–31.

Stark, S. W. (2011). Blind, deaf, and dumb: Why elder abuse goes unidentified. *Nursing Clinics of North America, 46*(4), 431–4366.

Thobaben, M. (1996). Beyond physical care. Elder abuse and neglect. *Home Care Provider, 5,* 267–269.

Tomlin, S. K. (1989). *Abuse of elderly people: An unnecessary and preventable problem.* London, UK: British Geriatrics Society.

U.S. Administration on Aging (2010). Older American's Act. Retrieved from http://www.aoa.gov/AoA_programs/OAA/index.aspx

Vida, S., Monks, R. C., & Des Rosiers, P. (2002). Prevalence and correlates of elder abuse and neglect in a geriatric psychiatric service. *Canadian Journal of Psychiatry, 47,* 459–467.

Wierucka, C. & Goodridge, D. (1996). Vulnerable in a safe place: Institutional elder abuse. *Canadian Journal of Nursing Administration, 9*(3), 82–104.

Wilson, J. S. (1992). Granny dumping: A case of caregiver stress or a problem relative? *Home Healthcare Nurse, 10*(3), 69–70.

World Health Organization (n.d.). Elder abuse. Retrieved from http://www.who.int/ageing/projects/elder_abuse/en/

Zhang, Z., et al. (2011). *Neglect of Older Adults in Michigan Nursing Homes. Journal of Elder Abuse and Neglect, 23*(1), 58–74.

For a full suite of assignments and additional learning activities, see the access code at the front of your book.

LEARNING OBJECTIVES

At the end of this chapter, the reader will be able to:

> Explain what constitutes complimentary and alternative medicine (CAM).
> Explain each classification of CAM.
> Discuss nursing interventions associated with the most popular herbal products.
> Compare the benefits and drawbacks of the diets identified under natural products.
> Distinguish the differences between veritable and putative energy fields.
> Discuss why older adults may use CAM.
> Contrast Ayurveda and traditional Chinese medicine (TCM) systems.
> Discuss the benefits and supports for mind–body interventions.

KEY TERMS

Acupuncture

Ayurveda

Biofeedback

Chiropractic practice

Dosha

Guided imagery

Homeopathy

Massage therapy

Meditation

Mind–body medicine

Music therapy

Natural products

Naturopathic medicine

Pet-assisted therapy

Prayer

Putative energy field

Qi (chi)

Reiki

Sound energy therapy

Therapeutic (healing) touch

Traditional Chinese medicine

Veritable energy field

Yang

Yin

Chapter 24

(Competencies 8, 9,18)

Alternative Health Modalities

Carole A. Pepa

The use of complementary and alternative medicine (CAM) has been steadily increasing in both the United States and worldwide (National Center for Complementary and Alternative Medicine, [NCCAM], 2012e). Although the 2007 statistics do not breakdown CAM use by older adults specifically, the widespread use of CAM therapies among those 65 years of age or older previously was documented by Ness, Cirillo, Weir, Nisly, and Wallace (2005). The widespread use of CAM therapies requires healthcare providers to be knowledgeable about these modalities and to educate clients and patients about the safety of their use. See **Table 24-1** for a list of the most commonly used CAM therapies.

What Is Complementary and Alternative Medicine?

According to NCCAM, CAM "is a group of diverse medical and health care systems, practices, and products that are not presently considered part of conventional medicine" in the United States (NCCAM, 2012f, para. 2). In their classic article on unconventional medicine in the United States, Eisenberg et al. (1993) defined unconventional or alternative therapies as "medical interventions not taught widely at U.S. medical schools or generally available at U.S. hospitals" (p. 246). Although considered alternative or complementary in the United States, many of the modalities under this umbrella term are considered mainstream medicine in other countries (Bielory, 2002). In addition, the definition of what is complementary or alternative today may be considered a mainstream modality in the future (NCCAM, 2012f). CAM is used to treat illness and promote health and well-being, as well as to gain more control over one's health (Barnes, Bloom, & Nahin, 2008; National Institutes of Health [NIH] Senior Health, 2012).

TABLE 24-1	CAM Most Identified Mind-Body Therapies Ranked by Reported Use
Prayed for own health	52.1%
Others ever prayed for your health	31.3
Participate in a prayer group	23.0
Deep breathing exercises	14.6
Meditation	10.2
Yoga	7.5
Healing ritual for own health	4.6
Progressive relaxation	4.2
Guided imagery	3.0
Tai Chi	2.5
Hypnosis	1.8
Energy healing therapy (Reiki)	1.1
Biofeedback	1.0
Qi gong	0.5

Source: Barnes, P. M., Powell-Griner, E., McFann, K., & Nahin, R. L. (2004). CDC Advance data report # 343. Complementary and alternative medicine use among adults: United States, 2002. Betheseda, MD: Author.

Classifications of Complementary and Alternative Medicine

NCAAM classifies complementary and alternative medicine (CAM) into broad categories: (a) *natural products*, (b) manipulative and body-based practices, (c) *mind–body medicine*, and (d) other, which includes various energy fields and whole medical systems (NCCAM, 2012f; NIH Senior Health, 2012). These categories are somewhat different from how NCCAM had previously categorized the various CAM therapies. Since the categories are not mutually exclusive, some CAM practices may fit into more than one category. In addition, the categories are only broadly defined.

Natural Products

This broad category was previously referred to as biologically based therapies. It includes botanicals, animal-derived extracts, vitamins, minerals, fatty acids, proteins, prebiotics and probiotics, whole diets, and functional foods (NCCAM, 2012f). Vegetarian, macrobiotic, Atkins, Pritikin, Ornish, and Zone are examples of whole diets included in the biologically based category (see **Table 24-2**). Although some whole diet therapies may be used to prevent or treat health conditions, others may not provide all the micronutrients an individual may need. This is especially true of fad diets. Nurses should include questions about whole diet practices in their assessments.

Dietary supplements, which may include vitamins; minerals; herbs or other botanicals; amino acids; and substances such as enzymes, organ tissues, glandulars, and metabolites, are a subset of this category (Biologically Based Therapies, 2009; NCCAM, 2012f). According to Barnes, Bloom, and Nahin (2008), nonvitamins and nonmineral natural products were the most commonly used CAM therapies. Barnes et al. report that nearly 18% of adults who used complementary and alternative medicine within the past year used nonvitamin and natural products, while 3.6% used diet therapies. In 2002, 2.8% used megavitamin therapy; however, in 2007 use was too small to measure (Barnes et al., 2008). Because this category includes natural products, individuals, particularly the elderly, may have the mistaken belief that there are no side effects or concerns in using these products. However, caution must be taken in using these products with certain prescribed medications. The ingredients listed on the labels of dietary supplements may be long and printed in a font size difficult for the older adult to read easily. Consequently, ingredients with the potential for interactions with medications could be overlooked.

TABLE 24-2	Popular Diets Listed Under Biologically Based Therapies
Diet	**Description**
Atkins	Emphasizes low carbohydrates (40 g or less) with an increase in fat and protein (Barnes et al., 2004).
Macrobiotic	Low-fat diet emphasizes whole grains and vegetables and a decrease in fluid intake. Meat, dairy products, eggs, alcohol, sugar, sweets, coffee, and caffeinated tea are avoided.
Ornish	High-fiber, low-fat vegetarian diet promotes weight loss by restricting the types of food rather than calories.
Pritikin	Low-fat (10% or less) diet emphasizes consumption of foods with a large volume of fiber and water (low in calorie density). Diet includes many vegetables, fruits, beans, and unprocessed grains.
Zone	Each meal consists of 30% low fat protein, 30% fat, and 40% fiber-rich fruits and vegetables. The goal of this diet is to control key hormone production to alter metabolism.
Vegetarian	Diet excludes meat, fish, fowl, or products containing these foods.
Lacto-ovo-vegetarian	Diet is based on grains, vegetables, fruit, seeds, nuts, legumes, dairy products, and eggs. It excludes meat, fish, and fowl.
Lacto-vegetarian	Diet excludes eggs, meat, fish, and fowl, but includes dairy.
Vegan vegetarian	Diet excludes dairy, eggs, meat, fish, fowl, and other animal products.

Source: Mangels, Messina, & Melina, 2003.

Vitamins are compounds the body needs to maintain health. The concern, however, is that some individuals believe that "if a little is good, more must be better," and they take megadoses of vitamins. A list of potential risks of large doses of vitamins is found in **Table 24-3**. Vitamin deficiencies can also cause problems beyond those related to vitamin action. For example, older adults may have difficulty absorbing vitamin B_{12} from unfortified foods, but can absorb the vitamin from fortified foods and supplements. A vitamin B_{12} deficiency may mimic signs of dementia, including memory loss, disorientation, hallucinations, and tingling in the arms and legs (Office of Dietary Supplements, 2011). A daily vitamin from a reliable manufacturer that supplies nearly 100% of the daily requirements is a good choice for older adults.

Table 24-4 displays the 10 most commonly used natural products identified by those who used complementary and alternate medicine in the year preceding the 2007 National Health Interview Survey (NHIS). Actions, uses, and contraindications for these products are also included. In addition to those natural products listed in Table 24-3, other medicinal herbs also are popular. Valerian (or valerian root) is used as a sedative and sleep aid. It should not be used in conjunction with alcohol, sedatives, and antianxiety medication. Side effects include mild headache or upset stomach. It is not addictive, and should not be used by mothers who are breastfeeding (Zauderer & Davis, 2012). Kava (*Piper methysticum*) has been shown to relax skeletal muscles. It is used for anxiety, stress, restlessness, and insomnia; it is not addictive, and its use is contraindicated in individuals with liver disease or depression (Zauderer & Davis, 2012). It should not be used with antidepressives, alcohol, or tranquilizers. Side effects include dizziness, headache, drowsiness, and hepatic toxicity (Deglin & Vallerand, 2007). Saw palmetto has been used for treating

TABLE 24-3 Potential Side Effects of Large Doses of Vitamins	
Vitamin	**Side Effects of Large Doses**
A (retinol)	Nausea, vomiting, headache, dizziness, blurred vision, possible risk of osteoporosis (U. S. Food and Drug Administration, 2007). Beta carotene (a precursor to vitamin A) is less toxic than preformed A (retinol) at high levels of intake (Vitamins, 2007).
B_3 (niacin)	Flushing, redness of skin, upset stomach (U. S. Food and Drug Administration, 2007).
B_6 (pyridoxine)	Nerve damage to limbs (U.S. Food and Drug Administration, 2007).
C (ascorbic acid)	Upset stomach, kidney stones, increased iron absorption (U.S. Food and Drug Administration, 2007).
D (calciferol)	Nausea, vomiting, poor appetite, constipation, weight loss, confusion (U.S. Food and Drug Administration, 2007).
Folic acid (folate)	Hides signs of vitamin B_{12} deficiency (U.S. Food and Drug Administration, 2007).

TABLE 24-4   Ten Most Often Used Natural Products

Name	Actions/Use	Contraindications/Side Effects
Echinacea purpurea (Echinacea)	Anti-infective; stimulates immune response Uses: treatment and prevention of coughs, colds, flu, and bronchitis; wounds and burns; fevers	May interfere with immunosuppressant drugs; contraindicated in diseases related to immune response, multiple sclerosis, tuberculosis, AIDS, and autoimmune diseases Should not be used for more than 8-week intervals or immune system may be depressed (Deglin & Vallerand, 2007)
Panax ginseng (Asian ginseng) *Panax quinquefolius* (American ginseng)	Uses: improve physical and mental stamina; treatment of diabetes; sedative; aphrodisiac; increase immune response; increase appetite	May decrease effectiveness of warfarin; may interfere with MAO inhibitors; may have hypoglycemic effects; caffeine may increase herb effect; use with caution with estrogen; may increase risk of bleeding if used with antiplatelet herbs; may prolong QT interval if used with bitter orange; may interfere with immunosuppressant therapy Side effects: agitation, insomnia, tachycardia, depression, hypertension (Deglin & Vallerand, 2007)
Gingko biloba (Gingko) Standardized: 24% flavonoid glycosides 6% terpenela-ctones	Uses: symptomatic relief of organic brain dysfunction; intermittent claudication; vertigo and tinnitus (vascular origin); sexual dysfunction; improve peripheral circulation	Use with caution if individuals are on anticoagulant or antiplatelet therapy or have diabetes Contraindicated if individuals have bleeding disorders or increased blood sugars Side effects: headache, dizziness, GI disturbances
Garlic supplements	Vasodilator, antiplatelet properties Uses: hypertension, lowering cholesterol	May increase bleeding; not as effective in lowering cholesterol as other medications (Deglin & Vallerand, 2007)
Glucosamine	May stimulate cartilage growth Use: osteoarthritis	Contraindicated if shellfish allergy is present May interfere with glucose regulation in diabetics (Deglin & Vallerand, 2007)
St. John's wort (*Hypericum perforatum*)	Antidepressant; when used topically, may have antiviral, anti-inflammatory, antibacterial activity Uses: mild to moderate depression	Alcohol and other antidepressives may increase CNS side effects Side effects: dizziness, restlessness, sleep disturbance, hypertension, bloating, abdominal pain, flatulence (Deglin & Vallerand, 2007)

(continues)

TABLE 24-4   Ten Most Often Used Natural Products (*continued*)

Name	Actions/Use	Contraindications/Side Effects
Peppermint	Muscle relaxant, particularly in the digestive tract; reduces inflammation in nasal passages Uses: irritable bowel syndrome, nausea and vomiting, congestion related to colds and allergies	May cause choking feeling if applied to chest or nostrils of a child under 5; may intensify symptoms in hiatal hernia; avoid large doses if pregnant because it can relax uterine muscles Side effects: none identified (Supplements: Peppermint, n.d.)
Fish oils/omega fatty acids	May decrease risk of coronary artery disease; may protect against irregular heartbeats Uses: protect against heart disease	None
Ginger supplements	Inhibit platelets, prostaglandins; improve digestion, appetite; may be hypoglycemic Uses: nausea and vomiting; joint pain	Use with caution in patients with bleeding tendencies or on anticoagulant therapy or with diabetics
Soy supplements	Lowers total cholesterol and low-density lipoprotein (LDL)	Side effects: heartburn Controversy that isoflavones, a component of soy, are phytoestrogens, a weak estrogen, and may increase cancer risk; other evidence supports that soy may protect against breast cancer (Henkel, 2000)

benign prostatic hyperplasia (BPH), and early studies supported its efficacy (Ernst, 2002; Gordon & Shaughnessy, 2003; Wilt, Ishani, & MacDonald, 2002). However, in a systematic review, Tacklind, MacDonald, Tutks, Stanke, & Wilt (2009) determined that saw palmetto was no different than a placebo in controlling symptoms of BPH. Side effects of this herb include mild gastrointestinal upset; there are no reported drug interactions. The biggest concern about the use of saw palmetto is that individuals may self-medicate without verifying the diagnosis of BPH; because of this, more serious diseases of the prostate could be missed. Capsaicin cream, derived from hot peppers, is used topically to relieve pain from neuralgias, osteoarthritis, rheumatoid arthritis; back pain; and nerve pain, among other conditions. Capsaicin produces a stinging or burning sensation when initially used. Clients should be instructed to keep capsaicin away from the eyes and other sensitive areas of the body. Randomized control studies supported capsaicin use over the use of placebo (Wong, 2006).

Even though herbs are natural products, some medicinal herbs have side effects that could adversely affect the elderly. Yohimbe, for example, is used to treat impotence. Although it has been shown to be effective, it is not recommended by the U.S. Food and Drug Administration (FDA). When combined with tricyclic antidepressants, side effects include hypertension, renal failure, seizures, hypotension, tachycardia, and dizziness. Comfrey has been used for gastritis, gastrointestinal ulcers, rheumatism, bronchitis, internal bleeding, diarrhea, and sprains and pulled ligaments. Because of the potential side effect of liver toxicity, however, the FDA has identified comfrey as a possible health hazard. In 2001, the FDA required oral comfrey removed from all dietary supplement products. Although topical products containing comfrey are available, comfrey should not be applied to open wounds or on broken skin (University of Maryland Medical Center, 2007). The FDA also proposed a limit to the amount of ephedrine alkaloids in dietary supplements (ephedra, Ma Huang, Chinese ephedra). The use of ephedra has been linked with nervousness, dizziness, heart attack, stroke, seizures, and death (NCCAM, 2012b). Consumers must be instructed to read labels because ephedra may be an ingredient in supplements imported from other countries.

Although most herbal medications are safe when used as recommended, the concern is that many older adults do not tell their nurse practitioners, physicians, or other healthcare providers about the botanicals they are taking. This increases the possibility of drug interactions (Marinac et al., 2007). Also, many times healthcare providers do not ask their patients about what natural substances they are taking (Milden & Stokols, 2004). Patients taking prescription drugs such as blood thinners, blood pressure medications, cyclosporine, digoxin, hypoglycemic agents, phenytoin, theophylline, and antidepressants should avoid herbal medications (Kuhn, 2002; Williamson, Fletcher, & Dawson, 2003). In addition, many safety concerns and drug interactions are underresearched in the elderly. Consumers should be cautioned when using herbal remedies to buy only reputable products because the FDA does not regulate herbal manufacturing (see **Case Study 24-1**).

Case Study 24-1

Mr. Walters, 85 years old, is receiving home care following a hospitalization for an exacerbation of congestive heart failure (CHF). He is diagnosed with atrial fibrillation and peripheral vascular disease. His legs are dry with scales; they are discolored from mid-calf to the foot. Both feet are warm to the touch. He was sent home on oxygen at 3 liters with an oxygen concentrator. He is taking the following medications:

Lanoxin 0.125 mg daily

Enteric coated aspirin 325 mg daily

Enalapril 25 mg twice a day

Furosemide 40 mg each morning

Vitamin E 400 IU every day

Gingko biloba 120 mg leaf extract twice a day

Panax ginseng 200 mg every day

Capsaicin to his back and legs when he has been working in the garden

Questions

1. What assessments would the home health nurse make during home visits?

2. What instructions should Mr. Walters receive from the nurse?

3. What would be appropriate follow-up for the next visit?

Manipulative and Body-Based Practices

Manipulative and body-based practices primarily focus on the structures and systems of the body. These practices are not new; some are rooted in traditional medical systems and others have been practiced in the United States for over 150 years. Those practitioners of manipulation and body-based practices believe that parts of the body are interdependent and the body has the ability to heal itself. Chiropractic and osteopathic manipulation, massage therapy, reflexology, and rolfing are examples of practices from this category (NCCAM, 2012a). Both chiropractic care and massage were reported to be among the 10 most-used CAM therapies (Barnes et al., 2008).

Chiropractic practice is considered a holistic approach to health. It is thought to provide benefit by helping place the body in proper alignment. Many third-party payers for healthcare provide some reimbursement for chiropractic care. Although satisfaction with chiropractic care is high (Hertzman-Miller, 2002; NCCAM, 2012a) empirical evidence about the long-term efficacy is mixed (Cherkin, Sherman, Deyo, & Shekelle, 2003; Ernst & Canter, 2003; NCCAM, 2012a). A review of articles by Bryans and colleagues (2011) supported the use of chiropractic care to improve migraine and cervicogenic headaches. However, based on the evidence, the authors could not make a recommendation for the use of spinal manipulation for tension-type headaches (Bryans et al., 2011, p. 282).

Massage therapy dates back thousands of years. It includes various techniques that involve the manipulation of soft tissue through pressure and movement. Massage promotes circulation of blood and lymph, stimulates nerve endings, increases nutrients to the tissues, and removes waste products (Mitzel-Wilkinson, 2000). Many individuals use massage therapy to increase relaxation and reduce stress, recover from muscle stress and strain, heal injuries, and relieve pain. Satisfaction with massage treatments is very high. A Cochrane review by Hillier, Louw, Morris, Uwimana, and Statham (2010) reported that there is some evidence to support the use of massage therapy to improve quality of life for persons living with HIV/AIDS, especially when combined with other stress management modalities. In addition, research studies have supported the use of massage in a variety of situations (Billhult, Bergbom, & Stener-Victorin, 2007; Cutshall et al., 2010; Drackley et al., 2012; Furlan, Brosseau, Imamura, & Irvin, 2008; Gatlin & Schulmeister, 2007). Although massage is considered a low-risk intervention, it is contraindicated under several circumstances, including deep vein thrombosis, burns, skin infections, eczema, open wounds, bone fractures, and advanced osteoporosis (Gatlin & Schulmeister, 2007).

Mind–Body Interventions

Mind–body interventions are among the most widely used of the complementary/ alternative modalities (Barnes et al., 2008). Among the therapies included in this category are prayer, deep breathing, meditation, yoga, biofeedback, tai chi, and guided imagery (Table 24-1). Other modalities that would fit under this category are pet therapy and music therapy. Mind–body interventions acknowledge that emotional, mental, social, spiritual, and behavioral factors can directly affect health (NCCAM, 2012f). The mind–body connection entails two physiological pathways that involve the nervous, immune, and endocrine systems (Maier-Lorentz, 2004). The sympathetic-adrenal-medullary (SAM) pathway activates the autonomic nervous system; neurotransmitters and neuropeptides communicate with the immune cells. The hypothalamic-pituitary-adrenal (HPA) pathway signals the endocrine system to release hormones, particularly thyroid and adrenal, which have a direct effect on the immune system (Maier-Lorentz, 2004). The impact of stressors and hormones on the immune system is discussed in Chapter 6.

Several of the mind–body interventions have their roots in religious traditions, but in the report released by the 2007 National Center for Health Statistics, faith healing or prayer was not a part of this survey (Barnes et al., 2008). Although *prayer* is widely used and accepted by many, research studies as well as Cochrane reviews supporting the value of prayer and healing have led to inconclusive results (Candy et al., 2012; Gundersen, 2000; Maier-Lorentz, 2004; Roberts, Ahmed, Hall, & Davison, 2009; Sending Prayers, 2002; Sicher, Targ, Moore, & Smith, 1998). Difficulties in standardizing methods, including treating prayer, religion, and spirituality as the same concept, may be responsible for some of the mixed results (Gundersen, 2000; Maier-Lorentz, 2004; Roberts et al., 2009). Meditation is closely related to prayer; it is a conscious process that induces the relaxation response (NCCAM, 2010). According to the 2007 National Center for Health Statistics, 9.4% of adults who used CAM in 2006 participated in meditation; this was an increase from the 2002 report (Barnes et al., 2008). There are two common forms of *meditation*. In transcendental meditation (TM), the individual focuses on a mantra, sound, or visual image and is able to quiet the mind by concentrating on this focal point. It is derived from Hindu traditions. The second form of meditation, mindfulness or vipassana meditation, begins with the individual focusing on breathing and continues until he or she develops a nonjudgmental awareness of the present. This form of meditation has roots in Buddhism. Meditation can be practiced by individuals of all ages and has been used to reduce stress, promote relaxation, and remove pain as the main focus of an individual's mind (NCCAM, 2010).

The practice of yoga, which has its roots in India, integrates physical, mental, and spiritual health so that the individual can be in harmony with the universe. There are different schools of yoga, and each has a different focus, but basically yoga combines disciplined breathing, defined gestures, and specific postures (asanas) to achieve a sense of harmony. Although some studies have supported the benefits of yoga for a wide variety of medical conditions and a wide variety of ages (Okonta, 2012; Tilbrook et al., 2011), an integrative review by Li and Goldsmith (2012) indicated mixed results and a need for additional research with larger sample sizes.

Tai Chi is an ancient Chinese martial art. Although it can be used as a method of self-defense, it is practiced by many as an exercise to promote mental tranquility and improve physical fitness, balance, and relaxation (Jimenez, Melendez, & Albers, 2012). The movements in Tai Chi are "circular and rhythmic, and each of the postures moves slowly into the next posture following the sequence of form" (Field, 2011, p 141). A review of 43 articles supported that Tai Chi improved quality of life for participants, but to the same degree as other low to moderate-intensity activities (Jimenez et al., 2012). However Jimenez and associates (2012) indicated that many of the studies reviewed had methodological weaknesses in their designs, and more rigorous research should be conducted in this area. Field (2011) also supported participation in Tai Chi for a variety of mental and physical improvements, but identified methodological weaknesses in the studies reviewed.

Guided imagery is a "directed deliberate daydream that uses all senses to create a focused state of relaxation and a sense of physical and emotional well being" (Gonzales et al., 2010, p. 181). Sights, sounds, smells, or tastes can be used to create mental images to aid in relaxation and manage physical symptoms of stress and anxiety. These self-created mental images, called guided imagery, are considered a powerful self-help technique that is easy to learn and can be used by individuals of all ages (Menzies & Taylor, 2004; Miller, 2003). Guided imagery has been used by patients to decrease the side effects of chemotherapy treatments and to relieve stress and pain. A systematic review by Posadzki, Lewandowski, Terry, Ernst, and Stearns (2012) indicated that guided imagery was helpful in alleviating nonmusculoskeletal pain, but the findings were not conclusive. As with the other CAM therapies in this section, more rigorous research studies must be conducted to decrease the methodological weaknesses.

Biofeedback is now used in traditional therapies as well as complementary and alternative therapies. An individual uses machines to receive information about bodily functions such as skin temperature, brain waves (electroencephalography [EEG]), breathing, blood pressure, and heart rate. This information is in the form of audible or visual signals; the person is trained to focus on controlling the targeted bodily function with reinforcement coming in the form of the audible or visual signals. With practice, the individual becomes more skilled at controlling the targeted function. Eventually, the individual can control the function without the use of the machine to provide feedback. Some studies have demonstrated that biofeedback has been used successfully to control a variety of symptoms such as headaches, chronic pain, hot flashes, and incontinence (Kuhn, 1999). However Yucha et al. (2001) conducted a meta-analysis of 23 studies to determine the effectiveness of biofeedback on hypertension. The results indicated biofeedback resulted in a decrease in both systolic and diastolic blood pressures. However, the authors concluded that more research is needed with larger population sizes.

Another mind–body therapy not listed in the NCCAM categories is pet-assisted therapy, or pet-assisted visitation. *Pet-assisted therapy* and visitation is gaining in popularity, especially with children and older adults. A variety of animals (dogs, cats, horses, and rabbits) have been used to decrease stress and increase feelings of well-being. Although sometimes the terms are used synonymously, animal-assisted therapy is different from animal-assisted visitation. In animal-assisted visitation, certified therapy animals visit patients and families in a common room or at the bedside. A trained professional, on the other hand, performs animal-assisted therapy (Stanley-Hermanns & Miller, 2002). Research studies tend to support the effectiveness of pet-assisted visitation and therapy (Hooker, Freeman, & Stewart, 2002; Stanley-Hermanns & Miller, 2002). To initiate a pet therapy or visitation program, disease prevention strategies must be undertaken. Animals must be examined by a veterinarian to make sure they are free of any diseases or parasites and are up-to-date on vaccinations. Animals should be bathed within 24 hours before visiting and should be under the handler's control at all times (Stanley-Hermanns & Miller, 2002).

Music therapy is becoming more and more popular as a nonpharmacologic intervention to enhance the physical and psychological well-being of individuals in a variety of settings. Aldridge (1994) described two basic types of music therapy: active and passive. In active music therapy, the individual participates in singing or playing a musical instrument with the therapist. Passive music therapy is most often used in clinical settings in the United States. With passive music therapy, the individual listens to recorded music. This music may be chosen for the individual from selections known to provide a calming effect or the individual may make his or her own selections from music provided by the therapist or nurse. A third option is that the individual provides his or her own musical selections from personal favorites. The effect of music therapy on decreasing anxiety or reducing pain has been reported in the literature, and the findings are mixed. Vanderboom (2007) conducted an integrative review to determine if music should be used as an intervention to modify the anxiety-provoking stimuli experienced by patients undergoing interventional radiology procedures. The review identified that the music intervention may be effective in decreasing blood pressure and reducing the need for medication, but the evidence was limited. Richards, Johnson, Sparks, and Emerson (2007) and Daniel, O'Keefe, and Pepa (2002) each conducted reviews of current research related to the effect of music therapy on patients. Both groups of researchers concluded that although music may be helpful in reducing pain and anxiety, the evidence was limited and findings could not be generalized to all patient populations. These findings are consistent with the findings of the systematic review by Cepeda, Carr, Lau, and Alverez (2006), which stated that, although music reduced pain levels and the need for opioids, the magnitude of the benefits was small.

Whole Medical Systems

Whole medical systems "are complete systems of theory and practice that have evolved over time in different cultures and apart from conventional (allopathic) medicine" (NCCAM, 2012f, para. 18). Examples include homeopathic medicine, naturopathic medicine, Ayurvedic medicine, and traditional Chinese medicine.

Homeopathy originated with German physician Dr. Samuel Hahnemann's natural law of "like cures like" or the Principle of Similars (NCCAM, 2012c; Teixeira, 2011). According to homeopathic theory, when a person's vital force or self-healing response is out of balance, health problems will develop. The goal of homeopathy is to stimulate the body's own healing responses to prevent or treat illnesses (NCCAM, 2012c). Homeopathic remedies are prepared by diluting certain substances and then—gradually increasing the dilution until no actual measurement of the original substance exists. Although there are no active ingredients in a homeopathic solution, it helps the body to begin to heal itself by using its own defense mechanisms. Homeopathic remedies are recognized and regulated by the FDA. Remedies are also listed in the *Homoeopathic Pharmacopoeia of the United States.*

Homeopathy has been used to treat illnesses such as respiratory infections, headaches, ear infections, neck stiffness, postoperative infections, dental pain, flu, motion sickness, and general aches and pains as well as sprains, bruises, and burns. The use of homeopathy has been controversial because of how the remedies are created using the dilution process. Research studies designed to support the efficacy of homeopathic remedies have demonstrated mixed results (McCarney, Linde, & Lasserson, 2008; NCCAM, 2012c; Sinha et al., 2012).

Naturopathic medicine focuses on keeping the person healthy as well as treating diseases. It is practiced in Europe, Australia, New Zealand, Canada, and the United States (NCCAM, 2012d). Principles of naturopathy include "(a) the healing power of nature, (b) identification of the cause and treatment of disease, (c) the concept of 'do no harm,' (d) doctor as teacher, (e) treatment of the whole person, and (f) prevention" (NCCAM, 2012d). It encompasses a variety of healing practices, including diet and nutrition, hydrotherapy, spine and soft tissue manipulation, acupuncture and acupressure, herbs, exercise, counseling, and light therapy (NCCAM, 2012d). In naturopathy, if the body is supported and barriers to cure are removed, the body will heal itself. There are minimal isks to naturopathic medicine, but natural healing takes longer than traditional allopathic medicine. Therefore, symptoms may last longer before they are eradicated. Also, qualifications of naturopathy practitioners may vary, so, clients should be informed to check the credentials of the practitioners before choosing this CAM.

Traditional medical systems of non-Western cultures are also included under this category of CAM. Ayurveda and traditional Chinese medicine are examples of these systems. *Ayurveda* dates back 5,000 years and is rooted in the ancient Hindu medical texts alled Vedas. Sanskrit for "knowledge or science of life," Ayurveda is a comprehensive system that encompasses the body, mind, and consciousness connection and seeks to restore a person's harmony or balance. It emphasizes prevention and encourages maintaining health. Ayurveda includes geriatrics as one of eight medical divisions. Practices in Ayurveda medicine include (1) diet, (2) exercise, (3) meditation, (4) herbs, (5) massage, (6) exposure to sunlight, (7) controlled breathing, and (8) detoxification (Sharma,

Chandola, Singh, & Basisht, 2007a). According to Ayurveda, five elements make up all things: (1) space or ether, (2) air, (3) fire, (4) water, and (5) earth. These elements are not static, but rather are always in flux. In addition to the five elements, Ayurveda identifies three types of energy, or *doshas*: vata is the energy of movements and comes from ether and air, pitta is the energy of digestion and comes from fire and water, and kapha comes from water and earth and is the energy of lubrication and structure, which keeps the cellular body together (Sharma et al., 2007a). In Ayurvedic medicine, each person has a unique energy pattern. Disease is caused by an imbalance in the body, or disorder. Diagnosis is made through symptomatology rather than through traditional laboratory diagnostics, with the goal of treatment to bring the body into balance. Although the Ayurvedic physician has many treatments available, most of the research evaluated by the Agency for Healthcare Research and Quality (AHRQ) focused on herbal remedies (Sharma, Chardola, Singh, & Basisht, 2007b). Sharma et al. (2007b) also state that clinical trials should be used to study other Ayurvedic approaches as well.

Traditional Chinese medicine (TCM) dates back in written form to 200 B.C. Korea, Japan, and Vietnam all have medical systems based on the traditional medical systems in China. Traditional Chinese medicine consists of six primary branches: acupuncture, herbal medicine, massage, exercise (such as Tai Chi), dietary therapy, and lifestyle modifications (Smith & Bauer, 2012). According to TCM, the body is a balance of two opposing forces: yin and yang. *Yin* represents the cold, slow, darkness, or passive principle, usually considered the female aspect. *Yang*, on the other hand, simulates fire and is the hot, excited, active principle, usually considered the male aspect. In this tradition of medicine, health is balance. Disease is seen as an imbalance between yin and yang; this imbalance impedes the flow of vital energy (*qi or chi*) and blood along pathways called meridians (Smith & Bauer, 2012). The system of qi forms the basis for diagnosis and treatment of illness as well as for promoting health and preventing illness (Chen, 2001). Diagnosis of disharmony is made on the basis of a patient's complaints and report of the experience of being sick (Fan, 2003). The evaluation of the quality of the pulse at nine particular points in the body and the appearance of the tongue are also taken into account when diagnosing disharmony.

Acupuncture is an integral part of TCM; it promotes the flow of qi through pathways in the body called meridians. There are 14 major meridians used in acupuncture; each meridian consists of an internal pathway, which often connects with an internal organ, and a corresponding external pathway. A total of 361 regular acupuncture points fall on the external pathways of the 14 meridians. An additional 40 acupuncture points fall outside the meridians (Lee, LaRiccia, & Newberg, 2004). Based on patient history and a physical examination, the acupuncturist determines which points on the external pathway of a meridian to stimulate and for how long (Lee et al., 2004). Very thin, solid, metallic needles are inserted at the appropriate acupuncture point to increase the circulation of qi and to bring the body back into balance. Nothing in allopathic medicine compares to the meridians in TCM.

Although acupuncture originated in China more than 2,000 years ago, it did not become well known in the United States until 1971, when a *New York Times* reporter wrote about how acupuncture eased his pain postoperatively (NCCAM, 2004). Burke, Upchurch, Dye, and Chyu (2006) reported that 4.1% of the adults in a 2002 National Health Interview Survey had used acupuncture at some time, and 1.1% had used acupuncture in the past year. According to the World Health Organization (WHO, 2003), there is support for the use of acupuncture to relieve postoperative pain, chemotherapy-induced nausea and vomiting, nausea associated with pregnancy, and dental pain. In a systematic review completed to determine the effects of acupuncture for individuals with neck pain, Trinh et al. (2006) found that there is moderate evidence that acupuncture relieves pain better than some sham treatments and moderate evidence that those who received acupuncture reported less pain at short-term follow-up than those on a waiting list. It is believed that acupuncture releases endogenous opioids, the same mechanism behind the use of transcutaneous electrical nerve stimulation (TENS) (Gloth, 2001). Promising results have been shown in the treatment of headache, stroke rehabilitation, osteoarthritis, low back pain, carpel tunnel syndrome, and asthma, but more research needs to be done to support the efficacy of acupuncture in treating these problems (National Institutes of Health Consensus Development Panel on Acupuncture, 1998).

Energy Medicine

Energy medicine encompasses two basic types of energy fields: veritable, which can be measured, and putative, which currently cannot be measured. Examples of *veritable energy fields* include mechanical vibration and electromagnetic forces, while *putative energy fields* (biofields) include the vital energy (qi or chi) of TCM; doshas in Ayurvedic medicine; ki in the Japanese Kampo system; and prana, etheric energy, fohat, orgone, odic force, and homeopathic resonance in other systems (NCCAM, 2007). Therapists claim they work with this energy to improve health by reducing pain, anxiety, and blood pressure; increasing wound healing; and providing a sense of well-being (NCCAM, 2007). Examples of practices using putative energy fields include Reiki, qi gong, healing (or therapeutic) touch, and prayer for the health of others (intercessory prayer). As a group, these are the most controversial of CAM practices because the energy fields cannot be measured, making traditional scientific research methodology difficult.

Also, there is an overlap between the CAM designations of mind–body medicine and putative energy fields. This can be confusing to consumers. It also illustrates that many of the CAM modalities cannot be investigated in isolation, but, rather, must be studied within the larger context. Those modalities that were covered under mind–body medicine, such as acupuncture, Ayurvedic medicine, homeopathy, and music therapy, will not be explained again.

Qi gong refers to exercises that improve health and increase a sense of harmony by manipulating qi (vital energy) through movement and meditation.

Currently, qi gong is considered an umbrella term for all energy exercises, such as yoga, Reiki, and meditation. It is widely practiced in Chinese hospitals and clinics, but there have been no large clinical trials outside China to support this practice. Studies, however, have demonstrated some evidence to support the influence of qi gong (Chen, Hassett, Hou, Staller, & Lichtbroun, 2006; Liu, Miller, Burton, Chang, & Brown, 2011; Sancier & Holman, 2004; Tsang, Fung, Chan, Lee, & Chan, 2006).

Therapeutic (healing) touch and Reiki both involve movement of a practitioner's hands over the patient's body to balance energy fields (Reiki, 2009). *Reiki* is a form of healing through the manipulation of ki (Japanese for life energy; similar to Chinese qi). Therapeutic touch may involve either physically touching the body or noncontact touch. When the body is not physically touched, the touch refers to the "touching" or movement of the individual's energy field (Eschiti, 2007). The purpose of therapeutic touch is to transfer life energy through the therapist's hands to the client, who will use the energy to rebalance and restore health. Certification in healing touch can be obtained through Healing Touch International, Inc.; healing touch classes are taught worldwide. Although anecdotal evidence and relatively small research studies tend to support therapeutic touch (Eschiti, 2007; Hardwick, Pulido, & Adelson, 2012; Wardell, Decker, & Engebretson, 2012), no large-scale controlled studies have been conducted with these therapies. A systematic review to determine the effects of therapeutic touch on the healing of acute wounds produced no evidence that therapeutic touch promotes the healing of wounds (O'Mathuna & Ashford, 2012).

Several electromagnetic fields, part of veritable energy medicine, have been used in conventional medicine. Magnetic resonance imagery, cardiac pacemakers, transcutaneous electrical nerve stimulators (TENS), and radiation therapy are all examples of the use of these fields. Another veritable energy modality is magnetic therapy, which is the use of static magnets to relieve pain or increase energy levels. Anecdotal reports support the efficacy of static magnets, but more scientific research is needed to support this therapy (NCCAM, 2007).

Sound energy therapy includes music therapy. The basis of sound energy therapy is that specific sound frequencies can facilitate the body's healing (NCCAM, 2007). Music therapy is also a mind–body modality, further supporting the overlap of mind–body interventions and energy medicine. Light therapy has been used to treat seasonal affective disorder successfully, but other uses do not have as much empirical support (NCCAM, 2007). This is an area for further research.

Reasons for Complementary and Alternative Medicine Use

Older adults use CAM for pain relief, to increase quality of life, and to maintain health and fitness (Astin et al., 2000; Cheung, Wyman, & Halcon, 2007; Williamson et al., 2003). Some view CAM as a return to a "kinder and gentler medicine" (Barrett et al., 2004); however, most use CAM in combination with conventional medication rather than as a primary source of treatment (Barnes et al., 2004; Bausell, Lee, & Berman, 2001). In addition, most rely on family and friends to provide information about choosing a modality (Chau, Wade, Kronenberg, Kalmus, & Cushman, 2006; Najm, Reinsch, Hoehler, & Tobis, 2003). As a rule, elders choose CAM because of the belief system behind the modality, not because of dissatisfaction with conventional care (Smith, 2004). However, the nurse cannot overlook the fact the some elders may use CAM because they have difficulty accessing traditional medical care or medications (Pagan & Pauly, 2005).

Nursing Interventions

When performing assessments, nurses must ask clients about their use of CAM, why particular modalities are used, the source of the therapy, and their knowledge of side effects (Marinac et al., 2007). These questions should be phrased in a nonjudgmental manner and should also be phrased in such a way as to cover the variety of modalities. Clients may not acknowledge they are taking herbal medicines, but may identify that they are taking natural products. This is particularly important when clients are on prescribed medications for blood thinning, blood pressure, depression, anxiety, or insomnia. Also, elders may not consider vitamins or minerals as medications because they are considered dietary supplements; however, if taken in conjunction with some prescribed medications or in large doses, vitamins may interfere with the actions of the medications and produce side effects. Good communication skills are a key to a thorough assessment of CAM use. Integrated care, a combination of allopathy and CAM, may be the best model of care for an older adult. The nurse must be a knowledgeable member of this integrated healthcare team to be able to provide comprehensive, holistic care (Killinger, Morley, Kettner, & Kauric, 2001). To facilitate cultural competency and to provide holistic care to clients and patients, nursing and medical schools have added content on complementary and alternative medicine to their curricula.

Summary

As CAM becomes more widely used by the elderly as well as by the general population, the nurse has a responsibility to be knowledgeable about the modalities clients may be using. The World Health Organization (WHO) estimates that 80% of the world's population uses some form of CAM (Bielory, 2002; Milden & Stokols, 2004), so knowledge of CAM may be considered part of culturally competent care (Cuellar, Cahill, Ford, & Aycock, 2003). Nurses should have basic knowledge of the most commonly used CAM therapies in order to provide holistic care to older adults who may wish to incorporate these modalities into their treatment plan. Remember that the effectiveness of some CAM therapies with the older population has not been well researched. Nurses will need to tailor their care to the needs of each individual.

Notable Quotes

"For a completely safe and effective form of balance training, I recommend tai chi, the slow-motion, patterned movements sometimes called 'Chinese shadow boxing' or 'swimming in air.' . . . Older people who practice tai chi are less likely to fall and less likely to suffer injury if they do fall."

—Andrew Weil, MD, from his bestselling book *Healthy Aging: A Lifelong Guide to Your Well-Being*, pp. 233–234

BOX 24-1   Research Highlight

Aim: This two-group randomized study examined the effects of guided imagery on pain perception, functional status, and self-efficacy in persons with fibromyalgia.

Methods: This longitudinal experimental study randomly assigned volunteer participants with fibromyalgia into two groups. The experimental group (n = 24) received usual care as well as three guided imagery audiotapes for a 6-week treatment phase and a 4-week follow-up phase. The control group (n = 24) received usual care. Demographic information was collected at baseline. Pain, functional status, and self-efficacy were measured at baseline, at week 6, and at week 10. Pain was measured by the Short-Form McGill Pain Questionnaire; functional status was measured by the Fibromyalgia Impact Questionnaire; and self-efficacy was measured by the Arthritis Self-Efficacy Scale. The self-efficacy scale was modified to be specific for persons with fibromyalgia.

Findings: The groups were similar on demographic and outcome variables at baseline.

Over time, the group receiving guided imagery showed significant improvements in functional status and self-efficacy for managing pain when compared to the group receiving usual care alone. There were no significant differences between the groups over time in perceived pain.

Application to practice: Although the perception of pain did not change over time for either group, guided imagery made a difference in the functional status and self-efficacy in the ability to manage pain in this population. This has implications for improving quality of life. More research needs to be done to provide a body of evidence to support the efficacy of guided imagery as a nonpharmacological intervention to assist patients living with chronic pain.

Source: Menzies, V., Taylor, A. G., & Bourguignon, C. (2007). Effects of guided imagery on outcomes of pain, functional status, and self-efficacy in persons diagnosed with fibromyalgia. *Journal of Alternative and Complementary Medicine, 12*, 23–30.

BOX 24-2   Resource List

General

The Cochrane Collaboration for systematic reviews:

http://www.cochrane.org

Institute of Medicine Board: Health Promotion and Disease Prevention. (2005). *Use of complementary and alternative medicine (CAM) by the American public*. Washington, DC: Author.

National Center for Complementary and Alternative Medicine (NCCAM):

http://nccam.nih.gov

University of Maryland Medical Center Complementary and Alternative Medicine Index (CAM):

http://www.umm.edu/altmed

University of Pittsburgh—The Alternative Medicine Homepage:

http://zone.medschool.pitt.edu/sites/StudentGroups/IHIG/Shared%20Documents/The%20Alternative%20Medicine%20Homepage.htm

Diet and Herbs

Alternative Medicine Foundation:

http://www.herbmed.org

Blumenthal, M. (Ed.). (1998). *The complete German commission E monographs: Therapeutic guide to herbal medicines*. Austin, TX: American Botanical Council.

(continues)

BOX 24-2 Resource List (*continued*)

Complementary/Integrative Medicine Program at the University of Texas M. D. Anderson Cancer Center:

http://www.mdanderson.org/CIMER

Pet Therapy

Delta Society:

http://www.deltasociety.org

Therapet Animal Assisted Therapy Foundation:

http://www.therapet.com

BOX 24-3 Web Exploration

Explore conferences, products, certifications, and careers in music therapy at American Music Therapy Association (AMTA):

http://www.musictherapy.org

Check out Canine Companions for Independence, an association that facilitates

the breeding, raising, and training of dogs to be working companions to those with disabilities:

http://www.cci.org/site/c.cdKGIRNqEmG/b.3978475/

BOX 24-4 Recommended Readings

Adams, L. L., Gatchel, R. J., & Gentry, C. (2001). Complementary and alternative medicine: Applications and implications for cognitive functioning in elderly populations. *Alternative Therapies in Health and Medicine, 7*(2), 52–61.

Astin, J. A. (1998). Why patients use alternative medicine: Results of a national study. *Journal of the American Medical Association, 279*, 1548–1553.

Barrett, B. (2003). Alternative, complementary, and conventional medicine: Is integration upon us? *Journal of Alternative and Complementary Medicine, 9*, 417–427.

Birch, S., Hesselink, J. K., Jonkman, F. A. M., Hekker, T. A. M., & Bos, A. (2004). Clinical research on acupuncture: Part I. What have reviews of the efficacy and safety of acupuncture told us so far? *Journal of Alternative and Complementary Medicine, 10*, 468–480.

Cartwright, T (2007). "Getting on with life": The experiences of older people using complementary health care. *Social Science and Medicine, 64*, 1692–1703.

Doherty, D., Wright, S., Aveyard, B., & Sykes, M. (2006). Therapeutic touch and dementia: An ongoing journey. *Nursing Older People, 18*(11), 27–30.

Dossey, L. (1993). *Healing words: The power of prayer and the practice of medicine.* San Francisco, CA: Harper.

Gloth, F. M. (2001). Pain management in older adults: Prevention and treatment. *Journal of the American Geriatrics Society, 49*, 188–199.

Jonas, W. B., Kaptchuk, T. J., & Linde, K. (2003). A critical overview of homeopathy. *Annals of Internal Medicine, 138*, 393–399.

Schofield, P., Smith, P., Aveyard, B., & Black, C. (2007). Complementary therapies for pain management in palliative care. *Journal of Community Nursing, 21*(8), 10, 12–14.

Steyer, T. E. (2001). Complementary and alternative medicine: A primer. *Family Practice Management, 8*(3), 37–42, 61–62.

Vangsness, S., Moffitt, R., & Herbold, N. H. (2005). Education and knowledge of dietetic interns regarding herbs and dietary supplements: Preparing for practice. *Topics of Clinical Nutrition, 20*, 269–276.

Critical Thinking Exercises

1. **Access the National Center for Complementary** and Alternative Medicine Web site (http://nccam.nih.gov) and explore one of the CAM therapies listed. Review the information presented from the perspective of a consumer with no medical knowledge. What is the reading level? Is the material easy to understand? What would you add and why? What would you delete and why?

2. **Interview several older adults and ask them** what supplements, vitamins, or herbals they use and why. During the course of conversation, ask them if they inform their healthcare providers about their practices and why. Discuss your findings with a group of nursing students. As a group, identify nursing interventions appropriate for the adults interviewed.

3. **In a group, critique research articles exploring** the efficacy of a CAM modality with research reports on clinical trials of allopathic medicines. Compare the levels of evidence of each report.

Personal Reflections

1. Think about what CAM therapies you have used personally. If you have not used any, think about one therapy you think you may want to try. Why did you use CAM or why would you use CAM? Think about patients that you have had who have used CAM. What was your reaction to the information? Have you changed your mind about CAM since reading the chapter? Did the patients use CAM for the same reasons you did or thought you may?

2. Look through your local newspaper for a week. What references to CAM do you find? How many references were directed at the older adult? Were you surprised by what you found?

References

Aldridge, D. (1994). An overview of music therapy research. *Complementary Therapies in Medicine, 2*, 204–216.

Astin, J. A., Pelletier, K. R., Marie, A., & Haskell, W. L. (2000). Complementary and alternative medicine use among elderly persons: One-year analysis of a Blue Shield Medicare supplement. *Journals of Gerontology, 55A*, M4–M9.

Barnes, P. M., Powell-Griner, E., McFann, K., & Nahin, R. L. (2004). *CDC advance data report #343. Complementary and alternative medicine use among adults: United States, 2002.* Bethesda, MD: Centers for Disease Control and Prevention.

Barnes, P. M., Bloom, B., & Nahim, R. L. (2008). *Complementary and alternative medicine use among adults and children: United States, 2007.* National Health Statistics Reports, 12, Hyattsville, MD: National Center for Health Statistics.

Barrett, B., Marchand, L., Scheder, J., Applebaum, D., Plane, M. B., Blustein, J.,…Capperino, C. (2004). What complementary and alternative practitioners say about health and health care. *Annals of Family Medicine, 2*, 253–259.

Bausell, R. B., Lee, W. L., & Berman, B. M. (2001). Demographic and health-related correlates of visits to complementary and alternative medical providers. *Medical Care, 39*, 190–196.

Bielory, L. (2002). "Complementary and alternative medicine" population based studies: A growing focus on allergy and asthma. *Allergy, 57,* 655–658.

Billhult, A., Bergbom, I., & Stener-Victorin, E. (2007). Massage relieves nausea in women with breast cancer who are undergoing chemotherapy. *Journal of Alternative and Complementary Medicine, 13,* 53–57.

Biologically Based Therapies. (2009). Merk Manual Home Health Handbook for Patients and Caregivers. Retrieved from http://www.merckmanuals.com/professional/special_subjects/complementary_and_alternative_medicine/biologically_based_practices.html

Bryans, R., Descarreaux, M., Duranleau, M., Marcoux,H., Potter, B., Ruegg, R., …White, E. (2011). Evidence-based guidelines for the chiropractic treatment of adults with headache. *Journal of Manipulative and Physiological Treatments, 34,* 274–289. doi: 10.1016/j.jmpt,2011,04.008.

Burke, A., Upchurch, D. M., Dye, C., & Chyu, L. (2006). Acupuncture use in the United States: Findings from the National Health Interview Survey. *Journal of Alternative and Complementary Medicine, 12,* 639–648.

Candy, B., Jones, L., Varagunam, M., Speck, P., Tookman, A., & King, M. (2012). Spiritual and religious intervention for well-being of adults in the terminal phase of disease. *Cochrane Database of Systematic Reviews, 5,* Art. No: CD007544.pub 2

Cepeda, M. S., Carr, D. B., Lau, J., & Alvarez, H. (2006). Music for pain relief. *Cochrane Database of Systematic Reviews, 2,* Art. No.: CD004843. doi: 10.1002/14651858.CD004843.pub2

Chau, M. T., Wade, C., Kronenberg, F., Kalmuss, D., & Cushman, L. F. (2006). Women's reasons for complementary and alternative medicine use: Racial/ethnic differences. *Journal of Alternative and Complementary Medicine, 12,* 719–722.

Chen, K. W., Hassett, A. L., Hou, F., Staller, J., & Lichtbroun, A. S. (2006). A pilot study of external qigong therapy for patients with fibromyalgia. *Journal of Alternative and Complementary Medicine, 12,* 851–856.

Chen, Y. (2001). Chinese values, health, and nursing. *Journal of Advanced Nursing, 36,* 270–273.

Cherkin, D. C., Sherman, K. J., Deyo, R. A., & Shekelle, P. G. (2003). A review of the evidence for the effectiveness, safety, and cost of acupuncture, massage therapy, and spinal manipulation for back pain. *Annals of Internal Medicine, 138,* 898–906.

Cheung, C. K., Wyman, J. F., & Halcon, L. L. (2007). Use of complementary and alternative therapies in community-dwelling adults. *Journal of Alternative and Complementary Medicine, 13,* 997–1006. doi: 10.1089/acm.2007.0527

Cuellar, N. G., Cahill, B., Ford, J., & Aycock, T. (2003). The development of an educational workshop on complementary and alternative medicine: What every nurse should know. *Journal of Continuing Education in Nursing, 34,* 128–135.

Cutshall, S. M., Wentworth, L. J., Engen, D., Sundt, T. M., Kelly, R. F., & Bauer, B.A. (2010). Effect of massage therapy on pain, anxiety, and tension in cardiac surgical patients: A pilot study. *Complementary Therapies in Clinical Practice, 16*(2), 92–95. doi: http://dx.doi.org.ezproxy.valp.edu/10.1016/j.ctcp2009.10.008

Daniel, C., O'Keefe, P., & Pepa, C. A. (2002, November). *The use of music therapy in selected clinical areas: An integrative review.* Paper presented at the 10th annual Northwest Indiana Nursing Research Consortium conference, Merrillville, IN.

Deglin, J. H., & Vallerand, A. H. (2007). *Davis's drug guide for nurses* (10th ed.). Philadelphia, PA: F.A. Davis.

Drackley, N. L., Degnim, A. C., Jakub, J. W., Cutshall, S. M., Thomley, B. S., Brodt, J. K., …Boughey, J. C. (2012). Effect of massage therapy for postsurgical mastectomy recipients. *Clinical Journal of Oncology Nursing, 16(2),* 121–124. doi: 10.1188/12.cjon, 121–124.

Eisenberg, D. M., Kessler, R. C., Foster, C., Norlock, F. E., Calkins, D. R., & Delbanco, T. L. (1993). Unconventional medicine in the United States. *New England Journal of Medicine, 328,* 246–252.

Ernst, E. (2002). The risk-benefit profile of community-used herbal therapies: Gingko, St. John's wort, ginseng, echinacea, saw palmetto, and kava. *Annals of Internal Medicine, 136,* 42–53.

Ernst, E., & Canter, P. H. (2003). Chiropractic spinal manipulation treatment for back pain? A systematic review of randomized clinical trials. *Physical Therapy Reviews, 8,* 85–91.

Eschiti, V. S. (2007). Healing touch: A low-tech intervention in high-tech settings. *Dimensions of Critical Care Nursing, 26*(1), 9–14.

Fan, R. (2003). Modern Western science as a standard for traditional Chinese medicine: A critical appraisal. *Journal of Law, Medicine and Ethics, 31,* 213–221.

Field, T. (2011). Tai Chi research review. *Complementary Therapies in Clinical Practice, 17,* 141–146. doi: 10.1016/j.ctcp.2010.10.002

Furlan, A. D., Brosseau, L., Imamura, M., & Irvin, E. (2008). Massage for low-back pain. *Cochrane Database of Systematic Reviews, 4,* Art. No.: CD001929. doi: 10:1002/14651858.CD001929.pub2

Gatlin, C. G., & Schulmeister, L. (2007). When medication is not enough: Nonpharmacologic management of pain. *Clinical Journal of Oncology Nursing, 11,* 699–704.

Gloth, F. M. (2001). Pain management in older adults: Prevention and treatment. *Journal of the American Geriatrics Society, 49,* 188–199.

Gonzales, E. A., Ledesma, R. J. A., McAllister, D. J., Perry, S. M., Dyer, C. A., & Maye, J. P. (2010). Effects of guided imagery on postoperative outcomes in patients undergoing same-day surgical procedures: A randomized, single-blind study. *AANA Journal, 78,* 181–188.

Gordon, A. E., & Shaughnessy, A. F. (2003). Saw palmetto for prostate disorder. *American Family Physician, 67,* 1281–1283.

Gundersen, L. (2000). Faith and healing. *Annals of Internal Medicine, 132,* 169–172.

Hardwick, M. E., Pulido, P. A., & Adelson, W. S. (2012). Nursing intervention using healing touch in bilateral total knee arthroplasty. *Orthopaedic Nursing, 31*(1), 5–11.

Henkel, J. (2000). Soy: Health claims for soy protein, questions about other components. *FDA Consumer Magazine.* Retrieved from http://permanent.access.gpo.gov/lps1609/www.fda.gov/fdac/features/2000/300_soy.html

Hertzman-Miller, R. P. (2002). Comparing the satisfaction of low back pain patients randomized to receive medical or chiropractic care: Results from the UCLA low-back pain study. *American Journal of Public Health, 92,* 1628–1633.

Hillier, S. L., Louw, Q., Morris, L., Uwimana, J., & Statham, S. (2010). Massage therapy for people with HIV/AIDS. *Cochrane Database of Systematic Reviews, Issue 1, ART No: C0007502.* doi:10.1002/14651858.CD001929.pub2

Hooker, S. D., Freeman, L. H., & Steward, P. (2002). Pet therapy research: A historical review. *Holistic Nursing Practice, 17*(1), 17–23.

Jimenez, P. J., Melendez, A., & Albers, U. (2012). Psychological effects of Tai Chi Chuan. *Archives of Gerontology and Geriatrics, 55,* 460–467. doi: 10.1016/j.archger.2012.02.003

Killinger, L. Z., Morley, J. E., Kettner, N. W., & Kauric, E. (2001). Integrated care of the older patient. *Topics in Clinical Chiropractic, 8*(2), 46–54.

Kuhn, M. (1999). *Complementary therapies for health care providers.* Philadelphia, PA: Lippincott Williams & Wilkins.

Kuhn, M. A. (2002). Herbal remedies: Drug-herb interactions. *Critical Care Nurse, 22*(2), 22–30.

Lee, B. Y., LaRiccia, P. J., & Newberg, A. B. (2004). Acupuncture in theory and practice Part I: Theoretical basis and physiologic effects. *Hospital Physician, 40*(4), 11–18.

Li, A. W., & Goldsmith, C. W. (2012). The effects of yoga on anxiety and stress. *Alternative Medicine Review, 17*(1), 21–35.

Liu, X., Miller, Y., Burton, N., Chang, J., & Brown, W. (2011). Qi gong mind-body therapy and diabetes control: A randomized trial. *American Journal of Preventive Medicine, 41,* 152–158.

Maier-Lorentz, M. M. (2004). The importance of prayer for mind/body healing. *Nursing Forum, 39*(3), 23–32.

Marinac, J. S., Buchinger, C. L., Godfrey, L. A., Wooten, J. M., Sun, C., & Willsie, S. K. (2007). Herbal products and dietary supplements: A survey of use, attitudes, and knowledge among older adults. *Journal of the American Osteopathic Association, 107,* 13–23.

McCarney, R. W., Linde, K., & Lusserson, L. (2008). Homeopathy for chronic asthma. *Cochrane Database of Systematic Reviews, 1,* ART NO: CD000353. doi: 10.1002/14651858.CD000353.pub 2

Menzies, V., & Taylor, A. G. (2004). The idea of imagination: An analysis of "imagery." *Advances in Mind Body Medicine, 20*(2), 4–10.

Milden, S. P., & Stokols, D. (2004). Physicians' attitudes and practices regarding complementary and alternative medicine. *Behavioral Medicine, 30,* 73–82.

Miller, R. (2003). Nurses at community hospital welcome guided imagery tool. *Dimensions of Critical Care Nursing, 22,* 225–226.

Najm, W., Reinsch, S., Hoehler, F., & Tobis, J. (2003). Use of complementary and alternative medicine among the ethnic elderly. *Alternative Therapies in Health and Medicine, 9*(3), 50–57.

National Center for Complementary and Alternative Medicine. (NCCAM). (2004). *Backgrounder. An introduction to acupuncture.* NCCAM Publication No. D003. Retrieved from http://nccam.nih.gov/health/acupuncture.htm

National Center for Complementary and Alternative Medicine. (NCCAM). (2007). *Backgrounder. Energy medicine: An overview.* NCCAM Publication No. D235. Retrieved from http://nccam.nih.gov/health/backgrounds/energymed.htm

National Center for Complementary and Alternative Medicine. (NCCAM). (2010). Backgrounder: Meditation: An Introduction. Retrieved from http://nccam.nih.gov/health/meditation/overview.htm

National Center for Complementary and Alternative Medicine. (NCCAM). (2012a). *Backgrounder: Chiropractic: An introduction.* Retrieved from http://nccam.nih.gov/health/chiropractic/introduction.htm

National Center for Complementary and Alternative Medicine. (NCCAM). (2012b). *Herbs at a glance: Ephedra.* Retrieved from http://nccam.nih.gov/health/ephedra

National Center for Complementary and Alternative Medicine. (NCCAM). (2012c). *Homeopathy: An introduction.* Retrieved from http://nccam.nih.gov/health/chiropractic/introduction.htm

National Center for Complementary and Alternative Medicine. (NCCAM). (2012d). *Naturopathy: An introduction.* Retrieved from http://nccam.nih.gov/health/naturopathy/naturopathyintro.htm

National Center for Complementary and Alternative Medicine. (NCCAM). (2012e). *Statistics on complementary and alternative medicine national health survey.* Retrieved from http://nccam.nih.gov/news/camstats/NHIS.htm

National Center for Complementary and Alternative Medicine. (NCCAM). (2012f). *What is complementary and alternative medicine?* Retrieved from http://www.nccam.nih.gov/health/whatiscam

National Institutes of Health Consensus Development Panel on Acupuncture. (1998). Acupuncture. *Journal of the American Medical Association, 280,* 1518–1524.

National Institutes of Health Senior Health. (2012). *CAM practices.* Retrieved from http://nihseniorhealth.gov/cam/campractices/01.html

Ness, J., Cirillo, D. J., Weir, D. R., Nisly, N. L., & Wallace, R. B. (2005). Use of complementary medicine in older Americans: Results from the health and retirement study. *The Gerontologist, 45,* 516–524.

Office of Dietary Supplements, National Institutes of Health. (2011). *Health professional dietary supplement fact sheet: Vitamin B12.* Retrieved from http://ods.od.nih.gov/factsheets/vitaminB12-HealthProfessional/

Okonta, N. R. (2012). Does yoga reduce blood pressure in patients with hypertension?: An integrative review. *Holistic Nursing Practice, 26,* 137–141.

O'Mathuna, D. P., & Ashford, R. L. (2012). Therapeutic touch for healing acute wounds. *Cochrane Database of Systematic Reviews, 6,* Art. No. CD002766. doi 10.1002/14651858.CD002766.pub 2

Pagan, J. A., & Pauly, M. V. (2005). Access to conventional medical care and the use of complementary and alternative medicine. *Health Affairs, 24,* 255–262.

Posadzki, P., Lewandowski, W., Ernst, E., & Stearns, A. (2012). Guided imagery for non-musculoskeletal pain: A systematic review of randomized clinical trials. *Journal of Pain and Symptom Management, 44,* 95–104. doi: 10.1016/j.painsymman.2011.07.014

Reiki: An Introduction. (2009). Retrieved from http://nccam.nih.gov/sites/nccam.nih.gov/files/D315_BKG.pdf

Richards, T., Johnson, J., Sparks, A., & Emerson, H. (2007). The effect of music therapy on patients' perception and manifestation of pain, anxiety, and patient satisfaction. *MEDSURG Nursing, 16,* 7–14.

Roberts, L., Ahmed, I., Hall, S., & Davison, A. (2009). Intercessary prayer for the alleviation of ill health. *Cochrane Database of Sytematic Reviews, 2,* Art. No.: CD000368. doi: 10.1002/46518858CD 000 368. Pub 3.

Sancier, K. M., & Holman, D. (2004). Commentary: Multifaceted health benefits of medical qigong. *Journal of Alternative and Complementary Medicine, 10,* 163–165.

Sending prayers: Does it help? (2002). *Harvard Health Letter, 27*(7), 7.

Sicher, F., Targ, E., Moore, D., & Smith, D. (1998). A randomized double-blind study of the effect of distant healing in a population with advanced AIDS: Report of a small scale sample. *Western Journal of Medicine, 169,* 356–363.

Sharma, H., Chandola, H. M., Singh, G., & Basisht, G. (2007a). Utilization of Ayurveda in health care: An approach for prevention, health promotion, and treatment of disease. Part 1—Ayurveda, the science of life. *Journal of Alternative and Complementary Medicine, 13,* 1011–1019.

Sharma, H., Chandola, H. M., Singh, G., & Basisht, g. (2007b). Utilization of Ayurveda in health care: An approach for prevention, health promotion, and treatment of disease. Part 2—Ayurveda in primary health care. *The Journal of Alternative and Complementary Medicine, 13,* 11-35-1150.

Sinha, M. N., Siddiqui, V. A., Nayak, C., Singh, V., Dixit, R., & Dewan, D. (2012). Randomized controlled pilot study to compare homeopathy and conventional therapy in acute otitis media. *Homeopathy, 101,* 5–12.

Smith, M. E., & Bauer, W. S. (2012). Traditional Chinese medicine for cancer-related symptoms. *Seminars in Oncology Nursing, 28,* 64–74. doi: 10.1016/j.sonen.11.007

Stanley-Hermanns, M., & Miller, J. (2002). Animal assisted therapy. *American Journal of Nursing, 102*(10), 69–76.

Supplements: Peppermint. (n.d.). Retrieved from http://www.wholehealthmd.com

Tacklind, J., MacDonald, R., Rutks, I., Stanke, J. U., Wilt, J. (2009) *Serenoa repens* for benign prostatic hyperplasia. *Cochrane Database for Systematic Reviews, 2, ART NO: CD001423.* doi: 10.1002/14651858. CD001423.pub 2

Teixeira, M. Z. (2011). New homeopathic medicines. Use of modern drugs according to the principle of similitude. *Homeopathy, 100,* 244–252.

Tilbrook, H. E., Hewitt, C. E., Kang'ombe, A. R., Chaung, L. H., Jayakody, S., Aplin, J. D., …Watt, I. (2011). Yoga for chronic low back pain: A randomized trial. *Annals of Internal Medicine, 155,* 569–578.

Trinh, K. V., Graham, N., Gross, A. R., Goldsmith, C. H., Wang, E., Cameron, I. D.,…Cervical Overview Group. (2006). Acupuncture for neck disorders. *Cochrane Database of Systematic Reviews, 3.* Art No.: CD004870. doi: 10.1002/14651858.CD004870.pub3.

Tsang, H. W. H., Fung, K. M. T., Chan, A. S. M., Lee, E., & Chan, F. (2006). Effect of qigong exercise programme on elderly with depression. *International Journal of Geriatric Psychiatry, 21,* 890–897.

University of Maryland Medical Center. (2007). *Comfrey.* Retrieved from http://www.umm.edu/altmed/articles/comfrey-000234.htm

U.S. Food and Drug Administration. (2007). *Fortify your knowledge about vitamins.* Retrieved on from http://www.fda.gov/CONSUMER/updates/vitamins111907.html

Vanderboom, T. (2007). Does music reduce anxiety during invasive procedures with procedural sedation? An integrative research review. *Journal of Radiology Nursing, 26,* 15–17.

Wardell, D. W., Decker, S. A., & Engebretson, J. C. (2012). Healing touch for older adults with persistant pain. *Holistic Nursing Practice, 24,* 194–202. doi: 10.1097/HNP.06013e31825852gd

Williamson, A. T., Fletcher, P. C., & Dawson, K. A. (2003). Complementary and alternative medicine: Use in an older population. *Journal of Gerontological Nursing, 29*(5), 20–29.

Wilt, T., Ishani, A., & MacDonald, R. (2002). Serenoa repens for benign prostatic hyperplasia. *Cochrane Database of Systematic Reviews, 2.* Art. No.: CD001423. DOI: 10.1002/14651858.CD001423.

Wong, C. (2006). What is capsaicin cream? Retrieved from http://altmedicine.about.com/od/completeazindex/a/capsaicin_cream.htm

World Health Organization [WHO]. (2003). Traditional medicine. Retrieved from http://www.who.int/mediacentre/factsheets/fs134/en/print.html

Yucha, C. B., Clark, L., Smith, M., Uris, P., La Fleur, B., & Duval, S. (2001). The effect of biofeedback in hypertension. *Applied Nursing Research, 14(1)*, 29–35.

Zauderer, C., & Davis, W. (2012). Treating post partum depression and anxiety naturally. *Holistic Nursing Practice, 26*, 203–209.

For a full suite of assignments and additional learning activities, see the access code at the front of your book.

LEARNING OBJECTIVES

At the end of this chapter, the reader will be able to:

> State the potential risks factors in transitioning across healthcare settings for older adults.
> Describe different evidence-based practice (EBP) care transition models used in different settings (acute/subacute care, long-term care, home care).
> Recognize the key roles and functions of the geriatric nurse in optimizing care across the continuum.
> Define terms utilized for care settings.
> Contrast and compare settings available for older adult living.
> Contrast settings of care in which nurses care for older adults.

KEY TERMS

Acute rehabilitation

Adult day services

Aging in place

Assisted living facility

Continuing care retirement community

Green House

Home health care

Hospice

Independent living

Long-term acute care hospitals (LTACHs)

Long-term care facility (LTCF)

Memory care

Naturally occurring retirement community

Respite care

Smart Homes

Transitional care

Chapter 25

(Competencies 4, 5, 8, 10,14)

Caring Across the Continuum

Carol Ann Amann
Raeann G. LeBlanc

Continuum of Care

Healthcare systems that collaborate, coordinate care, communicate, and anticipate patients' needs are essential to ensuring quality nursing care that is "safe, effective, patient-centered, timely, efficient, and equitable" (Institute of Medicine [IOM], 2001, p. 6). In addressing quality care across the continuum, it is critical to be familiar with the different settings of care. In understanding these settings, nurses can apply evidence-based practice models to ensure both safe transitions across the care continuum and quality outcomes. Nursing is about teamwork and collaboration. Care across the continuum asks that health professionals critically look at the setting of care and anticipate the needs of patients as these settings change.

Healthcare Policy

Influenced by policy changes reflected in the Patient Protection and Affordable Care Act (2010), programs that improve quality and reduce costs focus specifically on reducing avoidable hospital admissions and improving transfer of care interventions for chronically ill older adults. Transitions in setting of care (hospital, rehabilitation, long-term care, home) are considered to be vulnerable exchange points and contribute to the risk of poor health outcomes (Naylor, Aiken, Kurtzman, Olds, & Hirschman, 2011). This risk is especially true for older adults who may have several chronic diseases, cognitive dysfunction, sensory impairment, and functional decline that may coexist with acute and chronic illness.

Risk in Care Transitions

Care across the continuum requires attention to clients as they move across settings in how care is coordinated and communicated, and how complications are prevented. As older adults move across settings, they are in a vulnerable period. Older adults may transition between the care settings of hospital, rehabilitation, and home several times, even within a year. It important to address, in the promotion of optimal care, safe transitions across settings and prevention of avoidable adverse outcomes across the continuum of home, long-term care, acute care, and rehabilitation (Marek & Antle, 2008; Kripalani et al., 2007).

There are key risk factors that lead to poor outcomes in the transition of care across the continuum. These risks include inadequate education to the clients and their family in how to manage their illness, poor communication between care providers and clients, poor coordination of care among healthcare providers, inadequate assessment at the point of care, medication discrepancies, lack of follow up care, health literacy issues, lack of support systems, and cultural barriers.

In a study by Corbett, Setter, Daratha, Neumiller, and Wood (2010), 94% of participants transitioning from acute care to home had a medication discrepancy. Medication discrepancies are any difference between the discharge medication list and the medications patients report actually taking at home. In understanding the characteristics of transition care interventions, priority emphasis is given to medication management, symptom management, and early follow-up (Hennessey & Suter, 2011).

Information Exchange

Effective communication is essential in achieving the goals of remaining functional and stable on return to home. Communication breakdown in information exchange about medications and disease management reflect individual, population, and systematic problems that influence safety. Communication problems within the system of healthcare delivery include both miscommunication and the absence of communication about medications and disease management (Arora et al., 2010), all significant elements of risk for the home care population (Ellenbecker Frazier, & Verney, 2011). Communication insures optimal exchange of key patient information. Relationships between healthcare providers that promote information exchange improve safety (IOM, 2001).

BOX 25-1   Research Highlight

Aim: The authors wished to explore the benefits of transitions of care.

Methods: In a review of 21 randomized clinical trials focusing on transitional care interventions, 9 programs reflected robust evidence of the benefits of transitions care.

Findings: The majority of positive interventions designated a nurse, commonly an advanced-practice registered nurse (APRN), as the clinical leader.

Application: Health organizations that want to make a positive difference in transitional care outcomes should consider hiring an APRN.

Source: Naylor, M. D., Aiken, L. H., Kurtzman, E. T., Olds, D. M., & Hirschman, K. B. (2011). The importance of transitional care in achieving health reform. *Health Affairs, 30*(4), 746–754. doi: 10.1377/hlthaff.2011.0041

Transitional Care Models

Often, *transitional care* models emphasize self-care (Coleman, Parry, Chalmers, & Min, 2006) and therefore most of the research originates on cohorts of older adults who are able to manage their care independently or with informal caregiver supports. With very short-term education and coaching by nurses, this level of self-management is greatly improved. Gaps in transitional care interventions for the population of frail older adults include the absence of studies on cognitively impaired adults and medically underserved populations (Golden, Tweary, Dang, & Roos, 2010; Naylor et al., 2011).

Many innovations in transitional care interventions have been developed, and the majority focus on the transition from acute care hospital to home (BOOST, Care Transitions Program, Transitional Care Model). Other models focus on in-home assessments (GRACE) and additional models focus on long-term care (INTERACT). All models focus on the priority to reduce preventable rehospitalization and potentially avoidable hospitalizations.

Potentially preventable rehospitalizations can be broadly understood as a rehospitalization for a diagnosis or related diagnosis within 30 days of a hospital discharge (Institute for Health Care Improvement, 2010). Potentially avoidable hospitalizations are defined as specific conditions that could have been identified and treated in the setting of care, for example in the nursing home, that would then allow the resident to avoid the risks of hospitalization (see **Table 25-1**). The models of transitional care are developed based on the setting.

TABLE 25-1 Causes of Potentially Avoidable Hospitalizations of Residents in Long-Term Care
Congestive heart failure
Chest pain
Pneumonia
Bronchitis
Mental status change
Urinary tract infection
Sepsis, cellulitis
Dehydration
Gastrointestinal bleeding
Diarrhea
Musculoskeletal pain
Psychiatric problems
Adverse drug effect

Source: Adapted & summarized from Ouslander et al., 2010

Transitional Models in Acute Care

Several evidence-based care transition models focus on the older adult in the acute care environment. One robust example of the use of a transition intervention is provided from Mount Sinai Medical Center's Visiting Doctor's Program, where an advanced practice nurse serves as the clinical consultant for frail, elderly clients who are admitted to the hospital. In a process reflecting consistency of care, the nurse practitioner consultant process has shown significant improvement in medication safety, medication reconciliation, and medication adherence, as well as improved provider and patient satisfaction (Popejoy, 2011).

Better Outcomes for Older Adults through Safe Transitions (BOOST) has as its primary objective to reduce 30-day hospital readmission rates for older adults, improve patient satisfaction, identify high-risk patients to prevent adverse events, improve information exchange between inpatient and outpatient physicians, and better prepare the client and family for discharge (Society for Hospital Medicine, 2008). BOOST provides tools to support nurses in improving care transitions. One key element of BOOST is the strength of the education and communication tool components.

BOOST is a 30-day intervention that includes pre- and postdischarge interventions. The use of "teach-back" for discharge education is one example of a key intervention. Teach-back (Schillinger et al., 2003) is a tailored education process that begins by identifying the client's understanding, explaining in simple terms any misunderstandings, and then asking the client and or family to repeat back their understanding.

Physician Eric Coleman is a leader in the Care Transitions Program (2008). One of the main features of this model is the use of a Transitions Coach, who follows the client pre- and postdischarge from the hospital and for follow up. The coach's role encourages self-management and reinforces important aspects of care, including improved client–physician communication, offers strategies on how to respond to changes in health or important concerns, and engages clients in medication reconciliation. Coaches make one home visit postdischarge. The Four Pillars of this model are medication self-management, patient-centered health records, follow up with a medical provider, and negotiating emergent health concerns and changes in status. Outcomes from the use of this model indicate a decrease in hospital readmissions and an increase in client's self-indentified goals regarding symptom management (Coleman et al., 2006).

Arora and associates (2010) found that the majority of frail older adults report problems after discharge from the hospital to home. These problems were twice as likely to happen when the primary care provider was unaware of the hospitalization. Additional changes in the system of healthcare delivery point to further communication vulnerability, including "growing fragmentation of the multidisciplinary, multi-venue, and multilingual care environment" (Golden et al., 2010, p. 452).

Naylor's Transitional Care Model (TCM) (Naylor & Keating, 2008) is a nurse-led model that follows the client from hospital to home. The nurse acts as the main care manager, who consults with the client in hospital, at home within 24 hours of discharge, accompanies the client to postdischarge follow up visits and weekly home visits, and is on call 7 days a week for home visits and telephone consults. The emphasis of TCM is care coordination and continuity of care.

Coordination of care across specialties and multiple providers requires leadership in communication and interventions that identify this role as that of a coach and/or care manager (Coleman et al., 2006). A pilot nurse practitioner-led care program improved communication between the hospital and community care providers and facilitated timely transfer of important information (Kelly & Penney, 2011).

Transitional Model in Home Care

Community-dwelling older adults who meet the criteria for nursing home admission (needs assistance with both activities of daily living and independent activities of daily living, and who may have a skilled nursing requirement) may also require transitional care interventions, but within a supportive care management model versus a self-management care approach. The Geriatric Resources for Assessment and Care of Elders (GRACE) is a model to support optimal health at home (Counsell, Callahan, Buttar, Clark, & Frank, 2005). This model utilizes nurse practitioners and social workers to conduct home visits and collaborate with a geriatric interdisciplinary team (geriatrician, physical therapist, nurse) in the coordination and implementation of a care plan.

Safe, equitable, and quality care across the continuum for older adults is an important practice area for nurses. Evidence-based models can guide practice to improve quality and optimize care while being cost-effective. Of these models highlighted here, important leadership roles of the geriatric nurse are that of communicator, advocate, case manager, care coordinator, coach, and educator across settings of care (see **Box 25-2**).

BOX 25-2 Evidence-Based Practice Box

For information on an innovation to help older adults get the access they deserve to appropriate living arrangements and health care, explore this EBP link to http://www.innovations.ahrq.gov/content.aspx?id=2066. Read the innovation called "Team-Developed Care Plan and Ongoing Care Management by Social Workers and Nurse Practitioners Result in Better Outcomes and Fewer Emergency Department Visits for Low-Income Seniors."

Transitional Model in Long-term Care

Hospitalization can be physically and emotionally difficult for residents in long-term care. Interventions to Reduce Acute Care Transfers (INTERACT) is an evidence-based quality improvement program designed to improve the identification of, evaluation of, and communication about changes in resident status. Early identification, evaluation, and communication improve care through early intervention and prevention of complications and decrease the need to transfer the resident to the acute care hospital. INTERACT is a model used in long-term care settings. Clinical-based tools that support INTERACT include a decision-making algorithm to guide interventions and actions. Additional aspects of INTERACT support focused geriatric assessment and care pathways for common geriatric syndromes.

Healthcare Settings

Because of the nature of the aging process, it is highly likely that older adults will enter and exit healthcare systems at many different points throughout their lifespan. **Figure 25-1** presents the web of health care that often occurs when older adults enter the system related to illness or accidents. To better comprehend the nature of healthcare settings, the following offers a brief description of the most common settings of care.

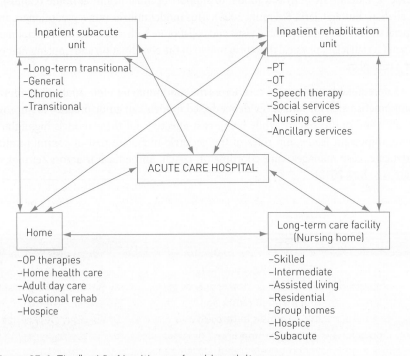

Figure 25-1 The "web" of health care for older adults.

Source: © Mauk, K.L., 2010. Gerontological Nursing: Competencies for Care, Second Edition. Jones and Bartlett Learning. Used with permission.

Acute Care Hospital

The acute care hospital is often the point of entry into the healthcare system for older adults. Due in part to the increasing older adult admissions for hospital care, it is essential that nurses have education specific to the needs of this specialty population. In the acute care setting, the primary focus of nursing care involves caring for acute illnesses, injuries, exacerbations of chronic diseases such as cardiopulmonary conditions, orthopedic problems, and various cancer treatments. Care of the older adult often begins in the emergency setting and may progress into critical care, general units, or to rehabilitative services. Regardless of the acute care setting, the optimal goal is to promote recovery and maintain the elder's optimal level of functioning through quality care and the prevention of complications.

Acute Rehabilitation

Rehabilitation services begin while in the acute care setting and extend throughout the continuum based on the needs of the older adult. *Acute rehabilitation* (rehab) is an appropriate option for those who will benefit from an intensive, multidisciplinary approach to care delivery. The typical rehab team consists of nurses, therapists, physicians, and other specialists who work collaboratively with the patient to maximize independence and optimal level of functioning. Additional services such as neuropsychology, speech, and respiratory therapy are also available for patients during their rehabilitation.

The level of intense therapy in a rehabilitation unit is greater than those services provided in acute or transitional care units and extended care facilities. Each patient admitted to an acute rehab unit receives a minimum of 3 hours of combined therapies per day to fulfill Medicare requirements for admission. Primary conditions necessitating a referral with subsequent admission to an acute rehabilitation facility include conditions such as stroke, head trauma, neurological diseases, amputation, spinal cord injury, and orthopedic surgery.

Transitional/Progressive Care Unit

Transitional or progressive care is a broad term that encompasses a variety of skilled nursing services, including subacute, skilled, and some rehabilitative care services. Medically stable patients requiring nursing care beyond the acute illness or injury phase can be managed in a hospital-based transitional care unit (TCU) or a skilled nursing facility (SNF) on a short-term basis. The terms *transitional care* and *skilled care* are often used interchangeably, but depending on the setting there can be wide variations (Jones & Foster, 1997). Transitional care bridges the gap for patients with complex or multiple problems who are not stable enough to return to a home setting, but not sick enough to require long-term nursing care. An example of the conditions included in admission to such a unit are general debility, wound care, gait training, and intravenous therapy.

In a hospital-based TCU setting, patients are transferred to a designated unit: from an acute bed to a designated skilled care bed. Hospital-based skilled nursing facilities exist as a distinct part of the hospital and are usually called transitional care units. Skilled care helps patients transition from illness to wellness—from dependence to self-care.

Long-Term Acute Care Hospital

Long-term acute care hospitals (LTACHs) or units furnish extended medical and rehabilitative care to individuals with clinically complex problems, such as multiple acute or chronic conditions, that need hospital-level care for relatively extended periods. The usual length of stay for patients admitted to this type of facility is generally about 25 days.

While LTACHs are often confused with nursing homes or rehabilitation facilities, there is a big difference. LTACHs treat patients who might be classified as intensive care patients at short-term hospitals. Some of these facilities are stand alone hospitals; however, nearly half of all LTACHs are "hospitals within hospitals" because they are hosted by an acute care hospital that leases a floor, wing, or other space to the LTACH (Butcher, 2007).

Home Health Care

One of the most sought-out options for older adults requiring observation or nursing care upon discharge from a medical facility may be for home health care services. *Home health care* is designed for those who are homebound due to severity of illness or immobility. For reimbursement of allowable expenses, home health services must be medically necessary and ordered by a healthcare provider.

There has been much growth in the recent past related to the number of home health agencies. This increase is due in part to the desire to be cared for in familiar surroundings by families and in-home caregivers. Providing care in the home improves the quality of life and increases the likelihood that the person receiving care will remain more active and independent.

Although physical, occupational, and speech therapy may be obtained through home care, a registered nurse must have initial contact, complete an in-depth assessment, evaluate the client, and develop a plan of care to assure the individual's health condition warrants the need for nursing services to qualify for home health services. The majority of home health care patients are older adults with a variety of nursing needs, such as wound care, intravenous therapy, management of newly diagnosed diabetes, and tube feedings.

Managing Long-Term Needs

In the United States, the demand for long-term care is expected to rise exponentially. There were approximately 1.9 million people aged 90 and older; by 2050, the ranks of people 90 and older may reach 9 million, according to the United States

Census Bureau report commissioned by the National Institute on Aging (NIA) at the National Institutes of Health (Cire, 2011). In light of these findings, an older person's likelihood of living in a nursing home (long-term care) increases sharply with age. "About 1% of the young elderly (aged 65–69 years) currently live in a nursing home or long-term care facility. The proportion rises to 3% for ages 75–79, 11.2% for ages 85–89, 19.8% at ages 90–94, 31.0% at ages 95–99, and up to 38.2% among centenarians" (Cire, 2011, p. 1). As providers of care to the older adult populations, it is essential that we have an understanding of potential living arrangements and options available to address the growing needs of the older adult.

An important consideration for every older adult is safe and affordable housing. While this is a difficult subject to broach, this topic must be eventually addressed by the individual, caregivers, and family members. As a large part of America's population enters into their advancing years, the need for proper housing increases. With the potential for decreased mobility and the increase in needed medical requirements, housing options need to be flexible in providing a safe living environment.

Housing must meet all the needs of a senior citizen, including physical, financial, and accessibility needs. There may be seniors who are no longer able to take care of themselves or a spouse by themselves, so other viable options need to be explored. Older adults, as well as individuals providing care, need to work collaboratively to find the most optimal solution. There are many senior care housing/facility options available today, some of which will be discussed below.

Long-Term Care Facility

Traditionally referred to as nursing homes, ***long-term care facilities (LTCFs)*** provide care primarily for older adults or any persons who have lost some or all of their ability for self-care due to illness, disability, or advanced dementia; to be able to operate, they have to follow guidelines and meet patients' needs to give proper care (SeniorHousing.Net, 2012). Most seniors who live in nursing homes have complex medical needs, so the best option is this type of facility. Medical assistance and care is given to those who qualify by nursing home directors and physicians. Nursing homes are often times thought of as end-of-life care; however, these facilities are also commonly utilized for rehabilitation, recovery from surgery, extended illnesses, wound care, and debility.

Registered nurses working in long-term care provide care planning and oversight of multiple residents, as well as direct and coordinate the care provided by licensed practical nurses and certified nursing assistants. The challenge for nurses in this environment is to maintain the nutritional status and functional ability of the resident while preventing complications such as immobility, pressure ulcers, and falls. Dementia care is often a substantial part of the nursing care provided, as is managing residents' chronic and acute medical conditions and medication regimens.

Alzheimer's/Memory Care Facilities

A growing trend in LTCFs is to offer dedicated units for the care of persons with middle-to-late stage Alzheimer's disease and other dementias. Alzheimer's facilities are long-term residences for individuals suffering from Alzheimer's disease and other types of memory loss or dementia. There are several long-term care options that may be appropriate for an Alzheimer's patient, depending on the stage to which the disease has progressed.

Often, family members can render the care that is required for their loved ones in the home setting during the early stages of the disease process. However, due to the progressive nature of the disease, once the person has entered the middle to late stages of dementia, the older adult usually cannot be left alone. As memory loss and increased needs on behalf of the elder become evident, home care givers often are overwhelmed and unable to provide the round-the-clock care that is necessary.

Memory care facilities are designed for seniors with Alzheimer's or other forms of dementia. As Alzheimer's disease or dementia progresses, the level of care and assistance a person requires increases (Seniorhomes.com, 2012). The goal of memory or dementia care is to preserve the functional status of the elder by providing supportive care that fosters self worth and socialization in a safe environment within the context of diminishing cognitive capacity. In times of placement, the decision for care can be a complex issue for the caregiver(s), who are often riddled with grief.

Eden Alternative

The Eden Alternative's principle-based philosophy, founded by Dr. William Thomas, empowers care partners to transform institutional approaches to care into the creation of a community where "life is worth living" (Eden Alternative, 2009, p. 1). The Eden Alternative positively impacts the physical environment, organizational structure, and psychosocial interactions of the older adults' living arrangements to improve conditions for older adults—in essence, providing them with a voice. This model is not only utilized in home settings, but extended care/skilled nursing facilities as well.

The approach is related to de-institutionalizing the current culture and environment of nursing homes and other care facilities by instituting older adults concerns, needs, and desires to recapture and maintain autonomy over their daily lives. By moving away from the top-down bureaucratic approach, structured scheduling of daily care, and familial restrictions related to how and when care should be completed, the older adult takes charge over their lives and home. "Edenizing" organizations are helping to support a meaningful life for their older adults.

Maintaining Independence: Living Options for Older Adults

Aging in place is the idea of providing stability for the older adult by working toward the common goal of either maintaining the current residence or living in a non-healthcare environment. Aging in place successfully requires planning on the part of the older adult, caregivers, and healthcare professionals. To accommodate physical, mental, and psychological changes that may accompany aging, varying changes may be required within the residence. This may be accomplished through the use of products, services, and conveniences that enable the older adult to remain in their current home setting without having to move as circumstances change (SeniorResource, 2012a).

To provide choices and informed decision making for older adults, it is imperative that nurses have the knowledge to assist the older adult through improved awareness of community services, availability of services, access points, eligibility for service, and affordability of quality care for older adults (Tang & Pickard, 2008). Some of the types of programs that promote aging in place will be discussed below.

Adult Day Services

Many older adults prefer to remain in their own homes as they age; however, many persons are faced with the decreased ability to maintain their independence because of age-related physical or cognitive impairments or chronic health conditions. For these individuals, *adult day services* (ADS) might be an ideal alternative to congregate residential care such as assisted living and nursing homes (Matthiesen & Schumaker, 2010). Adult day services create a partnership among caregivers, families, and professionals in managing the health and well-being of an individual to promote and support aging in place. An ADS program may provide health care, meals, activities, and care in a group setting for households where the caregiver might not be available to provide care at home during the day.

Adult daycare programs may be sponsored by a variety of organizations, including churches, hospitals, or healthcare systems, which includes extended-care facilities. These centers provide socialization, planned outings, nutritional diet-appropriate meals, supervised activity, medication administration, and a safe environment for older adults. Many ADS providers offer 6-, 8-, or 12-hour service options, which allows caregivers to continue working or have respite periods. The persons who may benefit from these services are those with chronic health conditions, cognitive impairments, limited mobility or physical disabilities, and safety concerns.

Notable Quotes

"The vast majority of older adults want to age in place, so they can continue to live in their own homes or communities" (AARP, 2011, p. 1). Retrieved from http://www.aarp.org/home-garden/livable-communities/info-11-2011/Aging-In-Place.html)

Assisted Living Facility

Assisted living facilities (ALFs) come in different shapes and sizes. Many residences are freestanding facilities, while others are a part of retirement communities that have long-term care facilities attached. Residents are older adults who can function on their own, but may need some assistance with activities of daily living (ADLs). Additionally, this living arrangement can also provide for a feeling of security for those who do not feel safe living alone.

The typical living arrangements for ALFs vary. In general, they replicate the typical apartment settings with various floorplans and sizes to accommodate the needs, finances, and desires of the renter. Assisted living facilities generally provide nutritious meals, planned activates, common rooms for entertainment, gardens, exercise, and game rooms for the residents whereby older adults can socialize with others in a safe and protected environment.

Unlike a nursing home, assisted living residences are not subject to federal standards or inspections. Individual states vary widely in quality standards, licensing requirements, level of assistance offered to residents, staffing, and monitoring of residents. It is advisable that older adults and their families review their current and future needs before choosing an assisted living facility. Depending on the level of assistance required, the older adult may choose a facility that is connected with a long-term care facility, so that as the need for care increases, they may progress to the next level of care available while essentially remaining in the same facility. The drawback of choosing a free-standing facility is that in the event the older adult's condition worsens, where he or she requires greater assistance and care, it may be necessary to find an alternative living arrangement, which then can lead to relocation stress and an increased financial burden.

Coming Home Project: Caring for Rural America

Coming Home: Affordable Assisted Living was a 13-year, $13 million national program created in 1992 by the Robert Wood Johnson Foundation (RWJF) and NCB Capital Impact to develop affordable assisted-living models, with a specific focus on underserved, low-income older adult populations in rural America. In this report, it is noted that rural communities within the United States contain the nation's highest concentrations of older people per capita. The primary mission of this project was to provide affordable assisted-living solutions that fulfill the growing need for housing, and to empower older adults in underserved communities (Murray, Maher, Jenkens, & Baldwin, 2009).

Older adults with chronic disabilities need health care, personal care, and social services that rural communities are often unable to provide in sufficient quantity or duration, especially for low-income seniors. Affordable assisted-living housing arrangements offer a nursing home alternative when older adults require more assistance than they can obtain in their home. In 1992, affordable assisted living was almost nonexistent in rural areas of the United States. As a consequence, many rural older adults were forced to leave their home communities or were prematurely institutionalized in nursing homes in order to receive needed services. Despite improvements for housing in these rural areas, we still have a long way to go.

Green House Concept

The Green House model of assisted living de-institutionalizes long-term care by restoring individuals to a home in the community. *Green House* projects support the most positive elderhood and work life possible, by combining small homes with the full range of personal care and clinical services expected in high-quality nursing homes and providing opportunities for meaningful engagements and relationships (The Green House Project, 2011). Endorsed by the Centers for Medicare & Medicaid Services, the Green House Model developed by geriatrician Dr. William Thomas, is becoming an increasingly popular alternative to traditional long-term care facilities (The Green House Project, 2011).

Green Houses look like other homes in a residential community. Larger than an average home, they may house about 10 residents, each with a private bedroom, but sharing a central living and kitchen area to foster a home environment. Workers in Green Houses received additional training, and staff turnover is significantly less than a nursing home setting (Haber, 2010).

The primary purpose of the model is to provide a place where elders can receive assistance and support with activities of daily living and clinical care without that assistance becoming the focus of their existence. Caregivers in Green Houses are empowered to provide individualized care to older adults who retain control over daily activities—in short, creating an environment that is a home (see **Figure 25-2**). Chapter 8 provides a more thorough discussion of Green Houses.

Independent Living

The term *independent living* can encompass a variety of settings, including home ownership, apartment dwelling, retirement communities, and subsidized government housing for seniors. Since a large majority of senior citizens rely on Social Security benefits as their main source of income, it is essential to take prudent financial considerations into place when selecting housing (Gonzales, 2011). Unfortunately, for the older adult on a limited income, advance planning is essential.

Green House Philosophy

The philosophy of The Green House long-term care model is to enhance elders' quality of life by:

- Creating small homes that offer intentional communities and high levels of care
- Recognizing and valuing individuality of elders and staff
- Supporting elders' dignity
- Honoring autonomy and choice
- Providing privacy
- Creating an atmosphere of security
- Promoting maximum functional abilities
- Facilitating physical comfort
- Offering opportunities for reciprocal relationships between elders and staff
- Fostering enjoyment by offering meaningful activities
- Fostering emotional and spiritual well-being
- Offering comprehensive care

Figure 25-2 The Green House philosophy.

Source: http://thegreenhouseproject.org/about-us/mission-vision/

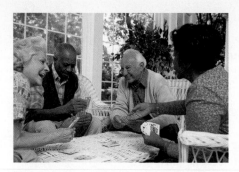

Figure 25-3 Independent and assisted living facilities provide opportunities for safety, comfort, and social networking.

Source: © Comstock Images/Alamy Images.

Subsidized housing, available through the United States Department of Housing and Urban Development (HUD), is limited in number, depending on locale, and may have waiting lists so long that it can take years to receive rent-controlled apartments. Other options for independent living will be discussed below (see **Figure 25-3**).

Continuing Care Retirement Community

Continuing care retirement communities (CCRCs) provide a continuum of care that spans independent living to skilled nursing care in a traditional nursing home setting, all within a single campus setting. Levels of care provided are based on the older adults' needs. Depending on the facility's business model, contractual services are provided often for an additional fee, or may be included in an upfront lump-sum type of payment plan.

Older adults can move seamlessly among the living settings, beginning with independent living, to assisted living and skilled or long-term care as their condition warrants. This type of facility make transition to a higher level of care somewhat easier for the resident since they remain within similar environments. Some CCRCs provide home health services while the resident maintains their current residence in independent or assisted living based on individual need and duration of need for the higher level of care. Nurses in this type of setting are valuable in assisting residents as they encounter various levels of care. However, one of the most important aspects of nursing care is that of health promotion and wellness, to assist the older adult in maintaining their highest level of functioning for as long as possible.

Foster Care or Group Homes

Group homes usually consist of many older adults living under one roof, all of whom have varying physical and medical needs. The majority of the residents are able to perform the majority of ADLs, but often have safety concerns and require cueing and assistance with activities such as bathing, dressing, or taking medications. The premise of this living arrangement is to provide the older adult with comfortable living accommodations in a safe, personalized, family-like environment. Depending on individual state requirements, these facilities may require licensing to operate or provide care.

Some persons offering this service have a small number of older adults in their home, whereas others have constructed or purchased a large home specifically for this purpose. These settings provide an alternative to nursing home care. Although nurses and other medical personnel may own and operate a group home, there is no requirement that a person have a healthcare background, nor is there a requirement that a nurse's services be available to the residents. It is imperative that those considering this type of setting thoroughly investigate the facility prior to placement. Social workers are a good resource to provide information regarding local foster or group homes.

Naturally Occurring Retirement Community

Naturally occurring retirement communities (NORCs) are living communities specifically for older adults. Most are duplexes, condominiums, apartments, trailers, or single-family homes that are all located in the same neighborhood. Residents typically have to be 55 years old or older, without children living with them, to purchase or lease this type of property. Currently, approximately 27% of older adults live in a NORC (SeniorResource, 2012b). The appeal for these communities is that they are geared to the needs of retirees and generally offer significant amenities and services that may include:

> Social and recreational programs
> Continuing education programs
> Information and counseling
> Outside maintenance and referral services
> Emergency and preventive healthcare programs
> Meal programs
> Transportation on a schedule

A Shift in Living Arrangements

When asked, over 80% of older adults state they want to live at home; however, this option may require healthcare assistance (Seniorcare.net, 2012). For America's 75 million aging adults, options for care decisions have traditionally involved relocating to a more "traditional" type of setting (University of Missouri-Columbia, 2011). However, with the advent of an aging in place strategy, a new model of care is being undertaken to make it possible for older adults to stay home, in an environment they feel comfortable in, utilizing advanced technology. Assistive domotics, also coined *Smart Home* Technology, is an application of home automation that focuses on enabling older adults or disabled persons to live at their home instead of a healthcare facility. Smart Home Technology is already being utilized in multiple areas and will continue to allow older adults to remain in their comfortable surroundings while assistance is provided via sensors that can manipulate the environment for comfort and anticipate the resident's needs.

Elder Cottage Housing Opportunity

Utilizing Smart Home technology, elder cottage housing opportunities (ECHOs) are free-standing, mobile, modular-type homes that can be transformed to be temporarily placed on a caregiver's property to maintain safety for the older adult requiring assistance while allowing for privacy and independence. Similar to a hospital room or studio-type apartment, this "pod" can remotely monitor the resident through sensors that alert caregivers to an occupant's fall, monitor telemetry remotely, and can utilize computer technology to remind the occupant to take medications. Based on the resident and caregiver requirements, the technology utilized is specialized based on specific needs of the individual. This same technology also provides entertainment, offering a selection of music, reading materials, and movies. It also contains a family communication center that provides telemetry, environmental control, and dynamic interaction to off-site caregivers through smart and robotic technology

(MEDcottage, 2012). Each unit comes minimally equipped with amenities to include living space, handicap accessible bathroom, and a kitchenette.

End-of-Life Care Options
Hospice Care

In its earliest days, the concept of hospice was rooted in the centuries-old idea of offering a place of shelter and rest, or "hospitality," to weary and sick travelers on a long journey. In 1967, Dame Cicely Saunders at Saint Christopher's Hospice in London first used the term "hospice" to describe specialized care for dying patients (American Cancer Society, 2011). Today, the concept of *hospice* is centered on the holistic, interdisciplinary care that helps the dying person "live until they die." A number of team members who specialize in thanatology and palliative care work together to provide quality care for patients in their final months, weeks, days, or hours of life. Pain management and comfort care are the standards upon which treatment is based to make death as comfortable and easy a transition as possible.

Hospice care can be found in a variety of facilities. Some hospices are stand-alone organizations with their own building. Home care agencies offers hospice services, and in some cases nursing homes may offer a hospice unit or utilize hospice nurses on the skilled unit from an outside agency. Whatever the setting, hospice care requires patience, compassion, caring, expertise, and interdisciplinary communication among the caregivers, the person, and loved ones.

Nursing Responsibility in Transitioning Care

Regardless of nursing care settings, it is a requirement that nurses contribute to the safety and continuity of care for their patients upon discharge or transfer to another care setting. Diligence on the part of the discharging nurse and the admission nurse of the receiving facilit, is essential to assure a lapse of care does not occur.

For interagency transfers, a detailed transfer form must be completed, as must a verbal report to the accepting facility, prior to discharge/transfer. The basic information to be included includes: a detailed assessment, treatments, wounds, current medications, allergies, level of independence, recent diagnostic testing, and primary care practitioner notification upon discharge and admission to the receiving facility. **Figure 25-4** depicts a typical transfer form one may encounter in practice.

Discharge to a home setting requires detailed discharge instructions for the patient and applicable caregiver. Timely education and planning are essential to ensure that the patient and caregiver are able to appropriately transition care without disruption. To achieve this, the nurse begins planning for discharge at the time of admission. With the ongoing trend for decreased length of stay in the acute care facility, time is of the essence. Teaching and understanding of the care needs must be undertaken to ensure optimal health maintenance is achieved. **Figure 25-5** is an example of discharge instructions utilized by healthcare facilities.

Purpose: To provide pertinent information for patients being discharged or transferred throughout the healthcare continuum.

Instructions: To be sent to the receiving facility upon discharge.

NAME: _____ **DOB** _____

Discharge to: ☐ home health ☐ long-term care ☐ rehabilitation ☐ outpatient services ☐ other:_____

Admit from: ☐ nursing home:_____ ☐ assisted living ☐ other:_____

Allergies/Reactions (include medications, food, latex, environmental etc.): ☐ No known allergies

_____

_____

Height: _____ ☐ cm ☐ inches **Weight:** _____ ☐ kg. ☐ lb. **Diabetes:** ☐ yes ☐ no

Pulse: _____ **Temperature:** _____ **Respiration rate:** _____ **Blood pressure:** _____

Adult assuming care: ☐ N/A Name: _____

Relationship:_____ Phone #: (_____)_____

Vision: ☐ adequate ☐ poor ☐ blind **Glasses/Contacts:** ☐ no ☐ yes ☐ with patient

Hearing: ☐ adequate ☐ poor ☐ deaf **Hearing aid:** ☐ right ☐ left ☐ with patient

Dentures: ☐ full ☐ upper ☐ lower ☐ partial ☐ with patient

Mental status: ☐ alert ☐ confused ☐ unresponsive **Oriented:** ☐ person ☐ place ☐ time

Behavior: ☐ cooperative ☐ uncooperative ☐ wandering ☐ noisy ☐ aggressive

Communication: ☐ speaks ☐ writes ☐ gestures **Understanding:** ☐ speaks ☐ writes ☐ gestures

Language: ☐ English ☐ other: _____ ☐ needs interpreter

Mobility aids: ☐ walker ☐ wheelchair ☐ cane ☐ other: _____

History of falls: ☐ yes ☐ no **Fall risk:** ☐ yes ☐ no **VITIES OF DAILY LIVING** (mark as appropriate)

Activities

Bowel incontinence: ☐ yes ☐ no Date of last bowel movement: _____

Bladder incontinence: ☐ yes ☐ no Last urine void: _____

Date Foley inserted/changed: _____ time: _____ If Foley discontinued, date: _____

Activities	Total Assist	Partial Assist	Self Care
Bowel			
Bladder			
Bathing			
Dressing			
Eating			
Turning			
Transfers			
Ambulation			

Type of infusion catheter: ☐ Peripheral IV ☐ PICC line Dialysis access: _____ Site:_____

Type of central line: Insertion date:_____ # Lumens:_____ Site:_____

Isolation precautions: ☐ MRSA ☐ VRE ☐ C-Diff ☐ Tuberculosis ☐ other:_____

Date Influenza vaccine given: _____ **Date Pneumococcal vaccine given:**_____

Patient aware of diagnosis: ☐ yes ☐ no, explain:_____

Physician Name Procedure/Service

Family/Designee aware of transfer: ☐ yes ☐ no, explain:

DNR: ☐ yes ☐ no **Advance Directive** ☐ yes ☐ no

Significant care issues/assessments (include psychosocial; fall interventions; Braden Score; full description of skin integrity including wounds, incision and ulcers and also including size (length and depth), location, color, drainage, odor and stage, if pressure ulcer; dressing, tubes, aspiration risk special equipment, etc.):

_____

_____

_____

Signature/Title: _____ Print Name: _____ Date: _____ Time: _____

Figure 25-4 Interagency nursing communication record.

Source: http://www.deha.org

DISCHARGE DATE:	University Hospital cares about your health. If you smoke, we strongly urge you to quit. See back for referrals.
DISCHARGE SUMMARY WILL BE DONE BY:	**PLEASE BRING THIS FORM WITH YOU TO YOUR DOCTOR'S OFFICE**
ATTENDING.	

DIAGNOSIS/PROBLEM LIST

You were in the hospital because:

MEDICATIONS

Medication reconciliation form reviewed ☐   Prescription given: ☐ Yes ☐ No

ACTIVITY

☐ No restrictions   ☐ Restricted

☐ Ask your doctor about your exercise program

DIET

☐ No restrictions   ☐ Restricted

WOUND CARE

☐ Keep your incision clean. You may shower and pat the incision dry.

If pain, redness or swelling at your incision site, or if you have a fever greater than 101, call your doctor.

☐ Other:

Education and handouts given: ☐ CHF ☐ AMI ☐ Diabetes ☐ Heart disease ☐ Other:

Follow up/Tests –to be followed up with your doctor

Appointments/Follow up	When	Phone Number

Home care instructions:

Symptoms to report to your physician- decreased activity tolerance, increased shortness of breath, difficulty breathing, chest pain, dizziness, 5lbs weight gain in 1 week, nausea, swelling in feet or legs.

I/We have received theses instructions and have been able to ask questions and am/are aware of whom to contact for questions after discharge.

Patient/individual receiving instructions   Relationship

Nurse signature   Date/Time   MD signature   Date/Time

Patient Label

DISCHARGE INSTRUCTIONS

White Copy – Medical Records   Yellow Copy - Patient

Figure 25-5 Discharge instructions.

Source: http://www.hospital-forms.com

Caring for the Caregiver
Respite Care

Caregiving for a dependent older adult can be a demanding task. Often caregivers need a break or respite from the daily responsibilities to relieve stress and prevent caregiver burnout. *Respite care* provides much-needed time off for family members who care for someone who is ill, injured, frail, debilitated, or demented. Respite care can be provided in an adult day facility, in the home of the person being cared for, or in an assisted living or long-term care facility.

Although there are different approaches to respite care, all have the basic premise: to provide caregivers with temporary, intermittent, or substitute care to allow for relief from the daily responsibilities of caregiving. Respite care is not covered by Medicare or Medicaid, unless the person receiving care is in hospice care, and, even so, the coverage is extremely limited. As nurses, it is necessary to learn of community resources that can be utilized, based on the older adult's needs, to assist the family, such as churches, synagogues, or service-based groups.

Summary

Gerontological nurses will care for older adults in a variety of care settings; as a result, they need to fully comprehend the various settings where care is implemented. It is imperative that the nurse recognize and institute appropriate client- and family-specific interventions to decrease the potential risk factors in transitioning across healthcare settings for older adults, as well as utilize various evidence-based practice care transition models used in the care settings discussed throughout this chapter (see **Box 25-3**).

BOX 25-3   Web Exploration

These weblinks connect to current and innvotive examples for solutions for senior care, some of which are discussed in this chapter. Visit these sites for some useful resources.

http://www.interact2.net/docs/INTERACT_II_Tool_Tablec.pdf

http://www.hospitalmedicine.org/ResourceRoomRedesign/RR_CareTransitions/PDFs/Project_BOOST_Fact_SheetFinal.pdf

http://www.caretransitions.org/

http://guidedcare.org/solution.asp

http://www.interact2.net/docs/INTERACT_II_Figurec.pdf

http://www.interact2.net/index.aspx

http://www.seniorresource.com/

http://www.seniorcare.net/

Critical Thinking Exercises

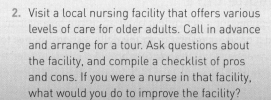

1. Visit the websites of the Transitional Care Models highlighted in this chapter; compare and contrast them. Discuss your findings with a student nurse in your clinical group.

2. Visit a local nursing facility that offers various levels of care for older adults. Call in advance and arrange for a tour. Ask questions about the facility, and compile a checklist of pros and cons. If you were a nurse in that facility, what would you do to improve the facility?

Personal Reflections

1. Have you or anyone close to you ever been hospitalized and discharged to home? What was it that they needed upon returning home? Was it difficult? What made the transition back to home go well or not so well?

2. Consider an older adult who may be in your family. As their care needs increase, what type of facility or services would you most likely incorporate? What alternatives to care could be provided? How difficult would it be to place a loved one in a long-term care facility?

Case Study 25-1

The Borkowskis are a close knit family of five whose grandfather, Papa B, has been living with them in their home since he was widowed 10 years prior. Papa B is 88 years old and has been recently diagnosed with middle-stage Alzheimer's disease. The family is having increasing difficulty in supervising and providing round-the-clock care for him. Unfortunately, it has gotten to the point where it is no longer safe for him to be home alone. The adult daughter of Papa B, with whom he resides, works full time, as does her husband. The three children are in school during the day.

The family desperately wants to keep Papa B at home, but do not know what resources may be available to them. As their nurse, they come to you for help and guidance.

Questions

1. What services might the Borkowski family use to help them keep Papa B at home? Do these services seem feasible at this time?

2. As his condition deteriorates further, what services discussed in this chapter might be necessary at various points in time?

References

American Cancer Society. (2011). *Hospice care.* Retrieved from http://www.cancer.org/ Treatment/FindingandPayingforTreatment/ChoosingYourTreatmentTeam/HospiceCare/ hospice-care-what-is-hospice-care

Arora, V. M., Prochaska, M. L., Farnan, J. M., D'Arcy, M. J., Schwanz, K. J., Vinci, L. M., … Johnson, J. K. (2010). Problems after discharge and understanding of communication with their primary care physicians among hospitalized seniors: A mixed methods study. *Journal of Hospital Medicine, 5*(2), 385–391. doi: 10.1002/jhm.668

Butcher, L., (2007). Hospitalists and LTACs: For some physicians, it's a perfect fit. *Today'sHospitalist.* Retrieved http://www.todayshospitalist.com/index.php?b=articles_read&cnt=321

Cire, B. (2011). *NIH-commissioned census bureau report describes oldest Americans—Is 90 the new 85?* National Institutes of Health-National Institute on Aging. Retrieved from http://www.nia.nih.gov/ newsroom/2011/11/nih-commissioned-census-bureau-report-describes-oldest-americans

Coleman, E. A., Parry, C., Chalmers, S., & Min, S. (2006). The care transitions intervention. *Archives of Internal Medicine, 166,* 1822–1828.

Corbett, C. F., Setter, S., Daratha, K. B., Neumiller, J. L., & Wood, L. D. (2010) Nurse identified hospital to home medication discrepancies: Implications for improving transitional care. *Geriatric Nursing, 31*(3),188–196.

Counsell, S. R., Callahan, C. M., Buttar, A. B., Clark, D. O., & Frank, K. I. (2005). Geriatric Resources for Assessment and Care of Elders (GRACE): A new model of primary care for low-income seniors. *Journal of the American Geriatric Society, 5*(7), 1136–1141.

Delaware Healthcare Association. *Form B: Interagency nursing communication record.* Retrieved from http://www.deha.org/Interagency%20Form-B%20%201-06%20Final.pdf

Eden Alternative (2012). *The Eden Alternative.* Retrieved from http://www.edenalt.org/

Ellenbecker, C. H., Frazier, S. C., & Verney, S. (2004). Nursing observations and experiences of problems and adverse effects of medication management in home care. *Geriatric Nursing, 25*(3), 164–170.

Golden, A., Tweary, S., Dang, S., & Roos, B. (2010). Care management's challenges and opportunities to reduce the rapid rehospitalization of frail community-dwelling older adults. *The Gerontologist, 50*(4), 451–458. doi:10.1093/geront/gnq015

Gonzales, C., (2011). *Congressional corner: By Representative Charles Gonzalez (20th-TX).* Retrieved from http://seniorsleague.org/2011/congressional-corner-by-representative-charles-gonzalez-20th-tx/

Haber, D. (2010). Promoting healthy Aging. In K. L. Mauk (Ed.) *Gerontological nursing: Competencies for care* (pp. 328–353). Sudbury, MA: Jones & Bartlett.

Hennessey, B., & Suter, P. (2011). The community-based transitions model: One agency's experience. *Home Healthcare Nurse, 29*(4), 218–230.

Hospital Forms.com. (2012). Retrieved from http://www.hospital-forms.com/index.html

Institute for Health Care Improvement (2010). *STAAR.* Retrieved from http://www.ihi.org/offerings/ Initiatives/STAAR/Documents/STAAR%20Issue%20Brief%20-%20Cross%20Continuum%20Teams .pdf

Institute of Medicine [IOM]. (2001). *Crossing the quality chasm: A new health system for the 21st century.* Washington, DC: National Academies Press.

Jones, A., & Foster, N. (1997). Transitional care: Bridging the gap. *MedSurg Nursing, 6*(1), 32–38.

Kelly, M., & Penney, E. (2011). Collaboration of hospital care managers and home care liaisons when transitioning patients. *Professional Case Management, 16*(3), 128–136.

Kripalani, S., LeFevre, F., Phillips C. O., Williams M. V., Basaviah, P, & Baker D. W. (2007). Deficits in communication and information transfer between hospital-based and primary care physicians: Implications for patient safety and continuity of care. *Journal of the American Medical Association, 297,* 831–841.

Matthiesen, S., & Schumaker, C., (2010). *Adult day services: Providing support and care for seniors and their families.* CARF International. Retrieved from http://www.carf.org/WorkArea/DownloadAsset .aspx?id=23809

Marek, K. D., & Antle, L. (2008). *Medication management of the community-dwelling older adult in patient safety and quality: An evidence-based handbook for nurses*. Rockville, MD: Agency for Healthcare Research and Quality.

MEDCottage. (2012). *About us*. Retrieved from http://medcottage.com/about.php

Murray, T., Maher, L., Jenkens, R., & Baldwin, C. (2009). *Coming Home*®: *Affordable assisted living*. Robert Woods Johnson Foundation.

Naylor, M. D., Aiken, L. H., Kurtzman, E. T., Olds, D. M., & Hirschman, K. B. (2011). The importance of transitional care in achieving health reform. *Health Affairs, 30*(4), 746–754. doi: 10.1377/hlthaff.2011.0041

Naylor, M., & Keating, S. A. (2008). Transitional Care: Moving patients from one care setting to another. *American Journal of Nursing, 108*, 58–63. doi: 10.109701.NAJ.0000336420.34946.3a

Ouslander, J. G., Lamb, G., Perlow, M. Givens, J. H., Kluge, L., Rutland, T., ... Saliba, D. (2010). Potentially avoidable hospitalizations of nursing home residents: Frequency, causes, and costs. *Journal of the American Geriatric Society, 58*, 627–635.

Patient protection and affordable care act. Public law 111–148. Retrieved from http://housedocs.house.gov/energycommerce/ppacacon.pdf

Popejoy, L. (2011). Complexity of family caregiving and discharge planning. *Journal of Family Nursing, 17*(11), 61–81.

Schillinger, D., Piette, J., Grumbach, K., Wang, F., Wilson, C., Daher, C., ...Bindman, A. B. (2003). Closing the loop: Physician communication with diabetic patients who have low health literacy. *Archives of Internal Medicine, 163*(1), 83–90.

SeniorCare.net. (2012). Retrieved from http://www.seniorcare.net/

SeniorHomes.com. (2012). *Senior housing options*. Retrieved from http://www.seniorhomes.com/

SeniorResource. (2012a). *Aging in place*. Retrieved from http://www.seniorresource.com/house.htm#hinplace

SeniorResource. (2012b). *What is a NORC?* Retrieved from http://www.seniorresource.com/ageinpl.htm#norc

Society for Hospital Medicine. (2008). *BOOSTing care transitions*. Retrieved from http://www.hospital-medicine.org/ResourceRoomRedesign/RR_CareTransitions/CT_Home.cfm

Tang, F., & Pickard, J. G. (2008). Aging in place or relocation: Perceived awareness of community-based long-term care and services. *Journal of Housing For the Elderly, 22*, 404–422.

The Green House Project: Caring homes for meaningful lives [SM]. (2011). Retrieved from http://thegreen-houseproject.org/

University of Missouri-Columbia. (2011). Aging in place preserves seniors' independence, reduces care costs, researchers find. *ScienceDaily*. Retrieved from http://www.sciencedaily.com/releases/2011/03/110307124816.htm

For a full suite of assignments and additional learning activities, see the access code at the front of your book.

LEARNING OBJECTIVES

At the end of this chapter, the reader will be able to:

> Identify historical influences and attitudes toward death and dying.
> Recognize the choices of older adults and their families in directing their end-of-life care as well as the nurse's role in support/implementation of the patient's choice of care.
> Compare curative care, hospice care, and palliative care.
> Examine the goals/objectives of curative, palliative, and hospice care at end of life.
> Discuss the nurse's role at end of life using the preceding concepts of care.
> Describe the nurse's role as a member of an interdisciplinary team focused on end-of-life care.
> Identify the fundamentals of pain and other symptom management.
> Discuss death in a contemporary multicultural society.
> Identify cultural traditions at end of life.
> Recognize the importance of spirituality at end of life.
> Describe some effects of grief and mourning on the elderly.
> Recognize caregiver/compassion fatigue.
> Describe ethical and legal issues common at end of life.
> Recognize several aspects of care contributing to a "good death."

KEY TERMS

Addiction

Advance directives

Allow natural death (AND)

Communicating bad news

Complementary therapies

Curative/acutecare

Dependence

Do not resuscitate (DNR)

End of life

Five Wishes

Good death

Grief

Hope

Hospice care

Interdisciplinary group/team (IDG/IDT)

Mourning

Pain scales

Palliative care

Physician's Orders for Life Sustaining
    Treatment (POLST)

SUPPORT study

Symptom management

Tolerance

Chapter 26

End-of-Life Care

Patricia Warring
Luana S. Krieger-Blake

Woody Allen once said, "It's not that I'm afraid to die, I just don't want to be there when it happens" (Allen, 1976, Act 1). "By excluding death from our life we cannot live a full life, and by admitting death into our life we enlarge and enrich it." This statement, written by a victim of the Holocaust, describes the powerful role that death has in human life (Hillesum, 1996, p. 155).

Reality tells us that every person will die. In 2009, less than 10% of U.S. citizens died suddenly, either from accidents, influenza and pneumonia, or intentional self-harm; the vast majority of Americans died after dealing with prolonged illness (Centers for Disease Control and Prevention [CDC], 2010).

The accumulation of experiences throughout a person's lifetime helps to clearly define the way he or she wishes to experience his or her own end of life. Familial and cultural factors, along with life events, often provide defining moments that influence a person's choices when facing the end of one's life and a death that will come sooner rather than later. Anthropologist Margaret Mead was quoted as saying, "When a person is born we rejoice, and when they're married we jubilate, but when they die we try to pretend nothing happened."

This chapter deals with the nurse's role in assisting a patient and family to identify the options for meeting end-of-life needs. It promotes the role of the nurse as a member of a team of professionals who focus on care and treatment of issues specific to the elderly as their health declines. It also offers practical assistance for nurses as they deal with various aspects of end-of-life care.

Historically, education about end-of-life issues and medical needs has been lacking. Initiatives including those by Last Acts and those encouraged by the Robert Wood

Johnson Foundation, such as Education in Palliative and End-of-Life Care (EPEC), End-of-Life Nursing Education Consortium (ELNEC), and Center to Advance Palliative Care (CAPC), are in place to address the need for additional information and research in this area.

One of the most demanding roles nurses undertake is that of caring for patients near the end of life. Nurses provide the most direct care for patients and families, and also help the family provide care that is competent, comprehensive, and compassionate. Therefore, nurses "must take the lead in integrating palliative and end-of-life care into the daily practice of every nurse, making it a core competency for all nurses who care for people with actual or potentially life-limiting illnesses... Nurses must advocate for and deliver this quality care—regardless of specialty" (Rushton, Spencer, & Johanson, 2004, p. 34).

Caring for dying patients and their families is a common component of the nurse's role, yet it can be particularly distressing for nursing students because very little classroom or clinical time is spent in this area. It has been suggested that because of the inherent richness in working with these patients, clinical rotations should be structured appropriately to include end-of-life experiences (Allchin, 2006). Partnering with local hospices and/or palliative care programs to provide educational opportunities and hands-on care of the dying would benefit the student by providing a relevant life experience.

Historical Attitudes Toward Death and Dying

With the advent of ever-increasing modern technology, especially following World War II, dying in the United States underwent a multitude of changes. In years past, Americans frequently lived in multigenerational homes, often in rural settings where living and dying experiences occurred commonly on the farms. Children were exposed to life and death issues as a matter of fact and grew to be adults having some experience of death before experiencing the death of someone close to them. As the ability to cure illnesses and to prolong life developed, technology took death to the hospital—to the sophistication of machines, antibiotics, chemotherapy, surgery, and such—and away from the comforts of home and family.

The role of nursing has changed along with the evolution of technology in administering end-of-life care in this country. For the most part, nurses shared the focus toward cure prevalent in the hospital setting. Training to care for the dying patient is often linked to the technical aspects of care and the physical preparation of the body after death (Krisman-Scott, 2003). A research and literature review performed by Benoliel for the period 1900–1960 revealed only 21 articles for nurses about caring for the dying patient: "There was little evidence that care of the dying was ever a major concern of nurses in this country" (Quint, 1967, p. 11).

As a result of the changes in our attitudes toward death and dying over time, some have said that the United States is a death-denying society. Kerry Crammer, MD, said, "In the Orient, dying is a requirement. In Europe, dying is inevitable. In America, dying appears to be an option" (Lewis, 2001, p. 24).

This death-denying attitude has created very expensive medical care. Spending on behalf of Medicare beneficiaries in their last year of life is five to six times as much as for other beneficiaries. Medicare expenditures are not distributed evenly across the last 12 months of life, but accelerate rapidly in the last few months, peaking at 20 times the amount for other beneficiaries in the last month of life as a result of inpatient hospital spending (Hogan, Lunney, Gabel, & Lynn, 2003).

Even though the expense of medical care at *end of life* is great, it does not necessarily follow that the needs of the elderly terminally ill are being met. The *SUPPORT study* (the Study to Understand Prognosis and Preferences for Outcomes and Risks of Treatment) conducted between 1989 and 1994 reported that nurses often were the first to recognize the impending death of a patient (Sheehan & Schirm, 2003). It also revealed that our healthcare system does not meet either the needs of patients with advanced chronic illnesses or the needs of dying, terminally ill patients (Quaglietti, Blum, & Ellis, 2004). Nor does the care we have come to accept meet the wishes of many Americans who are terminally ill. The National Hospice and Palliative Care Organization (NHPCO) reports that a great majority of Americans say their wish is to die at home, but of the 2.4 million Americans who die each year, less than 25% actually die at home. In comparison, of the nearly 1.6 million patients who received hospice care in 2010, almost 67% died at home (NHPCO, 2012).

Recently, dying is beginning to be seen in a newer, more realistic light. Ira Byock, a leading palliative care physician and advocate for improving care at end of life, has linked dying to an ongoing potential for growth. "Dying represents more than a set of problems to be solved; it represents an extraordinary opportunity—an opportunity for review, for restitution, for amends, for exploration, for development, for insight. In short, it is an opportunity for growth" (Kinzbrunner, Weinreb, & Policzer, 2002, p. 259). Instead of growing up, growing old, and dying, Dr. Byock suggests we grow up, grow old, and grow on. "Growing on takes place for both the terminally ill aged and their families. And although patients and their families will universally find growth producing deaths as important and positive, it may not be easy. Indeed there are typically many obstacles that must be overcome if the process of death is to unfold in a productive manner" (McKinnon & Miller, 2002, pp. 259–260).

Nurses have the opportunity and ability to influence the process of death by virtue of their proximity to patients and families. Nurses spend more time with patients and their families at end of life than any other member of the healthcare team (Ferrell, Grant, & Virani, 1999). Families and patients look to the nurse for support, education, and guidance at this difficult time, yet little education is provided to prepare nurses for this unique type of care. Nurses face end-of-life situations in almost all practice settings, including hospitals, hospices, long-term care facilities, home care, prisons, and clinics, but many remain uncomfortable providing care. Because of the importance of end-of-life care, nursing education is beginning to focus on care at this stage of life (Hospice and Palliative Nurses Association [HPNA], 2004b).

The focus of care at end of life should center on living with terminal illness—with medical care, support, and interventions geared toward quality of life and comfort, rather than on prolonging suffering or the dying process—if that is what the patient wants. In determining the wishes of patients for end-of-life care, their physical, emotional, psychosocial, and spiritual needs must all be addressed. The cumulative nature of these aspects of a person's life will impact the choices they make at this important time.

Communication About End of Life
Talking About Death and Dying

Talking about death and dying is often difficult for both nurses and patients. If the nurse doesn't respond in a way that encourages discussion, that discussion will likely not take place, and death will become the "elephant in the room"—something unavoidable and yet taboo (Griffie, Nelson-Marten, & Muchka, 2004; see **Box 26-1**).

Perhaps the easiest method of learning about a person's preferences is for the caregiver to simply ask them! However, these conversations are often not held because of fear—the elderly person's fear of being perceived as giving up, the family's fear of not wanting the elderly person to think they are wished to be dead, or perhaps the care provider's fear of not knowing what to say or how to discuss bad news. The societal attitudes about denying death are certainly a factor in whether these conversations are held. In hospice circles, it has been implied that most people would rather talk to their children about drugs and sex than to their elderly parents about terminal illness. There are resources designed to assist with these conversations, because not having the conversation may prohibit an individual from having the type of care they want, simply because they are not aware of the options.

Communicating Bad News

The Education in Palliative and End-of-Life Care (EPEC) Project, supported by the American Medical Association and the Robert Wood Johnson Foundation (Emanuel, von Gunten, & Ferris, 1999), as well as End-of-Life Nursing Education Consortium (ELNEC), view the communication of bad news as an essential skill for physicians. It is also an essential skill for nurses and other interdisciplinary team members who interact with the patients and families.

BOX 26-1   There's an Elephant in the Room

There's an Elephant in the Room

By Terry Kettering

There's an elephant in the room.

It is large and squatting, so it's hard to get around it.

Yet we squeeze by with, "How are you?" and, "I'm fine ..."

And a thousand other forms of trivial chatter.

We talk about the weather,

We talk about work.

We talk about everything else ...

Except the "elephant" in the room.

There's an elephant in the room.

We all know it is there,

We are thinking about the elephant

As we talk together.

It is constantly on our minds.

For, you see, it is a very big elephant.

It has hurt us all, but we do not talk about

The elephant in the room.

Oh, please, say her name.

Oh, please, say, "Barbara" again.

Oh, please, let's talk about

The elephant in the room.

For if we talk about her death,

Perhaps we can talk about her life.

Can I say, "Barbara" to you

And not have you look away?

For if I cannot,

Then you are leaving me alone—

In a room—

With an elephant!

Source: Reprinted with permission of Bereavement Publishing, Inc., (888) 604-4673, 4765 Carefree Circle, Colorado Springs, CO 80917

EPEC Project Module 2 presents a six-step approach to *communicating bad news* (Emanuel et al., 1999):

1. *Get started:* Plan what to say, confirm medical facts, create a conducive environment, determine who else the patient would like present, and allocate adequate time.
2. *Find out what the patient knows:* Assess his or her ability to comprehend bad news.
3. *Find out how much the patient wants to know:* Recognize and support patient preference to decline information and to designate someone else to communicate on his or her behalf; accommodate cultural, religious, and socio-economic influences.
4. *Share information:* Say it, then stop. Pause frequently, check for understanding, and use silence and body language; avoid vagueness, jargon, and euphemisms.
5. *Respond to feelings:* Expect affective, cognitive, and fight–flight responses; be prepared for strong emotions and a broad range of reactions. Give time

to react; listen, and encourage description of feelings. Use nonverbal communication of touch and eye contact.

6. *Plan/follow up:* Provide additional tests, symptom treatment, and referrals as needed. Discuss potential sources of support; assess the safety of the patient and home supports before he or she leaves. Repeat the news at future visits.

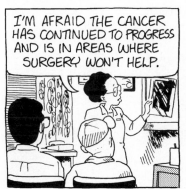

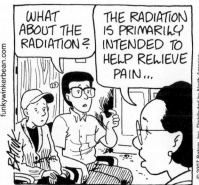

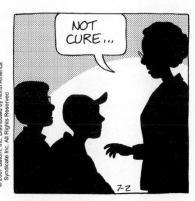

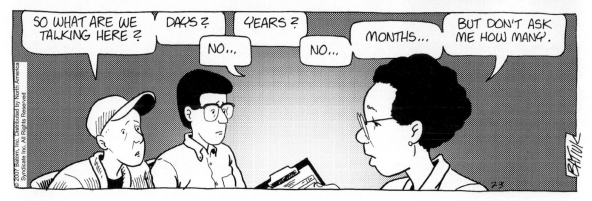

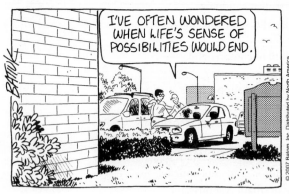

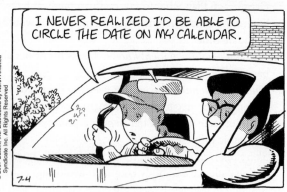

Source: ©BATOM, INC. NORTH AMERICAN SYNDICATE

Advance Directives

The Patient Self-Determination Act (PSDA), a federal law, requires healthcare providers to routinely provide information about *advance directives*. There are several nationally recognized advance directives to help an individual identify their personal wishes in a legal manner and to share that information with the people around them, including medical personnel. Durable power of attorney, living will, appointment of healthcare representative, *do not resuscitate (DNR)*, and life-prolonging procedures declarations are all legally recognized documents for indicating one's healthcare wishes. Additionally, *Five Wishes* (Towey, 2005), *allow natural death (AND)*, and the *Physician's Orders for Life Sustaining Treatment (POLST)* are three more recent options for stating end-of-life care wishes.

Five Wishes is a movement that encourages people to provide more specific instructions than those offered by a living will, including one's wishes in five categories:

> The person chosen to make decisions when the individual can no longer make them for himself or herself—a durable power of attorney for health care
> The kind of treatment the person wants or doesn't want—a living will
> How comfortable the person wants to be
> How the person wants to be treated by others
> What the person wants his or her loved ones to know

The Five Wishes documents are legal in 42 states and can be used as attachments to other documents, showing intent in the remainder of states (Aging with Dignity, 2007).

An AND order is considered a more descriptive and more positive order than a DNR. Its focus is on allowing death as nature takes its course at the end of an illness. Do not resuscitate implies taking something away, or not doing something for the patient (i.e., resuscitation), and can be viewed as a harsh and insensitive statement of medical care that promotes a feeling of abandonment by patients and families alike. In contrast, AND provides for comfort measures so that even with the withdrawal of artificially supplied nutrition and hydration, the dying process would occur as comfortably as possible (Meyer, 2001).

The POLST paradigm differs from an advance directive in that it is designed to instruct emergency personnel on what actions to take while the patient is still at home—before emergency treatment is given. It has segments concerning CPR, medical interventions, antibiotics, and artificially administered nutrition (Morrow, 2012). It was developed for seriously ill persons receiving treatments that were inconsistent with their stated wishes and designed to honor the person's end-of-life treatment preferences even when transferred from one care setting to another (Center for Ethics in Health Care, Oregon Health & Science University, 2008). While not recognized in every state, promotion of the paradigm is becoming more prevalent as its value is more widely demonstrated.

Advance directives can also be crafted for specific and personal concerns (e.g., for ongoing care for dependents or a pet). All advance directives should include a periodic review to ensure clarity and to reflect changing needs and concerns. Any documents relating to health care should be discussed and shared with physicians, family members, or decision makers and placed in the medical records held by each of the patient's physicians (see **Case Study 26-1**).

Options for End-of-Life Care
Curative/Acute Care

Curative, life-prolonging, and *acute care* options focus on cure. Despite the findings of the SUPPORT study, there are those patients, families, and cultures who choose the life-prolonging focus of care of a hospital death (see **Case Study 26-2**). Many of these deaths will take place in an ICU setting, with tubes, vents, and devices to do everything possible to preserve life. It is important that judgments not be made

---

Case Study 26-1: Family Disagreement With Advance Directives

Mary is 78, just home from the acute care hospital and the rehab unit at a local extended care facility for treatment of a cerebrovascular accident (CVA). She has come home with a feeding tube, placed at the urging of the hospital staff when she was unable to take solid foods. Mary's daughter, Sue, is the POA/HCR (power of attorney/healthcare representative)—the only remaining child, because her sibling died 2 years prior. Mary was widowed about 10 years ago.

Sue had been distraught when she received the call from Mary's neighbor and found that her mother had called 9-1-1. When Sue arrived at the hospital, Mary was in the ER, and was subsequently transferred to ICU. Mary was minimally responsive and therefore unable to speak, nor able to make her needs and wishes known. IV nutrition and hydration were implemented. Although Mary had an advance directive, indicating no use of tubes, her daughter Sue acquiesced to the physician's statement that "Starving to death is an awful way to die.... I wouldn't want that for MY

mother," and agreed to placement of a G-tube for feeding.

Mary survived and underwent a few weeks of rehabilitation therapy. She regained some abilities—but not the ability to speak or swallow without significant aspiration. Sue noted that Mary seemed very angry, sullen, and withdrawn. Sue was able to ascertain that Mary was very angry with her for the placement of the feeding tube against her wishes. Sue's attempts to explain the rationale for the placement did not make Mary any less angry. Sue was able to learn that Mary wanted the tube removed, and she contacted the primary physician to facilitate this. The physician contacted the visiting nurse agency seeking an evaluation of the situation, Mary's frame of mind, and requested objective assistance in helping determine a future plan of care for his patient.

Questions

1. As the evaluating nurse, what information would you want to reference?

2. How would you attempt to obtain input from Mary?

3. How would you respond to Sue's strong statements of guilt for having had the tube placed in spite of Mary's advance directive?

4. What would you begin to look for in evaluating appropriateness for hospice care?

Suggested Actions/Responses

The evaluating nurse asked to see Mary's advance directive and found it to be the typical state-approved document, but with some additional clauses that Mary had deemed important as part of her instructions to her family. In actuality, Mary had indicated three specific provisions that mirrored her perceptions of quality of life—the ability to smoke a cigarette, the ability to pet her dog, and meaningful verbal communication.

The evaluating nurse communicated directly with Mary using statements/questions that she could acknowledge with a yes/no nod of the head. The nurse decided, with Mary's nodded approval, to use the provisions of her advance directive to evaluate Mary's quality of life and to generate discussion about her end-of-life wishes. Mary agreed that she was unable to communicate in a meaningful way with her family. Her little dog was placed on her lap, and she was unable to pet it or caress it behind its ears. Her daughter lit a cigarette for her, and she was unable to puff on it. The nurse confirmed with Mary that this was a fair assessment of her wishes.

The nurse asked if Mary wanted to hear about the hospice option, and with an affirmative nod in response, explained the goals of comfort and dignity as nature took its course with her remaining life. The nurse further explained how Mary's illness might progress without the feeding tube, and Mary nodded her understanding. Mary indicated she wanted hospice care and confirmed, in her daughter's presence and with her daughter's tearful apology for her hasty decision in the hospital, that hospice was her choice for end-of-life care.

For Personal Reflection

How could this uncomfortable scenario have been avoided for Mary and Sue? Did Mary actually talk to her daughter about her wishes? Could Mary have taken Sue with her when she made the advance directive? Did Sue have a copy when she met Mary in the ER? Was there a family conference held to discuss options for care? Could the nurse taking care of Mary have helped Sue advocate by virtue of the advance directive when the physician pressed for tube placement?

Case Study 26-2: Hospital Death

Despite studies showing that the majority of people would prefer to die outside the hospital setting, there are those who find comfort in a more structured environment. Death in the hospital need not be a terrible or frightening event, as evidenced in this case study.

Jake is a 90-year-old man, diagnosed with end-stage dementia. He has been living in the home of his daughter and son-in-law, who are retired and in their 60s. His daughter is a power of attorney–healthcare representative. He has a living will in which he indicates an intentional

(continues)

Case Study 26–2: Hospital Death (continued)

nondecision about artificially supplied nutrition and hydration. In the past 2 years, he has become progressively weaker, unable to ambulate, unable to carry on a meaningful conversation, and increasingly incontinent of bowel and bladder. He was admitted to the hospital with dehydration and lethargy. A hydration IV has been started at 75 cc/hr. The physician has mentioned the possibility of a G-tube for feedings if the family so wishes. The certified nurse assistant (can) reports Jake moaned when she turned him during his bath, and he did not arouse when she attempted to feed him his breakfast.

You are the nurse caring for this patient. The daughter is in a quandary, stating, "I don't think Dad would want a tube in his stomach, but he never told me that for sure. My brother thinks we should do it so Dad doesn't starve to death. I tried to feed him his oatmeal this morning, but he seemed to choke. He's been coughing when he eats for a couple of months now." Your physical assessment reveals crackles throughout the lung fields, respiratory rate of 44 breaths per minute, edema to lower extremities, decreased level of consciousness, an irregular apical pulse, and a blood pressure of 76/48 mmHg.

Questions

1. What active symptoms affect the decision making for Jake?

2. What quality-of-life issues might also be involved in the decision making?

3. How would you help Jake's daughter understand the benefits and burdens of tube feedings?

4. How would your hospital-based team address the son's differing opinion?

5. What treatment would be appropriate for Jake's pain? His shortness of breath? The crackles in his lungs?

Suggested Actions/Responses

- Jake's symptoms clearly indicate an end-of-life process. You notify the physician of the family's quandary and request permission to set a family meeting for discussion of all the issues, including his terminal status.

- In answering the daughter's questions about G-tubes, you explain to her that sometimes a G-tube may be beneficial when the outcome is uncertain—for example, when there is potential for recovery as in a car accident or after a CVA. Dementia is a progressive disease, with little hope for improvement, and with an expectation of terminality at some point in time. When fluids are added to a failing body, the burdens may outweigh the benefits. These burdens might include increased congestion, edema, and nausea.

- The hospital social worker and/or chaplain might explore Jake's son's fears and feelings about Jake's end-of-life status. Quality-of-life issues might also be discussed in order to ascertain the importance of this family's cultural background in their decision making.

- Jake's nonverbal cues of pain must be addressed. Because dementia patients are often unable to report pain or its location, it is important for the nurse to observe behavior and treat appropriately. Because Jake is having difficulty swallowing, oral medications are not feasible. A low-dose opioid by IV or SQ route would be appropriate.

- The low-dose opioid initiated for pain would also help with his shortness of breath; supplemental oxygen may also be of benefit. Lowering or discontinuing the IV rate could improve the congestion and edema. The addition of hyoscine could also be helpful.

about these choices, but to note that other choices exist as well. Options for non-life-prolonging care at end of life are available and focus on comfort rather than cure.

Hospice Care

Hospice care provides one option for non-life-prolonging care and has the following philosophy:

Hospice provides care and support for persons in the last phases of incurable disease (and their families) so they may live as fully and comfortably as possible. Hospice recognizes dying as part of the normal process of living, and focuses on maintaining the quality of remaining life. Hospice affirms life and neither hastens nor postpones death. Hospice exists in the hope and belief that through appropriate care, and the promotion of a caring community sensitive to their needs, individuals and their families may be free to attain a degree of mental and spiritual preparation for death that is satisfactory to them. (NHPCO, 2012, para. 1)

Hospice care originated in order to provide comfort and dignity at end of life. Eligibility for hospice services is based on a life expectancy of 6 months or less, if an illness runs its normal course. Services are available as long as a patient is considered to be terminally ill, even though it may be longer than 6 months. Hospice utilizes a team approach to address the physical, emotional, social, and spiritual needs of the patient and (see **Figure 26-1**) family. Hospice care is discussed in more detail later in this chapter.

Palliative Care

Palliative care evolved from the hospice movement in the 1960s and 1970s. It assists increasing numbers of people who experience chronic, debilitating, and life-limiting illnesses, and can be practiced in a variety of settings, including hospitals, outpatient settings, community home health programs, and hospices (National Consensus Project for Quality Palliative Care, 2009).

Palliative care refers to the comprehensive management of the physical, psychological, social, spiritual, and existential needs of patients. It is especially suited to the care of people with incurable, progressive illnesses (Quaglietti et al., 2004). According to the *Clinical Practice Guidelines for Quality*

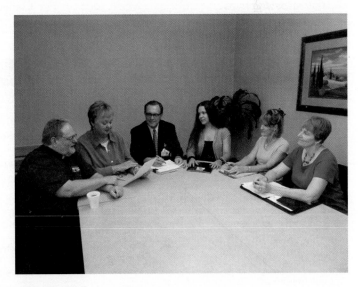

Figure 26-1 The interdisciplinary hospice team meets to discuss patient cases.

Palliative Care (2009), palliative care has become an area of special expertise within medicine, nursing, social work, pharmacy, chaplaincy, rehabilitation, and other disciplines. The goal of palliative care is to achieve the best possible quality of life for patients and their families. Control of pain, other symptoms, and of psychological, social, and spiritual problems is paramount. Palliative care has been found to not only promote improved quality of life, but to prolong life itself (see **Boxes 26-2** and **26-3**).

BOX 26-2   Ten Self-Care Tips for the Nurse Caring for Patients at End of Life

1. Become educated—knowledge is power! Develop expertise in symptom management. It lessens anxiety in working with patients and their families.

2. Maintain professional boundaries and relationships with patients and families.

3. Utilize the other palliative care or hospice team members. Each has a perspective and expertise to add to the case. The nurse does not have to do it all.

4. Develop an interdisciplinary care team in your palliative or end-of-life care setting or facility.

5. Utilize all facility staff/team members in their respective roles.

6. Find and maintain balance in your personal life.

7. Locate and use appropriate support persons for debriefing during and after a difficult case.

8. Allow yourself and all team members to grieve the death of your patient.

9. Include the other members of the team (including CNAs, housekeeping, and other staff who knew the patient) in rituals or memorial activities following the death of your patient.

10. Practice good self-care in your personal and professional life. Eat, sleep, play, laugh, cry (...enough!!), ... and wear comfortable shoes.

BOX 26-3   Death and Dying: A Simulation Exercise

This is a very effective guided reflection, with the facilitator reading the scenario and the participants listening, actively taking part with their responses to the slips of paper and subsequent instructions. The element of surprise is effective if the participants do not know the scenario before beginning the exercise. This exercise often provokes emotional responses, which can then be discussed and processed to incorporate into the learning experience.

Supplies: One packet of 12 slips of paper for each participant

Writing utensil

Overhead transparency of questions for class or small group discussion (optional)

Instructions: Slips of paper can be premarked with the following four topics (three slips for each topic):

• A person who is very dear to you

• A thing you own that you regard as very special

• An activity in which you enjoy participating

• A personal attribute or role of which you are proud

BOX 26-3 Death and Dying: A Simulation Exercise

Verbal instruction by facilitator:

Write one item per topic on each slip of paper.

Arrange the 12 slips of paper in front of you so that you can see all of them.

Get into a comfortable position; take a deep relaxing breath.

Listen without comment and follow the instructions given to you while I describe some happenings, some situations, and some people.

(Facilitator should develop the scenario carefully, allowing time for awakening all the senses.)

1. You are at your doctor's office; you hear the diagnosis—cancer.

   Please select and tear up three slips of paper. (Allow time [15–30 seconds] for selection and tearing ... brief pause ... facilitator or assistant may want to physically collect the papers and deposit them in a wastebasket for greater effect.)

2. You are back at home—who is there? Who do you want to be there? What do you say? What do you want to hear?
   Please tear up another three slips of paper. (Provide another appropriate-length pause. Collect and discard.)

3. It is now 2 months later. You are aware your symptoms are worsening and you are feeling weaker. Where are you? What is your lifestyle? What do you continue to do? What can you do? Tear up another two slips of paper. (Provide appropriate time between each phrase for reflection and for choices of paper to be discarded.)

4. Now, it is 4 months later—you are undeniably ill. The pain has increased considerably. Where are you? Who stays with you? Who visits you? Who are the people you want around you? Tear up another two slips of paper (discard).

5. Six months have now passed, and you find that even the smallest activity of daily living takes most of your energy. How do you feel about yourself? Where are you? Who is with you? Turn over the last two slips of paper in front of you.
   I will take one of them at random. (Facilitator takes one of the remaining slips from each participant and tears and discards.)

6. Facilitator says only: Tear up your last slip of paper ... you have died.

Discussion and Reflection:

May be discussed in small groups in the class setting.

Personal reflection:

- What issues arose for you from each scenario? Fears? Concerns?

- What were the easiest things to give up? Most difficult?

- What emotional reactions did you have with each scenario? (Possible responses: denial, bargaining, depression, acceptance, avoidance, relief, comfort, anger, feelings of unfairness, sadness with remembered real-life scenarios).

- What did you think/feel/experience when one of the slips was randomly taken from you?

- Did you anticipate the content of the last scenario?

- What were your thoughts/feelings/reactions to tearing up the last slip of paper?

Reflection in reference to the elderly:

- What different issues would arise for the elderly population? Fears?Concerns? (e.g., caregiving issues, financial concerns, being alone, lack of support, physical limitations)

(continues)

BOX 26-3   Death and Dying: A Simulation Exercise (*continued*)

- Might an elderly person have a harder/easier time giving up things in the four categories on the slips of paper? Why/why not for each category?

- Would the emotional responses of an elderly person be different from your own for each scenario? Why/why not?

Source: First used by Hospice of Bloomington in April 1986, provided by Rev. Dick Lentz from St. Vincent's Hospice, Indianapolis, IN; adapted for use with VNA Hospice of Porter County; further adapted for use in this book.

The Choice of End-of-Life Care

It can be very difficult for a patient and family to choose one of these options for care. A practical suggestion that may help the patient and/or family in weighing the choices is to encourage a frank discussion with the physician, which would include several important questions: What is the expected outcome if I do treatment option #1? What is the expected outcome if I do treatment option #2? What is the expected outcome if I do neither of these, and choose comfort care? Weighing the answers to each of these questions may help the individual make an informed choice, based on the differences between the expected outcomes and the individual's own philosophy about how to experience his or her end of life (see **Figure 26-2**).

Questions to Ask:
Is the hospice certified by Medicare?
Is the hospice certified by (JCAHO) or another recognized agency?
Does the hospice offer all levels of care: home care, continuous care, general inpatient care, respite care?
Does the hospice serve residents of long-term care facilities?
Is inpatient care provided in a dedicated unit manned by hospice-trained and employed staff?
Does the hospice allow the attending physician to continue to actively care for the patient?
Does the hospice have validated guidelines for pain and symptom management?
Does the hospice have an active bereavement program?
Is the program supported by a recognized funding agency or other recognized institution?
Does the program provide care in both inpatient and home care settings?
If not, does the program have relationships to ensure that care can be provided in both settings?
Is the staff of the program specially trained in palliative care?
Choose a program that can assure YES answers to all or most questions.

Figure 26-2 Algorithm for choosing the proper end-of-life care provider.

Source: Kinzbrunner, B. M., Weinreb, N. J., & Policzer, J. S. (2002). *Twenty common problems in end-of-life care.* New York, NY: McGraw-Hill.

End-of-Life Hospice Care

Cicely Saunders, a nurse, social worker, and physician, started St. Christopher's Hospice in London in 1967. She incorporated a variety of team members to work together to help with the problems of care at end of life. The success of her type of care prompted expansion of hospice services to other parts of the world. Hospice care has existed in the United States since 1974, brought to the United States by Florence Wald of Yale University (Storey, 1996) (see **Case Study 26-3**).

The U.S. government, recognizing the cost-effectiveness of hospice care, incorporated hospice benefits into the Medicare program in 1983. Credentialing agencies require that hospices provide all of the mandated services in order to be licensed and/or certified by Medicare and Medicaid and to be recognized by other insurers and some states. Reimbursement to provider agencies is contingent upon this certification (Centers for Medicare and Medicaid Services [CMS], 2012).

According to the CMS *Conditions of Participation and Standards*, hospice services include, but are not limited to:

Case Study 26-3: Options for End-of-Life Care

Hospice care is appropriate when the plan of care shifts from cure to comfort. This case study exemplifies this process.

Dee is a 72-year-old woman with advanced chronic obstructive pulmonary disease (COPD) and a history of congestive heart failure (CHF). She has been a patient with a home care agency, receiving nursing and physical therapy services for the past 6 weeks. Dee has been unable to maintain the rigors of physical therapy due to her poor lung status. She is oxygen and steroid dependent, and homebound. Dee is dependent on her husband, Jay, also age 72, for all aspects of her care. He is in need of a knee replacement, but is unable to receive one due to his caregiving role. Until several years ago, Dee and Jay enjoyed socialization with friends and neighbors, going out to dinner, playing golf and cards, and attending her church on a regular basis. They have a supportive adult daughter who works, lives about 15 miles away, is attentive, and visits nearly every day. Their son lives out of state, calls frequently, and visits on occasion.

Dee voiced to her home care nurse the desire not to return to the hospital. "It doesn't do any good. I'm tired of living this way. Can't we do something at home?" In response to Dee's inquiry, the home care nurse indicates the possibility of hospice care at home because hospice is appropriate for any end-stage illness and because Dee's prognosis was determined to be 6 months or less by her attending physician (according to the National Hospice Organization's guidelines for non-cancer diagnoses). For end-stage lung disease, these symptoms include dyspnea at rest, poor response to bronchodilator therapy, and other debilitating symptoms such as decreased functional activity, fatigue, and cough. Dee has had multiple hospitalizations for these symptoms without significant improvement in her overall condition. Her appetite is fair to poor; constipation has been a problem; she is short of breath with any exertion; and has crackles to bilateral bases, with frequent complaints of mid-back pain. She has pedal edema; her hands and feet are cyanotic. Her current medications

(continues)

Case Study 26-3: Options For End-of-Life Care (continued)

include an ACE inhibitor, furosemide 40 mg qd, prednisone 5 mg qd, and O2 2 lpm/nc. Jay reports Dee is forgetful and cries "at the drop of a hat." Dee is admitted to hospice care at home.

Questions

1. As the admitting nurse, what are your recommendations after this initial assessment?

2. Which team members should be a part of Dee's care plan?

3. How can we determine Dee's goals for her end of life?

4. Evaluate Dee's emotional status; how does it affect her daily functioning? How does it affect her relationship with her husband? How can other team members assist with these issues?

5. What impact do Dee's spiritual life/beliefs have on her condition and functional ability?

6. How might we offer Jay assistance in meeting the physical care needs of Dee?

7. What can be done for Dee's shortness of breath?

8. What should be done for Dee's complaint of constipation?

9. How might one address Dee's back pain?

Suggested Actions/Responses

- The easiest way to determine a patient/family's goals is simply to ask them! Dee is in physical distress, so that is foremost on her mind. Addressing her physical needs first will allow her to be able to identify and concentrate on other goals as her comfort is increased.

- Based on physical and psycho-social-spiritual assessment, Dee and Jay are offered the services of the whole hospice team. They

know their individualized plan of care is under the direction of Dee's attending physician and managed by the interdisciplinary team, which includes the services of a hospice-skilled medical director. Although apparently overwhelmed by the admission process, Dee and Jay initially agreed to a nurse, social worker, and home health aide (HHA), and decide to consider a volunteer and chaplain.

- The primary nurse first attends to physical symptoms, because that is often the overwhelming need. Dee's shortness of breath is her primary complaint; after consultation with the attending physician, the nurse received orders to initiate liquid morphine 5 mg q4hrs prn. The nurse instructed and demonstrated the use of morphine to Dee and Jay, because he will be responsible for administration of medications.

- Depending on the underlying pathology of Dee's back pain, the liquid morphine may also help this complaint. A nonsteroidal anti-inflammatory drug (NSAID) was ordered for possible bone pain.

- Adding opioids contributes to additional constipation, so a stool softener/laxative was ordered on a scheduled basis.

- Because activities of daily living (ADLs) are an increasing problem, and in light of Jay's knee pain, hospice can assist with the physical care needs by interventions of an HHA as needed. Stand-by assistance to full bed-bath is available depending on Dee's condition on a given day.

- The social worker often accompanies the admitting nurse for the admission process. This enables the family to be exposed to the "team" from the very beginning, as well as allowing the social worker to hear the patient/family "story" from the beginning, as an aid to assessment. Initial assessment reveals Dee is somewhat tearful in describing her physical decline and realization that her illness is life-ending. However, she is adamant about staying at home, avoiding rehospitalization, and voices several times that she is "tired, not able to fight this anymore. I want to be comfortable. I want Jay to have help."

- When Dee's symptoms indicated she was near death, and when Jay could no longer physically provide her care, she was transferred to the hospice center for the last week of her life. She received around-the-clock symptom management and physical care, allowing Jay to change roles from that of caregiver to husband.

> Nursing services and coordination of care
> Physical therapy, occupational therapy, and speech-language pathology services
> Medical social services
> Home health aides and homemaker services
> Physician services/medical director
> Counseling services (dietary, pastoral, bereavement, and other)
> Short-term inpatient care
> Medical appliances and supplies
> Medications and biologicals

Focus on Symptoms

Among the nurse's primary responsibilities as a member of any interdisciplinary team is to coordinate the patient's care and to assist with *symptom management*. Patients and families want to know what to expect as they transition through the end-

Hospice Team

The *interdisciplinary group or team (IDG/IDT)* provides or supervises the care and services offered by the hospice, including ongoing assessment of each of the patient/caregiver/family's needs. Its members consist of:

- Doctor of medicine or osteopathy

- Registered nurse—coordinates the plan of care for each patient

- Social worker

- Pastoral or other counselor

Other team members who also are required include:

- Volunteers with training appropriate to their tasks—must contribute at least 5% of all staff hours

- Clergy/spiritual support and counseling

- Additional counseling (dietary, bereavement) (CMS, 2012)

Complementary therapies are not required but are often provided to enhance the patient/family care with services such as massage, healing touch, music therapy, pet therapy, and others. Many of these additional therapies are provided by volunteers skilled in these particular areas.

of-life process. Nurses must be informed to guide the patient and family and answer questions as they arise. The remainder of this chapter will provide practical assistance with managing the variety of symptoms frequently encountered at end of life.

Physical, Nonpain Symptoms

Respiratory

Dyspnea is a distressing difficulty in breathing. It is a symptom, not a sign. A patient may have difficulty breathing and have no abnormal physical signs. Dyspnea, like pain, is whatever the patient perceives it to be. Episodic shortness of breath is sometimes due to hyperventilation. Any patient with dyspnea is prone to episodes of anxiety or panic. Patients have described this complex, subjective, and distressing phenomena as a feeling of suffocation, which often severely impedes their quality of life. The goal of treatment for terminal dyspnea is to relieve the perception of suffocation or breathlessness (Brennan & Mazanec, 2011).

Opioid therapy is used to treat shortness of breath, as morphine reduces the inappropriate and excessive respiratory drive. A low dose is usually very effective— liquid morphine 2.5–5 mg PO every 4 hours is a good starting dose. It may also be given subcutaneously at one-third the oral dose if the patient is unable to swallow. It reduces inappropriate tachypnea (rapid breathing) and over-ventilation of the large airways (dead space). It does not cause CO_2 retention and can reduce cyanosis by slowing ventilation and making breathing more efficient. Morphine does not depress respirations when used judiciously and titrated appropriately. For patients who do not tolerate morphine, other opioids such as oxycodone and hydromorphone can be used (McKinnis, 2002).

Anxiety can be precipitated by the fear of suffocation, which worsens the perception of dyspnea, creating a vicious cycle. Antianxiety agents, such as lorazepam 0.5–2.0 mg every 4–6 hours PRN, will help with restlessness and thus often decrease respiratory effort. It can be given PO, sublingually, bucally, or rectally (McKinnis, 2002).

Oxygen may not be effective if hypoxemia is not the cause of dyspnea, but may have a placebo effect and decrease the individual's anxiety. Oxygen should be started at 2 lpm/nc; increase to 4 lpm/nc if needed.

Other helpful and practical techniques might include:

> Head of the bed elevated 30–45 degrees
> Cool, humidified air
> Relaxation techniques
> Fan at bedside or ceiling fan

Excess secretions, resulting from fluid overload from artificial hydration or from increasing inability to swallow secretions, allow a buildup in large airways and cause a rattling sound. This rattle may be more distressing to the family at bedside than uncomfortable for the patient. Scopolamine TD or SQ or hyoscyamine SL may be helpful in treating this condition (McKinnis, 2002).

Gastrointestinal

Constipation results from a variety of causes for persons at end of life. Nonmedical causes include inactivity and decrease in food and fluid intake. Exercise contributes to bowel motility, but persons with life-ending illnesses are often incapacitated by their disease processes. Medications used to control pain almost always have a constipating effect. Rather than withholding opioids, the constipating side effects of the medications must be treated. A combination softener/stimulant should be used, because use of a softener alone could lead to a soft impaction. Legend indicates that Dr. Cicely Saunders (mother of the modern hospice movement) gave a lecture in which every fourth slide read, "Nothing matters more than the bowels!" (Levi, 1991).

Nausea/vomiting, while common at end of life, may have multiple causes that may or may not be reversible. If a reversible cause is identified, appropriate measures should be taken. The VOMIT acronym is helpful in identifying the causes of vomiting and in choosing the appropriate treatment to address the underlying etiology.

V=Vestibular
> Receptors involved: cholinergic, histaminic
> Anticholinergic, antihistaminic medication such as scopolamine patches and promethazineare helpful

O = Obstruction of bowel, due to constipation
> Receptors involved: cholinergic, histaminic, 5 HT3
> Medications that affect the myenteric plexus, such as senna, are helpful

M = Mobility of the upper gut (lack of)
> Receptors involved: cholinergic, histaminic, 5HT3
> Prokinetic drugs that stimulate the 5HT receptors, such as metoclopramide, are helpful

I = Infection and inflammation
> Receptors involved: cholinergic, histaminic, 5HT3
> Anticholerginic and antihistaminic agents are helpful

T = Toxins stimulating the chemoreceptor trigger zone (opioids)
> Receptors involved: dopamine, 5HT3
> Antidopaminergic and 5HT3-antagonists are useful. Examples include prochlorperazine, haloperidol, and ondansetron (Enclara Health Hospice Pharmacy Services, 2011)

Nonpharmacological measures to help control nausea and vomiting include providing fresh air; loosening clothing; using a cool, damp cloth on the skin; relaxation and visualization techniques; deep breathing; improving oral care; eating small, frequent meals; serving cold food; and discouraging family from wearing strong perfume/deodorants.

Anxiety, Delirium, and Terminal Restlessness

Anxiety, a psychological and physiological state of distress, is characterized by physical, emotional, mental, and behavioral components. At end of life it can be caused by a variety of factors, including loss of control, loss of self-esteem, and loss of independence, which can be very distressing to a person who has previously been autonomous. A change in environment for the dying person may add to the anxiety. These changes may be large—as in a family caregiver, a place of care, or meeting new professional staff—or small, such as a change of bed or medication. Treatment for anxiety includes relieving physical symptoms that may be present, such as pain or shortness of breath. The simple presence of someone the dying person trusts can be very reassuring. Antianxiety medications may also be used in conjunction with these interventions (Wright, 2002).

Delirium is an acute, fluctuating cognitive disturbance, characterized by changes in mental status over a short period of time. It occurs in the last hours to days of life in a large percentage of dying patients. Delirium is especially devastating to family and friends because it can stand in the way of meaningful conversations and good-byes. The most common physical causes may include dyspnea, pain, constipation, or urinary retention, all of which can be treated. Other causes may include medication reactions, dehydration, hypoxia, anemia, infection, and metabolic and multisystem failure (renal failure, liver failure, hypercalcemia, hyponatremia, or hypoglycemia). Delirium at end of life is often referred to as terminal restlessness, occurring in approximately 25–85% of terminally ill patients at time of death (Brajtman, 2005).

Environmental comfort can be provided by reducing stimuli; reorientation, if possible; having familiar persons at the bedside; and interdisciplinary team members providing emotional, social, and spiritual support. Music therapy, therapeutic/healing touch, and nonmedical nursing interventions should be considered. Antianxiety medications, used cautiously, may also be helpful.

Uncontrolled restlessness may require pharmacological treatment options, including palliative/terminal sedation. Terminal sedation can be defined as the monitored use of medications to relieve the intractable suffering of imminently dying patients, which persists despite the use of usual multidisciplinary therapies (HPNA, 2003). It is designed to induce unconsciousness, but not death. Before initiating sedation, various factors must be considered and thoroughly discussed, demonstrating informed consent and documentation:

> Review plans for use of artificial hydration and nutrition, including wishes for continuation or stoppage
> Confirm any specific goals to be met prior to implementation of plan (e.g., visitors)
> Confirm patient/family wishes for spiritual support
> Assure a peaceful and quiet setting, anticipating few interruptions
> Review medication and treatment orders with physician
> Confirm that DNR order is written (Salacz & Wiseman, 2004)

Nutrition and Hydration

Declining appetite is a natural occurrence in the process of dying. This concept is one of the most difficult for caregivers to embrace, because our society tends to equate love with provision of food. When end of life nears, the body is less active and requires less nourishment. From the patient's perspective, food does not taste the same, so favorite foods may no longer provide comfort; appetite is easily satisfied by bites of food rather than regular portions. Caregivers should be encouraged to offer small amounts of a variety of foods. When a patient clenches his or her teeth to negate feeding attempts, it may be his or her way of exerting control.

The attempt to artificially hydrate may be detrimental to comfort, because the failing body may not be able to process the added fluids, contributing to fluid overload (see **Box 26-4**). In this case, thirst may be satisfied by providing small amounts of oral fluids, popsicles, or ice chips. Dry mouth may be successfully managed with meticulous mouth care (Kinzbrunner, 2002).

BOX 26-4   Evidence-Based Practice

Patients with advanced illness often experience a natural decline in appetite, a loss of interest in eating and drinking, and weight loss. Most patients at the end of life will be unable to take food and fluid by mouth, or will simply stop eating. This can be particularly distressing to family and caregivers, who may be concerned that the patient is hungry or starving. They may also perceive that dehydration can result in troublesome symptoms like thirst, dry mouth, headache, delirium, nausea, vomiting, and abdominal cramps.

Artificial hydration and nutrition (AHN) interventions were developed to provide short-term support for patients who were acutely ill, and are often used to provide sustenance until recovery or to meet therapeutic goals of prolonging life. There are very few studies examining the efficacy of AHN in meeting these goals.

An important goal of hospice and palliative care is to minimize suffering and discomfort. When AHN is used in a terminally ill person, evidence suggests these measures are seldom effective in preventing suffering. Artificial nutrition and hydration is a medical intervention that should be evaluated for each individual utilizing evidence-based practices reflecting the benefits and burdens, the clinical circumstances, and the overall goals of care. (See bullet points that follow.)

Possible side effects of ANH exist for patients with advanced illness. Studies have shown that tube feeding does not appear to prolong life, and complications from tube placement may increase mortality in certain populations. Furthermore, artificially delivered nutrition does not protect against aspiration and, in some patient populations, may actually increase the risk of aspiration and its complications. Tube feedings are associated with increased infections, fluid overload, and skin excoriation around the tube. Since many tube-fed patients are not offered food even if they are able to eat, they may be deprived of human contact and the pleasure of eating.

Artificial nutrition and hydration may lead to life-threatening fluid overload complications with regards to edema, increased secretions, ascites, and pleural effusions. Research has shown that artificial nutrition and nutritional supplements do not enhance frail elder strength and physical function. Finally, therapies such as ANH that require the use of tubes increase the likelihood that the patient will

(continues)

BOX 26-4   Evidence Based Practice (*continued*)

be restrained. Physical restraints are distressing and often increase patient agitation and skin breakdown.

Evidence to consider in the evaluation of ANH for use in hospice should:

- Support education of patient and family about the dying process and its effects on nutrition and fluid status.

- Teach caregivers to enhance the patient's comfort by providing frequent oral and skin care, effective and timely symptom management, and psychospiritual support.

- Support caregivers in coping with feelings of helplessness, loss, and fear.

- Recognize that in certain situations, ANH may be clinically beneficial: It may help with reversal of myoclonis and opioid toxicity. It might also be beneficial in functional patients with mechanical blockage of the mouth, esophagus, stomach, or bowel.

- A time-limited trial may be helpful for evaluation of efficacy; it can be stopped if the desired results are not achieved.

- Artificial nutrition and hydration may have symbolic importance and be related to the religion or culture of the patient and family. This importance should not be overlooked.

- Encourage nurses to collaborate with speech therapists, nutritionists, and other healthcare providers to identify and implement strategies that enable caregivers to provide oral nutrition and fluids safely and effectively as an alternative to ANH. Alternatives may include adaptations such as fluid thickeners, teaching swallowing techniques, and positioning.

- Acknowledge and support the legal and moral right of competent patients to refuse unwanted treatment, including ANH.

- Promote early discussions about the goals of care and treatment choices, including the expected benefits and burdens of possible end-of-life interventions before starting treatment, refusal, or withdrawal.

- Encourage policies that guide a decision-making process for resolving disagreements about care among patients, families, surrogates, and healthcare team members.

- Support research on the outcomes of ANH in hospice and palliative care patients.

Source: Hospice and Palliative Nurses Association [HPNA]. (2011). HPNA position statement: Artificial nutrition and hydration in advanced illness. Retrieved from www.hpna.org/PicView .aspx?ID=1527

Physical Pain Symptoms

Relevant Issues for the Elderly

Albert Schweitzer said, "We all must die. But if I can save him from days of torture, that is what I feel is my great and ever new privilege. Pain is a more terrible lord of mankind than even death himself." (1961, p. 62) (see **Boxes 26-5** and **26-6**).

Pain in the elderly is particularly problematic. "Unrelieved pain can contribute to unnecessary suffering, as evidenced by sleep disturbance, hopelessness, loss of control, and impaired social interactions. Pain may actually hasten death by increasing physiological stress, decreasing mobility, contributing to pneumonia and thromboemboli" (HPNA, 2004a, p. 62). Underreporting of pain is common, because the elderly learn to expect chronic pain and accept it as part of growing older. They may minimize pain to

BOX 26-5   Research Highlight

Aim: Palliative care, with its emphasis on management of symptoms, psychosocial support, and assistance with decision making, has the potential to improve the quality of care and reduce the use of medical services at end-of-life.

Method: One hundred fifty-one ambulatory patients with newly diagnosed metastatic non-small-cell lung cancer were enrolled in a nonblinded, randomized, controlled trial of early palliative care integrated with standard oncologic care, as compared with standard oncologic care alone, at Massachusetts General Hospital in Boston, MA. Known prognostic factors, including age, gender, ECOG performance status, known metastases, smoking status, and initial anticancer therapy were balanced between the study groups. Specific attention was paid to assessment of physical and psychosocial symptoms, establishing goals of care, assistance with decision making relative to treatment, and coordination of care on the basis of the individual needs of the patient. All participants received routine oncologic care throughout the study period. Health-related quality of life (physical, functional, emotional and social well-being) was measured, as was mood, including depression.

Findings: Despite receiving less aggressive end-of-life care, patients in the palliative care group had significantly longer survival by about 2 months, and "clinically meaningful improvements in quality of life and mood." Less aggressive end-of-life care did not adversely affect survival.

Application to practice: With earlier referral to a hospice program, patients may receive care that results in better management of symptoms, leading to stabilization of their condition and prolonged survival. Early outpatient palliative care for patients with advanced cancer, with its emphasis on symptom management, can alter the use of healthcare services, including care at the end of life. The results "offer great promise for alleviating distress in patients with metastatic disease and addressing critical concerns regarding the use of health care services at the end of life."

Source: Temel, J.S., Greer, J.A., Muzikansky, A., Gallagher, E. R., Admane, A., Jackson, V.A., … Lynch, T. J. (2010). Early palliative care for patients with metastatic non-small-cell lung cancer. *New England Journal of Medicine, 263*, 733–742.

BOX 26-6   Research Highlight: Suffering in Terminally Ill Dementia Patients

Aim: This study attempted to evaluate the suffering of terminally ill dementia patients over time, from admission to the hospital until death.

Method: The study included consecutive end-stage dementia patients who were dying in the hospital. Using the Mini Suffering State Examination (MSSE) scale, 71 patients in a 2-year period were evaluated weekly for level of suffering.

Findings: Using the MSSE scale, 63.4% of patients died with high levels of suffering, and 29.6% died with intermediate levels of suffering. The level of suffering actually increased during the hospital stay, which averaged about 38 days. Seven percent of patients died with a low level of suffering. The most significant aspects of suffering included restlessness, pressure sores, nutritional issues, and medical instability.

(continues)

BOX 26-6   Research Highlight: Suffering in Terminally Ill Dementia Patients (*continued*)

Application to practice: Despite traditional nursing and medical care, a significant portion of dying dementia patients experienced an increase in suffering as they approached death. New palliative measures need to be developed for dying dementia patients.

Source: Aminoff, B. Z., & Adunsky, A. (2004). Dying dementia patients: Too much suffering, too little palliation. *American Journal of Alzheimer's Disease and Other Dementias, 19*(4), 243–247.

avoid diagnostic testing or to protect families or themselves against a poor prognosis. They may also use softening words, such as discomfort, soreness, or aching, instead of the word "pain." In addition, healthcare providers may tend to underestimate and undertreat pain in this population, for fear of promoting addiction to pain medications.

Research has shown that approximately 25–50% of community-dwelling elders have significant chronic pain, and between 45% and 80% of nursing home residents have undertreated, substantial pain. The pain of those in nursing homes is generally "underappreciated, underreported, and undertreated" (Ferrell, 1991, p. 2).

Additionally, McCaffery and Pasero (1999) identify that there are many misconceptions about pain in the elderly.

> Pain is a natural outcome of growing old.
> Pain perception or sensitivity decreases with age.
> If an elderly person does not report pain, he or she does not have pain.
> If an elderly patient appears to be asleep or otherwise distracted, he or she does not have pain.
> Potential side effects of opioids make them too dangerous to use to relieve pain in the elderly.
> Alzheimer patients and others with cognitive impairments do not have pain, and their reports of pain are most likely invalid.

It is important that nurses recognize the many facets of pain in older dying adults. The plan of care should be guided by consideration of physical, psychological, and social aspects of pain. This interdisciplinary plan should evolve over time, in response to the patient's changing needs (Gibson & Schroder, 2001).

To successfully treat pain, the nurse must be able to assess the pain of the individual. "Pain is whatever the experiencing person says it is, existing whenever he says it does" (McCaffery, 1968, p. 95). However, individuals may require assistance in describing their pain. A commonly used *pain scale* is shown in **Figure 26-3**.

Treatment of pain in the elderly is very effective when based on a basic understanding of origins of pain and a systematic approach to treatment. Different types of pain require different treatments (see **Case Study 26-4**). Sometimes a combination

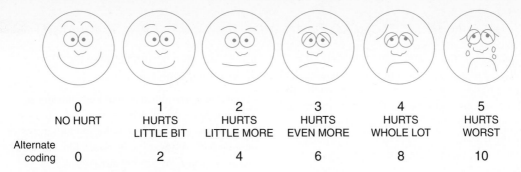

| 0 | 1 | 2 | 3 | 4 | 5 |
| NO HURT | HURTS LITTLE BIT | HURTS LITTLE MORE | HURTS EVEN MORE | HURTS WHOLE LOT | HURTS WORST |

Alternate coding   0   2   4   6   8   10

Figure 26-3 Wong-Baker FACES Pain Rating Scale.

Source: From Wong, D. L., Hockenberry-Eaton, M., Wilson, D., Winkelstein, M. L., Schwartz, P.: Wong's Essentials of Pediatric Nursing, 6/e, St. Louis, 2001, p. 1301. Copyrighted by Mosby, Inc. Reprinted with permission.

Case Study 26–4: Use of Medications for Treatment of Pain

Jane is an 84-year-old woman, diagnosed with breast cancer 2 years ago, now with metastases to the bone and lung. She has refused any further active treatment (i.e., chemotherapy and radiation) and has asked her healthcare representative daughter Patty to help her talk to her oncologist about her wishes. After this discussion, the patient, daughter, and physician have agreed upon a hospice evaluation.

Upon evaluation and subsequent admission to hospice services, the patient's most pressing need was adequate pain control. Previously, she had tried scheduled Tylenol without relief—her pain rated at an 8 on a 0–10 scale. Her oncologist then prescribed hydrocodone 7.5/750 mg, 1–2 tabs q 4 hrs as needed, which lowered her pain acuity to a 6.

Questions

1. As the admitting hospice nurse, you recognize that 8 on the pain scale greatly impairs Jane's quality of life. Using the World Health Organization (WHO) step approach, what would be your plan of intervention?

2. Knowing that Jane probably has two types of pain due to the metastases, what adjuvant might you consider for the bone pain?

3. Looking to the future, what other comfort issues might Jane face as her lung metastasis impacts her life?

4. How could you help Jane reach her goal of selected activities (e.g., shopping, lunch, church)?

Possible Solutions

The hospice nurse recognized that the maximum dose of Tylenol would be exceeded by the hydrocodone combination, and so short-acting morphine was initiated in place of hydrocodone. Using a conversion chart comparing the two medications, the nurse calculated the amount of morphine that could safely be given every 4 hours. Jane received "around the clock pain medication for her around the clock pain," to keep the pain from getting out of control. The starting dose was at a conservative starting point of 5 mg every 4 hours. The daughter was instructed to call hospice if the patient's pain was not managed at this dose. She was also educated that Jane may be sleepy for 24–48 hours until her body adjusted to the new medication, and this would be a temporary side effect and not an adverse reaction. The nurse made plans to visit daily until the pain was controlled.

(continues)

Case Study 26–4: Use of Medications for Treatment of Pain (continued)

Twenty-four hours later, Jane reported, "It's better; I'm at a 5 most of the time." Asking Jane about her acceptable level of pain, she indicated, "If I could just get it to a 2, I could do the things I would like to do." The dose was then taken to 10 mg q 4 hrs. After 48 hours, Jane reported, "You know, I think I could do a little shopping today and have some lunch with my daughter—of course she will have to drive." The hospice nurse then calculated the therapeutic amount of morphine used in 24 hours, which was 60 mg. The 60 mg was divided by 2, as long-acting morphine lasts for 12 hours. The therapeutic dose would be 30 mg of extended release morphine every 12 hours. A breakthrough dose of 10 mg (one-third of the 12-hour dose) immediate-release morphine is available for prn use in case pain occurs between the 12-hour doses during Jane's shopping trip.

At this point, an adjuvant might be considered for bone pain—possibly decadron, 2–4 mg daily—because steroids are helpful for the inflammation of bone pain. At this time in Jane's life, steroids are appropriate for use because her life expectancy is weeks or months rather than years, and long-term side effects are less of an issue.

If Jane experiences shortness of breath related to lung metastasis, the morphine and decadron are both helpful in alleviating this symptom.

A variety of interventions can improve the quality of Jane's life, allowing her the flexibility and freedom to continue some favorite activities.

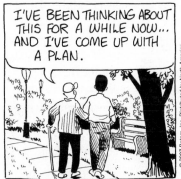
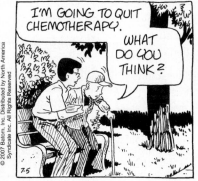
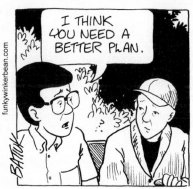

Source: ©BATOM, INC. NORTH AMERICAN SYNDICATE

of pain medication and adjuvants (such as antidepressants or anticonvulsants) can be more therapeutic than each used alone.

Pharmacological interventions remain the first line of treatment for unrelieved pain. Opioids are needed when pain does not respond to nonopioids alone. Some clinicians and patients avoid opioids due to fear of *addiction*. Nurses need to be able to understand and explain to patients and families the differences among addiction, *tolerance*, and physical *dependence*. Fear of addiction should not be a factor in pain control. The findings of several studies have shown that addiction as a result of using opioids for pain relief occurs in less than 1% of patients (McCaffery & Pasero, 1999) (see **Box 26-7**).

BOX 26-7 Tolerance of and Physical Dependence on Opioids

Tolerance of opioids and physical dependence on opioids are not the same as addiction to opioids, but these three terms are often confused. The following are the definitions used by the American Pain Society (1992):

- Opioid addiction is psychological dependence. It is "a pattern of compulsive drug use characterized by continued craving for an opioid and the need to use the opioid for effects other than pain relief" (McCaffery & Pasero, 1999, p. 50) or for nonmedical reasons. In other words, taking opioids for pain relief is not addiction, regardless of the dose or length of time on opioids.

- Physical dependence is the occurrence of withdrawal symptoms when the opioid is suddenly stopped or an antagonist such

as naloxone (Narcan) is given. Withdrawal symptoms usually are easily suppressed by gradual withdrawal of the opioid.

- Tolerance is a decrease in one or more effects of the opioid (e.g., decreased analgesia, sedation, or respiratory depression). Tolerance to analgesia may be treated with increases in dose. However, disease progression, not tolerance to analgesia, appears to be the reason for most dose escalations. Thus, tolerance to analgesia poses very few clinical problems.

Source: Reprinted from McCaffery, M., & Pasero, C. (1999). *Pain: Clinical manual* (2nd ed., p. 50). St. Louis, MO: Mosby. ©1999, with permission from Elsevier.

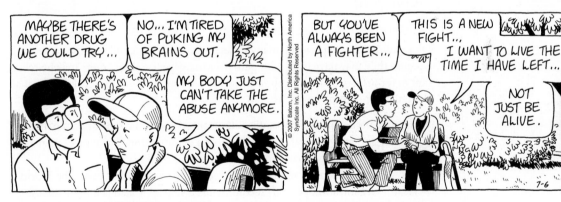

Source: ©BATOM, INC. NORTH AMERICAN SYNDICATE

Pain is divided into two major physiological types—nociceptive and neuropathic. Nociceptive pain is further divided into two types, somatic and visceral.

Somatic nociceptive pain typically involves the following symptoms and treatments:

> Tissue injury resulting in stimulation of afferent nerve endings
> The skeletal system, soft tissue, joints, skin, or connective tissue

> The patient typically can localize the pain, may be able to point to the specific area; may describe as dull, aching, throbbing, or gnawing in nature.
> Best treated with NSAIDs or steroids, though partially responsive to opioid therapy; may require a combination
> Examples: bone fracture, bone metastases, muscle strain

Visceral nociceptive pain typically involves the following:

> Activation of nociceptors
> Internal organs
> Patient often unable to localize; may use an open hand to show area affected because pain may be diffuse
> May describe as deep, aching, cramping, or sensation of pressure
> Very responsive to opioid therapy
> Examples: shoulder pain secondary to lung or liver metastases

Neuropathic pain typically involves the following:

> Injury to peripheral nerves or central nervous system
> May be described as shooting, stabbing, burning, or shock-like
> May be constant or intermittent
> Less responsive to opioids; responds best to anticonvulsants or tricyclic antidepressants
> Examples: herpes zoster or diabetic neuropathy (Weinreb, Kinzbrunner, & Clark, 2002)

Guidelines for Treatment of Pain in the Older Population

Older adults may experience many different types of pain, often at the same time. Because they may have lived with pain over many years, older adults may be reluctant to report new pain. The nurse must use appropriate assessment skills to get an accurate picture of the person's pain.

> As in all patient populations, it is important to assess the type of pain being treated: somatic, visceral, neuropathic, or a combination. The type of pain determines the appropriate medication to use.
> A systematic approach should be utilized in the treatment of pain. The World Health Organization [WHO] recommends a step approach (Lipman, 2006):
>   > Step 1: Mild pain (1–3 on 0–10 scale, with 0 being no pain and 10 being the worst possible imaginable pain). Acetaminophen and NSAIDs are the recommended medications for this step. Acetaminophen should be dosed at 4,000 mg/day or less. An adjuvant may also be used.
>   > Step 2: Moderate pain (4–6 on a 0–10 scale). Low-dose, short-acting opioids, in combination with acetaminophen and NSAIDs, are recommended in this step. Combination medications have a ceiling dose because of the nonopioid components of acetaminophen and NSAIDs. Opioid-naïve patients should be started at this level. If pain is uncontrolled with this combination, they may require a move to step 3. Adjuvants may also be used.

> Step 3: Severe pain (7–10 on a 0–10 scale). Opioids used at this step are not used in combination with Tylenol or NSAIDs, so there is no ceiling for dosing at this level. This allows for the use of higher doses of these opioids as the disease progresses. Nonopioids and adjuvants may also be used at this step.

> Oral medication is the route of choice and is well-tolerated in the geriatric population. However, other routes are acceptable when the patient is unable to swallow at the end of life. These routes may include sublingual, subcutaneous, intravenous, rectal, or topical, depending on the medication.

> To avoid possible adverse drug reactions, it is often recommended to prescribe half the dose usually prescribed to a younger person. However, even though the advice of "start low and go slow" is common, it may create the risk of undertreatment of pain. It is important to treat the individual and not the "geriatric population" (Perley & Dahlin, 2007).

> A study of opioid titration in people with cancer found that older persons required lower doses to achieve comfort. Opioid effects (including dose escalation, number of opioids, and route of administration) did not differ among age groups (Mercadante, et al., 2006)

> Special considerations for the geriatric population:

> > Acetaminophen is recommended for long-term use because it is well tolerated in the older population. It is especially therapeutic for musculoskeletal pain, a common source of pain in the older adult. Doses higher than 4,000 mg per day should be avoided. Be aware that acetaminophen may be in combination with other medications, and toxic dose ranges may be reached quickly in a person who is moving towards end of life.

> > NSAIDs are also useful in the treatment of pain. Older adults with a history of ulcer disease or congestive heart failure are more vulnerable to the side effects of these medications, however. In the palliative setting, the risk–benefit ratio helps determine the plan of care, and if prognosis is days–weeks, a trial of NSAIDs is acceptable.

> > Opioids are an acceptable option for older persons with moderate to severe pain (see **Box 26-8**). It is best to start with a short half-life agonist (e.g., morphine, hydromorphone, oxycodone) because they are generally easier to titrate than the longer half-life agonists (e.g., fentanyl patch, methadone).

> > Morphine is considered the "gold standard" and is the most commonly used opioid due to its cost and various routes of administration. The elderly population may develop sedation or confusion due to the metabolites of morphine after several days of use. If this happens, it might be wise to change to another opioid. (Remember, however, the patient may be drowsy or sleepy because their pain is controlled, and they are finally able to rest.) This side effect should subside in 48 hours. Assessment continues to be very important. Long-acting morphine should be used only after a several-day trial of short-acting morphine. Morphine is also therapeutic in the treatment of shortness of breath.

BOX 26-8 Research Highlight: Hospice Patients Live Longer

Aim: Some healthcare providers perceive that symptom control in hospice patients, especially the use of opioids and sedatives, may cause patients to die sooner than they otherwise might. Some evidence has suggested, however, that the lives of some patients might be extended through the use of hospice care. This study evaluated the effect of hospice care on elevating the longevity of terminally ill patients.

Method: In this retrospective cohort study, an innovative prospective/retrospective case control method and Medicare administrative data were used to measure time until death starting from dates narrowly defined within the data. Multiple regression models were used to evaluate the difference of survival periods of terminal illness for patients using hospices and those who did not.

Findings: The survival period was significantly longer for the hospice cohort than for the nonhospice cohort for those patients with congestive heart failure, lung cancer, and pancreatic cancer, and longer—but not statistically significant—for those with colon cancer.

Application to practice: Hospice may, indeed, have a positive impact on patients' longevity, or at least not hasten death. For certain well-defined terminally ill populations, patients who choose hospice care live an average of 29 days longer than similar patients who do not choose hospice. This pattern persisted over four of the six disease categories studied. The findings are important in helping to dispel the myth that hospice care hastens a patient's death. Some factors that may contribute to this longevity may include avoidance of the risks of overtreatment, improved monitoring and treatment, and that the psychosocial supports inherent in hospice care may tend to prolong life. Additional research would clarify the applicability of these findings to other patients and diseases, but nurses can assure patients and families that the use of hospice is not associated with hastening death.

Source: Connor, S. R., Pyenson, B., Fitch, K., Spence, C., & Iwasaki, K. (2007). Comparing hospice and nonhospice patient survival among patients who die within a three year window. *Journal of Pain and Symptom Management, 33*(3), 238–242.

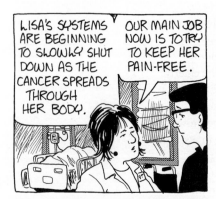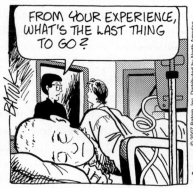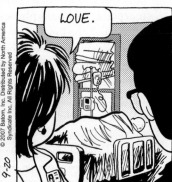

> Opioids other than morphine may also be used (e.g., oxycodone, transdermal fentanyl) using the same principle of a short-acting trial before initiation of a long-acting formulation.
> Opioids are constipating, so implementing a concurrent bowel program is essential. A stimulant and stool softener combination is recommended at the onset of opioid therapy (Derby & O'Mahoney, 2006).

Loss and Grief

The elderly are confronted with a variety of losses in many aspects of their lives, not just with the death of a spouse, family members, or long-time friends. Loss of bodily function occurs as illness becomes more prevalent. Loss of support systems occurs as companions die. Loss of independence is a factor as one's physical abilities wane, including loss of mobility, inability to make decisions, and limited access to various other support systems. Not only are the bodily functions lost, but the realization of never regaining these functions is particularly difficult. Primary losses are the loss of people close to them—spouses, children, parents, or siblings. Secondary losses are those resulting from the primary loss—companionship, roles the deceased assumed in the relationship (e.g., bill payer, cook), and independence.

Although the terms *grief* and *mourning* are frequently used interchangeably, each does have a specific meaning. *Grief* is the natural and normal response to loss of any kind and is experienced psychologically, behaviorally, socially, and physically. It involves many changes over time (Rando, 1993). *Mourning* is the cultural and/or public display of grief through one's behaviors. These include accepting the reality of the loss, reacting to the separation and finding ways to channel the reactions, handling the unfinished business, and transferring the attachment to the deceased from physical presence to symbolic interaction. It seeks to accommodate the loss by integrating its realities into ongoing life (Rando, 1993). Alan Wolfelt (2001) distinguishes mourning as the shared social response to grief—grief gone public.

In this author's experience with hospice bereavement support, the practical application of this information suggests a concept that seems logical and is acceptable to people who are mourning: The goal of grieving is not to "get over it" as much of our society encourages, but rather to figure out how to go on living without the loved one actively present in one's life—learning to better cope with the changes that occur.

Wolfelt (2004) suggests the following mourner's reconciliation needs:

> Acknowledge/accept the reality of the death.
> Embrace the pain of the loss.
> Convert the relationship of the person who died from one of presence to one of memory.
> Develop a new self-identity.
> Search for meaning.
> Receive ongoing support from others.

Wolfelt's reconciliation needs present some challenges for the elderly because of the limits they may experience physically and emotionally due to chronic or other illnesses. However, it is still important to emphasize reasonable versus unreasonable expectations—grievous loss will produce strong grief, and mourners must be allowed to experience the full dimensions of their unique process.

There are patterns to grief that help describe and show progression in the mourning process, regardless of age. Knowing patterns exist is sometimes comforting, but individualized responses must be acknowledged and affirmed. A reasonable goal is to find a personal balance in each of the aspects of grief patterns—physical aspects such as eating and sleeping and emotional aspects such as tears and stoicism, to name a few—as the mourner attempts to incorporate the loss into his or her daily life patterns.

The mourning process has been characterized by stages or phases. Although it is tempting to consider it as a neat and tidy progression, the concept of overlapping, retrogressing, and recurring jumbles of feelings and responses is probably more realistic. Phases include the period of numbness occurring at the time of the loss, which provides some emotional protection for a brief time. The period of yearning for the loved one's return tends to deny the permanence of the loss for a time and may include feelings of anger about a variety of aspects of the loss (including, for example, anger at the medical profession, at the person who died, and/or at God). The phase of disorganization and despair is one of difficulty in functioning in the environment, in which the mourner (see **Box 26-9**) begins to do the "figuring out" of how to function in each area of disarray. The phase of reorganized behavior is when one pulls life back together, and in which a new "normal" might be identified (Parkes & Bowlby in Worden, 1991).

BOX 26-9   Gone from My Sight: The Dying Experience

Summary of Guidelines for Impending Death

Recognizing that although each person approaches death in his or her own way, there are some identified patterns that assist in the recognition of end-stage status, noted in common language for ease of comprehension by patients and families.

One to three months:

- Withdrawal from the world and people

- Decreased food intake

- Increase in sleep

- Going inside of self

- Less communication

One to two weeks:

Mental changes:

- Disorientation

- Agitation

- Talking with the unseen

- Confusion

- Picking at clothes

Physical changes:

- Decreased blood pressure

- Pulse increase or decrease

- Color change (pale, bluish)

- Increased perspiration

- Respiration irregularities

- Congestion

- Sleeping but responding

- Complaints of body being tired and heavy

- Not eating, taking little fluid

- Body temperature hot/cold

Days or hours:

- Intensification of 1- to 2-week signs

- Surge of energy

- Decrease in blood pressure

- Eyes glassy/tearing/half open

- Irregular breathing

- Restlessness or no activity

- Purplish/blotchy knees, feet, hands

- Pulse weak and hard to find

- Decreased urine output

- May wet or stool the bed

Minutes:

- "Fish out of water" breathing

- Cannot be awakened

Source: Summary of Guidelines, pp. 12–23. Gone from My Sight: The Dying Experience, Barbara Karnes, RN, P.O. Box 189, Depoe Bay, OR, 97341. Copyright 1986.

There is no timetable for grief; this is one of the individualized differences in the grief/mourning process. Stages, commonly identified as denial, anger, bargaining, depression, and acceptance, are not meant to be a linear progression, but rather help frame and identify the feelings associated with the adjustments.

A brief review of the risk factors for complicated mourning provides special insight into the vulnerabilities of the elderly, especially in light of the secondary losses noted earlier. According to Rando (1993), there are seven high-risk factors in two categories that might predispose a person to complicated mourning.

Factors associated with the specific death:

> Sudden, unexpected (traumatic, violent, random)
> Overly lengthy illness (multidimensional stresses including anger, ambivalence, guilt, problems obtaining health care)
> Loss of a child, including adult children
> Perception of the death as preventable (lack of closure, attempt to regain control, search for reasons and meaning)

Antecedent and subsequent variables:

> Markedly angry/ambivalent/dependent relationship
> Unaccommodated losses/stresses/mental health problems
> Perception of lack of social support

Mourners must be given the opportunity to process the aspects of their grief, but in a context that is helpful to them. Nurses, who are likely to frequently encounter grieving patients, can facilitate the mourning process by being aware of the aspects of grief and mourning, and by advocacy with the people who surround the mourner. Alan Wolfelt (2012a) suggests a Mourner's Bill of Rights to help mourners sift out the unacceptable advice they are often given. This includes the right to:

> Experience unique grief, without the pressure of "shoulds/shouldn'ts"
> Talk about grief, or be silent as needed
> Feel a multitude of emotions, without feeling judgment
> Tolerate physical and emotional limits, and fatigue
> Experience sudden surges of grief
> Use rituals
> Embrace spirituality, or not
> Search for meaning, recognizing some questions may not have answers
> Treasure memories; share them
> Move toward grief and heal; avoid people who are intolerant of your grief
> Recognize that "grief is a process, not an event"

Other ways nurses can help include active listening without judging the mourner; having compassion and allowing the expression of feelings without criticizing; allowing the mourner to identify his or her own feelings without saying, "I know how you feel;" and offering presence over time (Wolfelt, 2012b).

Frequently, when an elderly person experiences the death of a spouse of long standing, the life expectancy of the remaining spouse may be shortened because of the inability to reconcile the needs of mourning, the complications of grief, and the lack of physical and emotional reserves to make the additional investment into a reconfiguration of one's own future. It is also important to note the potential for difference in mourning styles between men and women, and among various cultures.

Psychosocial, Emotional, and Spiritual Symptoms

Although we frequently attempt to distinguish among psychosocial, emotional, and spiritual issues, the reality is that the range and depth of being human make it nearly impossible to recognize where one aspect of being ends and another begins. It has been suggested to address these areas as a continuum, and to view the issues that arise in these aspects of our human functioning at end of life as opportunities, rather than as problems (McKinnon & Miller, 2002). "For those caring for the terminally ill, psychosocial and spiritual issues that in the past have been seen as problems can, with information and compassion, become opportunities—opportunities that will allow each of us to live fully until we say goodbye" (McKinnon & Miller, 2002, p. 273) (see **Box 26-10**).

Some issues that arise must be viewed in a practical light, because addressing them might assist in providing resources for the dying elderly to promote quality of life and dignity.

BOX 26-10 Psychosocial and Spiritual Opportunities Near the End of Life

The opportunity to:

Reframe society's view of dying: grow on!

Expand the definition of quality of life.

Focus on the individual, not the disease.

Address as a whole physical pain, psychosocial issues, and spiritual concerns

Move through fear to peace.

Move through confusion to meaning.

Move through despair to hope.

Move from isolation to community.

Come to terms with the physical body.

Move from loss to closure.

Adjust to new roles.

Get affairs in order.

Source: Kinzbrunner, B. M., Weinreb, N. J., & Policzer, J. S. (2002). *Twenty common problems in end-of-life care*. New York, NY: McGraw-Hill.

Psychosocial Issues

When family members are the primary caregivers of the elderly, role changes are very common. Caregivers may resist providing increasing physical care, not wanting to recognize the decline or not wanting to diminish the dignity of the patient. The patient may resist it as well, resenting the need for the increased level of care because it demonstrates yet more limitations and inabilities in level of independence. Caregivers may not comprehend the emotional changes and resistance of their elder, and may become frustrated with the increasing tasks of care and with the emotional burdens of its constancy.

It may be helpful for caregivers to view the last year of a person's life as a reversal of the first year of life. This revised perspective helps the caregiver see that the person is not intentionally increasingly helpless, or necessarily giving up certain functions. Rather, he or she may be losing abilities in a reverse order of that in which infants gain abilities over the first year of life. These may affect the areas of mobility, activities of daily living, cognition, and personal care needs. As physical ability declines, people begin to withdraw from activities, which may further increase dependence on persons around them and their sense of isolation.

Having sufficient physical care—whether from family, paid caregiver resources, or in assisted living or long-term care facilities—is important for those facing end of life. What constitutes sufficient care may vary with the individual, but it is always an aspect of end-of-life care that will become more important as the person's physical abilities decline. Although some elderly enjoy this increased dependence, very independent individuals often find this increasing caregiver need to be one of the hardest aspects of treatment to accept.

Many patients and families have financial concerns. The concerns are greater, of course, for individuals or families with few resources, or with only some resources.

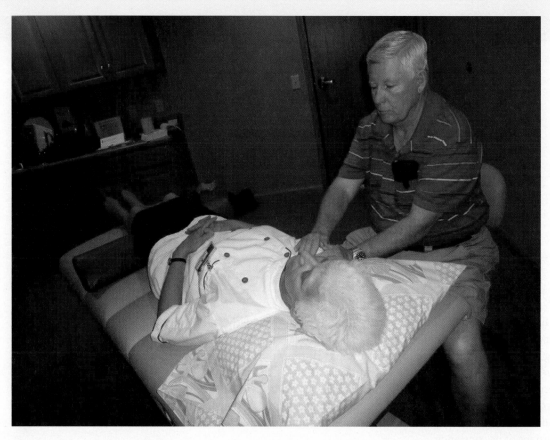

Figure 26-4 Therapeutic touch may be used by trained staff to promote comfort.

Although subsidies for some services are available, many people may not have the ability to access them. The palliative care or hospice team may be helpful in linking the patient and family with appropriate financial resources. Nurses may also want to have basic information available for possible referrals when access to other team members is not available. There are agencies and individuals available to augment the family's ability to provide care. Most require private pay resources, but some are government sponsored in order to keep people in their homes a bit longer (e.g., some Medicaid-sponsored hours to provide in-home support are available in some states for those individuals who financially qualify).

Emotional Issues

A person's place in the life cycle affects their reaction to end-of-life circumstances. As an elderly person faces death, the individual looks back upon life and reflects upon its experiences. There is an attempt to emotionally integrate all the aspects of one's life, including determination of its meaning and acceptance of its uniqueness (Rando, 1984). It is an unfair exaggeration to imply that the elderly are all at peace with their coming death. Some are and some are not. The elderly do appear to see death as an important issue, one they often think about and plan for. Caring intervention should continue to facilitate an appropriate death for the aged individual according to the patient's desires, not what the medical personnel deem appropriate.

Anticipatory grief is a process of adjustment during the course of the terminal illness that is faced by the patient as well as by the family/caregivers. It usually begins at the time of diagnosis and can be caused by a variety of adjustments and secondary losses experienced by and required of the individual. These might include loss of control, independence, productivity, security, various abilities, predictability and consistency, future existence, pleasure, ability to complete plans and projects, significant others, meaning, dreams, and hopes for the future (Rando, 1984).

Persons who are facing end of life often encounter feelings of hopelessness. They may find comfort and be helped to adjust to their changing condition by recognizing a changing focus of *hope*. "A patient can hear a terminal diagnosis and still have hopes for the type of life remaining" (Rando, 1984, p. 270). When a person is confronted with the possibility of a life-ending illness, usually the first response is: "I hope it's nothing serious or that it can be easily treated without much disruption in my life." As treatment is not successful and as the illness progresses, one might hope that "my family and I will have the opportunity to get things done … have closure … see my granddaughter get married."

When getting better or prolonging life is not feasible, one is often confronted with giving up hope altogether. That is how some people feel when they choose hospice or palliative care. That is, in fact, what some physicians imply when they say, "There is nothing more that can be done for you." Hospice and palliative care personnel believe that hope can continue—but the focus of hope moves away from that of getting better. One can hope for the appropriate help and support for themselves and their families through the transitions that end of life brings. They can hope that they will be provided with guidance and emotional comfort, and that their care will be provided with respect for their dignity through the dying process. They can hope that their passing will be comfortable and pain-free. They can hope that their families will receive the appropriate support before and after their death. They can hope to be treated holistically—as an individual with unique needs, wishes, and desires.

Four powerful statements proposed by Ira Byock provide a clear path to emotional wellness throughout a lifetime. They also provide a format for resolving some personal, emotional, and/or spiritual issues at end of life. They are:

1. Please forgive me.
2. I forgive you.
3. Thank you.
4. I love you (Byock, 2004, p. 3).

Spiritual/Cultural Issues

Spiritual issues may or may not be related to the person's relationship or lack thereof with an organized religion. Some may find great peace and comfort in a religion and its practices and rituals. Others are just as spiritual, without the link to religious ties and practices, perhaps finding comfort in nature or some other source.

Spiritual and cultural rituals may be important for some people at end of life. Nurses may be in a position to help patients and families to obtain access to the rituals that may be important as a person is nearing death. For some religions, this may mean obtaining appropriate clergy for confession, communion, and anointing. For others it may mean a more general ritual for commendation of the dying. In some cultures, certain foods, fasting, handling of the body, and placement in a certain position to facilitate burial may be important (Kirkwood, 1993) (see **Table 26–1**.) As in other aspects of individualized care, it is appropriate to ask the patient and/or family about these preferences.

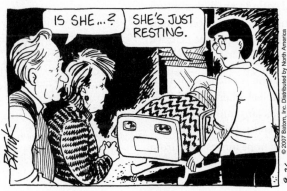
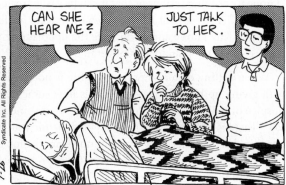
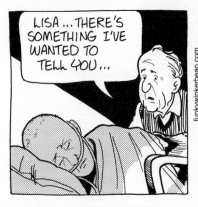
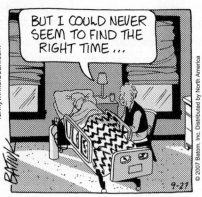
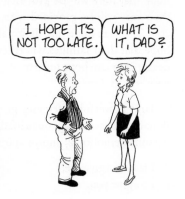

TABLE 26-1	Cultural and Religious Practices at End of Life		
Religion	**During Sickness**	**Dying/Death**	**After Dying**
Buddhism	Important to die in positive state of mind; organ donation permitted	Help die peacefully by encouraging forgiveness; position on right side, left hand on left thigh, legs stretched out; no special body preparations	Leave body alone as long as possible to avoid disturbing the consciousness during transition from death to new life
Hinduism	Family does daily care; father/oldest son makes health decisions; same-sex caregiver due to modesty	With terminal diagnosis, dying information given to family, not the patient; family decides how much info to share with the patient	Body washed, usually by eldest son, then cremated
Islam	Prayer five times per day; clean area of any body waste, including person and sheets; can use pitcher and basin provided; use clean sheet to cover patient during prayer. Best efforts provided to maintain life; hardship is a test from Allah; can remove life support; natural death will allow person to accept the will of Allah	Body on its side, facing Mecca; friends and loved ones pray for mercy, forgiveness, and blessings of Allah	Person of same gender prepares body for burial; same day as death if possible; cremation forbidden.
Jehovah's Witness	No blood transfusions; organ transplants per individual conscience	Respectful care for dying person and family; respond to their individual needs	Generally follow traditional state mandates for burial or cremation
Judaism	In serious illness, patient is not to be left alone—to be attended by family;		Cremation forbidden; focus on deceased and funeral; mourning occurs in the home for 7 days after the funeral.

(continues)

TABLE 26-1	Cultural and Religious Practices at End of Life (*continued*)		
Religion	**During Sickness**	**Dying/Death**	**After Dying**
Judaism	doctor's duty to prolong life unless death is imminent and certain; cannot hasten death	Autopsy not permitted unless required by law; organ donation only after person declared dead (not at all by Orthodox)	Orthodox: extend arms alongside the body, fingers outstretched; tubing, body fluids, sheets/blankets with blood are buried with the body; designated Orthodox Jew should clean the body. Someone stays with body, praying until body enters ground.
Christianity (general)	Respect and dignity for body; organ donation and autopsy allowed; if treatment is of no benefit or unreasonable burden, may forgo and allow natural death; decision up to patient/family	Open to pastoral care; some have a rite of anointing by a priest; some have service of commendation of the dying	Practices may vary by denomination, but commonly include a gathering with family and friends after the funeral or memorial service.
Orthodox Christianity	Fasting on certain days = no meat, milk, fish, eggs; no eating before communion; can use drugs to reduce pain/suffering; removing life supports done after prayer and discussion with family members, medical professional, and spiritual director; organ donation acceptable	Family encouraged to be at bedside; invite priest; Anointing of the Sick (Holy Unction)	Body buried in ground, w/coffin, grave liner, monument with image of the cross; cremation is not allowed.
Roman Catholicism	If possible, fast 1 hour before receiving Eucharist; moral obligation to use ordinary or proportionate means of preserving life (in judgment of patient)	Sacrament of Anointing of the Sick before surgery, for elderly in weakened condition, by a priest	May be cremated; cremains may be brought to funeral mass.

Source: Table generated from Handbook for Chaplains, by Mary M. Toole. Copyright 2006 by Mary M. Toole/Paulist Press, Inc, New York/Manwah, NJ. Reprinted by permission of Paulist Press, Inc. www.paulistpress.com

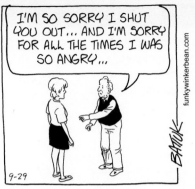
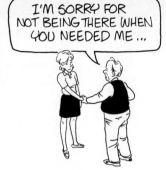
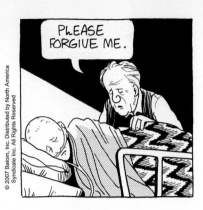

Source: ©BATOM, INC. NORTH AMERICAN SYNDICATE

To formalize this asking, several brief assessments have been developed for use by nurses to incorporate a spiritual component into their nursing plan of care. These are available for detailed review in *Spiritual Care in Nursing Practice* (Mauk & Schmidt, 2004) (see **Boxes 26-11, 26-12** and **26-13**). The assessments are easy to incorporate, using acronyms as reminders in obtaining the spiritual history content.

BOX 26-11   Suggested Resources

Albom, M. (1997). *Tuesdays with Morrie: An old man, a young man, and life's greatest lesson*. New York, NY: Doubleday.

Association for Death Education and Counseling (ADEC). (2010). Retrieved from http://www.ADEC.org

Byock, I. (2012). *The bestcare possible: A physician's quest to transform care through the end of life*. New York, NY: Avery.

Callanan, M., & Kelley, P. (1992). *Final gifts: Understanding the special awareness, needs, and communications of the dying*. New York, NY: Poseidon Press.

Ferrell, B.R., & Coyle, N., (2001). *Textbook of palliative nursing*. New York, NY: Oxford University Press.

Hospice Foundation of America. http://www.hospicefoundation.org

Journal of Hospice and Palliative Nursing. http://www.jhpn.com

National Hospice and Palliative Care Organization. http://www.nhpco.org

Nuland, S. B. (1993). *How we die: Reflections on life's final chapter*. New York, NY: Random House.

Project on Death in America. Open Society Institute. http://www.soros.org/initiatives/pdia

Smith, W. J. (2000). *The culture of death: The assault on medical ethics in America*. San Francisco, CA: Encounter Books.

Toole, M. M. (2006). *Handbook for chaplains: Comfort my people*. New York, NY: Paulist Press.

Webb, M. (1997). *The good death: The new American search to reshape the end of life*. New York, NY: Bantam Books.

Wit. (2001). A movie made for HBO and a Pulitzer Prize-winning play by Margaret Edson featuring a single-minded English professor, who in the face of imminent death learns the power and importance of simple acts of human kindness.

BOX 26-12   HOPE Model

H = Sources of hope, meaning, comfort, strength, peace, love, and connection: What do you hold on to during difficult times?

O = Organized religion: Importance? Helpful and nonhelpful aspects?

P = Personal spirituality and practice: Relationship with God? Most helpful aspects of spiritual practices?

E = Effects on medical care and end-of-life issues:

Has illness affected your ability to do the things that usually help you spiritually? Are there specific practices to be aware of in providing care? Can I help access resources helpful to you?

Source: Reproduced with permission from Spirituality and medical practice: Using the HOPE questions as a practical tool for spiritual assessment. January 1, 2001, *American Family Physician* ©2001 American Academy of Family Physicians. All rights reserved.

BOX 26-13   FICA Model

F = Faith or beliefs (What gives meaning to life?)

I = Importance and influence (Is faith important? How do beliefs influence behavior toward illness?)

C = Community (Is the spiritual orreligious community supportive? How? Person or people important to you? People you love?)

A = Address (How would you like healthcare providers to address these issues in your health care?)

Source: Puchalski, C., & Romer, A. L. (2000). Taking a spiritual history allows clinicians to understand patients more fully. *Journal of Palliative Medicine, 3*(1), 129–131.

The information obtained by the nurse may be useful for interventions with the patient and family by other members of the care team, regardless of the setting in which care is provided.

Caregiver Issues/Compassion Fatigue

Because providing care for a patient over an extended period of time is common in hospice and palliative care, it is important to recognize issues that may affect a person's ability to provide this care. In hospice care, the Social Work Assessment Tool (SWAT) has been developed to help measure not only the patient's adjustments to aspects of the dying experience, but also those of the caregivers. It encompasses decision making, anxiety about death, environmental preferences, safety, comfort, finances, anticipatory grief, and others. It is designed to show progression in the patient's and caregiver's adjustments over time (NHPCO, 2008.)

Nurses are at moderate-to-high risk for the development of compassion fatigue—a condition that is commonly present when a caregiver continues to provide compassionate care to others in stressful situations without practicing good self-care for her/himself. Stress, trauma, anxiety, life demands, and excessive empathy (caring more for patient's needs than their own) were key determinants of compassion fatigue risk. Because the risk is apparent, compassion fatigue is preventable and treatable (Abendroth & Flannery, 2006). Awareness is the first step in treatment of compassion fatigue. Authentic, sustainable self-care is possible with education, clarification of personal boundaries, healthy living choices (eating,sleeping, and exercise), stress management, and a healthy support system—living life in balance (Compassion Fatigue Awareness Project, 2012).

Components of Peaceful Dying

It may be possible to plan for a peaceful death, given the knowledge of having a terminal illness. "The key to peaceful dying is achieving the components of peaceful living during the time you have left" (Preston, 2000, p. 161). Some components are accomplished only by the individual, whereas others may require the assistance of family and medical providers, such as the following:

> Instilling good memories
> Uniting with family and medical staff
> Avoiding suffering, with relief of pain and other symptoms
> Maintaining alertness, control, privacy, dignity, and support
> Becoming spiritually ready
> Saying goodbye
> Dying quietly (Preston, 2000)

A *good death* is possible and can be facilitated by the nurse who advocates for and works to ensure that the patients, families, and caregivers are free from avoidable distress and suffering, that the process is in accord with the wishes of the patient and family, and that it is consistent with clinical, cultural, and ethical standards (Dobbins, 2005).

Postmortem Care
Pronouncing Death

Procedures for pronouncing the death of a person vary from state to state and institution to institution. In some states, nurses may be able to pronounce the death, whereas in others this is not allowed. In inpatient settings, policies differ and the individual institutional policies are followed. In hospice home care, generally a nurse makes a visit, determines the lack of vital signs, and contacts the physician who has already agreed to sign the death certificate because the death has been anticipated. The funeral home or mortuary is contacted for removal of the body.

In pronouncing the death, it is customary to identify the patient and note the following (Berry & Griffie, 2006):

> General appearance of the body
> Lack of reaction to verbal or tactile stimulation
> Lack of pupillary light reflex (pupils fixed and dilated)
> Absent breathing and lung sounds
> Absent carotid and apical pulses (in some situations, listening for an apical pulse for a full minute is advisable)

Physical Care of the Body

Care of the body is an important nursing function. It is not surprising that families often recall the actions of the nurse after the death of their loved one. Careful and gentle handling of the body communicates care and concern on the part of the nurse. The nurse should allow the family to spend time with the body if desired. Rituals and customs should have been identified before the death, to now be incorporated into this care, reflecting the patient/family wishes.

Family members should be allowed to touch the body if they so desire and are comfortable with this action. They may wish to select special clothes for their loved one's transfer to the funeral home. If they choose to remain present through the post-mortem care, they should be educated about the potential for some body changes. For example, there may be the sound of air escaping from the lungs when the body is turned (a sighing sound), and stool and urine may be present in a previously continent person, as the rectal and urinary bladder sphincters relax. Nursing care also includes the removal of drains, tubes, IVs, and any other devices. Family members may wish to participate in bathing and dressing the body; some may find comfort in the small details of "a favorite gown and the hair just right" (Berry & Griffie, 2006).

Summary

When death approaches for the elderly patient, the role of the nurse changes along with the patient's changing condition. The role moves from a fix-it focus to that of presence—the ability to be with the patient and with his or her family. This presence involves the provision of comfort measures, lending a listening ear, providing a peaceful environment, and compassionately educating patient and family about the dying process.

Nurses caring for the dying also need to care for themselves. The nurse's gratification does not come from curing (see **Box 26-14**), but rather from supporting the patient in a peaceful and dignified "good death."

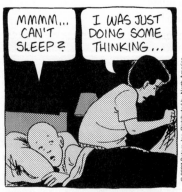
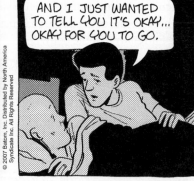
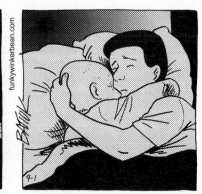

Source: ©BATOM, INC. NORTH AMERICAN SYNDICATE

BOX 26-14   Web Exploration

Explore the website for the Hospice Foundation of America at http://www.hospicefoundation.org and compare the contents with those at Ira Byock's website at http://www.dyingwell.com

Critical Thinking Exercises

1. Visit a funeral home and talk with the funeral home director(s) about their experiences. What are the major components of their job? How do they feel they provide a service to the community?

2. Review your local newspaper and read the obituaries. What are the ages of the persons who have died? Are most of them older or younger?

3. Recall a funeral for a family member that you may have attended in the past. What were the components of the service? How did religious and cultural aspects play a part in the funeral or memorial service? The burial? The grieving and mourning? How did family and friends grieve? How did they remember the loved one?

Personal Reflections

1. This chapter has provided a large amount of information on caring for older adults at end of life. Which portions of the chapter were you the least familiar with? Are there areas of your nursing practice that you need to further develop in order to provide effective care to the dying? List a few of those areas in which you could improve your practice.

2. If an older family member who is close to you was recently given a terminal diagnosis, how would you respond? What questions would you ask of him or her? What actions, if any, would you take?

3. Do you have advance directives or a living will for yourself? Why or why not?

4. Have you ever been with a person when they died? What was that experience like for you?

5. After learning the material in this chapter, will you view any aspects of end of life differently?

6. Have you ever provided postmortem care for a patient? If so, what was the most difficult aspect of that experience?

References

Abendroth, M., & Flannery, J. (2006). Predicting the risk of compassion fatigue: A study of hospice nurses. *Journal of Hospice and Palliative Nursing, 8*(6), 346–356.

Aging with Dignity. (2007). Five wishes: 2007 edition. Retrieved from http://www.agingwithdignity.org/catalog/product_info.php?products_id=28

Allchin, L. (2006). Caring for the dying: Nursing student perspectives. *Journal of Hospice and Palliative Nursing, 8*(2), 112–115.

Allen, W. (1976). *Without feathers, death* [Play]. Act 1. New York, NY: Ballantine Books.

American Pain Society. (1992). *Principles of analgesic use in the treatment of acute pain and cancer pain* (3rd ed.). Skokie, IL: Author.

Aminoff, B. Z., & Adunsky, A. (2004). Dying dementia patients: Too much suffering, too little palliation. *American Journal of Alzheimer's Disease and Other Dementias, 19*(4), 243–247.

Berry, P., & Griffie, J. (2006). Planning for the actual death. In B. R. Ferrell & N. Coyle (Eds.), *Textbook of palliative nursing* (pp. 561–577). New York, NY: Oxford University Press.

Brajtman, S. (2005). Helping the family through the experience of terminal restlessness. *Journal of Hospice and Palliative Nursing 7*(2) 73–81.

Brennan, C. W., & Mazanec, P. (2011). Dyspnea management across the palliative care continuum. *Journal of Hospice and Palliative Nursing, 13*(3) 130–139.

Byock, I. (2004). *The four things that matter most: A book about living.* New York, NY: Free Press.

Byock, I. (2012). *The best care possible: A physician's quest to transform care through the end of life.* New York, NY: Avery/Penguin.

Center for Ethics in Health Care, Oregon Health & Science University. (2008). Frequently asked questions about Physicians Orders for Life Sustaining Treatment Paradigm. Retrieved from http://www.ohsu.edu/polst/patients-families/faqs.htm

Centers for Disease Control and Prevention [CDC]. (2010). *Deaths and mortality.* Retrieved from http://www.cdc.gov/nchs/fastats/deaths.htm

Centers for Medicare and Medicaid Services (2012). Hospice payment system. Retrieved from http://www.cms.gov/Outreach-and-Education/Medicare-Learning-Network-MLN/MLNProducts/downloads/hospice_pay_sys_fs.pdf

Compassion Fatigue Awareness Project. (2012). *What is compassion fatigue?* Retrieved from http://www.compassionfatigue.org/pages/compassionfatigue.html

Connor, S. R., Pyenson, B., Fitch, K., Spence, C., & Iwasaki, K. (2007). Comparing hospice and non-hospice patient survival among patients who die within a three-year window. *Journal of Pain and Symptom Management, 33*(3), 238–246.

Derby, S., & O'Mahoney, S. (2006). Elderly patients. In B. R. Ferrell & N. Coyle (Eds.), *Textbook of palliative nursing* (pp. 639–640, 646–647). New York, NY: Oxford University Press.

Dobbins, E. H. (2005). Helping your patient to a "good death." *Nursing, 35*(2), 43–45. Retrieved from http://journals.lww.com/nursing/Fulltext/2005/02000/Helping_your_patient_to_a__good_death_.37.aspx

Emanuel, L. L., von Gunten, C. F., & Ferris, F. D. (1999). *Trainer's guide, module 2: Communicating bad news. The education for physicians on end-of-life care (EPEC) curriculum.* Princeton, NJ: Robert Wood Johnson Foundation.

Enclara Health Hospice Pharmacy Services. (2011). Management algorithmpharmacopoeia (MAP) handbook (3rd ed.). West Deptford, NJ: Enclara Health.

Ferrell, B. R. (1991). Pain in elderly people. *Journal of the American Geriatrics Society, 39*, 64–73.

Ferrell, B. R., Grant, M., & Virani, R. (1999). Strengthening nursing education to improve end-of-life care. *Nursing Outlook, 47*, 252–256.

Gibson, M., & Schroder, C. (2001). The many faces of pain for older, dying adults. *American Journal of Hospice and Palliative Care, 18*(1), 19–25.

Griffie, J., Nelson-Marten, P., & Muchka, S. (2004). Acknowledging the "elephant": Communication in palliative care: Speaking the unspeakable when death is imminent. *American Journal of Nursing, 104*(1), 48–58.

Hillesum, E. (1996). *An interrupted life: The diaries and letters from Westerbork*, p. 155. New York, NY: Henry Holt & Company.

Hogan, C., Lunney, J., Gabel, J., & Lynn, J. (2003). Medicare beneficiaries cost of care in the last year of life. *Health Affairs, 20*, 4.

Hospice and Palliative Nurses Association [HPNA]. (2003). Position paper: Palliative sedation at the end of life. *Journal of Hospice and Palliative Nursing, 5*(4), 235–237.

Hospice and Palliative Nurses Association [HPNA]. (2004a). Pain. Jou*rnal of Hospice and Palliative Nursing, 6*(1), 62–64.

Hospice and Palliative Nurses Association [HPNA]. (2004b). Value of the professional nurse in end-of-life care. *Journal of Hospice and Palliative Nursing, 6*(1), 65–66.

Karnes, B. (2001). *Gone from my sight: The dying experience* (pp. 12–13). Depoe Bay, OR: B. K. Books.

Kinzbrunner, B. M. (2002). Nutritional support and parenteral hydration. In B. M. Kinzbrunner, N. J. Weinreb, & J. S. Policzer (Eds.), *Twenty common problems in end-of-life care* (pp. 313–327). New York, NY: McGraw-Hill.

Kinzbrunner, B. M., Weinreb, N. J., & Policzer, J. S. (2002). *Twenty common problems in end-of-life care.* New York, NY: McGraw-Hill.

Kirkwood, N. A. (1993). *A hospital handbook on multiculturalism and religion: Practical guidelines for health care workers.* Harrisburg, PA: Morehouse.

Krisman-Scott, M. A. (2003). Origins of hospice in the United States: The care of the dying, 1945–1975. *Journal of Hospice and Palliative Nursing, 5*(4), 205–210.

Kubler-Ross, E., & Kessler, D. (2000). *Life lessons.* New York, NY: Simon and Schuster.

Levi, M. H. (1991). Constipation and diarrhea in cancer patients. *Cancer Bulletin, 43,* 412–422.

Lewis, L. (2001, July). Toward a good death in the nursing home: Pain management and hospice are key. *Caring for the Ages,* 24–26.

Lipman, A. G. (2006). Pharmacotherapy for pain control at end of life. In K. J. Doka (Ed.), *Pain management at the end of life: Bridging the gap between knowledge and practice* (pp. 156–158). Washington, DC: Hospice Foundation of America.

Mauk, K. L., & Schmidt, N. K. (2004). *Spiritual care in nursing practice.* Philadelphia, PA: Lippincott Williams & Wilkins.

McCaffery, M. (1968). *Nursing practice theories related to cognition, bodily pain, and man-environment interactions.* Los Angeles, CA: University of California at Los Angeles Student Store.

McCaffery, M., & Pasero, C. (1999). *Pain: Clinical manual* (2nd ed.). St. Louis, MO: Mosby.

McKinnis, E. A. (2002). Dyspnea and other respiratory symptoms. In B. M. Kinzbrunner, N. J. Weinreb, & J. S. Policzer (Eds.), *Twenty common problems in end-of-life care* (pp. 147–162). New York, NY: McGraw-Hill.

McKinnon, S. E., & Miller, B. (2002). Psychosocial and spiritual concerns. In B. M. Kinzbrunner, N. J. Weinreb, & J. S. Policzer (Eds.), *Twenty common problems in end-of-life care* (pp. 257–274). New York, NY: McGraw-Hill.

Mercadante, S., Ferrera, P., Villari, P., & Casuccio, A. (2006). Opoid escalation in patients with cancer pain: The effect of age. *Journal of Pain and Symptom Management, 32*(5) 413–419.

Meyer, C. (2001). Allow natural death—An alternative to DNR? *Hospice Patients Alliance.* Retrieved from http://www.hospicepatients.org/and.html

Morrow, A. (2012). What is POLST and do I need one? *About.com.* Retrieved from http://Dying.about.com/od/ethicsandchoices/f/POLST.htm

National Consensus Project for Quality Palliative Care (2009). Clinical practice guidelines for quality palliative care (2nd ed.). Retrieved from www.nationalconsensusproject.org/guideline.pdf

National Hospice and Palliative Care Organization [NHPCO]. (2008). Social work assessment tool. Retrieved from www.nhpco.org/files/public/nchpp/swat_assessment_tool.pdf

National Hospice and Palliative Care Organization [NHCPO]. (2012). *Hospice philosophy statement.* Paragraph 1. Retrieved from http://www.nhpco.org/i4a/pages/index.cfm?pageID=5308#2

Perley, M. J., & Dahlin, C. (Eds.). (2007). *Core curriculum for the advanced practice hospice and palliative nurse.* Washington, DC: Hospice and Palliative Nurses Association.

Preston, T. A. (2000). *Final victory: Taking charge of the last stages of life, facing death on your own terms.* Roseville, CA: Prima.

Puchalski, C., & Romer, A. L. (2000). Taking a spiritual history allows clinicians to understand patients more fully. *Journal of Palliative Medicine, 3* (1), 129–131.

Quaglietti, S., Blum, L., & Ellis, V. (2004). The role of the adult nurse practitioner in palliative care. *Journal of Hospice and Palliative Nursing, 6*(4), 209–213.

Quint, J. C. (1967). *The nurse and the dying patient.* New York, NY: Macmillan.

Rando, T. A. (1984). *Grief, dying and death: Clinical interventions for caregivers.* Champaign, IL: Research Press.

Rando, T. A. (1993). *Treatment of complicated mourning.* Champaign, IL: Research Press.

Rushton, C. H., Spencer, K. L., & Johanson, W. (2004). Bringing end-of-life care out of the shadows. *Nursing Management, 35*(3), 34–40.

Salacz, M. E., & Weissman, D. E. (2004). Controlled sedation for refractory suffering. End of life/Palliative education resource center. Retrieved from http:// www.eperc.mcw.edu/EPERC/FastFactsIndex/ ff_106.htm

Saunders, C. (1984). On dying well. *Cambridge Review,* 49–52.

Schweitzer, A. (1961). *On the edge of the primeval forest & more from the primeval forest: Experiences and observations of a doctor in equatorial Africa.* p. 62. UK: Macmillan.

Sheehan, D. K., & Schirm, V. (2003). End of life care of older adults. *American Journal of Nursing, 103*(11), 48–57.

Storey, P. (1996). *Primer of palliative care* (2nd ed.). Gainesville, FL: American Academy of Hospice and Palliative Medicine.

Temel, J. S., Greer, J. A., Muzikansky, A., Gallagher, E. R., Admane, A., Jackson, V.A., … Lynch, T. J. (2010). Early palliative care for patients with metastatic non-small-cell lung cancer. *New England Journal of Medicine, 263,* 733–742.

Toole, M. M. (2006). *Handbook for chaplains: Comfort my people.* New York, NY: Paulist Press.

Towey, J. (2005). *Five wishes: Questions and answers.* Retrieved from http://www.agingwithdignity.org/ five-wishes.php

Weinreb, N. J., Kinzbrunner, B., & Clark, M. (2002). Pain management. In B. M. Kinzbrunner, N. J. Weinreb, & J. S. Policzer (Eds.), *Twenty common problems in end-of-life care* (pp. 91–145). New York, NY: McGraw-Hill.

Wolfelt, A. D. (2001). *Healing a teen's grieving heart: 100 practical ideas.* Ft. Collins, CO: Companion Press.

Wolfelt, A. D. (2004). *The understanding your grief support group guide.* pp. 56–57, 77–79. Ft. Collins, CO: Companion Press.

Wolfelt, A. D. (2012a). The mourner's bill of rights. Retrieved from http://www.grieftogreatness.com/ professionalcommentaries.html#bill

Wolfelt, A. D. (2012b). *How to help the grieving.* Retrieved from http://www.grieftogreatness.com/ howtohelpthegrieving.html

Worden, J. W. (1991). *Grief counseling and grief therapy: A handbook for the mental health practitioner.* New York, NY: Springer.

Wright, J. B. (2002). Depression and other common symptoms. In B. M. Kinzbrunner, N. J. Weinreb, & J. S. Policzer (Eds.), *Twenty common problems in end-of-life care* (pp. 221–240). New York, NY: McGraw-Hill.

For a full suite of assignments and additional learning activities, see the access code at the front of your book.

LEARNING OBJECTIVES (WWW)

At the end of this chapter, the reader will be able to:

> Compare the aging policies of Japan, Germany, England, and Canada with those of the United States.
> Describe the effects of an aging population on health policy.
> Explain how morbidity and mortality can influence policies for the elderly.
> Analyze the benefits of social security.
> Contrast the Medicare and Medicaid programs.
> List the benefits and barriers to long-term care insurance.

KEY TERMS (WWW)

Benefit trigger
Copayment
Deductible
Delayed retirement credit (DRC)
Elimination period
Home care
Life expectancy

Long-term care
Medicaid
Medicare
Mortality
Nursing home
Social Security

Chapter 27

Global Models of Health Care

Carole A. Pepa

The aging of the population is a challenge worldwide (Sciegai & Behr, 2010). Comparing models of health care around the world may provide greater insights into how best to meet the challenges the growth in the aging population will create. Some countries, like Japan and the United States, have separate care models for the elderly, while other countries, like Canada and England, have healthcare delivery models that include all citizens.

International Models of Health Care
Japan

Japan has a universal healthcare system. Insurance is provided through the National Health Insurance, a variety of employer-based health insurance plans, and Health Insurance for the Elderly. Everyone in Japan must enroll in a health insurance plan.

There are several employer-based health insurance plans, which are based upon the size of the company. Premiums are fixed and shared between employers and employees. A 20% copayment is required for hospital costs, and a 30% copayment is required for outpatient costs (Kaiser.edu, 2010b). The National Health Insurance covers workers in agriculture, forestry, or fisheries; the self-employed; and those not employed, including students and retirees. Copayments are required for both inpatient and outpatient services and for prescriptions. As with the employer-based insurance plans, premiums are fixed and divided between employers and employees. If there is no employer, the government pays for that portion of the plan (Kaiser.edu, 2010b). Premiums are automatically deducted from pensions for those who are retired (Tomizuka & Matsuda, 2008). From 2000 until 2008, those over 65 years of age or 40–64 years of age with certain disabilities were covered by Health Insurance for the Elderly (Tamiya et al., 2011). In 2008, the government implemented a new insurance program for those 75 years of age and older, known as insurance for the Old-Old or Late Elders' Health Insurance. This scheme retains many of the characteristics and provisions of the previous scheme for the elderly, but its financial structure was intended to increase transparency: Half of the cost of the plan is covered by the general budgets of the three levels of government; the other half comes from premiums and subsidies from other insurance plans. Each insurance scheme contributes a fixed amount per enrollee to a central fund. These contributions cover 40% of the cost of this plan, as well as subsidize those individuals 65–74 years who belong to other plans (Ikegami et al., 2011, p. 1110). The elderly are to finance 10% of the cost of the program; this percentage will increase in the future as the number of younger contributors decreases (Tomizuka & Matsuda, 2008). Japan has one of the largest elderly populations in the world. In 2010, 23% of the population in Japan was over the age of 65 years (Ikeda et al., 2011). By 2020, the 65 years or older population will comprise 27% of the total population (Houde, Gautam, & Kai, 2007).

Since World War II, policies related to the elderly in Japan (see **Figure 27-1**) have undergone several changes. In 1954, the Pension Reform Act covered about 20% of the labor workforce; payments into the program were contributed by both the employee and the employer (Usui & Palley, 1997). Beginning in 1961, the National Pension Law provided coverage for the entire population, and in the 1970s, benefits for the elderly were expanded to include free medical care; pension benefits were also significantly increased (Usui & Palley, 1997). However, policies in place encouraged an overuse of acute care hospitals, and during the 1980s, Japan experienced a large increase in healthcare expenses (Usui & Palley, 1997). The Health Care for the Aged Law of 1982 terminated free medical care to the elderly; with this initiative, the elderly had to pay a small deductible for outpatient and hospital care. By 1985, coinsurance and *copayments* were also required. In addition to coinsurance and copayments, the 1985 act also discouraged the use of acute hospitals for long-term care. The law called for an increased use of intermediate nursing care, rehabilitation, and other lower-cost strategies to support discharged elderly patients (Usui & Palley, 1997). The Gold Plan of 1989 (formally called the Ten-Year Strategy to Promise Health and Welfare for the Aged) was a 10-year plan that targeted health promotion and welfare for the elderly while trying to control future cost escalation. The Gold Plan promoted three services: home help, short-stay institutions, and day services

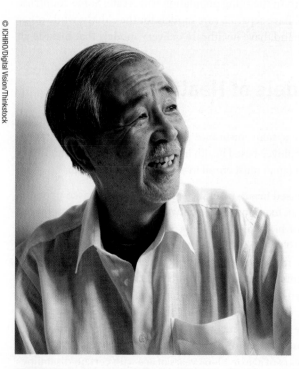

© ICHIRO/Digital Vision/Thinkstock

Figure 27-1 Japan has one of the largest elderly populations in the world.

(Usui & Palley, 1997). It also included education regarding normal aging to prevent misuse of health resources by persons acting as they thought elderly persons should act—for instance, many elderly were bedridden because they believed elderly people were supposed to be bedridden (Usui & Palley, 1997). The Gold Plan was modified in 1994 to place even more emphasis on community-based care, such as respite care for caregivers, daycare centers, short-stay nursing homes, and in-home care. On April 1, 2000, the Long-Term Care Insurance (LTCI) program was introduced. The purpose of the LTCI system was to "support the independence and quality of life for frail and impaired elderly persons by providing them with adequate health and welfare services" (Asahara, Momose, & Murashima, 2003, p. 770). Under this program, all those age 65 or older were entitled to receive long-term care according to their eligibility levels. The six levels of care were determined by physical and mental status; availability of family support was not considered when determining the level of care required (Ikegami, Yamauchi, & Yamada, 2003). To fund the program, everyone contributes to a designated fund based on income (Campbell, Ikegami, & Gibson, 2010). A 5-year review of LTCI revealed that both the number of certified users and *home care* users increased more than 100%; institutional users increased by 56% (Tsutsui & Muramatsu, 2007). Several reasons were posited for the increase in the use as well as the cost of the program. First, elders no longer had to meet a means test to be eligible for service, so elders who were not eligible in the past were able to secure services. Second, under the 2000 LTCI plan, it was less expensive for seniors to pay the copayment for a nursing home with food and around-the-clock care than to pay for rent and utilities for most apartments or copayment for community-based settings, such as a group home. However, institutional care costs the LTCI program more than three times the cost of community-based settings (Tsutsui & Muramatsu, 2007). Last, municipalities had little control over the type and quality of services provided. Originally, public health nurses were scheduled to act as care managers and create care plans based on a senior's certified need, but the shortage of public health nurses led to other health professionals with at least 5 years' experience being able to assume this role. These weaknesses were addressed with the 2005 reforms to the LTCI, one of which increased the standard copayment for a nursing resident by approximately 50%, effective in May 2005. Lower-income seniors are exempt from this increase. The goal of this increase is to lessen the gap in cost between institutional and community-based care.

The hallmark of Japan's long-term care insurance is that it does not offer monetary benefits; instead, it provides services to help relieve the stress on caregivers. These include community-based services such as help at home, adult day care, respite care, assistive devices, and visiting nurses (Campbell et al., 2010, p. 91). This long-term care approach has fostered a change in attitudes in Japan. Traditional Japanese values would neither allow a stranger into the home to provide care nor consider sending the elder out of the home for care (Tamiya et al., 2011).

As the community-based services have expanded, they have become more accepted (Tamiya et al., 2011).

With the emphasis on in-home caregivers for the Japanese elderly, combined with a growing elderly population, elder abuse has received additional attention. The Japan Federation of Bar Associations submitted a report to the Health, Labor and Welfare Ministry at the end of 2004 that included recommendations to assist both the victims and abusers (Roundup, 2005). According to the report, the elderly were reluctant to report abuse because they felt responsible when their children were the perpetrators because they raised them (Roundup, 2005). In 2006, Japan enacted the elder abuse prevention and caregiver support law (Nakanishi, Nakashima, & Honda, 2010) (see **Box 27-1**).

BOX 27-1   Research Highlight: Home-Based Needs of Japanese Long-Term Care Insurance Consumers

Aim: The purpose of this study was to clarify care receivers' needs for home care services or help at home. Another purpose was to identify those characteristics of elders most likely to need home care services. This study was conducted to assist public health nurses and home care agencies in their long-term planning to meet the needs of the elderly population in Japan.

Methods: For this descriptive study, care managers interviewed 300 clients from care levels 2, 3, 4, and 5. In addition to demographic data, the researchers evaluated a participant's ability to perform activities of daily living (ADL) using the Katz index of independence. Dementia was assessed using the Japanese Independence Index of Dementia established by the Ministry of Health and Welfare. Using the collected data, the researchers were then able to determine if the elder required daytime or nighttime services such as home help, home nursing and rehabilitation, or assistance with personal care. Descriptive analysis was used to describe the population and the findings. CHAID denograms were used to further explore the demographics of the group that required home help during the day and night.

Results: The results of the study suggested that there were large discrepancies between the number of people who need services and the number of people who are actually receiving them. In addition, the findings revealed that the discrepancies were especially large at night. A review of the characteristics of the elders needing services identified that for daytime need, the primary predictor of home help was cohabitation status. The primary predictor for home help at night was the need for assistance with ADLs.

Application to practice: The results of this study indicated that there is a need for additional professionals and trained nonprofessionals to provide needed services, especially at night. This information may assist public health nurses and home care agencies to better assess future needs and to better evaluate the effectiveness of the long-term care insurance program. The study also supported the need for future research regarding the barriers to using services.

Source: Naruse, T., Nagata, S., Taguchi, A., & Murashima, S. (2011). Classification tree model identifies home-based service needs of Japanese long-term care insurance consumers. *Public Health Nursing, 28*, 223–232. doi: 10.1111/j.1525-1446-2011.00915.x

Germany

Germany was the first country to establish a national healthcare program. Social insurance in Germany is a mandatory transfer system whereby employees and employers make equal contributions for long-term care (LTC), social health insurance, pension funds, unemployment, and worker's compensation (Kaiser.edu, 2010a). The German model of health care is based on the "solidarity principle," which states that "members of society are responsible for providing adequately for another's well-being through collective action" (Geraedts, Heller, & Harrington., 2000, p. 378). The statutory health insurance (SHI) covers about 90% of the population (Leiber, Greβ, & Manouguian, 2010) and provides a wide spectrum of services ranging from preventive care to inpatient hospital care. Prescription medications are also covered (Busse & Blumel, 2011). This insurance scheme is operated by over 150 competing sickness funds. Individuals have a choice of sickness funds and may change if not satisfied. The SHI covers the employee, pensioner, and dependents. Copayments are required for most services, and, although copayments are required for prescription medications, 5,000 medications are essentially free after adjustments in costs are made (Busse & Blumel, 2011, p. 57). The SHI is financed through compulsory contributions based on gross earnings (Busse & Blumel, 2011). In 2011, the insured employee (or pensioner) contributed 8.2% of the gross wage, and the employer (or pension fund) contributed 7.3% of gross wages (Busse & Blumel, 2011, p. 58).

The remaining population, including civil servants and the self-employed, are covered by private insurance. In addition, those with higher incomes can opt out of the SHI and choose private insurance. Once private insurance is chosen, the SHI is no longer an option; therefore, private insurance is regulated by the government so the insured are not faced with large premiums as they age and experience a decrease in income (Busse & Blumel, 2011).

In Germany, primary care physicians act as gatekeepers to hospital access, but German citizens can access specialists without a primary care referral. In turn, some of these specialists have direct hospital access, so it is possible to circumvent the primary care physician gatekeeping (Green & Irvine, 2001). Unlike some other countries' healthcare systems, there is little or no waiting for physician or care access in Germany.

Like many wealthy countries, the population in Germany is aging. Aware of the projected need, the German government integrated long-term-care (LTC) coverage into the social security system. Long-term care insurance (LTCI) is mandatory and is provided by the same public–private mix as the health insurance scheme (Busse & Blumel, 2011). In 2011, employers and employees shared a contribution of 1.9% of gross salary; those without children paid an additional 0.25% (Busse & Blumel, 2011). Everyone who has a need can apply for up to 2 years of benefits under LTCI. Applicants are assessed for need and, if need is determined, they are placed in one of three levels of care. Beneficiaries can choose between cash payment or in-kind services. LTCI covers about one-half of the costs of institutional care (Busse & Blumel, 2011). The goal of the LTC insurance law was to provide relief from the financial burden of long-term disability and illness (Geraedts et al., 2000). Before LTC insurance, 80% of the elderly in nursing homes depended on public assistance, funded by local communities (Geraedts et al., 2000). This situation created a financial strain for the local communities. In addition, more family members were fulfilling the role of informal caregivers. Mental strain, lack of support, and financial hardships, created when the caregiver was no longer employed outside the home, made family members reluctant to assume caregiving responsibilities. German citizens can also purchase private LTCI in place of the LTCI purchased with statutory health insurance. This private insurance is closely monitored because as citizens age, the premiums of private insurance increase as risk increases, and LTCI premiums may become unaffordable (Busse, 2002).

Although most aging Germans are still cared for by relatives, the LTCI provides incentives to establish additional home health care agencies, short-term institutional care facilities, and assisted living facilities (Geraedts et al., 2000). LTC insurance also provides cash to family caregivers and makes contributions to the pension fund if the caregiver provides more than 14 hours of caregiving a week (Campbell, Ikegami, & Gibson, 2010).

Quality of nursing homes and long-term care providers has been monitored since 2009. An independent institution is responsible for evaluating these agencies in 5 different areas with over 50 quality indicators (Busse & Blumel, 2011). Costs of the program have remained within the budget, but adjustments may be required in the future as the aging population increases and the younger population decreases.

England

The National Health Service (NHS) in England (Great Britain) was established in 1948. It is a universal system of health care based on clinical need rather than employment status; care is free at point of care. The NHS is divided into two basic sections: primary and secondary care. Primary care is usually the patient's first contact with a healthcare provider. Primary care providers are independent contractors with the NHS and may be general practitioners, dentists, pharmacists, or optometrists.

Over 75% of the funding for the health care comes from general taxes, with a little over 3% coming from user charges. A payroll tax imposed on all employees accounts for an additional 20% of funding (Harrison, Gregory, Mundle, & Boyle, 2011). Nearly 100% of the population of Great Britain has access to health services. The NHS covers comprehensive care, ranging from preventive services to inpatient and outpatient hospital care. Dental care, some eye care, mental health care, some long-term care, and rehabilitation are also covered (Harrison et al., 2011).

Primary Care Trusts (PCTs) control about 75% of the healthcare budget. These trusts are responsible for addressing the local needs of a community. It is the responsibility of the PCT to ensure that services are accessible, that collaboration occurs among services, and to commission services that best match the community's needs (Harrison et al., 2011; Holtz, 2008). PCTs also manage nurse-led walk-in centers. These centers are open past regular business hours and provide initial services available to anyone, without an appointment (Harrison et al., 2011; Holtz, 2008). General practitioners belong to PCTs and serve as the gatekeepers of the healthcare system. Although the general practitioners maintain ownership of their practices, they must belong to a PCT, and they can belong to only one. Physicians are paid by capitation, although there is some fee-for-service present. A patient in England can choose to see the general practitioner of choice as long as the physician has an opening for patients; the patient can also change physicians. The PCT website enables a resident to evaluate physicians based on outcomes, waits, and other criteria. If additional care is needed, the patient is referred to secondary care: specialists, the local hospital, or a regional or national hospital. Except in emergencies, general practitioners do not provide hospital services, but rather they must refer to the specialists. Specialists are also employees of the National Health Service.

Private health services are available in England, although they are much smaller than the National Health Service and serve about 12% of the population (Boyle, 2011). The private sector provides services similar to those offered by the National Health Service, but physicians in the private sector do not have to follow the national treatment guidelines nor do they have a focus on the health of the community (British Broadcasting System [BBC], 2008).

When the NHS was established in 1948, it was a leader in the provision of health care. By 2000, however, there was dissatisfaction with the system, as reflected by anecdotal evidence and public opinion polls. One of the leading reasons for dissatisfaction was the long waiting times (Monitor, 2005). These concerns were investigated, and changes were made in the system. First, additional financial resources were allocated to the NHS. In addition, Patient Choice was introduced. Under this system, the patients have a choice regarding which hospital they want to go to and can determine wait times (Monitor, 2005). In a review of survey data conducted on sicker adults in five countries to determine their concerns, British adults reported the most satisfaction with their healthcare system, even though they reported less satisfaction with hospital and dental services than other European Union countries (Boyle, 2011).

Long-term care, considered social care, has shifted from institutions to community-based care and from public to private sectors. Social care is not provided free as a universal right under the NHS. Charges for residential care are based on income and assets; charges for community-based care, if any, are determined by Councils with Adult Social Services Responsibilities (Boyle, 2011). The balance of public and private funding for LTC will be part of the policy discussions in the future.

Canada

The Canadian healthcare system, known as Medicare, provides universal coverage at no cost at the point-of-care access for physician and hospital services. Each of the 10 provinces is responsible for establishing, maintaining, and evaluating the provision of healthcare services within the province; their programs must follow national guidelines of universality, portability, ability to access, and public admin- istration (LaPierre, 2012). In addition, the services must be based on need, rather than ability to pay; sharing of best practices; accountability; and flexibility among provinces (Allin, Watson, & Commonwealth Fund, 2011). Therefore, even though each province has a slightly different coverage plan, a resident could receive covered care in another province if it wer necessary.

The healthcare system in Canada is funded primarily through tax monies. Although the federal government provides some money to the provinces, most of the costs are covered by the provinces themselves, which in turn levy taxes to pay for health care. Most physicians are in private practice, and they charge on a fee-for-service basis, though they cannot charge more than the negotiated fee. Hospitals are primarily private, not-for-profit institutions. In addition to medical services, most provinces and territories cover the cost of regular vision and dental care for children, seniors, and social assistance recipients. Also, most public drug plans cover seniors as well as those in low-income groups.

One criticism of the Canadian system has been the long waiting periods (LaPierre, 2012). In reality, in 2009, the self-reported median wait time for specialist physician visits for a new condition was 4.3 weeks (Canadian Minister of Health, 2011). Timely access to care is an area of priority for the National Health Service, and wait times have decreased in targeted areas. Also, the wait list is triaged by medically trained professionals who follow best medical practices, which helps ensures that more-ill patients can be moved to the top of the list (Canadian Minister of Health, 2011).

The Canadian Health Act does not guarantee coverage for care provided out of hospital or by providers other than physicians. Therefore, long-term care services and end-of-life care are considered "extended health services" (Allin et al., 2011, p. 24). Coverage for these services varies among provinces. Even when health services in resi- dential care facilities are covered, housing and meal costs are generally out-of-pocket unless the client meets a means test (Allin et al., 2011, p. 24). Individuals with financial resources are able to purchase long-term care services from private providers to offset the cost of care.

U.S. Health Care System and Policies
Effects of an Aging Society

The elderly population of the United States also is expected to increase, consistent with the increase in the elderly population worldwide. By the year 2035, 20% of the U.S. population will be over the age of 65 years, up from 13% in 2010. By 2050, it is expected that 25% of those over age 65 years will be 85 years or older (Sultz & Young, 2011). This increase in the elderly population is expected to bring challenges to policymakers, as the future population of the elderly is expected to be better educated, more active, and more culturally diverse than the current population

(Sultz & Young, 2011). This increase in the elderly population will create economic challenges, such as how to finance long-term care. In addition, interdisciplinary teams of healthcare providers with expertise in geriatrics will be needed to meet the physical and psychosocial consequences of the concomitant increase in chronic diseases (Sultz & Young, 2011). The shift in the demographic makeup of the population will create disequilibrium in the ratio between the working middle age population and the traditionally retired elderly population. Currently, there are 3.3 workers for every Social Security beneficiary; by the year 2030, there will be 2.2 workers for every beneficiary (Triest, 1997). More financial support will be needed. In response to these needs, creative healthcare delivery models will be required.

Effects of Mortality

Life expectancy, as a summary measure of *mortality*, is often used as an indicator of the health of a country (Health Center for Health Statistics, 2007). For a child born in 2012, life expectancy in the United States is 78.49 years; however, the United States is behind the countries of Monaco (the highest, at 89.68 years), Japan (83.91 years), Canada (81.48 years), France (81.46 years), Germany (80.19 years), and the United Kingdom (80.17 years). According to the Central Intelligence Agency (2012), the United States ranks 50th in life expectancy at birth out of the 221 countries listed.

Health practices in childhood and young adulthood influence the health of individuals as they age (Rowland, 2007). People are living longer, so measures that support health promotion and illness prevention in childhood and through young and middle adulthood may produce a healthier older adult population. An emphasis on preventing some chronic illnesses or decreasing their debilitating effects will help to decrease the cost of health care for the elderly. Currently, health expenditures by and for the elderly are disproportionate to the distribution of the elderly in the general population (Kramarow, Lubitz, Lentzner, & Gorina, 2007; Sultz & Young, 2011).

Social Security

During the Great Depression, unemployment affected nearly 25% of the of the American population (Social Security Administration, 2012a). Many middle- and upper-income individuals were affected as estate values and financial resources plummeted. It was during this time of financial stress that interest in an old-age pension was sparked. With the passing of the Social Security Act of 1935, the United States became one of the last industrial nations to establish a federal old-age pension program. However, the original Social Security Act did not provide benefits comparable to those provided by other industrial nations. The Social Security Act later was strengthened with the addition of survivors' and dependents' benefits (1939), disability insurance (1956), Medicare (1965), and automatic adjustment of benefits for inflation and supplemental income (1972). The Social Security Act provided a safety net of income in return for a lifetime of employment; it never was intended to be the sole source of retirement income. It also provided a standard age by which retirement could be defined (Social Security Administration, 2012a). Participation in the *Social Security* system is mandatory through payroll taxes called "contributions" (Social Security Administration, 2012a). No means test is required to receive benefits; rather, it is an earnings-related program. Benefits are financed by payroll taxes paid by employees and employers on income up to a certain level.

Basic benefits, available at full retirement age, are based on a worker's average indexed monthly earnings in covered employment (Social Security Administration, 2012a). For those individuals born before 1938, the full retirement age is 65 years, the age when one traditionally thinks of retirement. However, since 2003, the full retirement age has been rising. For example, a person born in 1955 will reach full retirement age at 66 years and 2 months; an individual born in 1960 will not reach full retirement age until 67 years (Social Security Administration, 2012b). If retiring before the age of full retirement, individuals may receive reduced Social Security benefits beginning at age 62; benefits are reduced by 1/180 for each month before full retirement age that an individual begins to collect benefits. Conversely, an eligible worker can increase full Social Security benefits through *delayed retirement credit (DRC)*. If a worker postpones retirement past full retirement age and up to age 70, the worker will receive more than the earned full benefit for which he or she was eligible for at age 65 (Social Security Administration, 2012b). Social Security has decreased poverty rates of the elderly, particularly for female elderly; one-half of the older women in the United States would live in poverty without their Social Security income (DeWitt, 2010). For unmarried women, including widows, Social Security comprises 49% of total income. This compares with 37% of unmarried elderly men's income and 32% of elderly couples' income ("Social Security is Important," 2012). Women represent 57% of all Social Security recipients 62 years of age and older; at age 85 years and older, women represent 68% of all Social Security recipients ("Social Security is Important," 2012).

Medicare

Medicare is Title XVIII of the Social Security Act; it was passed in 1965, after years of trying to provide some kind of universal health insurance. It is an insurance program for those 65 or over who have paid into the Social Security system, the railroad fund, or are diagnosed with end-stage renal disease. Those collecting Social Security Disability Insurance (SSDI) are eligible for Medicare after a 24-month waiting period. When Medicare was enacted, nearly one in three elderly were poor, and about half of America's elderly did not have hospital insurance (De Lew, 2000).

The Original Medicare Plan, managed by the federal government, provides Part A and Part B. Medicare Part A helps to cover inpatient hospital care, inpatient care in a skilled nursing facility (for transitional, but not custodial, care), hospice care, and some home healthcare services (Centers for Medicare and Medicaid Services [CMS], 2012). Financed by payroll taxes paid by the employer and employee, Medicare Part A is available without charge for those who are eligible to receive Social Security or Railroad Retirement benefits. If an individual is 65 years of age and has not worked

10 years (40 quarters) in a job that has paid Medicare taxes, he or she can still receive Medicare Part A by paying a premium. Part B, previously referred to as Supplemental Medical Insurance (SMI), is considered medical insurance. It covers some of the cost for laboratory services, home healthcare services, doctor services, some outpatient therapies, mental health services, and outpatient hospital services. Participation in Medicare Part B is not mandatory and is not funded by the Medicare trust fund. Participants may pay for Part B out of their Social Security checks. In 2012, premiums for Medicare Part B were based on income; for example, if an individual reported yearly income of $85,000 or below ($170,000 for a joint return) on his or her income tax return, the monthly premium was $99.90. This premium increases incrementally as income increases, to a high of $319.70 for individuals with a yearly reported income above $214,000 (above $428,000 for a couple). In addition to monthly premiums, beneficiaries must pay a yearly *deductible* ($146 for 2012, up from $135 in 2008) and 20% of the usual and customary charges (CMS, 2012). If a physician accepts Medicare assignment, then the physician must accept whatever Medicare provides as reimbursement. If the physician does not accept Medicare assignment, then the patient is responsible for any additional cost Medicare does not reimburse the physician. This is a question that all older adults should ask of their physicians prior to a visit.

For reimbursement purposes under Part A, Medicare establishes benefit periods, which consist of 90 days of inpatient hospital care. When a patient is admitted to a hospital for inpatient care, the benefit period begins. In 2008, for each benefit period, the beneficiary was required to pay a deductible of $1,156. If a patient were in the hospital for more than 60 days, a further charge of $289/day was incurred. If a patient was in the hospital for more than 90 days, then the beneficiary begins to use his or her lifetime reserve of 60 days, at a cost of $578 per day. All figures are amounts due in 2012; these charges have increased every year (CMS, 2012). If an individual requires additional skilled care in the transition from at least a 3-day inpatient hospital stay to home, Medicare Part A will cover the first 20 days of each benefit period in a skilled nursing facility for no out-of-pocket expense. However, for days 21–100, the 2012 out-of-pocket cost was $144.50/day. After 100 days in a skilled nursing facility, the individual is responsible for all costs in the benefit period (CMS, 2012).

In addition to the Traditional Medicare Plan with Parts A and B, Medicare also offers a plan called Medicare Advantage, also referred to as Medicare Part C. This option offers managed care plans like health maintenance organizations (HMOs) and preferred provider organizations (PPOs). Medicare Advantage plans provide all of the benefits of the hospital and medical insurance plans under original Medicare, but can charge different copayments and deductibles.

With the passing of the Medicare Prescription Drug Improvement and Modernization Act of 2003, Medicare Part D was added. This is the Medicare prescription option, and it offers multiple plans from which the beneficiary can choose. Each plan identifies the prescription medication it covers as well as the pharmacies, premium, deductible, and copayment. Consequently, the beneficiary must select the plan that covers most of the medications prescribed as well as determine whether to choose a higher premium or higher deductible. A beneficiary may change plans for the next year during the open enrollment period of the current year. Once enrolled, the beneficiary must remain on the chosen plan until the next open enrollment period. One criticism of Medicare Part D is the coverage gap, or what some call the doughnut hole: Once a beneficiary has spent a certain amount of money during a year, all medication costs are out of pocket until the beneficiary is eligible for catastrophic coverage. In 2012 during the coverage gap, as part of the Patient Protection and Affordable Care Act of 2010, beneficiaries received a 50% discount on covered brand-name prescriptions. The plan also pays 86% of the cost of generics. Choosing a prescription plan is very complex, and plans vary among states. In the booklet *Medicare & You*, plans and options are outlined so beneficiaries can determine which plans to contact for additional information (see **Box 27-2**). Even though this prescription option has saved the elderly money, medication costs can still be very expensive.

When Medicare was proposed, private sector insurance plans were used as the models for coverage, administration, and payment methods (De Lew, 2000). Initially, Medicare did not cover dental care, routine eye care and glasses, hearing aids, preventive services, prescriptions, or *long-term care*. Today, in addition to covering prescriptions with Part D, Medicare does reimburse for some screenings on a regular basis and a physical exam when the beneficiary first becomes eligible for Medicare services after the deductible has been met. Medicare also covers hospice care for those patients who have been certified by the physician as having 6 months or less to live, so long as the care is provided by a Medicare-certified hospice agency. Medicare also covers home care provided by a Medicare-certified agency (see **Box 27-3**). All of these services have criteria that must be met for reimbursement (CMS, 2012).

BOX 27-2   Web Link

Browse the free online version of *Medicare & You*, available at

http://www.medicare.gov/publications/pubs/pdf/10050.pdf.

BOX 27-3   Criteria for Medicare Reimbursement of Home Care Visits

1. Care must be provided by a Medicare-certified agency.

2. The plan of care must be certified by a physician every 60 days.

3. The client must be homebound.

4. The client must require intermittent skilled nursing care or physical, occupational, or speech therapy.

Medicaid

Medicaid is Title XIX of the Social Security Act. It is an assistance program that is jointly financed by the state and federal governments, but is administered by the state; therefore, coverage and eligibility differ from state to state. To qualify for Medicaid, an individual must fit into a category of eligibility and meet certain financial and resource standards. Medicaid provides three types of health protection: (1) health insurance for low-income families and people with disabilities, (2) long-term care (LTC) for older Americans and persons with disabilities, and (3) supplemental coverage for low-income Medicare beneficiaries for services not covered by Medicare (e.g., eyeglasses, hearing aids, prescription drugs) as well as Medicare Part B premiums and Medicare Parts A and B deductibles and copayments (Provost & Hughes, 2000).

Federal funding for Medicaid comes from the general revenues; there is no trust fund set up for Medicaid as there is for Medicare. The state Medicaid office directly pays the doctor, hospital, *nursing home*, or other healthcare provider. Not all physicians will accept Medicaid patients because physicians must accept as payment whatever Medicaid reimburses. In some instances, this reimbursement may be less than the cost to provide the service.

The elderly account for a disproportionate share of Medicaid costs. The fact that Medicaid is the primary reimbursement mechanism for long-term care explains this phenomenon (Provost & Hughes, 2000). In an attempt to decrease high-cost nursing home care, Medicaid instituted a waiver program to facilitate home and community-based care delivery (Indiana Home, 2008). Many states have instituted programs that support low-income elderly in their homes to prevent or delay nursing home placement. In another attempt to curtail Medicaid spending, many states have initiated a managed care model for Medicaid services.

Although eligibility for Medicaid is different in each state, each state does require an individual and family to use their own resources (spend down) before they can become eligible to receive Medicaid reimbursement for LTC. Usually, an unmarried individual is allowed a small amount of personal property (in Indiana, for example, this is $1,500). If the recipient of nursing home care is married, and the spouse is remaining in the couple's home, the spouse is allowed to keep one half of the total nonexempt resources jointly owned when the individual entered the nursing home. There are upper as well as lower limits to the amount the spouse can keep. Rules also cover property and other assets given away as gifts, so family members cannot give away resources that could be used to pay for care. The Patient Protection and Affordable Care Act of 2010 will have an impact on Medicaid coverage, as it provides incentives to states to increase home and community-based services.

Long-Term Care Insurance

Long-term care is expensive. For example, nursing home care averages $72,000 a year, assisted living facilities average $38,000 per year, and home care services average $21 per hour (Kaiser Commission on Medicaid Facts, 2011). Long-term care insurance (LTCI) is designed to cover those expenses of long-term care that are not covered by traditional health insurance or Medicare (U.S. Department of Health and Human Services [HHS], n.d.). Although it has increased in popularity, only about 10–15% of the elderly is covered by private LTCI. One barrier to long-term care insurance is the cost. For the elderly, because they are a population at high risk to use the benefits, the cost is high when compared with income. For instance, according to HHS (n.d.), the average cost of a comprehensive policy for an eligible person would be $2,207 per year for a policy that covered 4.8 years of benefit in the amount of $160 per day. Ideally, healthy middle-aged adults would be buying long-term care insurance against future need, but this is not happening to a large degree. Many employers are now offering long-term care insurance as an employee benefit. As a rule, companies offering long-term care insurance as a benefit do not contribute to offset the cost, but they do provide group rates for their employees (Sultz & Young, 2011).

Long-term care insurance can provide a wide spectrum of benefits; home care, assisted living, adult daycare centers, respite services, and nursing home care are among the care options that may be covered. Examples of services not included under these policies are care provided by a family member who is not an employee of a contracted service, care or services for which there would be no charge if insurance were not present, care for alcoholism and drug addiction, services usually covered by Medicare, and services or care for self-inflicted injury. Long-term care insurance policies can be complex, and it is important to understand how these policies work. Eligibility for long-term care under a policy begins with a *benefit trigger*, which consists of those criteria that are usually defined in terms of activities of daily living (ADLs) or cognitive impairments. Long-term care insurances refer to benefit amounts, and these range from $90/day to $500/day, with most individuals choosing $150–200/day (Shore, 2007). Benefits can be paid on either a daily basis or a monthly basis. If daily benefits are chosen, costs that exceed the daily amount would be paid out of pocket. For example, if a $90/day benefit were chosen, and the expenses for one day are $180, the $90 difference would be paid out of pocket. However, if a $360/month benefit were chosen, then expenses up to the monthly limit would be covered, regardless of when they were incurred during the month. Benefit periods refer to how long an individual wants the benefits to continue after they begin, usually a period of 5 years. If the total amount of coverage is not used during the benefit period, then the benefit period may be extended until the entire benefit amount is used. Long-term care insurance policies also have a waiting period called an *elimination period*, usually 30, 60, or 90 days. Some policies also state that the beneficiary must receive paid care or pay for services during this period. This is the time a beneficiary must pay out of pocket before the policy begins to cover expenses; the shorter the waiting period, the more expensive the policy premiums will be. Policies may also include an escalator to help cover the increase in care costs over time.

Depending on benefit amount, waiting or elimination period, and age of the purchaser, even with long-term care insurance, out-of-pocket expenses for long-term care services could be considerable. In addition, not everyone who would like to purchase long-term care insurance is eligible to do so. Anyone who is currently using long-term care services or who has a progressive health condition may be precluded from purchasing long-term care insurance.

Residents in most states have the opportunity to participate in state partnership programs. These programs link private insurance companies that offer Partnership Qualified (PQ) policies with Medicaid. Requirements for PQ policies vary, but most states require that the policies (a) offer comprehensive coverage, (b) be tax qualified, (c) provide certain specific consumer protections, and (d) include certain kinds of inflation protection (HHS, n.d.). Under these PQ policies, a beneficiary can apply for Medicaid under modified eligibility rules, including an "eligibility disregard" (HHS, n.d.). For instance, if the PQ policy protects $100,000 in assets, when the single beneficiary applies for Medicaid to help pay for long-term care, the beneficiary would be able to keep $100,000 in assets instead of the usual $1500-$2000 (HHS, n.d.).

According to Brown, Goda, and McGarry (2012), cost is not the only barrier to purchasing long-term care insurance. In their study, some respondents had concerns about the long-term financial viability of the insurers. Also, the respondents lacked trust that the insurers would continue coverage as promised into the future (Brown et al., 2012). All of these concerns have implications for policymakers.

Case Study 27–1

www,

Anne Swift, a retired school teacher, is a relatively healthy 72-year-old widow living alone in London, England. She visits her primary care physician for regular health visits. She is on a beta-blocker for mild hypertension. Mrs. Swift has been involved in an auto accident. At the scene, the emergency personnel determine that she has a possible broken arm, possible internal injuries, and she is complaining of a headache.

Questions

1. Explain how Mrs. Swift's care will proceed once she arrives at the hospital?

2. What will be Mrs. Swift's financial burden for her medical care?

3. Compare Mrs. Swift's financial and medical responsibilities in London with the financial and medical responsibilities of a 72 year old in the same situation in Chicago, Illinois, USA.

Summary

The international policies on aging within models of health care vary between countries. This chapter presented information on Japan, Germany, England, Canada, and the United States to provide comparisons and contrasts between care delivery systems. As the over-65 population increases worldwide, policymakers will review care delivery systems to determine the best practices. By understanding the different models of care (see **Case Study 27-1**), gerontological nurses will have the opportunity for input through research, analysis, and evaluation. Gerontological nurses also can assist patients and families to navigate the healthcare system by understanding reimbursement issues related to particular benefits (see **Box 27-4**).

Notable Quotes

"The secret of health for both mind and body is not to mourn for the past, nor to worry about the future, but to live the present moment wisely and earnestly."

—Buddha

BOX 27-4   Resource List

American Association for Long-Term Care Insurance:

http://www.aaltci.org

Centers for Medicare and Medicaid Services:

http://cms.hhs.gov

Department of Health and Human Services:

http://www.hhs.gov

U.S. Administration on Aging:

http://www.aoa.gov

Critical Thinking Exercises

1. In a small group, create a model for healthcare delivery for the year 2030. Identify which features would be present, why these features would be necessary, and how it would be financed. Explain the role of the professional nurse and the advanced practice nurse, as well as other healthcare providers.

2. In a small group, compare healthcare policies for the elderly in Japan, England, Canada, Germany, and the United States. Identify the strengths and weaknesses of each model.

3. **Box 27-5** lists some recommended readings. Choose one reference of interest to read, and share the information with a classmate.

BOX 27-5   Recommended Readings

Glasby, J., Martin, G., & Regen, E. (2008). Older people and the relationship between hospital services and intermediate care: Results for a national evaluation. *Journal of Interprofessional Care, 22,* 639–649.

Heijink, R., Noethen, M., Renaud, T., Koopmanschap, M., & Polder, J. (2008). Cost of illness: An international comparison of Australia, Canada, France, Germany and The Netherlands. *Health Policy, 88,* 49–61. doi:10.1016/jhealthpol.2008.02.012

Ikegami, N., Yoo, B., Hashimoto, H., Matsurnoto, M., Ogata, H., Babazono, A., ...Kobayashi, Y. (2011). Japanese universal health coverage: Evaluation, achievements, and challenges. *Lancet, 378,*1106–1115. doi: 10.1016/50140-6736(11)60828-3

Ikegami, N., & Anderson, G.F. (2012). In Japan, all-payer rate setting under tight government control has proved to be an effective approach to containing costs. *Health Affairs, 31,*1049–1056. doi: 10.1377/hlthaff.2011.1037

Sade, R. M. (2012). The graying of America: Challenges and controversies. *Journal of Law, Medicine, & Ethics, 40,* 6–9. doi:10.1111/j.1748-720x.2012.00639.x

Sparer, M.S., France, G., & Clinton, C. (2011). Inching toward incrementalism: Federalism, devolution, and health policy in the United States and the United Kingdom. *Journal of Health Politics, Policy and Law, 36,* 33–57. doi: 10.1215/03616878-1191099

Stone, R. I., & Reinhard, S. C. (2007). The place of assisted living in long-term care and related service systems. *Gerontologist, Special Issue 3,* 23–32.

Tsutsui, T., & Muramatsu, N. (2007). Japan's universal long-term care system reform of 2005: Containing costs and realizing a vision. *Journal of the American Geriatrics Society, 55,* 1458–1463.

Weil, T. P. (2011). Privatization of hospitals: Meeting divergent interests. *Journal of Health Care Finance, 38*(2), 1–11.

Personal Reflections

1. Interview someone who has come from another country. Explore with this person how the elderly were cared for in his or her country. Would that health policy be a viable model for the United States?

2. Interview an older adult in the United States. Explore with this person the perceived barriers and strengths of accessing health care and medications.

References

Allin, S., Watson, D., & The Commonwealth Fund (2011). The Canadian health care system. In S. Thomson, R. Osborn, D. Squires, & M .J. Reed (Eds.). *International profiles of health care systems, 2011* (pp. 21–31). The Commonwealth Foundation pub# 1562. Retrieved from http://www.commonwealthfund.org/Publications/Fund-Reports/2011/Nov/International-Profiles-of-Health-Care-Systems-2011.aspx

Asahara, K., Momose, Y., & Murashima, S. (2003). Long-term care insurance in Japan. Its frameworks, issues, and roles. *Disease Management & Health Outcomes, 11,* 769–777.

Boyle, S. (2011). United Kingdom (England) health system review. In A. Maresso (Ed.). *Health systems in transition* (pp. 1–486). Copenhagen, Denmark: World Health Organization. Retrieved from http://www.euro.who.int/__data/assets/pdf_file/0004/135148/e94836

British Broadcasting Corporation (BBC). (2008). *How the healthcare system works in England.* Retrieved from http://news.bbc.co.uk/dna/mbiplayer/plain/A2454978

Brown, J. R., Goda, G. S., & McGarry, K. (2012). Long-term care insurance demand limited by beliefs about needs, concerns about insurers, and care available from family. *Health Affairs, 31,* 1294–1302. doi:10.1377/hlthaff.2011.1307

Busse, R. (2002). Germany. In A. Dixon & E. Mossialos (Eds.), *Health care systems in eight countries: Trends and challenges* (pp. 48–60). Retrieved from http://www.hm-treasury.gov.uk/d/observatory_report.pdf

Busse, R., & Blumel, M. (2011). The German health care system, 2011. In S. Thomson, R. Osborn, D. Squires, & M. J. Reed (Eds.). *International profiles of health care systems, 2011* (pp. 57–64). The Commonwealth Fund pub# 1562. Retrieved from http://www.commonwealthfund.org/Publications/Fund-Reports/2011/Nov/International-Profiles-of-Health-Care-Systems-2011.aspx

Campbell, J. C., Ikegami, N., & Gibdon, M. (2010). Lessons from public long-term care insurance in Germany and Japan. *Health Affairs, 29,* 87–95. doi: 10.1377/hithaff.2009.D5-48

Canadian Minister of Health. (2011). *Healthy Canadians—A federal report on comparable health indicators 2010.* Retrieved from http://www.hc-sc.gc.ca/hcs-sss/pubs/system-regime/2010-fed-comp-indicat/index-eng.php

Centers for Medicare and Medicaid Services. (2012). Medicare & you 2012. Baltimore, MD: Author.

Central Intelligence Agency. (2012). The world factbook. Rank order: Life expectancy at birth. Retrieved from https://www.cia.gov/library/publications/the-world-factbook/rankorder/2102rank.html

De Lew, N. (2000). Medicare: 35 years of service. *Health Care Financing Review, 22*(1), 75.

DeWitt, L. (2010). The development of social security in America. *Social Security Bulletin, 70*(3), 1–26. Retrieved from http://www.socialsecurity.gov/policy/docs/ssb/v70n3/v70n3pl.pdf

Geraedts, M., Heller, G. V., & Harrington, C. A. (2000). Germany's long-term-care insurance: Putting a social insurance model into practice. *The Milbank Quarterly, 78*(3), 375–401.

Green, D. G., & Irvine, B. (2001). Health care in France and Germany: Lessons for the UK. London: Civitas.

Harrison, A., Gregory, S., Mundle, C., & Boyle, S. (2011). The English health care system 2011. In S. Thomson, R. Osborn, D. Squires, & M. J. Reed (Eds.), *International profiles of health care systems, 2011* (pp. 38–44). The Commonwealth Fund pub# 1562. Retrieved from www.commonwealthfund .org/Publications/Fund-Reports/2011/Nov/International-Profiles-of-Health-Care-Systems-2011.aspx

Health Center for Health Statistics. (2007). *Health, United States, 2007 with chartbook on trends in the health of Americans.* Hyattsville, MD: Author. Retrieved from http://www.cdc.gov/nchs/data/hus/ hus07.pdf

Houde, S. C., Gautam, R., & Kai, I. (2007). Long-term care insurance in Japan. *Journal of Gerontological Nursing, 33*(1), 7–13.

Ikegami, N., Yamauchi, K., & Yamada, Y. (2003) The long term care insurance law in Japan: Impact on institutional care facilities. *International Journal of Geriatric Psychiatry, 14*, 217–221.

Ikegami, N., Yoo, B. K., **Hashimoto**, H., Matsumoto, M., Ogata, H., Babazono, A., Watanabe, R....& Kobayashi Y. (2011). Japanese universal health coverage: Evolution, achievements, and challenges. Lancet. 17, 378, 1106-15. doi: 10.1016/S0140-6736(11)60828-3.

Ikeda, N., Saito, E., Kondo, N., Inoue, M., Ikeda, S., Satoh, T., ... Shibuya, K. (2011). What has made the population of Japan healthy? *Lancet, 378*, 1094–1105. doi:10.1016/S0140-50140-6736(11)61055-6

Indiana Home and Community-Based Services Waivers (2008). Retrieved from http://www.in.gov/fssa/ da/3476.htm

Kaiser Commission on Medicaid Facts. (2011). Medicaid and the Uninsured. Retrieved from http://www .kff.org/medicaid/upload/8050-05.pdf

Kaiser.edu. (2012a). *International health systems: Germany.* Retrieved from http://www.kaiseredu.org/ Issue-Modules/International-Health-Systems/Germany.aspx?p=1

Kaiser.edu. (2010b). International health systems: Japan. Retrieved from http://www.kaiseredu.org/ Issue-Modules/International-Health-Systems/Japan.aspx?p=1

Krammarow, E., Lubitz, J., Lentzner, H., & Gorina, Y. (2007). Trends in the health of older Americans, 1970- 20005. Health Affairs, 26, 1417–1425.

LaPierre, T. A. (2012). Comparing the Canadian and U.S. systems of health care in an era of health care reform. *Journal of Health Care Finance, 38*(4), 1–18.

Leiber, S., Greβ, S., & Manouguian, M. (2010). Health care system change and the cross-border transfer of ideas: Influence of the Dutch model on the 2007 German health reform. *Journal of Health Politics, Policy, & Law, 35*, 539–568. doi:10.1215/03616878-2010-016

Monitor. (2005). Securing an effective healthcare system for England. Retrieved from http://www .monitor-nhsft.gov.uk/sites/default/files/publications/Monitor_submission_to_DH_wider_review_ of_regulation.pdf

Nakanishi, M., Nakashima, T., & Honda, T. (2010). Disparities in systems development for elder abuse prevention among municipalities in Japan: Implications for strategies to help municipalities develop community systems. *Social Science & Medicine, 71*, 400–404. doi: 10.1016/j_socsimed.2010.03.046

Provost, C., & Hughes, P. (2000). Medicaid: 35 years of service. *Health Care Financing Review, 22*(1), 141.

Roundup: Japan seeks efforts to stem abuse of elderly (part one). (2005, January 10). Xinhua News Agency. Retrieved from Expanded Academic ASAP Plus database.

Rowland, T. W. (2007). Promoting physical activity for children's health: Rationale and strategies. *Sports Medicine, 37*, 929–936.

Sciegai, M., & Behr, R. A. (2010). Lessons for the United States from countries adapting to the consequences of aging populations. *Technology and Disability, 22*, 83–88. doi: 10.3233/TAD-2010-0283

Shore, R. M. (2007). Buying long-term care insurance? *The Maryland Nurse, 8*(3), 24.

Social Security Administration (2012a). *Historical background and development of Social Security.* Retrieved from http://www.socialsecurity.gov/history/briefhistory3.html

Social Security Administration. (2012b). *Understanding the benefits.* Retrieved from http://www .socialsecurity.gov/pubs/10024.html

Social Security is Important to Women (2012). Retrieved from http://www.socialsecurity.gov/pressoffice/ factsheets/women.htm

Sultz, H.A., & Young, K. M. (2011). *Health care USA: Understanding its organization and delivery* (7th ed.). Sudbury, MA: Jones & Bartlett Learning.

Tamiya, N., Noguchi, H., Nishi, A., Reich, M.R., Ikegami, N., Hashimoto, … Kawachi, I. (2011). Population aging and wellbeing: Lessons from Japan's long-term care insurance policy. *Lancet, 378*, 1183–1192. doi: 10.1016/50140-6736(11)61176-8

Tomizuka, T & Matsuda, R. (2008). New health insurance for the elderly. *Health Policy Monitor.* Retrieved from http://www.hpm.org/en/Surveys/Ritsumeikan_University_-_Japan/12/New_Health_Insurance_for_the_Elderly.html

Triest, R. K. (1997). Social security reform: An overview. New England Economic Review. Retrieved from Expanded Academic ASAP Plus database.

Tsutsui, T., & Muramatsu, N. (2007). Japan's universal long-term care system reform of 2005: Containing costs and realizing a vision. *Journal of the American Geriatrics Society, 55*, 1458–1463.

U.S. Department of Health and Human Services. (n.d.). National clearinghouse for long-term care information. Retrieved from http://www.longtermcare.gov/LTC/Main_Site/index.aspx

Usui, C., & Palley, H. A. (1997). The development of social policy for the elderly in Japan. *Social Services Review, 71*, 360–381.

For a full suite of assignments and additional learning activities, see the access code at the front of your book.

LEARNING OBJECTIVES

At the end of this chapter, the reader will be able to:

> Explain geriatric care as a continuum.
> Identify the types of models of care and services available to older adults, including acute care, transitional care, care coordination, community care, and nursing home care models.
> Describe appropriate coordination of the components of the healthcare system to provide better services to meet the needs of the older adult at different points in time.
> Understand the role of the nurse in new models of care.

KEY TERMS

Acute care of the elderly units (ACEs)
After Discharge Care Management of
    Low-Income Frail Elderly (AD-LIFE)
Adult daycare services
Acute geriatric units (AGUs)
Aging in place
Assisted living
Better Outcomes for Older Adults through
    Safe Transitions (BOOSTing)
Care Transitions Intervention (CTI)
Culture change
Eden Alternative
Geriatric resource nurse (GRN)
Geriatric Resource for Assessment and
    Care of Elders (GRACE)

Green House
Guided Care
Intergenerational care
Money Follows the Person (MFP)
National Transitions of Care Coalition
    (NTOCC)
Next Step in Care
Nurses Improving Care for the
    Hospitalized Elderly (NICHE)
Pioneer Network
Program of All-Inclusive Care for the
    Elderly (PACE)
Transforming Care at the
    Bedside (TCAB)
Transitional care model (TCM)

Chapter 28

(Competencies 4, 5, 8, 10, 14)

Using Current System Models to Guide Care

Valerie Gruss
Deborah Strickland

Many new models of care are focused on improving healthcare services for the older adult. The goal of these healthcare services is to provide a continuum of care across the life span and disease trajectory of the older adult. Understanding the use of the different healthcare models and identifying the types of models and services that are appropriate to meet the needs of the older adult at different points in time are essential to providing best care.

Components of these models of care include providing care for acute and chronic illness, health promotion, and health maintenance. These healthcare services are provided in a variety of settings and include care coordination during transition between healthcare settings.

As health care for the older adult has become more specialized, hospitals have developed units with staff specially trained in the care of the older adult and acute geriatric syndromes. Each hospital discharge involves transitioning a complex older adult to a different setting. Transitioning from acute care settings is associated with increased risk of subsequent health problems and potential negative outcomes. Better care coordination through transition care may diminish potential problems.

Home- and community-based services include many options, such as adult day centers, home care registries, home care agencies, and other innovative care coordination models that support elders with chronic illness or disabilities to remain independent in the community. There are also changes in nursing home models that support independence and homelike environments, providing person-centered care.

This chapter will introduce some of the care models that are enhancing the lives of the older adult and opening opportunities for innovative nurse care.

Acute Care Models and Programs

Acute Geriatric Units

Care of the older adult with acute medical conditions in *acute geriatric units (AGUs)* is more efficient than care provided in conventional hospital units and produces a functional benefit compared with conventional hospital care, thereby increasing the probability of the patient returning home (Baztán, Suárez-García, López-Arrieta, Rodríguez-Mañas, & Rodríguez-Artalejo, 2009). Additionally, AGU care has been found to reduce the hospital stays and hospital care costs (Baztán, Suárez-García, López-Arrieta, & Rodríguez-Mañas, 2011).

Acute Care of the Elderly Units

The *acute care of the elderly (ACE) unit* is a program developed through the work of *Nurses Improving Care for the Hospitalized Elderly (NICHE)* and the Frances Payne Bolton School of Nursing at Case Western Reserve University (Nurses for Improving Care for Healthsystem Elders [NICHE], 2012). An interdisciplinary team with special expertise in geriatric care and training in prevention of geriatric syndromes, as well as environmental adaptations to support the elderly, are used to prevent functional decline in the older adult in the acute care setting (Fulmer et al., 2002). Health systems wishing to improve the care of the older adult patient can implement any of the ACE unit concepts.

In addition to providing care in AGUs, over the past 10 years there has been movement to reduce re-admissions to the hospital. Rehospitalization rates among Medicare beneficiaries are high: 19.6% are rehospitalized within 30 days, and 34% are rehospitalized within 90 days (Jencks, Williams, & Coleman, 2009). To reduce rehospitalizations, new innovative models of care have been developed. These models of care posit that a continuum of care be provided across care settings as the older adults transitions between settings (hospital–home, hospital–nursing home, nursing home–hospital, nursing home–home).

Geriatric Resource Nurse

The *geriatric resource nurse (GRN)* role was developed to improve the care of the elderly by increasing the geriatric competency of the bedside nurse in acute care. The GRN receives training by a geriatric nurse specialist (GNS) in areas of geriatric syndromes such as falls, delirium, incontinence, and functional ability, as well as many other conditions commonly occurring in the elderly population (NICHE, 2012). The role of the GRN is to be the unit's "go-to" person for nurses on the acute care unit. GRNs also receive monthly training by the GNS. Fulmer and colleagues (2002) found significant improvement in the perceptions of nurses toward caring for elders who were acutely ill in health systems implementing this model.

Nurses Improving Care for the Hospitalized Elderly (NICHE)

NICHE is a program of the Hartford Institute for Geriatric Nursing at New York University College of Nursing. In 1992, NICHE began with a mission to create better care environments for the hospitalized older adult by improving nursing care. Nurse experts were convened to develop tools and processes that could be used to support individual health system efforts to improve care of the hospitalized elderly. In 1999, the NICHE toolkit was introduced, which included resources for the acute care facility to implement programs that educated nursing staff to the specialized care required of the acutely ill elderly patient.

Since 1996, NICHE has continued to work on programs to improve elder care, such as a Gerontological Nursing Certification Review Course, a national listserv, and a curriculum guide of best nursing practices. Boltz, Capezuti, and Shabbat (2010) found geriatric care models have the ability to increase the geriatric expertise of clinicians and transform the environment to be more supportive of the elderly. NICHE resources are available online (NICHE, 2012).

Transforming Care at the Bedside

Transforming Care at the Bedside (TCAB) is a national program of the Robert Wood Johnson Foundation (RWJF) and the Institute for Healthcare Improvement (IHI). TCAB provides a "How-to Guide" that builds upon research and published literature, and integrates what TCAB hospitals have learned as they strive to improve the quality of care for patients discharged from medical and surgical units within hospitals, discharged from the hospital to home, or to another healthcare facility. Although this guide specifically focuses on patients with heart failure (HF), the proposed changes for creating an ideal transition home can be generalized and adapted to improve the discharge process for all patients (Nielsen et al., 2008).

BOX 28-1   Evidence-Based Practice Highlight

Programs of All-Inclusive Care for the Elderly (PACE) serve the low-income, frail elderly. A central component of a PACE program is the interdisciplinary team that is responsible for the assessment and care oversight of each PACE participant. The nurse is a key member of this team. You can read about a very successful PACE program developed by the University of Pennsylvania School of Nursing.

Source: Sullivan-Marx, E., Bradway, C. & Barnsteiner, J. (2010) Innovative collaborations: A case study for academic owned nursing practice. *Journal of Nursing Scholarship 42*(1), 50–57.

Transitional Care Models and Programs

Transitional care focuses on transitions or movements between facilities for the elderly and chronically ill. The goal of transitional care is to provide patients with a seamless transition that does not result in this duplication of services or fragmented care. The care coordinator follows the patient through the healthcare system and facilitates open communication and collaboration among all providers. The primary focus is on maintaining continuity of care, enhancing patient and caregiver self-management activities, and preventing complications and rehospitalization.

Transitional care engages with patients while hospitalized and then intensively follows patients post-hospital discharge. The role of the nurse in these programs is to assist the older adult and their family in assuring that care is continued as planned after an acute care, long-term care, or rehabilitation admission. These transitional care programs normally have a shorter duration of care than a care coordination program.

The role and function of a nurse working in transitional care might include in-hospital assessment, in-home assessments, teaching patients about self-care, managing medications, symptom recognition, scheduling appointments and transportation for follow-up with primary care and specialists, coordination of information with primary care, medication reconciliation, development of a plan of care with elder/family, and follow-up phone calls.

Two models of transitional care programs that are well established are the Care Transitions Intervention (Coleman, Parry, Chalmers, & Min, 2006) and the Transitional Care Model (Naylor et al., 1999).

Care Transitions Intervention

Developed by Eric Coleman and colleagues at University of Colorado Health Sciences Center, *Care Transitions Intervention (CTI)* is a patient-centered intervention designed to improve quality of care and contain costs for patients with complex care needs as they transition across care settings. It is based on four pillars: assistance with self-management of medications; a patient-centered medical record that is kept by the patient; timely follow-up with primary physician or specialists; and a list of signs and symptoms that could indicate worsening of their condition (Coleman et al., 2006).

In this work, a transition coach (an advanced practice nurse [APN], registered nurse [RN], social worker, or occupational therapist) works with the older adult and family to be more actively engaged in the care transition, with a focus on self-management. The transition coach meets with the individual before discharge from the hospital, arranging a home visit within 48 to 72 hours postdischarge, and phoning or visiting weekly for 30 days posthospitalization to maintain continuity and support the patient and caregiver. More information and a training program

Notable Quotes

"One of the CDC's highest priorities as the nation's health protection agency is to increase the number of older adults who live longer, high-quality, productive and independent lives." (Centers for Disease Control and Prevention [CDC] & Merck Company foundation, 2007, p. 2)

for nurses and others interested in the Care Transitions Intervention is available at http://www.caretransitions.org/.

Transitional Care Model

Mary Naylor and colleagues developed the *Transitional Care Model (TCM)* (Naylor et al., 1999). This model includes a patient-centered intervention to improve quality of life, improve patient satisfaction, and reduce rehospitalizations. TCM was developed to address the needs of elders with chronic conditions after discharge from the hospital. Key components of this program include continuity of care at hospital discharge, focus on individual and caregiver understanding (including early symptom recognition), helping to manage chronic health issues and prevent decline, and medication management. Specific research-based nursing protocols were developed to assist the nurse.

The TCM model uses APNs experienced in serving older adults to provide discharge planning and home interventions for older adults who have been hospitalized. This model uses one care coordinator (CC) per 39 patients, with staff consisting of 3 APNs and RNs. The APN visits during the hospital stay (within 24 hours of admission and daily while hospitalized), in the home within 24 hours of discharge, and then as needed. The nurse also follows hospital discharge with a minimum of eight home visits (weekly during the first month, then biweekly during the second and third months) with the patient and/or family for a period of 3–6 months. Further information on Transitional Care Model training programs can be found at http://www.transitionalcare.info/.

Money Follows the Person

The *Money Follows the Person (MFP)* rebalancing demonstration program helps states to rebalance their long-term care systems by transitioning eligible Medicaid recipients from long-term care institutions back to the community. Each state's MFP program is individualized to meet that state's needs and specific goals.

The MFP initiative is based on the premise that many Medicaid beneficiaries residing in long-term care facilities would prefer to live in the community and would do so if they had adequate support and services. In addition, the MFP is based on the premise that it would cost less to care for and transition these individuals back into the community than what Medicaid currently spends on their long-term institutionalized care.

The goal of the MFP rebalancing program is to increase the states' ability to serve Medicaid recipients with long-term care needs in the community and reduce the use of institutionalized care. Once transitioned into the community, each MFP participant receives home- and community-based service (HCBS) benefits according to their individual needs and services required. The states receive a matching federal fund, Federal Medical Assistance Percentage (FMAP), for each participant they transition into the community. States are required to reinvest these FMAP funds into their long-term care systems. This is coined the "rebalancing initiative."

Forty-three states and the District of Columbia have implemented MFP programs. From spring 2008 through December 2010, nearly 12,000 people had transitioned back into the community through MFP programs (Mathematica Policy Research, 2011). The Patient Protection and Affordable Care Act of 2010 strengthens and further expands the Money Follows the Person program to more states; extends the MFP program through September 30, 2016; and appropriates an additional $2.25 billion over a 4-year period ($450 million for each FY 2012–2016).

Transitional Care Electronic Resources

National Transitions of Care Coalition

The *National Transitions of Care Coalition (NTOCC)* was formed in 2006, "bringing together thought leaders, patient advocates, and healthcare providers from various care settings dedicated to improving the quality of care coordination and communication when patients are transferred from one level of care to another" (National Transitions of Care Coalition, 2012, p.1). Its website provides consumer tools and resources with information for patients and caregivers. The website also provides healthcare-provider tools and resources, and best practices tips to enhance transitional care.

Next Step in Care

Next Step in Care provides information and advice to help family caregivers and healthcare providers plan safe and smooth transitions for patients. Next Step in Care's eight easy-to-use guides help family caregivers and healthcare providers work closely together to plan and implement safe and smooth transitions for chronically or seriously ill patients. More information is available at http://www.nextstepincare.org.

BOOSTing Care Transitions

The *Better Outcomes for Older Adults through Safe Transitions (BOOSTing)* Care Transitions resource site provides materials to help optimize the discharge process at any institution. This online resource was developed through support from the John A. Hartford Foundation. The program and tools are based on the principles of quality improvement, evidence-based medicine, and personal and institutional experiences. More information is available at http://www.hospitalmedicine.org/BOOST.

Care Coordination

Models of care coordination were first identified more than a century ago. As demographics shift and the number of older adults increases, the need has increased for models of care that support the older adult in the community. Komisar and Feder (2011) looked at promising models of healthcare delivery that coordinate across a continuum of care. Key components of successful models included: care that is "person-centered;" primary medical care core; an assessment of the older adults care needs, as well as the needs of the caregiver; coordination of both medical care and long-term care needs; a specific focus on transitional needs when moving in or out of a healthcare facility; ongoing relationship between the care coordinator and the primary care physician; and an ongoing relationship between the care coordinator and the older adult (Komisar and Feder, 2011).

Care coordination also encourages active patient participation in their care, promotes healthy lifestyle choices, and facilitates better self-management. The focus is on improving continuity of care across settings, promoting the use of effective preventive and community services, increasing accessibility to healthcare providers, and improving communication among the providers and the patient/family (Schraeder & Shelton, 2011).

Care coordination requires the nurse to work with the older adult as a coach and supporter. The goal of care coordination is to implement evidence-based guidelines for care management and to support the older adult in self-management of their health. Nurses in this role help the individual to focus on their personal health goals and support them through coaching and motivational techniques to reach these goals.

After Discharge Care Management of Low-Income Frail Elderly

An interdisciplinary approach to chronic care management, *After Discharge Care Management of Low-Income Frail Elderly (AD-LIFE)* uses medical and psychosocial care management models to coordinate care of older adults leaving acute care (Wright, Hazelett, Jarjoura, & Allen, 2007). In their pilot study, the interdisciplinary team included an APN, social worker, pharmacist, RN care manager, geriatrician, and other specialists as needed. An initial assessment by the APN prior to the older adult's discharge from acute care was shared with the interdisciplinary team. The team used evidence-based protocols to generate a care plan. The RN care manager working with the community-based primary care practitioner provided ongoing follow-up care to the older adult (Wright et al., 2007).

Guided Care

Chad Boult, MD, and his colleagues at Johns Hopkins developed the *Guided Care* model. The team sought to develop a model to improve the health care of older adults with multiple comorbidities by providing comprehensive health care by a nurse–physician team. Guided Care is based in a primary care office and uses registered nurses (RNs) trained in Guided Care principles to coordinate cost-effective care (Boyd et al., 2008). The Guided Care nurse curriculum includes training in areas such as promoting self-management, motivational interviewing, and patient-centered care planning, as well as additional techniques for visiting patients and working with physicians and community resources.

An initial assessment by the nurse focuses on the medical, functional, cognitive, nutritional, and environmental status of older adults in their home. This assessment also includes a depression scale, alcoholism scale, screening for hearing and vision impairment, and evaluation of risk for falls and incontinence (Boyd et al., 2007).

The nurse then works with the patient to develop a plan of care that focuses on the patient management of their chronic illness, including medication management, symptom monitoring, and nutritional and activity interventions. This plan of care is central to the care of the individual and used by the nurse in ongoing telephone visits, working with community resources, and if needed, communicating the older adults' needs during care transition between health care facilities.

Guided Care is a long-term care coordination program. The nurse can visit the home as needed, but manages much of the older adult's needs through routine and episodic phone calls. Nurses working in the Guided Care model are trained in this model and have responsibilities in the clinic environment as well as in the home. Evidence indicates that Guided Care improves quality of care, reduces caregiver strain, improves physician satisfaction, and suggests a reduction in use and cost of expensive services (Boult et al., 2008; Boult et al., 2011; Boyd et al., 2010).

Geriatric Resource for Assessment and Care of Elders

Dr. Steven Counsell and colleagues (2007) developed a model of primary care that focuses on improving the quality of care for low-income seniors by the longitudinal integration of geriatric and primary care services across the continuity of care. The *Geriatric Resource for Assessment and Care of Elders (GRACE)* uses a geriatric interdisciplinary team, including an APN and social worker in collaboration with a primary care physician and geriatrician. The team develops a plan of care and (with the primary care physician) modifies the plan if needed. The support team then meets with the patient to review and implement the plan of care. The team conducts an in-home assessment of the older adult and works with a geriatric interdisciplinary team, using care protocols to evaluate and follow common geriatric conditions.

Comprehensive primary care for these low-income older participants may be provided through a community health center (Boult & Wieland, 2010). The team uses resources such as pharmacy, mental health services, home health care, and other community-based services to meet the individual's needs. Ongoing support for the older adult occurs through monthly contacts and a home visit by the APN or social worker after any emergency room visit or hospitalization (Counsell et al., 2007). Nurses working in the GRACE model work as part of the interdisciplinary team, using care protocols to care for the elderly living in the community.

Community Care Models and Programs
Adult Daycare

Adult daycare centers provide supervised daily care in a nonresidential facility for the elderly and disabled. *Adult daycare services* are a growing source of nonresidential long-term care, with more than 4,600 adult daycare centers in the United States (National Adult Day Services Association [NADSA], 2012a). More than 150,000 care recipients receive care daily, and 260,000 care recipients and family caregivers are serviced annually through adult daycare centers throughout the United States.

Adult daycare provides social stimulation, recreational activities, and sometimes healthcare services for the care recipient and respite for the caregivers. Caregivers and care recipients typically select an adult daycare center based on the care needs of the recipients. One-half of all care recipients have some level of dementia, along with other chronic illnesses. Therefore, many adult daycare centers offer dementia care programs and have dementia-trained staff.

The National Adult Day Services Association (2012b) reports that 78% of adult day centers are operated on a nonprofit or public basis and average daily fees across the country are approximately $61. Funding comes from philanthropic or public sources, such as the local agency on aging. Third-party payers (Medicare Part B or health insurance) may cover skilled services or medical therapies. Many services are paid for privately by care recipients and families (NADSA, 2012b).

Aging in Place

According to the U.S. Centers for Disease Control and Prevention (CDC), *aging in place* is "the ability to live in one's own home and community safely, independently, and comfortably, regardless of age, income, or ability level" (CDC, 2012, p. 1). The ability to age in place and remain in one's own home and community requires resources and services to meet the changing needs of the older adult. Community resources and services may include provider and caregiving services; affordable, appropriate housing; assistive technologies such as telehealth; and home safety and security systems. Aging in place is promoted through the National Aging in Place Council at http://www.ageinplace.org/.

In addition to remaining in one's own home and community, there are specialized communities with an aging in place philosophy. One example is the Village model for aging. The Village model began in 2001 in Beacon Hill Village in Boston. The Village is a self-governed older adult community organization that relies on volunteers to provide assistance with transportation, housekeeping, and shopping—services that allow an older adult to continue to live independently in the community. Professional services such as healthcare services and home repairs are provided by vendors. As of 2010, there were over 50 Villages in existence, and close to 150 being developed.

Naturally occurring retirement communities (NORCS) are another source for older adults wishing to age in place. A NORC is a congregation of older adults living cooperatively. The NORC may offer social activities and social services. Funding support for NORCS are provided privately through foundations or through local, state or federal funding.

Assisted Living

More recently, aging in place includes institutional settings that provide a wide range of services. *Assisted living* facilities (ALFs) provide assistance and monitoring of older residential adults for whom independent living is no longer appropriate but who do not need 24-hour skilled nursing home care. In the United States, ALFs are regulated and licensed at the state level. More than two-thirds of the states use the licensure term "assisted living," and other licensure terms include supportive living facility (SLF), residential care home, and personal care homes.

Assisted living services vary by facility and recipient need. Independent apartments include handicap-accessible units with grab bars in bathrooms and wall-mounted emergency home response systems. Personal services may include assistance or supervision with activities of daily living (ADLs), medication management, coordination of healthcare-provider services, housekeeping services, financial management, meals provided, transportation to medical appointments, and trained medical staff.

Home Care Skilled Services

If a care recipient is receiving skilled nursing and/or therapy services in the home, Medicare (or private health insurance) may pay for home health services from a Medicare-certified agency on a short-term basis. Medicare requires the patient to be homebound and under the care of their physician to qualify for services.

When clients are receiving homemaker services or private duty services, private funds are typically required. Care recipients may qualify for funds through a long-term care insurance policy, entitled VA benefits, or through funds of some area agencies on aging.

Intergenerational Care

Intergenerational care centers are environments where "multiple generations receive ongoing services and/or programming at the same site, and generally interact through planned and/or informal intergenerational activities" (Goyer & Zuses, 1998, p. ix). Intergenerational care programs vary in style and scope but all provide ongoing services to multiple generations. These care programs include early childhood programs co-located with adult daycare services, an older adult community with onsite child care, or less common, housing for grandparents raising grandchildren.

Intergenerational care benefits the children, the older adults, and the community; these benefits, as determined by the U.S. Environmental Protection Agency's "Aging Initiative" (2012), are reported in **Box 28-2**. However, despite the evidence of the benefits of intergenerational programs, development of such programs is slow. There are many barriers to overcome in developing these programs, including regulatory conflicts (federal, state, and local), zoning and physical environmental barriers, liability issues, lack of training, and funding problems.

Even with these challenges, the movement to create intergenerational programs persists.

Here are three exemplary and diverse models:

> *Hope Meadows*, located in Rantoul, Illinois, was the first "planned neighborhood" of *Generations of Hope*, a nonprofit foster care and adoption agency. Lower-income senior residents live in reduced-rent housing in exchange for providing a minimum of 8 hours per week of support to children and their foster parents living in the community.
> The *Chicago Housing Authority Intergenerational Computer Learning Center* is a collaborative project between residents of Chicago Housing Authority's (CHA) Senior Housing and Chicago Public Schools. CHA's senior housing

---

BOX 28-2   Intergenerational Care Benefits

For Youth and Children:	Enhances social skills
	Improves academic performance
	Decreases drug use
	Increases stability
For Older Adults	Enhances socialization
	Stimulates learning
	Increases emotional support
	Improves health
For the Community	Strengthens community
	Maximizes human resources
	Maximizes financial resources
	Expands services
	Encourages cultural exchange
	Inspires collaboration

residents came together to create a computer-learning center to meet the needs of the surrounding community, electing to share their resource with local schoolchildren.

> *GrandFamilies House*, located in Dorchester, Massachusetts, is the first grandparents-raising-grandchildren housing program.

Program of All-Inclusive Care for the Elderly

The *Program of All-Inclusive Care for the Elderly (PACE)* originated in the early 1970s, when Marie Louise Ansak, a social worker, was hired to help families in the Chinatown section of San Francisco care for their elders. The mission of this program was to help older adults remain in the community. Now a Medicare- and Medicaid-reimbursed program, PACE has grown to 82 programs operating in 29 states (National Pace Association, 2011). Unlike other programs, PACE programs use an interdisciplinary team consisting of social workers, nurses, day center management, dietitians, a physician, physical and occupational therapists, recreational/activity therapists, as well as other disciplines to assess, plan, implement, and monitor interventions. Each discipline brings their own expertise, but they must be able to work as a team member, focusing on the goals of the older adult (Chinn, 2008). This can be challenging for team members whose disciplines are often passionate about their individual areas of study. Each team member assesses the older adult on enrollment into the program and then on a regular basis, at least annually. The team will work with the patient to develop a plan of care that focuses on the individual's needs and goals. PACE programs operate out of a day center that includes their primary care physician services, nursing services, nutritional and activity therapies, as well as assistance with activities of daily living. The PACE interdisciplinary team works with the patient to determine home care modification needs as well as home care assistance, then arranges the care. PACE programs also provide much-needed transportation services to and from the day center, as well as to medical appointments as needed. A nurse's role in this may be as a home care nurse, clinic nurse, or home care coordinator.

Nursing Home Care Models

Nursing homes are places of care for people with long-term disabilities who can no longer live independently in the community. Long-term care is associated with institutional nursing home settings, however long-term care services are also provided in community settings, including homes and apartments. This section will focus on changes within the institutional nursing home setting.

Culture Change

Culture change is a movement in long-term care facilities to deliver more person-centered care. The Pioneer Network, founded in 1997, is comprised of professionals who work in long-term care and wish to promote person-centered care for elders in long-term care, assisted living, or in the home and community. This network serves as a voice for culture change in policy and regulation development, and it is a resource for professionals on the road to a more person-centered environment. More about nursing home culture change is found in Chapter 26. The culture change movement is an overarching term for programs such as the Eden Alternative or the Green House.

Eden Alternative Model

Bill Thomas, MD, introduced the *Eden Alternative* in the 1990s. Dr. Thomas found in his work as a medical director in a nursing home that the residents suffered from more than just medical issues. He defined three plagues of nursing home residents: loneliness, helplessness, and boredom (Thomas, 2004). With his wife, Judith, he created a new type of nursing home care called the Eden Alternative. The model has been developed and implemented in nursing homes across the United States and many other countries. It is a framework for culture change that guides an organization to make changes necessary to provide more person-centered care based on the 10 guiding principles of the Eden Alternative (see **Box 28-3**).

The Green House

The *Green House* concept also originated with Dr. Thomas. This approach to providing nurturing, warm, loving places for elders to live together in small groups is

---

BOX 28-3   Eden Alternative Principles

1. The three plagues of loneliness, helplessness, and boredom account for the bulk of suffering among our elders.

2. An elder-centered community commits to creating a human habitat where life revolves around close and continuing contact with plants, animals, and children. It is these relationships that provide the young and old alike with a pathway to a life worth living.

3. Loving companionship is the antidote to loneliness. Elders deserve easy access to human and animal companionship.

4. An elder-centered community creates opportunity to give as well as receive.

5. An elder-centered community imbues daily life with variety and spontaneity by creating an environment in which unexpected and unpredictable interactions and happenings can take place. This is an antidote to boredom.

6. Meaningless activity corrodes the human spirit. The opportunity to do meaningful things is essential to human health.

7. Medical treatment should be the servant of genuine human caring, never its master.

8. An elder-centered community hones its elders by de-emphasizing top-down bureaucratic authority, seeking instead to place the maximum possible decision making authority in the hands of the elders or the hands of those closest to them.

9. Creating an elder-centered community is a never-ending process. Human growth must never be separated from human life.

10. Wise leadership is the lifeblood of any struggle against the three plagues. For it, there can be no substitute.

Source: Thomas, W. (2004). *What are old people for?* (p. 189). Acton, MA: VanderWyk & Burnham.

a concept considered long overdue by many who work in long-term care. Thomas (2004) states that we must abandon past practices. "A massive shift toward the deinstitutionalization of older people is called for, and the foundation for such a shift is being laid right now" (Thomas, 2004, p. 223).

The Green House is designed to be a homelike environment where elders can seek autonomy and dignity in their later years (Wilson, 2009). These homes employ workers who will fulfill several functions, such as acting as providers of personal care, leaders of activities, and cooks. The Eden Alternative philosophy is a guiding principle in these homes, which are designed to support the elder's needs. The nurse is still used in the Green House approach, but is no longer sitting at a nurse's station or pushing a medication cart. The care is individualized and more patient-centered. More information about the Eden alternative and the Green House concept is found in Chapter 31.

Pioneer Network

The *Pioneer Network* also supports other culture change initiatives and is working toward a new type of care for the elderly and chronically ill that better supports holistic, individualized care. Models in care of the elder have been developing at a pace not seen before. New career options for nurses have developed with these models. As nurses specializing in care of the elderly, the future has never held so much opportunity. **Box 28-4** provides resources for models to guide care.

Summary

This chapter has presented numerous systems that could be used to design care for older adults. These models can assist gerontological nurses in planning system or even city-wide care. The organizations and programs discussed in this chapter can be used by nurses to help support older adults to age in place and maintain quality of life in spite of health challenges.

BOX 28-4   Resource List

Area Agency on Aging (AAA)

Agency that gets state and federal funding to plan and coordinate services for people over age 60 years within a local area. In some cities, towns and states, the AAA is also known as Department for the Aging. AAAs run program such as National Family Caregiver Support Programs. To find the AAA in your area, call the Eldercare Locator at 1-800-677-1116 or visit the Department of Health and Human Services' Eldercare Locator.

Administration on Aging:

www.aoa.gov

Agency for Healthcare Research & Quality:

http://www.ahrq.gov

American Association of Homes and Services for the Aging:

http://www.aahsa.org

American Association for Long-Term Care Nursing:

http://www.aaltcn.org

American Nurses Association Council on Nursing Home Nurses:

http://www.nursingworld.org

Assisted Living Federation of America:

http://www.alfa.org/

Care Transitions Intervention:

http://www.caretransitions.org/

National Association of Area Agencies on Aging:

http://www.n4a.org

Center for Excellence in Assisted Living:

http://www.theceal.org

Guided Care:

http://www.guidedcare.org

Hartford Institute for Geriatric Nursing

http://www.hartfordign.org/

Institute for Healthcare Improvement:

http://www.IHI.org

National Adult Day Services Association:

http://www.nadsa.org

National Aging in Place Council:

http://www.ageinplace.org/

National Association of Home Care:

http://www.nahc.org

National Association of Professional Geriatric Care Managers (NAPGCM):

http://www.caremanagers.org

National Consumer Voice for Quality Long-Term Care (formerly the National Citizens Coalition for Nursing Home Reform):

http://www.theconsumervoice.org/

National Council on Aging:

http://www.ncoa.org

National Eldercare Locator:

http://www.eldercare.gov; 800-677-1116

National PACE Association:

http://www.npaonline.org

National Transitions of Care Coalition:

http://www.ntocc.org

Next Step in Care:

http://www.nextstepincare.com

Program of All-Inclusive Care for the Elderly:

http://www.npa.org

Pioneer Network:

http://www.pioneernetwork.net

Transitional Care Model:

http://www.transitionalcare.info/

Visiting Nurses Associations of America:

http://www.vnaa.org

Critical Thinking Exercises

Mrs. Barnes is a frail 98 year old widowed female who wishes to remain at home in spite of numerous falls and a recent hip fracture. Assuming all of the programs discussed in this chapter were available, answer the following:

1. Which program might be a best fit for Mrs. Barnes?

2. What additional information would you need to know before making a recommendation for one program versus another?

3. List, in order of priority, the three most appropriate programs for Mrs. Barnes.

Critical Thinking Exercises

1. This chapter identifies many new alternative and innovative programs developed for elders. Identify one model of care you learned about in this chapter that would benefit an elder who wishes to stay in a community or nonnursing-home setting. Search the Internet for organizations that provide this type of care in your area. Contact this organization and arrange a tour/information session for you and other nursing students.

2. Interview a family who is currently caring for an elderly family member. Listen to their challenges and successes. What did you learn from them? What needs did you identify that were unmet? Were there any innovative programs that were identified in this chapter that could benefit this family?

3. Meet with a social worker in your institution, or an institution that provides care for the elderly. What programs does this social worker often recommend?

Personal Reflections

1. What perceptions of nursing homes do you have?

2. Are these perceptions based on clinical experience or are your perceptions based on what you have heard from other healthcare professionals, family, or friends?

3. Have your current perceptions affected your thoughts about employment in this setting?

4. If you were to design a nursing home, what features would you include?

References

Baztán, J. J., Suárez-García, F. M., López-Arrieta, J., Rodríguez-Mañas, L., & Rodríguez-Artalejo, F. (2009). Effectiveness of acute geriatric units on functional decline, living at home, and case fatality among older patients admitted to hospital for acute medical disorders: Meta analysis. *British Medical Journal, 338*, b50. doi: 10.1136/bmj.b50

Baztán, J. J., Suárez-García, F. M., López-Arrieta, J., & Rodríguez-Mañas, L. (2011). Efficiency of acute geriatric units: A meta-analysis of controlled studies. *Revista Espanola Geriatria y Gerontologia, 46*(4), 186–192.

Boltz, M., Capezuti, E., & Shabbat, N. (2001). Building a framework for a geriatric acute care model. *Leadership in Health Services, 23*(4), 334–360.

Boult, C., Reider, L., Leff, B., Frick, K. D., Boyd, C. M., Wolff, J. L., Frey, K... Scharfstein, D. O. (2011). *Archives of Internal Medicine, 171*(5), 460–466. doi:10.1001/archinternmed.2010.540.

Boult, C., Reider, L., Frey, K. et al. (2008). Early effects of "Guided Care" on the quality of health care for multimorbid older persons: a cluster-randomized controlled trial. *Journal of Gerontological A Biol Sci Med Sci., 63* (3), 321–2327

Boult, C., & Wieland, G. D. (2010). Comprehensive primary care for older patients with multiple chronic conditions: "Nobody rushes you through." *Journal of the American Medical Association, 304*(17), 1936–1943. doi:10.1001/jama.2010.16223

Boyd, C. M., Boult, C., Shadmi, E., Leff, B., Brager, R., Dunbar, L., & Wegener, S. (2007). Guided care for multimorbid older adults. *The Gerontologist, 47*(5), 697–704.

Boyd, C. M., Shadmi, E., Conwell, L. J., Griswold, M., Leff, B., Brager, R., ... Boult, C. (2008). A pilot test of the effect of guided care on the quality of primary care experiences for multi-morbid older adults. *Journal of General Internal Medicine. 23*(5), 536–542.

Boyd, C. M., Reider, L., Frey, K., Scharfstein, D., Leff, B., Wolff, J., Groves, C., ... Marsteller, J. (2010). The effects of guided care on the perceived quality of health for multi-morbid older persons – 18-month outomces from a cluster-randomized controlled trial. *Journal of General Internal Medicine, 25*(3), 235–242. doi: 10.1007/s11606-009-1192-5.

Centers for Disease Control and Prevention [CDC]. (2012). *Health places terminology.* Retrieved from http://www.cdc.gov/healthyplaces/terminology.htm

Centers for Disease Control and Prevention [CDC] & Merck Company Foundation. (2007). *The state of aging and health in America, 2007.* Whitehouse Station, NJ: Merck Company Foundation.

Chinn, J. (2008). The PACE model: An Overview. Retrieved from http://www.google.com/url?sa=t&rct=j&q=&esrc=s&frm=1&source=web&cd=2&ved=0CDwQFjAB&url=http%3A%2F%2Fiom.edu%2F~%2Fmedia%2FFiles%2FActivity%2520Files%2FWorkforce%2Fagingamerica%2FChinHansenJennie.pptm&ei=kHYIUeavKY7tqAHxkYDYCA&usg=AFQjCNFw5mS6BhKVZGP1pgUpY7f8a3R6pA&bvm=bv.41642243,d.aWM

Coleman, E. A., Parry, C., Chalmers, S., & Min, S. J. (2006). The care transitions intervention. *Archives of Internal Medicine, 166,* 1822–1828.

Counsell, S. R., Callahan, C. M., Clark, D. O., Tu, W., Buttar, A. B., Stump, T. E., & Ricketts, G. D. (2007). Geriatric care management of low-income seniors: A randomized controlled trial. *JAMA, 298*(22), 2623–2632.

Fulmer, T., Mezey, M., Bottrell, M., Abraham, I., Sazant, J., Grossman, S., & Grisham, E. (2002). Nurses Improving Care for Health system Elders (NICHE): Nursing outcomes and benchmarks for evidenced-based practice. *Geriatric Nurse, 23*(3), 121–127.

Goyer, A. & Zuses, R. (1998). Intergenerational Shared-Site Project: A study of co-located programs and services for children, youth, and older adults: Final report. Washington, DC: AARP. Retrieved from www.gu.org/LinkClick.aspx?fileticket=rzlDauEh8eE%3D&tabid=157&mid=606

Jencks, S. F., Williams, M. V., & Coleman, E. A. (2009). Rehospitalizations among patients in the Medicare fee-for-service program. *The New England Journal of Medicine, 360,* 1418–1428.

Komisar, H. L. & Feder, J. (2011). *Transforming care for medicare beneficiaries with chronic conditions and long-term care needs: Coordinating care across all services.* Washington, DC: Georgetown University.

Mathematica Policy Research. (2011). *Money follows the person: Expanding options for long term care.* Retrieved from http://www.mathematica-mpr.com/health/moneyfollowsperson.asp

National Adult Day Services Association. (2012a). *The national voice for the adult day service community.* Retrieved from http://www.nadsa.org/

National Adult Day Services Association. (2012b). *Overview and facts.* Retrieved from http://www.nadsa.org/consumers/overview-and-facts

National Transitions of Care Coalition. (2012). *About NTOCC.* Retrieved from http://www.NTOCC.org

National PACE Association (NPA). (2011). *What is Pace?* Retrieved from http://www.npaonline.org/website/article.asp?id=12

Naylor, M. D., Brooten, D., Campbell, R., Jacobsen, B. S., Mezey, M.D., Pauly, M. V., & Schwartz, J. S. (1999). Comprehensive discharge planning and home follow up of hospitalized elders: A randomized clinical trial. *Journal of the American Medical Association, 281*(7), 613–620.

Nielsen, G. A., Bartely, A., Coleman, E., Resar, R., Rutherford, P., Souw, D., & Taylor, J. (2008). *Transforming care at the bedside how-to guide: Creating an ideal transition home for patients with heart failure.* Cambridge, MA: Institute for Healthcare Improvement.

Nurses for Improving Care for Healthsystem Elders (NICHE). (2012). *About NICHE.* Retrieved from http://www.nicheprogram.org/mission_vision_history

Schraeder, C. & Shelton, P. (2011). Comprehensive Care Coordination for Chronically Ill Adults. West Sussex, UK: Wiley-Blackwell.

Sullivan-Marx, E., Bradway, C. & Barnsteiner, J. (2010). Innovative collaborations: A case study for academic owned nursing practice. *Journal of Nursing Scholarship, 42*(1), 50–57.

Thomas, W. (2004). *What are old people for?* Acton, MA: VanderWyk & Burnham.

Transitional Care Model (TCM). (2008). Transitional Care Model. Retrieved from http://www .transitionalcare.info

U.S. Environmental Protection Agency. (2012). *Aging initiative.* Retrieved from http://epa.gov/aging

Wilson, K. (2009). Culture change: Definition and models. *Gerontology Special Interest Section Quarterly, 32*(3), 1–2.

Wright, K., Hazelett, S., Jarjoura, D., & Allen, K. (2007). AD-LIFE Trial: Working to integrate medical and psychosocial care management models. *Home Healthcare Nurse, 25*(5), 308–314. Retrieved from http://www.homehealthcarenurseonline.com

For a full suite of assignments and additional learning activities, see the access code at the front of your book.

Unit VIII
eChapters

IF YOU DO NOT HAVE AN ACCESS CODE, YOU CAN VISIT
HTTP://GO.JBLEARNING.COM/MAUK3E
TO PURCHASE ONE.

Glossary

21st century leadership: Characteristics of leadership need to transition from an industrial age to a "socio-technical age," adopting new strategies to meet the changing scene in health care.

a-adrenoceptors: Control vessel constriction.

Abandonment: Desertion of an older person by an individual who has assumed responsibility for providing care for the older adult, or by a person with physical custody.

Abuse: Harm or injury inflicted on another.

Accountability: Being held responsible for acts or omission of an action once a duty, or expected actions and obligations, have been established by the relationship between two parties.

Acculturation: The process by which people from particular ethnic backgrounds have incorporated the cultural attributes (e.g., values, beliefs, language, skills) of the mainstream culture, or a new cultural identity.

Acetylcholine: A neurotransmitter that plays an important role in learning and memory.

Acquired immunity: The branch of the immune system consisting of humoral immunity and cell-mediated immunity.

Actigraphy (ACTG): The measurement of movement activity data, which provides an objective measure of sleep over a 24-hour day, based on algorithms.

Actin: Protein within muscle that, together with myosin, is responsible for muscle contraction.

Activities of daily living (ADLs): Activities performed in the course of daily life; they include bathing, dressing, transferring, walking, eating, and continence.

Active memory: What you are thinking at any given moment.

Acupuncture: Insertion of very thin needles at pathways of meridians in the body to increase the flow of vital energy (qi).

Acute care of the elderly units (ACEs): In-hospital, acute interdisciplinary care provided specifically for older adults.

Acute geriatric units (AGUs): In-hospital, acute care geriatric specialty units run by specially trained elder care teams.

Acute pain: Temporary pain, experienced in a time-limited situation, with attainable relief.

Acute rehabilitation: Rehabilitation services offered in an acute care hospital or free-standing rehabilitation unit; patients must be able to tolerate 3 hours per day of therapy to be eligible.

Addiction: A primary, chronic, neurobiologic disease, with genetic, psychosocial, and environmental factors influencing its development and manifestation. It is characterized by behaviors that include one or more of the following: impaired control over drug use, compulsive use, continued use despite harm, and craving.

Adjuvant: Any drug that has a primary indication other than pain but has been found to have analgesic qualities.

Adrenal cortex: The outer portion of the adrenal glands.

Adrenal glands: Paired glands located above the kidneys.

Adrenal medulla: The inner portion of the adrenal glands.

Adrenocorticotropic hormone (ACTH): Pituitary hormone stimulating the release of glucocorticoids and sex hormones from the adrenal cortex.

Adult day care services: In-community, nonresidential group programs designed to meet the needs of older adults with cognitive and/or functional disabilities and provide respite to family caregivers.

Adult protective services (APS) agency: A social service agency designed to investigate and intervene when complaints of elder abuse or neglect are reported. APS agencies are generally organized as a division of local county government social service agencies.

Advance directives: Legal documents that record decisions regarding life-saving or life-sustaining care and actions to be taken in a situation where the patient is no longer able to provide informed consent.

Adverse drug reaction (ADR): Unwanted side effect of medication.

Advocacy: The act or process of pleading the case of another.

After Discharge Care Management of Low-Income Frail Elderly (AD LIFE): Interdisciplinary chronic care management program providing medical and social care for low-income older adults in the community.

Ageism: A negative attitude toward aging or older persons.

Age-related macular degeneration (ARMD): A condition associated with aging in which the macula of the eye deteriorates, causing loss of central vision.

Aging in place: The idea of providing stability for the older adult by working toward the common goal of either maintaining the current residence or living in a non-healthcare environment.

Agitation: Restlessness that may lead to negative behaviors or aggressive behavior.

Agnosia: Loss of ability to understand auditory, visual, or other sensations.

Agoraphobia: An anxiety disorder in which an individual has attacks of intense fear and anxiety. There is also a fear of being in places where it is difficult to escape, or where help might not be available.

Albumin: As a lab test, measures amount of protein in body.

Aldosterone: A mineralocorticoid targeting the kidneys and regulating fluid–electrolyte balance.

Alveoli: Tiny, spongy air sacs that are the functional units of the lungs and the site of gas exchange.

Allow natural death (AND): Used as an advance directive in some locations instead of a DNR (do not resuscitate) order; promotes a more positive approach to consideration of a person's wishes at end of life.

Alzheimer's disease (AD): A terminal neurological disorder characterized by deterioration of the brain leading to progressive forgetfulness and loss of independence.

American Indian: Many older American Indians prefer the term "Indian" to "Native American," believing that *anyone* born in the United States is a "Native American," and that the term "Indian" reflects the language used in treaties with the federal government. There are at least 558 different federally recognized tribes/nations and 126 tribes/nations applying for recognition in the United States.

Amino acid neurotransmitters: Glutamate is the major excitatory neurotransmitter and gamma- aminobutyric acid (GABA) is the major inhibitory neurotransmitter.

Andragogy: Related to the teaching of adults.

Andropause: Loss of androgen hormone such as testosterone in aging males.

Anemia: A disease characterized by a deficiency of erythrocytes.

Angina: Chest pain resulting from lack of oxygen to the heart muscle.

Anomia: Difficulty naming things.

Anorexia of aging: Age-related decline in food intake.

Anthropometric measures: Important indicators of an older adult's nutritional status; includes items such as body weight, BMI, triceps skin fold.

Antibodies: Antigen-attacking proteins of the immune system.

Anticholinergic: Medications that block acetylcholine and can cause or worsen confusion.

Antidepressant: A psychiatric medication used to alleviate mood disorders, such as depression, dysthymia, and sometimes anxiety disorders. Most antidepressants work by changing the levels of one or more of these naturally occurring brain chemicals.

Antigen: Any foreign substance invading the body.

Anxiety: A normal human emotion that everyone experiences. It can be expressed as irritability, nervousness, apprehension, or fear.

Anxiolytic: A medication used for the treatment of anxiety when it leads to psychological and physical symptoms.

Aphasia: Impaired ability to communicate.

Apnea: The absence of air flow for 10 seconds or longer at the nose and mouth.

Apolipoprotein E-e4: A protein that carries cholesterol in blood and that appears to play some role in brain function. Variants of this gene are associated with the development of Alzheimer's disease.

Apoptosis: A process of programmed cell death marked by cell shrinkage.

Apraxia: Inability to perform purposeful movements.

Arteries: Carry blood from the heart to the rest of the body or the lungs.

Asian/Pacific Islander (API): Persons from the continent of Asia, including China, Japan, India, Pakistan, Korea, Vietnam (including Hmong peoples), Laos, Thailand, Philippines, Pacific Islands (Hawaii, Samoa, Tonga), Micronesia (Marianas, Marshalls, Gilbert), or Melanesi (Fiji).

Assault: Threatening to harm.

Assimilation: See Acculturation.

Assisted living facility: In-community, independent living for older adults, which may provide assistance with certain ADLs or medications.

Assistive devices: Any item, piece of equipment, or product system, whether acquired commercially off the shelf, modified, or customized, that is used to increase, maintain, or improve functional capabilities of individuals with disabilities.

Assistive technologies: Technological tools used to access education, employment, recreation, or communication, enabling someone to live as independently as possible.

Atherosclerosis: Hardening and narrowing of the arteries to the heart from plaque buildup in vessel walls.

Atria: The two upper chambers of the heart; they receive blood from the venous system.

Attention: The ability to disengage, reengage, and sustain focus and vigilance.

Attitudes: Values, thoughts, and beliefs held by a person.

Atypical antidepressants: A psychiatric medication used to alleviate mood disorders in the class of antidepressants, but atypical antidepressants affect neurotransmitters including dopamine, serotonin, and norepinephrine. They work by changing the balance of these chemicals to help brain cells send and receive messages, which usually leads to improved mood.

Augmentative and alternative communication (AAC): All forms of communication that enhance or supplement speech and writing, either temporarily or permanently, or that involve the use of personalized methods or devices to aid a person's ability to communicate.

Autoimmunity: The immune system's attack of the body's own cells.

Autonomic nervous system: Part of the peripheral nervous system; contains the sympathetic and parasympathetic pathways.

Autonomy: Referring to self-governance or self-directing freedom; being in charge of one's own being; having moral independence.

Avoidable/unavoidable pressure ulcers: *Avoidable* means that a resident developed a pressure ulcer when the facility did not evaluate the resident's clinical condition and pressure ulcer risk factors; define and implement interventions consistent with the resident's needs, goals, and recognized standards of practice; or did not monitor and evaluate the impact of the intervention or did not revise the interventions as appropriate to the findings of the evaluation. *Unavoidable* means that a resident developed a pressure ulcer even though the facility had appropriately and comprehensively assessed the residents clinical condition and risk factors, implemented appropriated interventions, monitored and evaluated the effectiveness of these interventions, and revised them as indicated by the care plan.

Ayurveda: Traditional medical system of India.

B cells: Cells of the immune system that mature in the bone marrow and produce antibodies in response to antigen exposure.

b-adrenoceptors: Trigger vessel dilation.

Baby boomers: People born between the years 1946 and 1964, after World War II.

Background noise: Sound other than the voice or sound that is being listened to.

Barorecepter: Sensory nerve ending in vessels that responds to pressure changes.

Baroreflex: Reflex stimulated by baroreceptor activity.

Basic multicellular unit (BMU): Temporary anatomic structure composed of osteoblasts, osteoclasts, vasculature, nerve supply, and connective tissue; responsible for bone modeling and remodeling.

Battery: The act of touching without permission, as in the case of performing a procedure without consent.

Beers criteria: A list of potentially inappropriate medications for older adults.

Behavior theory: Comprised of four leadership styles, each with unique characteristics.

Beneficence: Doing or producing good.

Benefit trigger: Benign paroxysmal positional vertigo (BPPV); one of the more common and treatable causes of dizziness in older adults resulting from otoconia being displaced in the ear canal.

Benign prostatic hyperplasia (BPH): Enlargement of the prostate gland that often occurs with advanced age.

Beta-amyloid plaques: Deposits found in the spaces between nerve cells in the brain that are made of beta amyloid.

Better Outcomes for Older Adults through Safe Transitions (BOOSTing) Care Transitions: Transitional care program providing information and tools to help optimize the discharge process.

Bioelectrical Impedance Analysis: An in expensive, quick, and noninvasive tool used in clinical practice to estimate fat mass versus lean mass.

Biofeedback: Use of feedback from a machine to control target functions in the body with the mind; eventually the machine feedback is eliminated.

Biologically based practices: Use of those substances found in nature such as botanicals, vitamins, and minerals.

Biological therapies: Targeted therapies that affect the body's immune system, and may include interferons, interleukins, monoclonal antibodies, vaccines, and gene therapy.

Black American: Comprised of individuals of mixed ethnic and cultural heritage. The slave trade resulted in a diaspora (dispersion) from West and Central Africa; this group also includes immigrants from the West Indies, South America, Central America, Haiti, and other Caribbean Islands.

Bladder diary: A daily record of the time and volume of fluid intake, voiding, and incontinence episodes with associated activities.

Bladder training: An intervention that focuses on providing patients with the tools to delay urination and suppress urgency in order to establish more normal voiding intervals.

Body Mass Index (BMI): Used to determine body fat levels, with a BMI < 18.5 kg/m^2 indicating underweight and in increased risk of mortality; a BMI of 18.5 to 24.9 kg/m indicates normal weight, 25 to 29.9 kg/m^2 overweight, and >30 kg/m^2 obesity.

Bone mineral density (BMD): Screening test for osteoporosis.

Braden Scale for Pressure Ulcer Risk Assessment: Most widely used tool to assess pressure ulcer risk; a Braden score of 16 or less indicates a high risk of pressure ulcer development in the general population, while a score of 18 or less is indicative of high risk in older adults or persons with darkly pigmented skin.

Breakthrough pain: A transient, moderate to severe pain that increases above the pain addressed by the ongoing analgesics.

Broca's aphasia: Broken speech.

Brown bag assessment: Lay term for when patients bring in all their medications in a brown paper bag and a health professional reviews/assesses them.

Cachexia: Complex metabolic processes associated with an underlying terminal illness (e.g., cancer, end-stage renal disease) and is characterized by loss of muscle mass with or without loss of fat mass.

Calcitonin: A hormone of the thyroid gland that stimulates increased uptake of calcium by bone-forming cells.

Cancer: A malignant or invasive growth or tumor.

Capacity: The ability to make decisions.

Cardiac output: The amount of blood pumped by the heart per minute.

Cardiovascular disease (CVD): Includes hypertension, coronary heart disease, congestive heart failure, and stroke.

Caregiver burden: Emotional and/or physical illness associated with the demands of caring for an ill family member.

Care Transitions Intervention (CTI): Transitional care model (Coleman); patient centered to improve quality and contain costs for older adults with complex care needs.

Cartilaginous joints: Joints composed of two bones separated by a layer of cartilage.

Cataracts: A clouding of the lens of the eye, its capsule, or both.

Catecholamines: Hormones of the adrenal medulla released in response to sympathetic nervous system activity.

Catheter-associated urinary tract infection (CAUTI): A bladder infection caused by an indwelling urinary catheter.

Causation: Generally determined by a jury and answers the question: Did the defendant's action or failure to act cause, or significantly contribute to, the loss or injury?

Causative factors: Factors that influence pressure ulcer development such as (1) intensity of pressure, (2) duration of pressure, and (3) tissue tolerance, which is the ability of skin and its supporting structures to endure pressure.

CD34⁺ cells: The primary circulating progenitor stem cells.

Cell-mediated immunity: The branch of acquired immunity responsible for destroying intracellular antigens.

Centenarian: Someone who is 100 years of age or older.

Cerebrovascular accident (CVA): Stroke; brain attack.

Certification: A type of credential earned through meeting specific requirements that validate one's expertise and knowledge in a specialty area.

Cerumen: Ear wax.

Chemical restraint: A medication used to control behavior or to restrict the patient's freedom of movement and is not a standard treatment for the patient's medical or psychological condition.

Chemoreceptors: Receptors related to the abilities to smell and taste.

Chemotherapy: A systemic (entire body) therapy that uses chemicals to destroy cancer cells.

Chemotherapy-induced cognitive impairment: Also referred to as "chemo brain;" is a controversial symptom more recently noted in the survivor with cancer, manifesting as weakening or impairment of memory and/or cognitive function associated with cancer treatment, including chemotherapy and hormonal therapy.

Chiropractic practice: Manipulation of the skeletal system by trained practitioners to put the body back in balance.

Cholinergic neurons: Neurons that release the neurotransmitter acetylcholine, which plays a significant role in learning and memory in humans and animals.

Cholinesterase: An enzyme that degrades acetylcholine.

Cholinesterase inhibitor: A medication that inhibits cholinesterase and indirectly increases acetylcholine. Used as a treatment for Alzheimer's disease.

Chronic bronchitis: A type of COPD characterized by increased mucus production and scarring of bronchial tubes that obstructs airflow.

Chronic disease: A disease that is ongoing or recurring. Some types of cancer, as well as AIDS, have recently been designated as chronic diseases.

Chronic Disease Self-Management Program: A care model developed by Dr. Kate Lorig, at Stanford University, to facilitate self-management of chronic illnesses.

Chronic obstructive pulmonary disease (COPD): A group of diseases related to obstructed airflow in the lungs.

Chronic pain (nonmalignant): Pain that lasts a month or more beyond the usual expected recovery period or illness, or goes on for years.

Chronological aging: The process of physiological change caused only by the passage of time.

Circadian rhythm: Biologically or behaviorally-based functions that change systematically over each 24-hour day period, that can be modified or entrained to cycles of light/dark and sleep/wake.

Circadian rhythm disorders: Sleep disturbance pattern resulting from circadian timing system alterations or from endogenous circadian rhythm and exogenous factor misalignment, affecting sleep timing or duration.

Clonal expansion: A process through which B and T cells of the immune system multiply to produce cellular clones.

Codes of ethics: Codes of moral reasoning used by members of a profession to direct the moral behavior of their work.

Cognition: Group of mental processes including attention, awareness, judgment, memory, perception, and the like.

Cognitive behavioral therapy (CBT): A form of psychiatric treatment that focuses on examining the relationships among thoughts, feelings, and behaviors.

Cohort: A group of people with a similar characteristic, such as age or exposure to toxic chemicals, who are studied over time.

Colon: Another term for the large intestine; extends from the small intestine to the rectum.

Combativeness: Aggressive behavior and noncompliance.

Communicating bad news: Module 2 of Education in Palliative and End-of-Life Care (EPEC). This training for medical personnel promotes honest and compassionate discussion about end-of-life care and options for treating life-ending illnesses.

Communication: The giving and receiving of information.

Communication predicament of aging model: Speech modifications (such as elderspeak) may lead to negative outcomes for older adults.

Communication enhancement model: Provides direction for effective healthcare-provider communication; directs that the younger adult healthcare providers make an individualized assessment of the communication abilities of each older adult and only modify speech as needed to support effective communication with that individual.

Compensatory strategies: Focus on providing mechanisms to assist the person with the physical or neurological impairment.

Competence: Having the capacity to function or respond; having requisite or adequate abilities or qualities to perform a task or respond to a situation. Mental competence is evaluated to determine whether a person has adequate capacity to make informed decisions.

Complement system: A collection of proteins of the immune system involved in the destruction of antigens and initiation of the inflammatory response.

Complementary and alternative medicine: Alternative approaches to healing that may include acupuncture, biofeedback, guided therapy, healing touch, herbal and dietary supplements, Reiki, yoga, and the like.

Complementary and alternative therapy: A group of diverse medical and health-care systems, practices, and products that are not generally considered part of conventional medicine (also called Western or allopathic medicine).

Complexity leadership: Leadership is viewed as an interactive system of dynamic, unpredictable agents that interact with each other in complex feedback networks, which can then produce adaptive outcomes such as knowledge dissemination, learning, innovation, and further adaptation to change.

Conductive hearing loss: Occurs when the cause of hearing loss is located in the outer and/or middle ear.

Confidentiality: Being entrusted with confidences. Maintaining confidentiality is required to protect the right of privacy.

Conflict: Occurs when a choice must be made between two equal choices.

Conflict of interest: Conflict that arises from competing loyalties and opportunities. This may include conflicts between the nurse's value system and choices made by the patients, their families, other health care team members, the organization, or the insurance company, or when incentive systems or other financial gains create conflict between professional integrity and self-interest.

Conflict resolution: Encouraging collaborative decision making to move the team beyond the conflict.

Congestive heart failure (CHF): A chronic deficiency in the heart's ability to pump blood to the body.

Constipation: Sluggish bowels that result in hard stool and delay in normal bowel movements.

Continuing care retirement community: A community for the elderly that provides a continuum of care that spans independent living to skilled nursing care in a traditional nursing home setting, all within a single campus setting.

Continuity theory: The view that one's personality (and its influence on behavior) remain somewhat stable over the course of the lifespan.

Continuous bladder irrigation (CBI): Used after a TURP to flush the bladder.

Contracting: A specific agreement between the nurse and client in which a behavior change is described and a plan for the change is committed to paper.

Copayment: The amount of money one pays to a care provider in addition to what the insurance pays.

Core competencies: The essential skills and knowledge needed to provide quality care to older adults.

Core values: Basic beliefs and attitudes of an individual that reflects that individual's thoughts, behaviors, and culture.

Corneal ulcer: Irritation of the cornea that may be caused by stroke, infection, fever, or trauma, and often results in scarring.

Coronary artery disease (CAD): Also called coronary heart disease or ischemic heart disease; results from atherosclerosis.

Coronary heart disease (CHD): Includes myocardial infarction, angina, and other conditions.

Cortical bone: The outer layer of bone; also known as compact bone.

Corticotropin-releasing hormone (CRH): Hypothalamic hormone that stimulates release of adrenocorticotropic hormone from the pituitary gland.

Cortisol: The primary glucocorticoid in the human body and a hormone regulating the stress response.

Cultural awareness: Being mindful, attentive, and conscious of similarities and differences between cultural groups.

Cultural congruence: The understanding and application of acceptable beliefs, ideas, and practices that result in an interpersonal, social, and intercultural understanding and acceptance of differences and similarities of all peoples within a worldview.

Cultural diversity: Ethnic, gender, racial, and socioeconomic variety in a situation, institution, or group; the coexistence of different ethnic, gender, racial, and socioeconomic groups within one social unit.

Cultural humility: The identification of one's own biases and the acknowledgement that those biases must be recognized. Cultural humility acknowledges that it is impossible to be adequately knowledgeable about cultures other than one's own.

Cultural sensitivity: Being aware and sensitive to differences when working with others outside of our own culture.

Culture: Integrated patterns of human behavior that include the language, thoughts, communications, actions, customs, beliefs, values, and institutions of racial, ethnic, religious, or social groups.

Culture of safety: Safe and appropriate delegation of care.

Curative care: Medical care focused on healing/cure of disease.

Curative treatment: Interventions/medications aimed at eradicating disease.

Cystectomy: Surgical removal of the bladder.

Cytokines: Chemical messengers of the immune, hematopoietic, and other physiological systems.

Damages: Loss or injury.

Daytime sleepiness: An inability to stay awake and alert during the primary episodes of daytime wakefulness.

Declarative memory: Factual information that can be declared and is divided into three types: *episodic* (events), *semantic* (concepts), and *lexical* (word) *memory*.

Deductible: The amount of money one pays to a care provider before the insurance benefits are activated.

Deglutition: Act of chewing.

Dehydroepiandrosterone (DHEA): An adrenal sex hormone able to convert to a multitude of other hormones, primarily estrogen and testosterone.

Delayed retirement credit (DRC): Additional money one can earn in addition to full Social Security benefits if one works past age 65.

Delegation: Process for a nurse to direct another person to perform nursing tasks and activities.

Delirium: Acute confusion caused by physiological illness.

Dementia: A broad term referring to the symptoms associated with a progressive decline in cognitive function to the extent that it interferes with daily life and activities.

Demineralization: A decrease in the amount of minerals or inorganic salts in tissues, as occurs in certain diseases.

Demographic tidal wave: A term that describes the baby boomers; a large group about to "crash" into the resources of the United States.

Demyelination: Any disease of the nervous system in which the myelin sheath of neurons is damaged.

Dependence: Physical response to use of opioids, characterized by withdrawal symptoms when the opioid is stopped.

Depression: A mood disorder, common in persons with dementia.

Dermis: The intermediate layer of the skin.

Detrusor: Muscle in the bladder that assists with voiding.

Diabetic retinopathy: Impaired vision due to bleeding in the retina from ruptured vessels.

Diagnostic Related Groups (DRGs): Categories of care based on the diagnosis(es) applied to the patient.

Diaphragm: A sheet of muscle located across the bottom of the chest that aids in respiration through its contraction and relaxation.

Diarrhea: Loose, watery stool.

Diastole: Relaxation of ventricles when filling with blood.

Dietary Approaches to Stop Hypertension (DASH) diet: A diet promoted by the U.S. Department of Health and Human Services that has been proven to be palatable and effective in lowering blood pressure. It is rich in potassium, magnesium, and calcium, and low in salt.

Diet history review: A component of nutritional assessment in which the patient reports nutritional intake and behaviors.

Dilemma: Occurs when it appears there are no acceptable choices. To qualify as a dilemma, there must be active engagement in the situation that forces an evaluation of and need for choices. Actions are uncertain because alternatives are equally unattractive.

Direct physical abuse: Mistreatment that involves physical harm such as punching, beating, burning, and sexual abuse; involves the use of physical force to purposefully inflict pain or harm to another.

Diverticulitis: Inflammation of the intestinal diverticuli.

Do not resuscitate (DNR): A physician's written order instructing health care providers not to attempt cardiopulmonary resuscitation (CPR) in case of cardiac or respiratory arrest.

Dopaminergic system: Releases dopamine, affecting motor control.

Dosha: Energy in the Ayurvedic medical system.

Dry eyes: A lack of usual moisture in the eyes, sometimes associated with older age.

Dual sensory impairment: When one experiences a loss in both vision and hearing.

Due care: The specifics of what is expected of caregivers in their professional role.

Duty: Expected actions and obligations.

Dysarthria: Weakness of the musculature involved in speech.

Dysethethic: Any impairment of the senses, especially of the sense of touch.

Dyspareunia: Painful intercourse.

Dysphagia: Difficulty in swallowing.

Dysphagia diet: Particular diet that is safe for those with swallowing problems.

Dysthymia: A type of neurotic depression that is a mood disorder consisting of chronic depression, with less severe but longer lasting symptoms than major depressive disorder.

Eden Alternative: In-community, changing the culture of long-term care through ongoing training and continued dedication to creating a life worth living for those living there.

Elastic recoil: A measure of the lungs' ability to expand and contract.

Elder abuse: Mistreatment or harm to older adults via force to a vulnerable elder, whether physical, psychosocial, or financial; a single, or repeated act, or lack of appropriate action, occurring within any relationship where there is an expectation of trust which causes harm or distress to an older person.

Elder mistreatment: A preferred term to elder abuse; harm to older adults.

Elderly: Usually described as those persons age 65 or over.

Elderspeak: Speech that is overly caring and controlling and less respectful than normal adult-to-adult speech.

Emergency Nurse Association (ENA): Professional specialty organization for emergency nurses.

Emergency response system (ERS): A device that evaluates self-care and/or physiologic parameters and allows a person at high risk (for example, an older person who lives alone and has a health problem) to get immediate help in the event of an emergency.

Emergency Severity Index (ESI): Red flags that indicate a change in status.

Emphysema: A type of COPD that causes irreversible lung damage and results in decreased gas exchange at the alveolar level related to loss of elasticity.

Employee retention: Process and outcome in which a worker remains or is retained at a job.

End of life: Last stages of living; in this context usually caused by a terminal illness.

Environmental and situational factors: The institutional context of communication, including the focus on care tasks, lessened opportunities for communication, and intergenerational communication issues.

Environmental controls: Electronic systems that allow individuals to control lights, heating and cooling, and just about any electrical piece of equipment, such as curtains, garage doors, and gates, from a remote location.

Environmental hazards: Potential hazards in the environment that lead to falls, such as slippery floors, inadequate lighting, loose rugs, unstable furniture, and obstructed walkways.

Epidermis: The thin, outermost layer of the skin.

Epinephrine: A catecholamine of the adrenal medulla that regulates the body's stress response; also known as adrenaline.

Episodic memory: Ability to recall events.

Erectile dysfunction (ED): Impotence; the inability to attain or maintain an erection sufficient for intercourse.

Erythrocytes: Red blood cells.

Esophageal dysphagia: Trouble swallowing that results from motility problems, neuromuscular problems, or obstruction that interferes with the movement of the food bolus through the esophagus into the stomach.

Esophagus: Extends from the pharynx to the stomach.

Established incontinence: Incontinence that persists beyond resolution of acute causes or is longstanding.

Ethical principles: Guidelines that evolve from beliefs and values that facilitate decision making and guide practice.

Ethics committee: An interdisciplinary committee that provides insight into ethical issues and makes recommendations, but lacks formal legal authority.

Ethics of care: Ethical principles applied to health care situations.

Ethnocentrism: A universal tendency to believe that one's own culture and worldview are superior to another's.

Ethnogeriatrics: Health care for elders from diverse ethnic populations.

Excess disability: More disability or loss of function than can be explained by dementia alone.

Executive function: Higher level function of the cerebral cortex supporting abstraction, planning, sequencing, and decision-making ability.

Extrinsic aging: Aging due to chronic exposure to external factors such as smoking.

Extrinsic risk factors: Factors that contribute to a fall that are outside of the patient's body, such as a wet, slippery floor; rugs; IV poles; oxygen tubing; or lighting.

Facility acquired (FA) pressure ulcers: A pressure ulcer that did not exist prior to admission, but that was acquired in a healthcare facility.

Failure to rescue: Neglecting to take action or to recognize a preventable complication.

Fall: Unintentional incident of dropping to the ground or floor, which may or may not result in injury.

Fall injury risk factors: Factors that contribute to a fall injury that are related to a patient's body or health, such as taking warfarin, which increases the risk of bleeding.

Fall risk assessment: Evaluating the individual's risk factors for falling, such as intrinsic factors; extrinsic or environmental factors (in the home setting, e.g., loose rugs); medications that put the patient at risk; and a physical exam, such as strength, balance, and mobility.

Fast-twitch fibers: Muscle fibers that provide short bursts of energy but fatigue easily; used in activities of high intensity and low endurance.

Fatigue: Sense of tiredness.

Fidelity: The state of being faithful and loyal, referring to allegiance to another.

Fiduciary responsibility: An ethical obligation to good stewardship of both the patient's and the organization's funds.

Filipino Americans: Immigrants from the Philippines.

Financial abuse: Mistreatment of an older adult through stealing or misuse of his/ her money or property.

Financial exploitation: Using an older person and his or her worldly goods or money for personal gain.

Five Wishes: An alternative advance directive that gives additional information and explanation about a person's wishes for end-of-life care; not legally recognized in all states.

Follicle-stimulating hormone: Hormone released from the pituitary that stimulates follicle production in females and sperm in males.

Forced expiratory volume (FEV): The amount of air that can be forcefully expelled in 1 second.

Foreign-born: Born outside of the United States; not a U.S. citizen at birth.

Framingham Heart Study: A 50-year, longitudinal study of over 5,000 subjects designed to identify factors that cause and prevent cardiovascular disease.

Free radicals: Molecules with an unpaired electron in the outer shell of electrons that remain unstable until paired with another molecule.

Frequency: Number of vibrations that particles make in a certain period of time.

Functional decline: Decreased ability to independently perform activities of independent living or instrumental activities of daily living, such as dressing, bathing, shopping, and bill paying.

Functional incontinence: The genitourinary tract is functioning and incontinence is due to immobility or cognitive limitations.

Gallbladder: A small sac located below the liver that stores the bile sent from the liver.

Gastroesophageal reflux disease (GERD): When gastric acid and/or stomach contents come up into the esophagus.

Gastrointestinal immunity: Antibodies in the intestine that block antigens and bacteria in addition to neutralizing toxins.

General anxiety disorder (GAD): Extreme, excessive, unrealistic worry or nervousness and tension, even if there is minimal cause to provoke the anxiety. GAD is an anxiety disorder that is characterized by excessive, uncontrollable and often irrational worry about everyday things that is disproportionate to the actual source of worry. In the case of this disorder, symptoms must last at least 6 months. This excessive worry often interferes with daily functioning, with many individuals suffering GAD typically anticipating disaster and being overly concerned about everyday matters. Individuals often exhibit a variety of physical symptoms, including fatigue, fidgeting, headaches, nausea, numbness in hands and feet, muscle tension, muscle aches, difficulty swallowing, bouts of shortness of breath, difficulty concentrating, trembling, twitching, irritability, agitation, sweating, restlessness, insomnia, hot flashes, and rashes, as well as the inability to fully control the anxiety symptoms.

Geriatric assessment interdisciplinary team (GAIT): An interdisciplinary training model developed in Maryland as an elective for students from various health care disciplines.

Geriatric assessment team (GAT): An interdisciplinary team of professionals specializing in assessment of the elderly.

Geriatric evaluation and management (GEM): Defined inpatient units or services where the elderly are assessed and treated.

Geriatric interdisciplinary team training (GITT): An organized training program for professionals of various disciplines focused on learning about working in teams and the use of teams in gerontology.

Geriatric Resource for Assessment and Care of Elders (GRACE): In-community, model of primary care for low-income seniors.

Geriatric resource nurse (GRN): In-hospital, geriatric-trained acute care nurse.

Geriatrics: Medical care of the aged.

Geriatric syndrome: A common health condition in older adults that does not fit into the category of a discrete disease.

Gerogogy: Related to the teaching of older adults.

Gerontological nursing: A specialty within nursing practice where the clients/ patients/residents are older persons.

Gerontological rehabilitation nursing: Gerontological nursing care of older persons in which rehabilitation is emphasized; care for those with rehabilitation problems such as stroke, brain injury, neurological disorders, or orthopedic surgeries.

Gerontology: The study of aging or the aging process.

Geropharmacology: A specialty in medications and pharmacy of older adults.

Gerocompetencies: A set of standards or competencies to meet in order to provide quality care to older adults.

Glasgow Coma Score: Tool used to classify low-level brain injury/coma in three areas: best motor, best verbal, and best eye response.

Glaucoma: A group of degenerative eye diseases whereby vision is damaged by high intraocular pressure.

Global aphasia: Both receptive and expressive aphasia.

Glomerular filtration rate (GFR): Kidney filtration system for waste and toxins.

Glomeruli: Bundles of capillaries located in the kidneys.

Glucagon: A pancreatic hormone regulating blood glucose levels through stimulation of the release of stored glucose.

Glucocorticoids: Hormones of the adrenal cortex involved in both metabolic and anti-inflammatory functions.

Glucose tolerance: The ability to respond effectively to dramatic rises in blood glucose levels.

GLUT4: An insulin-mediated glucose transporter protein located within cytoplasmic vesicles.

Gonadotropin-releasing hormone (GnRH): Released by the hypothalamus and stimulates the synthesis and release of follicle-stimulating hormone (FSH) and luteinizing hormone (LH).

Gonioscopy: Tool to directly examine the eye.

Good death: Death free from avoidable distress and suffering, according to patient/ family wishes, consistent with clinical, cultural, and ethical standards.

Graying of America: Similar to the aging of America, referring to the increase in numbers of older Americans.

Green House: In-community, long-term skilled care model, providing care in small homes through self-managed team of cross-trained direct care workers.

Grief: A natural and normal reaction to a loss of any kind.

Growth hormone (GH): A pituitary hormone that stimulates amino acid uptake and synthesis of proteins.

Guided Care: In-community, model of comprehensive primary care provided by physician/nurse teams for older adult patients with complex chronic conditions.

Guided imagery: Use of imagery to elicit responses in the body.

Hallucinations: False sensory beliefs, such as seeing, hearing, feeling, tasting, or smelling things that others do not.

Hawaiian and other Pacific Islands ("the Pacific Rim" or "Oceania"): From Hawaii and/or Pacific Islands, including Samoa, Tonga, Micronesia, Fiji, Guam, Palau, and Marina and Marshall Islands.

Healthcare environment: The system in which care is provided, made up of multiple, intricate relationships between stakeholders. These relationships are built on needs and ability to meet those needs. The primary relationship is between providers and consumers.

Health disparities: A particular type of health difference that is closely linked with social, economic, and/or environmental disadvantage.

Health literacy: The degree to which individuals have the capacity to obtain, process, and understand basic health information and services needed to make appropriate health decisions.

Health policy: Decisive action chosen to respond to an issue in health care. This action includes the actual response to the healthcare issue and the plan to implement the response.

Health promotion: Activities aimed at improving or enhancing health.

Health screening: Population-wide efforts to detect early disease.

Health–illness continuum: The degree of client wellness that exists at any point in time, ranging from an optimal wellness condition (with available energy at the maximum) to death (which demonstrates total energy depletion).

Healthy People 2020: Launched in December 2010 to create an ambitious, yet achievable, 10-year agenda for health promotion and disease prevention activities aimed at improving the health of the United States.

Hearing aid: A device that amplifies sound.

Helicobacter pylori: A common bacterial contributor to symptoms of gastritis and peptic ulcers.

Hematopoiesis: The process of blood cell production.

Hemiparesis: Weakness of one side of the body.

Hemiplegia: Paralysis of one side of the body.

Herpes zoster: The virus that causes chicken pox and shingles.

High performance work team: A group of high-performing individuals who have brilliance and drive, with the ability to propose solutions to problems.

Hispanic/Latino: Includes the diversity of the subgroups of Mexican American, Cuban American, and Puerto Rican populations within a broader context. The U.S. Bureau of the Census uses the term "Hispanic" as an ethnicity category referring to persons who trace their origin or descent to Mexico, Puerto Rico, Cuba, Central or South America, or Spain, regardless of race. Hispanics/Latinos can trace their ancestry back to the indigenous people of North America as well as to Spanish/European, Asian, and African roots.

Histamine 2 (H2) blockers: Medications used for the treatment of GERD.

Holistic: Viewing, assessing, and treating the whole person; identifying equal value for the individual's status of mind, body, and spirit as a complex, dynamic entity.

Home care: Services provided in the home of a home-bound person; may include skilled nursing, therapy, and home health aides.

Home health care: Care provided in the home for those who are homebound due to severity of illness or immobility.

Homeopathy: Medical system that follows the natural law of "like cures like."

Homeostasis: The ability to maintain balance in the organ systems.

Homeostatic sleep drive/pressure: A building drive or pressure for sleep based on prolonged wakefulness.

Hope: To expect with confidence.

Hormones: Chemical messengers of the endocrine system.

Hospice care: A program to deliver palliative care to individuals in the final stages of a terminal illness; additionally provides personal support and care to the patient, and supports to the patient's family/caregivers while the patient is dying; provides bereavement support after the patient's death.

Humoral immunity: The branch of acquired immunity mediated by antibodies and responsible for defending the body against extracellular antigens.

Hwalek–Sengstock Elder Abuse Screening Test: A tool to use for screening for elder abuse or mistreatment.

Hyperactive form: Most recognized form of delirium that often presents with psychomotor agitation and a plethora of psychiatric symptoms, such as confusion, hallucinations, or delusions.

Hypersomnias: A group of sleep disorders with the main complaint of daytime sleepiness unrelated to other causes of sleep disturbance such as circadian rhythm or sleep-related breathing disorders, including narcolepsy; recurrent and idiopathic hypersomnias; hypersomnias due to medical conditions, drugs, or substances; and behaviorally-induced insufficient sleep syndrome.

Hypertension (HTN): Currently defined as a consistently elevated reading of 140/90 mmHg.

Hypoactive form: Delirium characterized by a flat affect or apathy; may mimic stupor or coma; often present in otherwise calm and seemingly alert patients.

Hypogeusia: Age-related decline in taste.

Hypophysiotropic: Acting on the pituitary gland.

Hypopnea: A reduced airflow of 10 seconds or longer in duration.

Hypothalamic-pituitary-adrenal (HPA) axis: Regulates glucocorticoid levels in the body and allows the body to respond to stressful conditions.

Iatrogenic harm/ iatrogenesis: Doctor- or healthcare-created harm.

Immigrant: An individual who moves into a country or region to settle there.

Immovable joints: Joints composed of collagen fibers that allow only minimal bone shifting; also known as fibrous joints.

Immunocompromise: A change or alteration of the immune system that normally serves to fight off infections and other illnesses.

Immunomodulation: The effects of various chemical mediators, hormones, and drugs on the immune system.

Immunosenescence: Aging of the immune system.

Incompetence: Lacking competence; this is a judgment of the court and limits the person's legal rights.

Incontinence: Involuntary loss of stool or urine.

Independent living: Older adults caring for themselves, but can occur in a wide variety of settings from the home to senior living apartments or CCRCs.

Indian Health Service: An agency of the Department of Health and Human Services that provides health services to American Indians and Alaskan Natives. It now serves over 1.9 million American Indians and Alaskan Natives in 35 states.

Infection: Invasion of pathogens in a bodily part or tissue.

Inflammatory response: Redness, swelling, and warmth produced in response to infection.

Informed consent: A legally binding and voluntary decision regarding a proposed treatment based on information regarding the risks, benefits, and alternatives to a procedure or treatment.

Inhibin B: Glycoprotein that suppresses FSH.

Injury Severity Score: Descriptors of anatomic injury to describe injury severity; help predict outcomes after injury.

Innate immunity: The branch of the immune system with which a person is born and that is the body's first line of defense against invading antigens.

Insomnia: Repeated difficulty with sleep initiation, duration, consolidation, or quality despite adequate time & opportunity for sleep; it is associated with some form of daytime impairment.

Institute of Medicine (IOM): An independent, nonprofit organization that works outside of government to provide unbiased and authoritative advice to decision makers and the public. The IOM asks and answers the nation's most pressing questions about health and health care.

Instrumental activities of daily living (IADLs): Activities related to independent living; they include meal preparation, money management, shopping, housework, and using a telephone.

Insulin: A pancreatic hormone regulating blood glucose levels through stimulation of glucose uptake.

Insulin resistance: A resistance to the actions of insulin.

Interdisciplinary collaboration: When a team of professionals from different disciplines collaborates around common goals.

Interdisciplinary group/team (IDG/IDT): Professional staff and volunteers who focus on physical, emotional, psychological, social, and spiritual aspects of a person in designing and/or implementing holistic care; common in hospice and palliative care and other care settings.

Interdisciplinary team: A team in which members of various disciplines interact, collaborate, and work together for common goals.

Intergenerational care: In the community, multiple generations receive ongoing services and/or programming at the same site, and interact through planned activities.

Internet: A vast collection of resources that includes people, information, and multimedia and is best characterized as the biggest labyrinth of computer networks on earth.

Interpretation: The oral conversion of verbal statement(s) said in one language to another language without adding, omitting, or distorting meaning.

Intractable pain: Chronic and persistent pain that can be psychogenic in nature and not relieved by ordinary medical, surgical, and nursing measures.

Intradisciplinary team: A team in which members are within a discipline but members may be at different levels of preparation; may also refer to members of various disciplines working with similar patients, but not necessarily with common goals.

Intraocular pressure (IOP): The amount of pressure inside the eye; normal is 9–21 mmHg.

Intrinsic risk factors: Factors that contribute to a fall that are related to a patient's physiology or current medical problems; anything the patient carries within his/her body.

Islets of Langerhans: Glandular cells of the pancreas.

Isolation: State of being alone or separated.

Justice: Conformity to principles of what is right and fair; establishment of rights following rules of equity.

Keratinocytes: Cells of the epidermis that produce the protein keratin.

Ketones: Acetone bodies in the urine indicating inadequate management of diabetes mellitus.

Killer T cells: T cells that directly attack and destroy infected cells within the body; also termed cytotoxic T cells.

Korean War: June 27, 1950, through Jan. 31, 1955.

Kotter's Change Model: A model that helps leaders generate positive feelings among employees toward change. It allows leaders to instill feelings of action in employees' hearts, by helping them to envision the problem and identify solutions to the problem.

Lack of opportunities: Fewer opportunities to communicate with peers and loved ones that often comes with advancing age.

Langerhans cells: Cells of the epidermis involved in immune response.

Language: The symbol system used by a shared group of people for communication.

Late-onset depression: Depression occurring for the first time in later life (after the age of 60); differs from early-onset (recurrent) depression, which is depression that occurs after the age of 60, but the individual has had a previous bout of depression at an earlier age.

Leaders: Visionaries who create the systems that managers manage and changes them in fundamental ways to take advantage of opportunities and to avoid hazards.

Legal nurse consultant: A nurse expert who provides analysis and informed opinion on legal matters related to health care.

Leptin: Clinical predictor of nutritional status in the elderly.

Leukocytes: White blood cells.

Lexical memory: Ability to store words.

Liability: Any legally enforceable obligation.

Life expectancy: How long one can expect to live based on statistical probability; usually calculated at birth and at age 65.

Lifelong learning: Learning that occurs throughout life, motivated by situational and developmental periods.

Limited English Proficiency (LEP): Individuals who do not speak English as their primary language and who have a limited ability to read, speak, write, or understand English.

Lipofuscin: An undegradable material that decreases lysosomal function; age pigment. A brown pigment found in aging cells relating to oxidative mechanisms.

Literacy: Ability to read/understand.

Liver: The largest gland in the body; secretes bile in the small intestine and screens blood from the stomach and intestines for toxins.

Living will: A document that provides information about the types of treatment the person would or would not wish to have if they were unable to speak for themselves.

Longevity: A long life.

Long-term acute care hospitals: Hospitals that furnish extended medical and rehabilitative care to individuals with clinically complex problems, such as multiple acute or chronic conditions, that need hospital-level care for relatively extended periods.

Long-term care: A variety of services to help persons with personal or health care needs over a period of time; usually custodial care in a nursing home type facility.

Long-term care facility: Also known as a nursing home; a facility in which care is provided primarily for older adults or any persons who have lost some or all of their ability for self-care due to illness, disability, or advanced dementia.

Long-term memory: Memory that is much more expansive than short-term memory; there is no limit as to how long information can be stored there.

Luteinizing hormone (LH): A hormone released from the pituitary that stimulates ovulation and corpus luteum growth in females; stimulates testosterone production in males.

Macrophage: An immune cell that acts as a scavenger, engulfing foreign substances, dead cells, and other debris through phagocytosis.

Macular degeneration: Loss of central vision, associated with aging; see also ARMD.

Major depression: A mood disorder characterized by an all-encompassing low mood accompanied by low self-esteem, and by loss of interest or pleasure in normally enjoyable activities and hobbies.

Malnutrition: The state of being poorly nourished.

Malpractice: Failure to meet the standard of care that results in harm to the patient.

Massage therapy: Manipulation of soft tissues in the body by kneading or other techniques.

Mauk model for poststroke recovery: A theoretical model derived using grounded theory methods that suggests a common process for stroke recovery and rehabilitation.

Mechanoreceptors: Receptors related to the ability to touch.

Medicaid: A government program first developed to provide care to the indigent elderly population and was expanded to include women and children living below the poverty level, as well as individuals with disabilities. Benefits are all-inclusive, requiring the recipients to seek out providers who take patients receiving Medicaid. Medicaid is funded through state and federal governments.

Medical anthropology: A subfield of anthropology that draws upon social, cultural, biological, and linguistic anthropology to better understand those factors that influence health and well-being (broadly defined), the experience and distribution of illness, the prevention and treatment of sickness, healing processes, the social relations of therapy management, and the cultural importance and utilization of pluralistic medical systems.

Medical interpreter: A trained staff member who is determined to have native knowledge of the target language and has undergone (typically) 45 hours of medical interpreter training to effectively provide verbal interpretation services in the healthcare field.

Medicare: A government program that pays for healthcare services for individuals over the age of 65, as well as for specific diagnoses to individuals who qualify. Benefits include acute care, outpatient services approved by the primary care physician, and hospice. Medicare also provides their recipients with a drug program that includes an additional expense for recipients to be covered.

Medication administration record (MAR): A strategy used to assess medication compliance; the patient (or family) lists the medications taken daily and tracks days 1–31 regarding what was taken at what time of day, including missed doses.

Medication-related problem (MRP): Drug-related problem that often results in negative outcomes and increased cost.

Meditation: A conscious process used to produce the relaxation response.

Melanin: A pigment produced by melanocytes and essential to protecting the body against ultraviolet radiation.

Melanocytes: Cells located within the epidermis that produce melanin.

Melatonin: A hormone produced by the pineal gland that is linked to sleep and wake cycles.

Memory care: Units designed for seniors with Alzheimer's or other forms of dementia.

Meniere's syndrome: A common cause of vertigo in the elderly characterized by dizziness and tinnitus.

Menopause: Cessation of menstrual cycles within the aging female.

Metastasis: Spreading of cancer to other organs beyond the primary site.

Mid-Upper Arm Circumference: A predictor of mortality in older adults living in long-term care facilities; the mid-point of the upper arm is measured with a tape measure placed snugly against the skin.

Mind–body medicine: Use of the powers of the mind to alter physical states in the body.

Mineralocorticoids: Hormones of the adrenal cortex involved in the regulation of extracellular mineral concentrations.

Minimum Data Set (MDS): Part of the U.S. federally mandated process for clinical assessment of all residents in Medicare or Medicaid-certified nursing homes.

Minor depression: A mood disorder that does not meet full criteria for major depressive disorder but in which at least two depressive symptoms are present for 2 weeks.

Minority: Subgroup within a population. In social science, it is used to identify a group that suffers subordination and discrimination within a society, usually because of their race, ethnicity, or national origin. The term is used by the federal government to describe protected and/or disadvantaged ethnic or racial populations.

Mitochondria: Parts of a cell that transform organic compounds into energy.

Mixed form: Delirium that presents with both hyperactive and hypoactive features.

Mixed hearing loss: Both conductive and sensorineural hearing loss are present.

Mixed urinary incontinence: The existence of urge and stress urinary incontinence symptoms at the same time.

Money Follows the Person (MFP): Transitional and community care, federal program which transitions eligible Medicaid recipients from nursing homes back to the community with community resources and services.

Monoaminergic system: Release of the neurotransmitters norepinephrine and serotonin.

Moral dilemma: Arises when two or more moral principles apply that support mutually inconsistent actions.

Moral distress: Occurs when someone wants to do the right thing but is limited by the constraints of the organization or society.

Moral principles: Those values, ethics, beliefs, and positions that guide behavior and thought.

Moral sensitivity: Responsiveness to moral principles and/or morality.

Moral uncertainty: The confusion surrounding situations in which a person is uncertain what the moral problem is or which moral principles or values apply to it.

Morbidity: Related to incidence of illness.

Mortality: Death.

Motor unit: The combination of a single nerve and all the muscle fibers it innervates.

Mourning: The outward demonstration of a person's grief responses to a loss.

Mucositis: Inflammation of the mucosa.

Multidisciplinary team: A team made up of members of various disciplines.

Muscle quality: Strength generated per unit of muscle mass.

Muscle strength: The capacity of muscle to generate force.

Music therapy: Use of music to enhance physical and psychological well-being.

Myelosuppression: The decrease in the production of blood cells.

Myocardial cells: Cells located in the heart; also known as cardiomyocytes.

Myocardial infarction (MI): Heart attack.

Myofascial: Muscle pain.

Myofibril: A contractile filament that comprises skeletal muscle fibers; composed of actin and myosin proteins.

Myosin: Protein within muscle that, together with actin, is responsible for muscle contraction.

Myth: Beliefs that evidence-informed research notes as false.

Nasogastric tube: A commonly used method of short-term enteral feeding in which a tube is passed through the nares into the stomach as a means to provide nutrition.

National Pressure Ulcer Advisory Panel (NPUAP): An expert group convened to develop a common classification systems for pressure ulcers.

National Transitions of Care Coalition (NTOCC): Transitional care tools and resources for providers, consumers, and caregivers.

Native-born: A citizen at birth.

Naturally occurring retirement community: Living communities specifically for older adults. Most are duplexes, condominiums, apartments, trailers, or single-family homes that are all located in the same neighborhood.

Natural killer (NK) cells: Cells of the immune system that attack and destroy infected cells.

Naturopathic medicine: A variety of healing practices that support the body to heal itself.

Nausea and vomiting: Symptoms of gastric upset and expelling gastric contents.

Nephrons: Located in the kidneys; combination of the Bowman's capsule and renal tubule with the glomerulus.

Nerve cells: Neurons within the nervous system that transmit chemical and electrical signals.

Neurofibrillary tangles: Collections of twisted tau found in the cell bodies of neurons; a symptom of Alzheimer's disease.

Neurogenesis: Formation of new neurons.

Neuropathic: A pathological change in the central or peripheral nervous system.

Neurotransmitters: Substances that carry nerve impulses across nerve synapses, such as norepinephrine.

Next Step in Care: Transitional care; eight easy-to-use guides to help family caregivers and providers plan and implement transitions.

Nociceptive: The process of detection and signaling the presence of a noxious stimulus.

Nocturia: The awakening from sleep to urinate more than once during the night.

Nondeclarative memory: Includes motor skills, cognitive skills, reflex responses, priming, and condition responses.

Nonmaleficence: Not committing harm or evil.

Nonrapid eye movement sleep (NREM): Refers to stages N1 through N3 of sleep.

Nonrestraint fall prevention interventions: Behavioral interventions in persons with agitation, having family or a sitter stay at bedside of high-risk fallers or those with cognitive impairment, or moving a patient closer to the nurse's station.

Nonstochastic theories of aging: Theories stating that a series of genetically programmed events occur to all organisms with aging.

Non-Hispanic White: Those who are of the White race and are not of Hispanic or Latino origin/ethnicity.

Nonverbal communication: Includes tone of voice and physical behaviors such as body language and eye contact.

Norepinephrine: A catecholamine of the adrenal medulla that regulates the stress response; also known as noradrenaline.

Nurse delegation: The National Council of State Board of Nurses addresses the circumstances under which a licensed nurse delegates a nursing function to an unlicensed person to carry out specific activities.

Nurse manager: Nurse who acts as administrative manager of a unit.

Nurse Manager Leadership Partnership Learning Domain Framework (NMLP): Describes essential functions of nurse managers and outlines opportunities that may be useful to achieve mastery of these functions. The framework includes three domains: (1) the leader within: creating the leader in yourself; (2) the art of leadership: leading people; and (3) the science of leadership: managing the business.

Nurses Improving Care for the Hospitalized Elderly (NICHE): In the hospital, tools and processes to educate nursing staff in specialized care of the hospitalized older adults.

Nursing home: A facility that provides daily help for residents with physical or other problems who are unable to live on their own.

Nursing informatics: A blending of computer, information, and nursing science designed to assist in the management and processing of nursing data, information, and knowledge to support the practice of nursing and the delivery of nursing care.

Nutrition Screening Initiative: A multidisciplinary effort led by the American Academy of Family Physicians and the American Dietetic Association to promote the integration of nutrition screening and dietary interventions into health care for the elderly.

Obsessive-compulsive disorder (OCD): Constant thoughts or fears that cause the individual to perform certain rituals repeatedly or follow certain routines. The disturbing thoughts are obsessive, and the routines or rituals are called compulsions. An example is a person with an unreasonable fear of germs who will not touch another person, washes his/her hands repeatedly, or who only uses plastic utensils (never using a utensil that another person has touched to eat).

Obstructive sleep apnea: A breathing disorder in which breathing repeatedly stops and starts during sleep.

Older adult: Person over the age of 65 years.

Oldest old: Someone 85 years of age or older.

Olfaction: The ability to smell.

Oncologic emergencies: An urgent, immediate event that results in medical care.

Oropharyngeal dysphagia: Trouble swallowing usually related to neuromuscular impairments affecting the tongue, pharynx, and upper esophageal sphincter.

Osteoarthritis: Deterioration of joints and vertebrae as a consequence of wear and tear.

Osteoblast: Bone cell responsible for formation of new bone and repair of damaged or broken bone.

Osteoclast: Bone cell responsible for bone resorption.

Osteocyte: Dormant osteoblast embedded in bone matrix.

Osteoporosis: Demineralization of the bones; decreased bone density.

Otoconia: "Stones" in the ear canal that affect balance.

Otosclerosis: Damage to the inner ear of unknown cause that leads to progressive deafness.

Overflow incontinence: Incontinence that occurs because the bladder has not been emptied and it has become overdistended.

Pacific Islanders: Person from consists of three distinct island groups in the Pacific Ocean: Micronesia, Melanesia, and Polynesia.

Pain: An unpleasant sensory and emotional experience associated with actual or potential tissue damage or described in terms of such damage.

Pain scales: Measurement options by which medical personnel can translate a person's self-assessment of pain for appropriate intervention decisions.

Palliative and hospice care team: A team whose focus is comfort and/or end of life care.

Palliative care: Concept of care designed to promote comfort and holistic management of symptoms at any stage of illness or disease.

Pancreas: A gland located below the stomach and above the small intestine; secretes pancreatic fluid that neutralizes stomach acid and breaks down large nutrients.

Panic attack: Feelings of terror that strike suddenly and repeatedly with no warning. Symptoms can include extreme nervousness, increased heart rate, increased blood pressure, sweating, chest pain, palpitations (irregular heartbeats), and a feeling of smothering or choking, which may make the person feel like he or she is having a heart attack or "going crazy."

Paranoia: False beliefs that others are conspiring against oneself; unfounded mistrust of others.

Parasomnias: Undesirable physical events or experiences that occur during entry into sleep, within sleep, or during arousals from sleep.

Parathyroid gland: A group of cells located at the back of the thyroid gland that secretes parathyroid hormone.

Parathyroid hormone (PTH): A hormone of the parathyroid gland involved in promoting elevation of blood calcium levels.

Parkinson's disease (PD): A neurological disorder characterized by lack of dopamine in the brain secondary to loss of neurons in the basal ganglia.

Pathophysiology: The study of the changes of normal mechanical, physiological, and biochemical functions, either caused by a disease or resulting from an abnormal syndrome.

Patient-centered communication: Consistent and clear communication between patient and clinician in which the patient is the center.

Patient Protection and Affordable Care Act of 2010 (PPACA): Also known as Obamacare, a comprehensive health reform law signed into law in 2010 in response to the need for healthcare reform. The intention of the Affordable Care Act was to provide affordable health care to enhance quality of life for all Americans.

Patient rights: Rights to which patients are entitled; usually defined or described by the organization charged with providing care or protecting patients.

Pelvic floor muscle exercises: Muscle exercises, often called Kegel exercises, that strengthen the pelvic floor, often use for the treatment of urinary incontinence.

Pelvic muscle rehabilitation: An exercise program designed to increase the strength, tone, and control of the pelvic floor muscles to facilitate a person's ability to voluntarily control the flow of urine and suppress urgency.

Percutaneous endoscopic gastrostomy: Invasive insertion of a feeding tube through the anterior abdominal wall in order to provide a vehicle for nutrition.

Periodic limb movements of sleep (PLMS): Repetitive, highly stereotyped, limb movements that occur during sleep.

Peripheral artery disease (PAD): A problem with blood flow in the arteries due to blockage or narrowing.

Peripheral neuropathy: A disorder of peripheral nerves in which symptoms (most often in the lower extremities) are often described as numbing, tingling, burning, and painful.

Peripheral vascular disease (PVD): The most common form of peripheral artery disease.

Personal amplification device: Devices that aid in hearing; can be developed to account for individual hearing loss.

Person-first language: Person-centered communication (such as "the person with diabetes" versus "the diabetic").

Personhood: The status of being a person; being human.

Pet-assisted therapy: Use of animals to decrease stress and increase feelings of well-being.

Phantom limb pain: Pain in an absent/amputated extremity.

Pharmacodynamics: How drugs work in the body, and a person's ability to manage medications.

Pharmacogenomics: A genetic, set-at-birth capacity to metabolize medications through numerous different pathways, each one working at a different rate in different people.

Pharmacokinetics: How drugs are absorbed, metabolized, and eliminated.

Pharynx: Connects the oral cavity to the esophagus.

Phobia: An intense fear of a specific object or situation, such as falling, spiders, heights, or flying. The behaviors associated with the level of fear are usually inappropriate to the situation and may cause the person to become avoid common, everyday situations or become isolated.

Photoaging: The process of change in skin structure and function resulting only from exposure to ultraviolet radiation.

Physical dependence: A state of adaptation that is manifested by a drug-class-specific withdrawal syndrome that can be produced by abrupt cessation, rapid dose reduction, decreasing blood level of the drug, and/or administration of an antagonist.

Physical restraint: Any manual method, physical or mechanical device, material, or equipment that immobilizes or reduces the ability of a patient to move his or her arms, legs, body, or head freely.

Physician's Orders for Life-Sustaining Treatment (POLST): A document that states what type of care a person wants at the end of life.

Pig in a python: Another descriptor of the baby boomers, as if they were a large lump inside a snake that is slowly moving along toward the tail; in other words, a bulge in population moving slowly through time.

Pineal gland: A small gland located deep in the brain that secretes melatonin.

Pioneer Network: A nonprofit organization formed in 1997 to advocate for person-directed care in long-term care.

Plaques: Made up of the amyloid b-peptide shown to be neurotoxic; occur outside of the neuronal cell and consist of gray matter with a protein core surrounded by abnormal neurites.

Plasma cell: An antibody-producing B cell.

Plasticity: The ability to form new neuronal connections onto available existing neurons.

Pluripotent stem cells: Cells possessing the ability to differentiate into cells of any other type.

Polydipsia: Excessive thirst.

Polyphagia: Excessive eating.

Polypharmacy: Concurrent use of multiple medications.

Polysomnography (PSG): The monitoring of sleep in detail (as in an overnight sleep study).

Polyuria: Excessive urination.

Posttraumatic stress disorder (PTSD): A severe anxiety disorder that develops after exposure to any significant traumatic event.

Power of attorney: Someone designated to make treatment decisions when a person is unable to express his or her wishes.

Prayer: A conversation with a higher being.

Prealbumin: A hepatic protein that may indicate a more recent change in nutritional status.

Precipitating factors: Those events or conditions that occur during hospitalization to trigger a delirium.

Predisposing factors: Those baseline vulnerabilities that are possessed by the patient prior to hospitalization.

Presbycusis: Age-related hearing loss that generally occurs at higher frequencies first.

Presbyopia: Age-related vision loss of objects at close range; known as farsightedness.

Prescribing cascade: When medication side effects are treated with other medications.

Pressure redistribution: The ability of a support surface to distribute load over the contact areas of the human body to reduce the overall pressure and avoid areas of focal pressure.

Pressure ulcer: "A pressure ulcer is localized injury to the skin and/or underlying tissue usually over a bony prominence, as a result of pressure, or pressure in combination with shear. A number of contributing or confounding factors are also associated with pressure ulcers; the significance of these factors is yet to be elucidated" (National Pressure Ulcer Advisory Panel [NPUAP] & European Pressure Ulcer Advisory Panel [EPUAP], 2009, p. 7).

Pressure ulcer management: Includes nursing assessment, accurate staging (classification) of the pressure ulcer, and documentation of the onset and assessed stage.

Pressure ulcer risk assessment: Evaluating for risk factors for pressure ulcer development including advanced age; immobility; malnutrition; incontinence; diminished level of consciousness; impaired sensation; history of pressure ulcers; multiple comorbidities such as diabetes, chronic obstructive pulmonary disease, renal disease, and arterial/vascular disease; medication history; and previous treatment with steroids, radiation, or chemotherapy.

Pressure ulcer staging system: Developed by the NPUAP to provide a common classification for wounds/pressure ulcers.

Primary prevention: Activities designed to completely prevent a disease from occurring, such as immunization against pneumonia or influenza.

Program of All-Inclusive Care for the Elderly (PACE): In-community, Medicare/Medicaid program that utilizes an interprofessional team that assesses, plans, implements, and monitors interventions for the older adult.

Proliferative retinopathy: The fourth and most advanced stage of diabetic retinopathy in which abnormal and fragile vessels develop to compensate for blocked blood flow to the retina; this leads to visual disturbances and often blindness.

Prompted voiding (PV): A scheduled intervention aimed at helping the individual recognize and act effectively on the sensation of the need to void.

Prostate-specific antigen (PSA): A serum screening test for prostate cancer.

Psychological or emotional abuse: The infliction of anguish, pain, or distress through verbal or nonverbal acts.

Psychological or emotional neglect: Not providing for physical or emotional needs of an elder; may be present when a person receives good or adequate physical care, but is socially isolated.

Public policy: Programs and policies developed by the government in response to the needs of the members of the society that have been identified by the government or another entity.

Putative energy field: Vital energy that cannot be measured.

Qi: The circulating life energy that in Chinese philosophy is thought to be inherent in all things.

Quality of life: An individual's perception about the value and benefits of life.

Radiation therapy: Cancer treatment that uses special equipment to provide a precise dose of radiation to the tumor.

Radical prostatectomy: Surgical removal of the prostate as a treatment for cancer.

Radicular: Pertaining to a nerve root.

Rapid eye movement sleep (REM): Refers to Stage R of sleep, which is characterized by rapid eye movements and muscle atonia.

Reactive oxygen species (ROS): Short-lived, highly reactive products of mitochondrial oxidative metabolism that destroy proteins, lipids, and nucleic acids.

Reciprocity: Referring to a mutual exchange of privileges, such as the ability to be true to one's self while respecting and supporting the values and views of another.

Reiki: Holistic Japanese technique of stress reduction in which life force energy is transferred to the client through the practitioner's hands.

Religiosity: Refers to believing in a god, organized rituals, and specific dogma, related to a superior being.

REM behavior disorder (RSBD): A parasomnia characterized by abnormal behaviors emerging during REM sleep that cause injury or sleep disruption.

Replicative senescence: A phenomenon in which cells are able to undergo only a finite number of divisions.

Reproductive axis: Integration of the hypothalamus, pituitary, and gonad to control reproductive hormones.

Resource utilization groups (RUGs): Categories to determine reimbursement. The RUG scores are based on data collected from resident assessments (MDS 3.0), staffing data, and geographic location.

Respite care: Services that provide a break for caregivers by providing care in the home or a facility.

Respondeat superior: Transfers the liability to the employer, who then becomes the principal from whom the accuser hopes to recover a perceived loss.

Restless legs syndrome (RLS): A sensorimotor disorder characterized by a complaint of a strong, nearly irresistible, urge to move the legs.

Restorative strategies: Interventions that address rebuilding skills that are impaired.

Retinal detachment: Situation in which the retina becomes displaced due to trauma or illness and requires immediate medical attention to restore vision.

Revised Trauma Score: A tool to help identify physiological response to injury.

Risk management: An essential process that enables the facility to identify sources of loss, financial risk, and potential for liability.

Sadness: Mood associated with, or characterized by, feelings of loss, despair, helplessness, sorrow, fear, and rage.

Sanctity of life: The belief that all life is of value and that this value is not based on how functional or effective a person's life is, but rather that all have a right to life.

Sarcomere: Muscle compartments containing actin and myosin.

Sarcopenia: Age-related loss of muscle mass.

Sarcoplasmic reticulum: A portion of the endoplasmic reticulum; membrane network in the cell cytoplasm in striated muscle fibers.

Scatter laser treatment: Treatment for diabetic retinopathy in which a laser burns abnormal vessels away from the retina to reduce further vision loss.

Secondary prevention: Efforts directed toward early detection and management of disease, such as the use of colonoscopy to detect small, cancerous polyps.

Self-neglect: A behavior in which a person neglects to attend to their basic needs, such as personal hygiene (bathing and grooming), appropriate clothing, eating, or neglecting to care for their medical conditions.

Selective serotonin reuptake inhibitors (SSRIs): A psychiatric medication used to alleviate mood disorders in the class of antidepressants. SSRIs are called selective because they primarily affect serotonin, not the other neurotransmitters.

Selective serotonin-norepinephrine reuptake inhibitors (SNRIs): A psychiatric medication used to alleviate mood disorders in the class of antidepressants. SNRIs block the re-absorption (reuptake) of the neurotransmitters serotonin and norepinephrine in the brain.

Semantic memory: Concept memory.

Senescence: The process of growing old.

Seniors: Those age 65 years and older.

Sensorineural hearing loss: Damage that occurs in the inner ear and/or auditory nerve fiber.

Servant leadership: Focus is on the leader meeting the needs of the followers before the needs of the leader or the organization are met.

Sexual intimacy: Closeness experienced through acts related to sex.

Sexuality: The total experience of being a sexual being; more than sexual intercourse.

Short-term memory: Memory that is limited in capacity and information remains for only a few seconds.

Silver tsunami: Term referring to the large wave of older adults reaching older age as baby boomers retire.

Skeletal muscle: Muscle under voluntary control; comprises the majority of all muscle mass and is also known as voluntary or striated muscle.

Sleep architecture: Refers to the different stages of sleep and their relative amounts within the sleep cycle, and timing of the sleep cycle.

Sleep cycle: The combination of NREM and REM stages of sleep, usually a period of 90–110 minutes duration, occurring 3 to 5 times per night.

Sleep efficiency: The time spent asleep during the time spent in bed attempting to sleep; calculated as total sleep time $\times$ 100/time in bed and expressed as a percentage.

Sleep fragmentation: Systematic disturbance of the cumulative sleep process by brief periodic arousals, resulting in reduced restoration similar to that found following sleep deprivation.

Sleep quality: Variously defined, but often refers to the subjective perception of feeling rested or restored upon waking.

Sleep-related breathing disorders (SRBD): Syndromes characterized by disordered respiration during sleep, including central and obstructive sleep apnea syndromes, as well as sleep-related hypoventilation syndromes.

Sleep/wake disorders: Alterations of the sleep-wake cycle often resulting in lack of quality sleep.

Slow-twitch fibers: Muscle fibers that contract steadily but are not easily fatigued; used in activities of low intensity and high endurance.

Smart homes: Assistive domotics, which are an application of home automation that focuses on enabling older adults or disabled persons to live at their home instead of a healthcare facility.

Social cognitive theory (SCT): States that behavior, cognitive factors, and the environment influence outcome expectations; outcome expectations are a person's beliefs that when he or she engages in a certain behavior, certain outcomes will result.

Social determinants of health: The conditions in which people are born, grow, live, work, and age, including the health system.

Social networks: Social engagements that provide support and socialization.

Social policy: Programs and policies that impact members of a society through how goods and services are distributed among members of that society. The intent of social policy is to improve each individual's access to food, shelter, education, and health care.

Social Security: A federal program that provides financial assistance to the elderly and disabled; federal "old age" pension program.

Somatic: Pertaining to the body wall, in contrast to the viscera.

Sound energy therapy: Use of sound frequencies to facilitate healing.

Speech: Production of sounds used for communication.

Spiritual assessment: An integral part of comprehensive assessment, this is a dynamic record of the client's core values and beliefs based on his personal philosophy and meanings.

Spiritual baseline assessment: The initial documentation about the client's values and beliefs based on his personal philosophy, understanding, and meaning of life.

Spiritual resources: Internal and external assistance utilized to support efforts toward meeting optimal level of spiritual functioning.

Spiritual well-being: Wellness or health of all the inner resources of a person, which is the ultimate concern around which all other values (of the individual) are focused.

Spirituality: The feeling of connectedness with something higher than oneself, whether it be a god, nature, or another being.

Spiritually-centric: Taking the perspective that everyone else shares the same meaning and practice of spirituality as I do, because my spirituality is the only correct one.

Standards of care: The degree of care that can be expected of a reasonably prudent person of the same profession in a similar situation.

Staging: The objective description of the extent of the disease and the determination of whether the person's cancer has spread or not.

START criteria: Screening Tool to Alert doctors to the Right Treatment.

Stem cell progenitors: The progeny cells of pluripotent stem cells.

Stereotype: A simplified standardized conception, image, opinion, or belief about a person or group.

Stochastic theories of aging: Theories stating that random events occurring in one's life cause damage that accumulates with aging.

STOPP criteria: Screening Tool of Older People's potentially inappropriate Prescriptions.

Stress incontinence: Leaking of urine occurs during activities that increase abdominal pressure, such as laughing, sneezing, and exercising.

Stroke: An interruption of the blood supply to the brain.

Subcutaneous layer: The innermost layer of the skin.

Substance-induced anxiety disorder: A mood disorder in which a person exhibits anxious symptoms. Symptoms may include irritability, nervousness, apprehension, or fear.

Successful aging: Includes not only maintaining physical, cognitive, and functional abilities, but also maintaining engagement with others through communication.

Suicidal ideation: An individual who has thoughts about suicide, which may be as detailed as a formulated plan, without the suicidal act itself.

Suicide: The act of intentionally causing one's own death. Prevent death.

SUPPORT study: The Study to Understand Prognoses and Preferences for Outcomes and Risks of Treatment; it revealed deficiencies in care and treatment of the terminally ill in U.S. medical practices.

Suppressor T cells: T cells that suppress the immune response.

Supraciasmatic nucleus (SCN): The primary circadian rhythm pacemaker (in humans).

Surgery: Invasive procedure to treat an illness or disease, usually by removal of a diseased organ or part.

Survivor: A person living from the time of a cancer diagnosis for the balance of life.

Survivorship: The survivor in the transition from active treatment to surveillance care.

Symptom management: Focus on promotion of comfort and alleviation of a variety of symptoms.

Symptoms: Characteristics signs of disease or illness.

Synapses: Space between the dendrites on neurons where chemical signals via neurotransmitters are relayed to other neurons.

Synaptogenesis: Generation of new synapses.

Synovial fluid: Fluid secreted by the synovium that allows smooth, easy movement of the bones comprising a synovial joint.

Synovial joint: Joint connecting two bones containing smooth cartilage on their opposing ends.

Synovium: Synovial joint capsule membrane that secretes synovial fluid.

Systole: Contraction of the heart that forces blood into the aorta.

T cells: Cells of the immune system that mature in the thymus and play a critical role in cell-mediated immunity.

T-helper cells: T cells that regulate the immune system.

Tangles: Paired helical filaments and a few straight filaments that occur in the neuronal cell body; the main protein associated with neurofibrillary tangles is known as tau.

Task talk: Nurse–patient conversations in healthcare settings where heavy workloads and staffing shortages contribute to the communication with patients being almost exclusively about care tasks.

Teach-back method: After providing health information, have patients repeat back to them what information they have received.

Telomerase: An enzyme that regulates chromosomal aging by its action on telomeres.

Telomere: Repeated sequences of DNA that protect the tips of the outermost appendages of the chromosome arms.

Tertiary prevention: Efforts used to manage clinical diseases in order to prevent them from progressing or to avoid complications of the disease, as is done when beta blockers are used to help remodel the heart in congestive heart failure.

Theory of adult learning: Developed by Malcolm Knowles, applies principles to enhance learning in adults over 18 years old who have completed mandatory public education.

Theory of self-efficacy: The belief that one's actions influence outcomes; self-efficacy and outcome expectations affect behavior, motivation, thought patterns, and emotions.

Therapeutic (healing) touch: Movement of the practitioner's hands over a patient's body to balance its energy fields.

Thrombocytes: Blood platelets responsible for blood clotting.

Thrombocytopenia: An inadequate number of platelets.

Thyroid: A small, butterfly-shaped gland located in the lower front portion of the neck.

Thyroid-stimulating hormone (TSH): A pituitary hormone stimulating the synthesis and release of triiodothyronine and thyroxine.

Thyroxine (T4): A thyroid hormone involved in metabolic and thermal regulation.

Tinnitus: Ringing in the ears.

Titration: The gradual increase/decrease of medication to reduce or eliminate pain while allowing the body to accommodate the side effects or toxicity.

Tolerance: A state of adaptation in which exposure to a drug induces changes that result in a diminution of one or more of the drug's effects over time.

Tonometer: An instrument used to measure intraocular pressure.

Total lung capacity: The maximum volume to which the lungs can expand during the greatest inspiratory effort.

Total sleep time (TST): The total minutes of sleep, including all stages of NREM plus REM sleep.

Trabecular bone: The inner portion of bone; also known as spongy bone.

Traditional Chinese medicine: The medical system that balances the opposing forces of yin and yang.

Transactional leadership: Style in which leaders seek to engage individuals in the recognition and pursuit of a commonly held goal.

Transcultural: A term used widely in nursing to apply to people of diverse cultures.

Transformational or charismatic leadership: Transformational leaders seeking to attain a collective goal for the organization and stimulating innovative thinking to transform followers' beliefs. They understand the need for change in the organization and clearly communicate the vision to achieve the change.

Translation: The most accurate, written conversion of a written document from one language into another without adding, omitting, or distorting meaning.

Transforming Care at the Bedside (TCAB): In-hospital care model to improve the quality of care for patients discharged from medical and surgical units *within* hospitals, discharged from the hospital to home, or to another health care facility.

Transient ischemic attack (TIA): Stroke symptoms that last from minutes to less than 24 hours with no residual effects.

Transient (acute) urinary incontinence: Incontinence caused by the onset of an acute problem that once successfully treated will result in resolution of the UI.

Transitional care: Care that facilitates the move between healthcare settings with an emphasis on self-care.

Transitional Care Model (TCM): Patient-centered care model to improve quality of life, patient satisfaction, and reduce hospital readmissions (Naylor).

Transurethral resection of the prostate (TURP): Surgical intervention for BPH.

Treatment options: The range of interventions available.

Triage: Meaning "to sort" a system of classification of severity of illness, injury, or trauma.

Triceps Skin Fold: Measured using a skinfold caliper by measuring the mid-point between the acromion process and the alecranon process of the upper arm; reflects fat stores.

Triiodothyronine (T3): A thyroid hormone involved in metabolic and thermal regulation.

Triphasic model of human sexual response: Three phases of sexual response: excitement, plateau, and orgasm.

Tuberculosis (TB): Disease caused by *Mycobacterium tuberculosis;* can affect any body part, but particularly the lungs.

t-PA (tissue plasminogen activator): Used to treat acute ischemic stroke.

Ureters: Tubes connecting the kidneys to the bladder.

Urethra: Canal that leads from the bladder out of the body.

Urge suppression techniques: Strategies that help control bladder contractions and therefore minimize or resolve urgency.

Urge urinary incontinence: Associated with a strong, abrupt desire to void and the inability to inhibit leakage before reaching the toilet.

Urinary tract infection: Bacterial invasion of the bladder or urinary tract.

Urostomy: Stoma through which urine passes into a receptacle on the outside of the body; used when the bladder has been removed.

U.S. Preventive Services Task Force (USPSTF): A task force convened by the U.S. Public Health Service to systematically review the evidence of effectiveness of clinical preventive services. Its mission is to evaluate the benefits of individual services and to create age-, gender-, and risk-based recommendations about services that should routinely be incorporated into primary medical care.

Values: Beliefs and attitudes that reflect a person's thoughts and culture.

Vasopressin: A pituitary hormone responsible for regulation of blood and osmotic pressure.

Ventilatory rate: The volume of air inspired in a normal breath multiplied by the frequency of breaths per minute; also known as the minute respiratory rate.

Ventricles: The two lower chambers of the heart; the left ventricle expels oxygen-rich blood into the aorta to be delivered to the entire body excluding the lungs, and the right ventricle expels oxygen-poor blood into pulmonary arteries traveling to the lungs for re-oxygenation.

Veracity: To tell the truth.

Verbal communication: Relies on knowledge of a common language as well as the ability to produce words.

Veritable energy field: Energy that can be measured.

Veteran: A person who has served active duty in the armed forces (41.9% of persons over 65 years of age).

Veterans Administration: An agency of the federal government that provides benefits and services to veterans as well as survivors of veterans. The Veterans Administration operates acute care centers, clinics, and long-term-care facilities across the United States that provide medical, surgical and rehabilitation services.

Vicarious liability: A legal relationship between two entities, such as an employer and employee or independent contractor, where liability is shared.

Vietnamese: Immigrants from Vietnam, Laos, Cambodia, and Hmong (the mountainous regions of China, Vietnam, Laos, and Thailand).

Vietnam War: Aug. 5, 1964 (Feb. 28, 1961, for Veterans who served "in country" before Aug. 5, 1964), through May 7, 1975.

Violation of personal rights: Failure to acknowledge and enforce the rights of a competent older adult.

Visceral: Pertaining to a bodily organ.

Vital capacity: The maximum amount of air that can be expelled from the lungs following a maximum inspiration.

Vitrectomy: Evacuation of the vitreous humor in order to remove blood that has leaked from damaged vessels in diabetic retinopathy.

Wandering: Tendency to walk around that may result in elopement; a common symptom in individuals suffering from cognitive impairment, including delirium and dementia.

Weight loss: A decrease in body weight; can be predictive of mortality in older adults.

Wernicke's aphasia: Difficulty comprehending speech; fluent and rhythmic but lacks meaning.

Working memory: Memory that includes executive functions such as planning, attention, inhibition, encoding, and monitoring.

World War II: Dec. 7, 1941, through Dec. 31, 1946.

World Wide Web: A system of clients (Web browsers or software applications used to locate and display Web pages) and servers that use the Internet for data exchange.

Yang: One half of the principle of opposites; it represents the bright, active, upward, hot, male force in traditional Chinese medicine.

Yin: One half of the principle of opposites; it represents the cold, dark, weak, female force in traditional Chinese medicine.

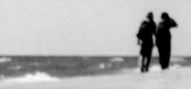

Index

In this index, *b* denotes box, *f* denotes figure, and *t* denotes table.